Atlas of Gastroenterology

Atlas of Gastroenterology

EDITED BY

Tadataka Yamada, MD

President, Global Health Program
Bill & Melinda Gates Foundation
Seattle, Washington;
Adjunct Professor
Department of Internal Medicine
Division of Gastroenterology
University of Michigan Health System
Ann Arbor, Michigan, USA

ASSOCIATE EDITORS

David H. Alpers, MD

William B. Kountz Professor of Medicine
Department of Internal Medicine
Division of Gastroenterology
Washington University School of Medicine
St Louis, Missouri, USA

Anthony N. Kalloo, MD

Professor of Medicine
Johns Hopkins University School of Medicine;
Director, Division of Gastroenterology and Hepatology
Johns Hopkins Hospital
Baltimore, Maryland, USA

Neil Kaplowitz, MD

Thomas H. Brem Chair, Professor of Medicine, Chief
Division of Gastrointestinal and Liver Diseases
Director, Liver Disease Research Center
Keck School of Medicine
University of Southern California
Los Angeles, California, USA

Chung Owyang, MD

Professor of Internal Medicine
H. Marvin Pollard Collegiate Professor and Chief
Division of Gastroenterology
University of Michigan Health System
Ann Arbor, Michigan, USA

Don W. Powell, MD

The Bassel and Frances Blanton Distinguished Professor of Internal Medicine
Professor, Neuroscience and Cell Biology
Program Director, General Clinical Research Center
Director, Division of Gastroenterology and Hepatology
The University of Texas Medical Branch
Galveston, Texas, USA

Fourth Edition

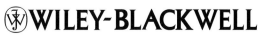

WILEY-BLACKWELL

A John Wiley & Sons, Ltd., Publication

This edition first published 2009, © 2009 by Blackwell Publishing Ltd

Blackwell Publishing was acquired by John Wiley & Sons in February 2007. Blackwell's publishing program has been merged with Wiley's global Scientific, Technical and Medical business to form Wiley-Blackwell.

Registered office: John Wiley & Sons Ltd, The Atrium, Southern Gate, Chichester, West Sussex, PO19 8SQ, UK

Editorial offices: 9600 Garsington Road, Oxford, OX4 2DQ, UK
    The Atrium, Southern Gate, Chichester, West Sussex, PO19 8SQ, UK
    111 River Street, Hoboken, NJ 07030-5774, USA

For details of our global editorial offices, for customer services and for information about how to apply for permission to reuse the copyright material in this book please see our website at www.wiley.com/wiley-blackwell

Library of Congress Cataloging-in-Publication Data

Atlas of gastroenterology / edited by Tadataka Yamada ; associate editors, David H. Alpers . . . [et al.]. – 4th ed.
    p. ; cm.
  Includes bibliographical references and index.
  ISBN 978-1-4051-6909-7 (alk. paper)
1. Gastroenterology–Atlases. 2. Gastrointestinal system–Diseases–Atlases. I. Yamada, Tadataka.
II. Alpers, David H.
  [DNLM: 1. Gastrointestinal Diseases–Atlases. WI 17 A87916 2009]
  RC801.T48 2009 Suppl.
  616.3′300222–dc22

                                                                                    2008040926

A catalogue record for this book is available from the British Library.

Set in 9/12 pt Meridien by SNP Best-set Typesetter Ltd., Hong Kong
Printed in Singapore by Fabulous Printers Pte Ltd

1 2009

Contents

Contents

PART 3 Diagnostic and therapeutic modalities in gastroenterology

A Endoscopic

Contents

Contributors

David A. Ahlquist, MD
Professor of Medicine
Consultant
Division of Gastroenterology and Hepatology
Mayo Clinic College of Medicine
Rochester, Minnesota, USA

Aijaz Ahmed, MD
Associate Professor of Medicine
Division of Gastroenterology and Hepatology
Stanford University Medical Center
Stanford, California, USA

Jacob Alexander, MD, DM
Senior Research Fellow
Division of Gastroenterology
University of Washington
Seattle, Washington, USA

Nathan M. Bass, MD, PhD
Professor of Medicine
Medical Director, Liver Transplantation Program
Division of Gastroenterology
University of California, San Francisco;
San Francisco, California, USA

Diane Bergin, MD
Assistant Professor of Radiology
Department of Radiology
University College Hospital
Galway, Ireland

Stephen J. Bickston, MD
Associate Professor
Department of Internal Medicine
Division of Gastroenterology and Hepatology;
Medical Director, Inpatient Digestive Health Center of Excellence
University of Virginia Health System
Charlottesville, Virginia, USA

Klaus Bielefeldt, MD, PhD
Associate Professor of Medicine
Division of Gastroenterology
University of Pittsburgh
Pittsburgh, Pennsylvania, USA

Adil E. Bharucha, MD
Professor of Medicine
Division of Gastroenterology and Hepatology
Clinical Enteric Neuroscience Translational and Epidemiological Research Program
Mayo Clinic College of Medicine
Rochester, Minnesota, USA

Elisa H. Birnbaum, MD
Associate Professor
Department of Surgery
Section of Colon and Rectal Surgery
Washington University School of Medicine at Barnes-Jewish Hospital
St. Louis, Missouri, USA

Lana Bistritz, MD, FRCPC
Gastroenterology Fellow
Division of Gastroenterology
University of Alberta
Edmonton, Alberta, Canada

David J. Bjorkman, MD, MSPH, SM (Epid)
Professor of Medicine and Dean
University of Utah School of Medicine
Salt Lake City, Utah, USA

Andres T. Blei, MD
Professor of Medicine
Division of Hepatology
Feinberg School of Medicine
Northwestern University
Chicago, Illinois, USA

Robert S. Bresalier
Chairman and Professor
Department of Gastrointestinal Medicine and Nutrition
University of Texas, M.D. Anderson Cancer Center
Houston, Texas, USA

William R. Brugge, MD
Director, Gastrointestinal Endoscopy
Massachusetts General Hospital;

Professor of Medicine
Harvard Medical School
Boston, Massachusetts, USA

Randall W. Burt, MD
Professor of Medicine
Division of Gastroenterology
University of Utah School of Medicine;
Senior Director for Prevention and Outreach
Huntsman Cancer Institute
University of Utah
Salt Lake City, Utah, USA

Alejandro Busalleu, MD
Vice Rector for Academic Affairs
Principal Professor
Department of Pathology
Instituto de Medicine Tropical Alexander von Humboldt
Universidad Peruana Cayetano Heredia
Lima, Peru

Roger F. Butterworth, PhD, DSc
Director, Neuroscience Research Unit
Hôpital Saint-Luc
University of Montreal
Montreal, Quebec, Canada

Michael Camilleri, MD
Atherton and Winifred W. Bean
Professor of Medicine and Physiology
College of Medicine
Mayo Clinic
Rochester, Minnesota, USA

Marcia Irene Canto, MD, MHS
Associate Professor
Director of Clinical Research
Departments of Medicine (Gastroenterology) and Oncology
Johns Hopkins University School of Medicine
Baltimore, Maryland, USA

Mitchell S. Cappell, MD, PhD
Chief, Division of Gastroenterology
William Beaumont Hospital
Royal Oak, Michigan, USA

Contributors

David L. Carr-Locke, MB, BChir, FRCP, FASGE
Director, The Endoscopy Institute
Brigham and Women's Hospital
Boston, Massachusetts, USA

Albert J. Chang, MD
Division of Gastroenterology and Liver Diseases
Keck School of Medicine
University of Southern California
Los Angeles, California, USA

Wenliang Chen, MD
Advanced Laparoscopic Surgery Fellow 2006
Massachusetts General Hospital
Boston, Massachusetts, USA

Onpan Cheung
Gastroenterology and Hepatology Fellow
Medical College of Virginia
Virginia Commonwealth University
Richmond, Virginia, USA

Kyung J. Cho, MD
Professor
Division of Interventional Radiology
Department of Radiology
University of Michigan Health System
Ann Arbor, Michigan, USA

Russell D. Cohen, MD, FACG, AGAF
Associate Professor of Medicine
Co-director, Clinical Inflammatory
  Bowel Disease
The University of Chicago Medical Center
Chicago, Illinois, USA

Jonathan A. Cohn, MD
Professor of Medicine and Associate Professor of
  Cell Biology
Duke University Medical Center
Durham, North Carolina, USA

Steven M. Cohn, MD, PhD
Paul Janssen Professor of Medicine and
  Immunology
Division of Gastroenterology and Hepatology
Department of Medicine
University of Virginia Health System
Charlottesville, Virginia, USA

David H.B. Cort, MD
Digestive Disease Medical Consultant
St Louis, Missouri, USA

David W. Crabb, PhD
John B. Hickam Professor and Chair
Department of Medicine
Division of Gastroenterology and Hepatology

Indiana University School of Medicine
Indianapolis, Indiana, USA

Laurie D. DeLeve, MD, PhD
Professor of Medicine
Liver Disease Research Center
Division of Gastrointestinal and Liver Diseases
Keck School of Medicine
University of Southern California
Los Angeles, California, USA

Silvia Delgado-Aros, MD, MSc
Metge Adjunt Servei Digestiu
Hospital del Mar (IMAS)
Barcelona, Spain

Evan S. Dellon, MD, MPH
Assistant Professor
Center for Esophageal Diseases and Swallowing,
  and Center for Gastrointestinal Biology and
  Disease
University of North Carolina, School of
  Medicine
Chapel Hill, North Carolina, USA

John A. Donovan, MD
Assitant Professor of Clinical Medicine
Division of Gastrointestinal and Liver Diseases
Keck School of Medicine
University of Southern California
Los Angeles, California, USA

Grace H. Elta, MD
Professor
Department of Internal Medicine
Division of Gastroenterology
University of Michigan Health System
Ann Arbor, Michigan, USA

B. Mark Evers, MD
Professor, Departments of Surgery and
  Biochemistry & Molecular Biology
Robertson-Poth Distinguished Chair in General
  Surgery
Director, Sealy Center for Cancer Cell
  Biology
Director, UTMB Comprehensive Cancer
  Center
The University of Texas Medical Branch
Galveston, Texas, USA

George T. Fantry, MD
Associate Professor
Director, Heartburn and Dyspepsia Program
Department of Medicine
University of Maryland School of Medicine
Baltimore, Maryland, USA

Lori E. Fantry, MD, MPH
Associate Professor
Department of Medicine

University of Maryland School of Medicine
Baltimore, Maryland, USA

James J. Farrell, MD
Director of Pancreaticobiliary Endoscopy
Assistant Professor of Medicine
Division of Digestive Diseases
David Geffen School of Medicine
University of California, Los Angeles
Los Angeles, California, USA

Richard N. Fedorak
Professor of Medicine
Division of Gastroenterology
University of Alberta
Edmonton, Alberta, Canada

Robert S. Fisher, MD
Gastroenterology Section
Department of Medicine
Temple University Hospital
Philadelphia, Pennsylvania, USA

Elliot K. Fishman, MD, FACR
Professor of Radiology and Oncology
Department of Radiology
Johns Hopkins Medical Institutions
Baltimore, Maryland, USA

Robert J. Fontana, MD
Associate Professor
Department of Internal Medicine
Division of Gastroenterology
University of Michigan Health System
Ann Arbor, Michigan, USA

Frank K. Friedenberg, MD, MS (Epi)
Gastroenterology Section
Department of Medicine
Temple University Hospital
Philadelphia, Pennsylvania, USA

Guadalupe Garcia-Tsao, MD
Professor of Medicine
Section of Digestive Diseases
Yale School of Medicine
New Haven, Connecticut;
Veterans Affairs Connecticut Healthcare System
West Haven, Connecticut, USA

Robert M. Genta, MD
Clinical Professor of Pathology and Medicine
  (Gastroenterology)
University of Texas Southwestern Medical
  Center;
Director of Academic Affairs
Caris Diagnostics
Irving, Texas, USA

Marc G. Ghany, MD
Staff Physician, Liver Diseases Branch
National Institute of Diabetes and Digestive and
  Kidney Diseases
National Institutes of Health
Bethesda, Maryland, USA

Ralph A. Giannella, MD
Mark Brown Professor of Medicine
Division of Digestive Diseases
University of Cincinnati College of Medicine
Cincinnati, Ohio, USA

Francis M. Giardiello, MD
Professor of Medicine and Oncology
Johns Hopkins University School of Medicine
Baltimore, Maryland, USA

Robert G. Gish, MD
Associate Professor
Department of Medicine
University of California, San Francisco;
Medical Director, Liver Disease Management and
  Transplant Program
California Pacific Medical Center
San Francisco, California, USA

Robert E. Glasgow, MD, FACS
Associate Professor
Department of Surgery
University of Utah
Salt Lake City, Utah, USA

Eric Goldberg, MD
Assistant Professor of Medicine
Division of Gastroenterology and Hepatology
University of Maryland School of Medicine
Baltimore, Maryland, USA

Christopher P. Golembeski, MD
Department of Pathology
University of Michigan Medical School
Ann Arbor, Michigan, USA

Sugantha Govindarajan, MD
Professor, Department of Pathology
Keck School of Medicine
University of Southern California
Los Angeles, California, USA

David Y. Graham, MD
Professor of Medicine and Molecular Virology
  and Microbiology
Michael E. DeBakey Veterans Affairs Medical
  Center
Baylor College of Medicine
Houston, Texas, USA

Leah M. Gramlich
Associate Professor of Medicine
Department of Medicine

University of Alberta
Edmonton, Alberta, Canada

Richard J. Grand, MD
Children's Hospital Boston
Gastroenterology/Nutrition Department
Boston, Massachusetts, USA

Edward G. Grant, MD
Professor and Chairman
Department of Radiology
Keck School of Medicine
University of Southern California
Los Angeles, California, USA

Peter H.R. Green
Professor of Clinical Medicine
Columbia University College of Physicians and
  Surgeons
New York, USA

C. Prakash Gyawali, MD, MRCP
Associate Professor
Associate Program Director
Division of Gastroenterology
Washington University School of Medicine
St Louis, Missouri, USA

E. Jenny Heathcote, MB, BS, MD, FRCP, FRCPC
Professor
Department of Medicine
University of Toronto;
Staff Gastroenterologist
Department of Medicine
Toronto Western Hospital
Toronto, Ontario, Canada

Gail A. Hecht, MD, MS
Professor of Medicine; Microbiology and
  Immunology
Chief, Section of Digestive Diseases and Nutrition
University of Illinois
Chicago, Illinois, USA

David G. Heidt, MD
Clinical Lecturer/Fellow
Department of Surgery
University of Michigan Health System
Ann Arbor, Michigan, USA

Hans Herlinger, MD
Professor of Gastrointestinal Radiology
Late of University of Pennsylvania Health System
Philadelphia, Pennsylvania, USA

Ikuo Hirano, MD
Associate Professor of Medicine
Division of Gastroenterology
Northwestern University Feinberg School of
  Medicine
Chicago, Illinois, USA

Richard A. Hodin, MD
Professor of Surgery, Harvard Medical School;
Massachusetts General Hospital
Boston, Massachusetts, USA

Akira Horiuchi, MD
Department of Gastroenterology
Showa Inan General Hospital
Komagane, Japan

Karen M. Horton, MD
Associate Professor
Department of Radiology
Johns Hopkins Medical Institutions
Baltimore, Maryland, USA

Matilde Iorizzo, MD, PhD
Clinical Fellow
Department of Dermatology
University of Bologna, Italy

Russell F. Jacoby, MD
Director, Colon Cancer Prevention Program
University of Wisconsin Comprehensive Cancer
  Center;
Associate Professor of Medicine
Section of Gastroenterology
University of Wisconsin Medical School
Madison, Wisconsin, USA

Sanjay B. Jagannath, MD
Assistant Professor of Medicine
Division of Gastroenterology
Johns Hopkins University School of Medicine
Baltimore, Maryland, USA

Stephen P. James, MD
Director, Division of Digestive Diseases and
  Nutrition
National Institute of Diabetes and Digestive and
  Kidney Diseases
National Insititutes of Health
Bethesda, Maryland, USA

Edward N. Janoff, MD
Chief, Infectious Diseases;
Director, Colorado Center for AIDS Research
University of Colorado at Denver and Health
  Sciences Center
Denver, Colorado, USA

R. Brooke Jeffrey Jr, MD
Professor
Department of Radiology
Associate Dean for Academic Medicine
Stanford University School of Medicine
Stanford, California, USA

Contributors

Robert T. Jensen, MD
Chief, Cell Biology, Digestive Diseases Branch
National Institute of Diabetes and Digestive and
Kidney Diseases
National Institutes of Health
Bethesda, Maryland, USA

Nirag C. Jhala
Gastrointestinal Pathology Program
Department of Pathology and Laboratory
Medicine
University of Alabama at Birmingham
Birmingham, Alabama, USA

Pamela T. Johnson, MD
Assistant Professor of Radiology
Department of Radiology
Johns Hopkins Medical Institutions
Baltimore, Maryland, USA

Joseph L. Jorizzo, MD
Professor and Former (Founding) Chair
Department of Dermatology
Wake Forest University School of Medicine
Winston-Salem, North Carolina, USA

Peter J. Kahrilas, MD
Gilbert H. Marquardt Professor of Medicine
Department of Medicine
Division of Gastroenterology
Feinberg School of Medicine
Northwestern University
Chicago, Illinois, USA

Robert A. Kane, MD
Professor
Department of Radiology
Harvard Medical School;
Director, Ultrasound Section
Radiology Department
Beth Israel Deaconess Medical Center
Boston, Massachusetts, USA

Gary C. Kanel, MD
Professor of Clinical Pathology
Keck School of Medicine
University of Southern California;
Associate Pathologist
LAC+USA Medical Center and USC University
Hospital
Los Angeles, California, USA

Sergey V. Kantsevoy, MD, PhD
Associate Professor of Medicine
Department of Medicine
Division of Gastroenterology
Johns Hopkins University School of Medicine
Baltimore, Maryland, USA

Mototsugu Kato, MD, PhD
Division of Endoscopy
Hokkaido University School of Medicine
Sapporo, Japan

Emmet B. Keeffe, MD, MACP
Professor of Medicine Emeritus
Division of Gastroenterology and Hepatology
Stanford University Medical Center
Stanford, California, USA

Paul Knechtges, MD
Clinical Assistant Professor
Associate Chair of Quality Assurance
Department of Radiology
University of Michigan Health System
Ann Arbor, Michigan, USA

Cynthia W. Ko, MD, MS
Associate Professor
Department of Medicine
University of Washington
Seattle, Washington, USA

Kris V. Kowdley, MD, FACP
Clinical Professor of Medicine
Director, Center for Liver Disease
Virginia Mason Medical Center
University of Washington School of Medicine
Seattle, Washington, USA

Richard A. Kozarek, MD
Clinical Professor of Medicine
University of Washington;
Executive Director
Digestive Disease Institute
Virginia Mason Medical Center
Seattle, Washington, USA

Jacob C. Langer, MD
Professor of Surgery
University of Toronto;
Chief of General Surgery
Hospital for Sick Children
Toronto, Ontario, Canada

Shawn D. Larson, MB, ChB
General Surgery Resident
Department of General Surgery
University of South Florida
Tampa, Florida, USA

Igor Laufer, MD
Professor of Radiology
University of Pennsylvania School of Medicine
Philadelphia, Pennsylvania, USA

Anne R. Lee, MSEd, RD, CDN
Nutritionist
Celiac Disease Center
Columbia University
New York, USA

Sum P. Lee, MD, PhD
Chair, Professor of Medicine, and Dean
University of Hong Kong
Li Ka Shing Faculty of Medicine
Hong Kong

William M. Lee, MD, FACP
Professor of Internal Medicine
The University of Texas Southwestern Medical
Center at Dallas
Dallas, Texas, USA

**Yuk Tong Lee, MD, FRCP (Edin),
FHKCP, FHKAM**
Honorary Clinical Associate Professor
Department of Medicine and Therapeutics
The Chinese University of Hong Kong
Shatin, New Territories, Hong Kong

Wai K. Leung, MD, FRCP
Department of Medicine and Therapeutics
The Chinese University of Hong Kong
Shatin, New Territories, Hong Kong

Marc S. Levin, MD, AGAF
Professor
Department of Medicine
Washington University School of Medicine;
Staff Physician
St Louis Veterans Affairs Medical Center and
Barnes-Jewish Hospital
St Louis, Missouri, USA

Joel S. Levine, MD
Professor of Medicine
Division of Gastroenterology and Hepatology
University of Colorado Health Sciences Center
Denver, Colorado, USA

Marc S. Levine, MD
Professor of Radiology
Chief, Gastrointestinal Radiology
Advisory Dean
University of Pennsylvania Medical Center
Philadelphia, Pennsylvania, USA

Ellen Li, MD, PhD
Professor
Department of Microbiology
Cornell University
Ithaca, New York, USA

T. Jake Liang, MD
Chief, Liver Diseases Branch
National Institute of Diabetes and Digestive and
Kidney Diseases
National Institutes of Health;
Chief Staff Physician
Hepatology Service
National Institutes of Health Clinical Center
Bethesda, Maryland, USA

Suthat Liangpunsakul, MD, MPH
Assistant Professor of Clinical Medicine
Department of Medicine
Division of Gastroenterology and Hepatology
Indiana University School of Medicine and the
    R.L. Roudebush Veterans Affairs Medical
    Center
Indianapolis, Indiana, USA

Mark L. Lloyd, MD
Private Practice
Meridian, Idaho, USA

John D. Long, MD
Associate Professor of Medicine
Section of Gastroenterology
Wake Forest University School of Medicine
Winston-Salem, North Carolina, USA

James D. Lord, MD, PhD
University of Washington Medical Center
Department of Medicine
Division of Gastroenterology
Seattle, Washington, USA

Mark A. Lovell, MD
Associate Professor of Pathology
University of Colorado School of Medicine;
Acting Chief of Pediatric Pathology
Department of Pathology
The Children's Hospital
Denver, Colorado, USA

Shelly C. Lu, MD
Professor
Department of Medicine
Division of Gastroenterology and Liver
    Diseases
Keck School of Medicine
University of Southern California
Los Angeles, California, USA

**Finlay A. Macrae, MB, BS, MD,
FRACP, FRCP**
Professor
Department of Medicine
University of Melbourne;
Head, Colorectal Medicine and Genetics
The Royal Melbourne Hospital
Parkville, Victoria, Australia

Marlyn J. Mayo, MD
Assistant Professor of Internal Medicine
The University of Texas Southwestern Medical
    Center at Dallas
Dallas, Texas, USA

Alec J. Megibow, MD, MPH
Professor of Radiology
New York University Medical Center
New York, USA

**Raphael B. Merriman,
MD, MRCPI**
Assistant Professor of Medicine
Division of Gastroenterology
University of California, San Francisco
San Francisco, California, USA

Carlos G. Micames, MD
Associate in Medicine
Division of Gastroenterology
Duke University Medical Center
Durham, North Carolina, USA

Rebecca M. Minter, MD
Assistant Professor
Department of Surgery
University of Michigan Health System
Ann Arbor, Michigan, USA

Martin Montes, MD
Assistant Professor
Department of Pathology
Instituto de Medicina Tropical Alexander von
    Humboldt
Universidad Peruana Cayetano Heredia
Lima, Peru

Elizabeth Montgomery, MD
Professor of Pathology
Johns Hopkins University School of Medicine;
Pathologist, Johns Hopkins Hospital
Baltimore, Maryland, USA

Richard H. Moseley, MD
Professor, Department of Internal Medicine
Division of Gastroenterology, University of
    Michigan Health System;
Chief, Medical System
Ann Arbor Veterans Affairs Medical Center
Ann Arbor, Michigan, USA

Michael W. Mulholland, MD, PhD
Professor and Chair
Department of Surgery
University of Michigan Health System
Ann Arbor, Michigan, USA

Sean J. Mulvihill, MD
Professor and Chairman
Department of Surgery
University of Utah School of Medicine;
Senior Director, Clinical Affairs
Huntsman Cancer Institute
Salt Lake City, Utah, USA

Anil B. Nagar, MD
Associate Professor of Internal Medicine
Section of Digestive Diseases, Yale University;
Endoscopy Director
West Haven Veterans Affairs Medical Center
West Haven, Connecticut, USA

Enders K.W. Ng, MD
Professor
Department of Surgery
The Chinese University of Hong Kong;
Department of Surgery
Prince of Wales Hospital
Shatin, New Territories, Hong Kong

Jeffrey A. Norton
Professor
Department of Surgery
Stanford University Medical Center
Stanford, California, USA

**Timothy T. Nostrant, MD, FACP,
FACG, AGAF, FASGE**
Professor
Department of Internal Medicine
Division of Gastroenterology
University of Michigan Health System
Ann Arbor, Michigan, USA

Ward A. Olsen, MD
Formerly Professor, Department of Medicine
University of Wisconsin;
Head, Gastroenterology Section
Department of Medicine
University of Wisconsin Hospitals and Clinics;
Chief, Gastroenterology Section
William S. Middleton Veterans Hospital
Madison, Wisconsin, USA

Stephen J. Pandol, MD
Professor
Staff Physician, Department of Veterans Affairs
Department of Medicine
University of California, Los Angeles
Los Angeles, California, USA

Julián Panés, MD
Assistant Professor
Department of Medicine
University of Barcelona;
Consultant, Department of Gastroenterology
Hospital Clinic
Barcelona, Spain

Sareh Parangi, MD, FACS
Assistant Professor, Department of Surgery
Harvard Medical School;
Attending Surgeon, Department of Surgery
Beth Israel Deaconess Medical Center
Boston, Massachusetts, USA

Henry P. Parkman, MD
Professor
Temple University School of Medicine
Gastroenterology Section
Philadelphia, Pennsylvania, USA

Marion G. Peters, MD
John V. Carbone MD Endowed Chair in Medicine
Chief of Hepatology Research, Department of
    Medicine

Contributors

Division of Gastroenterology, University of California;
Attending Physician, Department of Medicine
Moffit-Long Hospital
San Francisco, California, USA

Josep M. Piqué, MD
Associate Professor
Department of Medicine
University of Barcelona;
Chief, Department of Gastroenterology
Hospital Clinic
Barcelona, Spain

Cyrus Piraka, MD
Clinical Lecturer
Department of Internal Medicine
Division of Gastroenterology
University of Michigan Health System
Ann Arbor, Michigan, USA

John C. Rabine, MD
LtCol, U.S. Air Force;
Chief, Division of Gastroenterology
David Grant Medical Center
Travis Air Force Base
Fairfield, California, USA

David S. Raiford, MD
Professor of Medicine
Director, Liver Service
Vanderbilt University Medical Center
Nashville, Tennessee, USA

Philip W. Ralls, MD
Professor and Vice Chair
Department of Radiology
Keck School of Medicine
University of Southern California
Los Angeles, California, USA

Satish S.C. Rao, MD, PhD, FRCP (Lon)
Professor
Division of Gastroenterology and Hepatology
Department of Internal Medicine
University of Iowa Carver College of Medicine,
Iowa City, Iowa, USA

David W. Rattner, MD
Professor of Surgery
Harvard Medical School;
Chief, Division of General and Gastrointestinal Surgery
Massachusetts General Hospital
Boston, Massachusetts, USA

Jean-Pierre Raufman, MD
Moses and Helen Golden Professor of Medicine
Head, Division of Gastroenterology and Hepatology

University of Maryland School of Medicine
Baltimore, Maryland, USA

Howard A. Reber, MD
Chief, Gastrointestinal Surgery
Professor of Surgery
Division of General Surgery
David Geffen School of Medicine at UCLA
Los Angeles, California, USA

Joel E. Richter, MD, MACP
Richard L. Evans Chair and Professor
Department of Medicine
Temple University School of Medicine
Philadelphia, Pennsylvania, USA

Michelle L. Robbin, MD
Professor
Chief of Ultrasound
Department of Radiology
University of Alabama at Birmingham
Birmingham, Alabama, USA

Lewis R. Roberts, MB, ChB, PhD
Associate Professor of Medicine
College of Medicine, Mayo Clinic;
Colnsultant in Gastroenterology and Hepatology
Mayo Clinic
Rochester, Minnesota, USA

Hugo Rosen, MD, FACP
Waterman Professor of Medicine and Immunology
Endowed Chair in Liver Research
Division Head, Gastroenterology and Hepatology
University of Colorado Health Sciences Center
Aurora, Colorado, USA

Stephen E. Rubesin, MD
Professor
Department of Radiology
University of Pennsylvania School of Medicine;
Radiologist
Department of Radiology
Hospital of the University of Pennsylvania
Philadelphia, Pennsylvania, USA

Deborah C. Rubin, MD
Professor
Department of Medicine, Division of Gastroenterology
Department of Developmental Biology
Washington University School of Medicine
St Louis, Missouri, USA

Anil K. Rustgi, MD
T. Grier Miller Professor of Medicine and Genetics
Chief of Gastroenterology
Department of Medicine

University of Pennsylvania
Philadelphia, Pennsylvania, USA

Sammy Saab, MD, MPH
Head, Outcomes Research in Hepatology
Associate Professor of Medicine and Surgery
David Geffen School of Medicine at UCLA
Los Angeles, California, USA

Arun J. Sanyal, MB, BS, MD
Charles Caravati Professor of Medicine
Chairman, Division of Gastroenterology, Hepatology and Nutrition
Department of Internal Medicine
Virginia Commonwealth University
Richmond, Virginia, USA

Michael G. Sarr, MD
J.C. Masson Professor of Surgery, Mayo Medical School;
Consultant, Division of Gastroenterology and General Surgery
Mayo Clinic
Rochester, Minnesota, USA

Drew B. Schembre, MD
Chief of Gastroenterology
Virginia Mason Medical Center
Seattle, Washington, USA

Frank V. Schiødt, MD
Associate Professor
Department of Hepatology, University of Copenhagen;
Rigshospitalet
Copenhagen, Denmark

Janak N. Shah, MD
Assistant Clinical Professor of Medicine
University of California, San Francisco;
Director of Endoscopy
San Francisco Veterans Affairs Medical Center
San Francisco, California, USA

Nicholas J. Shaheen, MD, MPH
Associate Professor of Medicine and Epidemiology;
Director, Center for Esophageal Diseases and Swallowing
University of North Carolina School of Medicine
Chapel Hill, North Carolina, USA

Fergus Shanahan, MD
Professor and Chair
Department of Medicine and Director, Alimentary Pharmabiotic Centre
University College Cork
National University of Ireland;
Professor
Department of Medicine
Cork University Hospital
Cork, Ireland

Diane M. Simeone, MD
Lazar J. Greenfield Professor of Surgery
Chief, Gastrointestinal Surgery
University of Michigan Health System
Ann Arbor, Michigan, USA

Phillip D. Smith, MD
Mary J. Bradford Professor in Gastroenterology
Professor of Medicine and Microbiology
University of Alabama at Birmingham
Birmingham, Alabama, USA

Ronald J. Sokol, MD
Professor and Vice Chair
Chief, Pediatric Gastroenterology, Hepatology and
    Nutrition
Department of Pediatrics
Director, Colorado Clinical and Translational
    Sciences Institute
University of Colorado Denver School of
    Medicine;
The Children's Hospital
Aurora, Colorado, USA

Samuel L. Stanley Jr, MD
Professor
Department of Medicine
Washington University School of Medicine;
Vice Chancellor for Research
Washington University
St Louis, Missouri, USA

William F. Stenson, MD
Nicholas V. Costrini Professor of Gastroenterology
    and Inflammatory Bowel Disease
Department of Medicine
Division of Gastroenterology
Washington University School of Medicine
St Louis, Missouri, USA

Jung W. Suh, MD, MPH
Division of Gastroenterology and Liver Diseases
Keck School of Medicine
University of Southern California
Los Angeles, California, USA

Weijing Sun, MD
Associate Professor of Medicine
Director of Gastrointestinal Medical Oncology
    Program
Department of Medicine
Division of Hematology/Oncology
University of Pennsylvania
Philadelphia, Pennsylvania, USA

Joseph J.Y. Sung, MD, PhD
Professor of Medicine
Chairman of the Department of Medicine and
    Threapeutics
The Chinese University of Hong Kong
Prince of Wales Hospital
Shatin, New Territories, Hong Kong

Mimi Takami
Assistant Professor
Department of Internal Medicine
Division of Gastroenterology
University of Michigan Health System
Ann Arbor, Michigan, USA

Stephen R. Targan, MD
Director, Division of Gastroenterology
Inflammatory Bowel Disease Center and
    Immunobiology Institute
Cedars-Sinai Medical Center;
Professor
David Geffen School of Medicine at UCLA
Los Angeles, California

Phillip I. Tarr, MD
Melvin E. Carnahan Professor of Pediatrics
Professor of Molecular Microbiology
Director, Division of Gastroenterology and
    Nutrition
Department of Pediatrics and St Louis Children's
    Hospital
Washington University School of Medicine
St Louis, Missouri, USA

Ryan M. Taylor, MD
Fellow
Department of Internal Medicine
Division of Gastroenterology
Department of Internal Medicine
University of Michigan Health System
Ann Arbor, Michigan, USA

Dwain L. Thiele, MD
Professor and Vice Chair
Department of Internal Medicine
The University of Texas Southwestern Medical
    Center at Dallas
Dallas, Texas, USA

**Anthony C. Thomas, MD, PhD,
FRCPath, FRCPA**
Associate Professor, Department of Anatomical
    Pathology
Flinders University of South Australia;
Senior Specialist and Head, Department of
    Anatomical Pathology
Flinders Medical Center
Bedford Park, South Australia, Australia

**Paul J. Thuluvath, MB, BS,
MD, FRCP**
Associate Professor of Medicine
Johns Hopkins University School of Medicine
Baltimore, Maryland, USA

William J. Tremaine, MD
Professor of Medicine
Mayo Clinic College of Medicine
Rochester, Minnesota, USA

Jerrold R. Turner, MD, PhD
Professor
Associate Chairman for Academic Affairs
Department of Pathology
The University of Chicago
Chicago, Illinois, USA

Javier Vaquero, MD
Postdoctoral Research Fellow
Neuroscience Research Unit
Hôpital Saint-Luc
University of Montreal
Montreal, Quebec, Canada

Arnold Wald, MD
Professor of Medicine
Section of Gastroenterology and Hepatology
University of Wisconsin School of Medicine and
    Public Health
Madison, Wisconsin, USA

Kymberly D.S. Watt, MD, FRCPC
Hepatology/Liver Transplantation
Mayo Clinic
Rochester, Minnesota, USA

Jerome D. Waye, MD
Clinical Professor of Medicine
Division of Gastroenterology
Director of Endoscopy
Mount Sinai Medical Center
New York, USA

Theodore H. Welling, MD
Assistant Professor of Surgery
Division of Transplantation
University of Michigan Health System
Ann Arbor, Michigan, USA

A. Clinton White Jr, MD
Paul R. Stalnaker Distinguished Professor and
    Director, Infectious Disease Division
Department of Internal Medicine
The University of Texas Medical Branch
Galveston, Texas, USA

Russell H. Wiesner, MD
Professor of Medicine
Mayo Clinic Transplant Center
Mayo Medical School;
Director of Viral Hepatitis, Liver Transplant
    Program
Mayo Clinic
Rochester, Minnesota, USA

C. Mel Wilcox, MD
Professor
Department of Medicine
Division of Gastroenterology and Hepatology
University of Alabama at Birmingham
Birmingham, Alabama, USA

Contributors

John W. Wiley, MD
Professor
Department of Internal Medicine
University of Michigan Health System;
Director, Michigan Clinical Research Unit
University of Michigan
Ann Arbor, Michigan, USA

Christopher B. Williams, MA, BM, BCh, FRCP
Endoscopy Unit
St Mark's Hospital for Colorectal and Intestinal
    Disorders
Harrow, London, UK

Field F. Willingham, MD, MPH
Clinical and Research Fellow in Medicine
Harvard Medical School
Massachusetts General Hospital
Boston, Massachusetts, USA

Francis Y.K. Yao, MD
Professor of Clinical Medicine and Surgery
Associate Medical Director, Liver Transplantation
University of California, San Francisco
San Francisco, California, USA

Graeme P. Young, MD, FRACP
Professor of Gastroenterology
Department of Medicine
Flinders University of South Australia;
Director, Department of Gastroenterology
Flinders Medical Centre
Adelaide, South Australia, Australia

Tonia M. Young-Fadok, MD, MS, FACS, FASCRS
Professor of Surgery
Chair, Division of Colon and Rectal Surgery
Mayo Clinic, Arizona
Scottsdale, Arizona, USA

Tony E. Yusuf, MD
Director, Gastrointestinal Endoscopy and
    Pancreatobiliary Center of Excellence
State University of New York Downstate
    Medical Center and Kings County Hospital
    Center;
Assistant Professor of Medicine
State University of New York Downstate College
    of Medicine
Brooklyn, New York, USA

Harvey A. Ziessman, MD
Professor of Radiology
Director of Nuclear Medicine Imaging
Division of Nuclear Medicine
Russell H. Morgan Department of Radiology and
    Radiological Sciences
The Johns Hopkins University
Baltimore, Maryland, USA

Ellen M. Zimmermann, MD
Associate Professor
Department of Internal Medicine
Division of Gastroenterology
University of Michigan Health System
Ann Arbor, Michigan, USA

Preface

Among the most important developments in clinical medicine in recent years has been the rapid advancement in imaging technologies. These technologies allow clinicians to gain better insight into the pathophysiological processes underlying their patients' illnesses. The practice of gastroenterology, perhaps more than any other in medicine, is a visual one and has been enriched by such advances. Modalities such as endoscopy, double-contrast radiography, computed tomography, isotopic scintigraphy, ultrasonography, magnetic resonance imaging, and positron emission tomography have facilitated greatly the approach to diagnosing gastrointestinal disorders. The imaging of tissues using standard microscopy has been augmented with newer methodologies such as immunohistochemistry, in situ hybridization, and confocal microscopy, not to mention even more experimental techniques. While we have included descriptions of these advances in the *Textbook of Gastroenterology*, the old adage that "a picture is worth a thousand words" could not be more applicable to anything other than to the teaching of gastroenterology. With this in mind, we have endeavored to provide the fourth edition of the *Atlas of Gastroenterology* with additional graphic material that enhances the reader's understanding of the written material in the *Textbook*. The fourth edition of the *Atlas* expands on the material presented in the third edition by the addition of figures to existing chapters and by the addition of chapters covering new subject matter. The written text in the *Atlas* provides only an abbreviated introduction to the graphic material, and the reader is referred to the *Textbook* for more detailed information. Although the *Atlas* is meant to be especially useful to the reader of the *Textbook*, the quality of many of the figures is unique and not to be found readily in existing publications. Thus, we hope that the *Atlas* will serve as a valuable educational resource for all readers, independent of their familiarity with the *Textbook*.

We are delighted to welcome Tony Kalloo to the editorial team for the fourth edition of the *Atlas of Gastroenterology*. His hands-on experience in the most modern procedural techniques of gastroenterology, in addition to his broad understanding of the discipline, have added immensely to this edition.

We are most pleased as well to have a new publisher, Wiley-Blackwell, for this edition. Their keen insight into the publishing industry and the way in which textbooks are utilized today has been the basis for some of the changes made to the *Atlas*. In addition, their knowledge of the international world of medicine will help us to distribute the contents of the *Atlas* to a global audience. The editors would like especially to thank Elisabeth Dodds at Wiley-Blackwell, whose commitment to excellence has contributed materially to the quality of the book, and Alison Brown and Oliver Walter, without whose assistance this fourth edition of the *Atlas* would not have been published.

Our efforts were especially facilitated by the expert assistance of Lori Ennis and Barbara Boughen, who collaborated as a team, complementing editorial talents with interpersonal skills to maintain the high quality of the text and deliver the manuscripts in a timely fashion. The editors are indebted to their administrative and secretarial assistants, Patricia Lai, Terri Astin, Jennifer Mayes, Sue Sparrow, Patty Pool, Gracie Bernal-Muñoz, and Maria L. Vidrio. In addition, the faculty and fellows of the Gastroenterology Divisions at the University of Michigan, Washington University in St. Louis, and the University of Texas Medical Branch in Galveston provided valuable assistance in reviewing the chapters in the third edition of the *Atlas* in preparation for this, the fourth edition.

Tadataka Yamada, MD

1 Approach to the patient with gross gastrointestinal bleeding

Grace H. Elta, Mimi Takami

Gastrointestinal (GI) bleeding is a common clinical problem that requires more than 300 000 hospitalizations annually in the United States. Most bleeding episodes resolve spontaneously; however, patients with severe and persistent bleeding have high mortality rates. Evaluation of a patient with bleeding begins with assessment of the urgency of the situation. Resuscitation with intravenous fluids and blood products is the first consideration. Once the patient's condition is stable, a brief history and physical examination will help determine the location of the bleeding. For probable or known upper GI bleeding, a nasogastric tube is placed to help determine the location of bleeding and to monitor the rapidity of the bleeding. The algorithm in Figure 1.1 is a general guideline for evaluation of nonvariceal upper GI bleeding. There is an important exception to this algorithm; endoscopy may be used urgently in *all* patients with upper GI bleeding regardless if their bleeding has stopped spontaneously, allowing triage of patients to outpatient, inpatient, or intensive care. This practice has been shown to be safe and to lead to significant cost saving as patients without risk factors such as coagulopathy, serious concomitant diseases, or bleeding stigmata do not require hospitalization.

Patients with liver disease or other causes of portal hypertension have a potential variceal source of hemorrhage.

Urgent diagnostic endoscopy is indicated to confirm the bleeding source, because between one-third and half of these patients have bleeding from nonvariceal sites, and future management is different for bleeding varices. The algorithm in Figure 1.2 is for the evaluation and management of variceal hemorrhage.

Lower GI bleeding is defined as bleeding from below the ligament of Treitz. When patients hospitalized for GI bleeding are identified, lower GI sources account for one-quarter to one-third of all bleeding events. When the location of bleeding is suspected to be the lower GI tract, a nasogastric tube and even upper endoscopy may still be needed to rule out an upper GI source of hemorrhage. It is important to remember that as many as 10% of patients with hematochezia have an upper GI source, and that results of nasogastric aspiration can be falsely negative when bleeding is duodenal and there is no duodenogastric reflux or when the bleeding has ceased. The algorithm in Figure 1.3 is for evaluation of lower GI bleeding. Unfortunately, some patients have both upper and lower GI bleeding sites that defy diagnosis despite the numerous diagnostic modalities available. They need repeated studies if bleeding recurs or becomes a management problem.

Atlas of Gastroenterology, 4th edition. Edited by Tadataka Yamada, David H. Alpers, Anthony N. Kalloo, Neil Kaplowitz, Chung Owyang, and Don W. Powell. © 2009 Blackwell Publishing, ISBN: 978-1-4051-6909-7

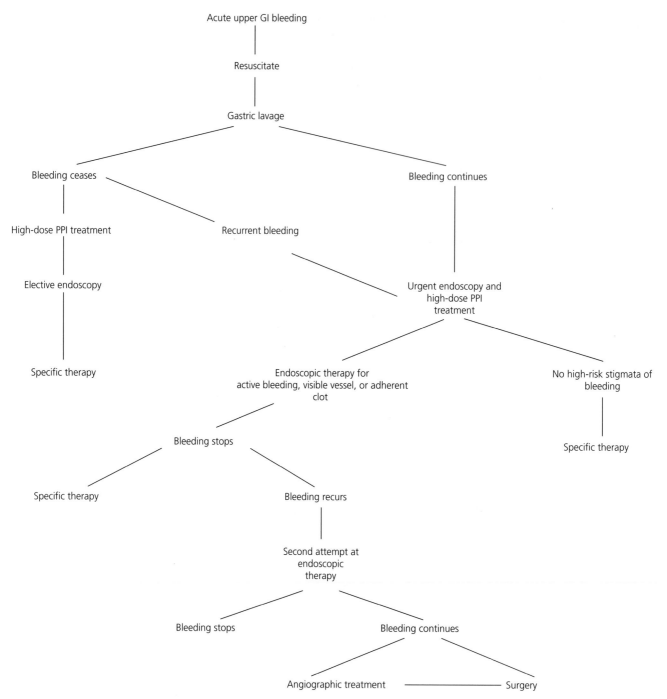

Figure 1.1 Algorithm for evaluation of nonvariceal upper GI bleeding. GI, gastrointestinal; PPI, proton pump inhibitor.

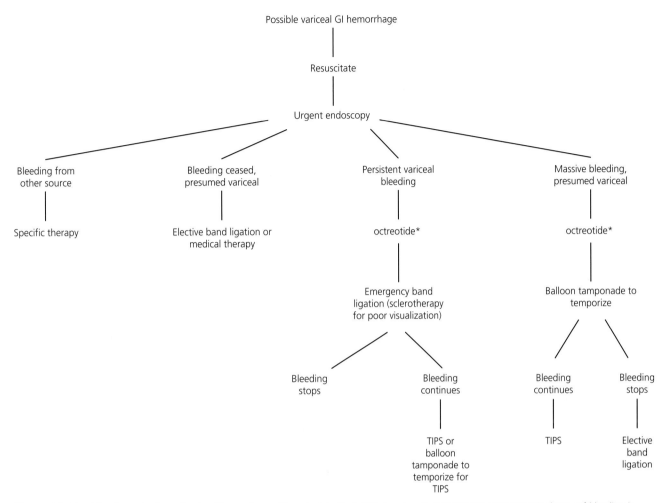

Figure 1.2 Algorithm for evaluation of variceal hemorrhage. GI, gastrointestinal; TIPS, transjugular intrahepatic portosystemic shunt. *If bleeding is persistent or massive, octreotide may be used prior to and concomitantly with endoscopy.

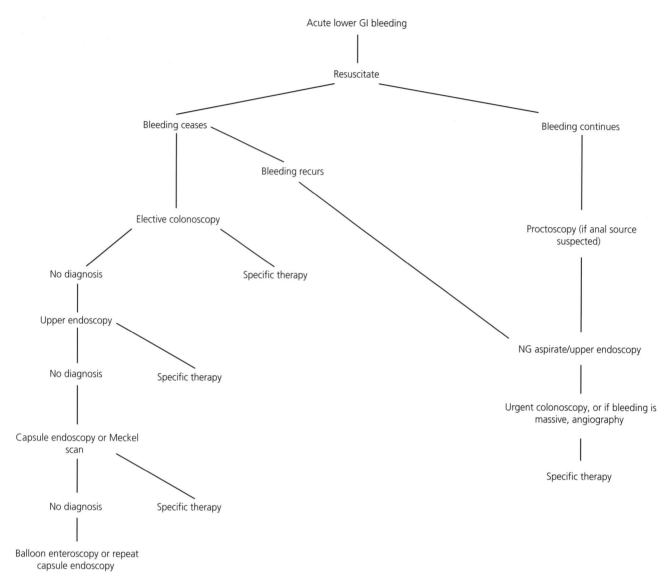

Figure 1.3 Algorithm for evaluation of lower GI bleeding. GI, gastrointestinal; NG, nasogastric.

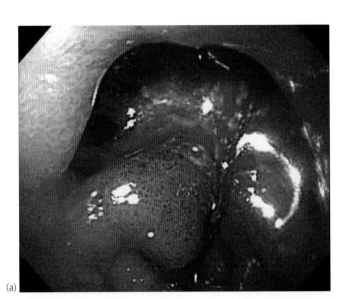
(a)

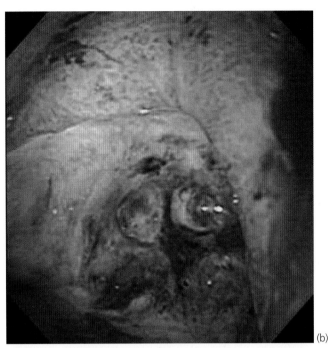
(b)

Figure 1.4 (a) An endoscopic view using a straight-viewing scope of a large posterior wall duodenal bulb ulcer in an elderly woman who had already required transfusion of 6 units of red blood cells. The entire ulcer could not be visualized adequately for endoscopic therapy. **(b)** Changing to a side-viewing duodenoscope gave excellent visualization of the crater base and a visible vessel, which was treated with epinephrine injection and multipolar coagulation. The patient had no further bleeding.

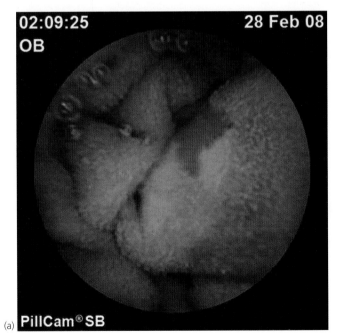
(a)

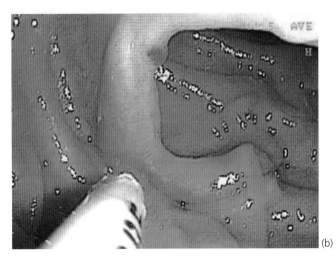
(b)

Figure 1.5 (a) An 80-year-old man with aortic stenosis presenting with intermittent melena and anemia requiring a weekly transfusion. Two upper endoscopies, two colonoscopies, and a small bowel barium study did not reveal an etiology. Capsule endoscopy revealed multiple medium to large arteriovenous malformations in the distal jejunum and proximal ileum. **(b)** These lesions were treated with argon plasma coagulation during double balloon enteroscopy.

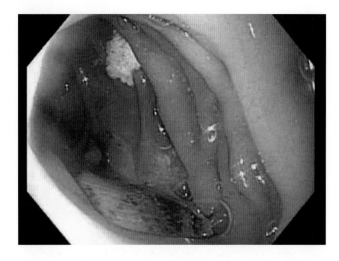

Figure 1.6 A 60-year-old man with a prior history of an aortic aneurysm repair presented with hematochezia. An upper endoscopy revealed visible aortic graft with distal oozing of blood in the third portion of the duodenum.

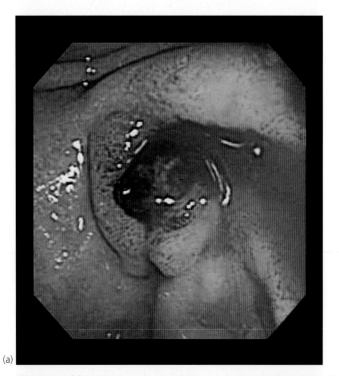

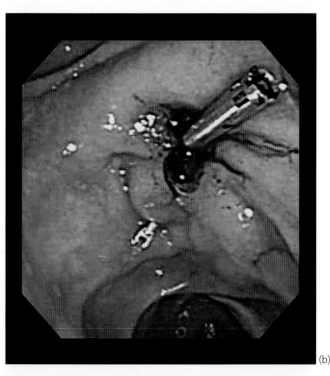

(a)

(b)

Figure 1.7 (a) Duodenoscopic view of the ampulla 1 week after biliary sphincterotomy in a patient who had restarted anticoagulation therapy and presented with melena. **(b)** After careful identification of the biliary and pancreatic orifices, the bleeding site was noted to be between these two sites, fairly close to the pancreatic orifice. Thermal therapy would require protective pancreatic stenting. Therefore, the choice for therapy was epinephrine injection followed by placement of a single clip. No further bleeding occurred.

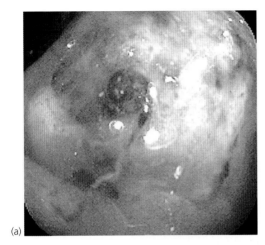

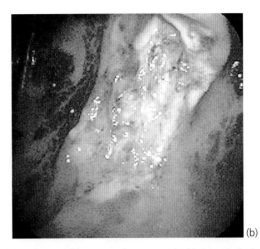

(a)

(b)

Figure 1.8 (a) Sigmoid colon view of a polypectomy site with a visible vessel in a 65-year-old woman who presented with hematochezia 3 days after polypectomy of a sessile polyp with snare electrocautery. **(b)** Sigmoid colon view of the postpolypectomy site after treatment with multipolar electrocoagulation.

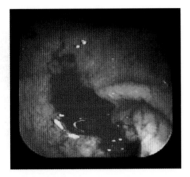

Figure 1.9 Duodenal bulb view of an actively bleeding Dieulafoy lesion in the distal bulb. After cleansing, there was no associated erosion or ulcer. This lesion was managed successfully with electrocautery. (Courtesy of W.D. Chey.)

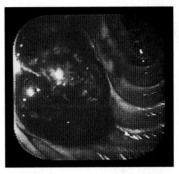

Figure 1.11 A 57-year-old woman with known metastatic carcinoma of the breast presented with melena and light-headedness. This lesion in the second portion of the duodenum was found at biopsy to be metastatic adenocarcinoma. (Courtesy of W.D. Chey.)

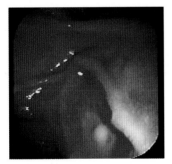

Figure 1.10 A 52-year-old man without a history of abdominal pain presented with his third episode of hematemesis in 5 months. Two previous upper endoscopic examinations did not show a bleeding source. At a third endoscopic examination, blood was found in the second portion of the duodenum, and examination with a side-viewing duodenoscope revealed hemobilia. Subsequent endoscopic retrograde cholangiopancreatography revealed a small stone in the distal common bile duct. The stone was removed after sphincterotomy.

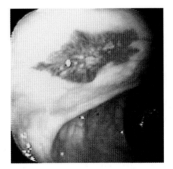

Figure 1.12 An 82-year-old man presented with an episode of hematochezia that lasted for 24 hours, along with mild anemia. Colonoscopy after preparation revealed vascular ectasia in the right colon.

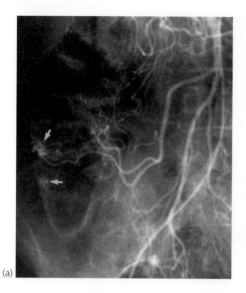

(a)

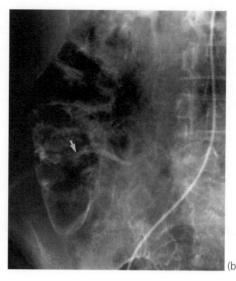

(b)

Figure 1.13 (a) Angiographic demonstration of two vascular tufts (arrows) consistent with cecal angiodysplasia. **(b)** Venous image from the same arteriogram demonstrated early venous filling (arrow), reflecting arteriovenous communication through a dilated vascular ectasia.

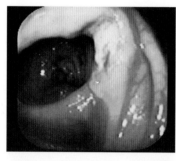

Figure 1.14 A 32-year-old man presented with maroon stools 4 days after running a marathon. Colonoscopy revealed two ulcers in the right colon. Biopsy findings were consistent with ischemia. The patient denied a history of use of nonsteroidal antiinflammatory drugs. Courtesy of W.D. Chey.

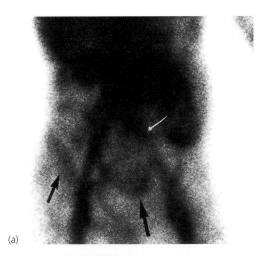

(a)

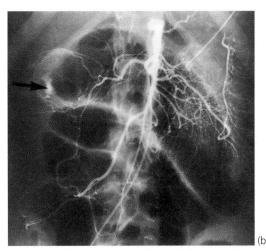

(b)

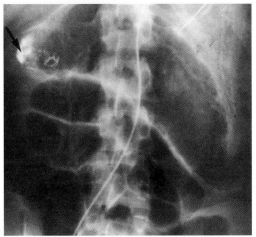

(c)

Figure 1.15 (a) Five-minute image from a technetium-99m pertechnetate-labeled red cell scan of a 23-year-old woman postpartum with diffuse intravascular coagulation and gross hematochezia. The radioactivity appears to extend from the hepatic flexure to a location distal to the splenic flexure (arrows). **(b)** Angiographic injection of the superior mesenteric artery of the same patient as in (a) immediately after the scintigraphic study demonstrated active bleeding in the hepatic flexure area of the colon (arrow). **(c)** Later image during the angiographic study shows persistent extravasation of contrast medium in the lumen of the colon (arrow).

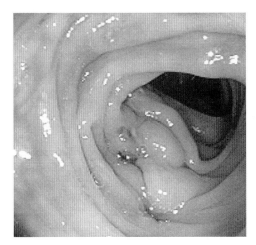

Figure 1.16 Sigmoid colon view of a bleeding diverticulum in a 68-year-old man on one aspirin per day after the bleeding was controlled with injection of 8 mL of 1:10 000 epinephrine.

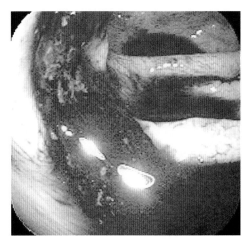

Figure 1.17 Sigmoid colon view of a bleeding diverticulum at 35 cm in a 58-year-old woman. The bleeding stopped after injection of diluted epinephrine and treatment with multipolar coagulation. The diverticula were limited to the sigmoid and descending colon. Hematochezia recurred 4 days later and a sigmoid colectomy was performed.

2 Approach to the patient with occult gastrointestinal bleeding

David A. Ahlquist

Occult gastrointestinal (GI) bleeding is, by definition, not apparent on inspection of stools. Its presence is either suggested indirectly, by the finding of iron deficiency with or without associated microcytic anemia, or directly, by a fecal blood test. As with overt GI bleeding, occult bleeding may be acute or chronic, intermittent or continuous. Occult GI bleeding may arise at any level from the oropharynx to the distal rectum, and there are many causes. As such, the clinician's judgment is challenged when faced with occult GI bleeding.

Iron deficiency anemia is the critical metabolic consequence of chronic occult GI bleeding. Occult GI bleeding may lead to iron deficiency in patients of any age, but is by far the most frequent etiology in men and postmenopausal women. Iron deficiency is exceedingly common, with a worldwide prevalence estimated at 15%; an appreciation of its causal association with occult GI bleeding is important.

Occult GI bleeding ranges from small physiological losses of 1–2 mL per day to marked pathological elevations. As much as 200 mL blood may be lost from the upper GI tract and remain occult. Generally, average blood losses of 5–10 mL per day or more are required to overcome compensatory mechanisms, deplete iron stores, and eventuate in anemia.

Occult GI bleeding involves a defect in the continuity of the epithelium and thus may be caused by inflammatory, neoplastic, infectious, vascular, or traumatic mechanisms. Most clinically important occult bleeding arises from the upper GI tract. As a group, acid peptic disorders are the most common cause of occult bleeding and anemia in industrialized countries. Malignant tumors of the GI tract represent another frequent cause: colorectal and gastric cancers are most common. On a global scale, however, hookworm infestation accounts for the largest number of persons with anemia from occult GI bleeding. Medications, especially aspirin and related nonsteroidal antiinflammatory drugs, commonly induce occult bleeding. Other causes of occult bleeding include the heterogeneous array of acquired and inherited vascular malformations, large hiatal hernias with associated Cameron erosions, inflammatory bowel disease, and certain endurance sports, especially long-distance running.

Because clinically significant lesions do not always bleed and not all occult bleeding results in iron deficiency, hematological and fecal blood assessment are complementary diagnostic tests and can be interpreted only in the context of all clinical information about the patient. In patients with new onset iron deficiency and occult GI bleeding, a hemorrhagic GI lesion should be aggressively sought.

Several types of tests for detection of fecal occult blood are available. These tests assay different portions of the hemoglobin molecule. Because the hemoglobin constituents, globin and heme, are altered during digestive transit, immunochemical- and guaiac-type tests, which respectively target these analytes, often fail to detect proximal gut bleeding. In contrast, the heme–porphyrin test is unaffected by the anatomic level of bleeding. As such, each type of test has advantages and disadvantages according to the clinical indication. For colorectal cancer screening, guaiac- or immunochemical-based tests may be preferable because of their simplicity, qualitative nature, and insensitivity for upper GI bleeding. For the evaluation of iron deficiency, the heme–porphyrin based test is most ideal because detection is quantitative and includes occult bleeding from all potential sites.

Effective treatment is dictated by the type of lesion found. The combination of extended upper endoscopy and colonoscopy will successfully identify the culprit lesions in more than 80%–90% of instances. However, the diagnostic evaluation may be complex in the remaining small proportion. The extent of evaluation in cases of obscure occult bleeding must be weighted by the refractoriness of anemia, presence of comorbidities, and other factors. Most obscure GI bleeding occurs as a result of vascular malformations occurring in the small intestine.

Atlas of Gastroenterology, 4th edition. Edited by Tadataka Yamada, David H. Alpers, Anthony N. Kalloo, Neil Kaplowitz, Chung Owyang, and Don W. Powell. © 2009 Blackwell Publishing, ISBN: 978-1-4051-6909-7

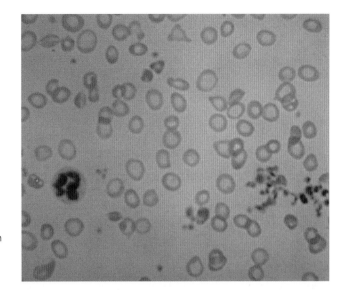

Figure 2.1 Peripheral blood smear from a patient with iron deficiency anemia. The red cells are small (microcytic), low in hemoglobin content (hypochromic), and variable in shape (anisocytic). However, these morphological features may occur with other conditions, including anemia of chronic disease, thalassemia, sideroblastic anemia, the presence of hemoglobin E, and copper deficiency. Iron stores should be assessed when microcytic anemia is discovered. Because anemia is a late manifestation of iron deficiency, iron stores are always low when anemia is caused by iron deficiency.

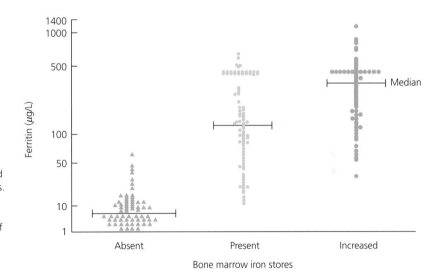

Figure 2.2 Relation between histologically assessed marrow iron stores and serum ferritin concentrations. All patients with ferritin values in the shaded region have absent storage iron. Thus, a low serum ferritin level is pathognomonic for iron deficiency. Causes of microcytic anemia other than iron deficiency are associated with normal or increased iron stores and ferritin levels.

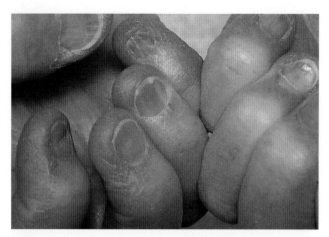

Figure 2.3 Koilonychia. These nail changes are characteristic of iron deficiency and consist of spooning concavity, longitudinal ridging, and brittleness. This patient had profound iron deficiency anemia caused by chronic occult bleeding from watermelon stomach.

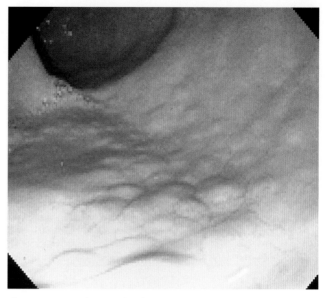

Figure 2.5 Antral mucosal nodularity with *Helicobacter pylori* gastritis. *H. pylori* gastritis may be associated with iron deficiency even in the absence of endoscopically demonstrated erosions or ulcerations. Collectively, peptic diseases of the esophagus, stomach, and duodenum are the most common cause of occult gastrointestinal bleeding and iron deficiency in adults from industrialized countries.

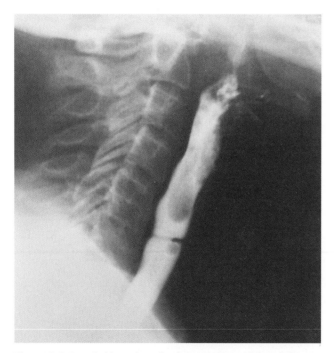

Figure 2.4 Postcricoid esophageal web in a patient with iron deficiency anemia (Plummer–Vinson or Paterson–Kelly syndrome). These webs are eccentric, sometimes multiple, proximally located, and more common among women. They may resolve with iron replacement.

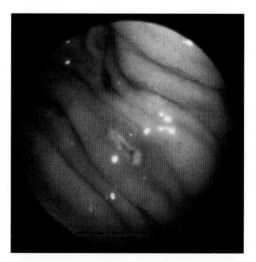

Figure 2.6 Endoscopic photograph of a Cameron erosion. This characteristic gastric mucosal lesion may accompany large hiatal hernias, which are found in as many as 10% of adults with iron deficiency anemia. Chronic occult bleeding results from these longitudinal erosions that straddle the diaphragmatic hiatus. Cameron erosions are probably caused by mechanical trauma from breathing.

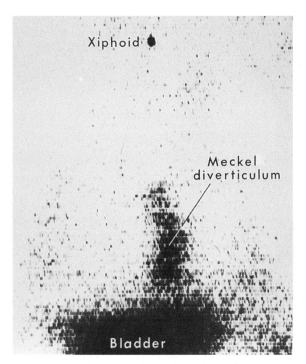

Figure 2.7 A pertechnetate scintigram shows abnormal tracer accumulation in Meckel diverticulum. Although commonly a cause of overt bleeding among children and young adults, Meckel diverticulum may produce chronic occult blood loss and anemia, as was the case for this 38-year-old woman.

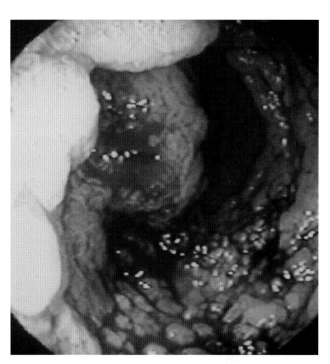

Figure 2.9 Hemorrhagic gastric adenocarcinoma in an elderly woman with profound iron deficiency anemia and negative immunochemical fecal blood test results. Because the globin portion of hemoglobin is digested by upper gastrointestinal peptidases, immunochemical tests may fail to detect occult bleeding from the proximal gut.

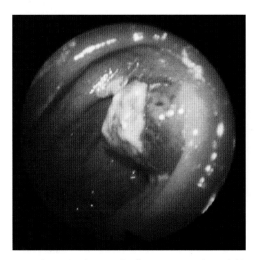

Figure 2.8 Endoscopic photograph of a rare cause of occult bleeding. This ulcerated lipoma in the descending colon caused occult bleeding in a patient taking long-term anticoagulant therapy. Elevated fecal blood levels for a patient taking anticoagulants usually reflect underlying gastrointestinal disease.

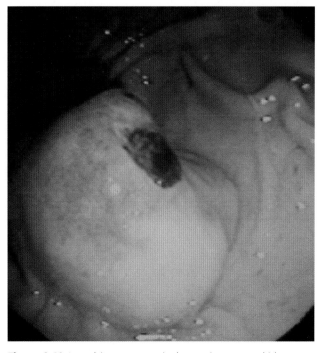

Figure 2.10 Large leiomyosarcoma in the gastric antrum, which presented with occult gastrointestinal bleeding and iron deficiency anemia. Such lesions are characteristically smooth walled with a central depressed ulceration.

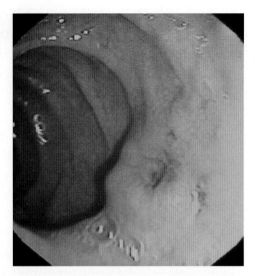

Figure 2.11 Ulcerated leiomyoma in the proximal jejunum, found on extended upper endoscopy. The initial evaluation in this 40-year-old man with iron deficiency and occult gastrointestinal bleeding included a negative upper endoscopy, colonoscopy, and small bowel barium radiograph.

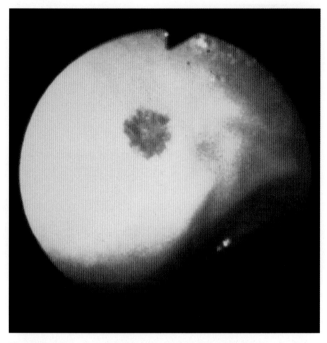

Figure 2.12 Endoscopic photograph of mulberry-type gastric vascular malformation. Vascular malformations of the gastrointestinal tract are heterogeneous in size, number, configuration, and location. Together they may explain 0.4%–6.0% of all iron deficiency anemias among adults in the Western world. Even when producing transfusion-dependent anemia, bleeding from vascular malformations remains occult in nearly one-half of cases.

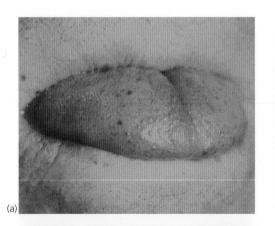

(a)

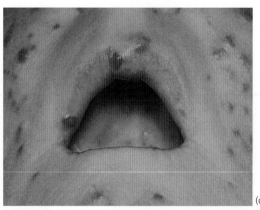

(c)

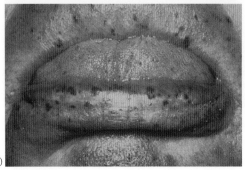

(b)

Figure 2.13 Hereditary hemorrhagic telangiectasia (Osler–Weber–Rendu) syndrome. Characteristic circumoral and lingual telangiectasia may be subtle **(a)**, moderately dense **(b)**, or florid **(c)**. Similar-appearing lesions occur throughout the gastrointestinal (GI) tract, especially in the gastroduodenal region. Gastrointestingal bleeding, usually occult, often becomes problematic in middle-aged patients.

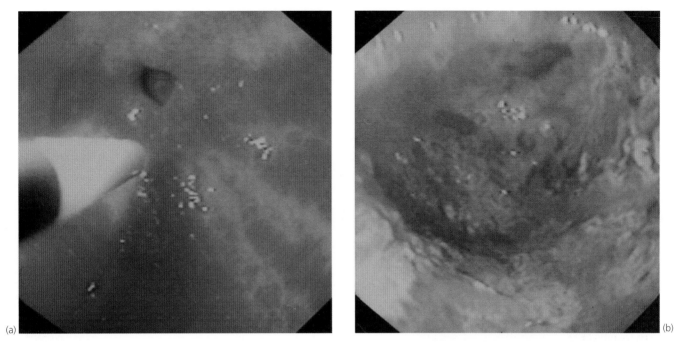

(a)

(b)

Figure 2.14 Watermelon stomach. Linearly arrayed vascular tissue radially distributed in the antrum looks like watermelon stripes **(a)**. Painless occult gastrointestinal bleeding with anemia in an elderly woman is the most typical presentation. This lesion is amenable to endoscopic thermal ablation, and the lesion shown was treated by argon plasma coagulation **(b)**.

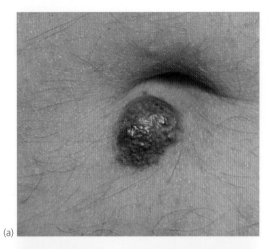

(a)

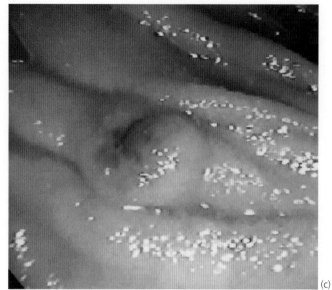

(c)

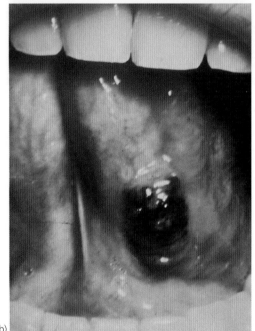

(b)

Figure 2.15 Blue rubber bleb nevus syndrome. This rare syndrome associated with occult gastrointestinal (GI) bleeding is characterized by congenitally acquired bluish hemangiomas that may occur on the skin **(a)** and mucous membranes of the mouth **(b)** or GI tract **(c)**. The GI lesions are amenable to endoscopic thermal ablation if they can be reached.

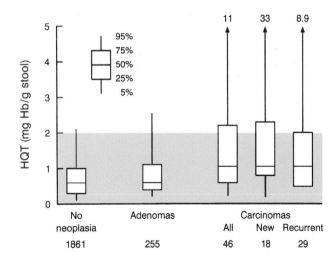

Figure 2.16 Fecal blood distribution measured by means of the HemoQuant test (Mayo Medical Laboratories, Rochester, MN) among persons without symptoms who are undergoing routine postoperative surveillance. The presence or absence of colorectal neoplasia was established by means of imaging (normally colonoscopy but occasionally sigmoidoscopy plus barium enema). The shaded zone represents the normal range as defined by the HemoQuant assay at a reported specificity of 95%.

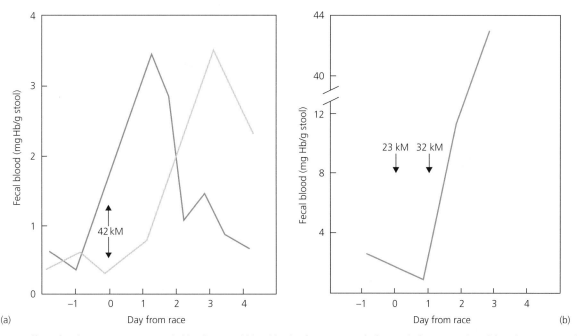

(a)

(b)

Figure 2.17 Effect of endurance sports on occult bleeding. Fecal blood levels of two runners before and after a marathon **(a)** and one runner after consecutive days of long-distance races **(b)**. Occult gastrointestinal bleeding may contribute to the relatively common finding of iron deficiency among endurance runners.

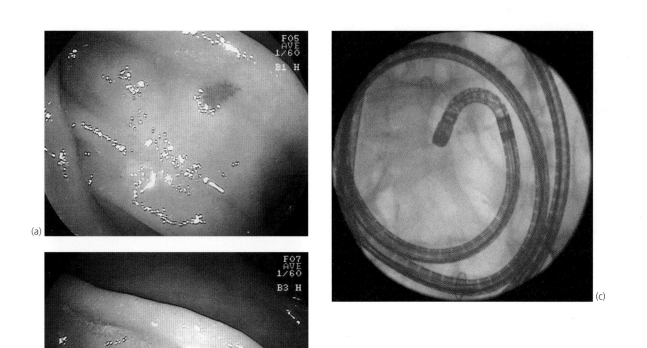

(a)

(b)

(c)

Figure 2.18 Double-balloon enteroscopy (DBE). This new endoscopic tool allows controllable lumenal imaging and therapeutic application to the full length of the small intestine. In a patient with refractory iron deficiency and consistently positive stool occult blood tests, DBE **(a)** revealed a vascular ectasia in the distal jejunum and **(b)** delivered definitive ablative coagulation. Fluoroscopy **(c)** demonstrates the deep insertion of the endoscope during this procedure.

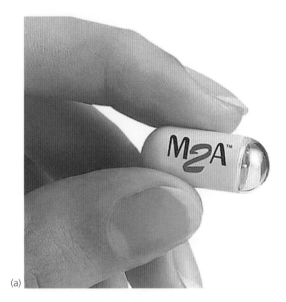

AVM

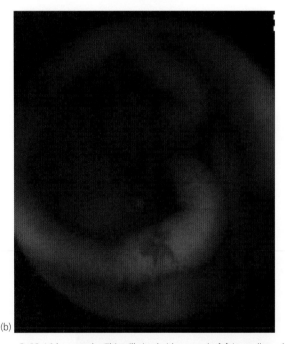

(a)

(b)

Figure 2.19 Videocapsule. This pill-sized videocapsule **(a)** is swallowed to transmit images of the gastrointestinal tract during its oro–anal transit. (Courtesy of Given Images, Inc., Norcross, Georgia) A videocapsule image of a small intestinal vascular ectasia **(b)** is shown. (Courtesy of Dr Elizabeth Rajan, Mayo Clinic.) This tool has become a feasible minimally invasive approach to inspect the small intestine, which is unreachable by conventional endoscopy.

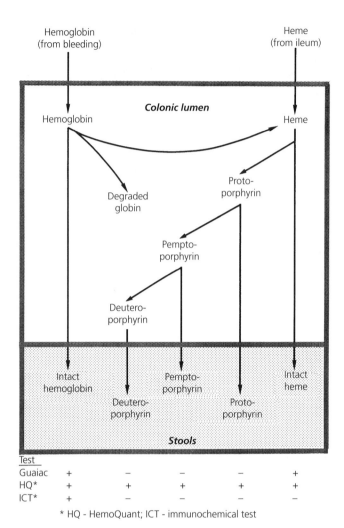

Test					
Guaiac	+	–	–	–	+
HQ*	+	+	+	+	+
ICT*	+	–	–	–	–

* HQ - HemoQuant; ICT - immunochemical test

Figure 2.20 The fate of hemoglobin and heme in the large bowel, the products found in feces, and the products detected by means of each of the three main occult blood test technologies. Upper box: Events occurring in the colonic lumen. Bottom shaded box: Derivatives found in stools. Dietary heme transiting through the ileum or hemoglobin arising from bleeding is composed of protoheme. Fecal bacteria act on the heme to remove the iron and modify the side chains, producing a range of heme-derived porphyrins. Hemoglobin itself in the feces is subject to degradative action by bacteria, which release the heme for further modification and degrade the globin. Degraded globin loses its immunoreactivity. Bottom panel: derivatives found in stools that are detected with the various fecal occult blood tests. Courtesy of Graeme Young, MD.

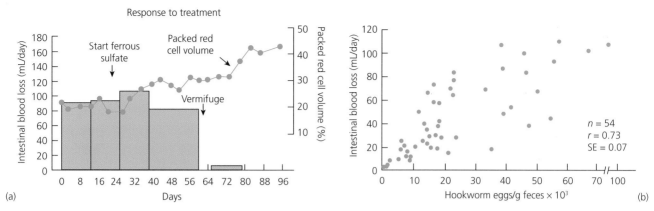

(a)

(b)

Figure 2.21 Hookworm infestation. **(a)** Hookworm-induced occult bleeding and response to vermifuge therapy. **(b)** Relation between fecal blood loss and hookworm burden. More than 600 million persons are host to this infestation, which is the most common reason for blood loss anemia worldwide.

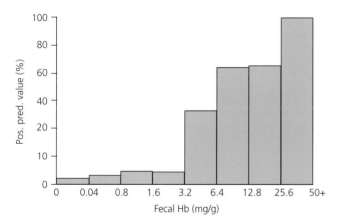

Figure 2.22 Positive predictive value of fecal hemoglobin (Hb) for presence of hemorrhagic gastrointestinal (GI) lesions. The positive predictive value increases in proportion to the fecal Hb level. Values are based on Mayo Clinic data from 1000 patients tested by the quantitative HemoQuant assay prior to GI investigation. Lesions included ulcers or erosions, vascular malformations, and malignancies.

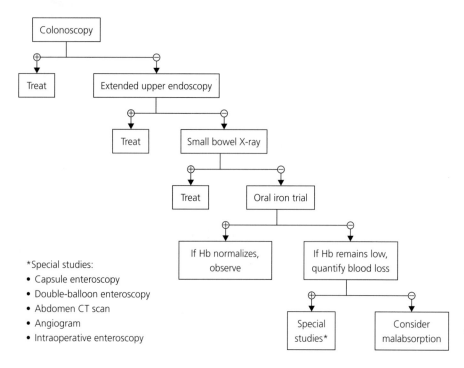

*Special studies:
- Capsule enteroscopy
- Double-balloon enteroscopy
- Abdomen CT scan
- Angiogram
- Intraoperative enteroscopy

Figure 2.23 Suggested algorithm for evaluation of an asymptomatic adult patient with iron deficiency anemia and occult gastrointestinal bleeding.

3 Approach to the patient with acute abdomen

Rebecca M. Minter, Michael W. Mulholland

The term *acute abdomen* describes a syndrome of sudden abdominal pain with accompanying symptoms and signs that focus attention on the abdominal region. It is clinically useful to limit the discussion to cases in which the pain has been present for less than 24 h. Associated symptoms such as nausea, vomiting, constipation, diarrhea, anorexia, abdominal distention, and fever often are present and sometimes are confusing. Although operative therapy is not required for all cases of acute abdomen, unwarranted operative delay can have serious, potentially fatal consequences. Successful management is based on a careful initial assessment that incorporates history taking and physical examination; delineation of clinical priorities; and concurrent resuscitation, diagnosis, and therapy.

The treatment of patients with acute abdominal processes differs in a fundamental way from the care delivered to patients with long-term problems. The potential for pathological processes to be rapidly progressive and for serious adverse consequences to result from therapeutic delay places a time constraint on diagnosis and treatment. An accurate diagnosis should lead promptly to specific therapy. A complete and accurate history and physical examination are the most important requirements for success.

The treating physician should first focus on the nature and timing of the abdominal pain. The pattern of onset and the progression of pain provide valuable clues to the cause. The pain associated with perforation of a duodenal ulcer or rupture of an abdominal aortic aneurysm is incapacitating, begins suddenly, and quickly reaches peak intensity. Because the onset of pain is so dramatic, patients may be able to provide detailed information about the time of onset or their activities at that moment. In contrast, pain associated with appendicitis increases over a period of one to several hours. Similarly, pain caused by acute cholecystitis increases over hours before reaching a steady intensity. The duration of painful symptoms is important. Biliary colic typically lasts for several hours before rapidly resolving, presumably as a result of dislodgment of the offending stone from the cystic duct. Pain caused by acute pancreatitis is unrelenting. Patients with mechanical obstruction of the small intestine initially may feel remarkably well between episodes of intense and debilitating colic.

The physical examination should be conducted in a systematic and unhurried manner. A complete abdominal examination requires unhindered visualization of the area between the nipples and the midthigh, anteriorly and posteriorly. The examination begins with observation of the patient's expression and behavior. A patient with serious intraperitoneal abnormalities usually has an anxious, pale face. Sweating, dilated pupils, and shallow breathing are common. In the presence of chemical or bacterial contamination of the peritoneum, the patient tends to lie immobile to minimize movement of inflamed viscera against the parietal peritoneum. Knees may be flexed, the abdomen scaphoid, breathing shallow. Inhaling deeply or coughing aggravates the pain. With ureteral colic or mesenteric ischemia, by contrast, the patient may appear restless with frequent changes in posture in an attempt to relieve discomfort. During inspection, the location of all surgical scars, masses, external hernias, and stomas is determined.

Auscultation precedes abdominal palpation. All four quadrants are auscultated for tone and quantity of bowel sounds and the presence of vascular bruits. Bowel sounds are considered to be absent only if no tones are heard over a 2-min period of auscultation.

Next, the abdomen is palpated. To determine areas of tenderness and the vigor with which palpation may be pursued, it is useful first to ask the patient to demonstrate the point of maximal discomfort. Palpation begins in the abdominal quadrant farthest from the area of suspected pathological change. Gentle pressure to elicit tenderness and muscular resistance ensues. Progressively deeper palpation is attempted to delineate masses. Intentional efforts to reproduce abdominal pain by means of deep palpation and rapid release of pressure, termed *rebound tenderness,* are not helpful and *should not be attempted.* Production of rebound tenderness

Atlas of Gastroenterology, 4th edition. Edited by Tadataka Yamada, David H. Alpers, Anthony N. Kalloo, Neil Kaplowitz, Chung Owyang, and Don W. Powell. © 2009 Blackwell Publishing, ISBN: 978-1-4051-6909-7

provides no information that is not available through gentle examination, causes the patient to guard voluntarily, and eliminates the possibility of meaningful serial abdominal examinations. The best evidence of a localized inflammatory process is demonstration of point tenderness, caused by movement of the parietal peritoneum against the inflamed surface of a diseased viscus. Point tenderness is sought by palpating the area of maximal discomfort, but also may be elicited by grasping the patient's hips and gently rocking the pelvis; the movement of the inflamed peritoneum is pre-sumed to cause pain. A stethoscope may be used to palpate the abdominal quadrants.

Every patient must undergo a digital rectal examination. If an inflamed appendix lies deep within the pelvis, point tenderness may sometimes be elicited only by means of palpation through the right rectal wall. Stool is tested for guaiac positivity. For female patients, manual and speculum vaginal examinations are required; vaginal secretions are obtained for Gram stain and culture. All external stomas, wounds, and fistulae are explored digitally.

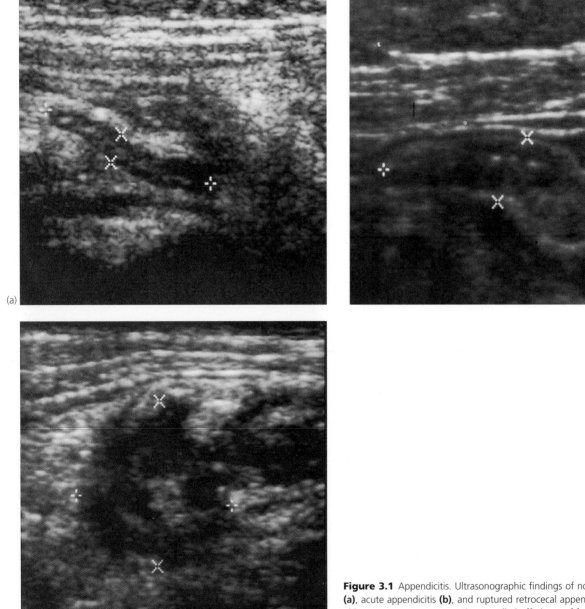

(a)

(b)

(c)

Figure 3.1 Appendicitis. Ultrasonographic findings of normal appendix **(a)**, acute appendicitis **(b)**, and ruptured retrocecal appendix with phlegmonous mass representing a walled-off abscess **(c)**. The retrocecal appendix (middle two cursors) is surrounded by echogenic amorphous material, representing the phlegmon.

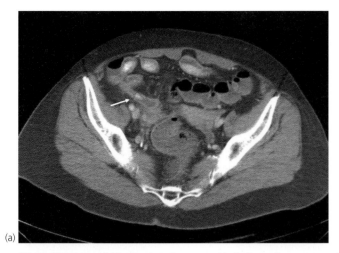

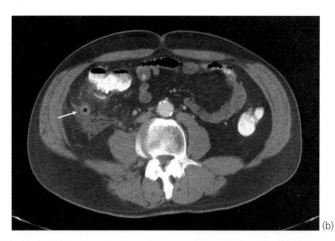

(a)

(b)

Figure 3.2 Appendicitis. Computed tomographic findings of acute appendicitis. Oral and i.v. contrast-enhanced computed tomography scan shows a thickened, fluid-filled appendix with an appendicolith (arrow) visualized within the lumen **(a)**. Cross-sectional image of a thickened, inflamed appendix with adjacent periappendiceal fat stranding **(b)**.

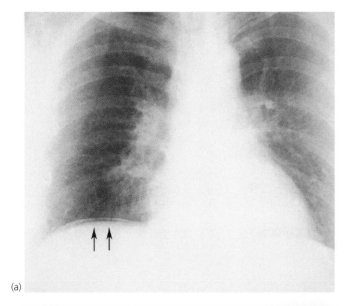

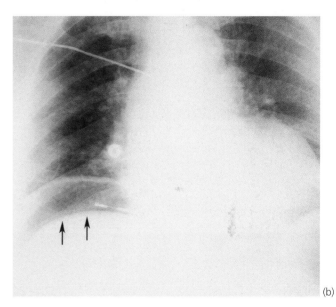

(a)

(b)

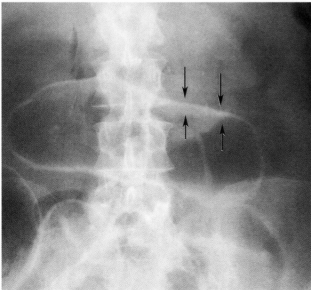

Figure 3.3 Pneumoperitoneum. **(a, b)** Upright chest radiographs of patients with pneumoperitoneum demonstrate minimal and large collections of air (arrows) under the right hemidiaphragms. **(c)** Flat abdominal radiograph demonstrates the double-wall sign of pneumoperitoneum (arrows). Free intraperitoneal air outlines the serosal surface of the bowel, and intralumenal gas outlines the mucosal surface.

(c)

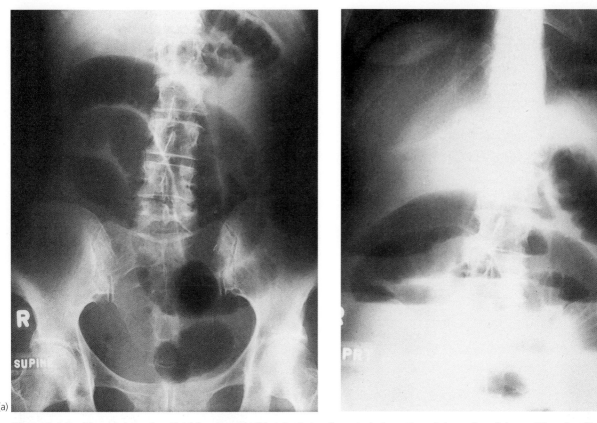

(a)   (b)

Figure 3.4 Small bowel obstruction. Flat **(a)** and upright **(b)** abdominal radiographs in the setting of obstruction of the small intestine. Distended, air-filled loops of small bowel and multiple air–fluid levels are present (b), and air is absent in the colon.

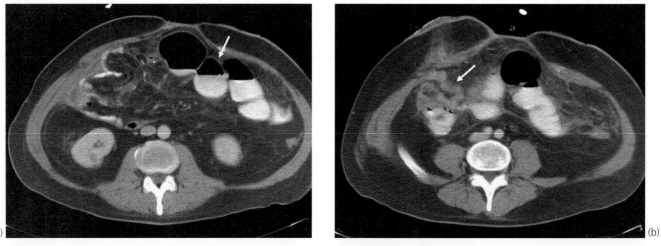

(a)   (b)

Figure 3.5 Small bowel obstruction. Computed tomographic findings of a complete small bowel obstruction following exploratory laparotomy for a perforated cecal mass. **(a)** Proximal small bowel is dilated and multiple air–fluid levels are noted (arrow). **(b)** A clear transition point is noted with decompressed small bowel distally (arrow). Contrast did not pass beyond this point.

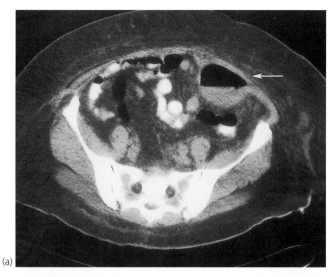

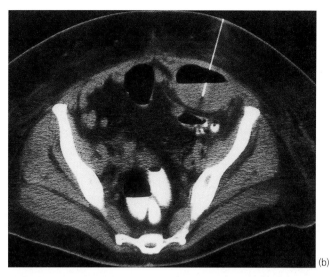

Figure 3.6 Diverticulitis. **(a, b)** Computed tomograms of a patient with sigmoid diverticulitis and associated pericolic abscess (arrow). The abscess was amenable to percutaneous drainage. **(b)** Needle aspiration of the abscess preparatory to drain placement.

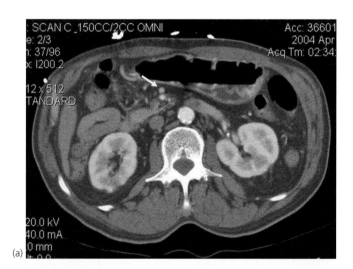

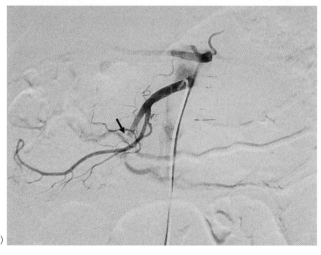

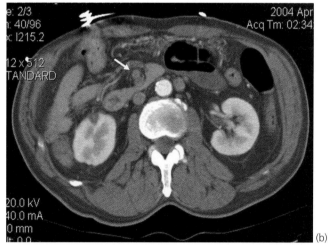

Figure 3.7 Acute mesenteric ischemia. Computed tomographic angiogram of a patient with abdominal pain out of proportion to physical examination and a history of atrial fibrillation. **(a, b)** The first image demonstrates patency of the proximal superior mesenteric artery (SMA) as evidenced by the presence of intralumenal i.v. contrast (arrow), followed in the sequential image by a large embolus within the lumen of the SMA (arrow) and an absence of intraarterial contrast. **(c)** Selective superior mesenteric angiogram verified the diagnosis, and demonstrates an abrupt cut-off at the level of the SMA embolus (arrow).

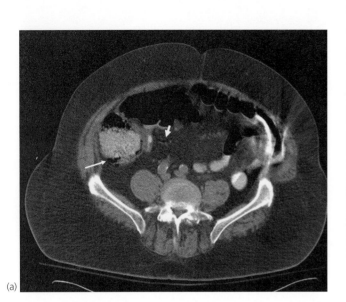

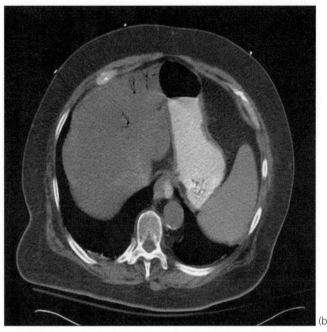

(a)

(b)

Figure 3.8 Intestinal ischemia. Computed tomograms of a patient with severe acidosis and localized peritonitis on examination. **(a)** Cecal pneumatosis intestinalis is noted in the dependent portion of the bowel wall (long arrow) with adjacent mesenteric venous air (short arrow). **(b)** Portal venous air was also noted within the liver.

4 Approach to the patient with ileus and obstruction

Klaus Bielefeldt

Ileus and obstruction are among the most common reasons for hospitalization owing to gastrointestinal problems. Though different in the pathology, both are characterized by stasis of lumenal contents and secondary changes, such as bacterial overgrowth, translocation, and systemic shifts in fluids and electrolytes (Fig. 4.1). If history and physical findings suggest the presence of ileus or obstruction, diagnostic evaluations are needed to differentiate between a generally impaired motor function of the intestinal tract (ileus) and the consequences of a mechanical obstruction to lumenal transit, the site must be localized, the cause identified, and possible complications anticipated.

Plain abdominal radiographs are often the first step. They may show dilated loops of the small or large intestine (Fig. 4.2). The plain film relies on air within the intestinal lumen as the natural contrast. Thus, dilated, fluid-filled loops of bowel may not be seen, limiting the sensitivity of this test. Moreover, conventional abdominal radiographs often cannot localize the site and determine the nature of an obstruction. The only exceptions are the classic image of a sigmoid volvulus (Fig. 4.3) or radioopaque foreign bodies, which can be readily recognized (Fig. 4.4).

Computed tomography (CT) has proven superior and is largely supplanting the abdominal radiograph as the initial method of evaluation of choice. CT scanning does not require air to visualize dilated loops of bowel, and thus has a higher sensitivity than conventional imaging. As is true for plain radiographs and contrast studies, a combination of clues from anatomical location, lumenal diameter, and the presence of haustrations or valvulae conniventes generally allows differentiation of the small bowel from the colon involved in the disease process (Fig. 4.5). The imaging of soft tissue structures and surrounding organs also allows identification of potentially underlying causes (Figs 4.6 and 4.7). In the absence of distinct abnormalities, such as inflammatory masses or tumors, the presence of an abrupt transition from dilated to collapsed loops of the bowel should lead us to suspect adhesive disease, which is the most common cause of small bowel obstruction in Western countries (Fig. 4.8). Computed tomography also has a higher sensitivity for identifying complications, such as ischemia, perforation, or pneumatosis intestinalis (Fig. 4.9).

Contrast studies play a minor role in the diagnosis of obstruction. In the case of partial small bowel obstruction, they may be able to identify underlying problems (Fig. 4.10). However, barium-containing contrast can trigger severe peritonitis in cases of perforation and can inspissate, which should be considered prior to performing the test. Conversely, water-soluble contrast typically is diluted significantly in the often distended and fluid-filled loops of intestine, limiting lumenal opacification and diagnostic gain (Fig. 4.11).

In easily reachable regions of the proximal and distal gastrointestinal tract, endoscopic studies can diagnose and at times treat obstructions. Dilation of pyloric or anastomotic strictures often suffices as therapy and avoids the need for surgery. Malignant stenoses can be dilated but require stenting to remain patent, which allows palliation of symptoms or improves results of more definitive surgical interventions in patients presenting with malignant obstructions (Fig. 4.12).

Atlas of Gastroenterology, 4th edition. Edited by Tadataka Yamada, David H. Alpers, Anthony N. Kalloo, Neil Kaplowitz, Chung Owyang, and Don W. Powell. © 2009 Blackwell Publishing, ISBN: 978-1-4051-6909-7

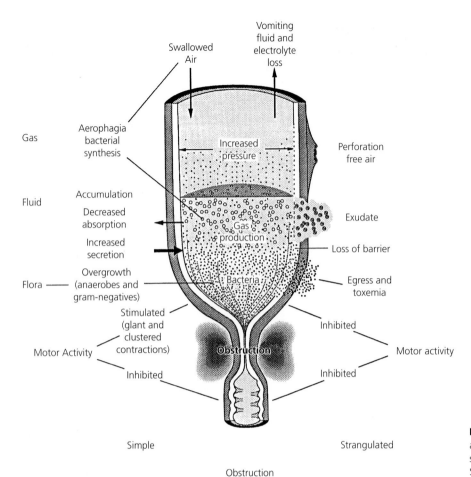

Figure labels for Figure 4.1:

Swallowed Air

Vomiting fluid and electrolyte loss

Gas

Aerophagia bacterial synthesis

Increased pressure

Perforation free air

Fluid

Accumulation

Decreased absorption

Gas production

Exudate

Increased secretion

Loss of barrier

Flora

Overgrowth (anaerobes and gram-negatives)

Bacteria

Egress and toxemia

Motor Activity

Stimulated (glant and clustered contractions)

Obstruction

Inhibited

Motor activity

Inhibited

Inhibited

Simple

Strangulated

Obstruction

Figure 4.1 Pathophysiology of simple (left) and strangulated (right) obstruction in the small intestine. Courtesy of Robert W. Summers.

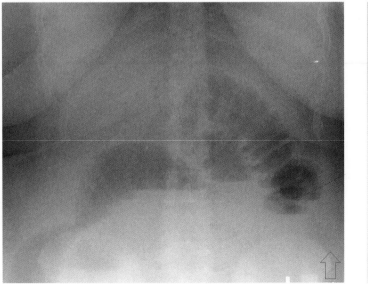
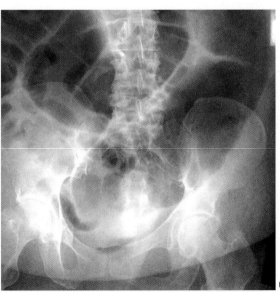

(a)

(b)

Figure 4.2 Plain abdominal films showing the typical appearance of small bowel loops **(a)** with closely spaced valvulae conniventes, whereas haustrations of the distended colon **(b)** are further apart from each other and are often not circumferential.

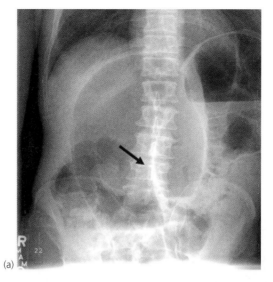

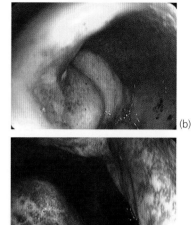

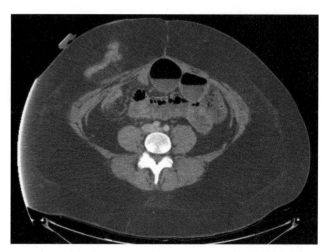

Figure 4.3 The plain abdominal radiograph **(a)** shows a sigmoid volvulus with a very distended loop of colon extending to the right upper quadrant and a distinct midline crease (arrow). The mucosa had a dusky and edematous appearance with spiraling folds as the colonoscope approached the distal end of the segment **(b)**. Advancement of the scope into the dilated segment revealed a congested, ischemic mucosa **(c)**.

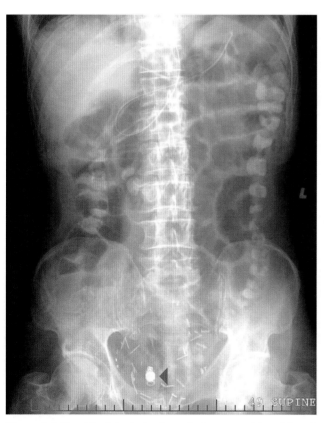

Figure 4.5 The section of an abdominal computed tomography scan shows dilated bowel loops with multiple small air bubbles trapped between valvulae conniventes ("string of beads").

Figure 4.4 The plain abdominal radiograph shows a partial small bowel obstruction in a patient after capsule endoscopy for obscure gastrointestinal bleeding. The dilated loops of the small bowel are surrounded by a decompressed colon, which is opacified by a residual oral contrast used during a preceding computed tomography scan. The red arrowhead points at the retained capsule. Multiple surgical clips and a nasogastric tube can be seen.

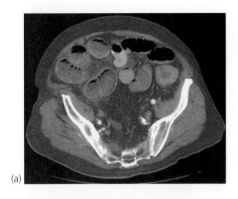

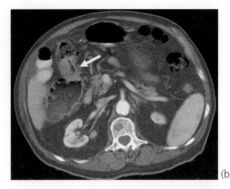

(a)

(b)

Figure 4.6 Sections of an abdominopelvic computed tomography scan showing dilated loops of small bowel with "string of beads" sign **(a)** and wall thickening with lumenal narrowing (as demonstrated by the arrow) in the ascending colon **(b)**. These findings are consistent with a partial small bowel obstruction owing to a proximal colonic malignancy.

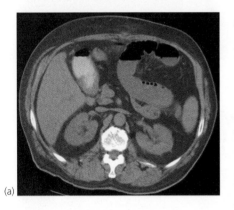

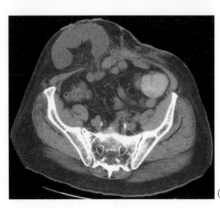

(a)

(b)

Figure 4.7 Sections of an abdominopelvic computed tomography scan showing dilated loops of small bowel with "string of beads" sign **(a)** and large incisional hernia as the cause of the small bowel obstruction **(b)**.

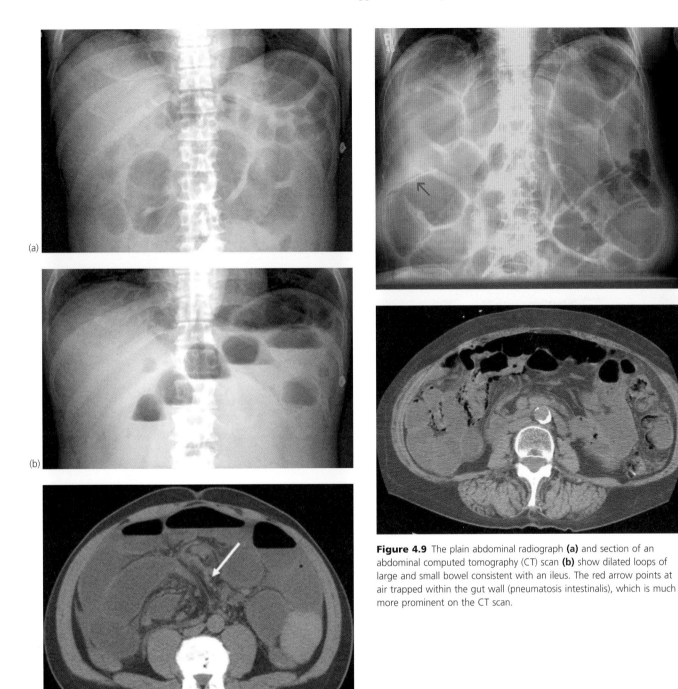

(a)

(b)

(c)

Figure 4.8 The supine **(a)** and upright **(b)** plain abdominal films show dilated loops of small bowel with multiple air–fluid levels. This is consistent with the computed tomography scan **(c)**, which demonstrates a collapsed colon (arrow). As the patient had previously undergone abdominal surgery, and imaging studies did not reveal intestinal wall thickening, lumenal foreign bodies, or soft tissue tumors causing extralumenal obstruction, these findings suggest the presence of adhesive disease.

(a)

(b)

Figure 4.9 The plain abdominal radiograph **(a)** and section of an abdominal computed tomography (CT) scan **(b)** show dilated loops of large and small bowel consistent with an ileus. The red arrow points at air trapped within the gut wall (pneumatosis intestinalis), which is much more prominent on the CT scan.

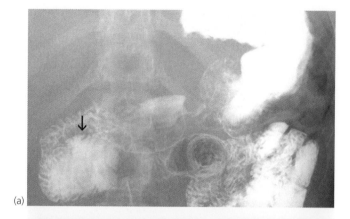

(a)

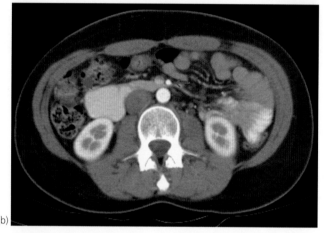

(b)

Figure 4.10 Barium contrast study **(a)** and computed tomography scan **(b)** show a dilated proximal duodenum (black arrow in (a) and red arrowhead in (b), respectively) due to extrinsic compression between the aorta and superior mesenteric artery (red arrow).

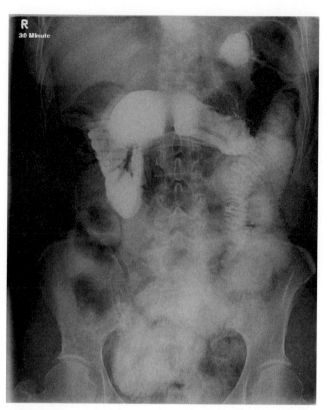

Figure 4.11 Contrast study with water-soluble contrast medium in a patient with partial small bowel obstruction owing to adhesive disease. The patient had previously undergone vertical banding gastroplasty. The prolonged retention of contrast in the gastric pouch demonstrates a problem with transit through the narrow pouch outlet. However, the dilated loops of the small bowel are only poorly opacified because of dilution of the contrast medium.

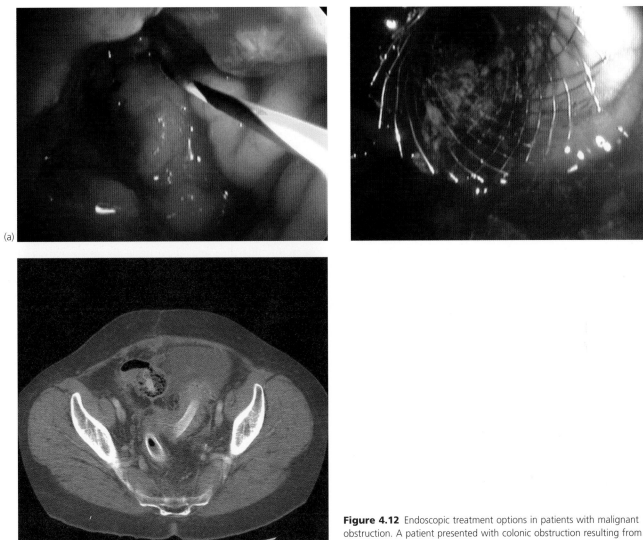

(a)

(b)

(c)

Figure 4.12 Endoscopic treatment options in patients with malignant obstruction. A patient presented with colonic obstruction resulting from cancer of the distal colon. After insertion of a guidewire **(a)**, the obstruction was successfully treated with stenting **(b and c)**. Courtesy of Dr. A Slivka.

5 Approach to the patient with diarrhea

Don W. Powell

Diarrheal diseases have quite different prevalences and outcomes in developed and developing countries. Although infant and child mortality rates have decreased in developing nations from 5 million per year in 1987 to 3.5 million per year in 1995, the infant mortality rate from diarrheal diseases in the United States is stable at 300 to 500 deaths per year. The death rate from diarrhea among persons older than 74 years in the United States is nearly 10 times that of infants, children, and younger adults.

Diarrhea (stool volumes greater than 200 mL/24 h) results from alterations in water and electrolyte transport mediated through changes in intracellular messengers or from unabsorbed osmotic solutes that retain fluid within the intestinal lumen. During inflammatory diarrhea, exudation of plasma from an ulcerated mucosa may add to the fluid loss.

Acute diarrhea is defined as having a duration of less than 2–3 weeks and most commonly being caused by infections. Consolidation of the food industry, the increased number of and use of fast-food restaurants and a change in eating habits in industrialized nations has led to a marked increase in foodborne illness and diarrheal disease. Various algorithms have been made to guide physicians in the investigation and management of acute diarrhea. The various bacteria each have specific antibiotics to which they are most sensitive.

Chronic diarrhea is that which lasts longer than 3 to 6 weeks. It may be caused by malabsorption, intestinal electrolyte transport abnormalities or intestinal inflammation. The classic example of a malabsorptive disease is celiac sprue. Steatorrhea is the clinical hallmark of malabsorption. Malabsorption of carbohydrate alone causes watery diarrhea. The most common causes of carbohydrate malabsorption are lactose intolerance and the use of the nonabsorbable carbohydrate sorbitol to sweeten dietetic chewing gum, candy, and liquid medicine (*elixir diarrhea*). Fructose is the primary sugar in fruit juice and is often used as a sweetener for soft drinks; some persons also malabsorb fructose.

Secretory diarrhea may be caused by toxin activation of various endogenous regulating systems, factitious ingestion of laxatives, use of drugs, or endocrine tumors. Neuroendocrine tumors are fairly rare, but they result in devastating, high-volume secretory diarrhea because of the elaboration of secretory hormones. Octreotide therapy can be useful to control symptoms, pending surgical intervention.

Stool electrolyte measurements and the response to fasting may be helpful in sorting out the cause of diarrhea. Secretory diarrheas generally do not decrease on fasting to volumes less than 200 mL/24 h unless the secretory state is mild, as in collagenous or microscopic colitis.

Determination of the osmotic gap in the stool can be useful in differentiating secretory from osmotic diarrhea. Specific congenital diarrhea can be suspected in infants and children because of changes in stool chloride or sodium content.

Many causes of diarrhea can be diagnosed on the basis of history, physical examination, and routine blood tests. A stool examination for microorganisms, blood, and fat and a colonic biopsy bring the diagnostic yield to between 75% and 80%. The remaining 20% of cases are elusive diarrheas that necessitate hospitalization and extensive testing.

The first principle in the management of diarrhea is to pay attention to the fluid and electrolyte status. It is dehydration and electrolyte imbalance that is the major cause of serious morbidity and mortality in this disease complex. The management of mild diarrhea can be safely supplemented with drugs, such as opiates, that alter intestinal motility. The somatostatin analogue octreotide has been shown to be useful in the management of neuroendocrine tumors and many other severe diarrheal states.

Atlas of Gastroenterology, 4th edition. Edited by Tadataka Yamada, David H. Alpers, Anthony N. Kalloo, Neil Kaplowitz, Chung Owyang, and Don W. Powell. © 2009 Blackwell Publishing, ISBN: 978-1-4051-6909-7

Table 5.1 Clinical diagnosis of foodborne illness by incubation period and symptoms

Predominant symptom	Incubation period			
	<2 h	1–7 h	8–14 h	>14 h
Upper intestinal, nausea/ vomiting	Heavy metals, chemicals, mushrooms	*Staphylococcus aureus*, *Bacillus cereus*, *Anisakis*	*Anisakis*	Norwalk agent
Noninflammatory, diarrhea, no fecal leukocytes			*Clostridium perfringens*, *B. cereus*	Enterotoxigenic *Escherichia coli*, *Vibrio cholerae*, *Giardia lamblia*, Norwalk agent
Inflammatory, ileocolitis				*Salmonella*, *Shigella* sp, *Campylobacter* sp, invasive *E. coli*, *Vibrio parahaemolyticus*, *Entamoeba histolytica*
Extragastrointestinal, neurological	Insecticides, mushroom and plant toxins, monosodium glutamate, shellfish, scombroid	Shellfish, ciguatera	Botulism	

From Aucott JN. Food poisoning. In: Blaser MJ, et al., eds. Infections of the gastrointestinal tract. New York: Raven Press, 1995:237.

Table 5.2 Naturally occurring fish and shellfish toxins

Poisoning	Toxin	Clinical syndrome
Ciguatera	Dinoflagellate toxin from reef algae ingested by tropical fish: amberjack, snapper, grouper, and barracuda	Gastrointestinal (diarrhea, nausea, vomiting, abdominal pain) and neurological symptoms (hot–cold inversion, muscle aches, perioral numbness and tingling, metallic taste, weakness, paresthesias, dizziness, and sweating)
Diarrheic shellfish poisoning	Okadaic acid, in certain marine phytoplankton ingested by bivalve mollusks (mussels, clams, oysters, scallops) in Japan, Spain, and Chile	Gastrointestinal symptoms (diarrhea, nausea, vomiting, abdominal pain)
Paralytic shellfish poisoning	Dinoflagellates ingested by bivalve "mollusks" in New England waters and Alaska, Washington, and California	Neurological symptoms (hot–cold inversion, muscle aches, perioral numbness and tingling, metallic taste, weakness, paresthesias, dizziness, and sweating). Severe and possibly proceeding to respiratory paralysis and death
Neurotoxic shellfish poisoning	Brevetoxin in red tide algae in Gulf of Mexico	Neurological symptoms as above but milder and transient (hours or days)
Estuarine toxin or *Pfiesteria piscicida* poisoning	Toxin of the dinoflagellate *Pfiesteria piscicida* ingested by fish in the Albemarle–Pamlico estuary of the southeastern United States	Neurological symptoms as above. (hot–cold inversion, muscle aches, perioral numbness and tingling, metallic taste, weakness, paresthesias, dizziness, and sweating) Effects on humans only now (1998) being clarified
Puffer fish poisoning	Tetrodotoxin contained in puffer fish eaten predominantly in Japan	Neurological symptoms as above. May cause respiratory paralysis and death (20–200 deaths per year)

Adapted from Ahmed FE, (ed.) Seafood safety. Washington, DC National Academy Press, 1991, and Morris JG Jr. Natural toxins associated with fish and shellfish. In: Blaser MJ, et al. (eds) Infections of the gastrointestinal tract. New York: Raven Press, 1995:251.

Table 5.3 Toxin-related food poisoning

Cause	Food	Incubation period	Duration	Vomiting	Diarrhea	Fever
Preformed toxin						
Staphylococcus aureus	Meat, egg salad, pastries	1–6 h	<12 h	Present	Rare	Rare
Bacillus cereus (emetic)	Fried rice	1–6 h	<12 h	Present	Rare	Rare
Toxin production in vivo						
B. cereus (diarrheal)	Meat, vegetables	6–24 h	<24 h	Rare	Present	Rare
Clostridium perfringens	Meat, gravy	6–24 h	<24 h	Rare	Present	Rare
Vibrio cholerae	Shellfish	16–72 h	5–7 days	Rare	Present	Absent
ETEC	Vegetables, meat	16–72 h	3–5 days	Rare	Present	Rare
EHEC	Meat, dairy products	1–8 days	3–6 days	Rare	Present	Rare

EHEC, enterohemorrhagic *Escherichia coli;* ETEC, enterotoxigenic *E. coli.*
From Afgani B, Stutman HR. Toxin-related diarrheas. Pediatr Ann 1994;23:549.

Table 5.4 Signs and symptoms of dehydration among patients with diarrhea

| Examination | Outcome | | |
	No signs of dehydration	Some dehydration	Severe dehydration
Look at:			
Mental status	Well, alert	Restless, irritable[a]	Lethargic or unconscious; floppy infant[a]
Eyes	Normal	Sunken	Very sunken and dry
Tears	Present	Absent	Absent
Mouth, tongue	Moist	Dry	Very dry
Thirst	Drinks normally, not thirsty	Thirsty, drinks eagerly[a]	Drinks poorly or not able to drink[a]
Feel:			
Skin pinch	Goes back rapidly	Goes back slowly[a]	Goes back very slowly[a]
Pulse	Normal	Faster than normal[a]	Very fast, weak, or nonpalpable[a]
Fontanelle	Normal	Sunken	Very sunken
Decide degree of dehydration	*No* signs of dehydration, 2.5% of body weight	If two or more of these signs exist, including at least one important[a] sign, then there is *some* dehydration, 2.5%–10% of body weight	If two or more of these signs exist, including at least one important sign, then there is *severe* dehydration, >10% of body weight

a Important signs and symptoms for assessment of dehydration.
Adapted from Swerdlow DL, Ries AA. Cholera in the Americas. JAMA 1992;267:1495.

Table 5.5 Composition of some currently experimental oral rehydration solutions

Solution	Na⁺ (mmol/L)	K⁺ (mmol/L)	Cl⁻ (mmol/L)	HCO₃⁻ (mmol/L)	Citrate (mmol/L)	Glucose (mmol/L)	Rice derivative or glucose polymer	Osmolality (mOsm/kg)
WHO (formula C)[a]	90	20	80	–	10	111	–	311
WHO (formula B)[a]	90	20	80	30	–	111	–	331
BP 1993[b]	90	20	80	–	10	111	–	311
USP 23[c]	90	20	80	–	10	111	–	311
Diocalm Junior[d] (Smith–Kline Beecham, Philadelphia)	60	20	50	–	10	111	–	251
Dioralyte[d] (Rhone Poulenc Rorer, Collegeville, PA)	60	20	60	–	10	90	–	240
Elecrolade[d] (Searle, Chicago, IL)	50	20	40	30	–	111	–	251
Gluco-Lyte[d] (Eastern, Smithtown, PA)	35	20	37	18	–	200	–	310
Infalyte[e] (Cupal, UK)	50	25	45	–	34	–	30[i]	200
Pedialyte[e] (Mead Johnson, Princeton, NJ)	45	20	35	–	30	139	–	269
Rapolyte[d] (Jannsen, UK)	60	20	50	–	10	111	–	251
Rehidrat[d,f] (Searle, UK)	50	20	50	20	9	91	–	336
Rehydralyte[e] (Ross)	75	20	65	–	30	139	–	329
Resol[e] (Wyeth-Ayerst, Philadelphia)	50	20	50	–	34	111	–	265
Experimental rice-based solution[g]	60	20	60	–	10	–	17.4[j]	140
Experimental glucose polymer-based solution[h]	60	20	60	–	10	–	18[k]	168
Glucose plus glycine	120	15	72	–	48	110 (20) plus 110 glycine	–	–

a WHO/UNICEF universal solution.
b From the British Pharmacopeia.
c From the US Pharmacopeia/National Formulary.
d Currently available in the United Kingdom (British National Formulary 1996).
e Currently available in the United States.
f Also contains sucrose (94 mmol/L) and fructose (2 mmol/L).
g Rice-based experimental polymer oral rehydration solution used by Thillainayagam et al.
h An experimental polymeric oral rehydration solution used by Thillainayagam et al.
i Rice syrup solids (g/L).
j Ground rice powder (g/L).
k A defined glucose polymer of mean chain length five glucose molecules (mmol/L).
UNICEF, United Nations International Children's Emergency Fund; WHO, World Health Organization.
From Thillainayagam AV, Hunt JB, Farthing MJ. Enhancing clinical efficacy of oral therapy: is low osmolality the key? Gastroenterology 1998;114:197 and Nalin DR, Hirschborn N, Grennough W, et al. Clinical concerns about reduced-osmolarity oral rehydration solution. JAMA 2004;291:2632.

Table 5.6 Patients who receive antimicrobial therapy for infections accompanied by diarrhea

Patients who have mild disease or who are improving should not be treated
All who are debilitated:
Leukemia and lymphoma
Malignancies, especially those receiving chemotherapy
Immunosuppressed (AIDS, congenital, steroids, transplant)
Abnormal cardiovascular system (valve prosthesis or disease, aneurysms or vascular grafts)
Orthopedic prostheses
Hemolytic anemia
Extremes of age (old or young)
All who have prolonged symptoms or who relapse

AIDS, acquired immunodeficiency syndrome.

Table 5.7 Frequently overlooked items may contain gluten

Broth	Malt, malt flavoring, vinegar
Breading	Modified food starch
Brown rice syrup	Nondairy creamer
Coating mixes	Pastas
Couscous	Peanut butter
Croutons	Processed meats and poultry
Caramel color	Salad dressings
Cereal products	Sausage products
Catsup and mustard	Sauces
Candy bars	Some brands of ice cream
Cheese spreads	Soup bases
Chip and dip mixes	Soy sauce
Flavoring in meat products	Stuffings
Hydrolyzed meat protein	Tomato sauce
Hot chocolate mixes or cocoa	Vegetable gum
Imitation bacon or seafood marinades	Vegetable protein (thickener)
Instant coffee and tea	Yogurts with fruit

From Abdulkarim AS, Murray JA. Celiac disease. Curr Treat Options Gastroenterol 2002;5:27.

Table 5.8 Companies that make gluten-free products

Dietary Specialties, Inc.	Kingsmill Foods Company, Ltd.
P. O. Box 227	1399 Kennedy Road, Unit 17
Rochester, NY 14601	Scarborough, ON M1P 2L6 CANADA
(800) 544-0099	(416) 755-1124y
Ener-G Foods, Inc.	Med-Diet, Inc.
P. O. Box 84487	3050 Ranchview Lane
Seattle, WA 98124	Plymouth, MN 55447
(800) 331-5222	(800) 633-3438
Fearn Natural Foods	Miss Ruben's
P. O. Box 09398	P. O. Box 1434
Milwaukee, WI 53209	Frederick, MD 21702
(414) 352-3333	(800) 891-0083
Gluten-Free Delights	Pamela's Products, Inc.
P. O. Box 284	335 Allerton Avenue
Cedar Falls, IA 50613	South San Francisco, CA 94080
(319) 266-7167	(650) 952-4546
The Gluten-Free Pantry, Inc.	Sterk's Bakery
P. O. Box 840	3866 23rd Street
Glastonbury, CT 06033	Vineland, ON LOR 2CO CANADA
(860) 633-3826	(800) 608-4501

From Abdulkarim AS, Murray JA. Celiac disease. Curr Treat Options Gastroenterol 2002;5:27.

Table 5.9 Celiac disease support and resource groups in the United States and Canada

American Celiac Society	Celiac Sprue Association/USA, Inc.
58 Musano Court	P. O. Box 31700
West Orange, NJ 07052	Omaha, NE 68131
(973) 325-8837	(402) 558-0600
	URL: www.csaceliacs.org
Canadian Celiac Association	Midwest Gluten Intolerance Group
190 Britannia Road East, Unit 11	4007 Forest Road
Mississauga, ON L4Z 1W6	St. Louis Park, MN 55416
CANADA	(612) 925-6136
(905) 507-6208	
Celiac Disease Foundation	Gluten Intolerance Group of North
13251 Ventura Blvd., #1	America
Studio City, CA 91604	P. O. Box 23053
(818) 990-2354	Seattle, WA 98102
www.celiac.com[a]	(206) 325-6980
	URL: www.celiac.org
	www.celiacdatabase.org[b]

a Comprehensive website with many links and useful information for the experienced patient with celiac disease (CD). May overwhelm patients with newly diagnosed CD.
b Useful website where a food product's gluten-free status can be checked using the UPC code or EAN code.
From Abdulkarim AS, Murray JA. Celiac disease. Curr Treat Options Gastroenterol 2002;5:27.

Table 5.10 Causes of enteropathic arthritis

Whipple disease
Ulcerative colitis
Crohn's disease
Shigellosis
Salmonellosis
Yersinia enterocolitis
Campylobacter colitis
Post-small intestine bypass (for obesity)

From Feldman M. Southwestern Internal Medicine Conference: Whipple's disease. Am J Med Sci 1986;291:59.

Table 5.11 Central nervous system symptoms and signs in Whipple disease

Symptoms	Signs
Mental and personality changes	Dementia
Lethargy, coma	Papilledema
Headache	Ophthalmoplegia
Convulsions	Hemiparesis
Motor weakness	Sensory loss
Numbness	Myoclonus
Slurred speech	Hyperreflexia (± positive Babinski sign)
Visual difficulties (diplopia, blurring)	Ataxia
	Pupillary abnormalities
Incoordination	Nystagmus
Dizziness	Ptosis
Tinnitus	Muscle rigidity
Hearing loss	Loss of vibratory and position sense
Muscular jerks and twitches	Hearing loss
Stiff neck	
Facial pain	
Sleep disorders	
Polydipsia	

From Feldman M. Southwestern Internal Medicine Conference: Whipple's disease. Am J Med Sci 1986;291:59.

Table 5.12 Comparison of clinical features of malabsorption caused by mucosal disease (celiac sprue) with impaired intralumenal digestion (chronic pancreatic insufficiency)

Clinical manifestations	Celiac sprue	Pancreatic insufficiency
Symptom or sign		
Sex	F > M (2:1)	M > F (3:1)
Age at onset (%)	<3; 20–40	30–60
Diarrhea (%)	70–90	70–90
Weight loss (%)	60–90	90
Flatulence and bloating (%)	40	0
Weakness and lethargy (%)	95	4
Anorexia (%)	30–50	0
Oral aphthous ulcers, recurrent (%)	60	0
Severe abdominal pain (%)	0	64
Increased appetite (%)	15	70
Oil separated from stool (%)	0	57
Extraintestinal symptoms		
Tetany, bone pain, hemorrhagic diathesis, edema or ascites, nocturnal polyuria (%)	20–50	0–10
Laboratory tests		
Stool fat, g/24 h	25 (range 3.5–87)	48 (range 8–180)
Stool fat concentration, g/100 g stool (%)	<9.5	>9.5
Total serum protein <6 g/dL (%)	71	14
Anemia (%)	21	0

Adapted from Evans WB, Wollaeger EE. Incidence and severity of nutritional deficiency states in chronic exocrine pancreatic insufficiency: comparison with nontropical sprue. Am J Dig Dis 1966;11:594; and Bo-Linn GW, Fordtran JS. Fecal fat concentration in patients with steatorrhea. Gastroenterology 1984;87:319.

Table 5.13 Dietary factors, disease states, and drugs affecting standard oral D-xylose tests

Factor	5-h urine excretion of D-xylose	1-h serum level of D-xylose
Delayed gastric emptying	May decrease	May decrease
Dietary fiber or glucose	May decrease	May decrease
Meat	May increase	May increase
Renal disease		
Not requiring dialysis	Decreases	No decrease
Requiring dialysis		Decreases
Portal hypertension	Decreases	Decreases
Ascites	Decreases	May decrease
Myxedema	Decreases	No decrease
Drugs		
Aspirin and indomethacin	May decrease	May decrease
Neomycin	May decrease	May decrease
Glipizide	May decrease	May decrease

From Craig RM, Atkinson AJ. D-Xylose testing: a review. Gastroenterology 1988;95:223.

Table 5.14 Sorbitol content of "sugar-free" products and various foods

Food	Sorbitol content
"Sugar-free" gum	1.3–2.2 g/piece
"Sugar-free" mints	1.7–2.0 g/piece
Pears	4.6 g[a]
Prunes	2.4 g[a]
Peaches	1.0 g[a]
Apple juice	0.3–0.9 g[a]

a Expressed as grams of sorbitol per 100 g dry matter or per 100 g juice. Dry weight equals approximately 15% of fresh weight.
From Hyams JS. Sorbitol intolerance: an unappreciated cause of functional gastrointestinal complaints. Gastroenterology 1983;84:30.

Table 5.15 Symptoms associated with sorbitol and lactulose ingestion

	Dose of sorbitol[a]			Lactulose (g)
Symptom	5	10	20	10
Gas	3/7	5/7	5/7	5/7
Bloating	3/7	5/7	5/7	5/7
Cramps	0/7	1/7	4/7	2/7
Diarrhea	0/7	1/7	4/7	2/7

a No. patients with symptom/no. patients tested.
From Hyams JS. Sorbitol intolerance: an unappreciated cause of functional gastrointestinal complaints. Gastroenterology 1983;84:30.

Table 5.16 Common features and symptoms of patients with factitious diarrhea

Features
Predominantly women (>90%)
Multiple previous examinations
Exploratory laparotomies
Psychological abnormalities

Symptoms
Severe, chronic, watery diarrhea
Abdominal pain
Weight loss
Nausea and vomiting
Peripheral edema
Generalized weakness and hypokalemia

From Ewe K, Karbach U. Factitious diarrhea. Clin Gastroenterol 1986;15:723.

Table 5.17 Findings suggestive of factitious diarrhea

Investigation	Characteristic findings	Cause
Sigmoidoscopy	Melanosis coli	Anthraquinones
Barium enema	"Cathartic" colon	Diphenolic laxatives and anthraquinones
Stool electrolytes and osmolality (if volume > 500 mL/d and other causes are excluded)	$(Na^+ + K^+) \times 2 <$ osmolality	Osmotic laxatives, urine contamination
	$(Na^+ + K^+) \times 2 =$ osmolality	Secretory laxatives (anthraquinone and diphenolic laxatives)
	Osmolality < 200 mOsm/L	Addition of water to stool

From Ewe K, Karbach U. Factitious diarrhea. Clin Gastroenterol 1986;15:723.

Table 5.18 Hormones produced by carcinoid tumors and medullary thyroid carcinoma

Hormone	Carcinoid tumors	Medullary thyroid carcinoma	Stimulatory effect on intestinal fluid secretion or motility
Serotonin	+	+	+
5-Hydroxytryptophan	+		+
Histamine	+		+
Kallikrein→bradykinin	+	+	+
Calcitonin	+	+	+
Noncalcitonin peptide		+	?
Calcitonin gene-related peptide		+	?
Katacalcin		+	?
Motilin	+	+	+
Substance P	+	+	+
Tachykinin-like immunoreactivity	+		+
Neurotensin	+	+	+
Bombesin and gastrin-releasing peptide	+	+	+
Glucagon, enteroglucagon	+		+
Gastrin	+		+
Prostaglandins E and $F_2\alpha$	+		+
Dopamine	+		−
Norepinephrine	+		−
Peptide YY	+		−
Somatostatin	+	+	−
β-Endorphin		+	−
Nerve growth factor		+	?
γ-Trace		+	?
Helodermin		+	?

From Rambaud JC, Hautefeuille M, Ruskone A, Jacquenod P. Diarrhea due to circulating agents. Clin Gastroenterol 1986;15:603.

Table 5.19 Hormone products found in carcinoid tumors

Serotonin	Somatostatin
Tachykinins	Adrenocorticotropic hormone
Histamine	Growth hormone
Substance P	Gastrin-releasing peptide
Substance K	Gastrin
Pentagastrin	Insulin
Pancreatic polypeptide	Melanocyte-stimulating hormone

From O'Neil BH, Venook AP. Carcinoid tumors and the carcinoid syndrome. Clin Perspect Gastroenterol 2001:279.

Table 5.20 Tests used in the examination of patients with endocrine diarrhea

Gastrinoma
Gastric acid secretion
Plasma gastrin
Secretin provocative test

VIPoma
Gastric acid secretion
Serum calcium
Fasting plasma glucose, glycosuria
Plasma VIP and calcitonin
Plasma and urinary catecholamines and metabolites

Somatostatinoma
Gastric and exocrine pancreas secretions
Fasting plasma glucose, glycosuria
Plasma somatostatin

Carcinoid syndrome
Blood serotonin
Urinary 5-HIAA

Medullary thyroid carcinoma
Plasma calcitonin
Serum carcinoembryonic antigen

Hyperthyroidism
Plasma triiodothyronine, thyroxine, and thyroid-stimulating hormone

5-HIAA, 5-hydroxyindoleacetic acid; VIP, vasoactive intestinal peptide; VIPoma, vasoactive intestinal peptide-secreting tumor.
From Rambaud J-C, Hautefauille M, Ruskone A, Jacquenod P. Diarrhea due to circulating agents. Clin Gastroenterol 1986;15:603.

Table 5.21 Factors affecting stool electrolyte and osmolality measurements

	Temperature (°C)	Time after collection (H)	Osmolality (mOsm)	Sodium (mEq/L)	Potassium (mEq/L)	Osmotic gap[a] (mOsm)
Storage temperature	25	0	281	54	115	−57
		24	417	54	115	79
	25	0	300	40	101	18
		24	453	40	101	153
	25	0	291	76	38	63
		24	389	77	43	149
Antibiotics						
Oral neomycin	25	0	285	3	20	239
	25	48	281	3	22	231
Triple therapy	25	0	305	5	19	257
	25	48	304	5	18	258

a Osmotic gap = measured osmolality − 2 × (Na + K).
From Shiau Y-F, Feldman GM, Resnick MA, Coff PM. Stool electrolyte and osmolality measurements in the evaluation of diarrheal disorders. Ann Intern Med 1985;102:773.

Table 5.22 Characteristics of patients with secretory and osmotic diarrhea and results of stool osmolality and electrolyte measurements

Patient	Diagnosis or treatment	Effect of fasting on diarrhea	Osmolality (mOsm)	Sodium (mEq/L)	Potassium (mEq/L)	Osmotic gap[a] (mOsm)
1	Carcinoid syndrome	Persisted	320	98	90	−56
	Carcinoid syndrome[b]	Persisted	345	135	54	−33
2	Acute diarrhea	Persisted	281	54	115	−57
3	Idiopathic pseudoobstruction	Persisted	285	139	14	−21
4	Secretory diarrhea	Persisted	284	47	108	26
5[c]	Secretory diarrhea	Persisted	300	40	101	18
6	Diabetic diarrhea	Persisted	330	82	24	118
7[d]	Diabetic diarrhea	Persisted	348	115	25	68
8	Pseudomembranous colitis	Persisted	285	92	15	71
9	Pancreatic insufficiency	Resolved	291	76	38	63
10	Two days after discontinuation of lactulose		298	45	49	110
	Taking lactulose[e]	Resolved	285	3	20	239
11	Taking lactulose	Resolved	285	21	38	167
12[e]	Taking lactulose	Resolved	305	5	19	257

a Osmotic gap = measured osmolality − 2 × (Na + K)
b Serum Na concentration was 167 mEq/L.
c Measurements were done 4 h after stool collection.
d Serum Na, 144 mEq/L; blood urea nitrogen, 80 mg/dL; and glucose, 360 mg/dL.
e Patients were receiving antibiotic agents.
From Shiau Y-F, Feldman GM, Resnick MA, Coff PM. Stool electrolyte and osmolality measurements in the evaluation of diarrheal disorders. Ann Intern Med 1985;102:773.

Table 5.23 Fecal electrolyte composition, osmolality, and pH in congenital chloride diarrhea compared with normal state and with different types of secretory diarrhea (values are mean ± SEM)

	Volume (mL)	Na$^+$ (mmol/L)	K$^+$ (mmol/L)	Cl$^-$ (mmol/L)	HCO$_3^-$ (mmol/L)	Osmolality (mOsm/kg)	pH
Normal adults		31 ± 2	75 ± 2	16 ± 1	40 ± 2	376 ± 8	7.0 ± 0.1
Congenital chloride diarrhea	943 ± 86	60 ± 3	40 ± 3	140 ± 5	3 ± 0.5	307 ± 6	5.9 ± 0.1
Congenital sodium diarrhea	1470 ± 159	104 ± 3	57 ± 4	46 ± 2	59	291 ± 2	7.1 ± 0.9
Pancreatic cholera syndrome	2764 ± 745	76 ± 10	54 ± 8	47 ± 13	66	284 ± 6	7.7
Cholera		126 ± 1	19 ± 1	94 ± 1	47 ± 1		

SEM, standard error of the mean.
Values are given at age 6–12 years for congenital chloride diarrhea and 6–8 years for congenital sodium diarrhea; all other values are for adults.
From Holmberg C. Congenital chloride diarrhea. Clin Gastroenterol 1986;15:58.

Table 5.24 Various definitions of diarrhea

- Too frequent passage of too loose stools, often with urgency or abdominal discomfort
- Normal frequency: three times a week to three times a day
- Consistency: stool is 60%–85% water (use weight as a surrogate for consistency – normal <200 g/day)
- Acute diarrhea: <3 weeks duration (rarely 6–8 weeks)
- Chronic diarrhea: >3 weeks duration (usually >6–8 weeks)

Table 5.25 Types of diarrhea

Chronic diarrhea
    Steatorrhea (malabsorptive diseases)
    Watery diarrheas
    Inflammatory diarrheas
Prolonged and postinfectious diarrhea
AIDS diarrhea
Acute diarrhea
    Traveler's diarrhea
    Food- and waterborne diarrhea
    Day-care diarrhea
    Sexually transmitted diarrhea (gay bowel syndrome)
    Antibiotic-associated diarrhea
    Elixir and chewing gum diarrhea
    Nosocomial (hospital) diarrhea
    Runner's diarrhea

Table 5.26 Causes of acute diarrhea

Ingested material (~20%)
Medications
Carbohydrates (lactose, fructose)
Food intolerances
Poisons/toxins

Infections (~80%)
Toxin-producing organisms
Adherent organisms
Invasive organisms

Table 5.27 Antidiarrheal agents for mild diarrhea

Kaopectate: Poor efficacy
Bismuth subsalicylate: Effective, but less so than opiates, safe for most
Opiates:
    Natural – codeine
    Tincture of opium
    Synthetic – diphenoxylate atropine (central effects), loperamide (drug of choice, poor passage of blood–brain barrier, large first pass metabolism)

Table 5.28 History and physical examination findings in watery diarrhea

Severity of diarrhea
    Number of stools
    Volume
    Nocturnal incontinence
    Hypokalemia
    Dehydration
Medication
CHO ingestion, food intolerance
Previous surgeries
Long-standing diabetes or alcoholism
Flushing or skin manifestation of endocrine tumor
Thyromegaly, signs of hyperthyroidism

Table 5.29 History and physical examination findings in malabsorptive diarrhea

Classic diarrhea
Bulky
Greasy
Foul-smelling stool or floating stools
With flatulence
Weight loss

No diarrhea but signs/symptoms of malnutrition
Vitamin D – bone disease, tetany
Vitamin K – hemorrhagic diathesis
Iron, folate, B-12 – anemia, glossitis
Vitamin A – night blindness and dermatitis
B vitamins – cheilosis, dermatitis, neuropathy
Protein/calorie – amenorrhea, infertility, impotence

Table 5.30 History and physical examination findings in inflammatory diarrhea

- Watery or bloody stools (occult blood)
- Fever
- Abdominal pain and tenderness – generalized or focal
- Oral apthous ulcers
- Polymigratory arthritis
- Uveitis and scleritis
- Pyoderma or erythema nodosum
- Vasculitis
- Edema from protein-losing enteropathy

Table 5.31 Characteristics of celiac disease (nontropical sprue) and tropical sprue.

Nontropical sprue
Malabsorption
Villus atrophy
Progressive if untreated
Highest incidence in temperate climates
Responds to gluten-free diet
Clinical and morphological deterioration on rechallenge with gluten

Tropical sprue
Malabsorption
Villus atrophy
Progressive if untreated
Contracted in the tropics
Responds to folic acid, tetracycline

From Westergaard H. Am J Med Sci 290;249:1985.

Table 5.32 Genetics of celiac disease

High prevalence in first-degree relatives (10%–20%)
Concordance in monozygotic twins (70%)
Two or more recessive genes
    One on chromosome 6 – HLA locus
    HLA-DQ2, 95% of celiac patients, extended haplotypes DR3, DR5, and DR7
    HLA-DQ8 (DR4), most of remainder
Because HLA-DQ2 present in 25%–30% of population without celiac disease; non-HLA genes may be more important
Chromosome 15q26, insulin-dependent diabetes mellitus locus
5q and possibly 11q
Another on short arm of 6

From Sollid LM. Annu Rev Immunol 2000;18:53.

Table 5.33 Gastrointestinal and liver manifestations of celiac disease

Gastrointestinal disease
False positive FOBT ~50%
Lymphocytic and autoimmune atrophic gastritis
Microscopic (lymphocytic) colitis
Ulcerative proctitis/colitis
Irritable bowel syndrome, diarrhea predominant
Gastroesophageal reflux disease

Liver disease
Isolated hypertransaminasemia ("transaminitis")
Primary biliary cirrhosis[a]
Autoimmune hepatitis[a]
"Overlap" syndrome[a]

a Probable
FOBT, fecal occult blood test.

Table 5.34 Extraintestinal manifestations of celiac disease: skin and mouth

Dermatitis herpetiformis
Alopecia areata
Aphthous stomatitis
Dental enamel hypoplasia
Sjögren syndrome
Follicular keratosis[a]
Psoriasis[a]

a Probable.

Table 5.35 Extraintestinal manifestations of celiac disease: endocrine

Type 1 diabetes mellitus
Autoimmune thyroid diseases
Osteopenia (rickets and osteomalacia)
Osteoporosis
Dental enamel hypoplasia
Addison disease

Table 5.36 Extraintestinal manifestations of celiac disease: hematological

Iron-deficiency anemia
Folate-deficiency anemia
Combined (dimorphic) anemia
Hyposplenism
    Howell–Jolly bodies
    Thrombocytosis
Autoimmune aplastic anemia

Table 5.37 Extraintestinal manifestations of celiac disease: neuropsychiatric

Neurological disease
Neuropathies – peripheral, polyneuropathy, mononeuritis multiplex
Cerebellar ataxia
Epilepsy, with or without posterior cerebral (occipital) calcifications
Myasthenia gravis[a]

Psychiatric disease
Depression
Schizophrenia[a]

a Probable.

Table 5.38 Extraintestinal manifestations of celiac disease: rheumatological

Arthralgia
Arthropathy
Sjögren syndrome
Rheumatoid arthritis
Systemic lupus erythematosus[a]
Polymyosis[a]

a Probable.

Table 5.39 Extraintestinal manifestations of celiac disease: pulmonary

Fibrosing alveolitis
Lung cavities
Pulmonary hemosiderosis
Sarcoidosis
Cystic fibrosis

Table 5.40 Extraintestinal manifestations of celiac disease: cardiac and miscellaneous

Cardiac disease
Pericarditis, recurrent
Dilated cardiomyopathy[a]
Congenital heart disease[a]
Miscellaneous disease
Chronic fatigue syndrome
Selective IgA deficiency
IgA nephropathy

a Probable.
IgA, immunoglobulin A.

Table 5.41 Extraintestinal manifestations of celiac disease: congenital and genetic

Down syndrome
Turner syndrome
Williams syndrome
Congenital heart disease
IgA deficiency
IgA nephropathy

IgA, immunoglobulin A.

Table 5.42 Extraintestinal manifestations of celiac disease: pregnancy-related

Amenorrhea
Infertility (celiac men also have poor sperm motility)
Severe anemia during pregnancy
Intrauterine growth retardation
Low birth weights (observed in offspring of celiac fathers also)
Symptomatic presentation during puerperium

From Norgard B, et al. Am J Gastroenterol 1999;94:2435; Gasbarrini A, et al. Lancet 2000;356:399; Eliakim R, Sherer D. Gynecol Obstetr Invest 2001;51:3; Ludvigsson JF, Ludvigsson J. Gut 2001;49:169.

Table 5.43 Pitfalls of histological diagnosis of celiac disease

Disease is patchy and sometimes mild in the duodenum: Take multiple biopsies, preferably from 2nd and 3rd portion of duodenum. Repeat endoscopy/biopsy may be necessary in difficult cases.
Tangential sectioning will alter villous/crypt ratio: Orient biopsies when fixed, take care in sectioning.
Review biopsy with clinician when serology and histology do not agree.

Table 5.44 Imaging in celiac disease

Contrast studies
Lumen dilation
Flocculation of barium
Hypersecretion
Thickened folds
Ultrasound
Fluid-filled small intestine
Flaccid and dilated small bowel
Slight diffuse thickening
Increased peristalsis
Enlarged mesenteric nodes
CT – above plus (rarely)
Hyposplenism
Cavitary mesenteric lymph nodes
Nodular masses by any technique
Consider lymphoma or adenocarcinoma

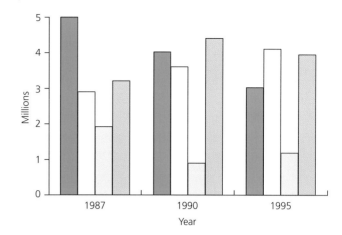

Figure 5.1 Diarrheal disease death rates (▪) among children younger than 5 years old compared with death rates from acute respiratory infections (□), measles (□), and other causes (□).

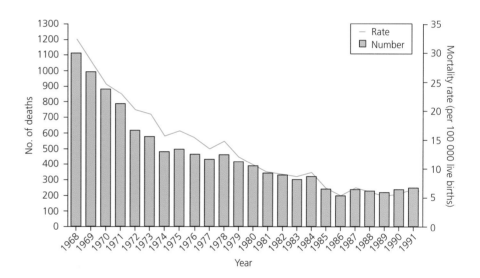

Figure 5.2 Diarrheal disease death rates (solid line) and annual number (bar) among US infants.

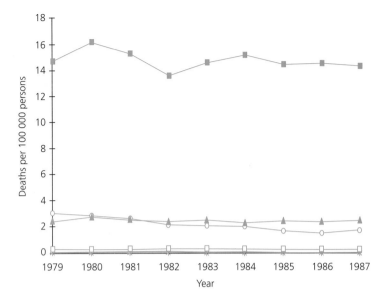

Figure 5.3 Diarrheal death rates in the United States. ○, age < 4 years; *, age 5–24 years; □, age 25–54 years; ▲, age 55–74 years; ■, age > 74 years.

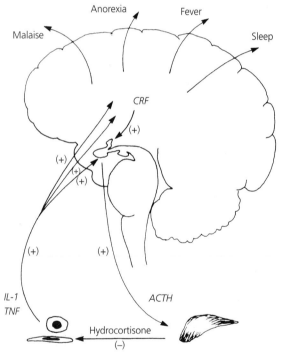

Figure 5.4 The systemic manifestations of severe intestinal inflammation are caused primarily by release of interleukin-1 (*IL-1*) and tumor necrosis factor (*TNF*), which have effects in the central nervous system. These agents also stimulate the pituitary-adrenal axis and initiate the glucocorticoid stress response. Glucocorticoids, through a negative feedback action, down-regulate the inflammatory cells in the lamina propria and decrease IL-1 and TNF release. ACTH, adrenocorticotropic hormone; CRF, corticotropin-releasing factor.

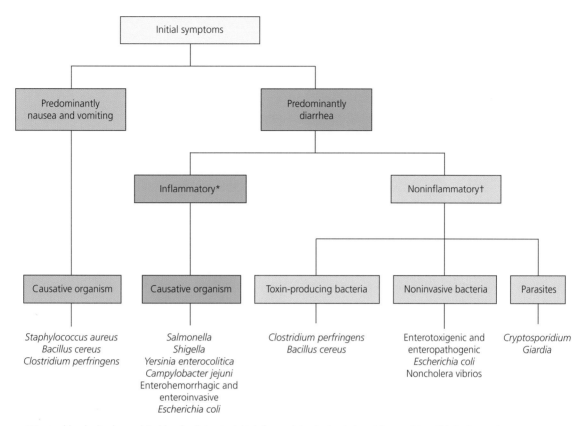

Figure 5.5 Differential diagnosis of food poisoning.

*Causes bloody diarrhea, white blood cells in stool, high fever, abdominal pain (consider empiric antibiotic therapy)
†Causes watery diarrhea, mild abdominal pain, low-grade fever

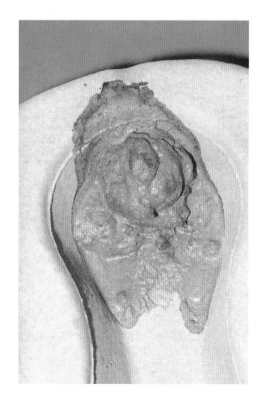

Figure 5.6 This steatorrheic stool is not easily confused with watery diarrhea. However, because fatty acids cause colonic secretion, malabsorption can present with watery diarrhea rather than steatorrheic diarrhea.

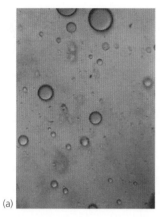
(a)

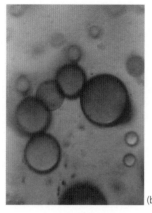
(b)

Figure 5.7 The hallmarks of abnormal findings at qualitative fecal fat examination are an increase in the number and, more importantly, an increase in the size of fat droplets. **(a)** This specimen has 1% triglyceride content and is equivalent to a quantitative stool fat level of 5 to 6 g/24 h. **(b)** This specimen has 5% triglyceride content and is equivalent to a quantitative stool fat level of 10 g/24 h.

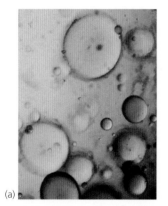
(a)

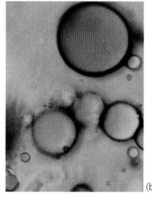
(b)

Figure 5.8 When fatty acids are present at usual stool pH, they are either ionized or in the form of soaps and will not readily take up Sudan stain. **(a)** At pH 5.6, fatty acids do not stain well with Sudan stain. **(b)** After acidification with two drops of acetic acid, the fatty acid droplets readily take up Sudan stain.

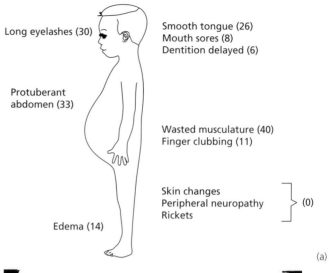

Long eyelashes (30)

Smooth tongue (26)
Mouth sores (8)
Dentition delayed (6)

Protuberant abdomen (33)

Wasted musculature (40)
Finger clubbing (11)

Skin changes
Peripheral neuropathy } (0)
Rickets

Edema (14)

(a)

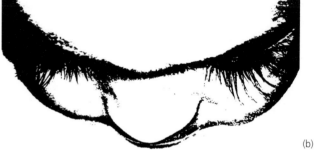

(b)

Figure 5.9 (a) Clinical presentation of children with celiac sprue. The number in parenthesis represents the number of patients demonstrating this finding out of a total of 42 patients. **(b)** The severe malnutrition of sprue leads to abnormalities of hair growth. This is manifested among children by the development of extremely long eyelashes.

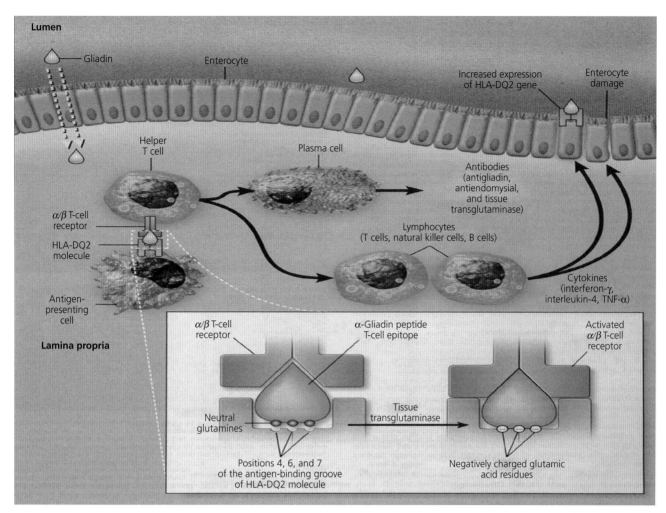

Figure 5.10 Pathogenesis of celiac disease.

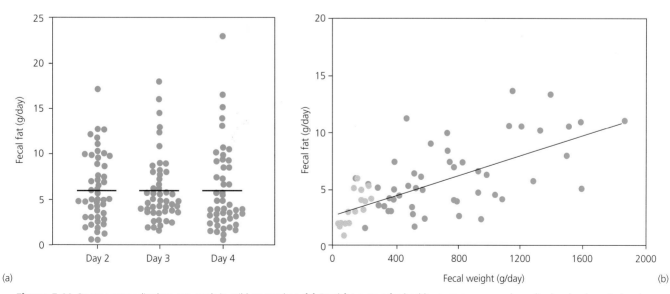

(a)

(b)

Figure 5.11 Severe watery diarrhea can result in mild steatorrhea. **(a)** Fecal fat output for healthy persons among whom diarrhea has been induced with MgOH$_2$ plus phenolphthalein (combined osmotic plus secretory diarrhea) can exceed 6 g/24 h. **(b)** Fecal fat output exceeds this value among more than 50% of persons if the diarrhea is severe; that is, fecal weight is more than 800 g/24 h.

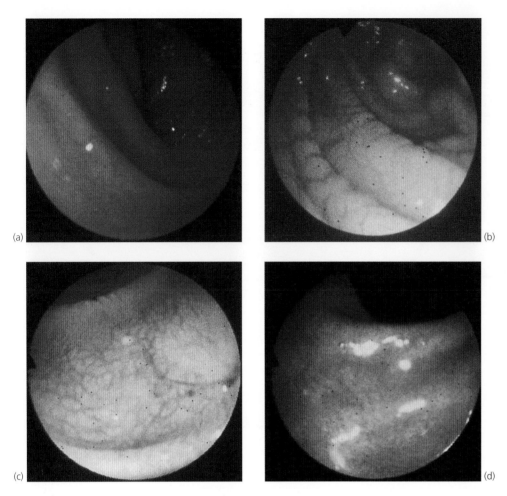

(a)

(b)

(c)

(d)

Figure 5.12 Duodenal biopsy specimen obtained means of upper gastrointestinal endoscopy can be diagnostic for intestinal causes of malabsorption. One disease that can be diagnosed on the basis of gross endoscopic appearance is celiac sprue. **(a)** Normal duodenal mucosa is smooth, velvety, and reddish. **(b)** Scalloped valvulae conniventes in the duodenum of a patient with celiac sprue. **(c)** Mosaic pattern of visible vasculature and scalloped valvulae conniventes is seen best on the edge of the valvula. **(d)** Mucosal appearance of the duodenal mucosa in a patient treated for sprue has returned toward normal with revision.

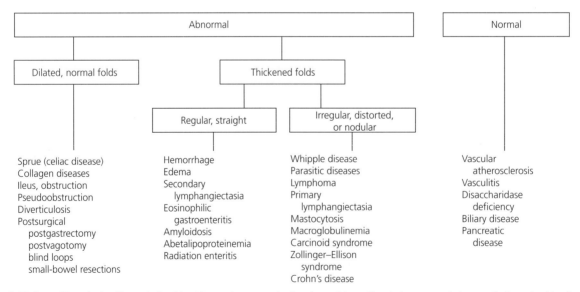

Figure 5.13 A small-intestinal radiograph should not be a primary examination for malabsorption, but may reveal changes that can lead to diagnosis of the cause.

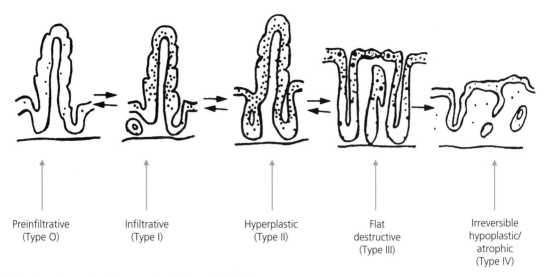

Preinfiltrative
(Type O)

Infiltrative
(Type I)

Hyperplastic
(Type II)

Flat
destructive
(Type III)

Irreversible
hypoplastic/
atrophic
(Type IV)

Figure 5.14 Marsh grading system for mucosal pathology of celiac disease.

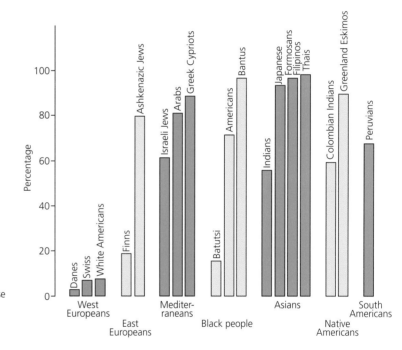

Figure 5.15 The prevalence of low lactase levels or lactose intolerance in various populations ranges from less than 10% among Western Europeans and their descendants to 80%–90% in other races and countries.

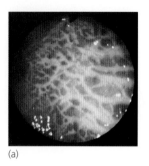

(a)

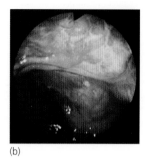

(b)

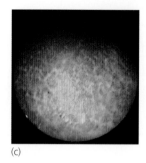

(c)

Figure 5.16 Melanosis coli develops from chronic use of anthracene cathartic agents. The endoscopic appearance of melanosis coli can be quite varied. It may also occur in patients with inflammatory bowel disease.

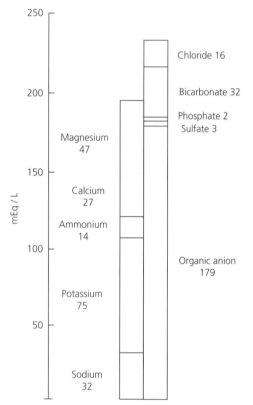

Figure 5.17 Human stool electrolyte concentrations obtained by means of fecal dialysis.

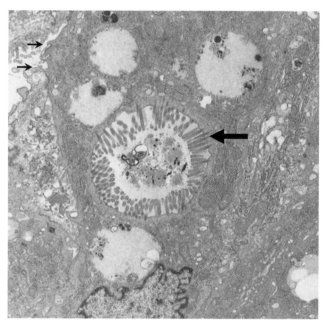

Figure 5.18 Microvillus inclusion disease is an autosomally transmitted recessive disorder in which the epithelial cells of the small intestine, colon, and gallbladder display intracytoplasmic vacuoles (large arrow) that contain brush borders that are not expressed on the apical surface of the absorbing epithelial cells. The epithelial cells may have rudimentary microvilli (small arrows), as in this specimen. In some epithelial cells, however, the microvilli are closer to normal than shown here. These patients have severe secretory diarrhea and need parenteral fluid replacement if they are to live beyond infancy.

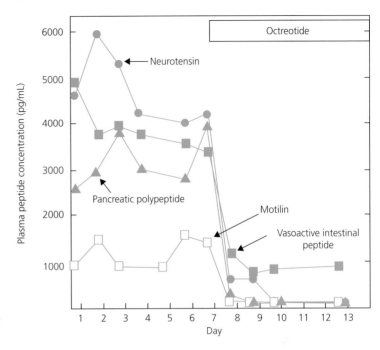

Figure 5.19 The somatostatin analogue octreotide significantly reduces tumor secretion of various hormones.

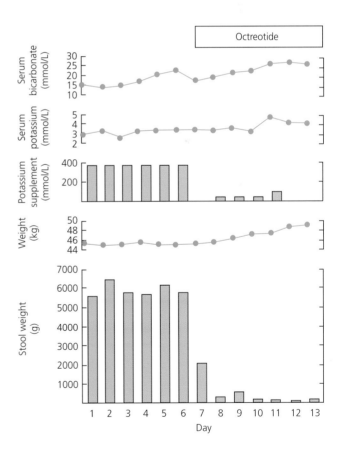

Figure 5.20 Octreotide also significantly reduced the diarrhea of this patient with a neuroendocrine tumor. This reduction in diarrhea is largely caused by the ability of the somatostatin analogue to reduce hormone secretion by the tumor.

6

Approach to the patient with suspected acute infectious diarrhea

John D. Long, Ralph A. Giannella

Acute diarrhea by definition lasts less than 2–3 weeks and is usually caused by infections. The causes of acute diarrhea are numerous but can be narrowed down by the clinical presentation and the country of origin (Table 6.1). In the United States, day-care centers are a common setting for acute infectious diarrhea (Table 6.2). A foodborne source for acute infectious diarrhea is being increasingly recognized, in which diarrhea results from the ingestion of either preformed toxins or specific microorganisms (Tables 6.3–6.5). The specific etiology of acute infectious diarrhea may be determined by assessing epidemiological features (Table 6.6), presenting symptoms and signs (Table 6.7), and the presence of inflammation in the stool (Table 6.8); the presence of inflammation is determined by the presence or absence of fecal leukocytes (Table 6.9). However, a definitive diagnosis of a specific viral, bacterial, or protozoal pathogen requires analysis of stool or, less commonly, aspiration of small bowel contents or mucosal biopsy (Table 6.10). Unfortunately, the yield of standard stool culture for the detection of bacterial pathogens is quite low, especially in

hospitalized patients (Table 6.11). The determination of the presence and severity of dehydration is a critical aspect of patient management (Table 6.12). Acute diarrhea in general may only require symptomatic treatment in the form of rehydration (Table 6.13) and antidiarrheal agents (Table 6.14). In specific clinical situations, antimicrobial therapy may be indicated (Table 6.15). Traveler's diarrhea is a specific form of acute diarrheal disease that requires a different approach (Table 6.16). Certain infectious pathogens may result in long-term complications (Table 6.17). Diagnostic algorithms are presented for patients with acute infectious diarrhea (Fig. 6.1) and suspected foodborne diarrhea (Fig. 6.2). Treatment algorithms are presented for patients with traveler's diarrhea (Fig. 6.3) and acute persistent diarrhea (Fig. 6.4). *Campylobacter* and *Salmonella* are the most common bacterial pathogens identified across all age groups (Fig. 6.5). Figures 6.6 through 6.11 include examples of the endoscopic and/or histopathological features of several pathogens that might be identified by endoscopic biopsy.

Table 6.1 Clinical presentations and likely causes of acute diarrheal disease in an outpatient setting

Clinical syndrome	Percentage of patients	Likely cause in industrialized countries	Likely cause in resource-poor countries
Watery diarrhea	90%	Rotavirus, other viruses	Rotavirus, ETEC, EPEC, *C. jejuni*
Dysentery	5%–10%	*Shigella, C. jejuni*, EIEC	*Shigella, C. jejuni*, EIEC, *E. histolytica*
Persistent diarrhea (>14 days)	3%–4%	*Giardia, Yersinia*, EPEC, EAEC	*Giardia*, EPEC
Severe purging, with rice-water stool	1% (higher in cholera endemic areas)	*Salmonella*, ETEC	*V. cholerae*, ETEC
Hemorrhagic colitis	<1%	EHEC	EHEC

C. jejuni, Campylobacter jejuni; E. histolytica, Entamoeba histolytica; EAEC, enteroadherent *E. coli*; EHEC, enterohemorrhagic *Escherichia coli*; EIEC, enteroinvasive *E. coli*; EPEC, enteropathogenic *E. coli*; ETEC, enterotoxigenic *E. coli. V. cholerae, Vibrio cholerae*.
Adapted from DiJohn D, Levine MR. Treatment of diarrhea. Infect Dis Clin North Am 1988;2:719.

Atlas of Gastroenterology, 4th edition. Edited by Tadataka Yamada, David H. Alpers, Anthony N. Kalloo, Neil Kaplowitz, Chung Owyang, and Don W. Powell. © 2009 Blackwell Publishing, ISBN: 978-1-4051-6909-7

Table 6.2 Causes of diarrhea in day-care centers in the United States

Organism	Primary attack rate (%)	Secondary attack rate (%)
Rotavirus	71–100	15–79
Shigella	33–73	26–46
Campylobacter jejuni	20–50	?
Clostridium difficile	32	?
Giardia lamblia	17–90	12–50
Cryptosporidium	50–65	14

Adapted from Guerrant RL, Hughes JM, Lima NL, et al. Diarrhea in developed and developing countries: magnitude, special settings, and etiologies. Rev Infect Dis 1990;12(Suppl 1):541.

Table 6.3 Naturally occurring fish and shellfish toxins

Poisoning	Toxin location	Clinical syndrome
Ciguetera	Dinoflagellate toxin from reef algae ingested by tropical fish: amberjack, snapper, grouper, and barracuda	Gastrointestinal – diarrhea, nausea, vomiting, abdominal pain. Neurological – hot–cold inversion, perioral numbness and tingling, metallic taste, myalgias, weakness, paresthesias, dizziness, sweating
Diarrhetic shellfish poisoning	Okadaic acid in certain marine phytoplankton ingested by bivalve mollusks: mussels, clams, oysters, scallops. Location – Spain, Japan, Chile	Gastrointestinal – diarrhea, nausea, vomiting, abdominal pain
Paralytic shellfish poisoning	Dinoflagellates ingested by bivalve mollusks. Location – New England, Alaska, Washington, California	Neurological – hot–cold inversion, perioral numbness and tingling, metallic taste, myalgias, weakness, paresthesias, dizziness, sweating; may progress to respiratory paralysis and death
Neurotoxic shellfish poisoning	Brevetoxin in red tide algae. Location – Gulf of Mexico	Neurological – same as above except milder and transient (hours to days)
Estuarine toxin or *Pfiesteria piscicida* poisoning	Dinoflagellate toxin from this organism ingested by fish. Location – Albemarle-Pamlico estuary of southeastern United States	Neurological – same as above
Puffer fish poisoning	Tetrodotoxin from puffer fish. Location – Japan	Neurological – same as above but may progress to respiratory paralysis and death (20–200 deaths per year)

Adapted from Morris JG, Jr. Natural toxins associated with fish and shellfish. In: Blaser MJ, et al., (eds). Infections of the gastrointestinal tract. New York: Raven Press, 1995 p. 251.

Table 6.4 Clinical diagnosis of foodborne illness by predominant symptoms and incubation period

Predominant symptom	Incubation period			
	<2 h	1–7 h	8–14 h	>14 h
Upper intestinal (nausea, vomiting)	Heavy metals Chemicals Mushrooms	*Staphylococcus aureus* *Bacillus cereus* Anisakis	Anisakis	Norwalk agent
Noninflammatory diarrhea (no blood or fecal leukocytes)			*Clostridium perfringens* *B. cereus*	Norwalk agent ETEC *Vibrio cholerae* *Giarda lamblia*
Inflammatory, ileocolitis (bloody or positive leukocytes)				*Salmonella* *Shigella* *Campylobacter* EIEC EHEC *V. parahaemolytic* *Entamoeba histolytica*
Extraintestinal Neurological	Insecticides Mushrooms Monosodium glutamate Shellfish Scombroid	Shellfish Ciguatera	Botulism	

EHEC, enterohemorrhagic *E. coli*; EIEC, enteroinvasive *E. coli*; ETEC, enterotoxigenic *E. coli*.
Adapted from Aucott JN. Food poisoning. In: Blaser MJ, et al. (eds). Infections of the gastrointestinal tract. New York: Raven Press, 1995 p. 237.

Table 6.5 Clinical features of toxin-related food poisoning syndromes

Cause	Food	Incubation period	Duration	Fever	Vomiting	Diarrhea
Preformed toxin						
Staphylococcus aureus	Meat Egg salad Pastries	1–6 hours	<12 hours	Rare	Common	Rare
Bacillus cereus (emetic)	Fried rice	1–6 hours	<12 hours	Rare	Common	Rare
Toxin production in vivo						
B. cereus	Meat Vegetables	6–24 hours	<24 hours	Rare	Rare	Common
Clostridium perfringens	Meat Gravy	6–24 hours	<24 hours	Rare	Uncommon	Common
Vibrio cholerae	Shellfish	16–72 hours	5–7 days	Rare	Uncommon	Common
ETEC	Meat Vegetables	16–72 hours	3–5 days	Rare	Uncommon	Common
EHEC	Meat Dairy products	1–5 days	3–6 days	Rare	Uncommon	Common

EHEC, enterohemorrhagic *E. coli*; ETEC, enterotoxigenic *E. coli*.
Adapted from Afgani B, Statman HR. Toxin-related diarrheas. Pediatr Ann 1994;23:549.

Table 6.6 Epidemiological clues to the etiology of acute infectious diarrhea

Clue	Potential pathogens
Water (including foods washed in contaminated water)	Norwalk agent, *Vibrio cholerae*, *Giardia*, *Cryptosporidium*
Foods	
Poultry	*Salmonella, Campylobacter*
Beef	Enterohemorrhagic *Escherichia coli*
Pork	*Yersinia enterocolitica*, tapeworm
Seafood/shellfish	*Vibrio cholerae, Vibrio parahemolyticus*
Eggs	*Salmonella*
Cheese, milk	*Listeria* species
Mayonnaise-containing food and pies	*Staphylococcus aureus, Clostridium perfringens*
Fried rice	*Bacillus cereus*
Canned vegetables/fruits	*C. perfringens*
Unpasteurized fruit juice	Enterohemorrhagic *E. coli*
Fresh berries	*Cyclospora*
Sprouts	Enterohemorrhagic *E. coli, Salmonella*
Exposures	
Animal-to-person (pets & livestock)	*Salmonella, Campylobacter, Giardia, Cryptosporidium*
Person-to-person	All enteric viruses, most bacteria and parasites
Day-care center	*Shigella, Campylobacter, Clostridium difficile, Giardia, Cryptosporidium*, viruses
Hospital	*Clostridium difficile*
Antibiotics and chemotherapy	*C. difficile*
Swimming pool	*Giardia, Cryptosporidium*
Foreign travel	*E. coli* (ETEC, EAEC, EIEC), *Salmonella, Shigella, Campylobacter, Giardia, Cryptosporidium, E. histolytica*

EAEC, enteroadherent *E. coli*; EIEC, enteroinvasive *E. coli*; ETEC, enterotoxigenic *E. coli*.
Adapted from Parks SI, Giannella RA. Approach to the adult patient with acute diarrhea. Gastroenterol Clin North Am 1993;22:483.

Table 6.7 Clinical clues to the etiology of acute infectious diarrhea

Clues	Potential pathogens
Fever	*Salmonella, Shigella, Campylobacter, Yersinia*
Severe or persistent abdominal pain	*Campylobacter, Salmonella, Shigella, Yersinia, Aeromonas, Clostridium perfringens*, enterohemorrhagic *Eschericha coli*
Rectal pain, tenesmus	*Campylobacter, Salmonella, Shigella, Entamoeba histolytica, Gonococcus, Herpes, Chlamydia*
Bloody stools	Enterohemorrhagic *E. coli, Salmonella, Shigella, Campylobacter, Clostridium difficile, E. histolytica*

Modified from Aranda-Michel J, Giannella RA. Acute diarrhea: A practical review. Am J Med 1999;106:670.

Table 6.8 Small bowel and colonic pathogens

Pathogen	Small bowel (noninflammatory[a])	Colon (inflammatory[b])
Bacteria	*Staphylococcus aureus*	*Campylobacter*
	Bacillus cereus	*Shigella*
	Clostridium perfringens	Salmonella*
	Enterotoxigenic *Escherichia coli* (ETEC)	*Clostridium difficile*
	Vibrio cholerae	Enteroinvasive *E. coli* (EIEC)
	Salmonella[c]	Enterohemorrhagic *E. coli* (EHEC)
	Aeromonas hydrophila	*Yersinia enterocolitica*
		Vibrio parahemolyticus
		Plesiomonas shigelloides
Viruses	Rotavirus	Cytomegalovirus
	Norwalk agent	Herpes simplex
		Adenovirus
Protozoa	*Giardia lamblia*	*Entamoeba histolytica*
	Cryptosporidium parvum	
	Cyclospora	
	Isospora belli	
	Microsporidia	

a Noninflammatory – Watery, large-volume diarrhea; usually no fever or fecal leukocytes.
b Inflammatory – Bloody, small-volume diarrhea, may have fever and toxicity, may have fecal leukocytes.
c Salmonella may cause both syndromes.
Adapted from Parks SI, Giannella RA. Approach to the adult patient with acute diarrhea. Gastroenterol Clin North Am 1993;22:483.

Table 6.9 Fecal leukocytes in intestinal infections

Present	Variable	Absent
Shigella	Salmonella	*Staphylococcus aureus*
Campylobacter	*Yersinia enterocolitica*	*Bacillus cereus*
Enteroinvasive *Escherichia coli* (EIEC)	*Vibrio parahemolyticus*	*Clostridium perfringens*
	Clostridium difficile	Enterotoxigenic *E. coli* (ETEC)
		Enteropathogenic *E. coli* (EPEC)
		Enterohemorrhagic *E. coli*
		Vibrio cholerae
		Giardia lamblia
		Cryptosporidium parvum
		Cyclospora
		Rotavirus
		Norwalk agent
		Coronavirus
		Adenovirus

Adapted from Thorne GM. Diagnosis of infectious diarrheal diseases. Infect Dis Clin North Am 1988;2:747.

Table 6.10 Materials required for microbiological testing performed by gastroenterologists

Pathogen	Specimen	Collection	Media/other needs
Bacteria	Stool[a]	Sterile specimen cup	Use Cary–Blair media for rectal swabs
			Nonbacteriostatic saline
	Mucosal biopsy (colon)	Sterile specimen cup	[a]For infectious proctitis, may need special media for gonococcus, Chlamydia, and herpes
			Culture for aerobes and anaerobes
	Jejunal aspirate	Sterile specimen cup	
Parasites	Stool[a]	Sterile specimen cup	Can refrigerate for up to 2 h
			[a]Use fixatives if >2-h interval from collection and analysis
	Jejunal aspirate	Sterile specimen cup	Same for string test
Mycobacteria and fungi	Stool	Sterile specimen cup	
	Mucosal biopsy	Sterile specimen cup	Nonbacteriostatic saline
Viruses	Stool	Viral transport media[b]	Swab of stool or rectum
	Mucosal biopsy	Viral transport media[b]	

a Similar requirements to process stool for bacterial toxin and protozoal antigen assays.

b Some viral transport media contain temperature-sensitive antibiotics and should be kept frozen until immediately before use.

Adapted from Tarr PI, Surawicz CM, Clausen CR. Microbiologic studies. In: Yamada T, Alpers DH, Laine L, et al., (eds). Textbook of Gastroenterology, 3rd edn. Philadelphia: Lippincott Williams & Wilkins, 1999.

Table 6.11 Prevalence of bacterial pathogens isolated by stool culture

Year	Author	Total # of specimens	# of positive specimens	Inpatient ≤3 days	Inpatient >3 days	Most common pathogen
1990	Siegel	1964[a]	40 (2.0%)	8/398 (2.0%)	0/997 (0%)	Campylobacter
1992	Bowman	505[a]	23 (4.6%)	NS	NS	Campylobacter
1993	Asnis	1097[a]	29 (2.6%)	29/530 (5.5%)[b]	0/567 (0%)	Campylobacter
1993	Fan	1743	47 (2.7%)	NS	NS	Salmonella
1995	Barbut	721	46 (6.4%)	41/377 (10.9%)	5/344 (1.5%)	Salmonella
1996	Chitkara	3072	319 (10.4%)	NS	NS	Campylobacter
1996	Valenstein	59 500[a]	3821 (6.4%)	564/18 179 (3.1%)	68/12 031 (0.6%)	Campylobacter
1997	Rohner	13 965[a]	856 (6.1%)	746/5913 (12.6%)[b]	110/8052 (1.4%)	Campylobacter
1999	Ozerek	4305	79 (1.8%)	NS	NS	Salmonella
2001	Bauer	3416	34 (1.0%)	20/598 (3.3%)	14/2818 (0.5%)	Salmonella
Total		90 288	5294 (5.7%)	1408/25 999 (5.4%)	197/24 809 (0.8%)	

a Included outpatient specimens.

b Outpatient specimens were included with inpatient specimens submitted ≤3 days.

NS, not specified.

Table 6.12 Symptoms and signs of dehydration among patients with acute diarrhea

Examination	Mild dehydration (3%–5% of body weight lost)	Moderate dehydration (6%–9% of body weight lost)	Severe dehydration (>10% of body weight lost)
Look at:			
Mental status	Well, alert	Restless, irritable[a]	Lethargic or unconscious[a]
Thirst	Drinks normally, not thirsty	Drinks eagerly, thirsty[a]	Drinks poorly, not able to[a]
Eyes	Normal	Sunken	Very sunken
Tears	Present	Absent	Absent
Mouth, tongue	Moist	Dry	Very dry
Feel:			
Skin turgor	Goes back rapidly	Goes back slowly[a]	Goes back very slowly[a]
Fontanelle	Normal	Sunken	Very sunken
Pulse	Normal	Faster than normal[a]	Tachycardia[a]
			Weak or nonpalpable
Blood pressure	Normal	Normal to low[a]	Shock[a]
Determine degree of dehydration	No signs of dehydration	If two or more of these signs are present, including at least one important sign, then there is *moderate* dehydration	If two or more of these signs are present, including at least one important sign, then there is *severe* dehydration

a Important symptoms and signs for assessment of dehydration.
Adapted from Swerdlow DL, Ries AA. Cholera in the Americas. JAMA 1992;267:1495.

Table 6.13 Composition of selected oral rehydration solutions

Solution	Na+ (mEq/L)	K+ (mEq/L)	Cl− (mEq/L)	Citrate (mmol/L)	Glucose (mmol/L)	Rice (g/L)	Osmolarity (mOsm/kg)
WHO 1975	90	20	80	10	111	–	311
WHO 2002[a]	75	20	65	10	75	–	245
Pedialyte (Mead-Johnson)	45	20	35	30	139	–	269
Rehydralyte (Ross)	75	20	65	30	139	–	329
Reosol (Wyeth-Ayerst)	50	20	50	34	111	–	265
Ceralyte 50 (Cera Products)	50	20	40	30	–	40	235

a Currently recommended reduced-osmolarity solution.
WHO, World Health Organization.
Adapted from Thillainayagam AV, Hunt JB, Farthing MJG. Enhancing clinical efficacy of oral rehydration therapy: is low osmolality the key? Gastroenterology 1998;114:197, and Duggan C, Fontaine O, Pierce NF, et al. Scientific rationale for a change in the composition of oral rehydration solution. JAMA 2004;291:2628.

Table 6.14 Antidiarrheal agents for the symptomatic treatment of acute diarrhea

Pharmacological agent	Indication/perspective	Dose/administration
Loperamide (Imodium)	Fever is absent or low grade Dysentery is not present Central opiate effects – minimal Preferred drug for patients with nonfebrile, nondysenteric diarrhea	Two tablets (4 mg) initially, then one tablet (2 mg) after each unformed stool Maximum of eight tablets once daily (16 mg) Duration of ≤2 days OTC available Forms – tablet, capsule, liquid
Diphenoxylate with atropine (Lomotil)	Fever is absent or low grade Dysentery is not present Central opiate effects – yes (with overdose potential) Atropine may cause side effects without offering antidiarrheal effects	Two tablets (5 mg) three to four times a day Maximum of six to eight tablets once daily (15–20 mg) Duration of ≤2 days Prescription only Forms – tablet, liquid
Tincture of opium (Paregoric)	Fever is absent or low grade Dysentery is not present Central opiate effects – yes Occasionally useful in HIV-associated diarrhea when loperamide fails	0.5–1.0 mL every 4–6 h Maximum of 6 mL once daily Duration of ≤2 days Prescription only Form – liquid
Bismuth subsalicylate (Pepto-Bismol)	Any form of acute diarrhea Cannot be combined with antibiotics Less effective than loperamide Should not be used in HIV-associated diarrhea	Two tablets (525 mg) or 30 mL every 30 min Maximum of eight doses once daily Duration of ≤2 days OTC available Forms – chewable tablet, liquid

OTC, over the counter.
Adapted from Dupont HL and Practice Parameters Committee of the American College of Gastroenterology. Guidelines on acute infectious diarrhea in adults. Am J Gastroenterol 1997;92:1962.

Table 6.15 Relative indications for use of antimicrobial agents in diarrheal disease of established cause

Clearly indicated	Indicated in some situations	Not indicated
Shigellosis	Nontyphoidal salmonellosis[b]	EHEC
ETEC[a]	Campylobacteriosis	EPEC
Cholera	EIEC	Rotavirus
Giardiasis	Yersinia[c]	Other viruses
Amebiasis	Noncholera Vibrio infection	
	Clostridium difficile	

a Enterotoxigenic *Escherichia coli* (ETEC) is the most common cause of acute traveler's diarrhea but should only be treated with antibiotics if moderate-to-severe.
b Indications for treatment of nontyphoidal salmonella gastroenteritis include: (1) age <12 months or >50 years; (2) predisposing medical conditions such as prostheses, valvular heart disease, severe atherosclerosis, cancer, uremia, immunocompromised, pregnancy; and (3) any patient with severe diarrhea.
c Indications for treatment of Yersinia gastroenteritis include: (1) severe diarrhea; (2) bacteremia; and (3) immunocompromised.
Adapted from DiJohn D, Levine MR. Treatment of diarrhea. Infect Dis Clin North Am 1988;2:719.

Table 6.16 Pharmacological self-therapy for traveler's diarrhea based on clinical features

Clinical syndrome	Probable cause	Recommendations
Vomiting, minimal diarrhea	Viruses, preformed toxins	Bismuth subsalicylate
Diarrhea in infants (<2 years old)	Bacteria	Fluids and electrolytes
Diarrhea in pregnant women	Bacteria	Fluids and electrolytes
		Can consider attapulgite: 3 g initially, repeated after each unformed stool or every 2 h (whichever comes first), for total dosage of 9 g once daily
Watery diarrhea (no fever or dysentery)	Noninvasive bacteria	Antibacterial drug plus (for adults) 4 mg of loperamide initially, then 2 mg after each unformed stool, not to exceed 16 mg once daily
Dysentery (passage of bloody stools with tenesmus) or fever >101.3	Invasive bacteria	Antibacterial drug without loperamide
Diarrhea despite trimethoprim-sulfamethoxazole prophylaxis	Unknown, probably drug-resistant bacteria	Fluoroquinolone, with loperamide if no fever or dysentery
Diarrhea despite fluoroquinolone prophylaxis	Unknown	Bismuth subsalicylate

Adapted from Dupont HL, Ericsson CD. Prevention and treatment of traveler's diarrhea. N Engl J Med 1993;328:1821.

Table 6.17 Potential long-term complications of acute intestinal infections

Complication	Potential pathogens
Hemolytic-uremic syndrome	Enterohemorrhagic *Escherichia coli*, Shigella
Toxic megacolon	Shigella, Salmonella, Campylobacter, Yersinia, *Clostridium difficile*, enterohemorrhagic *E. coli*
Reiter syndrome (arthritis, urethritis, and conjunctivitis in HLA-B27 individuals)	Shigella, Campylobacter, Yersinia
Guillain–Barré syndrome	Campylobacter
Postinfectious irritable bowel syndrome	Campylobacter, Shigella, Salmonella, *C. difficile*

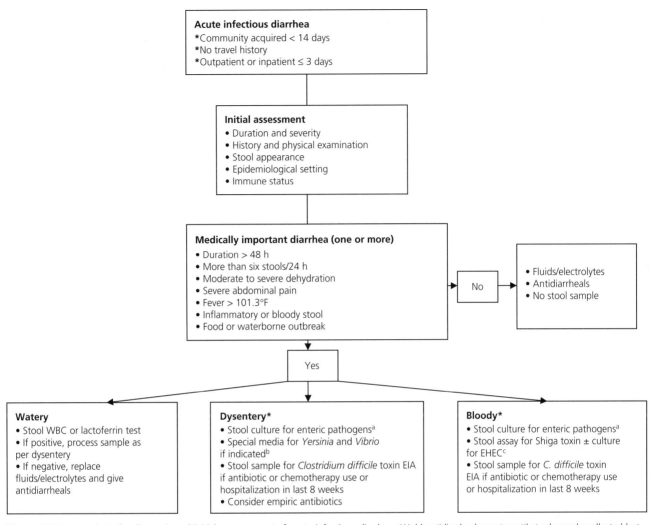

Figure 6.1 Approach to the diagnosis and initial management of acute infectious diarrhea. *Hold antidiarrheal agents until stool sample collected but may then be used in conjunction with antibiotics for patients with dysentery. [a]Enteric pathogens are Salmonella, Shigella, and Campylobacter. [b]Yersinia requires cold enrichment, vibrios require TCBS (thiosulfate citrate bile sucrose) agar. [c]EHEC (enterohemorrhagic *Escherichia coli*) requires special media. EIA, enzyme immunoassay; WBC, white blood cell.

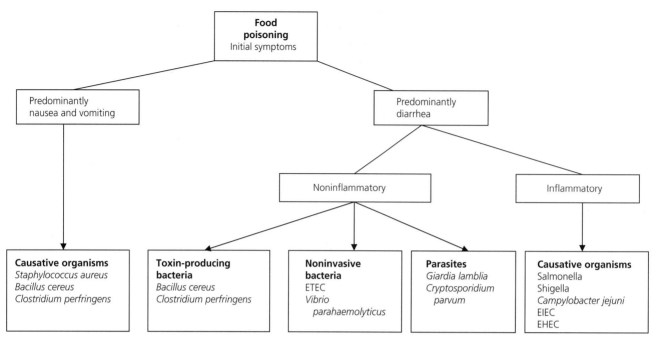

Figure 6.2 Differential diagnosis of bacterial food poisoning. EHEC, enterohemorrhagic *Escherichia coli*; EIEC, enteroinvasive *E. coli*; EPEC, enteropathogenic *E. coli*; ETEC, enterotoxigenic *E. coli*.

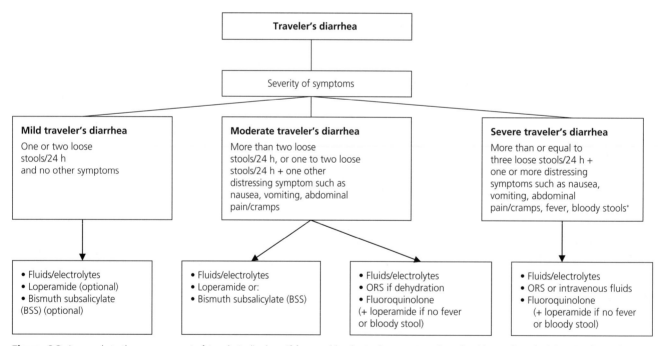

Figure 6.3 Approach to the management of traveler's diarrhea. If fever or bloody stools present, patient should consult a physician. Stool sample should be sent for analysis of enteric pathogens, ova, and parasites should be sent. ORS, oral rehydration solution.

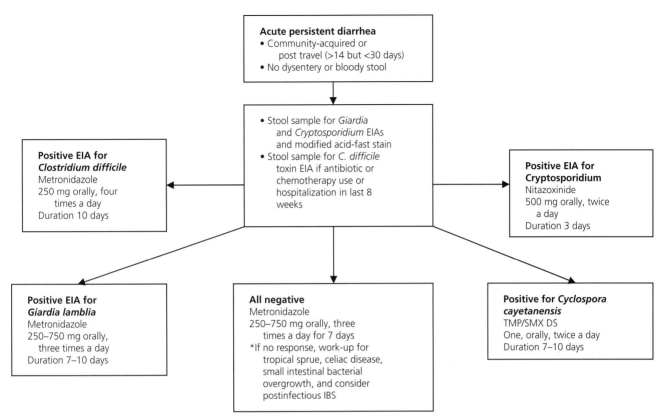

Acute persistent diarrhea
• Community-acquired or
   post travel (>14 but <30 days)
• No dysentery or bloody stool

• Stool sample for *Giardia*
   and *Cryptosporidium* EIAs
   and modified acid-fast stain
• Stool sample for *C. difficile*
   toxin EIA if antibiotic or
   chemotherapy use or
   hospitalization in last 8
   weeks

Positive EIA for
Clostridium difficile
Metronidazole
250 mg orally, four
   times a day
Duration 10 days

Positive EIA for
Cryptosporidium
Nitazoxinide
500 mg orally, twice
   a day
Duration 3 days

Positive EIA for
Giardia lamblia
Metronidazole
250–750 mg orally,
   three times a day
Duration 7–10 days

All negative
Metronidazole
250–750 mg orally, three
   times a day for 7 days
*If no response, work-up for
   tropical sprue, celiac disease,
   small intestinal bacterial
   overgrowth, and consider
   postinfectious IBS

Positive for *Cyclospora
cayetanensis*
TMP/SMX DS
One, orally, twice a day
Duration 7–10 days

Figure 6.4 Approach to the management of acute persistent diarrhea. EIA, enzyme immunoassay. IBS, irritable bowel syndrome; TMP/SMX, trimethoprim/sulfamethoxazole.

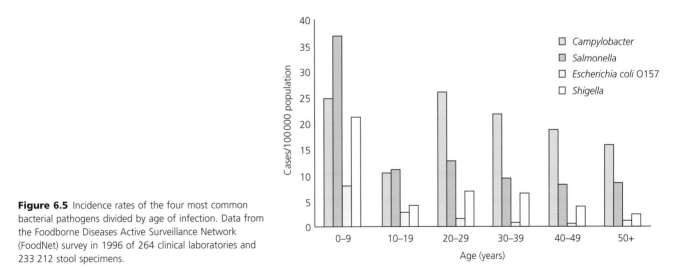

Figure 6.5 Incidence rates of the four most common bacterial pathogens divided by age of infection. Data from the Foodborne Diseases Active Surveillance Network (FoodNet) survey in 1996 of 264 clinical laboratories and 233 212 stool specimens.

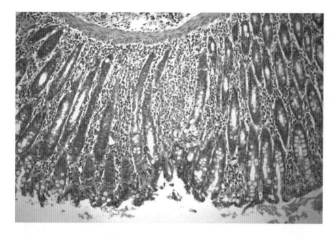

Figure 6.6 Biopsy specimen of colorectal mucosa from a patient with acute, self-limited, infectious-type colitis. Notice the preserved crypt architecture, acute lamina propria inflammation, and cryptitis.

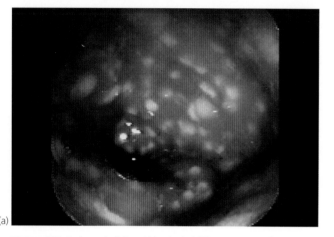

(a)

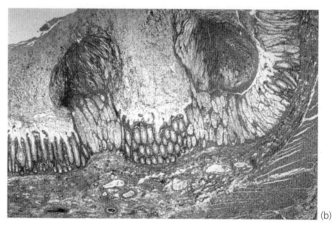

(b)

Figure 6.7 Endoscopic **(a)** and histological **(b)** appearance of pseudomembranous colitis due to *Clostridium difficile*. (a) Multiple scattered, yellowish plaques consistent with pseudomembranous colitis. (b) Denudation of the superficial epithelium and disruption of the mucosal surface in a mushrooming pattern along with a neutrophilic infiltrate in the lamina propria.

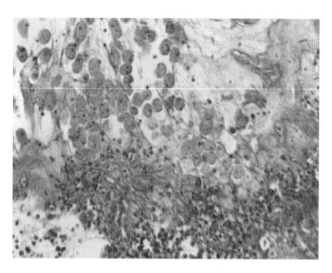

Figure 6.8 Biopsy specimen of colorectal mucosa from a patient with amebic colitis. Notice the abundant trophozoites of *Entamoeba histolytica* in the surface mucus. (H & E stain; original magnification x 100.)

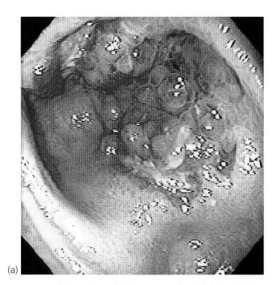 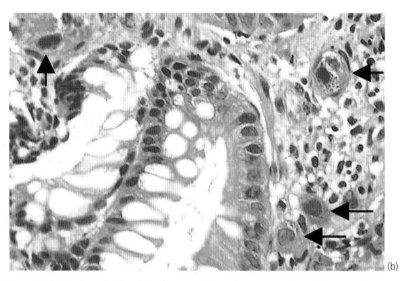

(a)

(b)

Figure 6.9 Endoscopic **(a)** and histological **(b)** appearance of cytomegalovirus (CMV) colitis. (a) Colonoscopic view showing an ulcerated lesion with pseudopolyps in the cecum. (b) Biopsy specimen of colorectal mucosa from a patient with CMV infection showing scattered typical CMV intranuclear inclusions (black arrows). (Low power, original magnification × 100.)

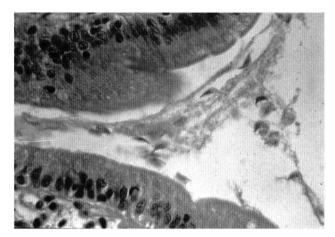

Figure 6.10 Biopsy specimen of duodenal mucosa from a patient with giardiasis. Notice the trophozoites of *Giardia lamblia* lining the lumenal surface of the enterocytes between two villi. (H & E stain; original magnification × 400.)

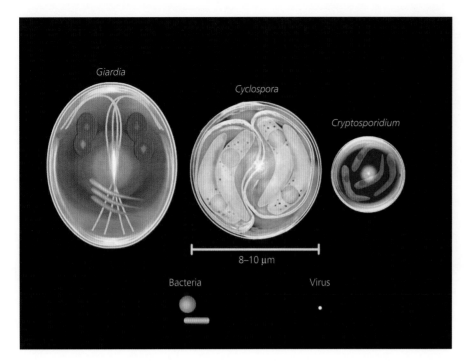

Figure 6.11 The appearance and relative sizes of protozoan cysts. The *Giardia lamblia* cyst (11–12 μm), *Cyclospora cayetanensis* oocyst (8–10 μm), and *Cryptosporidium parvum* oocyst (4–5 μm) are depicted. From Herwaldt BL. Cyclospora cayetanensis: A review, focusing on the outbreaks of cyclosporiasis in the 1990s.

7 Approach to the patient with constipation

Satish S.C. Rao

Constipation is a polysymptomatic, multifactorial disorder of the colon and anorectum. It comprises a constellation of symptoms, such as excessive straining, passage of hard pellet-like stools, decreased stool frequency, feeling of incomplete evacuation, feeling of blockage in the anorectal region or use of digital maneuvers to facilitate defecation. It affects approximately 15%–20% of the population, and places substantial burden on health-care resources. It predominantly affects women and the elderly. Broadly, constipation can be divided into two groups: primary constipation and secondary constipation.

Primary constipation

Primary constipation results from colonic and anorectal neuromuscular dysfunction as well as disordered regulation of brain–gut interactions. A well-known cause of constipation is Hirschsprung disease that is mostly seen in children. Primary constipation consists of at least three subtypes with a significant overlap. *Slow transit constipation* is characterized by prolonged delay of stool transport through the colon. This is either due to a dysfunction of colonic smooth muscle (myopathy) or its neurological intervention (neuropathy), and can also be secondary to an evacuation disorder. *Evacuation disorders* are characterized by either difficulty or inability with stool expulsion from the anorectum. The most common problem is dyssynergic defecation, and less commonly structural disorders, such as a rectocele or rectal prolapse, may cause constipation. The third group, *constipation predominant irritable bowel syndrome*, comprises patients who often have normal transit and normal evacuation; however, up to 60% exhibit rectal or visceral hypersensitivity.

Atlas of Gastroenterology, 4th edition. Edited by Tadataka Yamada, David H. Alpers, Anthony N. Kalloo, Neil Kaplowitz, Chung Owyang, and Don W. Powell. © 2009 Blackwell Publishing, ISBN: 978-1-4051-6909-7

Secondary constipation

Secondary constipation results from several mechanisms that include diet, drugs, behavioral, endocrine, metabolic, neurological and other disorders. Likewise, a number of drugs cause secondary constipation.

Evaluation of constipation

Constipation is best evaluated through a detailed medical, surgical, diet, and drug history. This will detect most organic and secondary causes of constipation. Because symptoms alone are poor predictors of underlying pathophysiology, physiological evaluation of colonic and anorectal function can provide useful mechanistic insights. These, together with patient history and physical examination findings, can facilitate a more accurate diagnosis of chronic constipation. The following tests are routinely performed and considered to be useful: colonic transit study, anorectal manometry, balloon expulsion test, and defecography. Because constipation is a heterogeneous condition that is caused by multiple pathophysiological mechanisms, a single test is inadequate to identify the subtype of chronic constipation.

A colonic transit study provides an objective measurement of the time taken to move stools through the colon. It is useful because a patient's recall of stool habit is often inaccurate. Currently, three methods are available:

1 Radiopaque marker test consists of ingestion of radiopaque markers followed by radiographs of the abdomen.

2 Scintigraphic colonic transit test consists of ingestion of radioisotopes followed by scintigraphic assessment of the geometric center of the isotope.

3 Ambulatory capsule manometry (SmartPill) test consists of ingestion of a pressure–pH capsule (SmartPill) followed by an assessment of the time taken for the capsule to move through the various segments of the gut. Additionally, it provides information on gut motility.

Anorectal manometry provides an assessment of the resting and squeeze sphincter pressures together with an assessment of rectal sensation, recto-anal reflexes and rectal compliance. Manometry is useful for a diagnosis of dyssynergic defecation and Hirschsprung disease. It is performed by placing a solid-state or water-perfused manometry probe into the anorectum.

The balloon expulsion test provides a simple bedside assessment of a subject's ability to expel an artificial stool. It is often performed by placing a 50-mL water-filled balloon in the rectum and allowing privacy for the subject to expel this device. Most normal subjects can expel a water-filled balloon in less than 1 min.

Defecography provides information regarding the morphological and functional changes of the anorectum, such as rectocele or dyssynergic defecation. It is performed by obtaining video fluoroscopic images after injecting barium paste into the rectum.

Colonic manometry provides comprehensive assessment of the overall motor activity in the colon during rest, sleep, after waking, and after provocative stimuli such as drugs, meal (gastrocolonic response), or following balloon distention. It is performed by placing a solid-state or water-perfused manometry probe into the colon under endoscopic or fluoroscopic guidance.

Rectal sensation, tone and compliance tests are best performed by placing a highly compliant balloon into the rectum, which is connected to a computerized pressure-distending device (Barostat). Subsequently, stepwise graded balloon distentions are performed to assess the sensorimotor responses.

Diagnostic tests are often indicated for identifying structural or functional causes of constipation in patients with either alarm symptoms or signs, or in patients with a clinical suspicion of dyssynergia or in those who do not respond to empirical therapy. There is good evidence that physiological tests such as anorectal manometry or colonic transit study can facilitate a diagnosis of the subtype of chronic constipation, and thereby guide treatment.

Table 7.1 Assessing colonic transit: strengths and drawbacks of current methods

	Radiopaque markers	Scintigraphy	Colon manometry	SmartPill
Radiation	Mild	Moderate	Mild	No
Invasive	No	Mildly	Moderately	No
GET and SBTT	No	Yes	No	Yes
Can assess colonic transit time	Yes	Yes	No	Yes
Identify myopathy/ neuropathy	No	No	Yes	?
Availability	Widely	Only 2 centers	Available	Available

GET, gastric emptying time; SBTT, small bowel transit time.

This table summarizes the strengths and drawbacks of current methods of assessing colonic motor function. Radiopaque marker tests provide an assessment of whole-gut and, primarily, colonic transit time, and involves radiation. However, it is noninvasive and does not provide an assessment of gastric emptying or small bowel transit. Although widely available, it does not identify colonic myopathy or neuropathy. Radionuclide scintigraphy provides a noninvasive assessment of gastric emptying and small bowel transit along with colonic transit time; however, it involves modest radiation, is not widely available and does not identify colonic neuropathy or myopathy. Colonic manometry is invasive, identifies the presence of colonic myopathy and neuropathy, and can facilitate optimal surgical treatment of constipation, but involves minimal radiation. The ambulatory pH and pressure capsule test (SmartPill) provides measurement of gastric emptying, small bowel transit time, colonic transit time and whole-gut transit time, as well as segmental gut motility, but does not involve radiation and is noninvasive.

Table 7.2 Trial design and key findings of four large randomized controlled trials of biofeedback therapy in the management of patients with chronic constipation and dyssynergic defecation

	Chiaironi et al. 2006	Rao et al. 2007	Chiaironi et al. 2005	Heymen et al. 2007
Trial design	Biofeedback vs PEG 14.6 g	Biofeedback vs standard vs sham biofeedback	Biofeedback for slow transit vs. dyssynergia	Biofeedback vs diazepam 5 mg vs placebo
Subjects and randomization	104 women, 54 biofeedback, 55 polyethylene glycol	77 (69 women), 1:1:1 distribution	52 (49 women), 34 dyssynergia, 12 slow transit, 6 mixed	84 (71 women), 30 biofeedback, 30 diazepam, 24 placebo
Duration and number of biofeedback sessions	3 months and 1 year, five, weekly 30 min training sessions performed by physician investigator	3 months, biweekly, 1 h, maximum of six sessions over 3 months, performed by biofeedback nurse therapist	Five, weekly 30-min training sessions, performed by physician investigator	Six biweekly, 1-h sessions
Primary outcomes	Global improvement of symptoms: Worse = 0, No improvement = 1, Mild = 2, Fair = 3, Major improvement = 4	(1) Presence of dyssynergia, (2) Balloon expulsion time, (3) Number of complete spontaneous bowel movements, (4) Global satisfaction	Symptom improvement: None = 1, Mild = 2, Fair = 3, Major = 4	Global symptom relief
Dyssynergia corrected or symptoms improved	79.6% reported major improvement at 6 and 12 months. 81.5% reported major improvement at 24 months	Dyssynergia corrected at 3 months in 79% with biofeedback vs. 4% sham and 6% in standard group; CSBM = Biofeedback group vs Sham or standard, p <0.05	71% with dyssynergia and 8% with slow transit alone reported fair improvement in symptoms	70% improved with biofeedback compared with 38% with placebo and 30% with diazepam
Conclusions	Biofeedback was superior to laxatives	Biofeedback was superior to sham feedback and standard therapy	Biofeedback benefits dyssynergia and not slow transit constipation	Biofeedback is superior to placebo and diazepam

CSBM, complete spontaneous bowel movement.

This table summarizes the trial design and the key findings of four large randomized controlled trials of biofeedback therapy in the management of patients with chronic constipation and dyssynergic defecation. Although the studies differed in their methodology, all four studies concluded that biofeedback was superior to alternative therapies such as laxatives, placebo or sham feedback therapy.

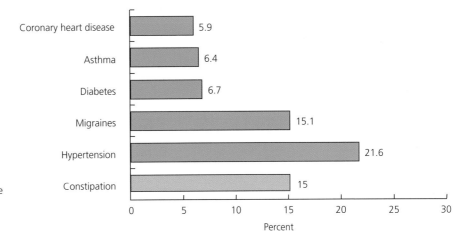

Figure 7.1 This figure compares the prevalence of various common diseases in the United States. It can be seen that chronic constipation is one of the most common disorders.

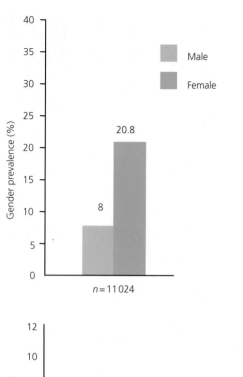

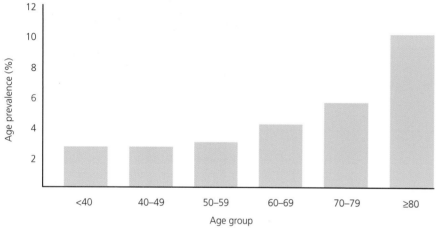

Figure 7.2 This shows the prevalence of chronic constipation based on gender and age. Constipation is more prevalent in women and the elderly.

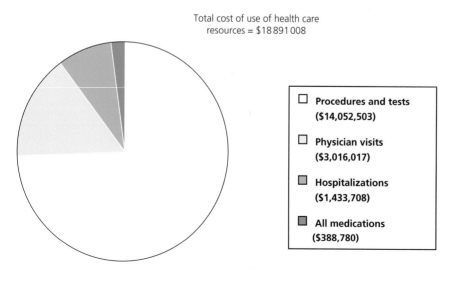

Total cost of use of health care resources = $18 891 008

☐ **Procedures and tests ($14,052,503)**

☐ **Physician visits ($3,016,017)**

☐ **Hospitalizations ($1,433,708)**

☐ **All medications ($388,780)**

Figure 7.3 This summarizes the total health-care costs, for patients with constipation that were incurred in a Medi-Cal population. It illustrates that constipation consumes a significant amount of health-care resources in the United States. There were 76 854 patients assessed and they did not have supplementary insurance. They enrolled in Medi-Cal. The average cost per patient was $246.

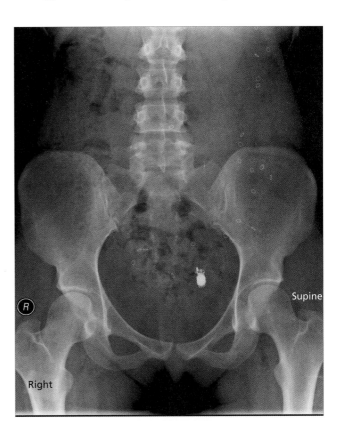

Figure 7.4 This plain radiograph of the abdomen shows an example of measuring colonic transit time with radiopaque markers. Here, a single SitzMark capsule containing 24 ring-shaped, radiopaque markers was swallowed on day 0 and a plain abdominal radiograph was obtained on day 5 (120 h later). The presence of five or fewer markers indicates normal colonic transit. In this example, several markers can be seen in the left colon and rectosigmoid region. Although the test identifies patients with slow transit constipation, it cannot differentiate whether the delayed transit is secondary to colonic neuromuscular dysfunction or dyssynergic defecation.

Wireless motility capsule

Figure 7.5 This graphic display was obtained after swallowing an ambulatory pressure, pH, and temperature sensing capsule (wireless motility; shown in the insert). This test provides a measurement of gastric emptying time, small bowel transit time, colonic transit time, and whole gut transit time. The capsule's location is judged by observing the pH profile. After ingestion, the pH is between 1 and 2, indicating that the capsule is located in the stomach. After 4 h, there is an abrupt increase in pH indicating the capsule's exit from the stomach and entry into the small bowel and where the contents are more alkaline. After another 4 h, there is a sustained and significant decrease in pH profile (≥1 unit). This corresponds with the arrival of the capsule in the cecum. After 120 h, the capsule was ejected. The values for gastric emptying time, small bowel transit time, and colonic transit time are displayed. This patient demonstrates delayed gastric emptying, normal small bowel transit time, and delayed colonic and whole gut transit time.

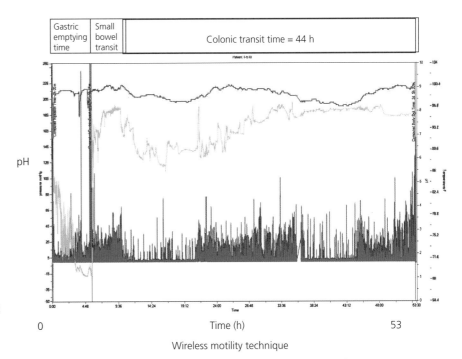

Gastric emptying time	Small bowel transit	Colonic transit time = 44 h

Wireless motility technique

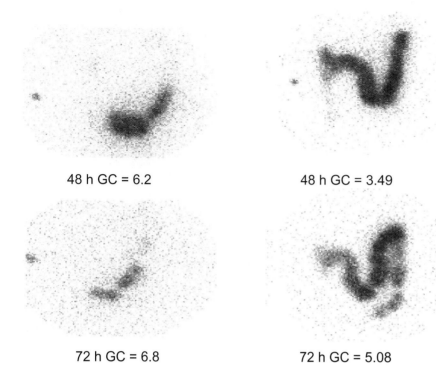

48 h GC = 6.2

48 h GC = 3.49

72 h GC = 6.8

72 h GC = 5.08

Figure 7.6 These sets of images were obtained by performing nuclear scintigraphy following oral ingestion of [111]indium-diethylenetriamine-pentaacetic acid radioisotope. As can be seen, in contrast to a healthy individual shown on the left, where the geometric center (GC) of the isotope at 48 h is 6.2 and at 72 h is 6.8, in a patient with chronic constipation **(right)** the geometric center is significantly lower indicating greater retention of the isotope. Also, the isotope is located in the distal left colon in the healthy subject, whereas it is distributed in the transverse colon or proximal left colon in the constipated subject. Courtesy of Dr Alan Maurer and Dr Henry Parkman, Temple University School of Medicine, Philadelphia.

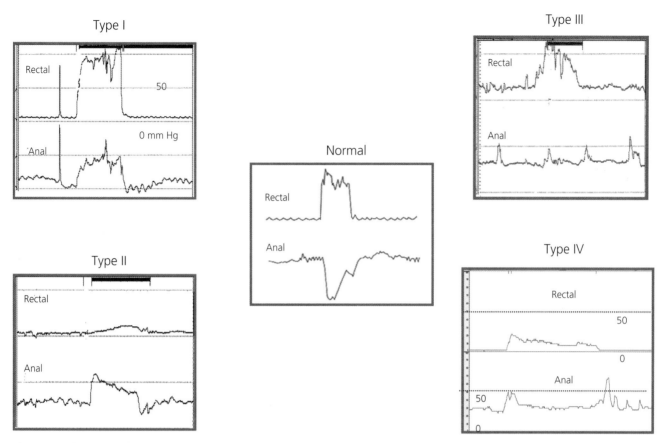

Figure 7.7 These series of images reveal the manometric patterns that are commonly seen during attempted defecation in a normal healthy individual (Normal) and in patients with dyssynergic defecation. These manometric tracings were obtained after placing a multisensor solid state manometry catheter into the rectum; to improve clarity, changes from a single sensor in the rectum and one from the anal canal are shown. It can be seen that the "normal" subject can generate a good pushing force (increase in intrarectal pressure) and simultaneously there is relaxation of the anal canal. In contrast, patients with dyssynergic defecation exhibit one of four abnormal patterns of defecation. In type I dyssenergia, the subject can generate an adequate propulsive force (rise in intrarectal pressure ≥40 mmHg) along with paradoxical increase in anal sphincter pressure. In type II dyssynergia, the subject is unable to generate an adequate propulsive force; additionally there is paradoxical anal contraction. In type III dyssynergia, the subject can generate an adequate propulsive force but there is either absent relaxation (a flat line) or incomplete (≤ 20%) relaxation of anal sphincter. In type IV dyssynergia, the subject is unable to generate an adequate propulsive force together with an absent or incomplete relaxation of anal sphincter.

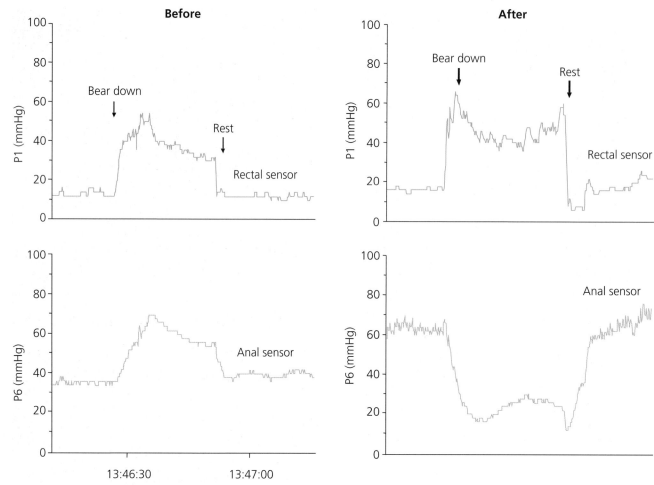

Figure 7.8 These figures show typical examples of intralumenal manometric pressure changes in the rectum and anal canal from a patient with chronic constipation and dyssynergic defecation, both before and after neuromuscular training with biofeedback therapy. The "before" graphs show an example of dyssynergia; when the patient attempts to bear down, the intrarectal pressure increases from 10 to 50 mmHg.

Simultaneously, the intraanal pressure also rises from 35 to 60 mmHg, revealing an abnormal and paradoxical increase in anal sphincter pressure. After biofeedback therapy, the patient has learned to coordinate the push effort. This is demonstrated by a rise in intrarectal pressure that is coordinated with anal sphincter pressure relaxation from 60 to 20 mmHg.

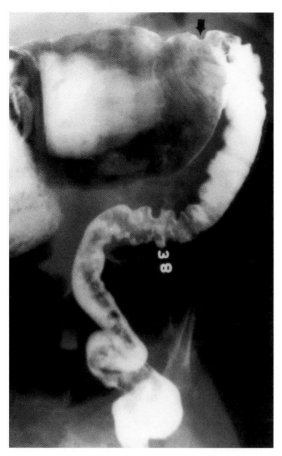

Figure 7.9 Hirschsprung disease. Barium enema radiograph of a child with Hirschsprung disease. A narrow section extends to the splenic flexure (arrow) with proximal dilation of the bowel. Courtesy of the Department of Radiology, Children's Hospital of Pittsburgh.

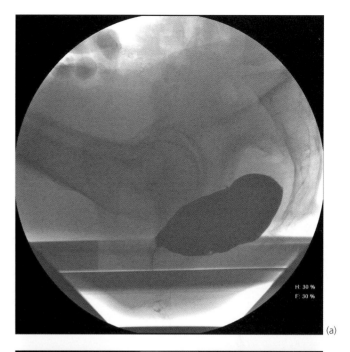

(a)

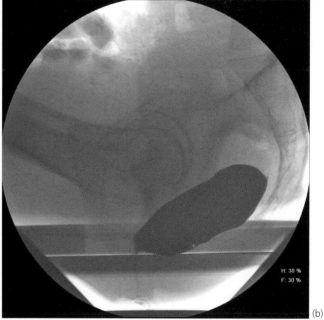

(b)

Figure 7.10 These radiographs reveal findings from a defecography study. In this study, usually 150 mL of barium paste is infused into the rectum with a caulking gun. Subsequently, the subject is asked to sit on a special chair and perform the following maneuvers; squeeze, cough and evacuate; simultaneously, lateral video fluoroscopic images are obtained. **(a)** The resting profile is shown with an anorectal angle of 100°. **(b)** Changes shown during attempted defecation. When the patient attempts to push and bear down, there is minimal perineal descent as indicated by the downward movement of the rectum and anal canal, there is mild ballooning of the rectal ampulla, but the patient exhibits paradoxical contraction of the anal sphincter or dyssynergia. Consequently, the patient is unable to expel the barium paste.

Healthy controls
100%: mean incidence/day = 10.1

Constipation
43%: mean incidence/day = 1.7

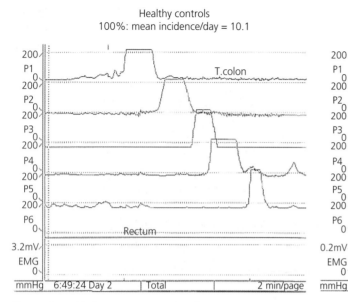

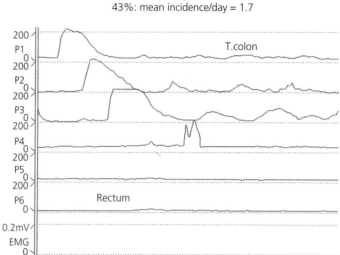

Figure 7.11 This figure shows examples of colonic high amplitude propagated contractions (HAPCs) in a healthy subject and a constipated patient. The mean incidence of HAPCs in healthy controls were ~10 per day and in constipated patients 1.7. 43% of patients had no HAPCs over 24 h. The HAPCs are characterized by high amplitude (≥105 mmHg) and prolonged duration (≥20 s), propagating pressure waves that commenced in the proximal colon and migrated into the rectum. They are akin to the mass movements seen in radiological studies. Patients with chronic constipation either had absent or fewer HAPCs or they aborted prematurely within the colon.

Figure 7.12 This figure shows colonic manometric pressure changes in a healthy individual in panel A and in a patient with chronic constipation in panel B, during baseline, and immediately 1–2 h after ingestion of a 1000 kcal meal. The study is performed by placing a 6-sensor solid-state manometry catheter, with the most proximal sensor P1 located at the hepatic flexure, the second sensor P2 located in the mid transverse colon, the third sensor at the splenic flexure, the fourth sensor in the mid descending colon, the fifth sensor in the sigmoid colon, and the sixth sensor P6 in the rectum. During the baseline period, occasional, sporadic, non-propulsive pressure activity can be seen. Immediately after ingestion of a meal, there is a robust increase in intralumenal pressure activity in all six channels in the healthy subject which comprise propagated and simultaneous contractions, and occasional high amplitude propagated contractions. In contrast, there is only sparse and short-lived increase in colonic motor response, which completely dissipates within 90 min in a patient with slow transit constipation. This impaired gastrocolonic motor response is a hallmark of severe slow transit constipation and is indicative of colonic neuropathy.

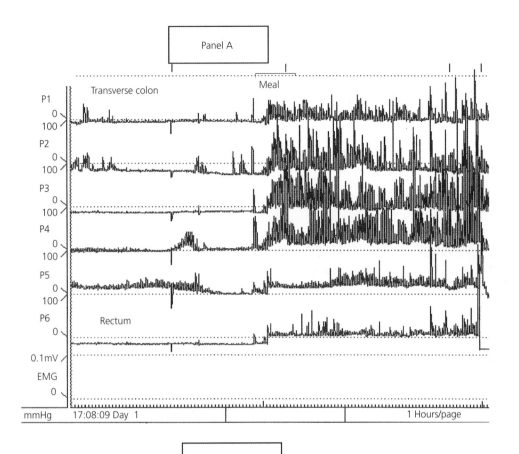

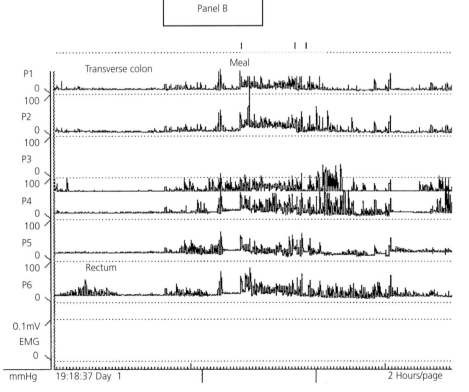

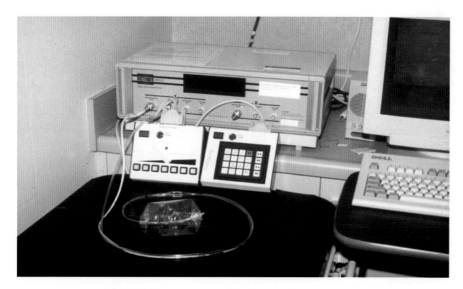

Figure 7.13 This figure shows a barostat, a computerized pressure-distending device. It is ideally suited for the assessment of sensation, tone and compliance of hollow lumenal organs, such as the rectum, colon or stomach. Also shown is a highly compliant balloon mounted on a catheter; these are often used. The perception panel enables the subject to score the severity of sensation.

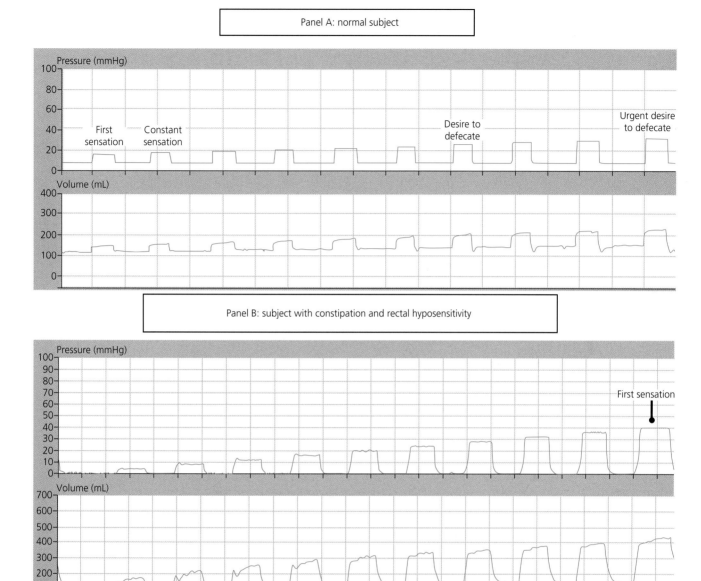

Figure 7.14 The graphs displayed reveal intraballoon pressure and volume changes from a healthy normal subject **(panel A)** and a patient with rectal hyposensitivity and constipation **(panel B)**. As can be seen, the normal subject reports first sensation, at rectal balloon distention pressure of 15 mmHg, a desire to defecate at 28 mmHg, and an urgent desire to defecate at 36 mmHg pressure distention. In contrast, a patient with constipation reports first sensation at a pressure distention of 40 mmHg, revealing severe rectal hyposensitivity. Simultaneously, the changes in intraballoon volume provide an assessment of rectal tone or compliance. As can be seen, the rectum is also more compliant in a patient with hyposensitivity, as demonstrated by higher intrarectal balloon volumes. By plotting the changes in rectal volume (dV) against the changes in intrarectal pressure (dP), it is possible to calculate a compliance curve for the assessment of rectal wall distensibility.

8 Approach to the patient with abnormal liver chemistries

Richard H. Moseley

Since the advent of routine automated serum testing, a common problem in gastroenterology has been the determination of the cause, and thus the importance, of abnormalities in liver chemistries. At first, such evaluations may be frustrating because of the lack of any well-defined diagnostic algorithms. However, armed with an understanding of the diverse panel of available measurements of liver function and serum markers of hepatobiliary disease, and knowledge of the patterns by which specific hepatobiliary disorders typically present themselves, the clinician can usually approach these diagnostic challenges in an orderly and selective manner. The normal values of certain laboratory tests that either lead to or assist in diagnosis are listed in Table 8.1, with ranges or reference intervals in traditional units and Système International d'Unités (SI).

Drug-associated abnormalities in liver chemistries are frequently encountered. Although familiarity with the hepatic side effects of all drugs used is not possible, knowledge of the potential for and clinical pattern of hepatic injury associated with commonly used agents is extremely useful. Representative drugs and their typical pattern of hepatic injury are listed in Table 8.2. Scales for scoring the probability of drug-induced hepatoxicity have been developed, such as the Council for International Organizations of Medical Sciences (CIOMS) system (Table 8.3).

The use of alternative medicine, particularly herbal medicine, is increasing and hepatotoxicity is a recognized complication of these preparations. A representative list of these remedies and their reported hepatotoxicity is provided in Table 8.4.

A thorough occupational history may provide important clues to an otherwise cryptic case of abnormal liver chemistries. A representative list of industrial and environmental hepatotoxins is provided in Table 8.5.

Elevated serum aminotransferase levels can be observed among patients with any type of liver disease, and among patients with cardiac and skeletal muscle disorders. All too commonly, serum aminotransferase elevations are incorrectly ascribed to alcoholic liver injury. Alternative diagnoses, such as autoimmune hepatitis, viral and drug-induced hepatitis, nonalcoholic steatohepatitis, hemochromatosis, Wilson disease, α_1-antitrypsin deficiency, and celiac sprue should always be considered (Fig. 8.1). The highest serum elevations of serum aminotransferases are seen in patients with viral, toxin-induced, and ischemic hepatitis. In alcoholic liver disease, serum aspartate aminotransferase (AST; SGOT [serum glutamic–oxaloacetic transaminase]) and alanine aminotransferase (ALT; SGPT [serum glutamic–pyruvic transaminase]) levels are typically less than 300 IU/L, and the ratio of AST to ALT is greater than two. In the case of acetaminophen (paracetamol) hepatotoxicity involving a patient with alcoholism, this ratio is maintained. The serum aminotransferase elevation is striking in this setting, reaching, and often exceeding, levels typically associated with toxic, ischemic, or viral injury. Diagnosis of acute viral hepatitis requires appropriate application of serological tests (Table 8.6). The typical course of chronic hepatitis B and C infections are illustrated in Figs 8.2 and 8.3, respectively.

Elevation of serum alkaline phosphatase levels occurs primarily in cholestatic disorders, but the degree of elevation does not help one differentiate extrahepatic from intrahepatic causes. In the face of findings inconsistent with extrahepatic obstruction, intrahepatic cholestasis (whether drug induced or from disorders such as primary biliary cirrhosis) as well as infiltrative processes (such as tuberculosis, sarcoidosis, and metastatic carcinoma) should be considered (Fig. 8.4). Granulomatous processes involving the liver may present with infiltrative features and the number of differential diagnoses of these is quite extensive. A partial listing of some of these disorders is provided in Table 8.7.

Atlas of Gastroenterology, 4th edition. Edited by Tadataka Yamada, David H. Alpers, Anthony N. Kalloo, Neil Kaplowitz, Chung Owyang, and Don W. Powell. © 2009 Blackwell Publishing, ISBN: 978-1-4051-6909-7

Table 8.1 Normal values of laboratory tests used in the approach to the patient with abnormal liver chemistries

Reference interval			
		Conversion	
Test	Present	SI	Factor
Alanine aminotransferase	0–35 U/L	0.0–0.58 µkat/L	00.01667
Albumin	4.0–6.0 g/dL	40–60 g/L	10.0
Alkaline phosphatase	30–120 U/L	0.5–2.0 µkat/L	00.01667
α1-Antitrypsin	150–350 mg/dL	1.5–3.5 g/L	10.0
α-Fetoprotein	0–20 ng/mL	0–20 µg/L	01.00
Ammonia (venous)	10–80 µg/dL	5–50 µmol/L	00.5872
Aspartate aminotransferase	0–35 U/L	0.0–0.58 µkat/L	00.01667
Bile acids, total	Trace–3.3 µg/mL	Trace–8.4 µmol/L	02.547
Cholate	Trace–1.0 µg/mL	Trace–2.4 µmol/L	02.448
Chenodeoxycholate	Trace–1.3 µg/mL	Trace–3.4 µmol/L	02.547
Deoxycholate	Trace–1.0 µg/mL	Trace–2.6 µmol/L	02.547
Lithocholate	Trace	Trace	02.656
Bilirubin, total	0.1–1.0 mg/dL	2–18 µmol/L	17.10
Bilirubin, conjugated	0.0–0.2 mg/dL	0–4 µmol/L	17.10
Ceruloplasmin	20–35 mg/dL	200–350 mg/L	10.0
Copper, serum	70–140 µg/dL	11.0–22.0 µmol/L	00.1574
Ferritin	18–300 ng/mL	18–300 µg/L	01.00
γ-Glutamyltransferase	0.0–30 U/L	0.0–0.50 µkat/L	00.01667
Iron, serum			
Men	80–180 µg/dL	14–32 µmol/L	00.1791
Women	60–160 µg/dL	11–29 µmol/L	00.1791
Iron-binding capacity	250–460 µg/dL	45–82 µmol/L	00.1791

The Système International d'Unités (SI) was adopted by the World Health Organization in 1977 in an attempt to bring international uniformity to laboratory measurements. The table lists the normal range or reference interval of laboratory values in traditional units and the multiplication factor necessary to convert to SI units. Certain values listed are method dependent and therefore verification of the reference interval for a given clinical laboratory may be necessary.

Table 8.2 Partial list of drug-induced abnormalities in liver chemistries

Hepatocellular injury (aminotransferase elevations)
Acetaminophen
Isoniazid
α-Methyldopa
Ketoconazole
Amiodarone
Labetalol
Ampicillin
Lovastatin
Clozapine
Methotrexate
Dantrolene
Nicotinic acid
Dapsone
Nitrofurantoin
Diclofenac
Propylthiouracil
Disulfiram
Rifampin
Etoposide
Tacrine
Fluconazole
Terbutaline
Glyburide
Trazodone
Heparin

Cholestatic injury (bilirubin or alkaline phosphatase elevations)
Androgenic anabolic steroids
Griseofulvin (e.g., methyltestosterone, danazol)
Haloperidol
Amoxicillin/clavulanic acid
Imipramine
Atenolol
Methimazole

Captopril
Penicillin
Chlorpropamide
Phenothiazines
Ciprofloxacin
Piroxicam
Cyclosporine
Propafenone
Dicloxacillin
Thiabendazole
Erythromycin
Ticlopidine
Estrogenic steroids
Tolazamide
Flurazepam
Tolbutamide
Floxuridine
Trimethoprim–sulfamethoxazole
Gold salts
Warfarin

Mixed hepatocellular and cholestatic injury
Azathioprine
Sulfonamides
Flutamide
Terbinafine
Phenylbutazone
Valproic acid
Phenytoin

Granulomatous infiltration (alkaline phosphatase elevation)
Allopurinol
Diltiazem
Carbamazepine
Phenytoin

Table 8.3 Council for International Organizations of Medical Sciences (CIOMS) scale for evaluating drug-induced hepatotoxicity

	Hepatocelluar type			Cholestatic or mixed type		Assessment
1. Time to onset						
Incompatible	Reaction occurred before starting the drug or more than 15 days after stopping the drug (except for slowly metabolized drugs)			Reaction occurred before starting the drug or more than 30 days after stopping the drug (except for slowly metabolized drugs)		Unrelated
Unknown	When information is not available to calculate time to onset, then the case is:					Insufficient data

	Initial treatment	Subsequent treatment	Initial treatment	Subsequent treatment	Score
From the initiation of the drug					
Suggestive	5–90 days	1–15 days	5–90 days	1–90 days	+2
Compatible	<5 or >90 days	>15 days	<5 or >90 days	>90 days	+1
From cessation of the drug					
Compatible	≤15 days	≤15 days	≤30 days	≤30 days	+1

2. Course

	Difference between the peak of ALT and upper limit of normal values	Difference between the peak of alk. phos. (or TB) and upper limit of normal values	
After cessation of the drug			
Highly suggestive	Decrease ≥50% within 8 days	Not applicable	+3
Suggestive	Decrease ≥50% within 30 days	Decrease ≥50% within 180 days	+2
Compatible	Not applicable	Decrease <50% within 180 days	+1
Inconclusive	No information or decrease ≥50%, after the 30th day	Persistence or increase or no information	0
Against the role of the drug	Decrease <50%, after the 30th day or recurrent increase	No situation	
If the drug is continued			
Inconclusive	All situations	Not applicable	−2
		All situations	0

3. Risk factors

	Ethanol	Ethanol or pregnancy	
Presence			+1
Absence			0
Age of the patient ≥55 years			+1
Age of the patient <55 years			0

4. Concomitant drug(s)

None or no information or concomitant drug with incompatible time to onset	0
Concomitant drug with compatible or suggestive time to onset	−1
Concomitant drug known as hepatotoxin and with compatible or suggestive time to onset	−2
Concomitant drug with evidence for its role, in this case (positive rechallenge or validated test)	−3

Continued

Table 8.3 *Continued*

5. Search for non-drug causes		
Group 1 (6 causes): Recent viral infection with HAV (IgM anti-HAV antibody) or HBV (IgM anti-HBc antibody) or HCV (anti-HCV antibody) and circumstantial arguments for nonA–nonB hepatitis); Biliary obstruction (ultrasonography); alcoholism (AST/ALT ≥2); acute recent hypotension history (particularly if underlying heart disease)	All causes – groups I and II – reasonably ruled out	+2
Group II: Complications of underlying disease(s); clinical and/or biological context suggesting CMV, EBV or Herpes virus infection	The six causes of group I ruled out	+1
	The five or four causes of group I ruled out	0
	Less than four causes of group I ruled out	−2
	Nondrug cause highly probable	−3

6. Previous information on hepatotoxicity of the drug	
Reaction labeled in the product characteristics	+2
Reaction published but unlabeled	+1
Reaction unknown	0

7. Response to readministration			
Positive	Doubling of ALT with the drug alone	Doubling of AP (or TB) with the drug alone	+3
Compatible	Doubling of ALT with the drugs already given at the time of the 1st reaction	Doubling of AP (or TB) with the drugs already given at the time of the 1st reaction	+1
Negative	Increase of ALT but less than N in the same conditions as for the first administration	Increase of AP (or TB) but less than N in the same conditions as for the first administration	−2
Not done or not interpretable	Other situations	Other situations	0

Total (add the encircled figures)

Scores may range from −5 to 14: <0, relationship excluded; 1–2, unlikely; 3–5, possible; 6–8, probable; >8, highly probable.
Adapted from Danan G, Benichou C. Causality assessment of adverse reactions to drugs. J Clin Epidemiology 1993;46:1323 and 1331.

Table 8.4 Herbal hepatotoxins

Liver injury	
Agent	**Pattern**
Greater celandine (*Chelidonium majus*)	Cholestatic hepatitis
Hydrazine sulfate	Submassive bridging necrosis
Chaparral (*Larrea tridentata*)	Cholestatic hepatitis
Kava (*Piper methysticum rhizoma*)	Acute and chronic hepatitis; acute liver failure
Jin Bu Huan (*Lycopodium serratum*)	Hepatitis with microvesicular steatosis
Germander (*Teucrium chamaedrys*)	Hepatitis
Pyrrolizidine alkaloids	
Comfrey tea (*Symphytum* species)	Venoocclusive disease
Crotolaria	
Senecio	
Heliotropium	

Table 8.5 Occupational and environmental hepatotoxins

Liver injury		
Agent	**Setting**	**Pattern**
Dimethylformamide	Organic solvent; used in many industrial applications including manufacture of polyurethane products and acrylic fibers	Hepatocellular
2-Nitropropane	Organic solvent; used in many industrial applications including manufacture of water-resistant coatings, printing inks, and adhesives	Hepatocellular
1,1,1-Trichloroethane	Organic solvent; widely used in industry	Hepatocellular
Trichloroethylene	Organic solvent; widely used in industry, including dry cleaning	Hepatocellular
5-Nitro-o-toluidine	Aromatic compound used as a raw material in azo dyes	Hepatocellular
Vinyl chloride	Polyvinyl chloride production	Infiltrative
Beryllium	Used in the manufacture of electrical equipment	Infiltrative

Table 8.6 Serological tests in acute viral hepatitis

Viral type	Serological test
Hepatitis A	IgM anti-HAV
Hepatitis B	HbsAg and IgM anti-HBc
Hepatitis C	HCV RNA
Hepatitis D	HbsAg and anti-HDV

Table 8.7 Hepatic granulomas

Infectious processes
   Tuberculosis
   Atypical mycobacterial infections
   Brucellosis
   Coccidiomycosis
   Histoplasmosis
   Candidiasis
   Q fever
   Syphilis

Hepatobiliary disorders
   Primary biliary cirrhosis

Miscellaneous disorders
   Drugs
   Berylliosis
   Sarcoidosis

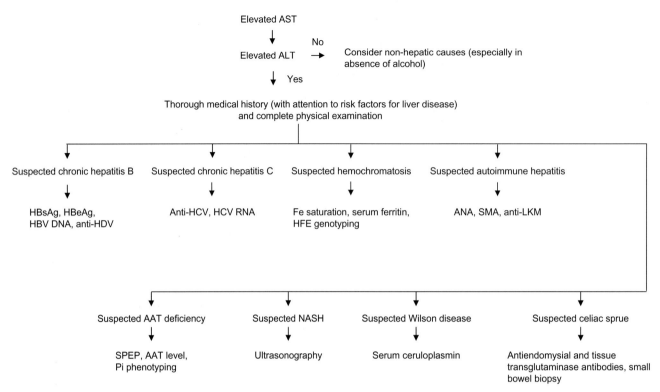

Figure 8.1 Algorithm for diagnosing the patient with elevated serum aminotransferase levels. Liver biopsy should be considered in most cases to confirm suspected disorders. AAT, alpha-1-antitrypsin; ALT, alanine aminotransferase; ANA, antinuclear antibody; AST, aspartate aminotransferase; DNA, deoxyribonucleic acid; HBeAg, hepatitis B e antigen; HBsAg, hepatitis B surface antigen; HBV, hepatitis B virus; HDV, hepatitis D virus; anti-LKM, antibody to liver kidney microsomes; NASH, nonalcoholic steatohepatitis; RNA, ribonucleic acid; SMA, smooth muscle antibody; SPEP, serum protein electrophoresis.

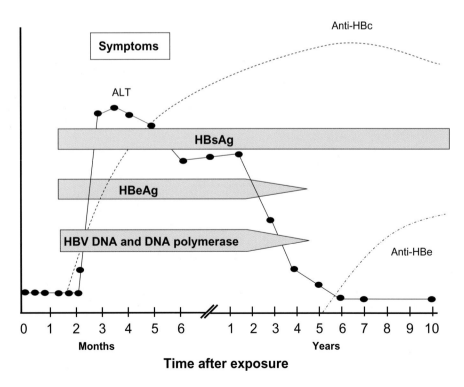

Figure 8.2 Typical course of chronic hepatitis B infection. ALT, alanine aminotransferase; anti-HBc, antibody to hepatitis B core antigen; HBeAg, hepatitis B e antigen; HBsAg, hepatitis B surface antigen; HBV, hepatitis B virus.

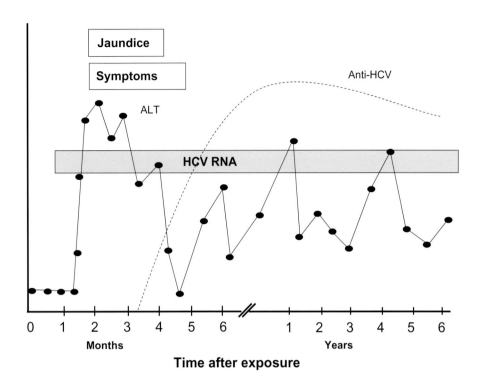

Figure 8.3 Typical course of chronic hepatitis C infection. ALT, alanine aminotransferase; HCV, hepatitis C virus; RNA, ribonucleic acid.

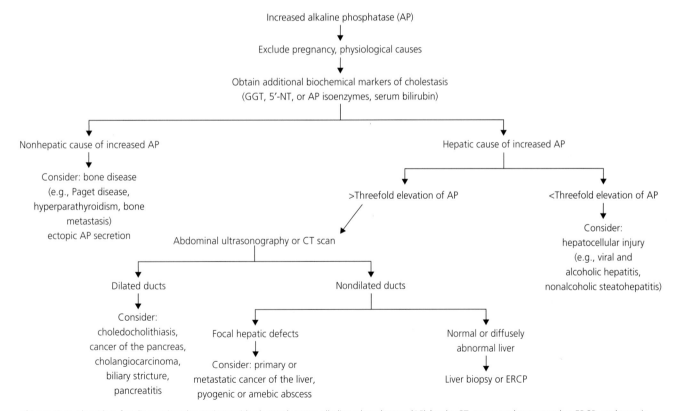

Figure 8.4 Algorithm for diagnosing the patient with elevated serum alkaline phosphatase (AP) levels. CT, computed tomography; ERCP, endoscopic retrograde cholangiopancreatography; GGTP, serum γ-glutamyl transpeptidase; 5'NT, 5'nucleotidase.

9 Approach to the patient with jaundice

Janak N. Shah, Raphael B. Merriman, Marion G. Peters

Approach to the patient with jaundice

The investigation of a patient with jaundice begins with a thorough review of the history of presentation, medication use, past medical history, examination, and evaluation of liver-related laboratory tests (Table 9.1). Physicians are 80%–90% accurate in diagnosing extrahepatic disease by these means, but obstruction is often overdiagnosed. With an understanding of the pathophysiology of cholestasis, a systematic approach to the jaundiced patient can be applied. Identification of the correct diagnosis can lead to an appropriate therapeutic intervention. The implications of jaundice in certain conditions can be life-threatening, and thus a timely diagnosis is important. When first evaluating a patient with hyperbilirubinemia, the physician must make a quick assessment of the emergency of the situation. Fever, leukocytosis, and hypotension point to ascending cholangitis, which requires immediate therapy. Asterixis, confusion, or stupor may indicate severe hepatocellular dysfunction or fulminant hepatic failure and mandates immediate therapy. After immediate life-threatening causes of hyperbilirubinemia have been excluded, a systematic approach to the patient helps to make the diagnosis.

Diagnostic approach

Figures 9.1 and 9.2 depict algorithms useful in the differential diagnosis and evaluation of a patient with jaundice, respectively. The initial step is to determine whether the jaundice is conjugated or unconjugated. The causes of conjugated hyperbilirubinemia range anatomically from the ampulla of Vater to the hepatocyte. If the history and physical examination do not provide a clue to the cause, the initial approach should be a right upper quadrant ultrasound to evaluate the liver, the biliary system, and the porta hepatitis. Laboratory tests can confirm suspicions formed during the

history and physical examination. Bilirubin remains normal until most of the bile ducts are obstructed. Alkaline phosphatase level is a more sensitive test for biliary obstruction than bilirubin.

Noninvasive tests

After the history, physical examination, and laboratory tests are obtained, further diagnostic tests include noninvasive tests, such as ultrasound, computed tomography (CT) or magnetic resonance imaging (MRI).

Ultrasound

Ultrasound (Fig. 9.3) is the first test used to detect biliary obstruction. Ultrasound is of low cost, widely available, noninvasive and easy to perform. The diagnostic accuracy ranges from 77% to 94%, and the result is most accurate when the bilirubin level exceeds 10 mg/dL. The variability in sensitivity reflects limitations from overlying bowel gas, obesity, site and size of the stones, and presence or absence of duct dilation. Ultrasound is inconsistent in determining the site or cause of obstruction, partly because of its inability to see the distal duct well in 30%–50% of patients. Despite these caveats and the fact that ultrasound is operator dependent, it remains the preferred initial screening test for evaluating biliary obstruction.

Computed tomography

Computed tomography imaging (Fig. 9.4) has a sensitivity of 60%–90%, and results rely less on the operator's proficiency. Computed tomography is not impeded by fat. Advances in CT technology (multidetector CT and helical CT) have resulted in superior quality imaging compared with prior-generation CT, and provide high accuracy in evaluating causes of biliary obstruction.

Magnetic resonance imaging

Magnetic resonance imaging (MRI) (Fig. 9.5) relies on the physical properties of unpaired protons in tissues to generate images, without use of ionizing radiation. Magnetic resonance imaging is sensitive and specific for the detection and

Atlas of Gastroenterology, 4th edition. Edited by Tadataka Yamada, David H. Alpers, Anthony N. Kalloo, Neil Kaplowitz, Chung Owyang, and Don W. Powell. © 2009 Blackwell Publishing, ISBN: 978-1-4051-6909-7

evaluation of focal and malignant lesions, and avoids the potentially nephrotoxic contrast agents used with CT imaging. This is particularly relevant in patients with jaundice or cholestasis. The MRI characteristics of stationary and mobile liquids make MR cholangiopancreatography (MRCP: Fig. 9.6) and MR angiography powerful noninvasive diagnostic tools. Bile duct calculi are seen particularly well with MRCP and should be used in those with negative sonography and a high index of suspicion. With MRI, imaging of the biliary tree is feasible both proximal and distal to the site of obstruction. Magnetic resonances cholangiopancreatography is more accurate than ultrasound in disease staging and evaluation of distal common bile duct lesions. Use of ultrasound and MRCP has decreased the use of diagnostic endoscopic retrograde cholangiopancreatography (ERCP) (Fig. 9.7) and aided in identifying patients who require therapeutic ERCP or surgery.

Invasive tests

Invasive tests currently used include ERCP, percutaneous transhepatic cholangiography (PTC), endoscopic ultrasound (EUS), and liver biopsy. Endoscopic retrograde cholangiopancreatography and PTC use cholecystographic dye and radiography to visualize the biliary tree. They are excellent tests to verify ductal dilation and permit concomitant therapeutic intervention. The decision to pursue ERCP, PTC, or EUS should depend on the presumed site of obstruction, the presence of coagulopathy or ascites, and the local expertise of the radiologists and gastroenterologists. Percutaneous transhepatic cholangiography and ERCP rarely are used in combination. Benign strictures should be differentiated from cholangiocarcinoma, which often requires cytological analysis or biopsy of the lesion.

Percutaneous transhepatic cholangiography

Figure 9.8 visualizes the biliary tree in 90%–100% of patients with dilated ducts and localizes the site of obstruction in 90% of cases. It requires a prothrombin time of less than 16 seconds, a platelet count of greater than 50 000, and the absence of ascites. Percutaneous transhepatic cholangiography is useful for intrahepatic intervention in patients with Roux-en-Y anastomoses or no navigable common bile duct strictures.

Endoscopic retrograde cholangiopancreatography

Endoscopic retrograde cholangiopancreatography (ERCP) (Fig. 9.9) can localize the site of obstruction in more than 90% of patients. Therapeutic procedures (e.g., stent placement, stone extraction) can also be performed when needed. However, the morbidity rate is 2%–3%, somewhat less than with PTC. The most common complications include pancreatitis, bleeding, and cholangitis. Given the complication rate with ERCP and the high diagnostic capability and better safety profiles of other tests (e.g., CT, MRI, EUS), ERCP should be reserved for patients with high suspicion of requiring a therapeutic intervention. Endoscopic retrograde cholangiopancreatography may not be an option in patients with prior surgery (e.g., Roux-en-Y loop).

Endoscopic ultrasound

Endoscopic ultrasound combines endoscopy with real-time, high-resolution ultrasound and provides excellent sonographic visualization of the biliary tree without bowel gas interference. It is superior to ultrasound and CT for diagnosing bile duct stones and is comparably accurate but safer and less expensive than ERCP for detecting choledocholithiasis. Moreover, EUS (Fig. 9.10) is also as accurate as, if not more accurate than, ERCP in detecting pancreatic tumors, and is more successful and safer in obtaining a tissue diagnosis. If available, EUS is preferred over ERCP in the initial evaluation of extrahepatic biliary obstruction, particularly if ERCP is mainly being performed for diagnostic purposes. The widespread use of EUS has altered the diagnostic approach and management of extrahepatic biliary obstruction, especially when caused by extrabiliary disease, permitting real-time imaging and sonographic-guided sampling.

Liver biopsy

If high-grade extrahepatic obstruction has been excluded or hepatocellular disease is strongly suspected, a liver biopsy should be performed. Liver biopsy can correct 20% of errors in clinical diagnosis. In the workup of a patient with hyperbilirubinemia, a liver biopsy can be useful if other diagnostic tests are unrevealing. If the ERCP result is nondiagnostic, a liver biopsy should be performed. Five percent of the cases of extrahepatic cholestasis are diagnosed by liver biopsy because of inadequate clinical suspicion of obstruction or an inability to visualize the ducts adequately. For 15% of cases, a liver biopsy is not helpful in determining the cause of the hyperbilirubinemia.

The decision tree that the clinician follows depends to a great extent on pretest probability (see Fig. 9.2). If there is a low suspicion of extrahepatic obstruction and the ultrasound scan is negative, further evaluation of possible dilated ducts probably is not warranted and intrahepatic disease would be assessed with liver biopsy. Clinical instinct should not be ignored, however, if the radiographic tests do not confirm the physician's suspicions, and further assessment with MRCP or CT should be performed. Judgment based on the patient's history and physical examination is dependable in evaluating patients with jaundice. Diagnostic accuracy with subsequent adequate care relies on the judicious use of appropriate confirmatory tests and radiographic studies.

Complications of cholestasis

Pruritus is commonly associated with cholestasis and may limit activity, cause anxiety, disturb sleep patterns, and result in a typical rash (Fig. 9.11) and even secondary skin infection. Table 9.2 outlines current management options for pruritus. *Hepatic osteodystrophy* is the metabolic bone disease that occurs in patients with chronic liver disease, particularly cholestatic disease, and can lead to pain and immobility owing to the development of fractures. The management of hepatic osteodystrophy is outlined in Table 9.3. Bone mineral density assessment using dual-energy X-ray absorptiometry (DEXA) is used to screen for fracture risk and should be performed in all patients with cirrhosis, especially in those with cholestatic liver disease. *Fat-soluble vitamin deficiency* is common in patients with prolonged cholestasis, and its management is outlined in Table 9.4. Oral or parenteral replacement will depend on the extent of deficiency and response to therapy. Care should be taken to inform patients of the risks and benefits of therapy, including the need for assessment of hypercalciuria after therapeutic intervention.

age of its α-methene bridge to form biliverdin, a reaction catalyzed by heme oxygenase. The enzyme is a monooxygenase, and O_2 and NADPH are required for the cleavage reaction. The reaction releases CO, iron, and biliverdin. The CO binds to hemoglobin and is excreted through the lungs, and most of the iron is reincorporated into new heme proteins. The second step in heme catabolism is the reduction of biliverdin IXα to bilirubin IXα by biliverdin reductase and nicotinamide adenine dinucleotide phosphate (NADPH). The result is unconjugated bilirubin. After bilirubin IXα is formed, it is released into the bloodstream, where it rapidly binds to plasma proteins, especially albumin. These complexes are poorly filtered by the glomerulus. Bilirubin is rendered more soluble in the liver by conjugation: the attachment of sugar residues, such as glucuronates, to its propionate side chains. This reaction requires the enzyme bilirubin UDP glucuronosyltransferase (bilirubin UGT).

Bilirubin metabolism

Bilirubin metabolism is shown in Fig. 9.1. The first step in the degradation of the heme group to bilirubin is the cleav-

---

Table 9.1 Causes of conjugated hyperbilirubinemia

Congenital conjugated hyperbilirubinemias	Idiopathic adult ductopenia
Rotor syndrome	Autoimmune (overlap) cholangiopathies
Dubin–Johnson syndrome	Infections
	Bacterial
Intrahepatic cholestasis	Fungal
Familial and congenital	Parasitic
Progressive familial intrahepatic cholestasis,	HIV-related
type I to III	Miscellaneous causes
Benign recurrent intrahepatic cholestasis	Postoperative sepsis
Cholestasis of pregnancy	Pregnancy
Choledochal cysts, Caroli disease	Total parenteral nutrition
Congenital biliary atresia	Cholestasis after liver transplantation
Hepatocellular conditions	Drug hepatotoxicity
Alcohol-related disorders	
Viral hepatitis	*Extrahepatic cholestasis*
Autoimmune disease	Inside bile ducts
Cirrhosis	Calculi
Drug-related disorders	Parasites
Wilson disease	Inside wall
Hereditary hemochromatosis	Stricture
Infiltrative conditions	Cholangiocarcinoma
Granulomatous	Sclerosing cholangitis
Carcinoma	Choledochal cysts
Hematological malignant disease	Outside duct wall
Amyloidosis	Tumor in porta hepatis
Cholangiopathies	Tumor in pancreas
Primary biliary cirrhosis	Pancreatitis, acute or chronic

Table 9.2 Management of pruritus of cholestasis

Topical therapy
Lower bathing water temperature and use fewer or lighter clothing
  and bed coverings
Minimize dry skin by using moisturizing soaps (e.g., Dove) and
  applying topical moisturizers liberally (e.g., Eucerin cream)

Anion-exchange resins
Cholestyramine or colestipol: start with 4 g (one scoop or packet)
  p.o. b.i.d., starting before and after breakfast, and increasing to six
  packets or scoops daily, separated from other medications by 2 h
  (esp. ursodeoxycholic acid)

Bile salts
Ursodeoxycholic acid, 15 mg/kg q.d. p.o.
Doxepin mast cell stabilizer
25–50 mg PO daily taken at night (q.h.s)

Hepatic microsomal enzyme induction
Rifampin, 150 mg, p.o., 2–3 times daily

Opioid receptor antagonists
Naltrexone, 12.5 mg p.o. daily, increasing slowly to 50 mg p.o. daily
Naloxone and nalmefene are only commonly available for parenteral
  use

b.i.d., twice a day; p.o., orally; q.d., once daily; q.h.s., once at night.

Table 9.3 Management of hepatic osteodystrophy

Baseline DEXA scanning
Normal (T Score):   < SD below the mean
Osteopenia: 1–2.5 SD below the mean
Osteoporosis: > 2.5 SD below the mean and/or one or more
                    fragility fractures (thoracolumbar radiographs
                    should be performed to screen for compression
                    fractures)

Laboratory testing
Baseline: 25-OH vitamin D level (normal range 10–55 mg/mL),
calcium, phosphate, thyroid function tests, intact parathyroid
hormone (free serum testosterone in men and estradiol and
luteinizing hormone in women)

Treatment
(Relative contraindication: patients with history of renal stones)
Adequate calcium (1.0–1.5 g q.d.), protein calorie nutrition and
  regular exercise
Before transplantation: calcifediol (Calderol), 20–50 µg three times
  weekly
After transplantation: calcifediol (Calderol), 20–50 µg weekly
If coexistent renal disease, calcitriol (Rocaltrol), 0.25–0.5 µg p.o. q.d.
Estrogen replacement (if no contraindications exist) or selective
  estrogen receptor modulators
If bone density worsens rapidly or if there is evidence of osteoporosis
  or symptomatic fractures, treat with bisphosphonates or calcitonin

Monitoring
DEXA
  For osteoporosis: repeat 6 months after treatment initiated and
    then yearly
  For normal study: repeat every 2 years
    Repeat 25-OH vitamin D and 24-h urine calcium yearly and treat
    accordingly

DEXA, dual-energy X-ray absorptiometry; p.o., orally; q.d., once daily;
SD, standard deviation.

Table 9.4 Management of fat-soluble vitamin deficiency in prolonged cholestasis

Monitoring fat-soluble vitamins
25-OH vitamin D level (normal range, 10–55 mg/mL) (if renal disease, check 1,25-(OH)$_2$ vitamin D)
Vitamin A level (normal range, 360–1200 μg/L)
Vitamin E level, with fasting total lipid profile (normal range, 5.5–17.0 mg/L) (total lipids = cholesterol plus triglycerides [in grams]. To calculate vitamin E level: serum vitamin E [mg]/total lipid [g]. If ≥ 0.8, normal; if < 0.6, supplement)
Vitamin K: measure prothrombin time (normal range, 11.4–13.2 s)

Replacement
Vitamin D: calcium, 1–1.5 g p.o. q.d.
Calcifediol (Calderol) 20–50 μg p.o. three times weekly, before transplantation (coexistent renal disease, use calcitriol [Rocaltrol®] 0.25–0.5 μg p.o. q.d.)
Vitamin A: β-carotene 15 mg (25 000 U vitamin A) p.o. q.d. or Aquasol A 50 000 U IM q.d. for 2 weeks
Vitamin E: Liquid E (D-α-tocopherol), water-soluble, 100 IU p.o. q.d.
Vitamin K: 10 mg subcutaneously daily for 3 days then monthly if cholestatic
ADEK p.o. 1–2 q.d.

Evaluation of therapy
After 3 months: 24-h urine calcium (normal range, 50–250 mg/day)
Yearly: 25-OH vitamin D (1,25-(OH)$_2$ vitamin D if renal disease), vitamins A and E, and prothrombin time

p.o., orally; q.d., once daily.

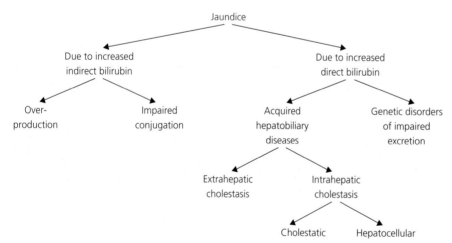

Figure 9.1 Differential diagnosis of the jaundiced patient.

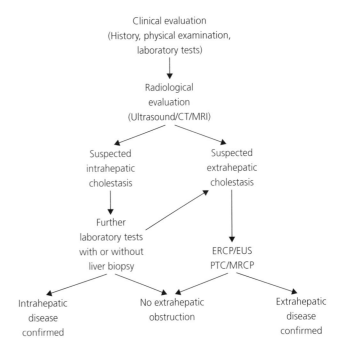

Clinical evaluation
(History, physical examination,
laboratory tests)

↓

Radiological
evaluation
(Ultrasound/CT/MRI)

Suspected
intrahepatic
cholestasis

Suspected
extrahepatic
cholestasis

Further
laboratory tests
with or without
liver biopsy

ERCP/EUS
PTC/MRCP

Intrahepatic
disease
confirmed

No extrahepatic
obstruction

Extrahepatic
disease
confirmed

Figure 9.2 The evaluation of the jaundiced patient.

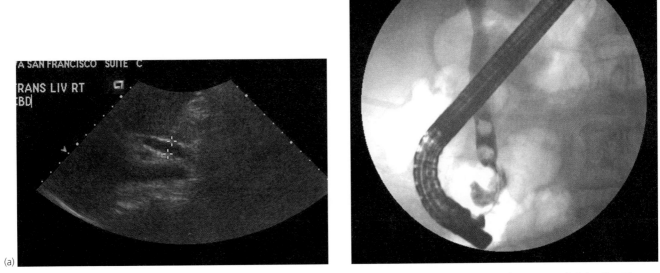

(a)

(b)

Figure 9.3 (a) Transabdominal ultrasound reveals a dilated common hepatic duct (1 cm) but without an apparent site or cause of obstruction. The distal biliary system was obscured by overlying bowel gas. **(b)** Subsequent endoscopic retrograde cholangiopancreatography (ERCP) performed in this same patient with high clinical suspicion for choledocholithiasis reveals two stones in the distal common bile duct. Stones were extracted at ERCP.

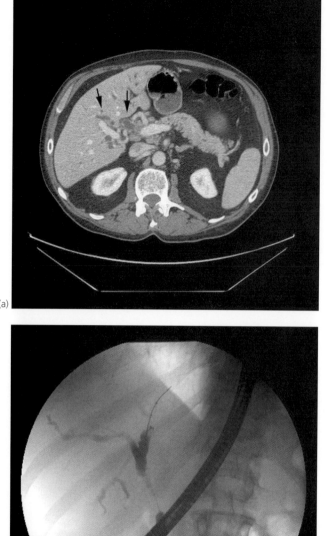

(a)

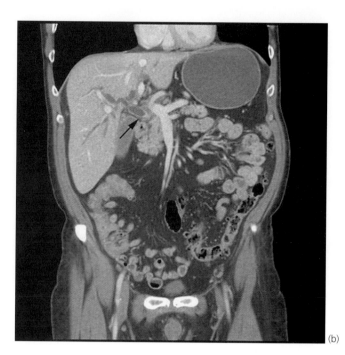

(b)

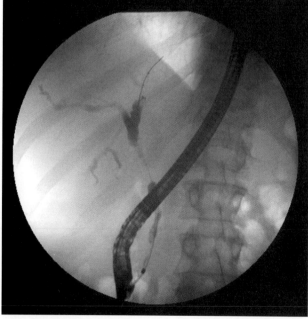

(c)

Figure 9.4 (a) Axial computed tomography (CT) image from a patient with painless, obstructive jaundice demonstrates a dilated intrahepatic biliary system and dilated common hepatic duct. **(b)** Computed coronal reconstructions from the thin-slice multidetector CT acquisition reveals a dilated biliary system with an abrupt transition at the level of the distal common hepatic duct (arrow). A focal enhancing mass suspicious for cholangiocarcinoma was seen on other CT images (not shown).
(c) Endoscopic retrograde cholangiopancreatography (ERCP), performed for tissue sampling in this high-surgical risk candidate, confirms a malignant-appearing, 1.5-cm-long, mid-extrahepatic duct stricture (cytology brushings positive for malignancy).

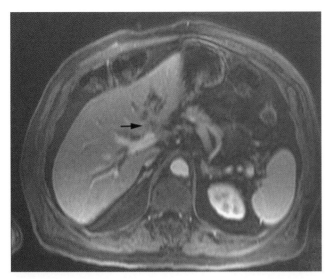

Figure 9.5 T2-weighted magnetic resonance imaging (MRI) reveals a small round mass (1.6 cm) near the origin of the left hepatic duct (arrow) suspicious for cholangiocarcinoma. Proximal intrahepatic ducts are dilated (left greater than right).

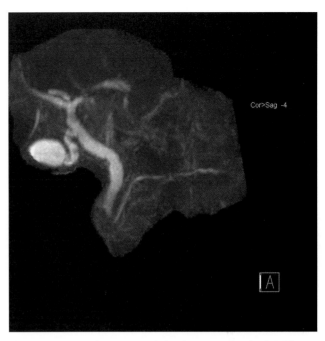

Figure 9.7 Magnetic resonance cholangiopancreatography (MRCP) was performed in this asymptomatic patient with persistent mild elevation of serum liver tests. The patient had a prior history of cholangitis and had undergone endoscopic retrograde cholangiopancreatography (ERCP) with biliary sphincterotomy and stone extraction (cholecystectomy not performed owing to advanced age of the patient). Magnetic resonance cholangiopancreatography reveals a mildly dilated common bile duct (age appropriate), but no suggestion for choledocholithiasis or biliary stricture. Magnetic resonance cholangiopancreatography obviated the need for ERCP, and evaluation of intrahepatic causes of cholestasis was initiated.

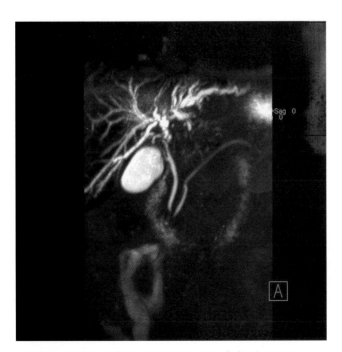

Figure 9.6 Corresponding magnetic resonance cholangiopancreatography (MRCP) image from the same patient as in Fig. 9.5 shows a dilated intrahepatic biliary system (left greater than right) with a transition point near the bifurcation (at location of mass).

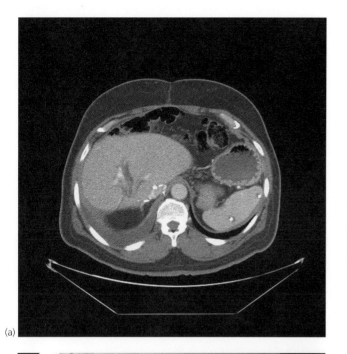

(a)

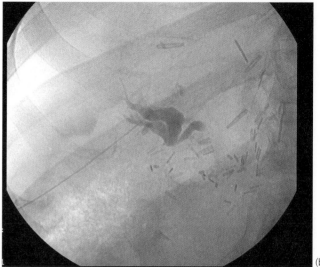

(b)

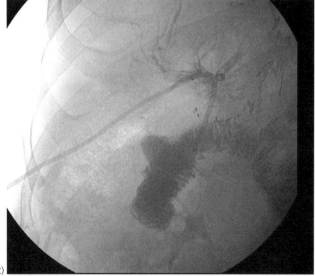

(c)

Figure 9.8 (a) Axial computed tomography image reveals dilated right intrahepatic ducts in a patient with Roux-en-Y hepaticojejunostomy, after left hepatectomy for metastatic colon cancer. **(b)** Percutaneous transhepatic cholangiography (PTC) performed for further evaluation and treatment of biliary obstruction reveals dilated biliary system with abrupt cut-off at hepaticojejunal anastomosis consistent with anastomotic stricture. **(c)** Percutaneous biliary drain traverses anastomosis and allows biliary decompression and ongoing access for subsequent interventions for stricture remediation (e.g., dilation, stenting).

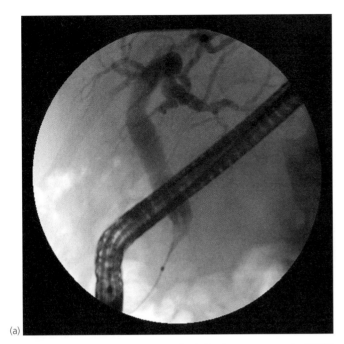

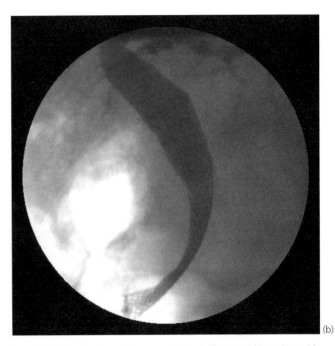

(a)

(b)

Figure 9.9 (a) Endoscopic retrograde cholangiopancreatography (ERCP) reveals a distal biliary stricture with proximal ductal dilation in this patient with known, unresectable pancreatic cancer. **(b)** A self-expanding metallic biliary stent was placed for palliation of obstructive jaundice.

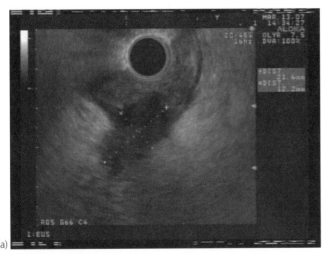

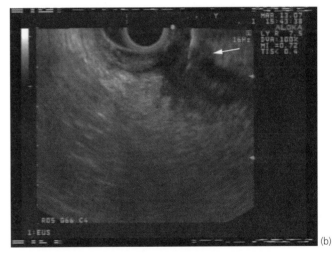

(a)

(b)

Figure 9.10 (a) Endoscopic ultrasound (EUS) detects a small hypoechoic (dark) mass measuring 2 cm in the head of the pancreas in this patient with obstructive jaundice. Although prior computed tomography demonstrated biliary dilation to the level of the distal common bile duct, a specific cause of obstruction was not found. **(b)** EUS guided fine needle aspiration (EUS-FNA) revealed pancreatic adenocarcinoma. The patient subsequently underwent surgical resection without requiring preoperative ERCP (endoscopic retrograde cholangiopancreatography).

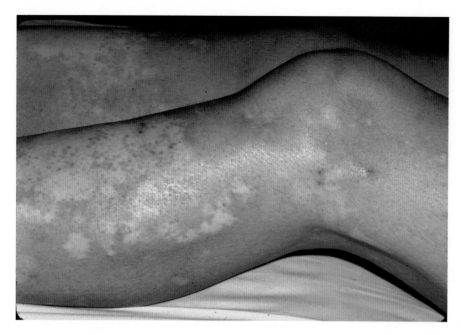

Figure 9.11 The lower limb of a patient with primary biliary cirrhosis showing vitiligo and the typical rash resulting from pruritus.

Approach to the patient with ascites and its complications

Guadalupe Garcia-Tsao

Ascites is the accumulation of fluid in the peritoneal cavity. The most common causes of ascites are cirrhosis, peritoneal malignancy, and heart failure.

In patients with cirrhosis, ascites is one of the complications that marks the transition from a compensated to a decompensated stage. Initially, ascites is "uncomplicated," that is, it responds well to diuretics and is not infected. As cirrhosis progresses and the mechanisms that lead to ascites formation worsen, ascites ceases to respond to diuretics (refractory ascites). Bacteria may infect ascites, an entity known as spontaneous bacterial peritonitis (SBP) that occurs mainly in hospitalized patients with severe liver disease. With further progression of cirrhosis, the patient with ascites may develop hyponatremia and functional renal failure (hepatorenal syndrome). The hemodynamic alterations that lead to ascites and refractory ascites are the same as those that lead to hyponatremia and hepatorenal syndrome, differing only in the degree of abnormality, with the latter complications denoting a more deranged circulatory status. The approach to a patient with ascites depends on the setting surrounding its presentation.

Suspected ascites

In a patient with suspected ascites (by history and physical examination) the least invasive and most cost-effective method to confirm the presence of ascites is *abdominal ultrasonography*. This test can be accompanied by Doppler examination of the hepatic venous system; this is an important initial test to rule out the presence of hepatic vein obstruction, which is a frequently overlooked cause of ascites.

New onset ascites

In a patient with new onset ascites, the priority is to determine the etiology of ascites as this will determine its man-

agement. A diagnostic paracentesis should be the first test performed in such a patient. The serum–ascites albumin gradient (SAAG) and the ascites total protein are two inexpensive tests that, taken together, are most useful. The three main causes of ascites (cirrhosis, peritoneal pathology [malignancy or tuberculosis] and heart failure) can be easily distinguished by combining the results of SAAG (a measure of sinusoidal pressure) and ascites total protein. In cirrhosis, the SAAG is high (>1.1 g/dL) and ascites protein is low (<2.5 g/dL); in peritoneal disease, the SAAG is low and ascites protein is high; in heart failure, both the SAAG and the ascites protein are high. The decisive test to determine the source of ascites (sinusoidal or not) is by measuring the hepatic venous pressure gradient. When the source is likely to be peritoneal (carcinomatosis or tuberculosis), the decisive test is a laparoscopy with peritoneal biopsy, culture, and histological examination.

Cirrhotic ascites

In a patient with cirrhotic ascites, management depends on the phase of ascites at which the patient with cirrhosis is situated, from the patient with uncomplicated ascites to the patient with hepatorenal syndrome.

Therapy of cirrhotic ascites is not an emergency as the risk of death is not implicit unless the fluid is infected. The mainstay of therapy is aimed at achieving a negative sodium balance (i.e., sodium restriction and diuretics). Diuretic treatment should only be initiated in the patient with cirrhosis in whom complications, such as gastrointestinal (GI) hemorrhage, bacterial infection, and renal dysfunction, are absent or have resolved. In a patient with tense ascites who experiences not only abdominal discomfort, but also respiratory distress, a single large-volume paracentesis (LVP) should be performed prior, or concomitant to, starting diuretics. Diuretic therapy should be spironolactone based, either with spironolactone alone (initial dose of 100 mg in a single daily dose, increased to a maximum of 400 mg/day) or in combination with furosemide (range of 20–160 mg/day). Both schedules are equally effective; however, dose adjustments

Atlas of Gastroenterology, 4th edition. Edited by Tadataka Yamada, David H. Alpers, Anthony N. Kalloo, Neil Kaplowitz, Chung Owyang, and Don W. Powell. © 2009 Blackwell Publishing, ISBN: 978-1-4051-6909-7

are needed more frequently in patients in whom treatment is initiated with combination therapy.

Before considering that ascites is refractory to diuretics, it is necessary to ascertain whether the patient has adhered to the prescribed sodium-restricted diet and has restrained from using nonsteroidal antiinflammatory drugs.

Refractory ascites

First line therapy for patients with refractory ascites is serial LVP, adding albumin (6–8 g/L of ascites removed) if more than 5 L are removed at once. In patients in whom 5 L or less are being removed, a plasma volume expander can be utilized. To increase the time between paracenteses, patients should continue on maximally tolerated diuretic dose provided that the urinary sodium is >30 mEq/L. In patients requiring more than two or three LVPs per month or in those in whom ascites is loculated and cannot be entirely removed with a single LVP, evaluation for TIPS placement should be undertaken. In general TIPS should not be performed in patients with serum bilirubin >3 mg/dL, a CTP score >11, age >70 years or evidence of heart failure, as these factors are associated with a poorer survival and a poorer shunt function. Although studies on TIPS for refractory ascites were performed using uncovered stents, covered stents should be used because of the lower rate of shunt dysfunction and potential benefits regarding development of encephalopathy and survival. In patients who are requiring frequent LVP and who are not TIPS candidates, a peritoneovenous shunt (PVS) should be considered. Refractory ascites is often associated with *type 2 hepatorenal syndrome*, a moderate renal failure (serum creatinine between 1.5 and 2.5 mg/dL), with a steady or slowly progressive course.

Hepatic hydrothorax

Hepatic hydrothorax should be treated in the same way as cirrhotic ascites, that is, the mainstay of therapy is sodium restriction and diuretics. Before determining that hydrothorax is refractory, a trial of in-hospital diuretic therapy should be attempted. In patients with refractory hepatic hydrothorax, other therapeutic options such as repeated thoracenteses, TIPS, or pleurodesis should be considered.

Spontaneous bacterial peritonitis

Spontaneous bacterial peritonitis (SBP) is the most common type of bacterial infection in hospitalized cirrhotic patients and occurs mainly in patients with low ascites protein and severe liver disease. Spontaneous bacterial peritonitis should be suspected in patients with symptoms/signs of SBP (fever, abdominal pain or tenderness, and leukocytosis) and in those with unexplained encephalopathy, jaundice or worsening renal failure. A diagnostic paracentesis, as well as simultaneous blood and urine cultures and chest radiograph should be obtained. The diagnosis of SBP is established with an ascites polymorphonuclear leukocyte (PMN) count >250/mm³. Intravenous antibiotics proven to be effective in SBP are cefotaxime (2 g every 12 h), ceftriaxone (1–2 g every 24 h) and the combination of amoxicillin and clavulanic acid (1 mg/0.2 g every 8 h). In patients with baseline serum bilirubin >4 mg/dL and serum creatinine >1 g/dL albumin should be used to prevent renal dysfunction. The dose of albumin used is arbitrary, 1.5 g/kg of body weight during the first 6 h, followed by 1 g/kg on day 3, with a maximum of 100 g/day. Patients surviving an episode of SBP should be started on indefinite antibiotic prophylaxis (norfloxacin 400 mg orally every day).

Acute renal failure

In hospitalized patients with cirrhosis, the most common cause of acute renal failure is prerenal (accounting for 60%–80% of the cases), resulting from any factor that will further decrease the effective arterial blood volume of the patient with cirrhosis. Therefore, it can result from (a) factors that cause hypovolemia, such as GI hemorrhage, overdiuresis or diarrhea; (b) factors that worsen vasodilatation, such as sepsis, use of vasodilators and the postparacentesis circulatory dysfunction; and (c) factors that cause renal vasoconstriction, such as nonsteroidal antiinflammatory drugs or intravenous contrast agents. These factors account for up to 80% of the causes of prerenal failure. Hepatorenal syndrome (HRS) is a type of prerenal failure as it results from hemodynamic abnormalities (extreme vasodilatation) leading to renal vasoconstriction.

In a patient with cirrhosis who presents with an acute deterioration in renal function, as evidenced by a doubling of serum creatinine to >2.5mg/dL within a 2-week period, the main concern is to rule out type 1 HRS. Diuretics should be discontinued and volume expanded with albumin intravenously. Spontaneous bacterial peritonitis (a common precipitant of HRS), other bacterial infections, and GI hemorrhage should be excluded and treated if present. If creatinine does not improve or continues to worsen, the diagnosis HRS-type 1 is suspected. The main differential at this point is with acute tubular necrosis (ATN), particularly in the presence of a history of a hypotensive event. Although urine osmolality (<350 mOsm/kg in ATN, >500 in HRS) and urinary sodium concentration (>40 mEq/L in ATN, <20 in HRS) may help distinguish prerenal failure (including HRS) from ATN, their usefulness is not absolute. In patients with ATN, renal function must be supported with hemodialysis until resolution of tubular function.

In patients with suspected type 1 HRS, diuretics should continue to be withheld to prevent further decreases in effective arterial blood volume. Although liver transplant is the only curative treatment for HRS, treatment with vasoconstrictors plus albumin can be used as a bridge to transplantation as this treatment leads to reversal of HRS-1 in about one-third of the patients, improving outcomes after liver transplant. The best evidence supports the use of terlipressin at a dose 0.5–2 mg intravenously every 4–6 h. Dose should probably be adjusted according to the mean arterial blood pressure (an indirect indicator of vasodilatation). This method has been used for adjusting the dose of midodrine (7.5–12.5 mg three times a day) plus octreotide (100–200 mcg s.c. three times a day). Albumin (20–40 g/day) should be administered together with the vasoconstrictor. Limited evidence favors the use of TIPS in responders to vasoconstrictors and the use of extracorporeal albumin dialysis in HRS; however, further trials are awaited.

Table 10.1 Etiology of ascites and classification by the serum–ascites albumin gradient (SAAG) and ascites protein: main etiological factors of ascites

	SAAG	Ascites protein
Cirrhosis and/or alcoholic hepatitis	High	Low
Congestive heart failure	High	High
Peritoneal malignancy	Low	High
Peritoneal tuberculosis	Low	High

Table 10.2 Other etiologies of cirrhosis (account for <2% of all cases)

	SAAG	Ascites protein
Massive hepatic metastases	High	Low
Nodular regenerative hyperplasia	High	Low
Fulminant liver failure	High	Low?
Budd–Chiari syndrome (late)	High	Low
Budd–Chiari syndrome (early)	High	High
Constrictive pericarditis	High	High
Venoocclusive disease	High	High
Myxedema	High	High
Nephrogenous (dialysis) ascites	High	High
Mixed ascites (cirrhosis + peritoneal malignancy)	High	Variable
Pancreatic ascites	Low	High
Serositis (connective tissue disease)	Low	High
Chlamydial/gonococcal	Low	High
Biliary	Low	High?
Ovarian hyperstimulation syndrome	Low?	High
Nephrotic syndrome	Low	Low

Those assessments followed by a question mark are theoretical and have not been confirmed by data in the literature.

Table 10.3 Analysis of ascitic fluid

Routine analysis of ascitic fluid
Gross appearance
Total protein
Albumin (with simultaneous estimation of serum albumin) so that the ascites–albumin gradient can be calculated by subtracting the ascitic fluid value from the serum value
White blood cell count and differential
Bacteriological cultures

Focused analysis of ascitic fluid
Cytology (to exclude malignant ascites)
Amylase (if pancreatic ascites is suspected)
Acid-fast bacilli smear and culture and adenosine deaminase determination (if peritoneal tuberculosis is suspected)
Glucose and lactic dehydrogenase (if secondary peritonitis is suspected in a patient with ascites PMN >250/mm^3)
Triglycerides (if the fluid has a milky appearance, i.e., chylous ascites)
Red blood cell count (if the fluid is bloody)

PMN, polymorphonuclear leukocytes.

Table 10.4 Differential of ascites based on HVPG measurements

Cause of ascites	WHVP	FHVP	HVPG
Cirrhosis	Increased	Normal	Increased
Cardiac ascites	Increased	Increased	Normal
Peritoneal malignancy or TB	Normal	Normal	Normal

FHVP, free hepatic venous pressure; HVPG, hepatic venous pressure gradient; TB, tuberculosis; WHVP, wedged hepatic venous pressure.

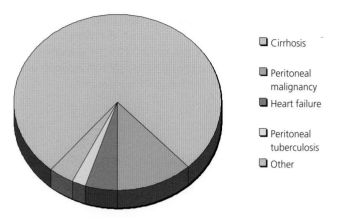

Figure 10.1 Causes of ascites. Cirrhosis is the most common cause of ascites, accounting for 80% of cases. Peritoneal malignancy, heart failure, and peritoneal tuberculosis are also common, accounting for another 15% of the cases. Less common causes of ascites include massive hepatic metastases, pancreatitis, nephrogenic ascites, and the Budd–Chiari syndrome. Of the most common causes, cirrhosis and heart failure are portal sinusoidal hypertensive causes of ascites, whereas peritoneal malignancy and tuberculosis are nonportal hypertensive causes.

- Cirrhosis
- Peritoneal malignancy
- Heart failure
- Peritoneal tuberculosis
- Other

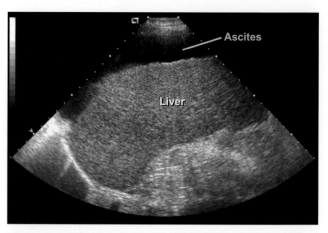

Figure 10.2 Ultrasound demonstrating the presence of ascites (dark area). Physical examination is relatively insensitive for detecting ascitic fluid, particularly when the amount is small or the patient is obese. The initial, most cost effective and least invasive method to confirm the presence of ascites is abdominal ultrasonography. It is considered the gold standard for diagnosing ascites as it can detect amounts as small as 100 mL.

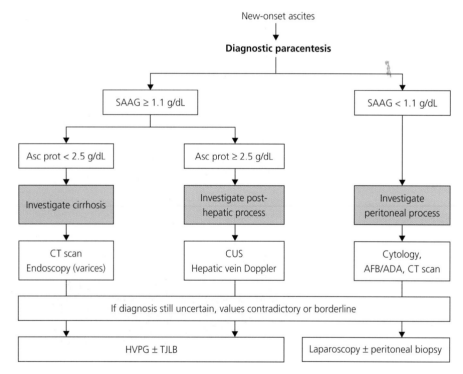

Figure 10.3 Approach to the patient with new onset ascites. ADA, adenosine deaminase; AFB, acid-fast bacillus; Asc Prot, ascites protein; CAT, computed axial tomography; HVPG, hepatic venous pressure gradient; SAAG, serum–ascites albumin gradient; TJLB, transjugular liver biopsy.

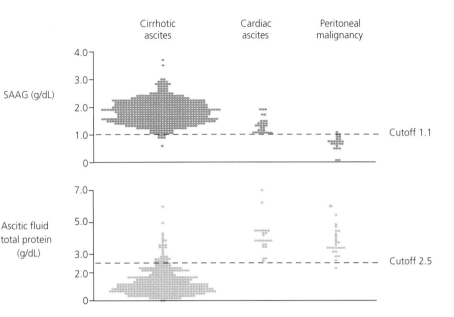

Figure 10.4 Serum–ascites albumin gradient (SAAG) and ascites protein levels help distinguish the most common causes of ascites. The three main causes of ascites (cirrhosis, right-sided heart failure and peritoneal pathology [malignancy or tuberculosis]), can be easily distinguished by combining the results of both the SAAG (top panel) and ascites total protein content (lower panel). The cutoffs for SAAG and ascites protein levels are 1.1 g/dL and 2.5 g/dL, respectively. Cirrhotic ascites is typically high SAAG and low protein; cardiac ascites is high SAAG and high protein; and ascites secondary to peritoneal malignancy is typically low SAAG and high protein. SAAG is obtained by subtracting ascites albumin from serum albumin in samples obtained almost simultaneously.

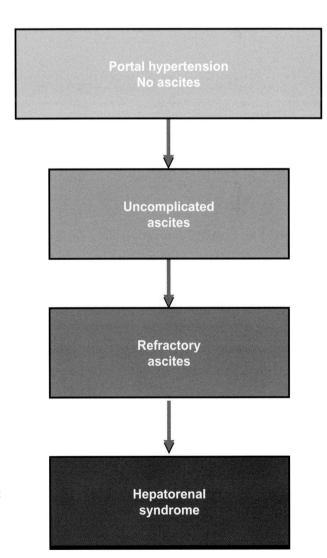

Figure 10.5 Natural history of cirrhotic ascites. The patient with cirrhosis develops portal hypertension. Initially, even though the patient has portal hypertension, it has not yet reached the minimal pressure threshold necessary for the formation of ascites. Later, and once this threshold is reached and hemodynamic alterations lead to sodium retention, the patient develops ascites, which is initially well controlled with diuretics. Later on in the natural history, the patient no longer responds to diuretics (refractory ascites) and, at its most severe, in addition to sodium retention there is renal vasoconstriction that leads to hepatorenal syndrome.

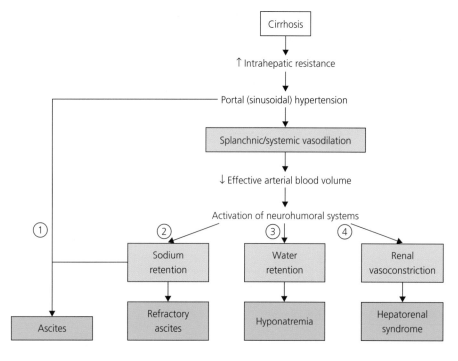

Figure 10.6 Common pathogenesis of ascites, hyponatremia, and hepatorenal syndrome. Cirrhosis leads to increased intrahepatic resistance and thereby to an increased sinusoidal pressure. In addition, portal hypertension leads to splanchnic and systemic arteriolar vasodilation, decreased effective arterial blood volume, up-regulation of sodium-retaining hormones, sodium and water retention and, consequently, plasma volume expansion. With progression of cirrhosis and portal hypertension, the systemic arteriolar resistance is more pronounced, leading to further activation of the renin–angiotensin–aldosterone and sympathetic nervous systems. The resulting increase in water and sodium retention can lead to refractory ascites and hyponatremia, whereas the increase in renal vasoconstriction can lead to a functional renal failure, the hepatorenal syndrome.

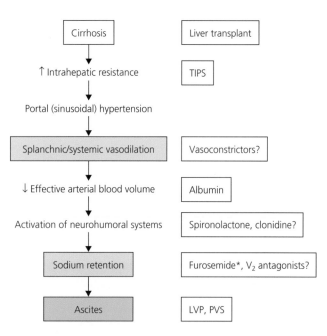

Figure 10.7 Site of action of different therapies for ascites. *Furosemide should only be used in conjunction with spironolactone. LVP, large-volume paracentesis; PVS, peritoneovenous shunt; TIPS, transjugular intrahepatic portosystemic shunt; V2, vasopressin type 2.

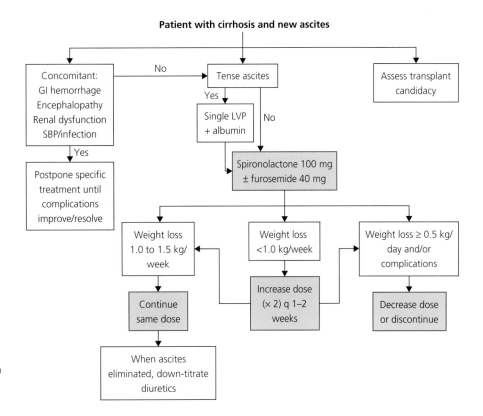

Figure 10.8 Approach to the patient with cirrhosis and uncomplicated ascites. LVP, large-volume paracentesis.

Figure 10.9 Meta-analysis of five randomized controlled trials of large-volume paracentesis (LVP) vs transjugular intrahepatic portosystemic shunt (TIPS) for refractory ascites. This meta-analysis shows that TIPS is more effective than LVP in preventing recurrence of ascites; however, the risk of encephalopathy was higher in patients treated with TIPS. Results on mortality were heterogeneous but once an outlier trial (Lebrec et al) was excluded there was a slight tendency for an improvement in survival in patients treated with TIPS. LVP, large-volume paracentesis; TIPS, transjugular intrahepatic portosystemic shunt.

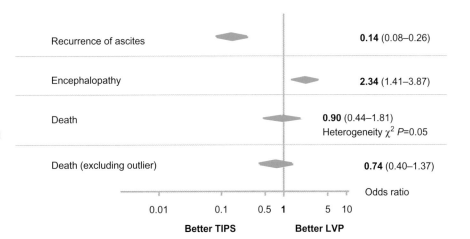

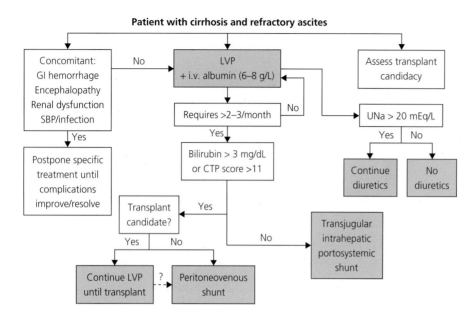

Patient with cirrhosis and refractory ascites

Figure 10.10 Approach to the patient with cirrhosis and refractory ascites. CTP, Child–Turcotte–Pugh; GI, gastrointestinal; i.v., intravenous; LVP, large-volume paracentesis; SBP, spontaneous bacterial peritonitis; UNa, urinary sodium.

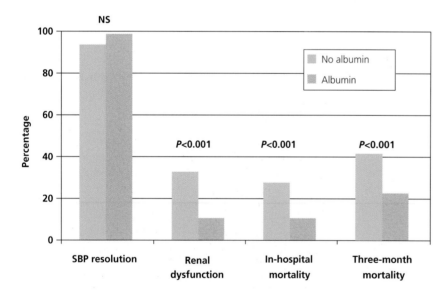

Figure 10.11 Albumin decreases renal dysfunction and short-term mortality in spontaneous bacterial peritonitis (SBP). A prospective randomized nonblinded study that compared cefotaxime + albumin vs cefotaxime alone showed that patients who received albumin had significantly lower rates of renal dysfunction and this was associated with a reduction in hospital mortality and 3-month mortality rates. The subgroup of patients that appear to benefit most from albumin are those with a baseline creatinine >1 g/dL, blood urea nitrogen >30 mg/dL or bilirubin >4 mg/dL.

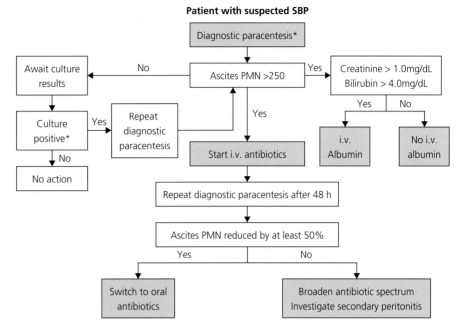

Figure 10.12 Approach to the patient with suspected SBP. *A diagnostic paracentesis should be performed in any patient with symptoms or signs suggestive of SBP, any patient with unexplained renal dysfunction or encephalopathy and in any hospitalized patient with cirrhosis and ascites. i.v., intravenous; PMN, polymorphonuclear leukocytes.

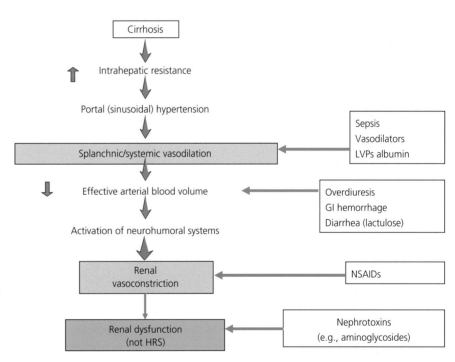

Figure 10.13 Causes of renal dysfunction in patients with cirrhosis. These causes need to be excluded before a diagnosis of hepatorenal syndrome can be established. GI, gastrointestinal; HRS, hepatorenal syndrome; LVP, large-volume paracentesis; NSAID, nonsteroidal antiinflammatory drug.

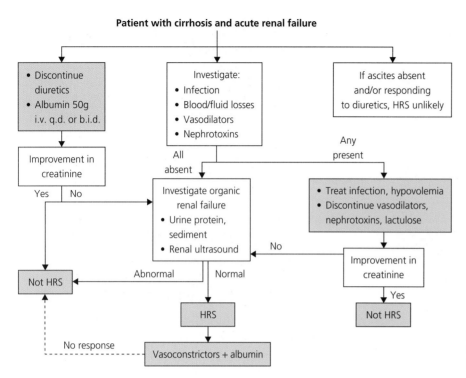

Figure placement — Patient with cirrhosis and acute renal failure flowchart

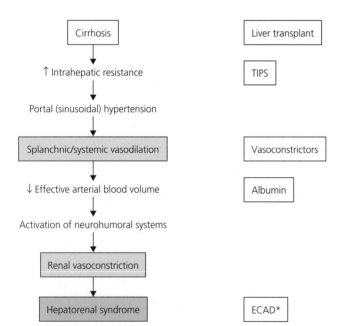

Figure 10.14 Approach to the patient with cirrhosis and acute renal failure. HRS, hepatorenal syndrome.

Figure 10.15 Site of action of different therapies for hepatorenal syndrome. *ECAD stands for extracorporeal albumin dialysis, an experimental therapy that seems to improve hepatorenal system (HRS) that probably acts by decreasing the amount of circulating vasodilators. TIPS, transjugular intrahepatic portosystemic shunt.

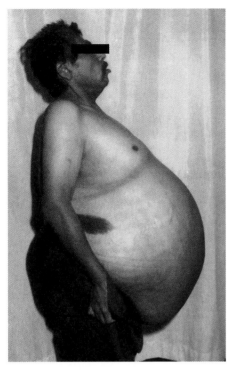

Figure 10.16 A man with alcoholic cirrhosis and ascites that was so massive it caused a gait disturbance. Courtesy of T.B. Reynolds.

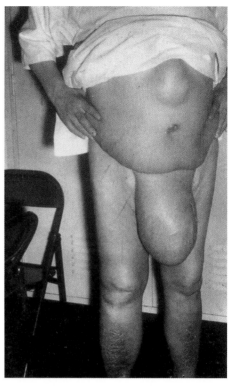

Figure 10.18 A man with large umbilical hernia and massive inguinal hernia. Courtesy of T.B. Reynolds.

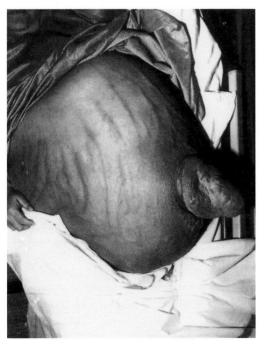

Figure 10.17 A woman with cryptogenic cirrhosis who did not seek medical attention until her umbilical hernia almost touched the floor when she was sitting. Courtesy of T.B. Reynolds.

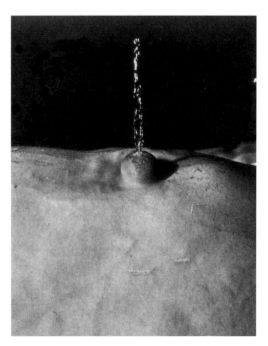

Figure 10.19 Ruptured umbilical hernia – one of the most feared complications of ascites. Courtesy of T.B. Reynolds.

11 Approach to the patient with acute liver failure

Ryan M. Taylor, Christopher P. Golembeski, Robert J. Fontana

Introduction

Acute liver failure (ALF) is an uncommon but potentially devastating illness owing to its unpredictable and variable natural history, including the frequent development of cerebral edema, sepsis, and multiorgan failure. In a patient without pre-existing liver disease, ALF can cause a rapid deterioration in hepatic function within 8–26 weeks of illness onset, leading to mental status changes and coagulopathy (i.e., international normalized ratio (INR) >1.5). Overall, ALF is rare in the general US population with an estimated 2300–2800 cases per year. Treatable etiologies of ALF include a multitude of infectious, metabolic, infiltrative, toxic, and vascular causes (Table 11.1). However, up to 20% of ALF cases are of indeterminate etiology with a low likelihood of spontaneous recovery (Fig. 11.1).

Acetaminophen toxicity

Therapeutic doses of acetaminophen (paracetamol) are metabolized by hepatic glucuronyl transferases and sulfotransferases to conjugated metabolites that are predominantly excreted in the urine (Fig. 11.2). A small fraction of a therapeutic acetaminophen (APAP) dose is also oxidatively metabolized by the cytochrome P-450 enzyme system to a reactive intermediate termed NAPQI (N-acetyl-p-benzoquinone imine). With therapeutic dosing, this highly reactive electrophile is conjugated by glutathione transferases to a stable metabolite excreted in the urine as mercapturic acid. However, if excessive doses of acetaminophen are ingested (i.e., >4 g/day), a larger amount of NAPQI is generated through oxidative metabolism. Under these cir-

cumstances, NAPQI can covalently bind to intracellular proteins and lead to hepatocyte necrosis manifested by an increase in serum aminotransferase levels and detectable serum acetaminophen-cysteine adducts (Fig. 11.3). In addition, if cytochrome P-450 enzyme activity is induced via chronic alcohol use or medications (e.g., dilantin, isoniazid) the high rate of NAPQI formation may deplete intrahepatic glutathione stores resulting in liver toxicity. Theoretically, depletion of glutathione stores via prolonged fasting may also increase the risk of acetaminophen hepatotoxicity but supporting evidence in humans has been difficult to establish.

In the United States, acetaminophen hepatotoxicity has emerged as the leading cause of ALF. In a recent report of 275 consecutive acetaminophen ALF cases, nearly 50% were nonintentional overdoses in patients taking a variety of acetaminophen-containing products for therapeutic indications. Prescription narcotic analgesics containing variable quantities of acetaminophen were identified in 63% of the nonintentional overdose patients. Currently, there are several hundred over-the-counter and prescription medications that contain acetaminophen (Table 11.4). Therefore, physicians should always take a careful and detailed medication history in all patients presenting with unexplained ALF and administer N-acetylcysteine if acetaminophen overdose is suspected (Tables 11.2, 11.3, Fig. 11.4).

In a case of nonintentional acetaminophen overdose, a 23-year-old woman presented 4 days after an elective tonsillectomy. She reported ingesting approximately 150 mL of Vicodin elixir (500 mg APAP/5 mg Hydrocodone per 15 ml is the same as 5 g APAP) and up to 6 g of standard acetaminophen in the 48 h prior to admission. Her initial alanine aminotransferase (ALT) level was 10 184 IU/L, INR 4.4, and creatinine 1.7 mg/dL. Treatment with N-acetylcysteine was initiated but her mental status rapidly deteriorated leading to stage IV encephalopathy necessitating mechanical intubation and pressors. The patient developed progressive cerebral edema refractory to medical management over a 48-h period (Fig. 11.5). Neurological examination while off

Atlas of Gastroenterology, 4th edition. Edited by Tadataka Yamada, David H. Alpers, Anthony N. Kalloo, Neil Kaplowitz, Chung Owyang, and Don W. Powell. © 2009 Blackwell Publishing, ISBN: 978-1-4051-6909-7

sedation demonstrated fixed and dilated pupils. She was declared brain dead and she died 4 days after admission from cerebral herniation. At autopsy, her brain was diffusely swollen and demonstrated evidence of cerebral edema (Fig. 11.6). In addition, her liver demonstrated extensive pericentral necrosis characteristic of severe acetaminophen hepatotoxicity (Fig. 11.7).

Cerebral edema in acute liver failure

Cerebral edema is a potentially devastating manifestation of ALF that significantly contributes to the morbidity and mortality of this disorder. The underlying pathophysiology is unknown, but there is evidence to support the "glutamine hypothesis" wherein astrocyte conversion of glutamate to glutamine can lead to increased brain tissue osmolarity with resultant parenchymal fluid retention. In addition, advanced cerebral edema is often associated with a loss of intracerebral vascular autoregulation that can further exacerbate increased intracranial pressure. Prompt recognition and treatment of elevated intracranial pressures is critical to prevent long-term sequelae such as irreversible ischemic brain damage and brain death from uncal herniation. Head CT scans are notoriously insensitive in detecting early cerebral edema. Management relies upon a combination of clinical assessment and various treatments which are optimally delivered when direct pressure measurements are available (Table 11.5). However, intracranial pressure monitoring has not been widely adopted owing to concerns from catheter placement in the setting of severe coagulopathy. (See Table 11.6 for management of coagulopathy.)

A 39-year-old male with a history of bipolar disorder ingested an unknown quantity of acetaminophen, zolpidem, and lamotrigine in a suicide attempt 48 h prior to presentation. His initial acetaminophen level was 87 μg/mL, ALT >9000 IU/L, INR 8.9, and factor V level <15%. He also had a severe lactic acidosis with hypotension, requiring pressors and intubation. The initial head CT showed no evidence of cerebral edema and he was listed for transplantation (Fig. 11.8). On his second day in hospital, an ICP monitor demonstrated an opening pressure of 12–15 mmHg. Liver transplantation was accomplished without immediate complications but the patient did not wake up postoperatively. A repeat head CT on his fourth day in hospital showed diffuse changes of worsening cerebral edema. Additionally, the foramen magnum was blurred, suggestive of transforaminal herniation. Magnetic resonance imaging of the brain also showed diffuse brain swelling with transforaminal herniation (Fig. 11.9). As shown in Figure 11.10, a technetium 99 (^{99}Tc) hexamethylpropyleneamine oxime nuclear medicine scan showed no intracranial activity compatible with brain death. Two days after his liver transplant, life support was withdrawn and the patient died from cerebral edema.

Autoimmune hepatitis

Autoimmune hepatitis (AIH) most commonly presents in female patients with mild to moderate serum aminotransferase elevations and less frequently as severe hepatitis with ALF. A diagnosis of fulminant AIH can be difficult to establish even with liver histology. The AIH scoring system (Table 11.7) uses objective laboratory and clinical criteria. Treatment of AIH consists of corticosteroids (Fig. 11.12) and other immunosuppressants and in rare instances, liver transplantation. A pretreatment score of >15 or a posttreatment score of >17 is consistent with a "definite" diagnosis of AIH while a pretreatment score of 10–15 and a posttreatment score of 12–17 is considered "probable" AIH.

Drug-induced liver injury

Drug-induced liver injury (DILI) is increasingly recognized as an important cause of ALF in the United States and worldwide. The diagnosis of DILI-related ALF can be challenging given the numerous prescription and over-the-counter medications on the market today, use of multiple medications, and unknown mechanism and risk factors for idiosyncratic DILI (Fig. 11.13). In addition, there are no objective laboratory or confirmatory tests for DILI, which is largely a diagnosis of exclusion. Therefore, clinicians must rely upon (1) the temporal association between medication use and injury onset (usually <12 months), (2) prior reports of hepatotoxicity owing to the suspect agent, (3) clinical features and biochemical profile in other patients with suspected hepatotoxicity, and (4) exclusion of competing causes of liver injury. Although liver biopsy can be helpful, a characteristic histological pattern as a result of a given drug may not be present.

Herpes hepatitis

Disseminated herpes simplex virus (HSV) infection leading to herpes hepatitis has a predilection for pregnant women and immunosuppressed hosts, but previously healthy individuals may be afflicted also. Patients may have a vesicular papular rash or mucocutaneous involvement at presentation (Fig. 11.14) but up to 50% have no skin findings. Serologies for HSV including anti-HSV IgM (immunoglobulin M)are notoriously nonspecific, while direct viral methods, such as polymerase chain reaction (PCR), increase the sensitivity and specificity and are preferred for diagnosis. Liver histology shows extensive nonzonal necrosis in a "patternless" distribution and the characteristic intranuclear inclusions of HSV may be difficult to find. In response to a high case fatality rate, treatment with intravenous acyclovir should be promptly initiated if ALF resulting from disseminated HSV infection is suspected.

Wilson disease

Wilson disease is an autosomal recessive disorder characterized by excessive copper accumulation in the body due to failure to excrete free copper through the biliary tract. Wilson disease frequently presents in young, previously healthy individuals with hepatic or neurological features. The disorder is rare, occurring in 1:30 000 in the general population. Patients with ALF as a result of Wilson disease are frequently cirrhotic at presentation, and mortality is nearly universal without liver transplantation. The diagnosis of Wilson disease is largely clinical in nature. Serum ceruloplasmin is characteristically low but as many as 10% of patients may have normal or elevated levels. A 24-h urine collection is helpful if it exceeds >100 μg/dL but other cholestatic liver diseases can also increase urine copper levels. Ocular findings of Wilson disease include Kayser–Fleischer rings (Fig. 11.15), which usually require a slit lamp examination by an experienced ophthalmologist to detect. In addition, approximately 50% of patients presenting with hepatic Wilson disease do not have Kayser–Fleischer rings. Other clinical clues include the presence of a Coomb's negative hemolytic anemia, low alkaline phosphatase–bilirubin ratio, and elevated aspartate aminotransferase (AST)/ ALT ratio. Liver biopsy in fulminant Wilson disease frequently demonstrates cirrhosis but it is the quantitative hepatic copper of >250 μg per dry weight that assists in making the diagnosis. Treatment of Wilson disease is focused on copper chelation. However, in fulminant Wilson disease, prompt listing for transplantation should be pursued owing to the high mortality rate with supportive medical therapy (Fig. 11.16).

Budd–Chiari syndrome

Budd–Chiari syndrome results from hepatic venous outflow obstruction at the level of the hepatic veins. Clinically, the disorder is characterized by right upper quadrant tenderness, hepatomegaly, and new onset ascites. In 70% of patients, Budd–Chiari syndrome is associated with a primary hypercoagulable state such as malignancy, hematological disorders, and other identifiable thrombophilias. The diagnosis of hepatic outflow obstruction can be made from liver ultrasound with Doppler, magnetic resonance angiography, or a direct hepatic angiogram. Liver biopsy demonstrates characteristic sinusoidal dilation with central vein congestion (Fig. 11.17). Treatment consists of anticoagulation and preferably heparin or low molecular weight heparin in the acute setting. Rarely liver transplantation may be required, with careful consideration to both perioperative and long-term anticoagulation.

Other rare causes of acute liver failure

Primary Epstein–Barr virus

Primary Epstein–Barr virus (EBV) infection can rarely present as a fulminant hepatitis (Fig. 11.18). The diagnosis is made with a combination of serologies, PCR testing for EBV-DNA, and characteristic findings on liver biopsy. Treatment is directed towards dampening the overly exuberant immune response to EBV antigens with use of corticosteroids and antivirals such as acyclovir. Outcomes following liver transplantation are generally favorable but the number of patients studied is limited.

Acute infiltrative hematological malignancies

Acute infiltrative hematological malignancies and lymphomas (Fig. 11.19) can rarely present as acute liver failure.

Pregnancy

Pregnancy can be associated with several unusual causes of ALF (Table 11.8). Acute fatty liver of pregnancy (AFLP), pre-eclampsia, and HELLP (Hemolysis, Elevated Liver enzymes, and Low Platelets) can occur in the third trimester of pregnancy. Patients with AFLP may have only modest elevation in serum aminotransferase and bilirubin levels, leukocytosis, hypoglycemia, and renal failure. Defects in long chain 3-hydroxyl CoA dehydrogenase (LCHAD) or carnitine palmitoyltransferase are thought to cause AFLP. Pre-eclampsia can present with elevations in serum aminotransferase levels, right upper quadrant (RUQ) pain, and disseminated intravascular coagulation (DIC). Complications include HELLP syndrome, hepatic infarction due to occlusion of hepatic sinusoids, subcapsular hematoma and rarely hepatic rupture due to ischemia. HELLP syndrome presents with marked elevation in transaminases, RUQ pain, nausea and vomiting, and weight gain. HELLP and AFLP may worsen within 48 h of delivery, and both may recur in subsequent pregnancies.

Table 11.1 Treatable causes of acute liver failure

	Etiology	Evaluation	Treatment
Viruses	Hepatitis B (HBV)	HBsAg, anti-HBc IgM, HBV-DNA by PCR	Lamivudine, entecavir
	Hepatitis D (HDV)[a]	HDV-RNA, anti-HDV IgM, HDV antigen	Lamivudine, entecavir
	Cytomegalovirus (CMV)	CMV-DNA PCR, CMV-IgM, biopsy	Ganciclovir, valganciclovir
	Epstein–Barr virus (EBV)	EBV-DNA PCR, serology, biopsy	Steroids, acyclovir
	Herpes simplex virus (HSV)	HSV-DNA PCR, anti-HSV IgM, biopsy	Acyclovir
Metabolic	Wilson disease	Ceruloplasmin, urinary and hepatic copper, slit-lamp examination	Chelating agents ?Plasmapheresis
	Acute fatty liver of pregnancy, HELLP syndrome	Preeclampsia findings (hypertension, edema, proteinuria)	Emergency delivery of infant
	Ischemic hepatitis	Systemic hypotension (cardiogenic shock, pulmonary embolism, hypovolemia)	Fluids reversal of hypotension, inotropes
	Autoimmune hepatitis	ANA, ASMA, IgG, IgM, IgA Liver biopsy	Steroids
Infiltrative	Metastatic malignancy	Imaging, liver biopsy	Chemotherapy
	Acute leukemia/lymphoma	Bone marrow aspiration, liver biopsy	Chemotherapy
Toxins	Acetaminophen toxicity	Medication history, serum APAP level ?APAP–cysteine adducts	*N*-acetylcysteine
	Idiosyncratic drug reaction	Temporal relationship	Withdraw suspect medication
	Amanita poisoning	Recent mushroom ingestion, severe gastrointestinal symptoms	Gastric lavage, charcoal, penicillin G, silymarin, hemodialysis
Other	Budd–Chiari syndrome	Thrombophilia work-up liver ultrasound with Doppler, angiogram	Heparin, warfarin

a Requires HBV coinfection.
ANA, antinuclear antibody; APAP, acetaminophen; ASMA, anti-smooth muscle antibody; HBc, hepatitis B core antigen; HBsAg, hepatitis B surface antigen; HELLP, hemolysis, elevated liver enzymes, and low platelet count; PCR, polymerase chain reaction.

Table 11.2 Diagnosis and management of acetaminophen overdose

Diagnosis

Ingestion of toxic dose of acetaminophen-containing product(s)

1 Review intake of all over-the-counter and prescription medications

2 More than 4 g acetaminophen in 24 h (usually > 10 g)

Consider diagnosis in all patients with unexplained serum ALT > 1000 IU/mL

1 Serum acetaminophen level (Rumack nomogram) if single dose ingestion

2 Check urine toxicology screen for other toxins or illicit substances

3 Bilirubin > 10 mg/dL may lead to false-positive serum acetaminophen levels

Management and treatment

Ipecac syrup/nasogastric lavage if within 4 h of ingestion

Activated charcoal 1 g/kg if within 4 h of ingestion

Admit to hospital if potential hepatotoxicity, coagulopathy, or altered mentation

Admit to ICU if encephalopathy

Liver biochemistries, electrolyte, arterial blood gas and lactate, PT/INR, and factor V levels at admission and q 12 h

Early transfer to transplant center if grade 2 encephalopathy or other adverse prognostic criteria[a]

Oral N-acetylcysteine (NAC):

  Loading dose: 140 mg/kg

  Maintenance dose: 70 mg/kg every 4 h for 17 doses or until INR < 1.5

  Mixing NAC with carbonated beverage can improve GI tolerance

  Nausea and vomiting in 20%, rare urticaria or bronchospasm

Intravenous N-acetylcysteine:

  Acetadote (Cumberland Phamaceuticals, Nashville, TN) is FDA approved for i.v. administration in acetaminophen overdose

  Telemetry monitoring recommended for infusion

  Indications: GI intolerance of oral NAC, ileus, pancreatitis or bowel obstruction, short gut syndrome, pregnancy

  Contraindications: known sulfa allergy

  Loading dose: 150 mg/kg in 250 mL D_5 over 1 h

  Maintenance dose: 50 mg/kg in 500 mL D_5 over 4 h then 125 mg/kg in 1000 mL D_5 over 19 h; 100 mg/kg in 1000 mL D_5 over 24 h × 2 days or until INR < 1.5

  Side effects: hypersensitivity or anaphylactoid reactions in 3%

  If mild hypersensitivity reaction, reduce infusion rate by 50% and consider i.v. diphenhydramine or steroids

a See text for further details.

ALT, alanine aminotransferase; D_5, 5% dextrose; FDA, US Food and Drug Administration; GI, gastrointestinal; ICU, intensive care unit; INR, international normalized ratio; PT, prothrombin time.

Table 11.3 Application of prognostic criteria to patients with acute liver failure

Prognostic scale	Positive predictive value (%)	Negative predictive value (%)	Predictive accuracy (%)
Acetaminophen hepatotoxicity			
King's College criteria[a]			
Arterial pH < 7.3	95	78	81
INR > 6.5, Cr > 3.4 mg/dL, grade 3/4 HE	67	86	83
Overall	84	86	85
King's College criteria and lactate[b]			
Overall	80	94	–
Non-acetaminophen acute liver failure			
King's College criteria[a]			
INR > 6.5	100	26	46
Any three of five variables[c]	96	82	92
Overall	98	82	94

a O'Grady JG, Alexander GJ, Hayllar KM, et al. Early indicators of prognosis in fulminant hepatic failure. Gastroenterology. 1989;97:439.

b Bernal W, Donaldson N, Wyncoll D, et al. Blood lactate as an early predictor of outcome in paracetemol-induced acute liver failure: a cohort study. Lancet 2002;359:558.

c INR > 3.5; jaundice to encephalopathy time >7 days, non-A, non-B hepatitis or drug-induced etiology; age <10 years or >40 years; serum bilirubin >17.5 mg/dL.

Cr, creatinine; HE, hepatic encephalopathy; INR, international normalized ratio.

Adapted from Rakela J, Lange SM, Ludwig J, et al. Fulminant hepatitis: Mayo Clinic experience with 34 cases. Mayo Clin Proc 1985;60:289.

Table 11.4 Prescription narcotic analgesics that contain acetaminophen

Trade name	Active ingredients[a]	Amount of APAP per tablet or dose
Anexsia	Hydrocodone + APAP	325–660 mg
Capital with Codeine Suspension	Codeine + APAP	120 mg/5 ml
Darvocet-N50	Propoxyphene + APAP	325 mg
Darvocet-N100	Propoxyphene + APAP	650 mg
Darvocet-A500	Propoxyphene + APAP	500 mg
Endocet	Oxycodone + APAP	325–650 mg
Esgic Plus	Butalbital + caffeine + APAP	500 mg
Fioricet	Butalbital + caffeine + APAP	325 mg
Fioricet with Codeine	Butalbital + caffeine + codeine + APAP	325 mg
Lorcet	Hydrocodone + APAP	325–750 mg, 500 mg/15 mL
Lortab	Hydrocodone + APAP	325–500 mg, 500 mg/15 mL
Maxidone	Hydrocodone + APAP	750 mg
Norco	Hydrocodone + APAP	325 mg
Panadol #3, and #4	Codeine + APAP	300 mg
Percocet/Oxycet	Oxycodone + APAP	325–650 mg
Phenaphen with Codeine	Codeine + APAP	325–650 mg
Roxicet	Oxycodone + APAP	325–500 mg, 325 mg/5 mL
Sedapap	Butalbital + APAP	650 mg
Talacen	Pentazocine + APAP	650 mg
Tylenol #2, #3, and #4	Codeine + APAP	300 mg
Tylox	Oxycodone + APAP	500 mg
Ultracet	Tramadol + APAP	325 mg
Vicodin	Hydrocodone + APAP	500 mg
Vicodin ES	Hydrocodone + APAP	750 mg
Vicodin HP	Hydrocodone + APAP	660 mg
Wygesic	Propoxyphene + APAP	650 mg
Zydone	Hydrocodone + APAP	400 mg

a Contact Poison Control Center or equivalent national poisons information service for exact dosage of constituents.

APAP, acetaminophen.

Table 11.5 Management of cerebral edema in acute liver failure

Grade 1 or 2 encephalopathy

Grade 1: Mild changes in mood and speech, disordered sleep

Grade 2: Inappropriate behavior, mild irritability, agitation, or somnolence

Hyperreflexia, clonus, asterixis may or may not be present

Transfer to ICU for frequent monitoring and neurological checks:

1 Quiet environment with minimal stimuli

2 Avoid sedatives/hypnotics

D_{10} drip with hourly blood glucose monitoring

Lactulose may be of benefit in selected patients (see text)

Grade 3 or 4 encephalopathy

Grade 3: Somnolent but arousable to verbal command, marked confusion, incoherent speech

Grade 4: Unarousable to painful stimuli

Avoid medications with sedative properties (e.g., narcotics, benzodiazepines) unless intubated

Elevate head of bed to 30° from horizontal

  Avoid Valsalva maneuvers, vigorous straining, or suctioning

  Use cooling blankets to keep core temperature ≤37°C

Elective intubation if hypoxia, respiratory failure, or to protect airway

  If intubated, propofol or midazolam sedation preferred

Head CT to rule out intracranial hemorrhage

Consider ICP monitor placement

  Correct coagulopathy (INR < 1.5) with FFP or rFVIIa

  ICP catheter type should balance risk of procedure vs benefit of accurate data (e.g., epidural vs subdural vs parenchymal)

Measures for elevated ICP

Maintain CPP above 50 mmHg (CPP = MAP − ICP)

Hyperventilate to P_{CO_2} of ~28–30 mmHg

If ICP >20 mmHg for >5 min, mannitol 0.5–1.0 mg/kg bolus over 5 min

Monitor serum osmolarity and osmolar gap

If persistently elevated ICP, pentabarbitol infusion with 100–150-mg bolus over 15 min followed by continuous infusion at 1–3 mg/kg/h

  May need pressors if pentobarbital used or CPP <50 mmHg

  Dopamine or levophed drips preferred

  Avoid vasopressin because of adverse effect on cerebral bloodflow[a]

  Moderate hypothermia (33°C–35°C) is investigational for refractory cerebral edema in ALF[a]

  Paralytic agent (atracurium) or propofol to prevent shivering

  Protocol for rewarming not established

Brain perfusion scan if prolonged increases in ICP to exclude brain death

a See text for discussion.
ALF, acute liver failure; CPP, cerebral perfusion pressure; CT, computed tomography; D_{10}, 10% dextrose; FFP, fresh frozen plasma; ICP, intracranial pressure; ICU, intensive care unit; INR, international normalized ratio; MAP, mean arterial pressure; rFVIIa, recombinant factor VIIa.

Table 11.6 Management of coagulopathy in acute liver failure

Multifactorial etiology

Hypoprothrombinemia caused by reduced hepatic synthesis of coagulation factors and DIC/hypofibrinogenemia

Thrombocytopenia caused by reduced hepatic thrombopoietin production, consumption, acute portal hypertension, and reduced marrow production (e.g., aplastic anemia, acute viral illness)

Vitamin K deficiency resulting from poor oral intake and jaundice/cholestasis

Assessment

PT/INR, PTT, CBC + platelet count, and fibrinogen q 12 h

  Serial INR and factor V levels have prognostic value

Clinically significant bleeding in ~10% of ALF patients

  Mucocutaneous hemorrhage, GI bleeding, and bleeding at insertion sites

Management

GI bleeding prophylaxis recommended in all patients with proton pump inhibitor or H_2 blocker

Vitamin K 10 mg subcutaneously for 3 days recommended for all patients

Prophylactic FFP infusions are NOT RECOMMENDED in absence of active bleeding

  Concerns of volume overload/worsening cerebral edema

  Lose prognostic value of INR

If active bleeding or planned procedure:

  FFP to keep INR <1.5

  Platelet infusion to keep platelet count >50 000 cells/mL

  Cryoprecipitate to keep fibrinogen >100 mg/dL

Consider rFVIIa only if contemplating invasive procedure such as ICP monitor placement and INR >1.5 after 4 units of FFP[a]

  Mechanism: enhances clot formation at areas of tissue factor release

  Contraindications: Budd–Chiari syndrome, malignancy, history of DVT/PE, pregnancy, thrombophilia

  Dose: administer as bolus rFVIIa at 80 μg/kg i.v. over 2–5 min

  Therapeutic window: half-life is 2–12 h for interventions

a Not approved by the US Food and Drug Administration for use in this setting.
CBC, complete blood count; DIC, disseminated intravascular coagulopathy; DVT, deep vein thrombosis; FFP, fresh frozen plasma; GI, gastrointestinal; INR, international normalized ratio; PE, pulmonary embolism; PT, prothrombin time; PTT, partial thromboplastin time; rFVIIa, recombinant factor VIIa.

Table 11.7 Diagnostic criteria for autoimmune hepatitis

Category	Factor	Score
Gender	Female	+2
Alkaline phosphatase: ALT	>3.0	−2
	<1.5	+2
Gamma globulin or IgG (× upper limit of normal)	>2.0	+3
	1.5–2.0	+2
	1.0–1.5	+1
	<1.0	0
ANA, SMA or anti-LKM1 titers	>1:80	+3
	1:80	+2
	1:40	+1
	<1:40	0
Markers of active viral infection	Positive	−4
	Positive	−3
	Negative	+3
HLA	DR3 or DR4	+1
Current immune disease	Any nonhepatic immune disease	+2
Other autoantibodies	Anti-SLP/LP, actin, LC1, pANCA	+2
Histological features	Interface hepatitis	+3
	Plasma cells	+1
	Rosettes	+1
	None of the above	−5
	Biliary changes	−3
	Atypical features	−3
Alcohol	<25 g/day	+2
	>60 g/day	−2
Hepatotoxic drugs	Yes	−4
	No	+1
Treatment response	Remission alone	+2
	Remission with relapse	+3

ALT, alanine aminotransferase; ANA, antinuclear autoantibodies; HLA, human leukocyte antigen; IgG, immunoglobulin G; LC1, liver cytosol; LKM1, liver kidney microsomes; LP, liver pancreas protein; pANCA, perinuclear antineutrophil cytoplasmic antibody; SLP, soluble liver protein; SMA, anti-smooth muscle autoantibodies.

Table 11.8 Features of acute liver failure in pregnancy

Disease	Dominant trimester	Findings/diagnosis	Histology	Treatment & outcome
Acute viral hepatitis (hepatitis A, B, C, E)	Any	Serologies	Portal and lobular inflammation	Supportive, HBIG and vaccination to the newborn of HBsAg+ mothers
Herpes hepatitis	Any, 2nd and 3rd most common	Serologies Vesicular rash in 50% High AST/ALT, mild hyperbilirubinemia – "anicteric liver failure"	Intranuclear inclusions	Acyclovir
Preeclampsia	2nd or 3rd	Hypertension Proteinuria Edema Elevated transaminases RUQ pain	Necrosis with infarction, periportal hemorrhage, fibrin deposition in sinusoids	Urgent delivery
HELLP Hemolysis, elevated liver enzymes, low platelets	3rd	Elevated AST/ALT, low platelets RUQ pain, nausea/vomiting, weight gain	Periportal/lobular necrosis, hyaline deposition	Urgent delivery
Hepatic infarction/rupture	3rd	Sudden abdominal pain, marked ⇑ AST/ALT Spiking fevers, anemia		Fluid resuscitation, surgical intervention or angiography
Acute fatty liver of pregnancy	3rd	⇑ AST/ALT, WBC, bilirubin	Microvesicular steatosis, Zone 3, overall hepatic architecture preserved	Urgent delivery Liver transplant, rarely May recur in subsequent pregnancies (genetic test for LCHAD deficiency)

AST/ALT, aspartate aminotransferase/alanine aminotransferase; HBIG, hepatitis B immunoglobulin; HBsAg, hepatitis B surface antigen; HELLP, hemolysis, elevated liver enzymes, and low platelet count; LCHAD, long chain fatty acid metabolic defect; RUQ, right upper quadrant; WBC, white blood cell count.
⇑, increase.

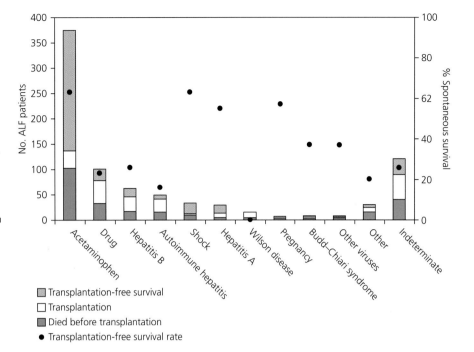

Figure 11.1 Etiologies and outcomes of acute liver failure in the United States, 1998–2005. Etiology and outcome in 838 consecutive adult patients with acute liver failure (ALF) enrolled at 23 sites comprising the Acute Liver Failure Study Group between 1998 and 2005. Patients with acetaminophen overdose and severe acute hepatitis A infection had the highest transplant-free survival rates of 63% and 55%, respectively. In contrast, subjects with idiosyncratic drug toxicity and indeterminate ALF had spontaneous survival rates of only 23% and 26%, respectively. (Will Lee, personal communication, December 2006.) NAPQI, N-acetyl-p-benzoquinone imine.

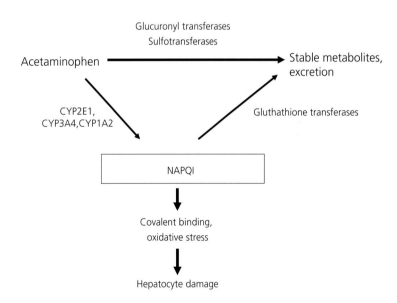

Figure 11.2 Pathways of acetaminophen metabolism in humans. CYP2E1, cytochrome P-450 2E1; NAPQI, N-acetyl-p-benzoquinone imine.

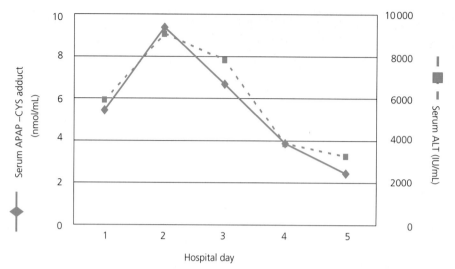

Figure 11.3 Serum acetaminophen–cysteine (APAP–CYS) adducts. A 23-year-old woman presented with nausea and vomiting after reportedly taking 30 tablets of Extra-Strength Tylenol (500 mg acetaminophen per tablet) as a suicide gesture 48 h previously. Initial serum acetaminophen level was 14 μg/dL, ALT 5920 IU/mL, INR 3.2, creatinine 0.8 μg/dL, and arterial pH 7.46. The patient was disorientated to place and time (Grade 1 encephalopathy). Oral N-acetylcysteine therapy was immediately initiated with ICU monitoring. Serum acetaminophen-cysteine adduct levels, a biomarker for acetaminophen mediated liver injury, were markedly positive on day 1 despite the low serum acetaminophen level and peaked on day 2 in parallel with serum alanine aminotransferase (ALT) levels. Serum acetaminophen-cysteine adducts appear to be a sensitive and specific biomarker for acetaminophen hepatotoxicity. Adduct levels courtesy of Laura James, MD, University of Arkansas.

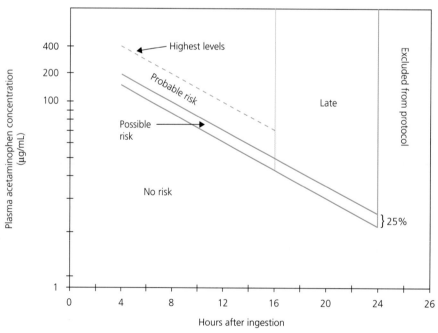

Figure 11.4 Rumack nomogram in acetaminophen overdose patients. The plasma acetaminophen levels at presentation in 662 patients who had ingested >7.5 g of acetaminophen and received N-acetylcysteine were determined. Hepatotoxicity defined by a serum ALT >1000 IU/mL was greatest in subjects whose plasma acetaminophen levels exceeded the probable risk line and varied from 7.7% between 4 and 10 h, 22.2% between 10 and 16 h, and 45.1% from 16 to 24 h after ingestion. The lower line was inserted to identify subjects with a "possible risk" of hepatotoxicity that varied from 3% to 13% within 24 h of presentation. It is currently recommended that all subjects with a single time point acetaminophen overdose and probable or possible hepatotoxicity receive N-acetylcysteine for 72 h in the hospital. For subjects with an acetaminophen level below the "Possible risk" line, N-acetylcysteine treatment beyond 24 h is likely not warranted unless there is evidence of progressive liver injury. Overdose patients presenting greater than 24 h from initial ingestion with elevated serum aminotransferase levels should be treated with N-acetylcysteine independent of their serum acetaminophen level. Courtesy of Barry Rumack.

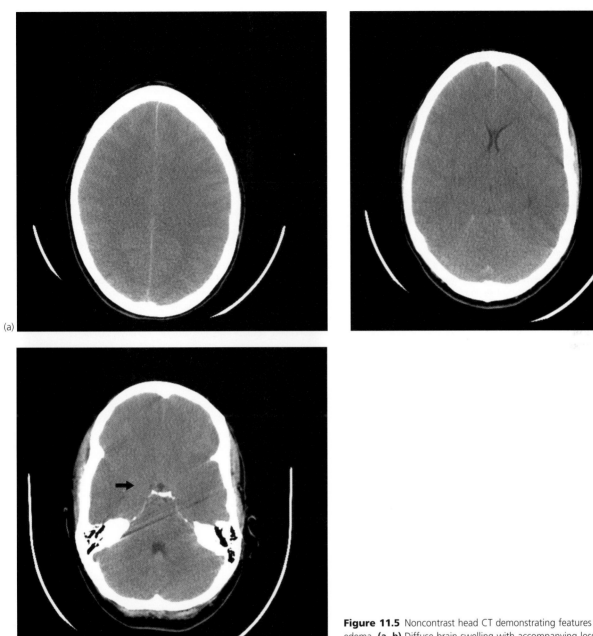

(a)

(b)

(c)

Figure 11.5 Noncontrast head CT demonstrating features of cerebral edema. **(a, b)** Diffuse brain swelling with accompanying loss of cortical sulci and reduced cerebral spinal fluid in the ventricles. **(c)** Effacement of the basal cisterns with loss of gray–white differentiation (arrow).

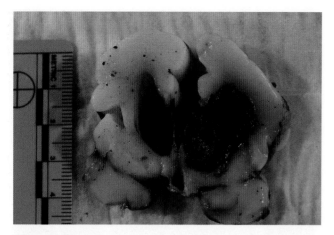

Figure 11.6 Patient with acute liver failure died from cerebral edema due to an acetaminophen overdose. Diffuse brain swelling led to flattening of the gyri and compression of the sulci in this patient. The cut surface of the brain has a glassy, monochromic appearance with an imperceptible interface between the white and gray matter. The left-sided intraventricular hemorrhage detected at autopsy presumably developed because of the underlying coagulopathy. Photograph at necropsy, courtesy of the University of Michigan Autopsy Gross Image Archive.

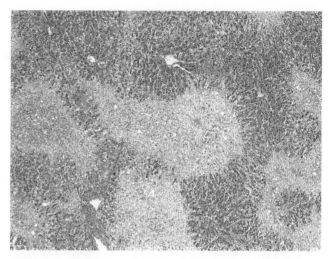

Figure 11.7 Liver injury secondary to acetaminophen. Acetaminophen hepatotoxicity leads to a characteristic pattern of pericentral hepatocyte necrosis. The well-preserved periportal zones and absence of significant inflammation in the extensive regions of necrosis is typical of a toxic liver injury such as acetaminophen overdose. (Photomicrograph at 4 × magnification, autopsy liver, hematoxylin and eosin stain.)

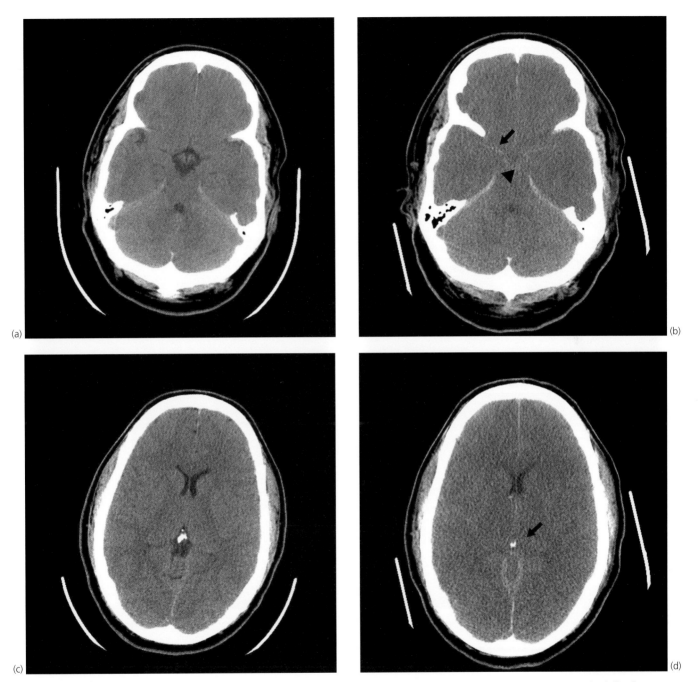

Figure 11.8 Radiological progression of cerebral edema. Noncontrast head CT scans were obtained at 72 h **(a, c)** and 24 h prior to death **(b, d)**. **(a, b)** Progressive loss of the gray–white matter interface with loss of the suprasellar cistern (arrowhead) and tightening of the fourth ventricle. Note the enhancement of the blood vessels ([b] arrow) due to progressive cerebral swelling. **(c, d)** Progressive loss of the gray–white differentiation and loss of cerebral spinal fluid in the pineal region despite successful interval liver transplantation ([d] arrow).

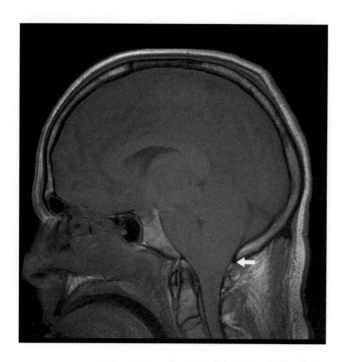

Figure 11.9 Transtentorial herniation of the cerebellum. Midline sagittal T1 MRI image reveals advanced cerebral edema as manifested by cerebellar tonsillar herniation (white arrow), deformed brainstem, and effacement of the basal cisterns. This image was obtained 24 h prior to declaration of brain death.

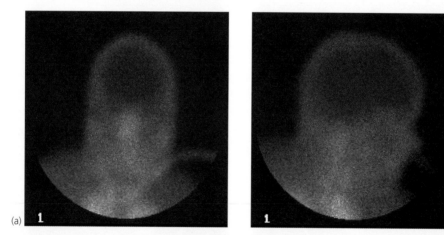

(a)

(b)

Figure 11.10 Nuclear medicine brain scan in terminal acute liver failure. Following intravenous administration of ^{99}Tc hexamethylpropyleneamine oxime, there was no intracranial signal detected, indicative of the absence of brain blood flow. Delayed static imaging reveals absence of tracer activity within the cerebrum and posterior fossa on both anterior **(a)** and lateral views **(b)**.

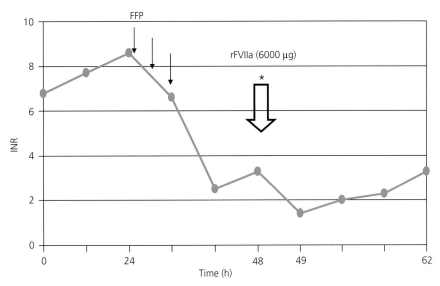

Figure 11.11 Use of recombinant factor VIIa (rF VIIa) in acute liver failure. A 21-year-old man with intentional acetaminophen overdose had an initial serum acetaminophen level of 105 µg/dL, ALT 460 IU/L, and INR 1.0. Despite receiving oral N-acetylcysteine, he developed rapidly worsening liver failure with ALT 10 000 IU/L and an international normalized ratio (INR) of 6.3. Owing to progressive obtundation, he was intubated for airway protection. A noncontrast head CT revealed effacement of the sulci consistent with cerebral edema and an intracranial pressure (ICP) monitor was planned. However, after 8 units of fresh frozen plasma (FFP), his INR remained elevated at 2.5. Following a bolus dose of 6000 µg of rF VIIa (80 µg/kg), his INR improved to 1.4 allowing the placement of an intracerebral monitor without complications. His ICP varied between 10 and 31 mmHg and he was treated with N-acetylcysteine, broad-spectrum antibiotics, and boluses of mannitol. His mental status slowly improved, allowing removal of the ICP monitor on day 7 and he was eventually discharged home on day 23 with no neurological sequelae.

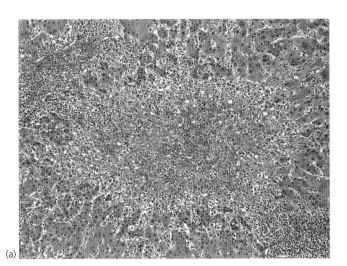

(a)

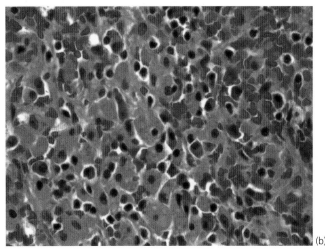

(b)

Figure 11.12 Fulminant autoimmune hepatitis. A 65-year-old woman with a history of systemic lupus, Sjogren syndrome, and rheumatoid arthritis presented with a 1-week history of fatigue, anorexia, and jaundice. Her antinuclear antibody was markedly positive at 1:1280, antismooth muscle antibody was positive at 1:20, and she had a polyclonal increase in gamma globulins. Initial serum ALT was 832 IU/L, INR 2.9, and bilirubin 8.9 mg/dL with a pretreatment autoimmune hepatitis (AIH) score of 17 (probable). She was treated with corticosteroids, but developed progressive encephalopathy leading to liver transplantation on her third day in hospital. The explanted liver revealed subfulminant necrosis that was focally pericentral. The extensive fibrosis is consistent with a clinical history of liver disease of several months' duration ([a] Photomicrograph at 20 × magnification, explanted liver, hematoxylin and eosin (H & E)). A higher power magnification demonstrates collections of residual plasma cells at the interface ([b] Photomicrograph at 60 ×, explanted liver, H & E).

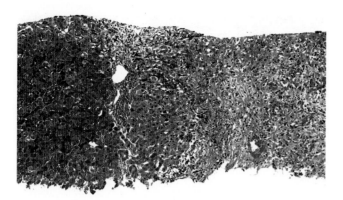

Figure 11.13 Idiosyncratic drug-induced liver injury leading to acute liver failure (ALF). A 33-year-old black woman received interferon beta-1a injections three times a week over 9 months for multiple sclerosis. She then presented with a 3-week history of jaundice and malaise and an AST of 681 IU/L, alkaline phosphatase 216 IU/L, bilirubin 25.3 mg/dL, and INR 2.2. Serological and radiological evaluation for identifiable etiologies of ALF were negative. A transjugular liver biopsy revealed predominantly central zone necrosis with large areas of collapse suggestive of a severe drug or toxin-induced liver injury. The collapsed region is replaced by scar (seen in blue) with a residual central vein **(right)** and entrapped biliary structures **(far right)**. The degree of scar is suggestive of a remote toxin exposure. The patient was managed expectantly but developed progressive sepsis and renal failure that ultimately led to her death from multiorgan failure. Prior reports have demonstrated severe hepatocellular injury leading to jaundice and rare fatalities in multiple sclerosis patients receiving interferon beta-1a. (Photomicrograph at 10 ×, liver core biopsy, Masson trichrome.)

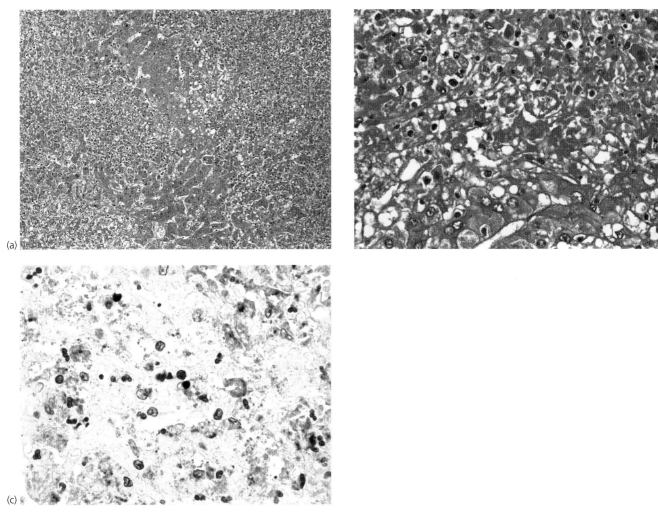

(a)

(b)

(c)

Figure 11.14 Fulminant herpes hepatitis. A 58-year-old white man presented with 9 days of high fevers and malaise. He had markedly elevated serum aminotransferases exceeding ~30 × the upper limit of normal, INR 1.7 and bilirubin of 6.4 mg/dL with vesicular lesions on his face and tongue. He was empirically started on high dose intravenous acyclovir for presumed disseminated herpes simplex virus (HSV) infection. Both his serum HSV IgG and IgM were positive as well as a HSV direct fluorescent antibody from the skin lesion. The patient's disease rapidly progressed, necessitating a liver transplant 3 days after presentation. The liver explant revealed massive hepatic necrosis secondary to HSV with intranuclear inclusions in infected necrotic hepatocytes. Unlike many toxin- and vascular-related liver insults, the necrosis of HSV is nonzonal, giving a "patternless" distribution on a low-power objective lens. **(a)** Photomicrograph at 10 × magnification, hematoxylin and eosin stain (H & E). A sea of hepatocyte "ghosts" typifies the extensive coagulative necrosis observed in primary HSV infections of the liver. A single hepatocyte **(top center)** contains a glassy intranuclear inclusion, and hepatocyte binucleation is evident **(top right)**. **(b)** Photomicrograph at 40 × magnification, H & E. Special staining for HSV-1 demonstrates characteristic intranuclear inclusion (seen in brown). **(c)** Photomicrograph at 40 × magnification, autopsy of the liver, immunohistochemistry.

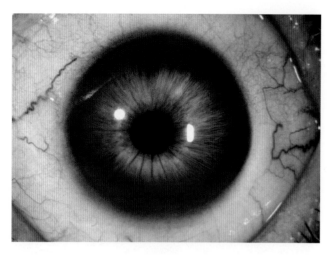

Figure 11.15 Kayser–Fleischer rings in Wilson disease. Slit lamp examination of a Wilson disease patient can reveal Kayser–Fleischer rings or sunflower cataracts. Kayser–Fleischer rings are characterized by a brown–green discoloration at the inferior and superior rims of the cornea, close to the surface. The deposits consist of fine granular copper complexed with sulfur located in Descemet's membrane. "Pseudo Kayser–Fleischer" rings can be seen also in other chronic cholestatic disorders including primary biliary cirrhosis and neonatal cholestasis owing to bilirubin deposition. Photograph courtesy of the Kellogg Eye Center, University of Michigan.

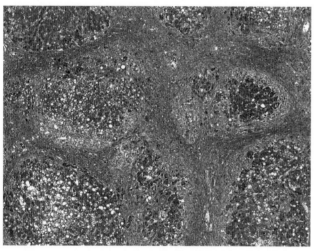

(a)

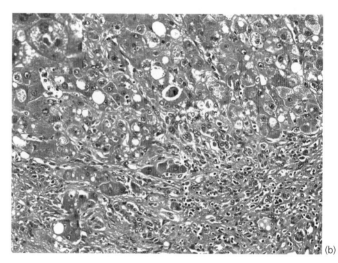

(b)

Figure 11.16 Liver histopathology in Wilson disease. A 22-year-old woman presented with a 1-week history of abdominal pain, malaise, and jaundice. On admission, her AST was 171 IU/L, ALT 82 IU/L, alkaline phosphatase 112 IU/L, total bilirubin 3.3 mg/dL, and INR 2.5. There was also evidence of hemolytic anemia with hemoglobin of 10.9 g/dL but no encephalopathy. Serum ceruloplasmin was low at 5.3 mg/dL (normal: 18-42 mg/dL) and a 24-h urine collection for copper was markedly positive at 1515 μg (normal <55 μg). Slit-lamp examination revealed Kayser–Fleischer rings. Despite treatment with zinc and trientene, the patient developed progressive renal failure and underwent liver transplantation on her tenth day in hospital. The explanted liver demonstrated thick bands of fibrosis (seen in blue) characteristic of micronodular cirrhosis and patchy steatosis and collections of ballooned hepatocytes. **(a)** Photomicrograph at 4 × magnification, explanted liver, Masson's

trichrome. The patchy steatosis and ballooned hepatocytes are more evident at higher magnification. In addition, there are scattered dead liver cells **(center)** and some hepatocytes have Mallory's hyaline **(insert upper left)**. Portal tracts contain mild lymphocytic inflammation. **(b)** Photomicrograph at 4 × magnification, explanted liver, hematoxylin and eosin stain. Note the bile ductular proliferation characteristic of cirrhosis at the periphery of portal regions **(lower right)**. No single histological feature is specific for Wilson disease; hence, diagnostic reports must be interpreted in the clinical context. While hepatocyte copper is the attributable injurious agent in Wilson disease, staining with rhodamine is not usually beneficial as the intensity and distribution are highly variable and hepatocyte copper can be seen with many liver diseases. Instead, quantitative hepatic copper determination is recommended to make a diagnosis of Wilson disease.

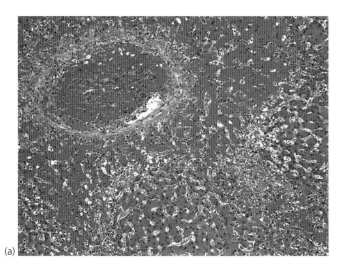

(a)

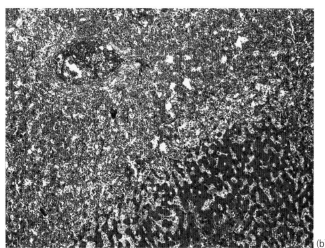

(b)

Figure 11.17 Histopathology of fulminant Budd–Chiari. A 20-year-old, previously healthy woman on oral contraceptives presented with a 1-week history of increasing abdominal pain and distention, weight gain, and nausea/vomiting. Initial AST was 598 IU/L, INR 1.5, and bilirubin 2.8 mg/dL. Ultrasound with Doppler revealed nonvisualization of the hepatic veins, reversal of flow in the portal venous system, diffuse abdominal ascites, and an enlarged hypoechoic caudate lobe. A transjugular portosystemic shunt was placed for acute Budd–Chiari syndrome but immediately clotted off, leading to emergent liver transplantation on her fourth day in hospital. Histopathology of the explanted liver revealed acute central vein thrombus accompanied by circumferential hepatocyte necrosis and intense hemorrhage into spaces of disease **(a)**. In addition, bridging necrosis was noted. The nonnecrotic liver parenchyma showed sinusoidal dilation. The central vein thrombus and surrounding hepatocyte necrosis are associated with minimal collagen deposition (seen in bright blue) because of the acuity of the thrombophilic event in fulminant Budd–Chiari. **(b)** Photomicrograph at 10 × magnification, explanted liver, hematoxylin and eosin, and Masson's trichrome.

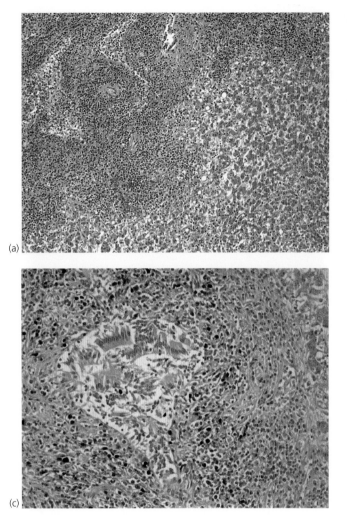

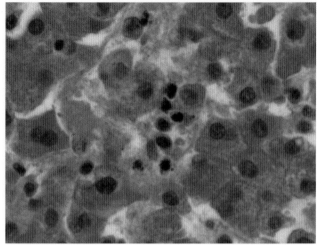

Figure 11.18 Epstein–Barr virus (EBV) hepatitis with hemophagocytic syndrome. An 18-year-old man with a 5-year history of Crohn's disease on 6-mercaptopurine developed a sore throat and high spiking fevers 3 weeks prior to presentation. He was diagnosed with mononucleosis 6 days prior to admission by monospot testing. He then presented a bilirubin of 11.1 mg/dL, alkaline phosphatase 1009 IU/L, ALT 116 IU/L, AST 334 IU/L, and INR 2.6. He was also noted to be anemic with hemoglobin 10.1 g/dL. Ultrasound revealed an enlarged liver as well as a markedly enlarged spleen. The patient was diagnosed with acute EBV hepatitis with hemophagocytic syndrome based on his clinical history and lack of other identifiable etiologies. Liver biopsy showed prominent portal lymphocytic inflammation with spillage across the interface into liver lobules. This appearance is unusually florid as the most common finding in EBV hepatitis is lobular hepatitis. **(a)** Photomicrograph at 10 × magnification, explanted liver, hematoxylin and eosin (H & E) stain. On higher power, a characteristic row of single-file lymphocytes can be seen within the hepatic sinusoid. **(b)** Photomicrograph at 40 × magnification, explanted liver, H & E stain. Strong nuclear staining of portal lymphocytes infected with Epstein–Barr virus (seen in blue) were also seen by in-situ hybridization. **(c)** Photomicrograph at 20 × magnification, explanted liver, Epstein–Barr virus encoded RNA (EBER) probe). The patient unfortunately progressed to septic shock, acute respiratory distress syndrome with diffuse alveolar hemorrhage, disseminated intravascular coagulation, and acute renal failure culminating in death 12 days after admission. EBV polymerase chain reaction (PCR) results obtained post-mortem revealed 1 237 000 copies/mL.

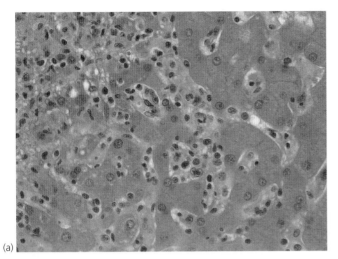

(a)

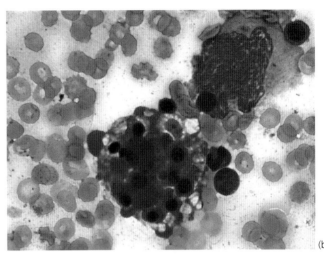

(b)

Figure 11.19 Liver biopsy in peripheral T-cell lymphoma. A 58-year-old man presented with upper respiratory symptoms that did not improve with 3 weeks of antibiotics. He subsequently developed high fevers, profound hemolytic anemia, and acute liver failure. A wedge liver biopsy showed an atypical lymphoid infiltrate involving portal tracts and central zones, with extension into liver sinusoids. Note the irregularity of nuclear contours with occasional prominent nucleoli and variability in size of the malignant cells. **(a)** Photomicrograph at 40 × magnification, liver wedge biopsy, hematoxylin and eosin (H & E) stain (photograph courtesy of Riccardo Valdez). A bone marrow biopsy also showed the presence of a peripheral T-cell lymphoma and evidence of the hemophagocytic syndrome. An epithelioid histiocyte is shown engulfing mature red blood cells and a variety of red blood-cell precursors. Erythrophagocytosis is a hallmark of T-cell lymphomas. **(b)** Photomicrograph under oil at 100 × magnification, bone marrow aspirate clot, Wright–Giemsa (photograph courtesy of Riccardo Valdez). Despite treatment with decadron and cyclophosphamide, the patient quickly succumbed to multiorgan failure with sepsis at 6 weeks from the onset of symptoms.

12 Approach to the patient with chronic viral hepatitis B or C

Sammy Saab, Hugo Rosen

Introduction

Chronic viral hepatitis can result in cirrhosis, hepatocellular carcinoma, and hepatic failure. Treatment is utilized to prevent these complications in susceptible people. However, the risks and benefits need to be compared and weighed by efficacy of available therapy, presence of comorbid conditions, costs, and potential cross-resistance.

Hepatitis B

The detection of hepatitis B surface antigen (HBsAg) for more than 6 months indicates chronic hepatitis B infection. Viral replication is suggested by the presence of hepatitis B e antigen (HBeAg) detection. However, patients can have precore and core mutant hepatitis B viruses with anti-HBe detected, and have low levels of viral replication. Molecular tests (i.e., HBV DNA) are the most accurate method to assess for viral replication. The viral load is also used to monitor treatment efficacy. One of the goals of antiviral therapy is to suppress viral replication.

Antiviral therapy should be considered in patients with elevated HBV viral loads and serum aminotransferases. There are currently six medications approved by the Food and Drug Administration (FDA) to treat hepatitis B, including four oral medications. The two injectable medications are interferon and pegylated interferon. The advantages of interferon over oral medications include a defined period of therapy, best probability of HBsAg loss, and no associated resistance. Unlike interferon, oral medications have little associated adverse effects and, as a result, are gaining popularity in clinical practice. However, the duration of treatment is not temporary and treatment is discontinued only after the viral replication is halted. Moreover, oral drugs may be

associated with cross-resistance. The dosages of these medications need to be adjusted according to creatinine clearance.

Lamivudine, a nucleoside analogue, was the first oral drug approved by the FDA in 1995. The major limitation of lamivudine is the development of resistance, which limits its use as a first line agent. Another nucleoside analogue is entecavir. The effectiveness and lack of resistance associated with entecavir make it a reasonable first line option in patients with compensated and decompensated liver disease who are lamivudine naive. Although entecavir is effective in lamivudine-experienced patients, cross-resistance may limit its use in this population. Adefovir is a nucleotide analogue with activity against hepatitis B. The advantages of adefovir are its long-term safety profile and low rate of resistance. The decrease in viral load with adefovir appears to be slower than with lamivudine and entecavir, but adefovir has been associated with lower resistance rates than lamivudine. Long-term therapy with adefovir is associated with cumulative viral suppression and infrequent viral resistance. The low resistant rates make adefovir particularly attractive in HBeAg-negative patients who are likely to require long-term therapy. Telbivudine is a nucleoside analogue that, although efficacious in suppressing viral replication, is associated with viral breakthrough, which limits its use in the clinical setting as monotherapy.

Hepatitis C

The diagnosis of hepatitis is suggested by the screening antibody test: the enzyme-linked immunosorbent assay (ELISA). However, diagnosis is confirmed by the detection of HCV viral load. A hepatitis C genotype estimates the likelihood of achieving a sustained virological response and the duration of antiviral therapy. A liver biopsy is helpful for assessing the degree of liver damage, determining the need for antiviral therapy, and estimation of prognosis.

The viral load is used to assess and predict response to therapy. Therapy is discontinued in patients who do not

Atlas of Gastroenterology, 4th edition. Edited by Tadataka Yamada, David H. Alpers, Anthony N. Kalloo, Neil Kaplowitz, Chung Owyang, and Don W. Powell. © 2009 Blackwell Publishing, ISBN: 978-1-4051-6909-7

reach certain milestones. For instance, therapy is discontinued in patients who do have at least a two-log drop in viral level at week 12 (early virological response [EVR]), or have a detectable viral level of any values at week 24. The viral load at the completion of treatment is known as the End of Treatment Response (ETR). The goal of therapy (the sustained viral response [SVR]) is defined by a nondetectable viral load 6 months after completing therapy.

Patients with genotype 1 have an estimated SVR of between 40% and 45%. Patients with genotypes 2 or 3 have SVR rates of between 70% and 80%. Current recommendations are that patients with genotype 1 exhibiting EVR should receive 48 weeks of peginterferon therapy with standard doses of ribavirin (1000–1200 mg/day), whereas patients with genotype 2 or 3 will need no more than 24 weeks (possibly shorter duration as discussed in the next paragraph) of therapy using a lower dose of ribavirin (800 mg/day). There is increasing interest in applying viral kinetics (i.e., the rate of viral decline) to help determine duration of therapy. Patients who achieve a rapid virological response may be considered for a shorter duration of therapy. Conversely, a longer course of therapy may benefit those who take longer to achieve a nondetectable viral level.

Unlike oral therapies for hepatitis B, interferon and ribavirin are associated with a number of signature adverse effects. Many adverse effects are predictable and most are manageable. Influenza-like symptoms (fever, myalgia, and rigors) occur in approximately one-half of treated patients and can be managed with acetaminophen (paracetamol) or nonsteroidal antiinflammatory drugs. Dose reductions (temporary or permanent) of either peginterferon or ribavirin may be necessary. However, efforts should be undertaken to prevent dose reductions, as they reduce the probability of achieving a SVR. Adherence to therapy may be improved with the use of antidepressant/anxiolytic medications and hemopoietic stem cell growth factors.

Table 12.1 Treatment algorithm recommendations for HBeAg-positive patients

HBeAg status	HBV DNA[a]	ALT[b]	Treatment strategy
Positive	<20,000	Normal	No treatment Monitor every 6–12 months[c] Consider therapy in patients with known significant histologic disease even if low-level replication
Positive	≥20,000	Normal	Low rate of HBeAg seroconversion for all treatments Younger patients often immune tolerant Consider liver biopsy examination, particularly if older than age 35–40 years; treat if disease present: in the absence of biopsy examination, observe for increase in ALT levels If treated, adefovir, entecavir, or peginterferon alfa-2a preferred[d]
Positive	≥20,000	Elevated	Adefovir, entecavir, or peginterferon alfa-2a are preferred first-line options[d,e] If high HBV DNA; adefovir or entecavir preferred over peginterferon alfa-2a

a Values shown in IU/mL (1 IU/mL is equivalent to approximately 5.6 copies/mL).
b The upper limits of normal for serum ALT concentrations for men and women are 30 IU/L and 19 IU/L, respectively.
c On initial diagnosis, every 3 months for every 1 year to ensure stability.
d Genotyping maybe useful to help decide between treating with peginterferon α-2a rather than with adefovir or entecavir (i.e., peginterferon has been shown to be more effective in patients with genotype A vs. D).
e Peginterferon α-2a and entecavir are preferred over lamivudine as they have been shown to be superior in randomized clinical trials, and lamivudine is limited by high rates of resistance.
From Keeffe EB, Dieterich DT, Han SH, et al. A treatment algorithm for the management of chronic hepatitis B virus infection in the United States: an update. Clin Gastroenterol Hepatol 2006;4:936.

Table 12.2 Treatment algorithm recommendations for HBeAg-negative patients

HBeAg status	HBV DNA[a]	ALT[b]	Treatment strategy
Negative	<2000	Normal	No treatment; majority inactive HBsAg carriers Monitor every 6–12 months[c] Consider therapy in patients with known significant histologic disease even if low-level replication
Negative	≥2000	Normal	Consider liver biopsy examination; treat if disease present; in the absence of biopsy examination, observe for increase in serum ALT levels If treated, adefovir, entecavir, or peginterferon alfa-2a are preferred[d]
Negative	≥2000	Elevated	Adefovir, entecavir, or peginterferon alfa-2a are preferred first-line options[d] Long-term treatment required for oral agents

a Values shown in IU/mL (1 IU/mL is equivalent to approximately 5.6 copies/mL).

b The upper limits of normal for serum ALT concentrations for men and women are 30 IU/L and 19 IU/L, respectively.

c On initial diagnosis, every 3 months for every 1 year to ensure stability.

d Lamivudine is not considered a reasonable treatment option because of the high risk for resistance with long-term therapy and proven inferiority to peginterferon α-2a and entecavir in randomized clinical trials.

From Keeffe EB, Dieterich DT, Han SH, et al. A treatment algorithm for the management of chronic hepatitis B virus infection in the United States: an update. Clin Gastroenterol Hepatol 2006;4:936.

Table 12.3 Treatment algorithm recommendations for compensated cirrhotic patients

HBeAg status	HBV DNA[a]	Cirrhosis	Treatment strategy
Positive or negative	<2000	Compensated	May choose to treat or observe Adefovir or entecavir preferred[b]
Positive or negative	≥2000	Compensated	Adefovir or entecavir are first-line options Long-term treatment required, and combination therapy may be preferred[c]

a Values shown in IU/mL (1 IU/mL is equivalent to approximately 5.6 copies/mL).

b Although there are no data available for peginterferon α-2a, it may be an option in patients with early, well-compensated cirrhosis.

c Combination therapy with lamivudine, or possibly entecavir, and adefovir has a theoretic advantage owing to the lower likelihood of the development of resistance.

From Keeffe EB, Dieterich DT, Han SH, et al. A treatment algorithm for the management of chronic hepatitis B virus infection in the United States: an update. Clin Gastroenterol Hepatol 2006;4:936.

Table 12.4 Treatment algorithm recommendations for decompensated cirrhotic patients

HBeAg status	HBV DNA[a]	Cirrhosis	Treatment strategy
Positive or negative	<200 to ≥200	Decompensated	Combination with lamivudine, or possibly entecavir, plus adefovir preferred[b,c] Long-term treatment required Waiting list for liver transplantation

a Values shown in IU/mL (1 IU is equivalent to approximately 5.6 copies/mL).

b No data available for entecavir; peginterferon α-2a contraindicated.

c Combination therapy with lamivudine (or possibly entecavir) and adefovir has a theoretic advantage owing to the lower likelihood of the development of resistance.

Data from Keeffe EB, Dieterich DT, Han SH, et al. A treatment algorithm for the management of chronic hepatitis B virus infection in the United States: an update. Clin Gastroenterol Hepatol 2006;4:936.

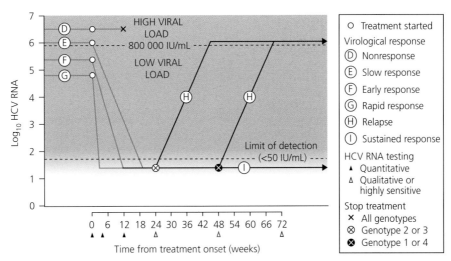

Figure 12.1 Monitoring treatment response with molecular testing of patients with chronic hepatitis C virus infection. The diagram shows four possible responses during treatment of chronic hepatitis C virus (HCV) infection and stopping rules. Suggested times for HCV RNA testing are shown along the same scale.

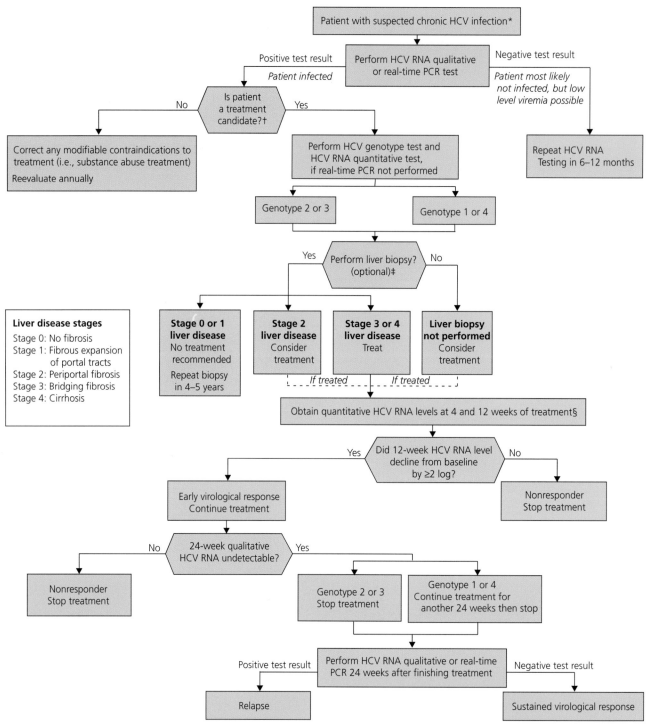

Figure 12.2 Algorithm for testing and treatment of chronic hepatitis C virus infection. HCV, indicated hepatitis C virus; PCR, polymerase chain reaction. *Chronic infection is suspected if a patient's most recent HCV exposure was more than 6 months before testing or if the patient does not have features of acute hepatitis C. †Treatment candidates include those without any absolute contraindications to treatment or those without relative contraindications that cannot be safely managed. ‡Liver biopsy is the most accurate method of determining the severity of liver disease. §If HCV RNA levels are negative at 4 weeks, there is a high probability of sustained virological response.

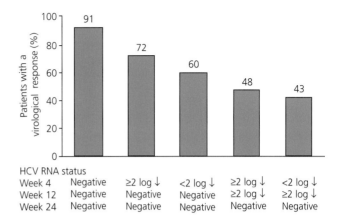

Figure 12.3 Rates of viral clearance predicts sustained virological response using pegylated interferon and ribavirin. The sooner viral clearance is achieved, the greater the likelihood of achieving a sustained virological response.

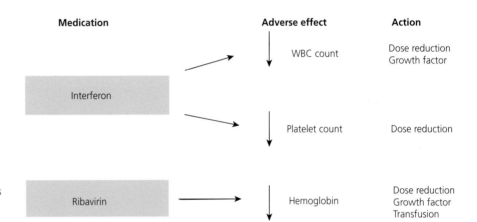

Figure 12.4 Hematological adverse effects from pegylated interferon and ribavirin are predictable and manageable.

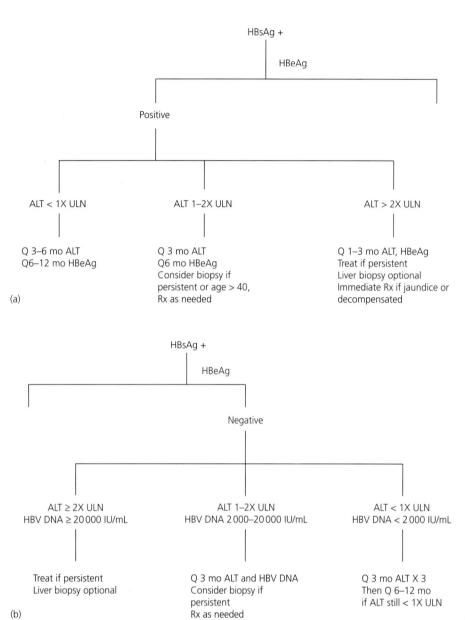

(a)

(b)

Figure 12.5 American Association for the Study of Liver Diseases Practice Guideline algorithm for follow-up of hepatitis B carriers who are hepatitis B e antigen (HBeAg) positive **(a)** or HBeAg negative **(b)**. ALT, alanine aminotransferase; HCC, hepatocellular carcinoma; Rx, treatment; ULN, upper limit of normal. *HCC surveillance if indicated.

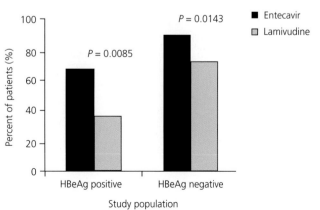

Figure 12.6 Efficacy of entecavir in suppressing hepatitis B virus (HBV) DNA in hepatitis B e antigen (HBeAg)-positive and negative treatment naive patients.

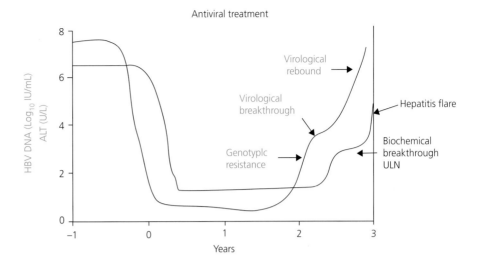

Figure 12.7 Serial changes in serum hepatitis B virus (HBV) DNA and alanine aminotransferase (ALT) levels in association with emergence of antiviral-resistant HBV mutants.

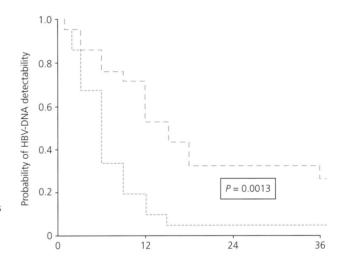

Figure 12.8 Significant earlier decline to nondetectable hepatitis B virus (HBV) DNA among hepatitis B e antigen (HBeAg)-negative chronic hepatitis B patients with baseline viral loads less than 10^7 copies/mL when adefovir used in lamivudine-resistant patients. Adefovir was used in combination with lamivudine or adefovir used as monotherapy.

Approach to the patient with a liver mass

John A. Donovan, Edward G. Grant, Gary C. Kanel

Discovery of a mass in the liver is cause for immediate concern and urgency. A correct diagnosis directs subsequent recommendations for additional study, indicates appropriate treatments, and guides future management. Masses in the liver are usually detected by abdominal imaging performed for the evaluation of right upper quadrant pain, the screening of the patient at risk for hepatocellular carcinoma and other malignancies, or by incidental discovery during the investigation of other medical or surgical conditions. Evaluation of the hepatic mass requires knowledge of both benign and malignant lesions affecting the liver. In the adult, benign lesions of the liver include hemangiomas, hepatic adenomas, focal nodular hyperplasia and a variety of other less common lesions, including bile duct adenomas, nodular regenerative hyperplasia, and focal fatty change.

Evaluation of the patient with a liver mass begins with a complete history, physical examination, and laboratory evaluation. Hepatic biochemistries are seldom of diagnostic importance or assistance. Characteristic radiographic findings, a confirmatory biopsy, or both, most often enable the accurate diagnosis of a benign liver lesion. Confirmation of a benign hepatic lesion usually confers an excellent prognosis and relieves the anxious patient.

Hepatic hemangioma

Hepatic hemangioma is the most common benign liver tumor in men and women. Most hepatic hemangiomas are incidentally discovered at the time of abdominal imaging performed for the evaluation of abdominal symptoms. Hepatic hemangiomas may range in size from less than 1 cm to greater than 20 cm in diameter and are more commonly located in the right hepatic lobe. Those measuring greater than 5 cm in diameter are classified as giant, or cavernous, hemangiomas. The natural history of the hepatic hemangi-

oma is usually benign. Rarely, more acute and diffuse abdominal pain results from the spontaneous or traumatic rupture of a larger hemangioma and hemoperitoneum.

Focal nodular hyperplasia

Focal nodular hyperplasia (FNH) is the second most common benign liver mass. The most common patient with FNH is a woman between 20 and 60 years old with this incidental finding. Often, FNH is solitary and typically measures less than 5 cm in its greatest dimension, although multiple and larger lesions may occur but more rarely. The usual FNH lesion does not cause symptoms. The incidental finding of FNH should not be an indication for therapeutic intervention. Importantly, if a suspected FNH lesion cannot be distinguished from hepatocellular carcinoma (HCC) in the patient at risk because of chronic liver disease, then surgical resection should be considered.

Hepatic adenoma

Hepatic adenomas (HAs) are benign hepatic lesions consisting normal appearing hepatocytes. Women more frequently (4:1) have HAs than men. A promoting effect of oral contraceptive medications and estrogens is well established. Seventy to eighty percent are solitary and two-thirds are located in the right lobe of the liver. More than 10 coexisting HAs defines adenomatosis. Most individuals with HAs are asymptomatic. Clinically, HAs are important because of the potential risks for intratumoral hemorrhage, rupture, and transformation to HCC. This potential for malignant transformation supports a policy of preemptive surgical resection, unless otherwise contraindicated.

Nodular regenerative hyperplasia

Nodular regenerative hyperplasia (NRH) is characterized by diffuse, or occasionally focal, nodules of regenerating hepa-

Atlas of Gastroenterology, 4th edition. Edited by Tadataka Yamada, David H. Alpers, Anthony N. Kalloo, Neil Kaplowitz, Chung Owyang, and Don W. Powell. © 2009 Blackwell Publishing, ISBN: 978-1-4051-6909-7

tocytes in the noncirrhotic liver. It appears that NRH occurs equally in men and women and is more prevalent with increasing age. If a patient is without evidence of chronic liver disease or cirrhosis but presents with unexplained complications of portal hypertension, NRH should be suspected. Nodules of regenerating hepatocytes are generally less than 4 mm in size but can coalesce to form larger nodules measuring up to 4 cm. in diameter. The diagnosis of NRH is more often dependent on the results of a diagnostic liver biopsy.

Biliary cystadenoma

Biliary cystadenoma of intrahepatic or extrahepatic bile duct is a rare cystic neoplasm of mesenchymal and Von Meyenberg complex origins that accounts for less than 5% of hepatobiliary tumors. Cyst aspiration characteristically yields a mucinous fluid. Carcinoembryonic antigen (CEA) or CA19-9 antibody may be elevated in the serum or found in the cyst fluid.

Biliary cystadenoma is a premalignant lesion. Percutaneous ablation or incomplete surgical resection are associated with recurrence. Treatment, and differentiation from biliary cystadenocarcinoma, is by a complete surgical resection.

Focal fatty change

Focal fatty change describes the localized and geometric deposit of macrovesicular fat in the liver. Focal fatty deposits are most often seen in he anteromedial portion of the medial segment of the left lobe (Couinard segment IV) and adjacent to the falciform ligament. Location near the gallbladder and portahepatis has also been reported. The subcapsular position of these lesions may result from local hyperperfusion that promotes the local accumulation of triglyceride in affected hepatocytes.

Dysplastic nodules

The discovery of regenerative and dysplastic lesions within the cirrhotic liver is of concern because of the association of these lesions with HCC. Microscopic foci of small cell dysplasia, characterized by nuclear crowding, nuclear polymorphism, and an increased nucleocytoplasmic ratio precede the development of low-grade and high-grade dysplastic nodules. The presence of high-grade dysplasia in the original dysplastic nodule is an independent predictor of eventual hepatocellular malignancy.

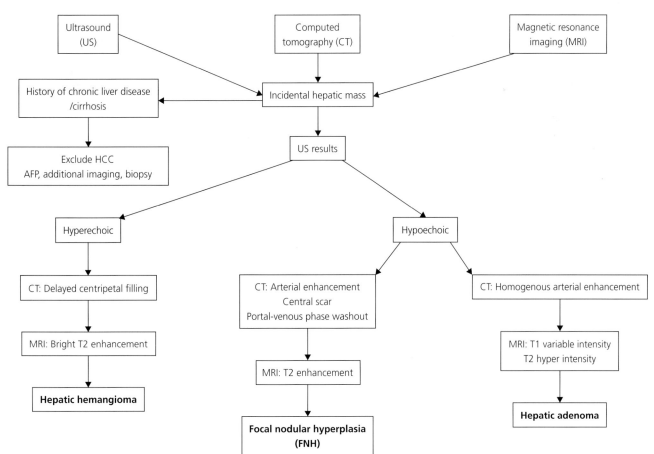

Figure 13.1 Clinical approach to the patient with a liver mass. AFP, α-fetoprotein; FNH, focal nodular hyperplasia; HCC, hepatocellular carcinoma.

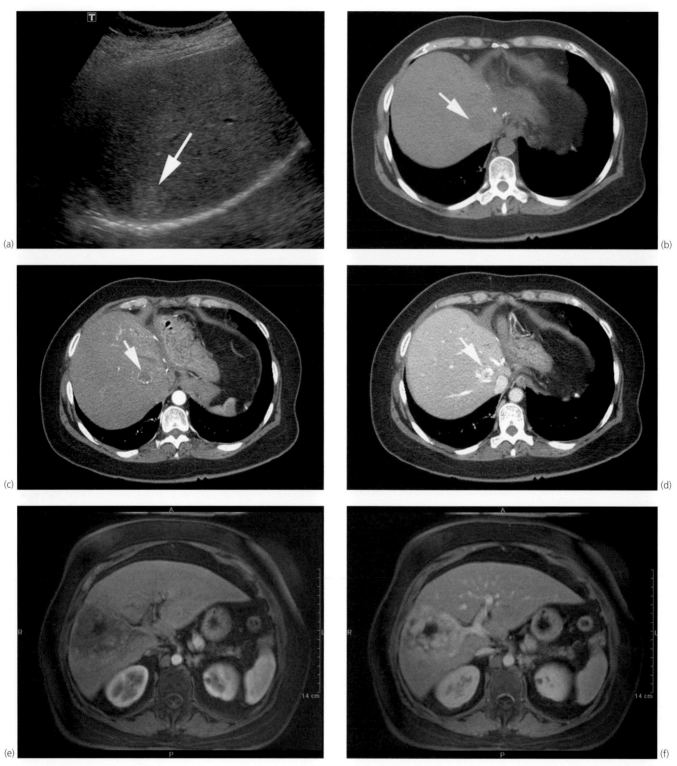

Figure 13.2 (a) Typical hyperechoic ultrasound appearance of a hepatic hemangioma (arrow) located in the posterior right lobe of liver adjacent to the diaphragm. Hepatic hemangioma in a 42-year-old woman after a previous left hepatic resection. Multiphase CT scanning images **(b)** include a well-defined, low density lesion in the medial right lobe of the liver seen on unenhanced images. Contrast enhanced arterial phase imaging **(c)** of the same lesion causes intense peripheral and nodular enhancement (arrow). Portal venous phase image **(d)** demonstrates delayed centripetal enhancement and accentuation of peripheral nodularity (arrow). Large hemangioma in an asymptomatic 48-year-old woman. MRI with contrast including arterial, portal venous and delayed sequences. Arterial imaging **(e)** shows a large, well-defined, heterogeneous, enhancing mass in the right hepatic lobe. The central, nonenhancing, region represents a scar or thrombosis. Portal venous phase imaging **(f)** shows peripheral nodular enhancement typical of a hepatic hemangioma. (*Continued on next page.*)

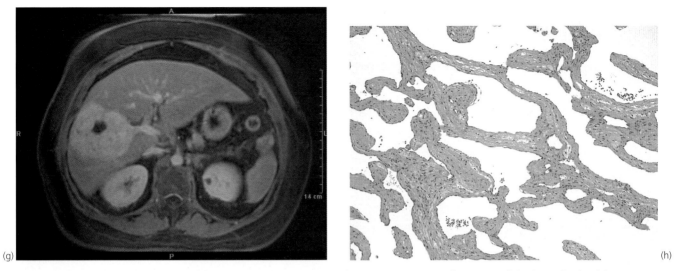

(g)

(h)

Figure 13.2 *Continued* Delayed imaging **(g)** demonstrates homogeneous enhancement, except centrally. In contradistinction to focal nodular hyperplasia this scar does not enhance. Microscopy of a cavernous hemangioma **(h)** shows enlarged vascular spaces with thick fibrous septa lined by flattened endothelial cells.

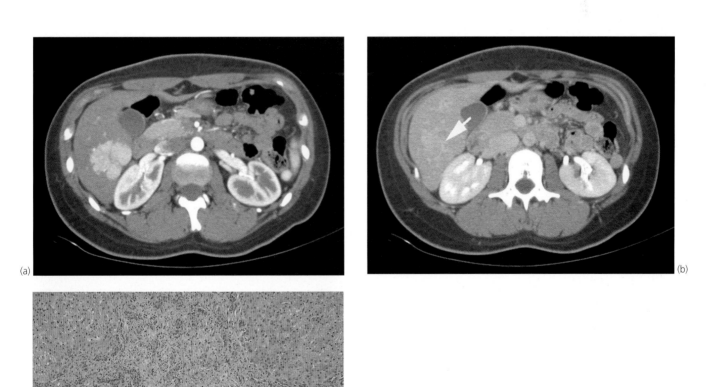

(a)

(b)

(c)

Figure 13.3 Focal nodular hyperplasia (FNH). Arterial and delayed phase axial CT imaging. **(a)** Arterial phase CT shows an intensely enhancing nodular mass with a central, nonenhancing scar. **(b)** Delayed imaging at three minutes shows the mass to have become isointense to the surrounding liver but demonstrates subtle enhancement of the central scar (arrow) that is unique to focal nodular hyperplasia. **(c)** The radiating fibrous septa within the center of the tumor shows a mild lymphocytic infiltrate. Numerous atypical ductules are present toward the border of the fibrous septa and the adjacent parenchyma composed of cytological benign hepatocytes.

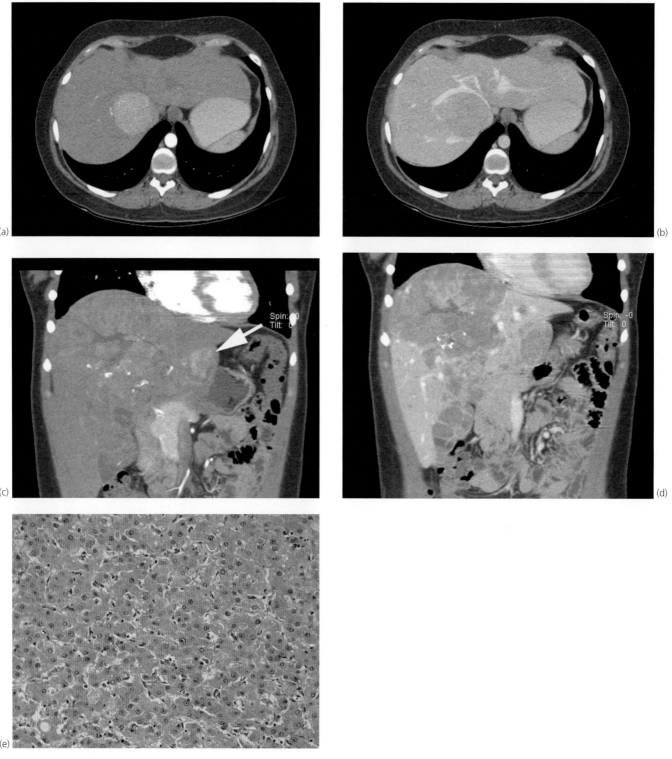

Figure 13.4 Hepatic adenoma. Axial arterial **(a)** and portal venous **(b)** phase CT imaging. Arterial phase imaging demonstrates a homogeneous, well-defined, intensely enhancing mass in the posterior segment of the right lobe of the liver. In the portal venous phase (b), this adenoma is isodense to the normal liver. The middle hepatic vein is displaced anteriorly. Hepatic adenomatosis in a 28-year-old female with a previous embolization procedure for hemorrhage. Coronal CT images in the arterial **(c)** and portal venous **(d)** phases. Arterial imaging demonstrates a large, inhomogeneous, enhancing mass beneath the dome of the right lobe of liver. Punctate high densities are from the previous embolization. A second smaller mass located in lateral portion of the lateral segment of the left lobe demonstrates intense enhancement (arrow). Several less well-defined, non-enhancing masses are also identified in the inferior right lobe. On portal venous phase imaging (d) the large lesion beneath the dome is hypodense when compared with the remaining liver. Note the presence of a large central scar in this adenoma, which is more often associated with FNH but may be seen in other benign lesions. Numerous additional low-density lesions are seen throughout the liver. **(e)** The liver cells of the hepatic adenoma show a normal nuclear–cytoplasmic ratio. Hepatic chords are one to two cells thick and lined by endothelial cells.

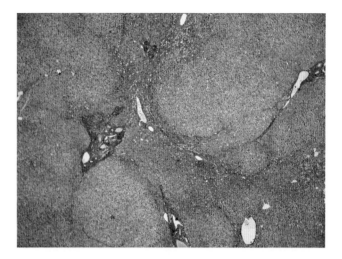

Figure 13.5 Nodular regenerative hyperplasia (trichrome stain). Low power shows irregular bulging nodules composed of regenerating hepatocytes. The portal tracts show only mild fibrosis, without evidence of bridging fibrous septa formation seen in cirrhotic nodules.

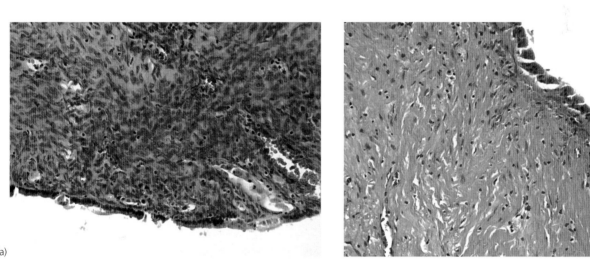

(a)
(b)

Figure 13.6 Hepatobiliary cystadenoma with mesenchymal stroma **(a)**. The cyst wall on high power shows prominent hypercellular mesenchymal spindle cells. The cyst wall is lined by a single layer of benign cuboidal duct epithelium. Hepatobiliary cystadenoma without mesenchymal stroma **(b)**. In contrast with (a) the cyst wall is composed of a fibrovascular stroma without any spindle mesenchymal cells. The cyst wall similarly is composed of a single layer of benign cuboidal duct epithelium.

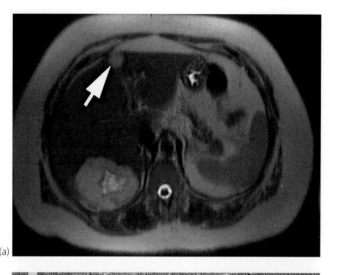
(a)

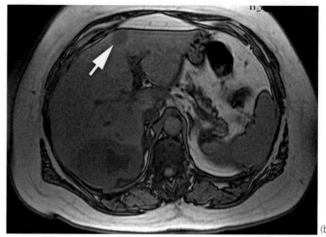
(b)

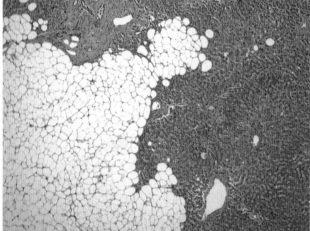
(c)

Figure 13.7 Focal fatty change. Location of this focal fatty lesion adjacent to the falciform ligament is typical. Axial T2 and in-phase MRI imaging. **(a)** A T2 sequence demonstrates a 1.5-cm high signal intensity lesion (arrow). **(b)** In-phase imaging shows a drop in signal intensity (arrow) confirming the presence of fat. The large lesion in the posterior right lobe of the liver was proven to represent a hemangioma with contrast imaging. Focal fatty change **(c)**. Low power demonstrates a large group of well-demarcated hepatocytes with prominent macrovesicular fatty change. In contrast to a benign liver cell adenoma containing fat, a normal hepatic architecture with small normal portal tracts is preserved.

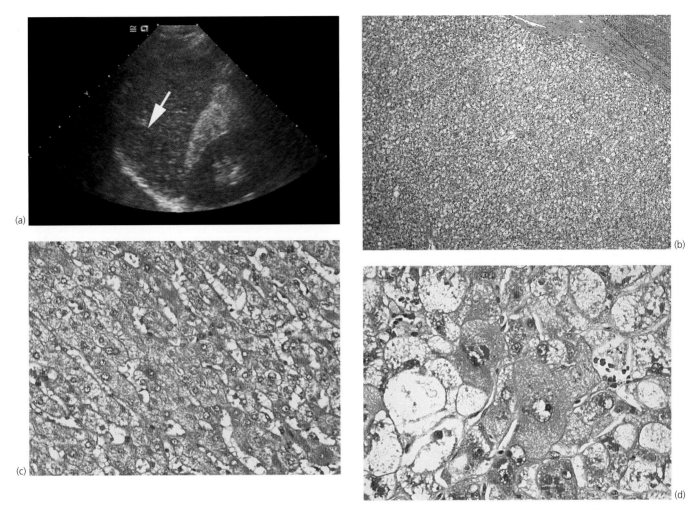

Figure 13.8 Regenerating nodule **(a)**. Ultrasound image of a right liver lobe mass with mixed echogenicity. Without contrast, ultrasound is nonspecific with regard to benign versus malignant masses in cirrhosis. Ultrasound-guided biopsy proved this lesion to be a regenerating nodule. Macroregenerative nodule **(b)**. A bulging regenerative nodule is seen on low power. The hepatocytes are more hydropic than the liver cells in the adjacent nodule which is smaller (upper right corner of the field). Macroregenerative nodule **(c)**. High power shows cytological benign hepatocytes forming cords no greater than two cells thick. Macroregenerative dysplastic nodule **(d)**. This high power image shows liver cells with ample cytoplasm and enlarged nuclei having prominent nucleoli. Some of the cells contain Mallory bodies (large cell dysplasia). Although difficult to fully appreciate on this hematoxylin–eosin stained specimen, the hepatic cords are no greater than two cells thick; a feature better depicted by a reticulin stain.

14

Esophagus: anatomy and developmental and structural anomalies

Ikuo Hirano

The majority of developmental and structural anomalies covered in this chapter are important although infrequently encountered. Certain entities, including esophageal heterotopic gastric mucosa (inlet patch) and Schatzki rings, are prevalent but only occasionally produce clinical manifestations. With the widespread use of upper endoscopy, recognition and understanding of both common and uncommon esophageal pathology is of relevance to clinical care. Esophageal biopsies obtained during endoscopy sample the squamous mucosa and only occasionally the submucosa that contains the lamina propria and muscularis mucosa. The histological evaluation of submucosal glands, Meissner and myenteric ganglia, and the muscularis propria depicted in Fig. 14.1 requires surgical biopsy. Endoscopic ultrasonography can evaluate the structural integrity and anomalies of these deeper structures. Extrinsic compression of the esophagus by adjacent mediastinal structures as shown in Fig. 14.2 is better appreciated on radiographic barium examination than endoscopy. Feline esophagus is depicted in Fig. 14.3 and can be mistaken for eosinophilic esophagitis. This is a transient phenomenon visualized with retching and may represent contraction of the muscularis mucosa.

Esophageal developmental anomalies include vascular lesions, duplications, and heterotopic gastric mucosa. Kartagener syndrome leads to right-sided rather than left-sided aortic arch esophageal compression (Fig. 14.4). Patients with dysphagia lusoria present with swallowing difficulties arising from extrinsic compression of the thoracic esophagus by an aberrant take-off of the right subclavian artery from the left side of the aortic arch (Fig. 14.5). Congenital venous malformations illustrated in Fig. 14.6 represent another vascular anomaly and are distinct from esophageal varices, as vascular obstruction and portal hypertension are not present in the former. Congenital esophageal duplications assume both tubular (Fig. 14.7) and cystic (Figs 14.8 and 14.9) forms. Although most are apparent before the age of 1 year, 25% can present in adults with symptoms of dysphagia. Heterotopic gastric mucosa (inlet patch), shown in Fig. 14.10, is a common congenital anomaly and has a prevalence of 4%

based on an autopsy series. Infrequently, this anomaly can lead to proximal esophageal stricture formation (Fig. 14.11) and cervical esophageal web formation (Fig. 14.12). Erosions resulting from acid secretion from heterotopic gastric mucosa could be the basis of some cases of Plummer–Vinson (also known as Paterson–Kelly) syndrome. Other uncommon developmental anomalies include esophageal atresia, congenital esophageal stenosis, and bronchopulmonary foregut malformations.

Structural esophageal anomalies include esophageal rings and webs, cricopharyngeal bar, and pharyngoesophageal and esophageal diverticula. The most widely recognized structural anomaly is the Schatzki ring found in 6%–12% of radiographic studies. It is one of the most common causes of dysphagia and food impaction, although the majority of Schatzki rings are asymptomatic. The inner diameter of the ring is a critical determinant for dysphagia and can be assessed on endoscopic retroflexed view (Fig. 14.13) or ingestion of a barium tablet of known diameter. Esophageal dilation is effective therapy, although recurrent dysphagia is not uncommon with long-term follow-up. A cricopharyngeal bar is found in 5%–19% of radiographic studies of the pharynx. Like Schatzki rings, the majority are not associated with dysphagia. Pathological and physiological studies support shared features between symptomatic cricopharyngeal bars and Zenker diverticula. The patient in Fig. 14.14 has both a cricopharyngeal bar (a) and small diverticulum (b). Therapeutic options of symptomatic cricopharyngeal bars and Zenker diverticula include both endoscopic and surgical approaches. Epiphrenic diverticula arise from the distal esophagus and are commonly associated with an underlying spastic esophageal motility disorder (Fig. 14.15). With time, the diverticula can increase in size resulting in food retention, bezoar formation, and symptoms of regurgitation (Fig. 14.16). Treatment for large or symptomatic epiphrenic diverticula is most commonly surgical and includes not only a diverticulectomy, but also treatment of the underlying motility disorder. Intramural pseudodiverticulosis is a rare finding best appreciated on barium esophagram rather than upper endoscopy as shown in Fig. 14.17. The disorder results from dilation on excretory ducts of submucosal esophageal glands and is associated with proximal esophageal strictures and esophageal candidiasis.

Atlas of Gastroenterology, 4th edition. Edited by Tadataka Yamada, David H. Alpers, Anthony N. Kalloo, Neil Kaplowitz, Chung Owyang, and Don W. Powell. © 2009 Blackwell Publishing, ISBN: 978-1-4051-6909-7

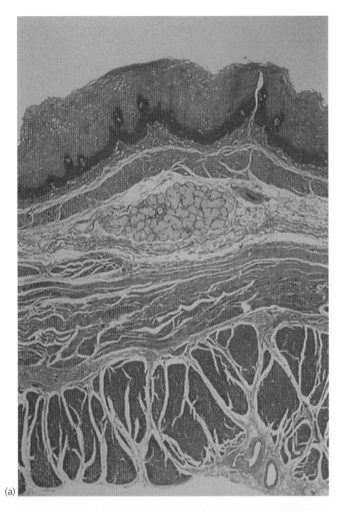

(a)

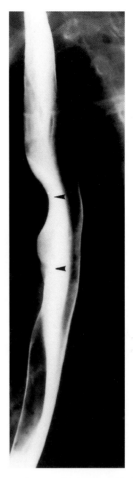

Figure 14.2 Barium esophagram shows normal indentation of the esophageal lumen by the aorta (top arrow) and left mainstem bronchus (bottom arrow).

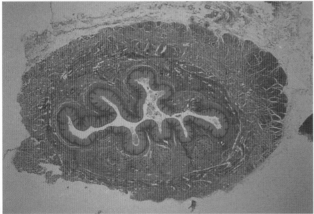

(b)

Figure 14.1 **(a)** Longitudinal section of esophageal wall (× 10). **(b)** This cross-section (× 2.5) from the middle third of the esophagus has a mixture of skeletal and predominantly smooth muscle in the muscularis propria. The submucosal glands are clearly shown. An esophageal cardiac gland in which a small focus of glandular epithelium interrupts the squamous mucosa is a normal finding, seen in at least 1% of all esophagi.

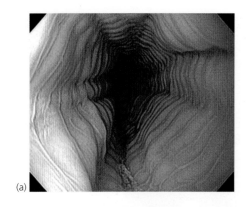
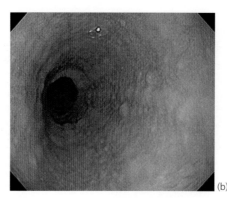

(a)   (b)

Figure 14.3 Feline esophagus **(a)** demonstrating rippling or plications of the esophageal mucosa. This is a transient occurrence and disappears with continued observation as shown in **(b)**. Eosinophilic esophagitis can present with a similar appearance but the rings persist with air insufflation and are less tightly spaced apart.

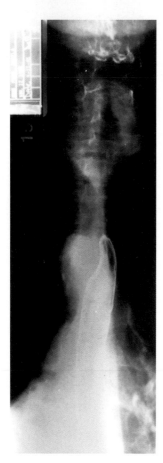

Figure 14.4 Barium esophagram of a patient with Kartagener syndrome, showing esophageal compression by the right-sided aortic arch and dextrocardia.

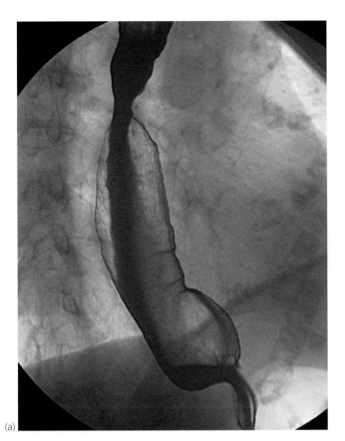

(a)

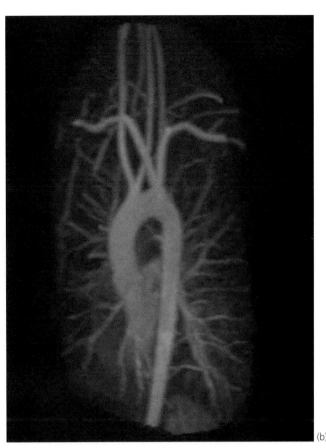

(b)

Figure 14.5 Dysphagia lusoria represents symptomatic esophageal compression by a vascular anomaly of the aortic arch, most commonly by an aberrant right subclavian artery. **(a)** Barium esophagram in a patient reveals thoracic esophageal compression by an aberrant right subclavian artery posterior to the esophagus. **(b)** Magnetic resonance angiography reveals an aberrant right subclavian artery arising from the aortic arch.

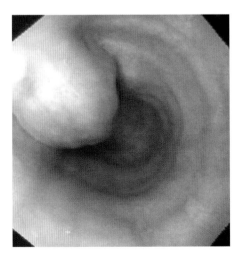

Figure 14.6 Congenital venous malformations as depicted may also be referred to as primary esophageal varices when no secondary cause, such as portal hypertension, can be identified. These venous structures rarely bleed spontaneously. Endosonography confirmed a conglomerate of venous channels in this case.

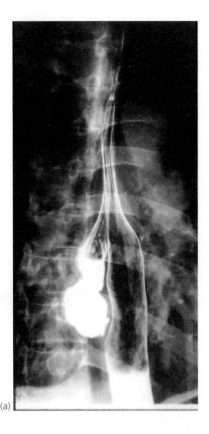

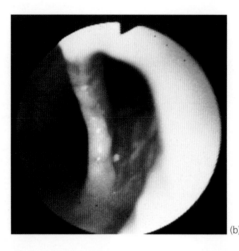

(a)

(b)

Figure 14.7 (a) Radiograph showing a large, congenital, tubular duplication of the esophagus. **(b)** Endoscopic view showing the opening to the tubular duplication (right) and esophageal lumen (left). Congenital esophageal duplications may be tubular or cystic.

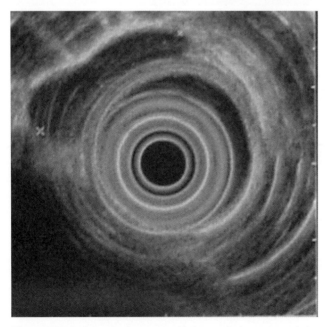

Figure 14.8 Endoscopic ultrasonographic image of a large, congenital esophageal duplication cyst. Duplication cysts are the second most common benign esophageal submucosal lesion, with stromal tumors being more common. Courtesy of Dr Rameez Alasadi.

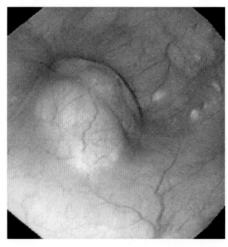

Figure 14.9 Small intramural cysts such as the bilobate type shown here are not symptomatic and are typically identified on barium esophagram or endoscopy for another indication. The cystic nature of the lesion can be confirmed using endoscopic ultrasonography. The differential diagnosis includes submucosal esophageal lesions and esophageal varices.

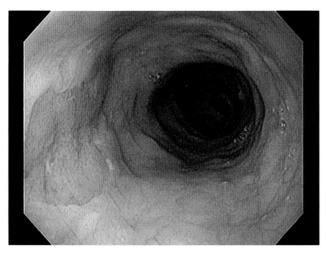

Figure 14.10 Heterotopic gastric mucosa (inlet patch) in the cervical esophagus. The reported prevalence approximates 4%. The lesions can be unifocal as in the case illustrated, multifocal, or circumferential.

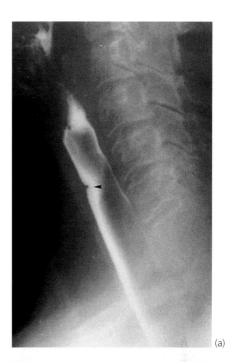

(a)

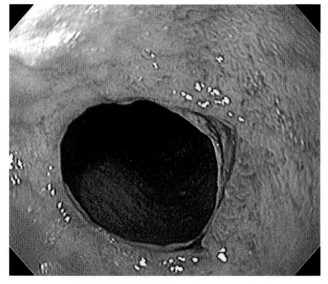

Figure 14.11 A large, circumferential focus of heterotopic gastric mucosa in the cervical esophagus associated with a circumferential mucosal web immediately distally. The web in this case likely represents a form of peptic stricture related to acid secretion from parietal cells within the inlet patch.

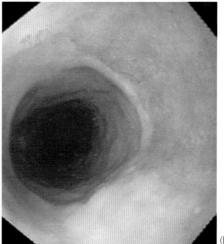

(b)

Figure 14.12 **(a)** Barium contrast radiograph showing a mucosal web in the cervical esophagus, often an incidental finding. **(b)** Corresponding endoscopic view of the cervical web from **(a)** demonstrates a proximal gastric inlet patch with web creating a shelf or lip at the distal aspect of the heterotopic gastric mucosa.

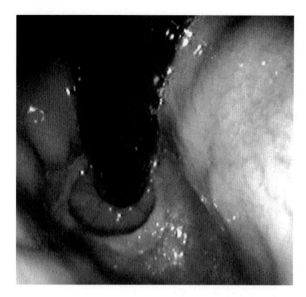

Figure 14.13 Retroflexed endoscopic view of a Schatzki ring. Schatzki rings are almost invariably seen in association with hiatal hernia, as is the case here. The inner ring diameter of a Schatzki ring is an important determinant of whether the ring is associated with dysphagia. The ring diameter can be estimated when viewed from the retroflexed position by referencing the ring to the known diameter of the endoscope.

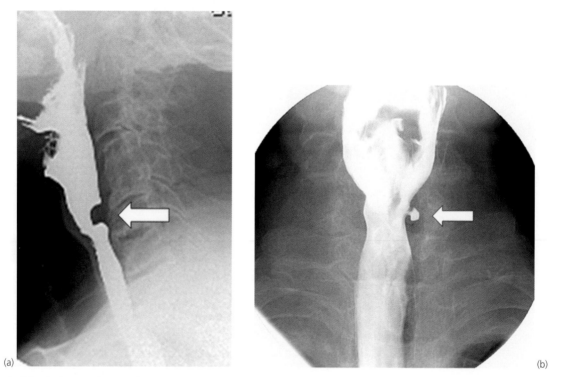

(a)

(b)

Figure 14.14 **(a)** A barium esophagram depicting a cricopharyngeal bar in an elderly patient presenting with dysphagia. The bar is a posterior indentation (arrow) arising from the cricopharyngeus muscle. **(b)** A small Zenker diverticulum (arrow) is seen in the same patient originating from the left lateral aspect of the posterior pharynx in this anteroposterior view. Physiological data links the pathogenesis of Zenker diverticula with increased intralumenal pressure that develops as a result of limited opening of the upper esophageal sphincter.

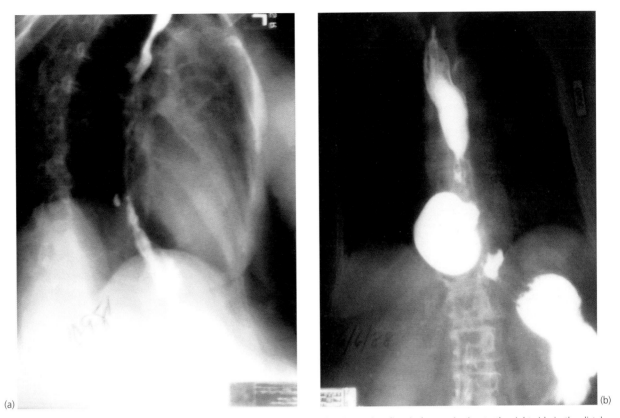

(a) (b)

Figure 14.15 (a) An esophagram of a 75-year-old woman obtained in 1981, showing a tiny diverticulum projecting to the right side in the distal esophagus. **(b)** By 1989, there was a marked increase in the size of the diverticulum and the patient developed symptoms of dysphagia and chest pain.

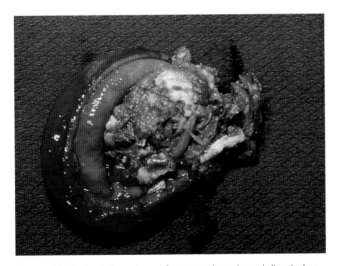

Figure 14.16 Surgical specimen of a resected esophageal diverticulum, which contained a large bezoar. Courtesy of Dr Thomas W. Rice.

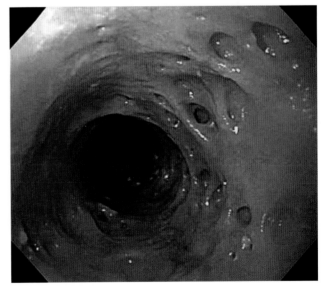

Figure 14.17 Endoscopic view of intramural pseudodiverticulosis with numerous small orifices in the esophageal mucosa. In other cases, the orifices can be punctuate and may be overlooked on endoscopy. Courtesy of Dr C. Prakash Gyawali.

15 Motility disorders of the esophagus

Ikuo Hirano, Peter J. Kahrilas

Dysphagia can be thought of as resulting from propulsive or structural abnormalities. *Propulsive* defects can result from the dysfunction of control mechanisms of the central nervous system, peripheral nerves, myenteric plexus, or intrinsic musculature; *structural* defects may arise from congenital anomalies, neoplasm, caustic injury, surgery, or trauma. In the esophagus, the physiological correlate of dysphagia, unrelated to intrinsic or extrinsic lumenal narrowing, is a peristaltic defect and failure of the propulsive mechanism may be intermittent or continuous. As distal esophageal contraction is mediated by the balance of activity between excitatory and inhibitory myenteric plexus neurons, peristaltic dysfunction may manifest as either simultaneous con-traction and failed lower sphincter relaxation in the case of an inhibitory defect or altered vigor of contractility with an excitatory defect. These defects characterize the major esophageal motor disorders of achalasia and esophageal spasm.

Refinements in the methodology for measuring intralu-menal pressure, advancements in radiological imaging along with improved computer technology have enhanced our understanding of these disorders. This chapter summarizes the pathophysiology, clinical manifestations, and diagnostic studies deemed most important to the evaluation and man-agement of these problems.

Atlas of Gastroenterology, 4th edition. Edited by Tadataka Yamada, David H. Alpers, Anthony N. Kalloo, Neil Kaplowitz, Chung Owyang, and Don W. Powell. © 2009 Blackwell Publishing, ISBN: 978-1-4051-6909-7

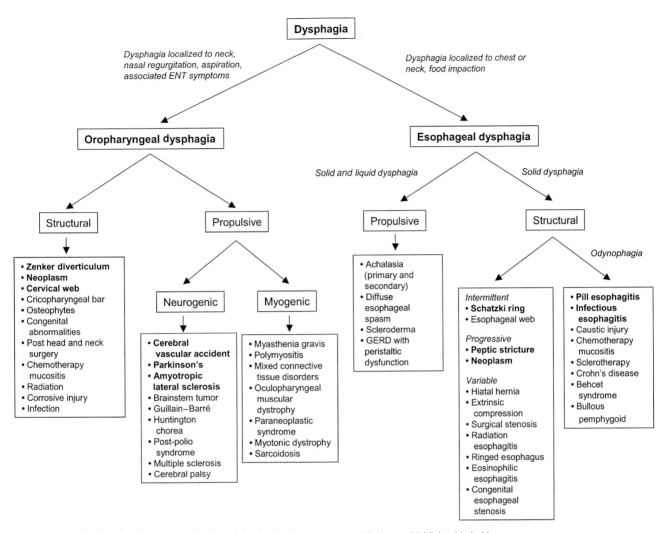

Figure 15.1 Algorithm for the conceptualization of dysphagia. More common etiologies are highlighted in bold.

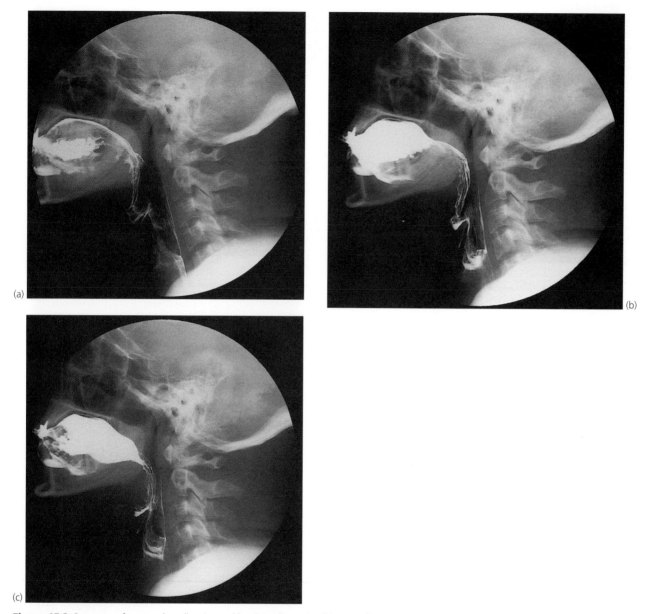

Figure 15.2 Sequence of a normal swallow imaged by cineradiography. **(a)** Preswallow tongue and pharyngeal surface contour is shown prior to administration of bolus. **(b)** With administration of barium, bolus propulsion begins with the loading phase of the tongue and bolus containment via adaptation of the lingual central groove. **(c)** Bolus is propelled into the pharynx with the tongue central groove exhibiting centripetal followed by centrifugal motion. (*Continued on next page.*)

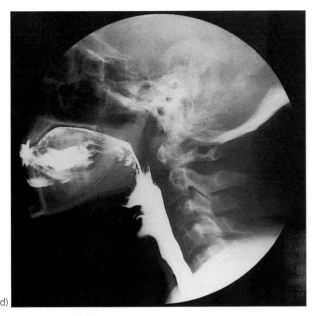

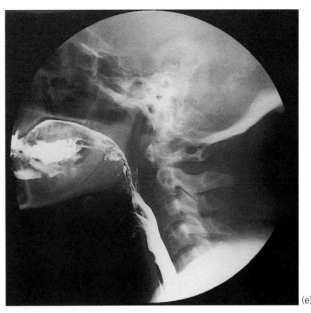

(d)

(e)

Figure 15.2 *Continued* **(d)** Nasopharyngeal closure is achieved by soft palate elevation and apposition to the posterior pharyngeal wall. Airway protection is realized by laryngeal elevation, vocal cord closure and arytenoid tilting. Upper esophageal sphincter (UES) opening occurs via relaxation of the sphincter and anterior hyoid traction with laryngeal elevation. **(e)** Pharyngeal clearance of ingested contents is achieved by profound shortening of the pharynx eliminating bolus access to the larynx and the propagating pharyngeal contraction. Although not shown, once the bolus has passed into the proximal esophagus, the epiglottis returns upright, the larynx reopens and the resting positions are resumed.

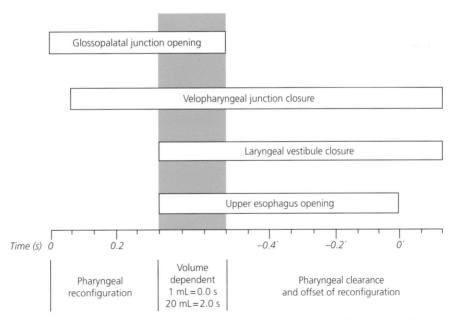

Figure 15.3 Time line showing the coordination and volume-induced modifications in the timing of events within the pharyngeal swallow. The horizontal lines depict the period during which each of the oropharyngeal valves is in its swallow configuration as opposed to its respiratory configuration. Note that events at the onset and offset of pharyngeal reconfiguration bear a fixed time relationship to each other regardless of swallow bolus volume. The stereotypy of these phases is demonstrated by referencing onset events from time 0 and counting forward or referencing offset events from time 0 and counting backward. This timing scheme defines the middle portion of the time line (shaded) as the volume-dependent section, which has a value of 0 s for 1 mL swallows and 0.2 s for 20 mL swallows. Therefore, the alteration in the timing of the swallow response with large volume swallows occurs by prolonging the persistence of pharyngeal reconfiguration without changing the synchrony of events at the onset or offset.

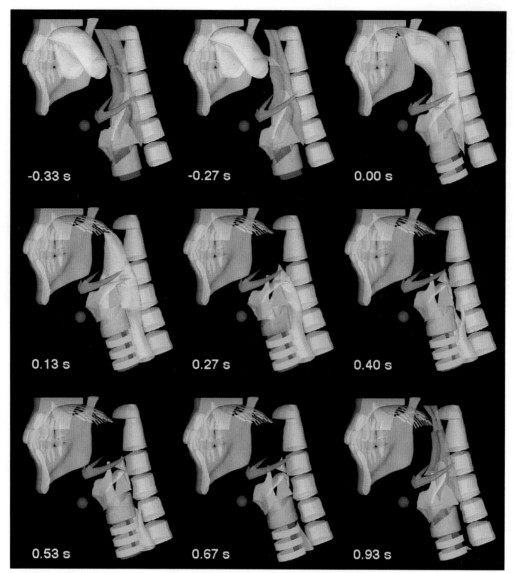

Figure 15.4 Three-dimensional modeling of the oropharynx during swallowing. This figure shows the reconstructions of nine representative pharyngeal configurations during a 10 mL swallow. In each image the bolus chamber is shown in white, the supraglottic airway is blue, the infraglottic airway is purple, the vertebrae are light tan, the hyoid is orange, the epiglottis is yellow, the arytenoid cartilage is dark green, the cricoid cartilage is dark pink, the tracheal rings are light blue, and the hemisected thyroid cartilage is light green. The times next to the images are referenced to the upper esophageal sphincter (UES) opening (time 0.0 s). Many mechanical events are encompassed during the act of deglutition. The preswallow configuration (–0.33 s) is characterized by the bolus chamber being dissociated from the airway by the sealed glossopalatal junction. At the time of velopharyngeal closure (–0.27 s), the nasopharynx is sealed from the bolus chamber by elevation of the soft palate and the bolus chamber expands to include the retrolingual space as the glossopalatal junction opens. The central groove of the tongue blade has deepened and the posterior oral portion of the pharyngeal propulsive chamber is forming. The larynx has begun elevating and the arytenoid is tilting toward the base of the epiglottis. At the instant of UES opening (0.00 s) the laryngeal vestibule has been obliterated by contact of the arytenoid against the epiglottic base. Note that the UES (at the inferior aspect of the cricoid cartilage) has elevated relative to its preswallow position and that the pharyngeal bolus chamber is fully formed. During lingual bolus propulsion (0.13 s), the volume of the bolus chamber is reduced by the centrifugal motion of the tongue surface and bolus expulsion results in full distention of the UES and proximal esophagus. The epiglottis is folded over the arytenoid and there is maximal pharyngeal shortening. The next four reconstructions, early pharyngeal clearance (0.27 s), mid pharyngeal clearance (0.40 s), late pharyngeal clearance (0.53 s), and UES closure (0.67 s), show the caudal progression of the pharyngeal contraction stripping the residua from the oropharynx into the esophagus. Ultimately, with airway reopening (0.93 s) the pharynx commences its return to the respiratory configuration as the larynx descends, the epiglottis flips up and the velopharyngeal junction reopens.

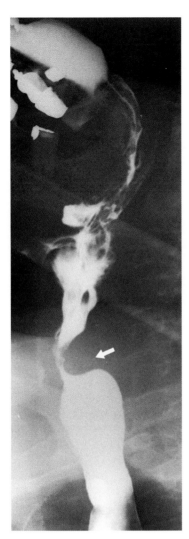

Figure 15.5 Cricopharyngeal bar in a patient with oropharyngeal dysphagia. This term refers to an impingement of the pharyngoesophageal junction seen at the level of cervical vertebra 4 or 5 (arrow) and is caused by a noncompliant cricopharyngeus muscle.

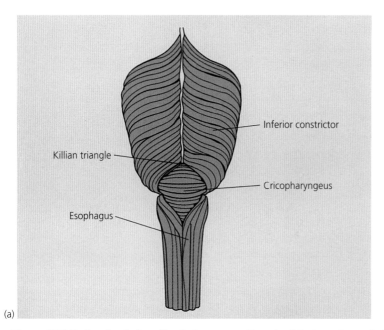

(a)

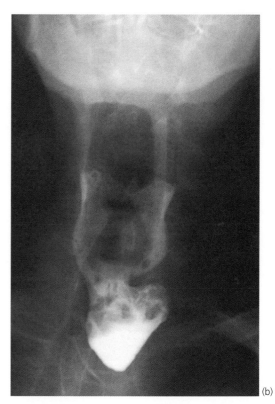

(b)

Figure 15.6 Zenker diverticulum. Diverticula can occur throughout the hypopharynx but when they are located posteriorly between the intersection of the transverse fibers of the cricopharyngeus and obliquely oriented fibers of the inferior pharyngeal constrictors (Killian dehiscence) **(a)** they are called Zenker diverticula **(b)**. Note the barium-filled outpouching of the pharynx.

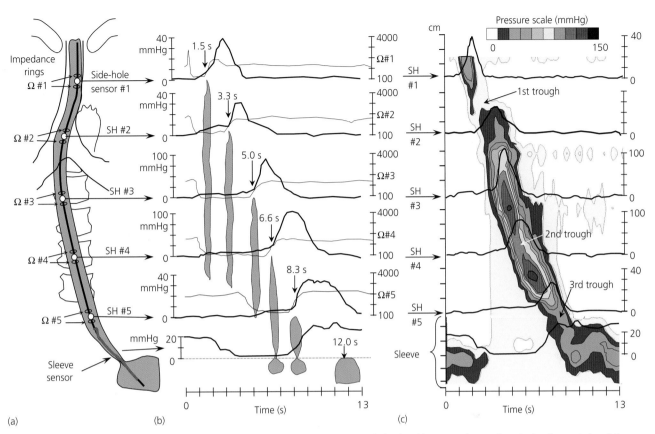

Figure 15.7 Representative physiological data, modified to illustrate the relationship between videofluoroscopic, manometric, impedance, and topographic representations of esophageal peristalsis.

(a) Schematic drawing of placement of a combined manometry/intralumenal impedance monitoring system with five manometric side holes (SH) spaced 4 cm apart and a 6 cm sleeve sensor placed just distal to the last manometric port. The impedance rings (Ω) are also spaced 4 cm apart with the rings straddling the manometric ports. The arrows to panel **(b)** point to the corresponding data tracings obtained from each combined manometry/impedance or sleeve recording site.

(b) Concurrent videofluoroscopic, manometric, and multichannel intralumenal impedance recordings of a 5-mL renograffin swallow that was completely cleared by one peristaltic sequence. Representative tracings from the videofluoroscopic sequence overlayed on the combined manometric/impedance tracing show the distribution of the bolus at the times indicated by the vertical arrows. At each recording site, the thick line intersecting the pressure scale (mmHg) on the left represents the manometric tracing and the fine line intersecting the impedance recording tracing in ohms (Ω) on the right represents the impedance recording tracing. Bolus entry at each combined manometry/impedance recording site is signaled by a subtle increase in pressure (intrabolus pressure) and a greater than 50% decrease in impedance. In this example, the bolus propagates past Ω#4 rapidly, indicated by an abrupt reduction in impedance in Ω#2, Ω#3, and Ω#4 at time 1.5 s. Lumenal closure and hence the tail of the

barium bolus is evident at each recording site by the upstroke of the peristaltic contraction and a 50% increase in recorded impedance. Hence, at 5.0 s, the peristaltic contraction was beginning at SH#3, corresponding to a 50% increase in impedance and the tail of the barium bolus at the same esophageal locus. Finally, after completion of the peristaltic contraction (time 12.0 s), all renograffin was in the stomach.

(c) Comparison of conventional manometry obtained with a sleeve assembly as depicted in (a) and high-fidelity manometry with recording sites at 1-cm intervals displayed topographically as an isocontour plot. The standard manometric recordings are superimposed on the isocontour plot at axial locations corresponding to the equivalent portion of the high fidelity manometry it represents. In the isocontour plot, brighter colors indicate higher pressures revealing four distinct pressure segments separated by three pressure troughs. Physiologically, the first trough is at the junction between striated and smooth muscle, the second is within the smooth muscle segment, and the third separates the peristaltic segment from the lower esophageal sphincter (LES). Note that LES relaxation is reliably recorded using either methodology, albeit somewhat differently. From the illustration one can see that the end of LES relaxation measured by the sleeve coincides with the peristaltic contraction contacting the proximal portion of the sleeve. In addition to measuring mean residual pressure, topographic analysis allows for more precise measurement of the transphincteric pressure gradient. Isocontour tracing courtesy of Ray Clouse.

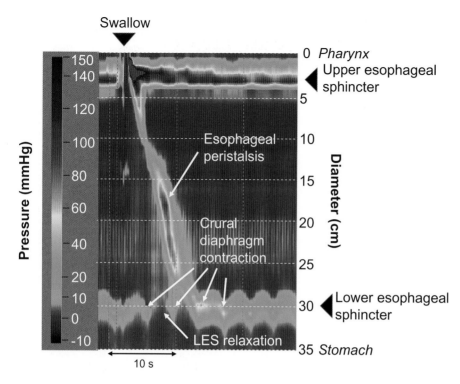

Swallow

Pressure (mmHg)

150
140
120
100
80
60
40
20
10
0
-10

Diameter (cm)

0 *Pharynx*
◀ Upper esophageal sphincter

5

Esophageal peristalsis

10

15

Crural diaphragm contraction

20

25

◀ Lower esophageal sphincter

30

LES relaxation

35 *Stomach*

10 s

Figure 15.8 High-resolution esophageal manometric recording during a water swallow. The recording was obtained using a manometric assembly incorporating 36 circumferential solid state pressure transducers spaced 1 cm apart and spans the entire length from the pharynx to the stomach. Again, note the segmental nature of esophageal peristalsis. Also note that crural diaphragm contraction is clearly evident as being superimposed on the lower esophageal sphincter (LES) and continues uninterrupted throughout the LES relaxation period.

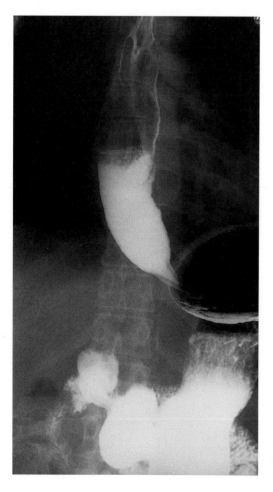

Figure 15.9 Barium esophagram in an untreated patient with achalasia. Note the classical radiological features of a dilated esophagus, retained barium and an intralumenal air fluid level with smooth tapering of the esophagogastric junction.

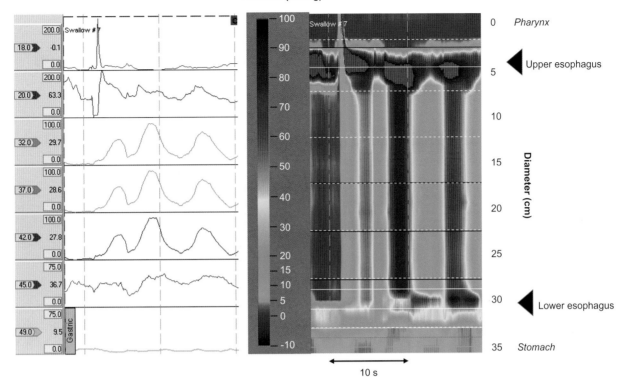

Figure 15.10 Esophageal manometric recording in a patient with achalasia. The left panel depicts a standard, seven-channel recording with sensors positioned in the pharynx, upper esophageal sphincter (UES), esophageal body (three sensors), lower esophageal sphincter (LES), and stomach. The three middle sensors recording activity within the distal esophageal body demonstrate isobaric wave forms contained within a "common cavity" sealed from above and below by higher amplitude, lumen-obliterating contractions of the upper and lower esophageal sphincters. The lower esophageal sphincter shows failed deglutitive relaxation. The right panel demonstrates a high-resolution esophageal manometry recording of the same water swallow. Within the esophageal body, the common cavity pressurization phenomena can be clearly visualized as three isobaric bars with coincident high amplitude contraction of the UES. Failed deglutitive relaxation of the lower esophageal sphincter is evident as is the development of an increased esophageal gastric pressure gradient.

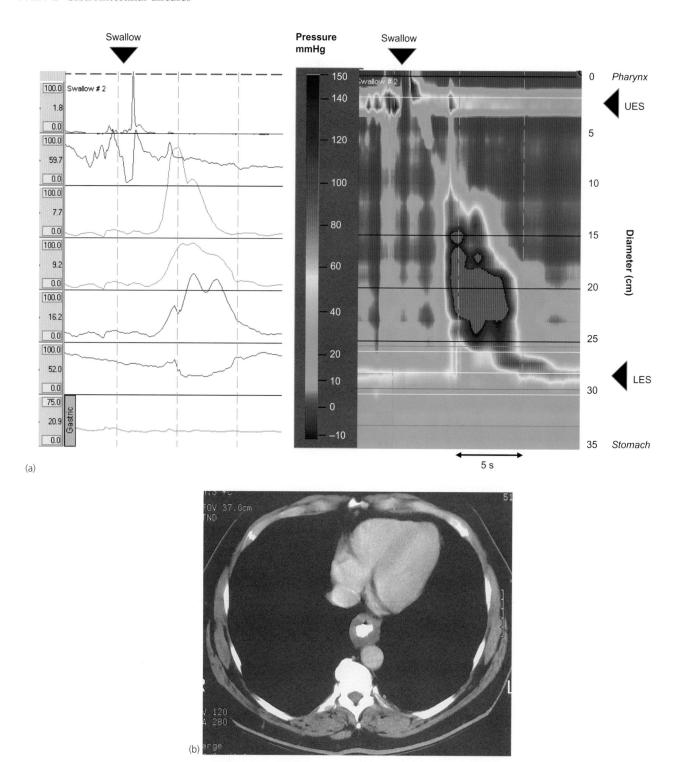

(a)

(b)

Figure 15.11 (a) Esophageal manometric recording in a patient with vigorous achalasia. The left panel shows a seven-channel line tracing in which simultaneous high-amplitude contractions (>100 mmHg) of varied morphology are evident. The basal lower esophageal sphincter (LES) pressure is 60 mmHg relative to intragastric pressure and shows minimal deglutitive relaxation. The corresponding high-resolution manometry depicts the same phenomena with bizarre morphology of the esophageal contractile activity apparent within the distal esophagus and paucity of activity within the proximal esophagus. An increased intrabolus pressure is evident proximal to the nonrelaxing LES. **(b)** Thoracic CT scan on a patient with vigorous achalasia demonstrating marked thickening of the distal esophageal wall. The esophageal lumen is not dilated although it is filled with contrast material.

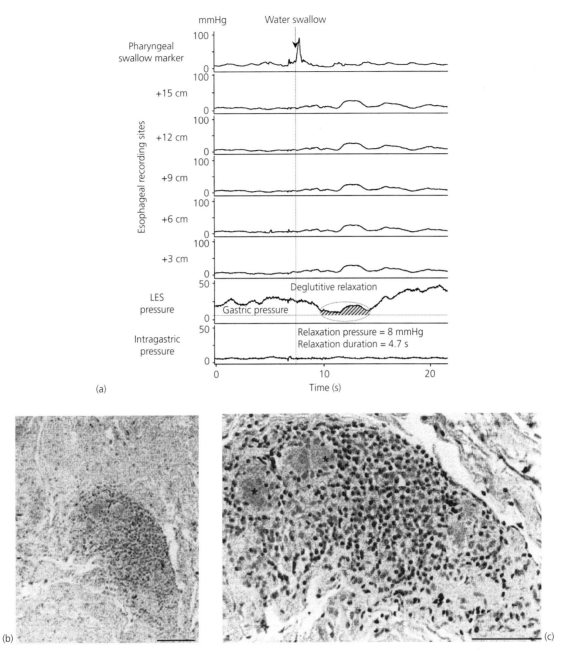

(a)

Figure 15.12 (a) Recording from a patient with a manometric variant of idiopathic achalasia. The recording demonstrates complete esophageal aperistalsis that is typical for classic achalasia. Atypical, however, is the finding of preserved deglutitive relaxation following a water swallow. The relaxation lower esophageal sphincter (LES) pressure was 8 mmHg. **(b)** Histological sections of the myenteric plexus of the patient whose manometric recording is illustrated in (a). Low (b) and high **(c)** power views of a myenteric ganglion showing nitric oxide synthase (NOS)-immunoreactive neurons (*). Numerous lymphocytes infiltrate this region suggesting ongoing chronic inflammatory activity of the myenteric plexus. Such inflammation may lead to the eventual destruction of the myenteric neurons that characterizes the pathophysiology of achalasia.

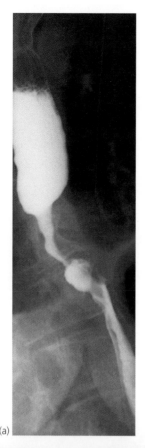

(a)

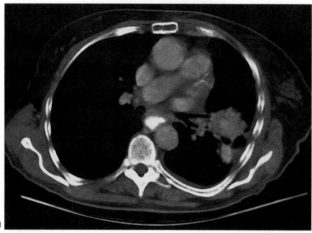

(b)

Figure 15.13 (a) Pseudo- or secondary achalasia. The tapering in the distal esophagus makes this barium esophagram difficult to distinguish from idiopathic achalasia. Note the dilated esophagus with intralumenal air fluid level. **(b)** Abdominal CT scan image in a patient with pseudo- or secondary achalasia. This CT image demonstrates a stellate pulmonary mass originating in the left lung invading the gastroesophageal junction.

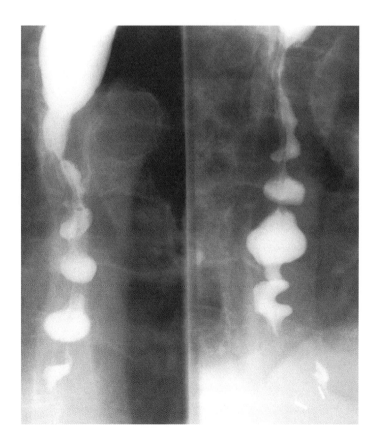

Figure 15.14 Simultaneous manometry and fluoroscopy showing minimal esophageal volume clearance with failed peristalsis and simultaneous contractions. As described in Figure 15.7, the tracings from the video images of the fluoroscopic sequence on the right show the distribution of the barium column at times indicated on the individual tracings and by arrows on the manometric recording. Pharyngeal injection of barium into the esophagus occurs at 3.4 s. Following this, esophageal peristalsis is initiated. At 7.0 s, the peristaltic contraction has stripped the barium from the esophagus proximal to that point. However, at 9.3 s, there is failed peristalsis and simultaneous contraction at the three distal sites. This results in impaired esophageal volume clearance and the appearance of retained barium at multiple locations in the esophagus that remain at 13.8 s. LES, lower esophageal sphincter; UES, upper esophageal sphincter.

Figure 15.15 Barium esophagram demonstrating esophageal spasm. The corkscrew appearance results from simultaneous nonpropulsive contractions of the esophagus occurring at multiple levels.

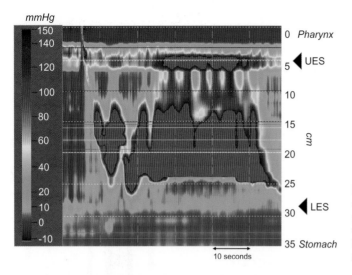

Figure 15.16 Manometric recording in a patient with diffuse esophageal spasm. The recording demonstrates high amplitude, prolonged duration esophageal contractions in the distal esophagus with lower esophageal sphincter (LES) hypotension. The esophageal body pressures in this patient are depicted off scale but were in excess of 500 mmHg.

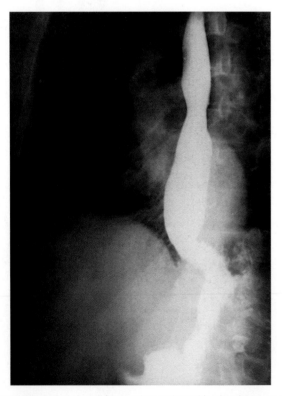

Figure 15.17 Barium esophogram in a patient with scleroderma. Note the dilated atonic esophagus yet patulous gastroesophageal junction.

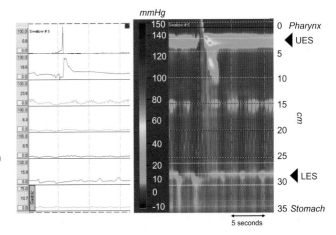

Figure 15.18 Manometric recording demonstrating a scleroderma pattern of esophageal contractility. The basal lower esophageal sphincter (LES) pressure is hypotonic and approximates intragastric pressure. There is a small focus of peristaltic activity visible for a few centimeters distal to the upper esophageal sphincter in response to a water swallow. Subsequent to this, no esophageal activity is apparent.

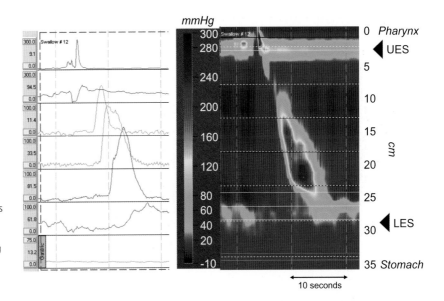

Figure 15.19 Esophageal manometry in a patient with "Nutcracker Esophagus." The recording depicts peristaltic esophageal contractions in response to a water swallow. The amplitudes of the esophageal contractions in channels 4 and 5 exceed 200 mmHg and are of mildly prolonged duration. The lower esophageal sphincter is normotensive and shows complete deglutitive relaxation.

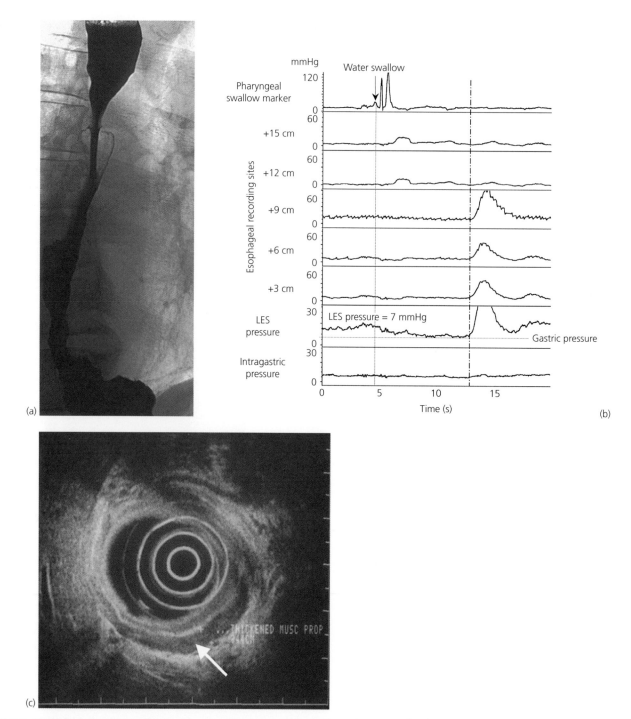

(a)

(b)

(c)

Figure 15.20 **(a)** Eosinophilic esophagitis. Barium swallow from an elderly patient who presented with progressive dysphagia. The radiograph depicts a mid-esophageal stricture with proximal dilation. A small amount of barium flows through the stenosis. **(b)** Esophageal manometry showing a hypotensive lower esophageal sphincter pressure and simultaneous contractions throughout the esophageal body. **(c)** Endoscopic ultrasound demonstrating diffuse, asymmetric thickening of muscularis propria of the esophagus. (*Continued on next page.*)

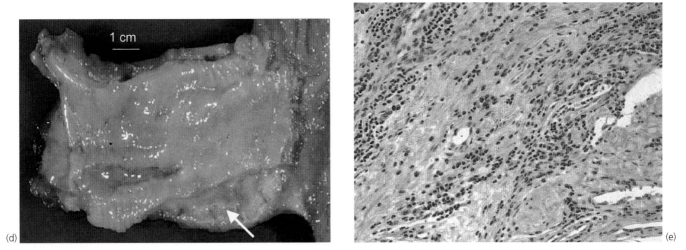

(d)

(e)

Figure 15.20 *Continued* **(d)** Surgical specimen depicting esophageal muscular hypertrophy. **(e)** Histopathology showing eosinophilic infiltration into the esophageal muscularis propria (H & E stain. original magnification ×100).

16 Gastroesophageal reflux disease

Joel E. Richter

Gastroesophageal reflux disease (GERD) is due to the failure of the normal antireflux mechanism to protect against frequent and abnormal amounts of gastroesophageal reflux; that is, the effortless movement of gastric contents from the stomach into the esophagus. Gastroesophageal reflux disease is a common problem. In a survey from Olmsted County Minnesota, the prevalence of heartburn and acid regurgitation in the past 12 months was 42% and 45%, respectively. Frequent symptoms (at least weekly) were reported by 20% of the respondents, with an equal gender distribution across all ages (Fig. 16.1).

The pathophysiology of GERD is complex. It results from an imbalance between *defensive factors* protecting the esophagus, including the antireflux barrier (Fig. 16.2), particularly the lower esophageal sphincter, hiatal hernia, lumenal clearance mechanisms (gravity, peristalsis, salivary bicarbonate) and tissue resistance, and *aggressive factors* from the stomach contents, including gastric acidity, volume, and duodenal contents (Fig. 16.3 and Table 16.1).

Gastroesophageal reflux disease (GERD) is recognized clinically by the development of classical symptoms of heartburn or acid regurgitation. Less common symptoms include dysphagia, water brash, odynophagia, burping, hiccups, nausea, and vomiting. Extraesophageal manifestations of GERD include chest pain, and pulmonary and ear, nose, and throat complaints. These latter symptoms result from either a vagally mediated reflex between the esophagus and bronchopulmonary tree or from microaspiration of acid (Fig. 16.4).

Multiple tests are available for evaluating the patient with suspected GERD or its complications. Upper endoscopy is the most sensitive and specific test in assessing tissue injury from reflux esophagitis (Fig. 16.5). It is the best test for identifying reflux esophagitis (Fig. 16.6), peptic stricture (Fig. 16.7),

Barrett esophagus (Fig. 16.8), or Barrett esophagus with associated adenocarcinoma (Fig. 16.9). Biopsies from the esophagus can help to confirm the presence of esophagitis (Fig. 16.10), especially when there is no erosive disease, and are required to make the diagnosis of specialized intestinal metaplasia that is characteristic of Barrett esophagus (Fig. 16.11). The barium esophagram helps in the evaluation of reflux patients with dysphagia. Good distention of the distal esophagus will bring out subtle strictures and rings (Fig. 16.12). Prolonged esophageal pH monitoring is helpful before antireflux surgery and among patients with difficult-to-manage typical or extraesophageal symptoms in whom the endoscopy is normal (Table 16.2).

The treatment of GERD involves the relief of symptoms, healing of esophagitis, and the prevention of relapses and complications. Lifestyle modifications are especially helpful in patients with mild symptoms or nocturnal complaints (Table 16.3). Patients with symptoms and no esophagitis can be treated with over-the-counter antacids, Gaviscon, histamine-2 receptor antagonists (H_2RAs), or prokinetic drugs. Patients with severe symptoms, esophagitis, or complications will need proton pump inhibitor (PPI) therapy or should be considered for antireflux surgery (Table 16.4).

Eosinophilic esophagitis is an increasingly common diagnosis; patients are usually young men, who present with a history of intermittent solid food dysphagia and who often have a history of food impaction. Many have associated asthma or food allergies, especially for milk, eggs, soy, melons, or peanuts. The diagnosis is suspected by the endoscopic findings of multiple rings (Fig. 16.13), longitudinal furrows, or pinpoint white exudates (Fig. 16.14). Esophageal biopsies of the proximal and distal esophagus should be undertaken, where histology will show basal cell hyperplasia and prolongation of rete pegs at lower power and hypereosinophilia at high power with >15–20 eosinophils per high-powered field (Fig. 16.15). The pathogenesis of eosinophilic esophagitis is unknown. Some suggest it is precipitated by foods and aeroallergens that stimulate a Th2 cytokine response, while other data suggest some patients have an

Atlas of Gastroenterology, 4th edition. Edited by Tadataka Yamada, David H. Alpers, Anthony N. Kalloo, Neil Kaplowitz, Chung Owyang, and Don W. Powell. © 2009 Blackwell Publishing, ISBN: 978-1-4051-6909-7

atypical variant of GERD. Eosinophils and symptoms will improve with oral or inhaled steroids or montelukast, a leukotriene D_4 antagonist. Patients with dysphagia and multiple rings may respond well to PPIs with careful bougie dilation. In this situation, some patients may experience a painful mucosal tear into the muscle, and sometimes will require narcotic pain relief as a result (Fig. 16.16). True perforations are rare. The natural history of eosinophils is poorly understood but has not been associated with esophageal cancer.

Table 16.1 Components of tissue resistance against acid injury to the esophagus

Preepithelial defenses
Mucous layer
Unstirred water layer
Surface bicarbonate ion concentration

Epithelial defenses
Structures
   Cell membrane
   Intercellular junctional complexes (tight junctions, glycoconjugates, or lipid)
Functions
   Epithelial transport
      Na^+/H^+ exchanger
      Na^+-dependent Cl^-/HCO_3^- exchanger
   Intracellular buffers
   Cell replication
Postepithelial defenses
   Blood flow
   Tissue acid–base status

From Orlando RC. Esophageal epithelial defenses against acid injury. Am J Gastroenterol 1994;89:S48.

Table 16.2 Guidelines for the clinical use of esophageal pH monitoring

Definite indications
To document abnormal esophageal acid exposure in an endoscopy-negative patient prior to antireflux surgery
To evaluate patients after antireflux surgery who are suspected of having persistent or recurring reflux symptoms
To evaluate patients with either normal or equivocal endoscopic findings and reflux symptoms refractory to PPIs

Possible indications
To evaluate patients for suspected extraesophageal symptoms of GERD

Not indicated
To detect or verify reflux esophagitis, which is best done using endoscopy with biopsies

GERD, gastroesophageal reflux disease; PPI, proton pump inhibitor. From Kahrilas PJ, Quigley EMM. Clinical esophageal pH recording: a technical review of practice guideline development. Gastroenterology 1996;110:1982.

Table 16.3 Lifestyle factors aggravating gastroesophageal reflux disease and their proposed mechanisms for heartburn

Lower LES pressure	Direct mucosal irritant	Increased intraabdominal pressure	Others
Certain foods	Certain foods	Bending over	Supine position
Fats	Citrus products	Lifting	Lying on right side
Sugar	Tomato-based products	Straining at stool	Red wine
Chocolate	Spicy foods	Exercising	Emotions
Onions	Coffee		
Carminatives	Tea		
Coffee	Cola drinks		
Alcohol	Medications		
Cigarettes	Aspirin		
Medications	NSAIDs		
Progesterone	Tetracycline		
Theophylline	Quinidine		
Anticholinergics	Aldreonates		
Diazepam	Potassium tablets		
Nitrates	Iron salts		
Calcium channel blockers			

GERD, gastroesophageal reflux disease; LES, lower esophageal sphincter; NSAIDs, nonsteroidal antiinflammatory drugs.

Table 16.4 Drug therapy for gastroesophageal reflux disease

Drugs	Dose	Mechanism of action
Antacids: liquid		
(e.g., Mylanta, Maalox, Riopan) Increase LESP	15 mL q.i.d. 1 and 3 h p.c., q.h.s. or p.r.n.	Buffers acid
Gaviscon	2–4 tablets q.i.d q.h.s. or p.r.n.	Viscous mechanical barrier Buffer HCl in esophagus
Prokinetics		
Bethanechol (Urecholine)	25 mg q.i.d. a.c. and q.h.s.	Increase LESP and acid clearance
Metoclopramide (Reglan)	10 mg q.i.d. a.c. and q.h.s.	Increase LESP Increase gastric emptying
H₂ receptor antagonists		
Cimetidine (Tagamet)	OTC: 200 mg p.r.n. Prescription dose: 800 b.i.d. or 400 q.i.d.	Decrease acid secretion and volume by inhibiting H_2 receptor
Ranitidine (Zantac)	OTC: 75 mg p.r.n. Prescription dose: 150 mg b.i.d. or q.i.d. Maintenance dose: 150 mg b.i.d.	Same
Famotidine (Pepcid)	OTC: 10 mg p.r.n. Prescription dose: 20 to 40 mg b.i.d.	Same
Nizatidine (Axid)	OTC: 75 mg p.r.n. Prescription dose: 150 mg b.i.d.	Same
Proton pump inhibitors[a]		
Omeprazole (Prilosec)	Acute: 20 mg q.d. in Am Maintenance: 20 mg q.d.	Blocks H^+,K^+-ATPase pump for HCl secretion
Lansoprazole (Prevacid)	Acute: 30 mg q.d. in Am Maintenance: 15 mg q.d.	Same Same
Rabeprazole (Aciphex)	Acute: 20 mg q.d. in Am Maintenance: 20 mg q.d.	Same Same
Pantoprazole (Protonix)	Acute: 40 mg q.d. in Am Maintenance: 20 mg q.d. IV: 40 mg q.d.	Same Same
Esomeprazole (Nexium)	Acute: 40 mg q.d. in Am Maintenance: 20 mg q.d.	Same Same

a For empiric trials of proton pump inhibitor therapy, higher, usually b.i.d., doses are used. The foregoing doses are those used in drug studies and the routine treatment of patients acutely (over 8–12 weeks) or for maintenance (long-term) therapy.
a.c., before meals; Am, the morning before breakfast; LESP, lower esophageal sphincter pressure; OTC, over the counter; p.c., after meals; p.r.n., as needed; q.h.s., at every bedtime.

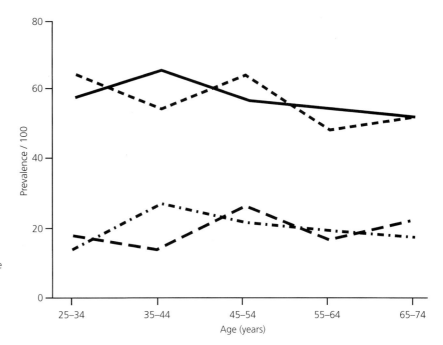

Figure 16.1 Age- and gender-specific prevalence rates (per 100) for any episodes of either heartburn or acid regurgitation and for at least weekly episodes among Olmsted County, MN, residents aged 25–74 years. Men any, weekly; women any, weekly.

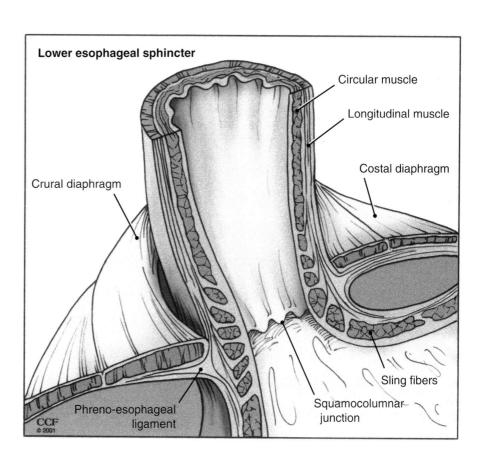

Figure 16.2 Anatomy of the gastroesophageal junction illustrating the major elements of the antireflux barrier.

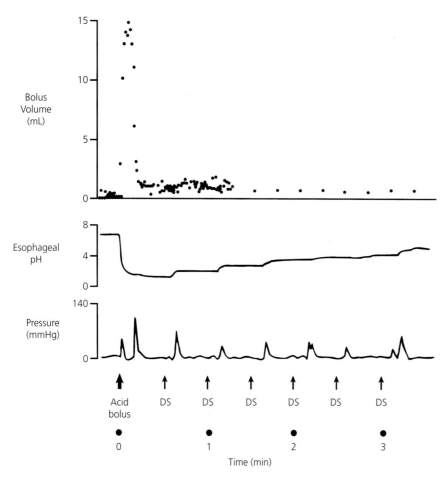

Figure 16.3 Relationship between esophageal peristalsis, distal esophagus pH, esophageal volume, and esophageal acid clearance in a healthy volunteer. Acid reflux is replicated by infusing radiolabeled 0.1 N HCl into the esophagus and scanning over the chest. The first peristaltic contraction clears all but about 1 mL of the infused fluid, but the esophageal pH remains unchanged. Stepwise increase in distal esophageal pH occurs, with subsequent swallows secondary to bicarbonate-enriched saliva.

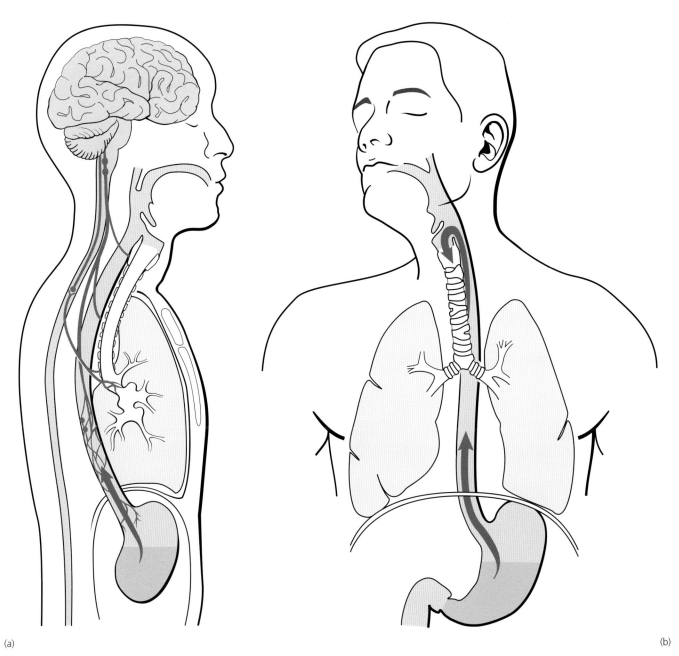

(a)

(b)

Figure 16.4 Proposed mechanisms for extraesophageal symptoms of gastroesophageal reflux disease. **(a)** Vagally mediated reflex arc between distal esophagus and bronchopulmonary tree. **(b)** Microaspiration of gastric acid.

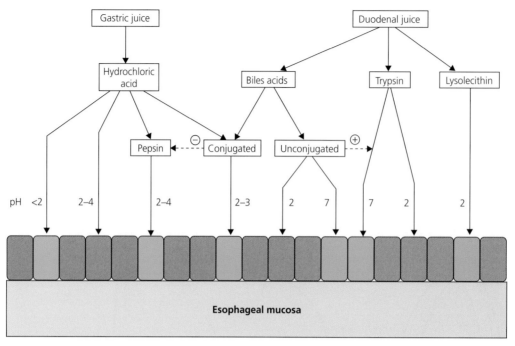

Figure 16.5 The postulated injurious agents responsible for esophageal mucosal damage. Mucosal injury is illustrated by the darker boxes representing the epithelial surface.

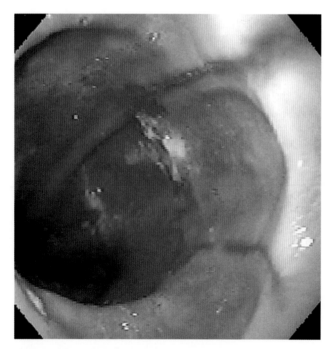

Figure 16.6 Los Angeles grade B esophagitis with mucosal breaks greater than 5 mm on multiple esophageal folds. These changes would be compatible with Savary–Miller and Hetzel grade II esophagitis.

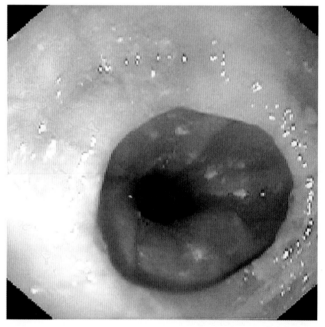

Figure 16.7 Smooth, thickened esophageal stricture at the squamocolumnar junction, just above a hiatal hernia. No esophagitis is seen.

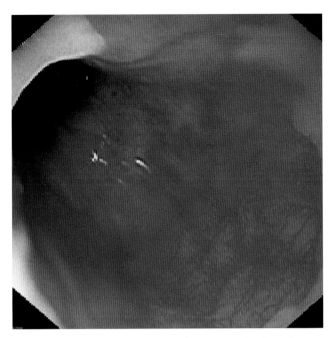

Figure 16.8 Long-segment Barrett esophagus measuring 4 cm above the hiatal hernia. The specialized intestinal metaplasia has a distinct reddish pink appearance in contrast with the glossy white squamous mucosa of the esophagus.

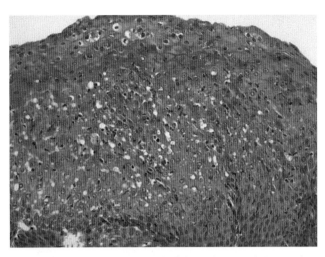

Figure 16.10 Esophageal biopsy of reflux esophagitis with increased neutrophils and eosinophils in the squamous mucosa.

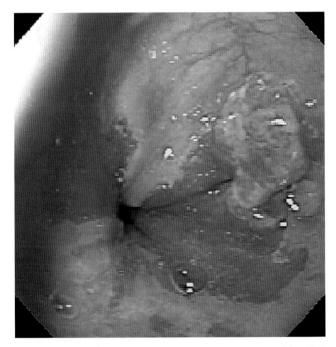

Figure 16.9 Barrett esophagus with an early adenocarcinoma identified on surveillance endoscopy.

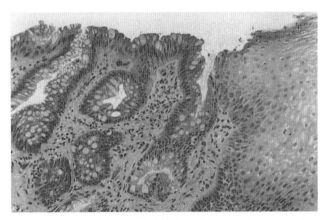

Figure 16.11 Esophageal biopsy at the new squamocolumnar junction in a patient with Barrett esophagus. Specialized intestinal metaplasia with goblet cells (left). The normal squamous mucosa (right).

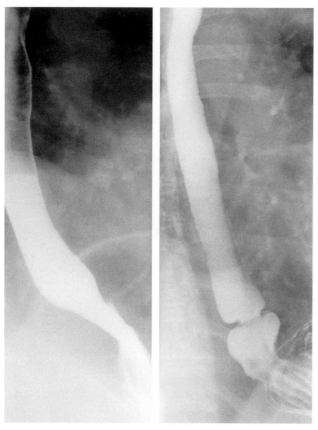

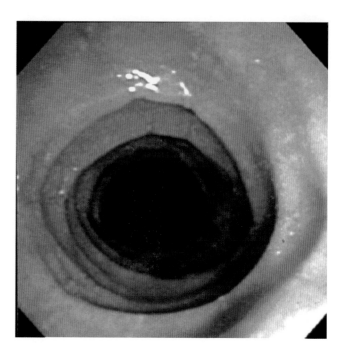

Figure 16.13 Multiple smooth rings throughout the esophagus in a patient with solid food dysphagia and eosinophilic esophagitis.

Figure 16.12 Barium esophagram in a patient with dysphagia. Left: the radiograph suggests a possible subtle stricture. Right: good esophageal distention by the Valsalva maneuver brings out a Schatzki ring with a small hiatal hernia.

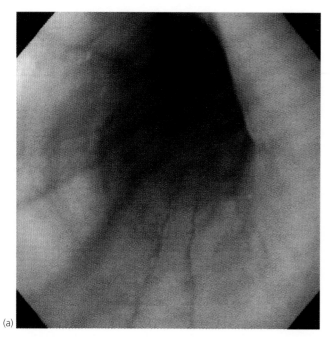

(a)

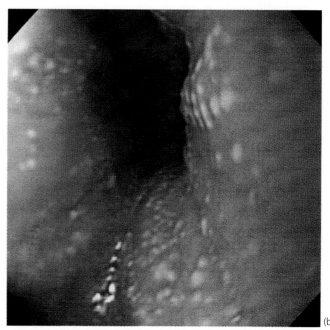

(b)

Figure 16.14 More subtle findings of eosinophilic esophagitis include **(a)** longitudinal shallow furrows and **(b)** white pinpoint exudates. The latter represent eosinophilic micro-abscesses that are more commonly seen in children.

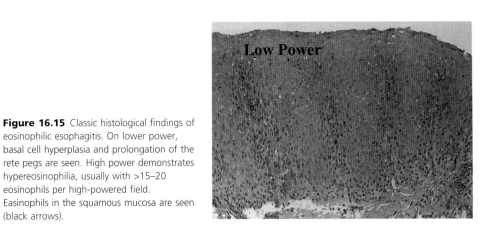

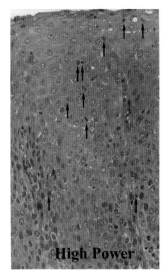

Figure 16.15 Classic histological findings of eosinophilic esophagitis. On lower power, basal cell hyperplasia and prolongation of the rete pegs are seen. High power demonstrates hypereosinophilia, usually with >15–20 eosinophils per high-powered field. Easinophils in the squamous mucosa are seen (black arrows).

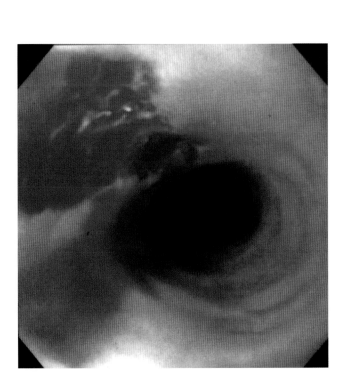

Figure 16.16 Painful mucosal tear into the esophageal muscle. The patient required overnight hospitalization to rule out a perforation and was administered narcotics for pain.

17

Esophageal infections and disorders associated with acquired immunodeficiency syndrome

C. Mel Wilcox

Although the acquired immunodeficiency syndrome (AIDS) epidemic was the major contributor to the witnessed upsurge in esophageal infections that was observed in the 1980s and 1990s, more recently, with the widespread availability of highly active antiretroviral therapy, these infections have become much less common. In addition, the adoption of antimicrobial prophylaxis for high-risk immunocompromised patients, such as those post organ transplantation, has also led to an overall fall in the incidence of infections, including those involving the esophagus. Despite these advancements, however, esophageal infections will remain important complications of immunodeficiency states.

Esophageal infections can be categorized by the infecting organism. Candida sp. are the most common fungal pathogens, with aspergillosis, histoplasmosis, and blastomycosis being very rare infections. Following fungi, viruses (herpes simplex virus [HSV] and cytomegalovirus [CMV]) are the most common cause of infection. Rare additional causes of esophagitis include bacteria, mycobacteria, and parasites. Odynophagia is the most common symptom of esophageal infection, with dysphagia being reported less frequently. Although barium esophagography is helpful in suggesting the presence of infectious esophagitis, these studies are not definitive. Endoscopy provides the highest diagnostic accuracy.

Candida albicans is the most common pathogen causing esophageal infection. Classically, barium radiographs of esophageal candidiasis reveal a "shaggy" appearance resulting from diffuse plaque material that coats the esophageal mucosa, mimicking ulceration (Fig. 17.1). The endoscopic appearance of *Candida* is well recognized and is essentially pathognomonic (Figs 17.2 and 17.3).

Candida rarely causes true ulceration; thus, the presence of esophageal ulcer associated with *Candida* esophagitis suggests an additional esophageal process (Figs 17.4 and 17.5).

Esophageal brushings have the highest diagnostic yield for candidal infection. Mucosal biopsies will be diagnostic when more severe disease is present, and should be performed in the presence of ulceration. Fungal cultures are not widely available and provide no additional information over the endoscopic and histological findings unless fungi other than *Candida* are suspected.

Other fungi rarely cause esophageal disease. Histoplasma is the most frequent fungal pathogen reported to involve the esophagus usually from mediastinal involvement (Fig. 17.6).

In contrast with *Candida* esophagitis, barium radiographs of viral esophagitis demonstrate ulceration. The ulcers are usually well circumscribed but may coalesce to form a superficial esophagitis. Ulcers associated with HSV infection typically are small and well circumscribed, whereas those associated with CMV have a greater propensity to form larger well circumscribed longitudinal or linear lesions. A diffuse viral esophagitis may result in a cobblestone or shaggy mucosal appearance similar to that observed in esophageal candidiasis (Fig. 17.7). Endoscopically, HSV ulcers correspond to the radiographic features appearing as well circumscribed small volcano-like lesions, likely the site of a vesicle (Fig. 17.8) or a shallow ulcers (Fig. 17.9); occasionally, when multiple and small, the lesions may mimic esophageal candidiasis (Fig. 17.10). Although esophageal ulcers caused by CMV may resemble HSV (Fig. 17.11), in general CMV causes larger or more extensive lesions that are often very deep in AIDS patients (Figs 17.12–17.14), leading to bleeding, stricture (Fig. 17.15), or, rarely, perforation. Multiple biopsies of the ulcer edge (for HSV) and ulcer base (for CMV) with careful histological examination of biopsy material should reveal the intranuclear (Cowdry type A) or cytoplasmic inclusions characteristic of HSV (Fig. 17.16) or CMV infection (Fig. 17.17), respectively.

Radiographic findings in esophageal tuberculosis are nonspecific but may show ulceration, stricture, or fistulae extending from the esophagus to the trachea, bronchi, or mediastinal lymph nodes (Figs 17.18 and 17.19).

Atlas of Gastroenterology, 4th edition. Edited by Tadataka Yamada, David H. Alpers, Anthony N. Kalloo, Neil Kaplowitz, Chung Owyang, and Don W. Powell. © 2009 Blackwell Publishing, ISBN: 978-1-4051-6909-7

An interesting disorder is the HIV-associated idiopathic esophageal ulcer, although its pathogenesis is not well defined. Characteristically, these lesions become manifest when immunodeficiency is severe (CD4 lymphocyte count <100/mm^3). The clinical, radiographic, and endoscopic manifestations are indistinguishable from CMV (Figs 17.20–17.22). These ulcers may be deep and result in esophago-esophageal fistula (Fig. 17.23). Other esophageal diseases seen in AIDS patients include parasites and, rarely, neo-plasms, such as Kaposi sarcoma or non-Hodgkin lymphoma (Fig. 17.24).

In summary, in most cases of infectious esophagitis the determination of the specific infection and the institution of appropriate therapy will result in mucosal healing and relief of symptoms. Endoscopy is the most sensitive and specific technique for establishing the etiology of esophageal infections.

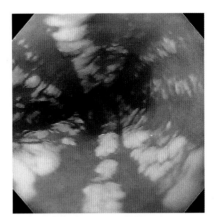

Figure 17.2 Multiple raised white plaques involving the esophagus with normal intervening mucosa. This would be classified as Grade II *Candida* esophagitis.

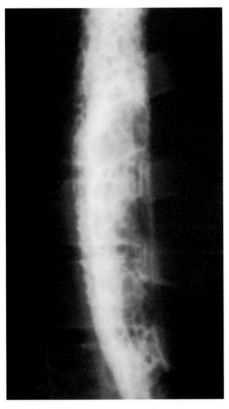

Figure 17.1 Barium esophagram shows multiple filling defects with irregularity of the mucosal surface resulting in a "shaggy" appearance owing to esophageal candidiasis.

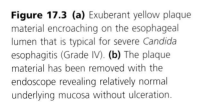

Figure 17.3 (a) Exuberant yellow plaque material encroaching on the esophageal lumen that is typical for severe *Candida* esophagitis (Grade IV). **(b)** The plaque material has been removed with the endoscope revealing relatively normal underlying mucosa without ulceration.

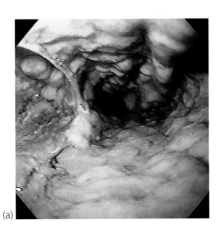

(a)

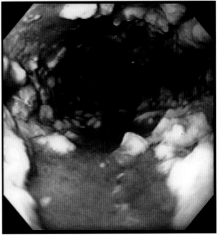

(b)

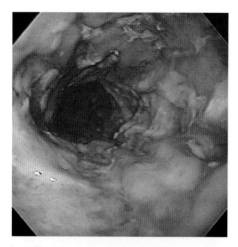

Figure 17.4 Diffuse ulceration with a serpiginous appearance with overlying candidal debris. This AIDS patient has cytomegalovirus esophagitis and *Candida* coinfection.

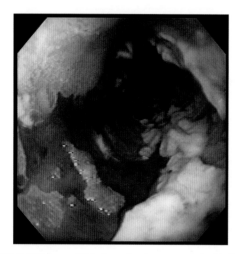

Figure 17.5 Diffuse candidal plaque has been removed with the endoscope revealing a shallow serpiginous ulceration, which, on biopsy, confirmed cytomegalovirus.

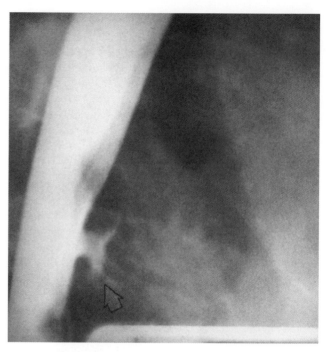

Figure 17.6 Ulcer seen in the mid-esophagus near the bronchus (arrow), caused by an infected lymph node from *Histoplasma capsulatum*. Courtesy of Robert Koehler, MD.

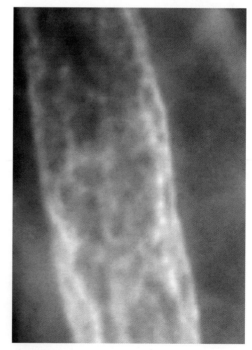

Figure 17.7 Barium esophagram showing diffuse mucosal irregularity resembling *Candida* esophagitis in a patient with AIDS. This patient had diffuse erosive esophagitis due to herpes simplex virus (HSV).

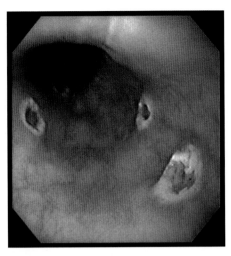

Figure 17.8 Small volcano-like ulcers due to herpes simplex virus (HSV).

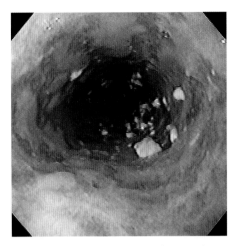

Figure 17.11 Shallow irregular ulceration with intervening areas of preserved but edematous squamous mucosa due to cytomegalovirus. Note also the candidal plaques in the distal esophagus. This endoscopic appearance is also compatible with herpes simplex virus esophagitis.

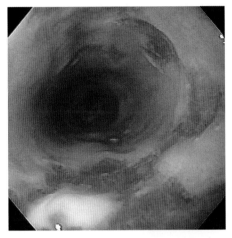

Figure 17.9 Multiple well-circumscribed, shallow esophageal ulcers due to herpes simplex virus esophagitis.

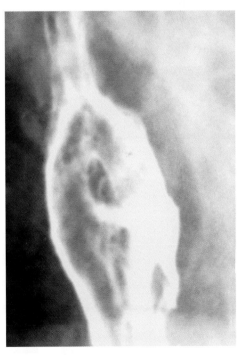

Figure 17.12 Barium esophagram shows large esophageal ulceration as a result of cytomegalovirus esophagitis in a patient with AIDS.

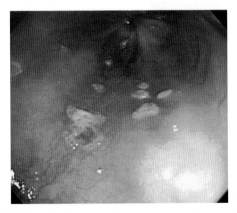

Figure 17.10 Small well-circumscribed areas of exudate resembling *Candida*. This is a classic appearance of mild herpes simplex virus esophagitis. This patient had neutropenia.

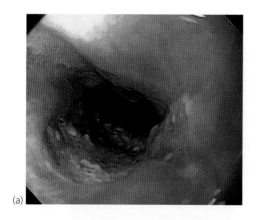

(a)

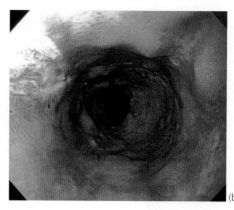

(b)

Figure 17.13 (a) Large, deep ulceration in the proximal esophagus due to cytomegalovirus in a patient with AIDS. **(b)** Ulcerations in the distal esophagus are smaller, more linear, and not as deep. Ulceration may not be uniform in the same patient.

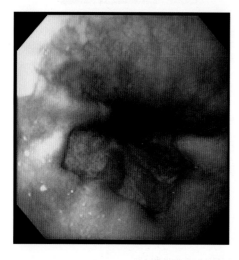

Figure 17.14 Solitary, deep, well-circumscribed ulcer at the gastroesophageal junction caused by cytomegalovirus.

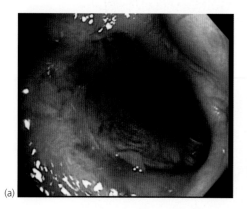

(a)

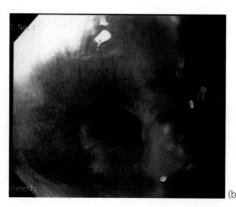

(b)

Figure 17.15 (a) Circumferential ulceration in the mid-esophagus caused by cytomegalovirus. **(b)** After therapy the ulcer healed, resulting in a tight esophageal stricture.

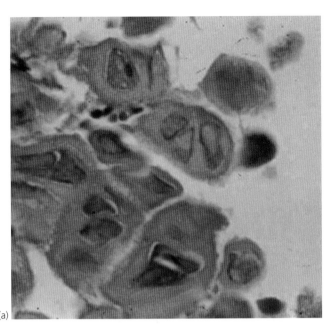

(a)

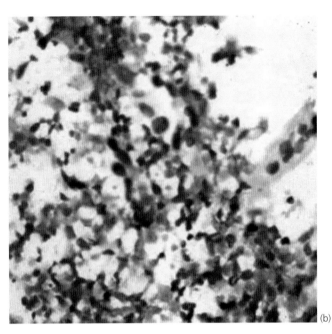

(b)

Figure 17.16 **(a)** Multinucleated giant cells in squamous mucosa, characteristic of herpes simplex virus infection. **(b)** Immunohistochemical staining shows herpes simplex virus antigens, thus confirming infection.

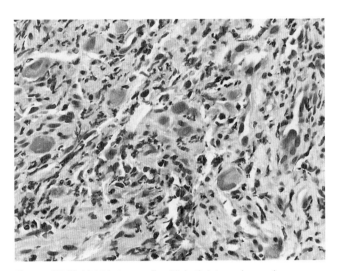

Figure 17.17 Multiple large cells with both intranuclear and intracytoplasmic inclusions, typical for cytomegalovirus viral cytopathic effect.

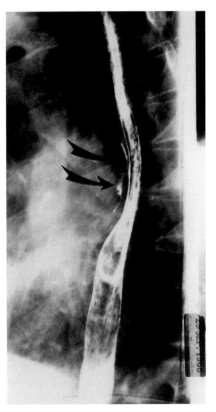

Figure 17.18 Barium esophagram reveals diffuse mucosal irregularity and a fistulous tract (arrows) to mediastinal lymph nodes in a patient with AIDS. This patient has tuberculosis. Endoscopy showed candidiasis and an ulcer at the opening of the fistulous tract. Courtesy of Dr R. DeSilva.

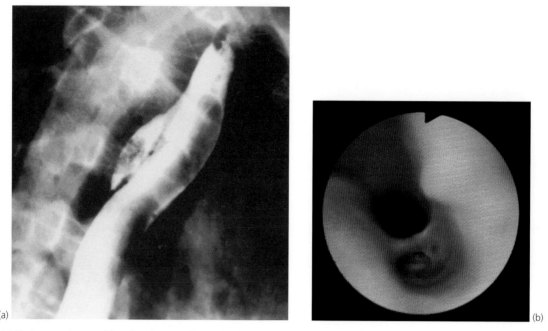

(a)

(b)

Figure 17.19 Barium esophagram **(a)** and endoscopic photograph **(b)** of an esophageal fistula in a man with AIDS, due to *Mycobacterium tuberculosis*. Courtesy of Dr. JP Raufman.

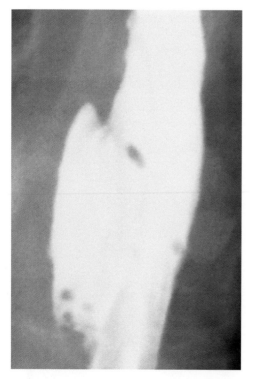

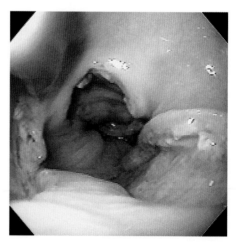

Figure 17.21 Three large deep ulcerations (idiopathic) in the distal esophagus in a patient with AIDS.

Figure 17.20 Barium esophagram showing large solitary ulceration in the mid-esophagus, which was idiopathic in a patient with AIDS.

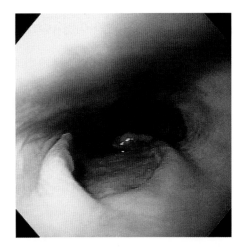

Figure 17.22 Solitary, large, well-circumscribed ulceration with a heaped-up appearance that is typical for the idiopathic esophageal ulceration of AIDS.

Figure 17.23 **(a)** Deep ulceration of the distal esophagus, resulting in an esophagoesophageal fistula. **(b)** Retroflex examination shows the opening from the gastroesophageal junction ulceration.

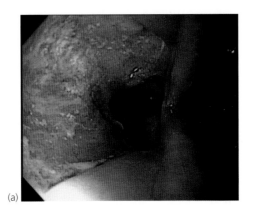 (a)

(b)

Figure 17.24 Heaped-up ulcerated lesions in the mid-esophagus, typical for non-Hodgkin lymphoma.

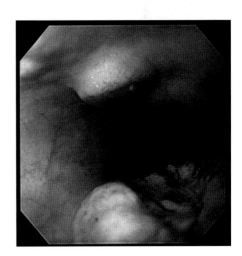

18

Esophageal neoplasms

Anil K. Rustgi, Weijing Sun

The most common malignant esophageal neoplasms are squamous cell carcinoma and adenocarcinoma, the latter typically arising in Barrett epithelium. Although esophageal squamous cell carcinoma is the more common of the two worldwide, adenocarcinoma is more frequent in the United States. Frequent symptoms resulting from lumenal masses include dysphagia, odynophagia, and weight loss, which require diagnosis by means of fiberoptic endoscopy with biopsy and cytology. On establishment of diagnosis, preoperative staging is needed before selection of therapy.

Esophageal squamous cell carcinoma occurs predominantly in lower socioeconomic groups within the United States, with predilection for African American males. Risk factors include tobacco and alcohol use, although in high-incidence areas of the world (northern China, India, Iran, southern Russia, South Africa, and some parts of South America) other factors appear more critical, such as exposure to nitrosamines and concomitant nutritional (minerals and vitamins) deficiencies. Clinical suspicion of squamous cell carcinoma merits performance of a barium esophagography. This may reveal an early cancer that manifests as a plaque-like lesion (Fig. 18.1) or, alternatively, advanced cancer with an ulcerated polypoid lesion (Fig. 18.2) or a circumferential annular lesion (Figs 18.3 and 18.4). Endoscopy with biopsies may demonstrate various stages: dysplasia, carcinoma in situ, or carcinoma (Fig. 18.5). Preoperative staging is necessary, with endoscopic ultrasound to determine esophageal wall invasion and lymph node involvement (Fig. 18.6). A computed tomography (CT) scan will exclude regional and distant metastases. Although surgical resection with esophagectomy and gastric interposition is preferred for cure of patients who are appropriate candidates, neoadjuvant therapy with chemotherapy and radia-

tion therapy followed by surgery has shown promise. Palliation is needed for patients who cannot undergo potentially curative therapy (Fig. 18.7).

Esophageal adenocarcinoma invariably develops in the setting of Barrett esophagus (Fig. 18.8a). An important factor in the development of Barrett esophagus is gastro-esophageal reflux, although other unidentified factors may be important. Because Barrett esophagus may progress from metaplasia to low- and high-grade dysplasia with eventual adenocarcinoma, endoscopic surveillance with a systematic protocol for biopsies is warranted. Initial suspicion and diagnosis of Barrett dysplasia and esophageal adenocarcinoma require barium esophagography (Fig. 18.9) and fiberoptic endoscopy (Fig. 18.8b). Pathology may reveal Barrett esophagus with varying degrees of dysplasia (Fig. 18.10) and adenocarcinoma (Fig. 18.11). As with squamous cell carcinoma, preoperative staging entails endoscopic ultrasound (Fig. 18.12) and CT scanning. Therapy may be surgical or multimodal (neoadjuvant chemotherapy and radiation therapy followed by surgery) if the patient is an appropriate candidate. Otherwise, palliative therapy is provided. It should be noted that both esophageal neoplasms could have associated complications, such as fistula formation (Fig. 18.13).

There are many other epithelial and nonepithelial esophageal neoplasms, both benign and malignant, but they are generally quite rare. An example of a benign nonepithelial tumor is leiomyoma, which is typically silent and patients are generally asymptomatic (Fig. 18.14). Rare malignant esophageal neoplasms include carcinosarcoma, metastatic cancer (melanoma, breast cancer), neuroendocrine tumors, and various sarcomas (Fig. 18.15).

Atlas of Gastroenterology, 4th edition. Edited by Tadataka Yamada, David H. Alpers, Anthony N. Kalloo, Neil Kaplowitz, Chung Owyang, and Don W. Powell. © 2009 Blackwell Publishing, ISBN: 978-1-4051-6909-7

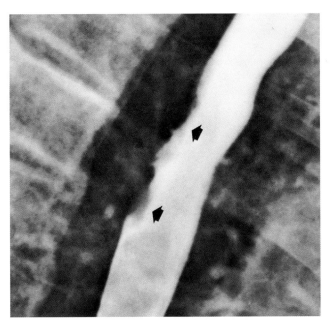

Figure 18.1 Early squamous cell carcinoma of the esophagus presenting as a plaque-like lesion (arrows) on the posterior wall.

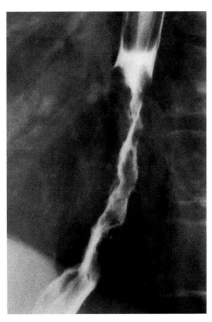

Figure 18.3 Esophagram shows extensive infiltrative lesion of the distal esophagus.

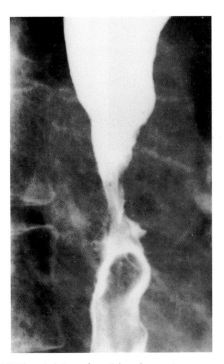

Figure 18.2 Ulcerated circumferential apple core-type squamous cell carcinoma.

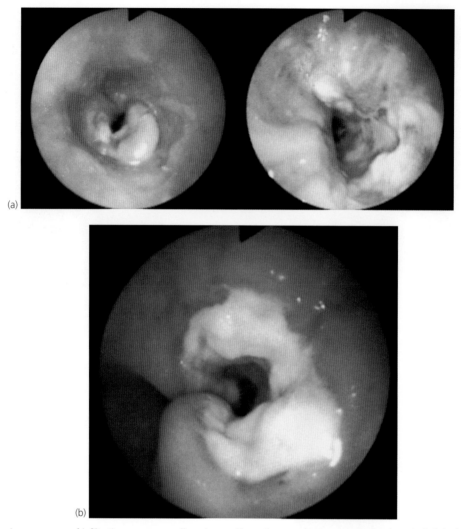

Figure 18.4 Endoscopic appearance of infiltrating squamous cell carcinoma. These three carcinomas have variously occluded the lumen and would present as dysphagia.

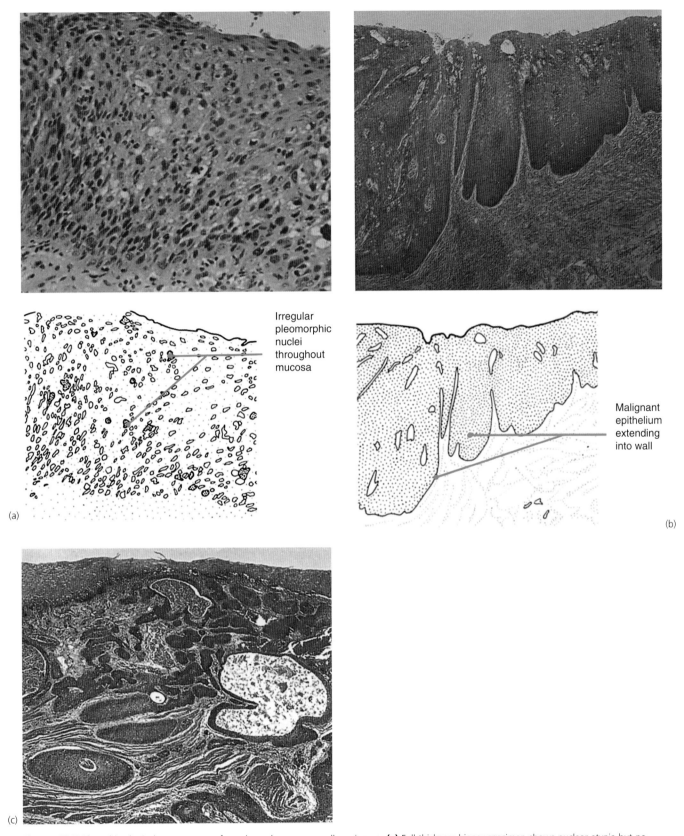

Figure 18.5 Three histological appearances of esophageal squamous cell carcinoma. **(a)** Full-thickness biopsy specimen shows nuclear atypia but no invasion. This is carcinoma in situ. **(b)** Specimen shows early invasive squamous cell carcinoma with downward extension of the tumor into the submucosa. **(c)** Established infiltrating, well-differentiated carcinoma. There are islands of malignant tissue under essentially normal squamous epithelium.

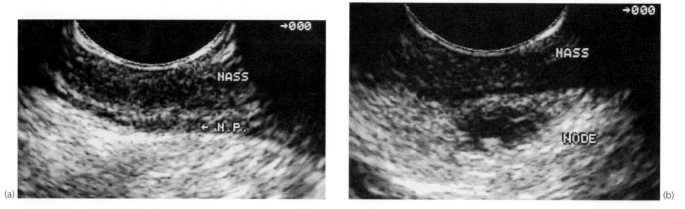

Figure 18.6 Endoscopic ultrasound images of different stages of esophageal cancer. Courtesy of William Brugge, MD.

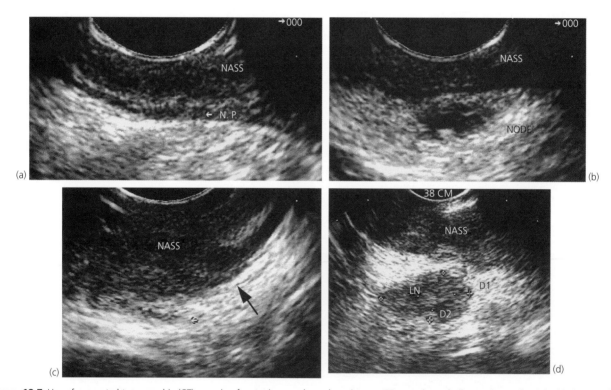

Figure 18.7 Use of computed tomographic (CT) scanning for staging esophageal carcinoma. CT scan shows bulky carcinoma (straight black arrows) essentially occluding the esophageal lumen (white arrow) and obliterating the fat plane adjacent to the aorta (curved black arrow). This obliteration of tissue planes indicates mediastinal extension of the lumen.

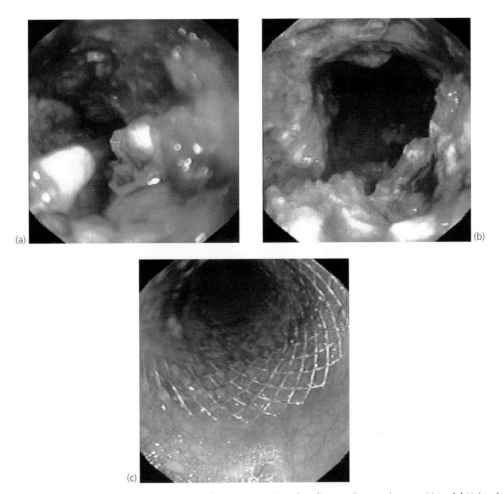

Figure 18.8 Photodynamic laser therapy for esophageal cancer after administration of porfimer sodium, a photosensitizer. **(a)** Light of 630 nm wavelength from a laser acts on cells that accumulate the photosensitizer. **(b)** After 6 days, there is some decrease in mass size. **(c)** After 12 days, the mass is markedly diminished in size, and a metallic endoprosthesis is inserted endoscopically. Courtesy of Norman Nishioka.

Figure 18.9 Barrett esophagus. **(a)** Upper endoscopy reveals short-segment Barrett esophagus. **(b)** Upper endoscopy reveals long-segment esophagus with inflammation and possible early cancer. Courtesy of David Katzka, MD.

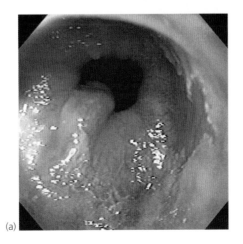 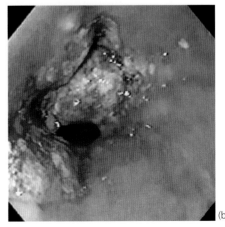

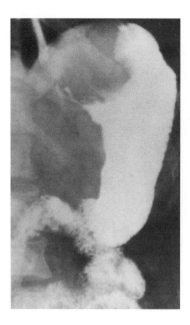
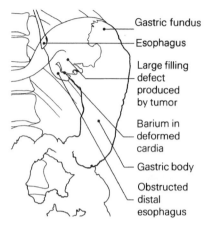

Figure 18.10 Adenocarcinoma of the distal esophagus may be difficult to differentiate from squamous cell carcinoma on the basis of radiographic appearance. However, as shown here, when the tumor extensively involves the fundus of the stomach, the diagnosis is more certain.

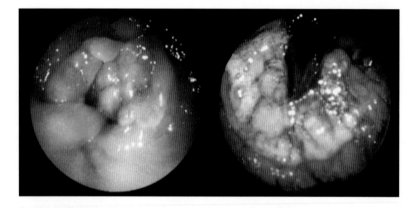
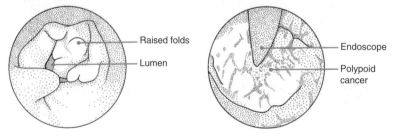

Figure 18.11 At endoscopy, adenocarcinoma may be difficult to differentiate from squamous cell carcinoma. Retroflexed views of the tumor from the stomach may help.

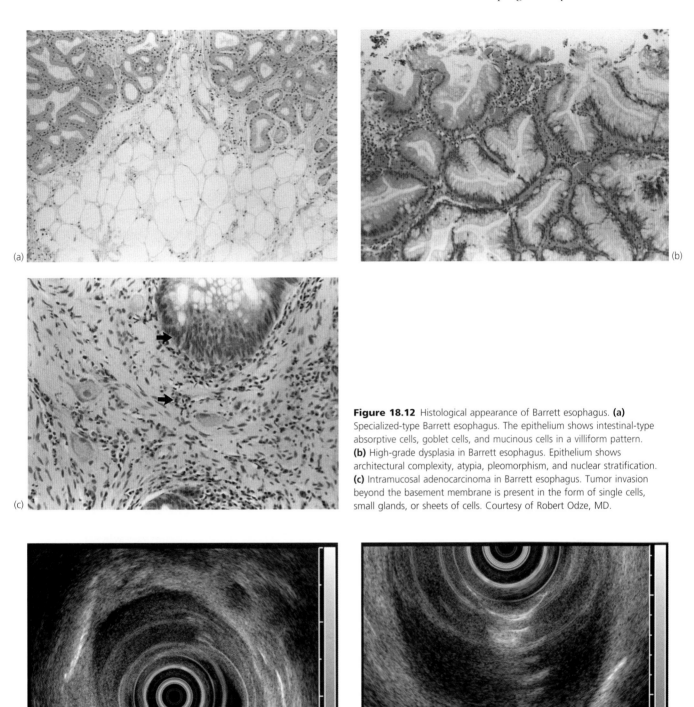

(a)

(b)

(c)

Figure 18.12 Histological appearance of Barrett esophagus. **(a)** Specialized-type Barrett esophagus. The epithelium shows intestinal-type absorptive cells, goblet cells, and mucinous cells in a villiform pattern. **(b)** High-grade dysplasia in Barrett esophagus. Epithelium shows architectural complexity, atypia, pleomorphism, and nuclear stratification. **(c)** Intramucosal adenocarcinoma in Barrett esophagus. Tumor invasion beyond the basement membrane is present in the form of single cells, small glands, or sheets of cells. Courtesy of Robert Odze, MD.

(a)

(b)

Figure 18.13 Endoscopic ultrasound (EUS). **(a)** An EUS demonstrates a T2N1 esophageal adenocarcinoma. **(b)** The lesion is invading the right pleura. Courtesy of Michael Kochman, MD.

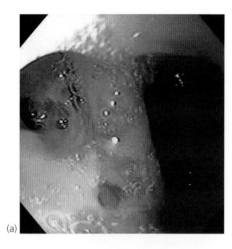

(a)

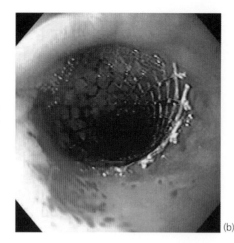

(b)

Figure 18.14 (a) An esophageal fistula complication of esophageal cancer. **(b)** A stent is inserted to seal the fistula. Courtesy of Michael Kochman, MD.

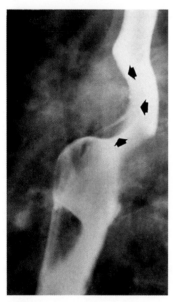

Figure 18.15 Leiomyoma usually presents itself as a smooth, rounded intramural defect (arrows) that encroaches on the barium column.

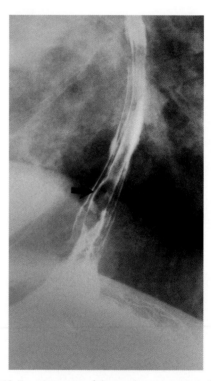

Figure 18.16 Kaposi sarcoma of the esophagus represented by a dumbbell-shaped submucosal mass (arrow) with superficial ulceration. Courtesy of Deborah Hall, MD.

19

Miscellaneous diseases of the esophagus: foreign bodies, physical injury, systemic and dermatological diseases

Evan S. Dellon, Nicholas J. Shaheen

This chapter presents images from a selection of diseases of the esophagus not illustrated elsewhere in the textbook, including foreign body impaction, trauma, corrosive and pill esophagitis, and rare manifestations of systemic and dermatological diseases.

As the portal to the gastrointestinal (GI) tract, the esophagus is the most common site of foreign body impaction. Accordingly, it is possible for a wide variety of objects to become lodged there. This may be owing to qualities of the object, such as sharp edges or a large size, or to underlying structural or motility abnormalities of the esophagus. When food bolus impaction is encountered, the bolus can often be gently advanced under endoscopic guidance into the stomach (Fig. 19.1). Frequently, examination of the cleared esophagus reveals a Schatzki ring or peptic stricture (Fig. 19.2).

Sharp bone fragments can also impale the esophageal wall, causing localized trauma (Fig. 19.3). Underlying strictures, in contrast, predispose solid objects, such as fruit pits, to become stuck if ingested (Fig. 19.4). Patients with psychiatric disease may swallow a panoply of unusual objects, including so-called "sporks," which are challenging to remove and can cause local ulceration (Fig. 19.5). Coins, most commonly swallowed inadvertently by pediatric patients, may also become lodged in the esophagus. Because they are radiopaque, an impacted coin can be detected and monitored with a plain radiograph, but if a coin does not spontaneously pass from the distal esophagus within 24 hours, endoscopic removal is warranted (Fig. 19.6).

Mallory–Weiss tears, mucosal lacerations at the gastroesophageal junction (GEJ) caused by a sudden rise in intraabdominal pressure during vomiting or retching, are common causes of upper GI hemorrhage. If either active bleeding or stigmata of recent bleeding is seen at endoscopy,

hemostatic treatment is recommended (Fig. 19.7). These tears can be subtle, and when suspected, careful antegrade and retroflexed examination of the GEJ is mandatory (Fig. 19.8).

Perforation of the esophagus following pneumatic dilation of the lower esophageal sphincter in achalasia or after bougie dilation of an esophageal stricture should be suspected with chest pain, fever, or the presence of subcutaneous air after dilation (Fig. 19.9). An esophagram with a water-soluble agent prior to the use of barium is recommended for initial diagnostic testing. Spontaneous rupture of the esophagus, Boerhaave syndrome (Fig. 19.10), is life-threatening, requiring immediate management.

Esophageal intramural hematomas represent another type of trauma to the esophagus, usually due to a mechanical insult. On endoscopic evaluation, a bluish or violet mass protruding into the esophageal lumen is seen, sometimes in association with superficial ulceration (Fig. 19.11). These often resolve spontaneously.

Purposeful or accidental ingestion of corrosive substances, particularly strong alkali solutions found in some cleaning products, can lead to caustic esophagitis with long-term sequelae of persistent esophageal strictures and increased risk of esophageal squamous cell carcinoma. Endoscopy can be useful in grading the injury, which ranges from mucosal erythema to sloughing, through ulceration of the mucosa, to frank esophageal necrosis (Fig. 19.12).

Pill esophagitis is also caused by a chemical irritant to the esophagus, specifically a medication tablet. Some medications may become stuck in the esophagus and cause local inflammation or erosions without any underlying esophageal structural or motility disorder. In other cases, however, an area of esophageal narrowing may be the underlying cause of pill esophagitis (Fig. 19.13).

A number of systemic diseases can affect the esophagus in rare instances, and in the case of Crohn's disease, the impact can be substantial. Owing to chronic transmural

Atlas of Gastroenterology, 4th edition. Edited by Tadataka Yamada, David H. Alpers, Anthony N. Kalloo, Neil Kaplowitz, Chung Owyang, and Don W. Powell. © 2009 Blackwell Publishing, ISBN: 978-1-4051-6909-7

inflammation, the esophagus can be narrowed with sinus tracts forming from deep ulcerations (Fig. 19.14). In some instances, esophagotracheal or esophagobronchial fistulae may develop, causing recurrent pneumonitis, pneumonia, or empyema, and requiring surgical management (Fig. 19.15).

Although graft-versus-host disease (GVHD) more commonly affects the lower GI tract and the liver, it can affect the esophagus also. Diagnosis is mostly decided from the biopsy result, which also excludes opportunistic infections in the immunosuppressed bone marrow transplant patient. Esophageal erythema or friability, as well as webs or strictures, can be seen on endoscopic examination (Figs 19.16 and 19.17). Behçet syndrome, characterized by oral and genital aphthous ulceration and ocular inflammation, is another systemic disease that rarely affects the esophagus (Fig. 19.18).

Finally, blistering dermatological diseases can rarely have esophageal involvement. Pemphigus vulgaris, as a result of autoantibodies acting against desmoglein-3 in keratinocytes, can cause esophageal blistering (Fig. 19.19). Benign mucous membrane pemphigoid (BMMP) is due to deposition of autoantibodies in the basement membrane of the esophageal mucosa, leading to tense blisters, with subsequent scarring and stricturing (Figs 19.20 and 19.21). Epidermolysis bullosa dystrophica (EPD), a heritable disease caused by a mutation in the collagen type VII gene, results in a cycle of recurrent blistering and scarring as a result of mild trauma. In the esophagus, the routine act of swallowing is enough to prompt this cycle, which leads to strictures, esophageal shortening, and dysmotility (Figs 19.22 and 19.23). Because endoscopy also induces trauma it is reserved for therapeutic dilation, making a barium esophagram the preferred diagnostic test in this condition.

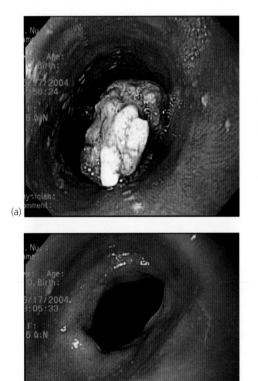

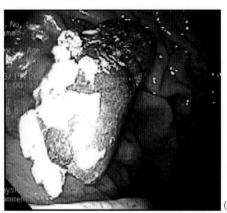

(a)

(b)

(c)

Figure 19.1 Food impaction in the distal esophagus **(a)**, which is cleared by gently advancing the bolus under direct endoscopic vision into the stomach **(b)**. A reexamination of the esophagus reveals a Schatzki ring as the underlying cause **(c)**.

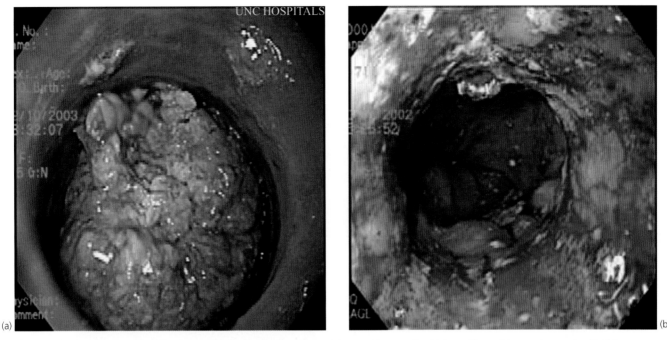

Figure 19.2 Another example of food impaction in the distal esophagus **(a)** caused by a peptic stricture with overlying erosive esophagitis **(b)**.

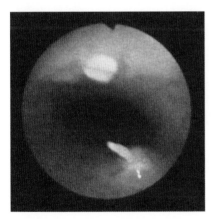

Figure 19.3 An endoscopic view of a fish bone lodged in the proximal esophagus. A contralateral ulcer is present in the 12 o'clock position. The patient sought treatment with severe neck pain after swallowing the bone. Courtesy of Douglas O. Faigel.

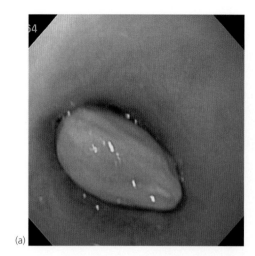

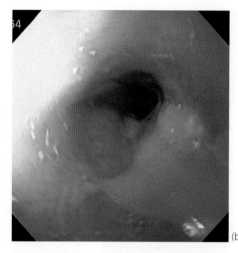

Figure 19.4 A fruit pit stuck in the esophagus **(a)** due to an underlying stricture **(b)**.

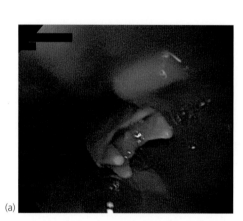

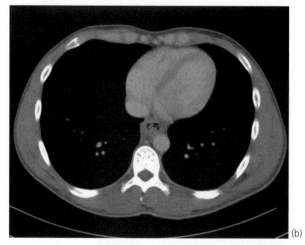

Figure 19.5 An endoscopic view of an impacted and folded plastic "spork" in the distal esophagus of a psychiatric patient **(a)**. On a computed tomography (CT) scan of the chest prior to the procedure, the foreign body can be seen in the distal esophagus, which is also thickened and mildly dilated **(b)**.

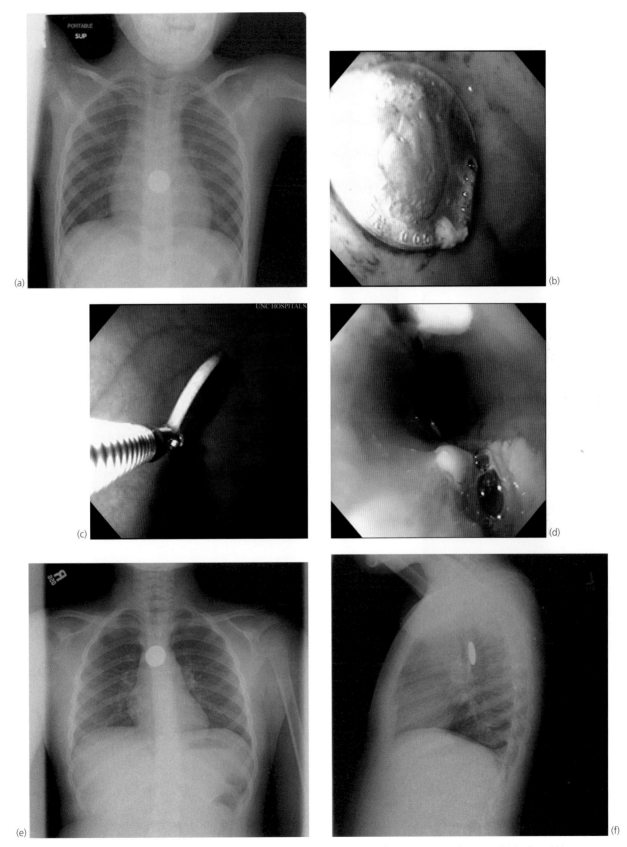

Figure 19.6 Images of coins impacted in pediatric patients. **(a)** Posteroanterior (PA) chest film showing a radiopaque disk in the midthorax. **(b, c, d)** Endoscopic views of the same patient, showing a penny in the esophagus with surrounding erosions, being removed by a pair of forceps, and the residual ulcerations left. **(e, f)** PA and lateral chest films showing a similar radiopaque disk, likely localizing to the esophagus and not passing after 24 hours. (*Continued on next page.*)

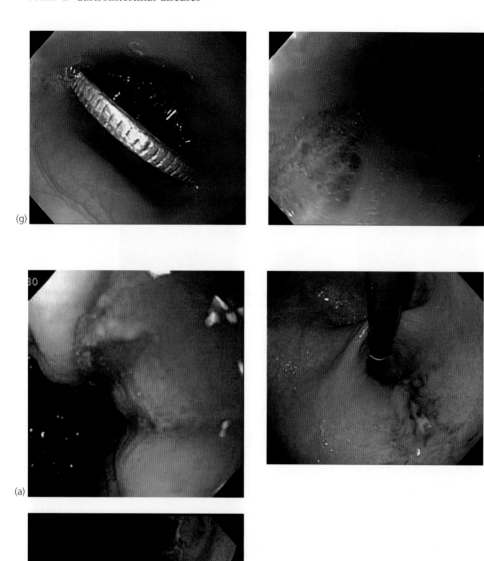

Figure 19.6 *Continued* **(g, h)** A dime is found lodged in the esophagus, with residual esophageal erosions after foreign body removal.

Figure 19.7 Examples of different morphologies of Mallory–Weiss tears in three different patients, seen in antegrade **(a)** and retroflexed **(b, c)** views in the proximity of the gastroesophageal junction.

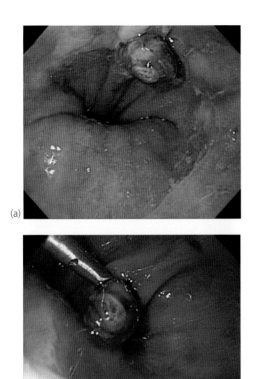

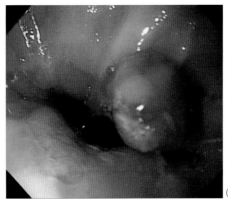

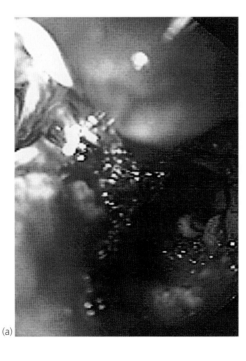

Figure 19.8 A Mallory–Weiss tear located at the gastroesophageal junction **(a)** with an overlying clot seen in close-up view **(b)**. Treatment with application of a clip at the base of the lesion achieved hemostasis **(c)**.

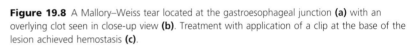

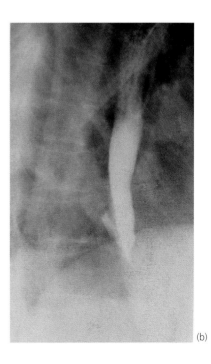

Figure 19.9 Endoscopic view of an esophageal perforation (seen between the 10 and 11 o'clock positions) after bougie dilation of the esophagus 2 days earlier **(a)**. A contained perforation was first demonstrated on barium swallow **(b)**. Courtesy of Douglas O. Faigel.

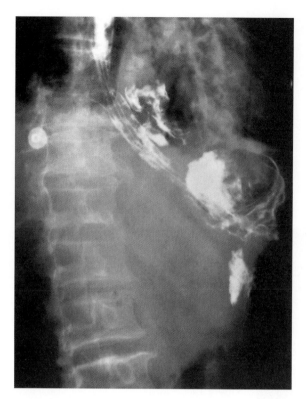

Figure 19.10 A barium swallow from a patient with Boerhaave syndrome shows extravasation of contrast material from the distal esophagus into the mediastinum. Courtesy of Douglas O. Faigel.

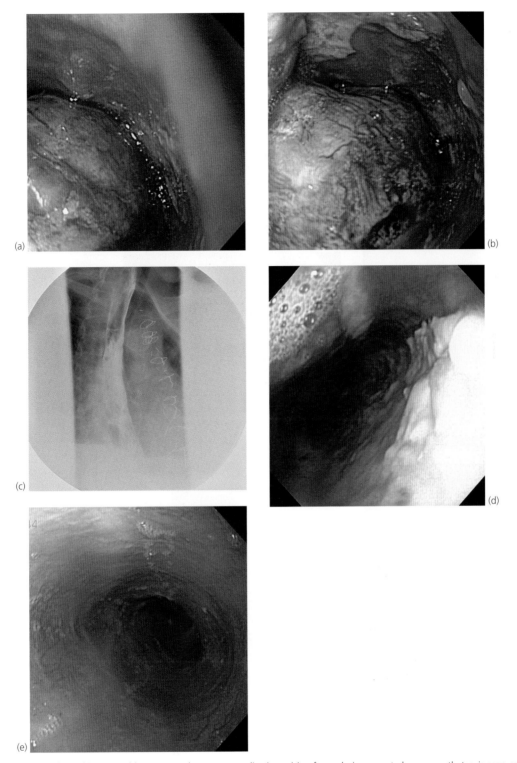

Figure 19.11 A large esophageal intramural hematoma, due to a complication arising from placing a central venous catheter, is seen endoscopically, nearly obstructing the lumen **(a)** with an overlying area of ulceration **(b)**. Barium swallow shows mucosal irregularity, a possible distal filling defect, and contrast that is slow to leave the esophagus **(c)**. On endoscopies over the subsequent 2 months **(d, e)**, the ulcerated area sloughs, the hematoma resorbs, and the mucosa heals with a mild stricture formed just above the gastroesophageal junction.

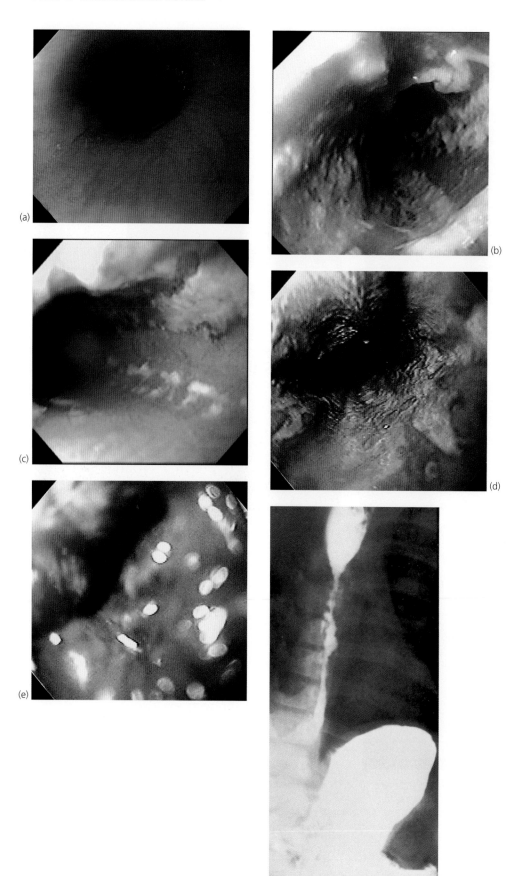

Figure 19.12 Examples of the range of caustic esophageal injury in several pediatric patients after ingestion of a household alkali cleaning agent. First-degree injury is manifest by mucosal erythema **(a)**, second-degree injury results in sloughing of the mucosa with ulceration **(b, c, d)**, and third-degree injury results in mucosal necrosis **(e)**. A long-term complication from severe injury is esophageal stricturing disease, seen here on a barium esophagram **(f)**. Figures **(d)** to **(f)** courtesy of Douglas O. Faigel.

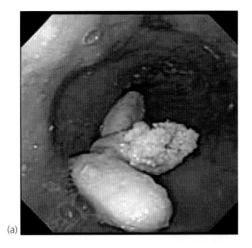

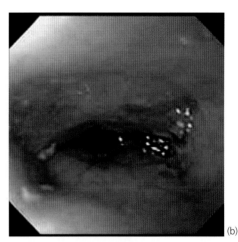

Figure 19.13 Three pill tablets (one partially dissolved) lodged in the midesophagus with nearby erosions **(a)**. After removal of the tablets, pill esophagitis and an underlying esophageal stricture are evident **(b)**. (a)

(b)

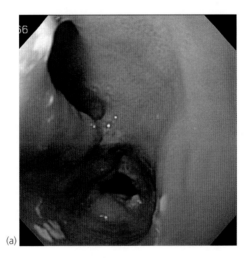

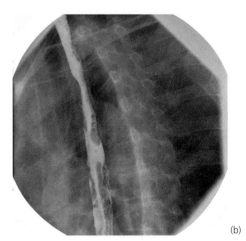

Figure 19.14 An endoscopic view of Crohn's disease of the esophagus with diffuse esophageal narrowing, a prominent sinus tract, and exudative plaques **(a)**. A barium swallow from the same patient shows esophageal narrowing, mucosal irregularity, ulceration, and nodularity, as well as sinus tracts parallel to the esophagus **(b)**. (a)

(b)

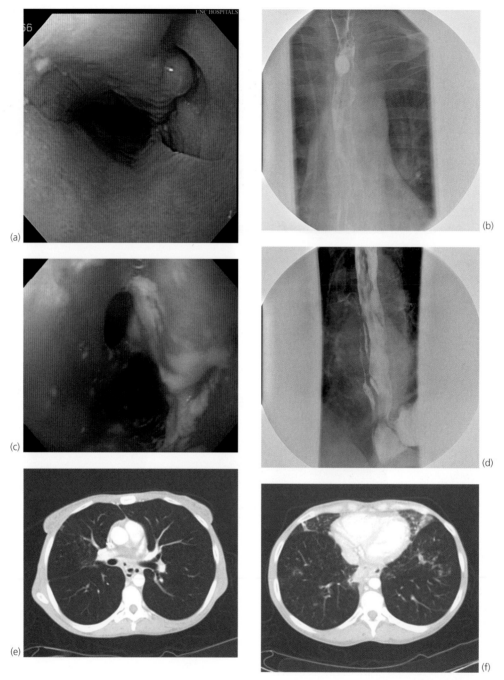

Figure 19.15 More examples of Crohn's esophagitis. Esophageal narrowing and deep sinus tracts again noted **(a)**, and on barium swallow, the barium tablet becomes lodged in the proximal esophagus **(b)**. Several fistulae with white exudate and possible *Candida* are seen opening from the esophagus. **(c)** Barium swallow confirms a thin fistulous tract from the area of the gastroesophageal junction (GEJ), extending caudally to the right mainstem bronchus **(d)**. On computed tomography (CT) scan, a thickened esophagus with multiple sinus tracts is readily apparent **(e)**, and just above the GEJ a fistulous tract is seen entering the lung **(f)**.

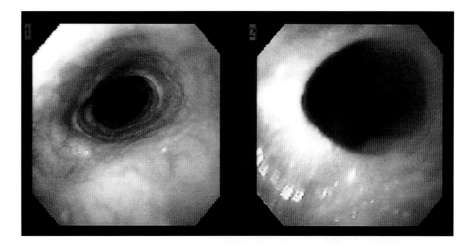

Figure 19.16 Graft-versus-host disease (GVHD) of the esophagus, with multiple fine mucosal webs present. Courtesy of Douglas O. Faigel.

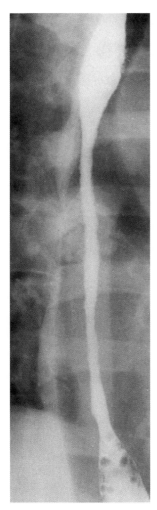

Figure 19.17 A long, tight stricture of the mid–distal esophagus in a patient with graft-versus-host disease (GVHD), involving the esophagus. Courtesy of Douglas O. Faigel.

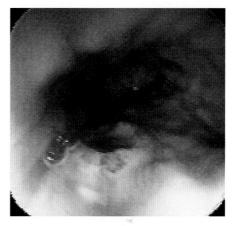

Figure 19.18 An endoscopic view of esophageal ulceration in a patient with Behçet disease. Courtesy of Douglas O. Faigel.

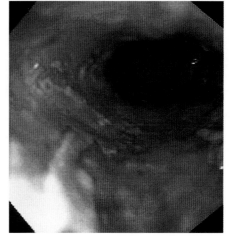

Figure 19.19 Desquamated esophageal mucosa in a patient with pemphigus vulgaris. Courtesy of Douglas O. Faigel.

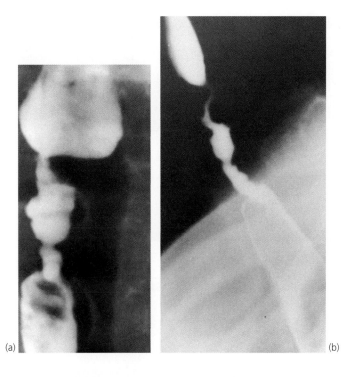

(a)

(b)

Figure 19.20 Benign mucous membrane pemphigoid. Postinflammatory scarring caused a long, irregular area of narrowing suggestive of a malignant process on a barium swallow.

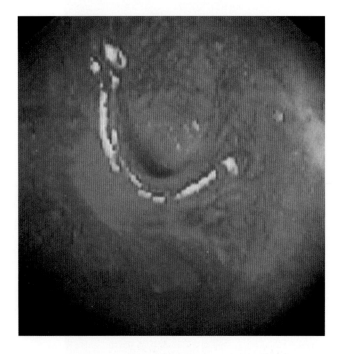

Figure 19.21 An endoscopic view of benign mucous membrane pemphigoid demonstrating a tight esophageal stricture. Courtesy of Douglas O. Faigel.

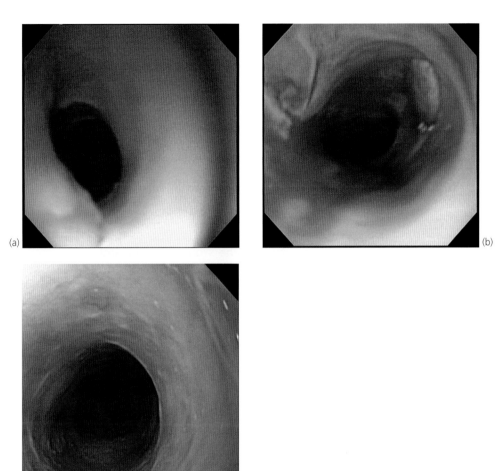

(a)

(b)

(c)

Figure 19.22 An endoscopic view of a tight esophageal stricture due to epidermolysis bullosa dystrophica before **(a)** and after **(b)** initial dilation. After multiple sessions of serial dilation, the stricture zone is much improved **(c)**.

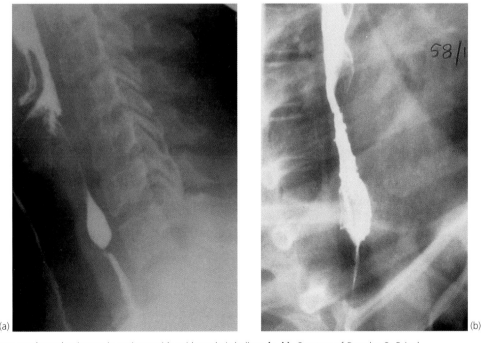

(a)

(b)

Figure 19.23 Severe esophageal strictures in patients with epidermolysis bullosa **(a, b)**. Courtesy of Douglas O. Faigel.

20

Stomach and duodenum: anatomy and structural anomalies

Jean-Pierre Raufman, Eric Goldberg

Normal gastric and duodenal anatomy

The tubular esophagus abruptly joins the sac-like stomach at the gastroesophageal junction (Fig. 20.1a). The cardiac region (Fig. 20.1b) and fundus (Fig. 20.1c) of the stomach abut the gastric side of the gastroesophageal junction. Like an accordion, the folds of the gastric body (Fig. 20.1d) permit distention of the stomach when full and contraction when empty. The smooth distal antrum (Fig. 20.1e) leads to the pyloric channel (Fig. 20.1f). The first portion or bulb of the duodenum (Fig. 20.1g) takes a turn into the tubular second and third portions (Fig. 20.1h) of the duodenum.

Vagal innervation and lymphatics of the stomach

Vagal fibers provide parasympathetic innervation to the stomach (Fig. 20.2). The branches of the anterior gastric nerve from the anterior vagal trunk innervate the cardia and provide a branch running to the right of the lesser curvature, known as the anterior nerve of Latarjet. The hepatic nerve, also a branch of the anterior vagus, innervates the liver, gallbladder, pylorus of the stomach, and proximal duodenum. The posterior vagal trunk divides into a celiac branch, which innervates the pancreas and other abdominal viscera, and posterior gastric branches, which innervate both surfaces of the stomach and form the posterior nerve of Latarjet. The anterior and posterior nerves of Latarjet course along the lesser curvature, give off branches to the fundus and body, and terminate in a "crow's foot" neural distribution to the antrum and pylorus (see Fig. 20.2). The gastric lymphatics (see Fig. 20.2) have a similar pattern to that of the arterial supply (Fig. 20.3), although flow is in the opposite direction. Lymph from the stomach drains into the celiac and gastric lymph nodes.

Vasculature of the stomach and duodenum

The stomach and duodenum derive their blood supply primarily from the celiac axis (see Fig. 20.3) and the superior mesenteric artery. The celiac artery branches off as the splenic, left gastric, and hepatic arteries (see Fig. 20.3). Branches from these vessels, including the right gastric and gastroduodenal artery from the hepatic artery and the short gastric arteries, and left gastroepiploic artery from the splenic artery, form a dense anastomotic network that encircles the stomach. The right gastric artery and superior pancreaticoduodenal artery, which also arise from the hepatic artery (see Fig. 20.3), supply the duodenum. In concert with the superior mesenteric artery, these vessels provide a rich blood supply to the stomach and duodenum.

The superior mesenteric artery derives from the aorta 3–4 cm below the celiac artery, just behind the body of the pancreas and the third to fourth parts of the duodenum (Figs 20.3 and 20.4). The inferior pancreaticoduodenal branch of the superior mesenteric artery supplies the distal stomach and the duodenum. Corresponding veins course with the arteries and ultimately drain into the portal vein.

Gastric mucosal cells

The organizational units of the glandular stomach (fundus and body) are the gastric glands that empty their contents into the gastric lumen through pits that stud the mucosal surface. These contents comprise an aqueous mixture of secretions primarily from mucous, parietal, and chief cells.

Mucous cells, which line the gastric surface, and, in larger number, mucous neck cells are the most common cell type in the upper third of the gastric glands (Fig. 20.5). The main secretory product of these cells is the glycoprotein mucin, which helps to protect the gastric epithelium from acid, pepsin, and other endogenous and exogenous injuriants. Parietal (oxyntic) cells, which secrete hydrochloric acid, are found predominantly in the midportion of the gastric glands. These cells are readily identified because of their concentric nuclei, abundant mitochondria, and eosinophilia (Fig. 20.6). Chief cells, which secrete the proenzyme pepsinogen, are found largely at the base of gastric glands. These polar,

Atlas of Gastroenterology, 4th edition. Edited by Tadataka Yamada, David H. Alpers, Anthony N. Kalloo, Neil Kaplowitz, Chung Owyang, and Don W. Powell. © 2009 Blackwell Publishing, ISBN: 978-1-4051-6909-7

basophilic cells are filled with zymogen granules at their apical poles. Numerous endocrine cells, such as the histamine-secreting enterochromaffin-like cells and somatostatin-secreting D cells are scattered throughout the lower two-thirds of the gastric glands close to their cellular targets.

Stimulation of parietal cells causes translocation of H^+,K^+-adenosine triphosphatase to the membrane of the expanded canaliculi. Activation of this enzyme, the so-called "proton pump," results in secretion of acid into the glandular lumen. Stimulation of chief cells results in movement of zymogen granules to the apical membrane, fusion of granule membranes with the apical membrane, and extrusion of pepsinogen into the glandular lumen. Hydrostatic forces "pump" glandular contents into the gastric lumen, where the acid environment catalyzes the hydrolysis of pepsinogen to the active acid protease pepsin.

When the stomach is empty, the mucosa and submucosa contract, creating thick folds called *rugae*. An endoscopic ultrasound image of the stomach and its rugal folds is shown in Fig. 20.7.

Embryology

The primitive foregut gives rise to the stomach and proximal duodenum. The distal duodenum, from the middle of the second part onward, is formed from the cephalic end of the midgut. During the fourth week of development, the stomach consists of a fusiform dilation in the foregut that, over subsequent weeks, rotates 90° clockwise around its longitudinal axis. The stomach ends with the left side anterior and the right side posterior (Fig. 20.8). The result of this rotation is that the left vagus nerve supplies the anterior wall of the stomach and the right vagus nerve supplies the posterior wall (see Fig. 20.2). The left wall of the stomach grows faster than the right, resulting in formation of the greater (left) and lesser (right) curvatures. Rotation of the developing stomach pulls the dorsal mesentery (mesogastrium) left to form the omental bursa (lesser sac) of the peritoneum (see Fig. 20.8). The ventral mesentery attaches the stomach and duodenum to the liver and antral wall. During gastric development, the duodenum enlarges rapidly to form a loop that projects ventrally, rotates right, and ends as a retroperitoneal organ.

The common bile duct and ventral pancreatic duct (Wirsung) enter the second portion of the duodenum via the posteromedially located ampulla of Vater. The accessory pancreatic duct (Santorini) enters the duodenum approximately 2 cm proximal to the ampulla of Vater via the minor papilla (Fig. 20.9).

Congenital abnormalities of the stomach and duodenum

Congenital abnormalities of the stomach include atresia, mucosal membranes, diverticula, duplication, teratoma, microgastria, and hypertrophic pyloric stenosis. Atresia and mucosal membranes in the antrum or pylorus probably result from failure of recanalization of the lumen, which is temporarily obstructed by the epithelium during normal embryogenesis. Membranes that contain either squamous or columnar epithelium encircle but generally do not occlude the lumen. Plain abdominal radiographs usually do not show mucosal membranes, but barium studies may demonstrate delayed emptying of contrast material and a sharply defined, bandlike defect in the prepyloric antrum that simulates a second duodenal bulb (Fig. 20.10). Gastric duplications, which contain mucosa, submucosa, and muscle, share a common wall and may communicate with the stomach (Fig. 20.11).

Intestinal malrotation, the most common cause of duodenal obstruction, may result in mesenteric bands or compression of the ligament of Treitz on the second or third parts of the duodenum (Fig. 20.12). Developmental abnormalities of adjacent organs, such as annular pancreas, preduodenal portal vein, or superior mesenteric artery syndrome may obstruct the duodenum.

In the superior mesenteric artery syndrome, this artery compresses the third portion of the duodenum against fixed retroperitoneal structures. This may result from acute angulation of the superior mesenteric artery, with the abdominal aorta associated with rapid childhood growth, weight loss, and immobilization, but the cause is not clear. Plain abdominal radiography of a patient with duodenal obstruction is unlikely to reveal the cause. Nevertheless, duodenal obstruction is suggested on these radiographs by a "double-bubble" sign (Fig. 20.13). In general, gastrointestinal barium contrast studies are more helpful in defining the abnormality. These radiographs typically show an abrupt cutoff of barium at the obstruction and proximal dilation. However, instillation of barium into the obstructed stomach or duodenum carries risk for aspiration of contrast medium. The stomach must be completely decompressed before administration of small, incremental amounts of barium, or a less risky modality, such as ultrasonography, should be used first. In superior mesenteric artery syndrome, abdominal aortograms in the lateral view may show narrowing of the angle between the superior mesenteric artery and the aorta.

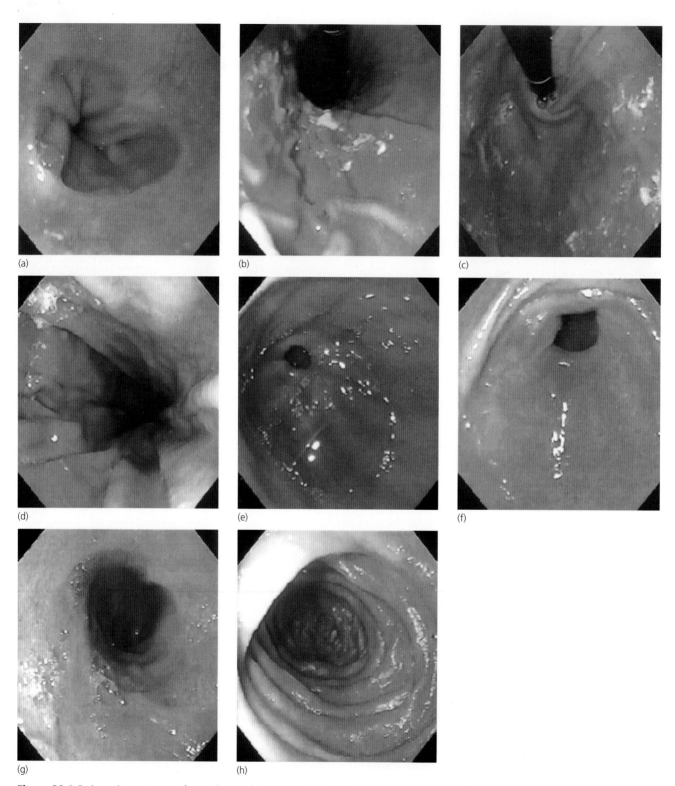

Figure 20.1 Endoscopic appearance of normal stomach and duodenum. **(a)** Gastroesophageal junction; **(b)** gastric cardia, **(c)** gastric fundus, **(d)** gastric body, **(e)** gastric antrum, **(f)** pylorus, **(g)** duodenal bulb, **(h)** second and third portions of duodenum.

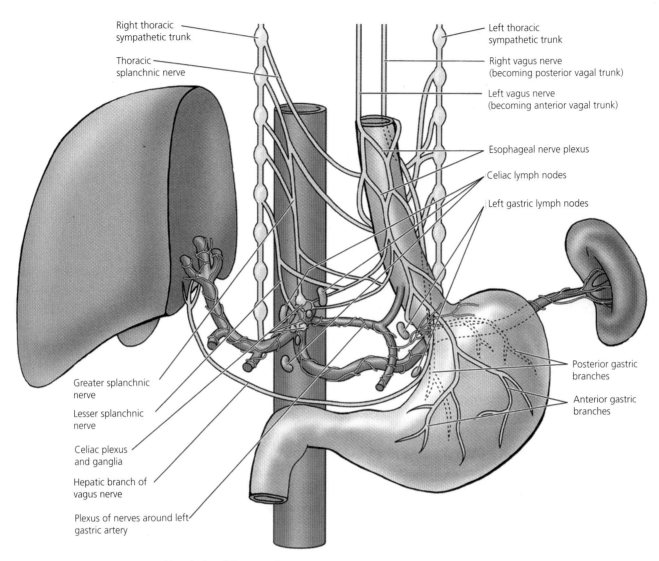

Right thoracic
sympathetic trunk

Thoracic
splanchnic nerve

Left thoracic
sympathetic trunk

Right vagus nerve
(becoming posterior vagal trunk)

Left vagus nerve
(becoming anterior vagal trunk)

Esophageal nerve plexus

Celiac lymph nodes

Left gastric lymph nodes

Posterior gastric
branches

Anterior gastric
branches

Greater splanchnic
nerve

Lesser splanchnic
nerve

Celiac plexus
and ganglia

Hepatic branch of
vagus nerve

Plexus of nerves around left
gastric artery

Figure 20.2 Vagal innervation and lymphatics of the stomach.

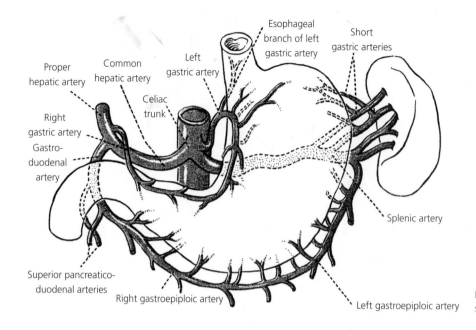

Figure 20.3 Arterial supply of the stomach and duodenum.

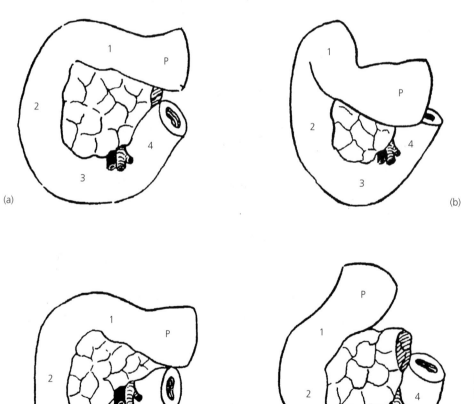

(a)

(b)

(c)

(d)

Figure 20.4 Normal variations in shape and orientation of the duodenum. Anatomic distinctions between the four parts of the duodenum become less distinct as one progresses from **(a)** to **(d)**. P, pylorus; 1–4, first to fourth portions of the duodenum.

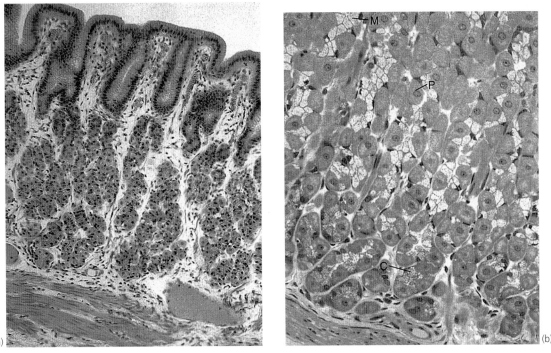

(a)

(b)

Figure 20.5 (a) Photomicrograph (original magnification ×132) of the mucosa of the fundic stomach. **(b)** Photomicrograph (original magnification ×270) of fundic glands. M, mucous neck cell; P, parietal cell; C, chief cell.

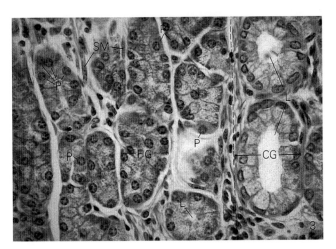

Figure 20.6 Comparison of fundic (FG) and cardiac (CG) gastric glands. Cardiac glands have larger lumens. Parietal cells (P) are eosinophilic with concentric nuclei. Unlabeled cells with more basophilic cytoplasm and basal nuclei are chief cells. Smooth muscle cells (SM) extend into the lamina propria from the muscularis mucosae. L, gland lumen.

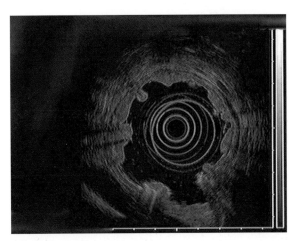

Figure 20.7 Endoscopic ultrasound image of the stomach and its rugal folds. Courtesy of Dr Peter Darwin.

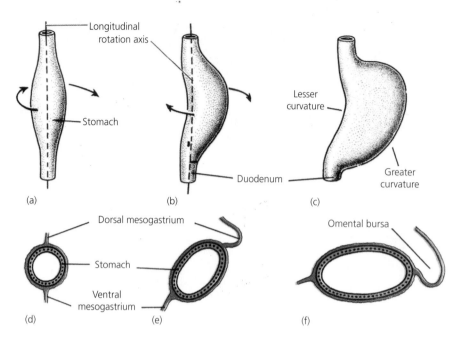

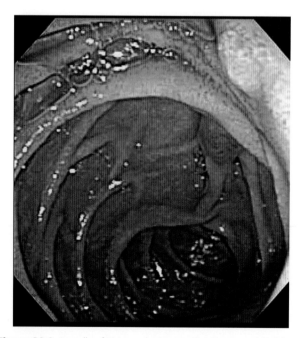

Figure 20.8 Development of the stomach and omental bursa (lesser sac). Fusiform dilation of the foregut during the fourth week enlarges and rotates clockwise around its longitudinal axis over subsequent weeks so that the original left side faces anteriorly and right side faces posteriorly.

Figure 20.9 Ampulla of Vater and minor papilla. Courtesy of Dr Eric Goldberg.

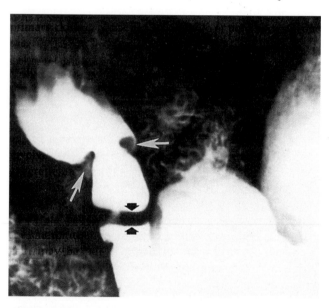

Figure 20.10 Barium contrast upper gastrointestinal series shows antral mucosal membrane (black arrows). White arrows point to the normal pylorus.

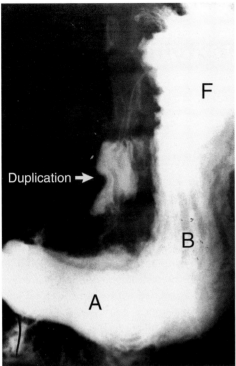

Figure 20.11 Barium contrast upper gastrointestinal series shows gastric duplication (arrow, rugal folds are present) communicating with the stomach. F, fundus; B, body; A, antrum. Courtesy of Dr Timothy Carter.

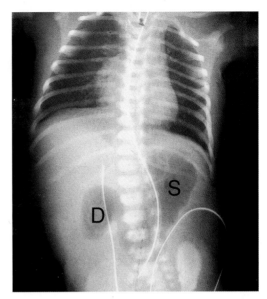

Figure 20.13 "Double bubble" sign on plain radiograph of the abdomen of an infant with duodenal atresia. Upper, larger "bubble" (S) represents gas in the stomach. Lower bubble (D) represents gas in the dilated duodenum proximal to the obstruction. Courtesy of Dr Timothy Carter.

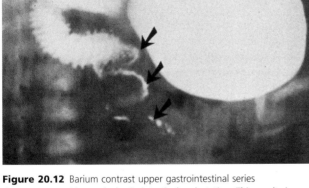

Figure 20.12 Barium contrast upper gastrointestinal series demonstrates midgut volvulus in intestinal malrotation. This results in dilation of the duodenal bulb and proximal duodenum, which terminates in a cone-shaped narrowing (upper arrow) and a "corkscrew" pattern of the distal duodenum and proximal jejunum (lower arrows).

21

Disorders of gastric emptying

Henry P. Parkman, Frank K. Friedenberg, Robert S. Fisher

Introduction

Gastric motility disorders include delayed gastric emptying (gastroparesis), rapid gastric emptying (as seen in dumping syndrome), and disorders with motor and sensory abnormalities (e.g., functional dyspepsia). Management of these patients requires an understanding of the pathophysiology, clinical tests, and treatment options.

Gastric motility

Gastric motility delivers ingested food into the duodenum at a rate that maximizes digestion and absorption. The motor activity of the stomach is generated by three different anatomic regions of the stomach: the proximal fundus, the distal antrum, and the pyloric sphincter, each with its own unique motility pattern. The proximal stomach accommodates to store the ingested meal; the distal stomach grinds down or triturates solid particles; and the pylorus allows emptying the meal in a regulated fashion into the duodenum. Thus, gastric emptying is a highly regulated process reflecting coordination between the propulsive forces of proximal fundic tone and distal antral contractions, and relaxation of the pylorus.

Gastroparesis

Gastroparesis is a disorder characterized by symptoms of, and evidence for, gastric retention in the absence of mechanical obstruction. Gastroparesis typically affects women, and has significant impact on quality of life. Although the true prevalence of gastroparesis is not known, it has been estimated that up to 4% of the population experiences symp-

tomatic manifestations of this condition. Diabetes mellitus is the most common systemic disease associated with gastroparesis. A similar number of patients present with idiopathic gastroparesis. Of interest, idiopathic gastroparesis was suspected of being associated with a previous viral infection in 23% of cases. Postsurgical gastroparesis, often with vagotomy or inadvertent damage to the vagus nerve, represents the third most common etiology of gastroparesis.

Symptoms of gastroparesis

The most frequently reported symptoms associated with gastroparesis include nausea, vomiting, early satiety, and postprandial fullness. Abdominal discomfort and pain also are noted by many affected patients and represent challenging symptoms to treat. Weight loss, malnutrition, and dehydration may be prominent in severe cases. In diabetics, gastroparesis may adversely affect glycemic control. Although it has been a common assumption that gastrointestinal symptoms can be attributed to delayed gastric emptying, most investigations have observed only weak correlations between symptom severity and the degree of gastric stasis. Symptoms that suggest delayed gastric emptying in patients with dyspeptic symptoms are primarily postprandial fullness, nausea, and vomiting. In patients with diabetes, symptoms that have been associated with delayed gastric emptying are abdominal bloating/fullness. A symptom questionnaire, the Gastroparesis Cardinal Symptom Index (GCSI), has been developed for quantifying symptoms in patients with gastroparesis (Table 21.1). The GCSI is based on three subscales (postprandial fullness/early satiety, nausea/vomiting, and bloating) and represents a subset of the longer patient assessment of upper gastrointestinal disorders-symptoms (PAGI-SYM).

Evaluation of gastroparesis

The diagnosis of gastroparesis is made when a documented delay in gastric emptying is present and endoscopic or radiographic testing exclude a mechanical blockage. The best accepted technique for measurement of gastric emptying is

Atlas of Gastroenterology, 4th edition. Edited by Tadataka Yamada, David H. Alpers, Anthony N. Kalloo, Neil Kaplowitz, Chung Owyang, and Don W. Powell. © 2009 Blackwell Publishing, ISBN: 978-1-4051-6909-7

scintigraphy, using an egg meal cooked with a technetium radiolabel. The gastric emptying test determines the percent gastric retention at both 2 and 4 h postprandially. Physicians from the American Neurogastroenterology and Motility Society with the Society of Nuclear Medicine have adopted the Tougas et al. low-fat, egg-white sandwich with jelly as a test meal and imaging at 0, 1, 2, and 4 h postprandially (Fig. 21.1). Imaging for gastric emptying up to 4 h, rather than 2 h, has been shown to increase the diagnosis of delayed gastric emptying and is now suggested as the standard in all tests to obtain reliable results for the detection of gastroparesis (Fig. 21.2). When gastric scintigraphy is performed for shorter durations, the test is less reliable because of larger variations in normal gastric emptying.

Gastric emptying scintigraphy measures only the net output of solids or liquids from the stomach and fails to define the pathophysiological mechanisms that may impair gastric emptying. Technical advances in scintigraphy provide information on fundic and antral abnormalities. Regional gastric emptying can be used to assess intragastric meal distribution and transit from the proximal to distal portion of the stomach (Fig. 21.3). Proximal retention has been described in gastroesophageal reflux disease (GERD), distal retention in functional dyspepsia, and global retention in gastroparesis. Dynamic antral contraction scintigraphy (DACS) with frequent imaging can visualize antral contractions (Fig. 21.4). Gastric mucosal labeling with single photon emission computed tomography (SPECT), which measures gastric volume as an index of accommodation, can be combined with a scintigraphic test that measures gastric emptying using two different radionuclides (Fig. 21.5). In this test, intravenous technetium 99m pertechnetate is used to image the gastric mucosa and an indium-111 radiolabeled solid meal is employed to measure gastric emptying.

Two new methods are available to measure gastric emptying. First, a recently Food and Drug Administration (FDA)-approved pH and pressure sensing capsule (SmartPill) can assess gastric emptying by recording the duration of acidity from capsule ingestion to the change in pH, from the acidic stomach to the alkaline duodenum (Fig. 21.6). This capsule can also record pressures as it passes through the gastrointestinal tract. Second, a ^{13}C-octanoate breath test (OBT) can be used for measuring gastric emptying, and has been shown to correlate significantly with gastric emptying for solids measured by scintigraphy. A muffin-based OBT is convenient, sensitive, and specific to detect delayed gastric emptying. Both of these new tests can be performed as an outpatient or as an inpatient in a hospital room.

Electrogastrography is the cutaneous recording of myoelectric activity of the gastric smooth muscle by means of superficial abdominal-wall electrodes overlying the stomach. The recorded signal is called an electrogastrogram (EGG) and usually consists of three cycles per minute (cpm) signal, reflecting gastric slow-wave (pacemaker) activity and the subsequent gastric contractions (Fig. 21.7). Abnormalities in the EGG signal have been demonstrated in patients with gastroparesis and functional dyspepsia (Fig. 21.8). A significant percentage of these patients may have very rapid, slow-wave frequencies (tachygastria) or slow-wave frequencies that are very slow (bradygastria). Multichannel EGG recording has been suggested as a way to assess gastric electrical slow-wave propagation velocity and to detect electromechanical uncoupling (Fig. 21.9). In this technique, the EGG is recorded using electrodes placed at different positions overlying the stomach. Multichannel electrogastrography may enhance the diagnostic utility of the test compared with traditional one-channel recording in detecting abnormalities, such as ectopic gastric pacemaker and abnormal coupling of the electrical slow waves.

Diabetic gastroparesis

Gastroparesis is a well-recognized complication of diabetes mellitus. Diabetic gastroparesis is clinically important because it causes gastrointestinal symptoms, alterations in glycemic control, and changes in oral drug absorption. It is associated with long-standing, insulin-dependent (type 1) diabetes mellitus (IDDM) with the complications of retinopathy, nephropathy, and peripheral neuropathy. Recent longitudinal studies suggest that delayed gastric emptying of solid or nutrient liquid meals is common, not only in 25%–40% of patients with long-standing type 1 diabetes, but also in 10%–20% of patients with type 2 diabetes, a more common condition.

Hyperglycemia, itself, may reversibly impair gastric motility by decreasing antral contractility, reducing antral phase III migrating motor complex activity, increasing pyloric contractions, stimulating gastric dysrhythmias (primarily tachygastria), and thus delaying gastric emptying. Normalization of serum glucose in hyperglycemic patients has been shown to improve gastric myoelectric activity, accelerate gastric emptying, and restore antral phase III activity in some patients. In addition, hyperglycemia reduces the effect of prokinetic agents.

Changes of gastric motility may also significantly affect postprandial blood glucose concentrations. In some diabetic patients, delayed gastric emptying may contribute to poor glucose control because of unpredictable delivery of food into the duodenum. Impaired gastric emptying with continued administration of exogenous insulin may also produce hypoglycemia. Conversely, acceleration of emptying has been reported to cause hyperglycemia. Problems with blood sugar control may be the first indication that a diabetic patient is developing a gastric motility disorder. Interestingly, in some of these patients, gastroparetic symptoms may be mild or absent.

In addition to abnormalities in gastric emptying, subjects with IDDM have an increased perception of gastric distention produced with a gastric barostat, perhaps resulting in exaggerated nausea, bloating, and upper abdominal pain. Increased sensitivity of the proximal stomach may be responsible for dyspeptic symptoms in the postprandial period during which the proximal stomach is distended by a meal. Thus, in some patients with diabetic gastroparesis, there is visceral hypersensitivity similar to that described in functional dyspepsia. There is also an overlap between idiopathic gastroparesis and functional dyspepsia, in that delayed gastric emptying has been described in approximately 35% of patients with functional dyspepsia. In these cases, one might be able to treat the gastroparesis with prokinetic agents or the dyspeptic symptoms with sensory modulating agents.

Treatment of gastroparesis

The goals of gastroparesis therapy include relief of symptoms, normalization of nutrition and hydration status, improvement of glycemic control in diabetics, and improvement of gastric emptying when appropriate. Treatment of gastroparesis includes dietary modifications, prokinetic and antiemetic medications, measures to control pain and address psychological issues, and endoscopic or surgical options in selected instances. The different therapeutic modalities may be offered alone or in different combinations as dictated by the needs of the individual patient.

Prokinetic agents enhance the motility of the upper gastrointestinal tract and accelerate the aboral movement of the intralumenal contents. In general, prokinetic agents increase gastric antral contractility, correct gastric dysrhythmias, and improve antroduodenal coordination. Current prokinetic agents for treatment include oral agents metoclopramide and erythromycin. Cisapride (Propulsid) and Tegaserod (Zelnorm) have been removed from the market because of cardiac side effects. Domperidone is not available in the United States, although it is available through the FDA Investigative New Drug (IND) program. Intravenous agents currently used to treat hospitalized patients include metoclopramide and erythromycin.

Gastric electrical stimulation with an implanted neurostimulator is an emerging therapy for treatment of refractory gastroparesis. It has been intensely investigated over the last two decades. Only in the last 5 years, however, have promising results been reported. There are several ways to electrically stimulate the stomach. First is gastric electrical pacing. Here, the goal is to entrain and pace the gastric slow waves at a higher rate than the patient's normal 3.0 cpm. Pacing at 10% higher than the basal rate has been shown to accelerate gastric emptying and improve dyspeptic symptoms. Second is neuromodulation using high-frequency stimulation at four times the basal rate (12 cpm). With these stimulation parameters, there may be improvement in symptoms with little change in gastric emptying. It has been suggested that this type of stimulation activates sensory afferent nerves to suppress symptoms. Finally, early studies in animals have used sequential circumferential direct muscle stimulation, employing bursts of very high frequency stimulation to sequentially induce direct muscle stimulation in a peristaltic fashion and accelerate gastric emptying.

Table 21.1 Gastroparesis Cardinal Symptom Index

	None	Very mild	Mild	Moderate	Severe	Very severe
1. Nausea (feeling sick to your stomach as though you might vomit)	0	1	2	3	4	5
2. Retching (heaving, as if to vomit, but nothing comes up)	0	1	2	3	4	5
3. Vomiting	0	1	2	3	4	5
4. Stomach fullness	0	1	2	3	4	5
5. Not able to finish a normal-sized meal	0	1	2	3	4	5
6. Feeling excessively full after meals	0	1	2	3	4	5
7. Loss of appetite	0	1	2	3	4	5
8. Bloating (feeling as though you need to loosen your clothes)	0	1	2	3	4	5
9. Stomach is visibly larger	0	1	2	3	4	5

The Gastroparesis Cardinal Symptom Index (GCSI) is a nine-symptom questionnaire that has been developed for quantifying symptoms in patients with gastroparesis.
From Revicki DA, Rentz AM, Dubois D, et al. Development and validation of a patient-assessed gastroparesis symptom severity measure: the Gastroparesis Cardinal Symptom Index. Aliment Pharmacol Ther 2003;18:141.

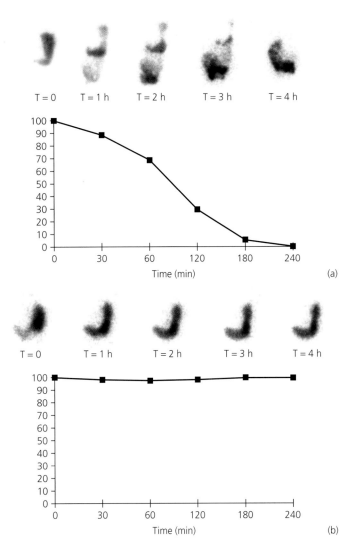

(a)

(b)

Figure 21.1 Gastric emptying scintigraphy. Gastric emptying scintigraphy using a technetium-99m-labeled egg sandwich. The percentages of gastric retention are shown for 0, 30, 60, 120, 180, and 240 min after meal ingestion. **(a)** Normal gastric emptying with only 30% retention at 2 h after meal ingestion (normal <50%) and complete emptying at 4 h (normal <10%). **(b)** Markedly delayed gastric emptying with little emptying at 4 h.

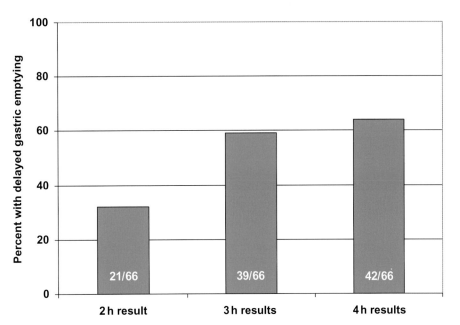

Figure 21.2 Gastric emptying scintigraphy with imaging up to 4 h. Imaging for gastric emptying up to 4 h increases the detection of delayed gastric emptying (see Chapter 23). Imaging up to 4 hours increased the diagnostic yield for delayed gastric emptying from 31% of patients at 2 h to 63% at 4 h.

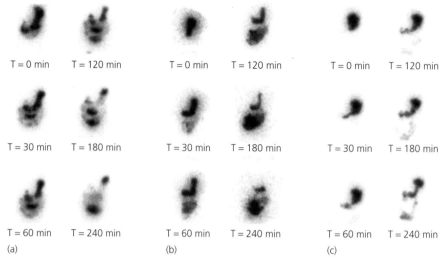

Figure 21.3 Regional gastric emptying scintigraphy. Regional gastric emptying abnormalities in gastroesophageal reflux disease, functional dyspepsia, and gastroparesis. **(a)** In patients with gastroesophageal reflux disease, there is retention of the radioactivity in the proximal portion of the stomach. **(b)** In patients with functional dyspepsia, there is retention of radioactivity in the distal portion of the stomach. **(c)** In patients with gastroesophageal reflux disease, there is retention in the distal portion of the stomach. In patients with gastroparesis, there is a global retention throughout the whole stomach.

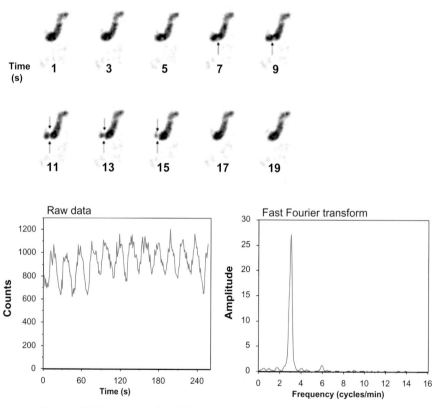

Figure 21.4 Dynamic antral scintigraphy. **(a)** Using dynamic (i.e., 1 s) acquisition, gastric antral contractions can be characterized noninvasively with scintigraphy; both the frequency and an estimate of the contractions can be obtained. An example of DACS with analysis is shown. **(b)** With a region of interest drawn around the mid antrum, the time activity curves show the counts oscillate at about three contractions per minute. The amplitude of the fast Fourier transform (FFT) analysis gives an approximation of the ejection fraction (contraction strength).

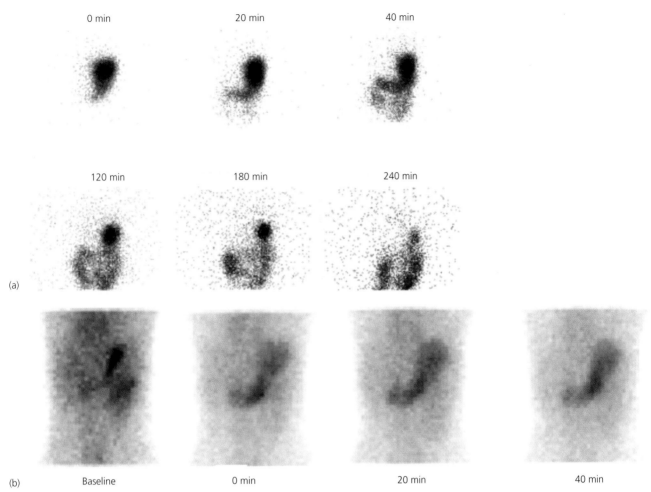

(a)

(b)

Figure 21.5 Simultaneous gastric emptying and gastric volume. Gastric mucosal labeling with SPECT imaging, which measures gastric volume as an index of accommodation, can be combined with a scintigraphic test that measures gastric emptying using two different radionuclides. In this test, intravenous technetium-99m pertechnetate is used to image the gastric mucosa and an indium-111 radiolabeled solid meal is employed to measure gastric emptying. **(a)** Gastric emptying of orally administered indium-111 labeled egg sandwich. **(b)** Gastric volume after intravenous technetium and orally administered egg sandwich. From Simonian HP, Kantor S, Knight LC, et al. Simultaneous assessment of gastric accommodation and emptying: Studies with liquid and solid meals. J Nuclear Med 2004;45:1155.

002003 Combined pressure and pH

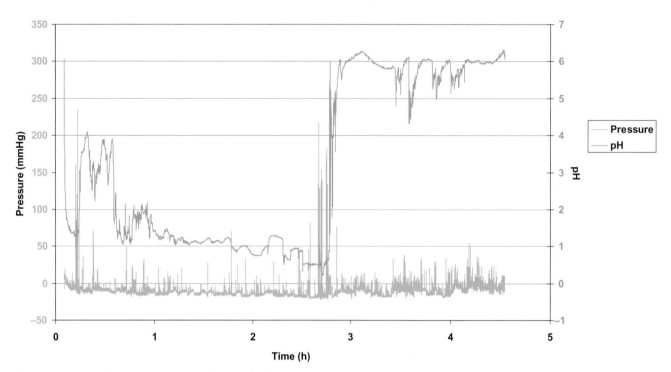

Figure 21.6 SmartPill pH and pressure recording capsule. The SmartPill, a recently FDA-approved pH and pressure sensing capsule, can assess gastric emptying by recording the duration of acidity from capsule ingestion to the change in pH from the acidic stomach to the alkaline duodenum. This capsule can also record pressures as it passes through the gastrointestinal tract. High-amplitude contractions precede the gastric emptying of the SmartPill at 2.75 h as indicated by the marked increase in pH.

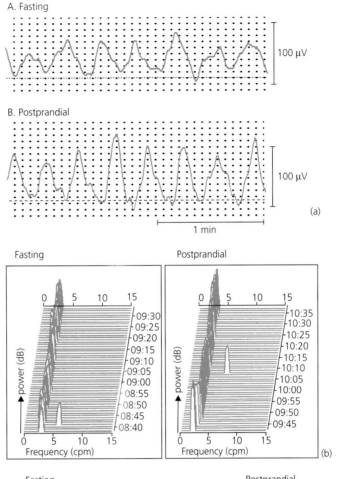

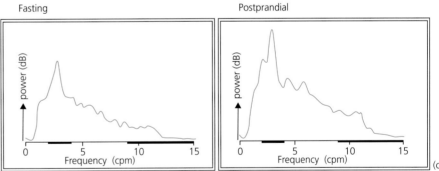

Figure 21.7 Single-channel electrogastrography. This figure shows the EGG tracings and computer analyses from a normal volunteer. The raw tracing **(a)** demonstrates a sinusoidal oscillation with a frequency of 3 cpm during both the fasting and postprandial periods. Signal amplitude increases with meal ingestion. Running spectral analysis **(b)** displays the dominant EGG frequencies as a function of time. Throughout the recording, the dominant frequency is in the frequency band 2–4 cpm. The power frequency spectrum **(c)** displays the dominant frequency for the entire fasting and postprandial periods (3 cpm). The increase in power with meal ingestion can be quantified using this analysis. Small peaks at harmonics of the dominant frequency are seen at 6 and 9 cpm.

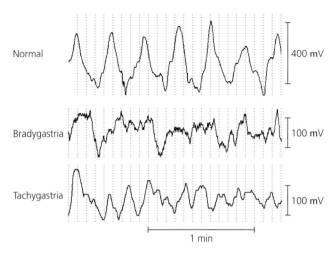

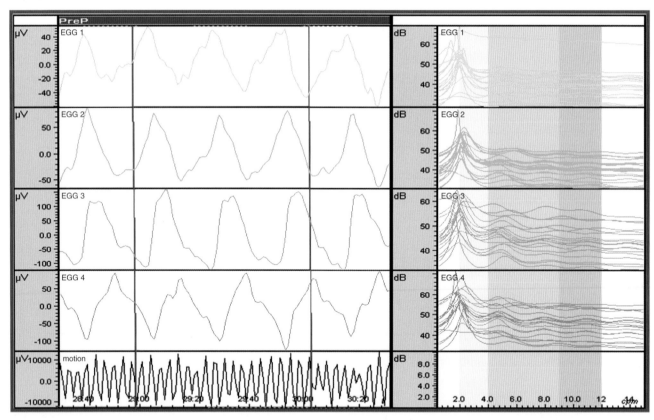

Figure 21.8 Gastric dysrhythmias recorded with electrogastrography (EGG). Representative EGG tracings showing examples of normal 3 cpm rhythm, bradygastria, and tachygastria.

Figure 21.9 Multichannel electrogastrography (EGG). Recently, multichannel EGG has been recorded using four cutaneous electrodes that are placed along the antral axis. This technique, as developed by Chen et al., can assess myoelectrical coupling between different leads. Coupling is defined as similar frequency in adjacent EGG leads. Multichannel EGG was used to assess electrical slow wave coupling in addition to the dominant frequency, power, and percent normal rhythm in normal subjects to define the normal parameters. Similar multichannel EGG values were observed among different genders and ages. Body mass and ethnicity may impact on some of the EGG values. The motion tracing shows normal 3 cpm activity among the four different EGG leads placed along the antral axis.

22

Peptic ulcer disease

David Y. Graham, Akira Horiuchi, Mototsugu Kato

Introduction

Peptic ulcer disease is an important cause of morbidity, and health-care costs (estimates of expenditures related to work loss, hospitalization, and outpatient care), excluding medication costs, are more than $5 billion per year in the United States. In general, ulcer disease results from an imbalance between aggressive factors (acid, pepsin, *Helicobacter pylori* and nonsteroidal antiinflammatory drugs [NSAIDs]) and the ability of the gastroduodenal mucosal to protect and heal itself. Other causes of peptic ulcer include pathological hypersecretory states (e.g., Zollinger–Ellison syndrome, mast cell disease), and other infections (herpes simplex) are rare.

Helicobacter pylori-related disease

Until recently, worldwide, *H. pylori* infection was the cause of the majority of duodenal (90%–95%) and gastric ulcers (60%–70%). *Helicobacter pylori* infection elicits an inflammatory response characterized by infiltration of both acute and chronic inflammatory cells, which tend to impair mucosal integrity. *H. pylori*, the host, and the environment interact with the environment to produce clinical disease. Ulcers tend to form at the sites of maximum inflammation. The virulence factors of *H. pylori* associated with production of proinflammatory virulence factors include the *cag*, such as the *cag* pathogenicity island, and the outer inflammatory protein, OipA. Important host factors include the intrinsic capacity to secrete acid and the presence of genetic polymorphisms leading to an enhanced inflammatory response to the infection (Fig. 22.1).

The location of *H. pylori*-associated ulcers can be either in the duodenum, the stomach, or both. Duodenal ulcers are associated with normal or higher than normal acid secretion.

The duodenal bulb typically contains areas of gastric metaplasia that serve as attachment sites for the organism. A critical variable in allowing duodenal ulcers to form, and in perpetuating their presence, is an increased duodenal acid load. The duodenal acid load has two components: increased acid secretion from the stomach and reduced ability of the duodenum to neutralize acid entering it (Table 22.1). The mechanism(s) that enables gastric ulcers to form, particularly as focal lesions, remains less clear. The more distal the ulcer, the more likely that acid secretion is increased.

The discovery that most peptic ulcers were curable manifestations of a mucosal infection changed the focus of approach to *H. pylori* eradication, and made enhancing mucosal integrity and suppression of acid subsidiary goals. *Helicobacter pylori* eradication cures *H. pylori*-induced ulcer disease whether or not specific therapy is directed toward ulcer healing.

Nonsteroidal antiinflammatory drug-induced ulcers

Nonsteroidal antiinflammatory drugs induce the gastrointestinal (GI) mucosal injury by direct toxic effects and by reducing mucosal prostaglandins that play a critical role in defense mechanisms and repair processes. They inhibit cyclooxygenase (COX), which is the rate-limiting enzyme required for the conversion of arachidonic acid to prostaglandins. Two COX isoforms have been identified and referred to: COX-1 and COX-2. The inducible COX-2 is an important regulator to generate prostaglandins that mediate inflammation and pain, whereas the constitutive COX-1 is responsible for maintenance of the integrity of gastric mucosa and platelet aggregation (Fig. 22.1).

The use of NSAIDs increased the risk of peptic ulcer by a factor of approximately 20. Risk factors for an ulcer or ulcer complication include a history of ulcer disease, old age, high doses of NSAID, multiple NSAID use and concomitant use of corticosteroids or anticoagulants. Figure 22.2 shows representative microscopic views of normal corpus and antral gland histology.

Atlas of Gastroenterology, 4th edition. Edited by Tadataka Yamada, David H. Alpers, Anthony N. Kalloo, Neil Kaplowitz, Chung Owyang, and Don W. Powell. © 2009 Blackwell Publishing, ISBN: 978-1-4051-6909-7

Figure 22.3 shows representative microscopic epithelial histology slides from patients with *H. pylori* infection. Although the organisms can be seen on routine hematoxylin–eosin stain, the use of a special stain provides superior results. (For further details, see "Chapter 23," Gastritis and gastropathy.) Documentation or demonstration of gastric or duodenal ulcer requires a structural study of the gastrointestinal tract. Traditional radiographic studies, such as a barium meal examination were the standard method for detecting gastric and duodenal lesions for more than half a century.

Figure 22.4 demonstrates an example of benign gastric ulcer and Fig. 22.5 shows a duodenal ulcer. The widespread availability of trained gastrointestinal endoscopists and diagnostic superiority of endoscopy over barium upper gastrointestinal examinations has led to a gradual replacement of barium studies by gastrointestinal endoscopy (Figs 22.6–22.32). Endoscopic examination of the stomach and duodenum provides a sensitivity and specificity of greater than 95% for detecting gastric and duodenal lesions. It also allows tissue diagnosis of suspicious lesions and documentation of the presence of *H. pylori* organisms.

Table 22.1 Factors that may increase the duodenal acid load and promote duodenal ulcer

Increase acid secretion
  Increased parietal cell mass
  Smoking
  Stress
  Abnormal downregulation of acid secretion by antral acidification
    or distention
Reduce ability of duodenum to neutralize acid load
  Duodenal mucosal inflammation
  Smoking
  Acid secretion by gastric metaplasia/heterotopia
  Small size of bulb
  Abnormal motility of bulb

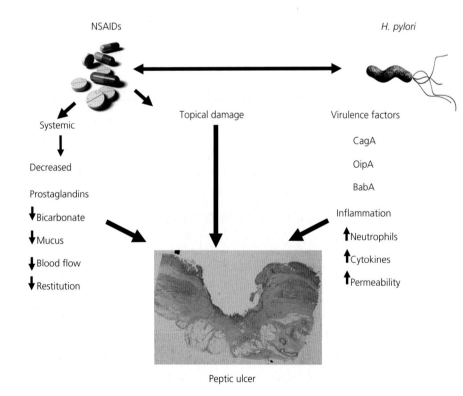

Peptic ulcer

Figure 22.1 The two main causes of peptic ulcer are use of nonsteroidal antiinflammatory drugs (NSAIDs) and infection with *Helicobacter pylori*. There is also interaction between the two major causes. Many NSAIDs have topical toxic effects by increasing mucosal permeability and permitting back diffusion of H⁺ ions because of acidic and unionized compounds, and are thus locally damaging. However, the primary effect is owing to the systemic activity of NSAIDs and is based on inhibition of cyclooxygenase I. Gastroduodenal mucosal prostaglandins play a critical role in defense mechanisms and repair processes (including blood flow, bicarbonate, and mucus secretion) and in the ability of the damaged mucosa to repair itself.

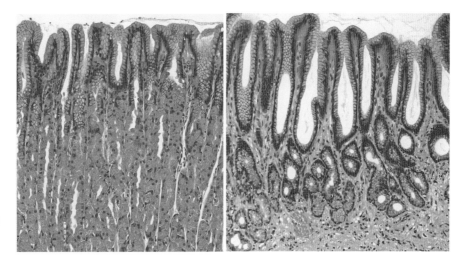

Figure 22.2 The left image shows normal pyloric (antral) gland histology. The right image shows normal fundic (body) gland histology with parietal and chief cells. Courtesy of Professor Hiroyoshi Ota, Department of Medical Technology, School of Allied Medical Sciences, Shinshu University, Matsumoto, Japan.

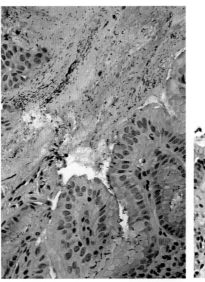

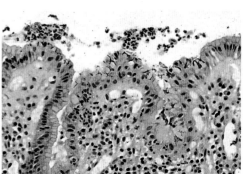

Figure 22.3 Left: gastric mucus with innumerable *Helicobacter pylori*. Organisms are seen both in the mucus and adhering to the antral mucosa. Right: surface epithelial damages caused by the adherence of *H. pylori*. Cells reduce or lose their apical mucin droplet, may take irregular cuboidal shapes and occasionally drop out, leaving small gaps that give the gastric epithelium a ragged, uneven appearance. Courtesy of Professor Robert Genta, MD, University of Texas Southwestern Medical School, Dallas, Texas.

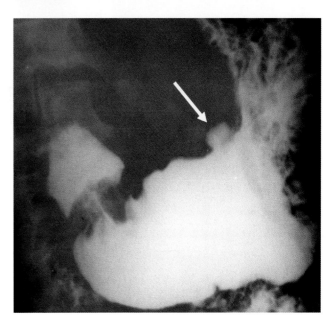

Figure 22.4 Barium study illustrating a benign gastric ulcer crater extending beyond the outlines of the stomach at the gastric angle.

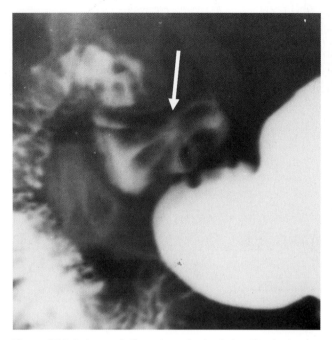

Figure 22.5 Barium study illustrating a duodenal ulcer. The duodenal folds are seen radiating toward the crater.

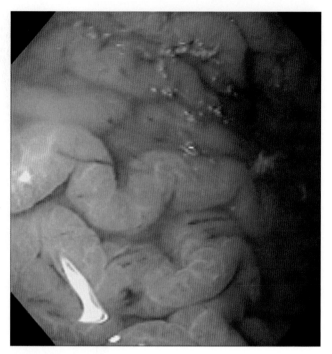

Figure 22.6 Endoscopic view of the greater curve of the body of the stomach, showing petechial hemorrhages that are leading blood into the lumen. This is a typical finding among aspirin/nonsteroidal antiinflammatory drug users. When the small amount of fluid is suctioned the fact that they communicate with the lumen is obscured and only "red dots" or "brown dots" are seen.

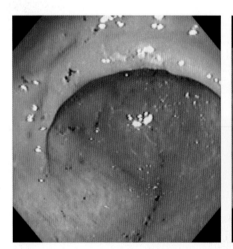

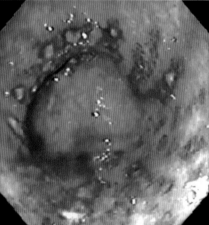

Figure 22.7 Nonsteroidal antiinflammatory drug (NSAID) gastropathy. The endoscopic view on the left shows a typical picture of an NSAID gastropathy with multiple tiny red and brown dots (superficial or intramucosal hemorrhage) and small superficial erosions. On the right there is more severe acute damage with many erosions with surrounding hemorrhage.

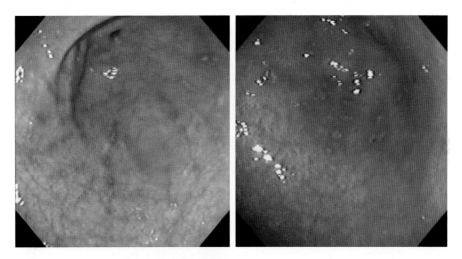

Figure 22.8 Typical endoscopic views of nonsteroidal antiinflammatory drug gastropathy with small superficial erosions in a linear pattern in the antrum. When the stomach is not distended, the erosions can be seen to typically line up along the tops of folds.

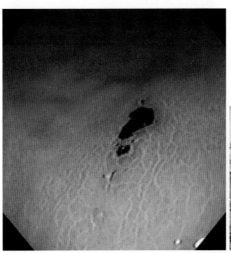

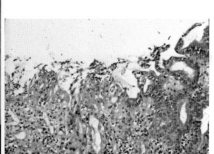

Figure 22.9 On the left, a large (3–4 mm) nonsteroidal antiinflammatory drug (NSAID)-induced erosion is seen with smaller erosions in a linear pattern. On the right the biopsy shows that the damage is very superficial involving only the upper mucosa. Erosions such as this are often scored as endoscopic ulcers in studies of antisecretory drug for the prevention of NSAID-induced damage.

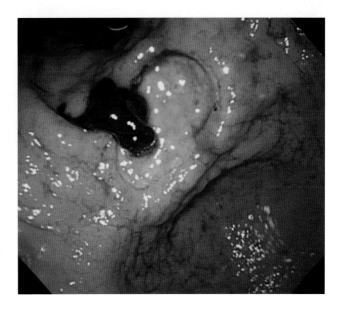

Figure 22.10 Benign gastric ulcers are typically found on the lesser curve at the gastric angle. This photograph shows a large and deep benign gastric ulcer at this typical location, with a large clot at the proximal margin.

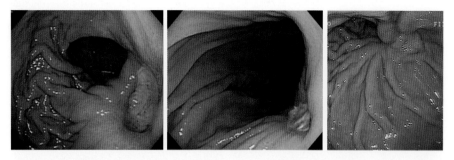

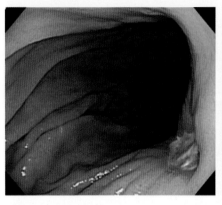

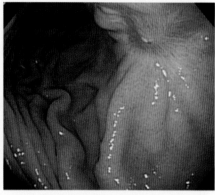

Figure 22.11 A large deep ulcer is seen in the distal gastric body on the posterior wall of the lesser curve. The three successive pictures show progressive healing of the ulcer with scar formation as shown by the increasing prominence of the radiating folds. In the third photograph, the ulcer is almost healed and the distal gastric body is significantly deformed.

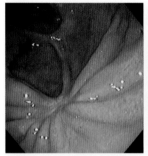

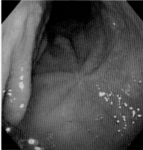

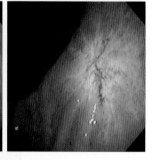

Figure 22.12 This shows a more proximal gastric body ulcer on the lesser curve. The photograph on the left shows the ulcer when first seen and the photograph on the right shows the ulcer after it was almost completely healed. The developing ulcer scar can be seen clearly along with surrounding deformity of the mucosa.

Figure 22.13 Endoscopic photographs of gastric ulcer scars during their evolution (from left to right). Over time, the degree of deformity and the radiating folds tends to decrease and after many years may become almost unapparent. The three scars are from different patients.

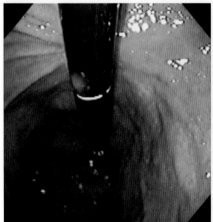

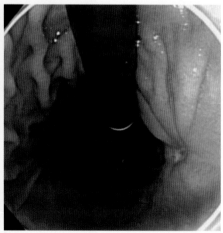

Figure 22.14 Lesser curve gastric ulcers can easily be missed as they are often covered by the endoscope in the retroflexed position. These photographs show that the practice of retroflexing in the antrum and then withdrawing the instrument into the fundus is not a good one. The mucosa of the stomach should be examined in detail both during entry and withdrawal. In this case, the careful observer will notice the radiating folds that disappear behind the shaft of the endoscope, signifying the presence of a scar, ulcer, or cancer. On the right, an ulcer is seen when the endoscope was moved to see what was behind it.

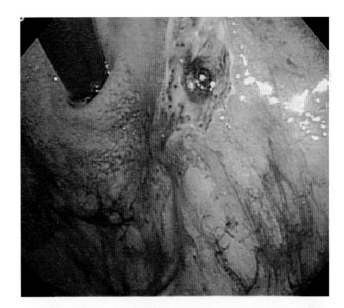

Figure 22.15 A gastric ulcer is seen adjacent to the gastroesophageal junction in a patient who presented with unexplained bleeding.

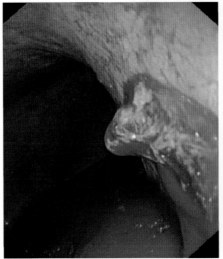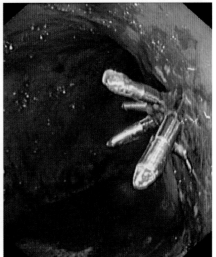

Figure 22.16 Gastric ulcer on the lesser curvature with a visible vessel/clot in a patient who has recently bled. The gastric pool consists largely of fresh blood. The picture on the right shows the ulcer site after endoscopic clipping, which successfully controlled the bleeding.

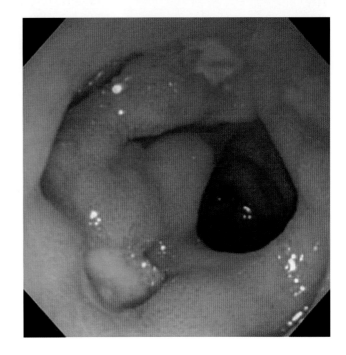

Figure 22.17 Prepyloric antral ulcers. Three small ulcers are seen in the prepyloric area, which is deformed.

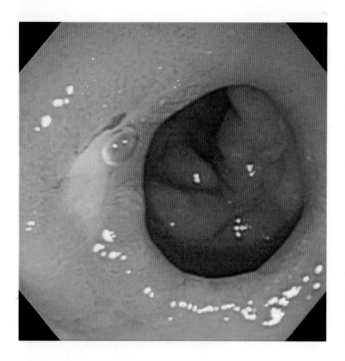

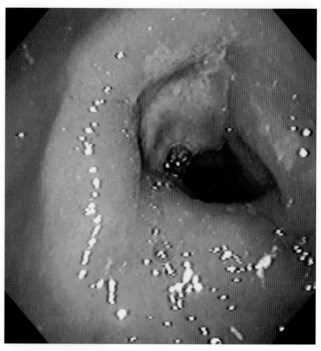

Figure 22.18 A prepyloric ulcer is seen on the anterior wall along with a duodenal ulcer seen through the pylorus on the posterior wall of the bulb.

Figure 22.19 A pyloric channel ulcer is seen that deforms the pylorus. There are also several small superficial erosions at the pylorus.

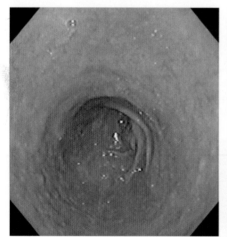

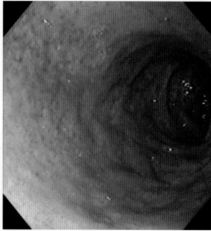

Figure 22.20 Two examples of normal duodenal bulbs are shown. Note that the normal duodenal bulb tends to be smooth and appears to be a relatively large structure, such that it is difficult to photograph an entire normal bulb in one image. These examples should be compared to the bulbs in Figs 22.21, 22.22, and 22.32, which are typical of duodenal ulcer patients, being shortened and deformed, with inflamed mucosa. These structural abnormalities result in abnormalities in motility and secretion of the duodenal bulb and contribute to the development of duodenal ulcers.

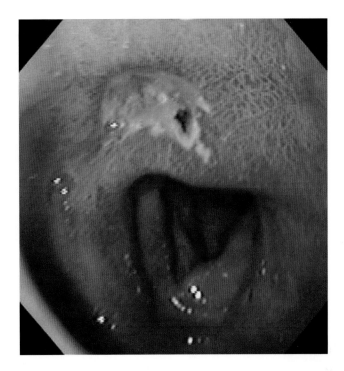

Figure 22.21 An apical duodenal ulcer. Note that the mucosa surrounding the ulcer appears inflamed and the villi that can be seen are enlarged. The bulb is foreshortened and deformed.

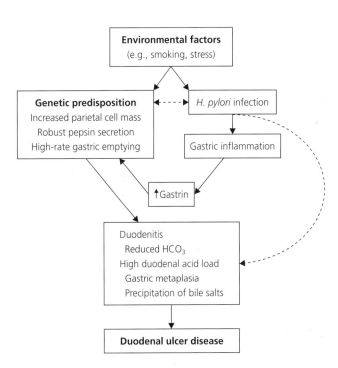

Figure 22.22 Hypothesis regarding the pathogenesis of duodenal ulcer disease showing the interaction of environmental, host and Hp factors, leading to an increased duodenal acid load, increased gastric metaplasia in the duodenum, and infection of that metaplastic epithelium, resulting in a duodenal ulcer.

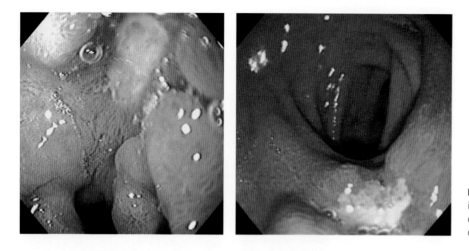

Figure 22.23 An apical **(left)** and an inferior **(right)** duodenal ulcer are seen with deformity of the bulb and abnormal, inflamed duodenal mucosa.

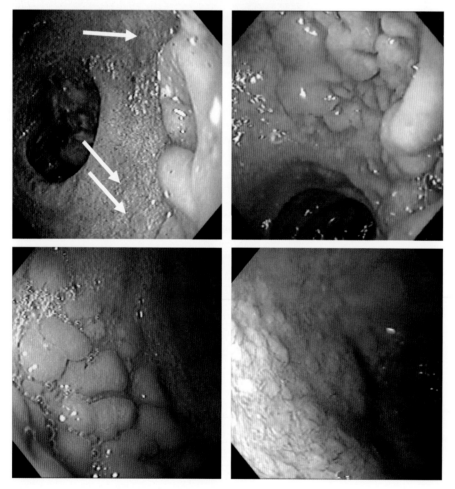

Figure 22.24 *Helicobacter pylori* are trophic for gastric epithelium and the duodenal bulb typically contains gastric epithelium either as a few isolated cells, and commonly as patches of gastric metaplasia, or heterotropic gastric mucosa. Here we show four different examples of different patterns of macroscopic gastric metaplasia. These are found most often adjacent to the pylorus, which often "curls" into the proximal duodenal bulb as shown in the first three photographs. Arrows on the upper left photograph also point out adjacent small patches of gastric metaplasia. The larger nodules typically contain parietal cells and are able to secrete acid into the duodenum, further increasing the duodenal acid load.

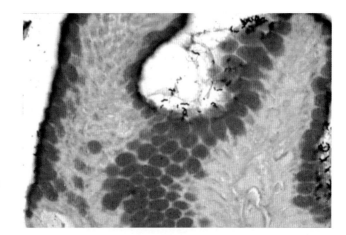

Figure 22.25 The use of an El-Zimaity dual stain consisting of periodic acid–Schiff solution (PAS) and a silver stain will show the presence of the gastric metaplastic cells and is particularly useful when one wishes to find patchy gastric metaplasia. The silver stain will also show whether *Helicobacter pylori* are present. They are to be expected in patients with infections in the stomach.

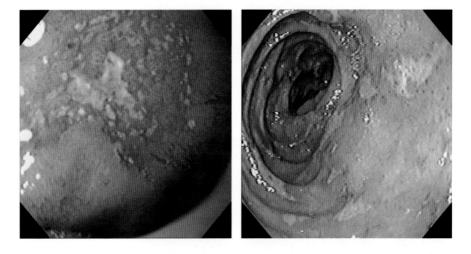

Figure 22.26 Diffuse duodenal erosions are seen on the anterior wall (left) and throughout the bulb and extending into the second portion of the duodenum. This is a typical finding of a nonsteroidal antiinflammatory drug duodenopathy.

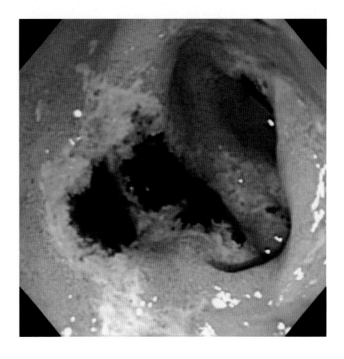

Figure 22.27 A severe case of chemical nonsteroidal antiinflammatory drug-induced injury to the bulb with deep acute ulcers/erosions extending from the bulb into the second portion of the duodenum.

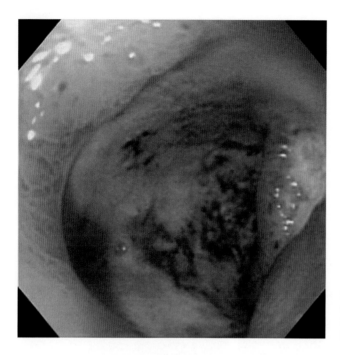

Figure 22.28 A giant duodenal ulcer that involves the entire anterior wall of the duodenum and extends to involve the posterior wall. One should consider Zollinger–Ellison syndrome and nonsteroidal antiinflammatory drug use in addition to *Helicobacter pylori* infection.

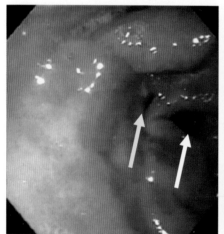 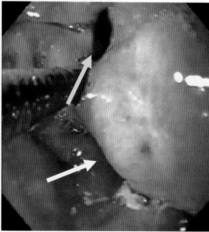

Figure 22.29 Double pylorus. In this instance a duodenal ulcer in the prepyloric area penetrated through the wall of the duodenum and into the duodenal bulb. The yellow arrow points to the opening of the false pylorus into the stomach. The white arrow points to the normal pyloric channel. The photograph on the right shows the use of a biopsy forceps to probe the false pylorus and show its patency.

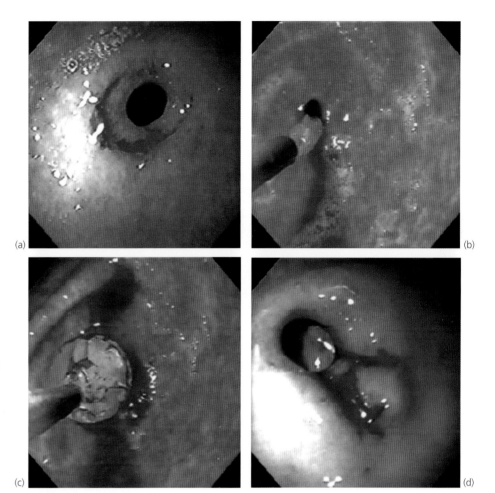

(a)

(b)

(c)

(d)

Figure 22.30 Pyloric stenosis. A series of photographs showing the presence of pyloric stenosis that resulted from the healing of a pyloric channel ulcer. **(a)** A ring of hemorrhage and an indentation where an attempt has been made to force an endoscope through. The next two photographs **(b and c)** show the insertion of a balloon dilator and its inflation. The final photograph **(d)** shows the result of the dilation with opening of the lumen and slight tearing of the mucosa where it would now allow entrance of the endoscope for examination of the duodenum.

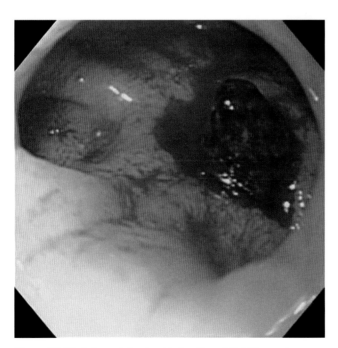

Figure 22.31 Deformed duodenal bulb with a clot/visible vessel inferiorly in a patient who had recently bled.

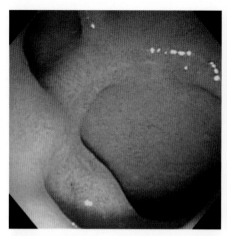
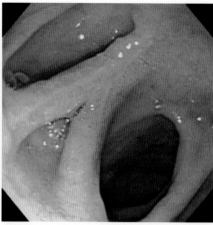

Figure 22.32 Deformed duodenal bulbs that show the residual of healed duodenal ulcers. One can easily imagine that barium would become trapped in the deformities and could confuse the radiologist regarding whether an active ulcer was present.

23

Gastritis and gastropathy

David Y. Graham, Robert M. Genta

Autoimmune gastritis

Autoimmune gastritis is a corpus-restricted chronic atrophic gastritis. It is usually associated with serum antiparietal cell and antiintrinsic factor antibodies and with intrinsic factor deficiency, with or without pernicious anemia. Most clinical manifestations of autoimmune gastritis result from the loss of parietal and chief cells of the oxyntic mucosa, and only become apparent in the florid or end-stage phases of the disease. Major effects include achlorhydria, hypergastrinemia, loss of pepsin and pepsinogens, iron deficiency with macrocytic anemia, vitamin B-12 deficiency with megaloblastic anemia, and increased risk of gastric neoplasms, particularly carcinoids.

Endoscopic appearance

In the corpus, the mucosa is usually thinner than normal (Fig. 23.1); this explains why few folds are left and fine submucosal vessels are easily recognized at endoscopic examination, especially in advanced stages of disease (Fig. 23.2). Figure 23.3 shows the appearance of an atrophic antrum.

Histopathological aspects

The main histopathological features of advanced autoimmune gastritis are the diffuse involvement of the oxyntic mucosa by chronic atrophic gastritis with moderate intestinal metaplasia and a normal gastric antrum (Fig. 23.4).

Enterochromaffin-like cell hyperplasia and dysplasia (Fig. 23.5), and multiple carcinoids are commonly found in association with an end-stage histopathological pattern. Hyperplasia of gastrin cells, secondary to achlorhydria, is often seen.

Intestinal metaplasia

Intestinal metaplasia is the replacement of the mucous cells that line the normal gastric mucosa with an epithelium similar to that of the small intestine. Intestinal metaplasia is found more frequently in *Helicobacter pylori*-positive subjects. The clinical significance of intestinal metaplasia is related to its association with dysplasia and adenocarcinoma. Recent studies suggest that the cell linage of intestinal metaplasia differs from that of gastric carcinoma and that it is either a dead end histologically or possibly transdifferentiation processes triggered by environmental stimuli.

Endoscopic appearance

The endoscopic feature most commonly associated with intestinalization is an irregular surface with patchy pink and pale areas (Figs 23.6 and 23.7). A technique that has encountered much favor in Japan, but which has not been found to be very reliable in either the United States or Europe, is the spraying of the gastric mucosa with indigo carmine, toluidine blue, or methylene blue. After the metaplastic mucosa sample is washed with saline, it maintains the characteristic blue color and may be differentiated from the nonmetaplastic areas.

Histopathological features

Some metaplastic areas look like normal small intestinal epithelium with an absorptive brush border and goblet cells that produce acidic mucins (Fig. 23.8); other areas are lined by a disorderly mixture of irregularly shaped goblet cells and immature intermediate cells that produce a wide spectrum of sialo- and sulfomucins. The most often used classification was proposed by Jass and Filipe: type I (brush border and no sialomucins); type II (no brush border, rare sulfomucins); type III (no brush border, cellular disarray, abundant sulfomucins). Follow-up studies have shown that repeat biopsy in the same area often shows a different type. Stains that were specifically used to determine the type of metaplasia by detecting sulfated mucins (such as high-iron Diamine) are being gradually replaced by immunohistochemical stains that identify proteins associated with particular

Atlas of Gastroenterology, 4th edition. Edited by Tadataka Yamada, David H. Alpers, Anthony N. Kalloo, Neil Kaplowitz, Chung Owyang, and Don W. Powell. © 2009 Blackwell Publishing, ISBN: 978-1-4051-6909-7

mucin-encoding genes. Although more than 20 such genes have been identified, in practice only a few (MUC1, MUC2, MUC5AC and MUC6) are used and the clinical relevance of mucin typing has not yet been established and is not recommended in clinical practice.

Helicobacter pylori gastritis

The thick mucous gel layer that normally covers the gastric mucosa often contains large numbers of bacteria (Fig. 23.9). When in contact with the epithelium, *H. pylori* organisms characteristically attach to surface mucous cells and cause distinctive epithelial changes: cells take irregular cuboidal shapes, reduce or lose their apical mucin droplet, and occasionally drop out, leaving small gaps that contribute to giving the epithelium a ragged, disorderly appearance (Fig. 23.10).

Mucosal neutrophils are the other distinctive histological feature of *H. pylori* infection. Neutrophils are seen in the lamina propria (mixed with mononuclear cells and eosinophils), within the surface and foveolar epithelium, and in more severe cases on the mucosal surface also (Fig. 23.10). After successful eradication therapy, neutrophils disappear rapidly; thus, their persistence is considered a good indicator of therapeutic failure. Gastric mucosa infected by *H. pylori* typically shows a mononuclear cell infiltrate, which is often subepithelial (chronic superficial gastritis) (Fig. 23.11). The intensity of mononuclear cell infiltrates declines slowly after successful eradication of the organism, and a portion of patients (estimated at 20%–30%) may retain the appearance of a chronic inactive gastritis for several years.

Detection of *Helicobacter pylori*
Helicobacter pylori infects both the antral and oxyntic mucosa, but in the cardia (narrowly defined as the transitional or antral-like mucosa found at the gastroesophageal junction) organisms tend to be more difficult to detect. In patients who use proton pump inhibitors *H. pylori* organisms tend to be rare or absent in the antrum and may also be more difficult to detect in the corpus, even in the presence of chronic active inflammation. In 70%–80% of gastric biopsy specimens from infected subjects, *H. pylori* organisms can be visualized by hematoxylin–eosin (H & E) stain (Fig. 23.12a). In the remaining 20%–30% of cases a special stain is needed, such as Giemsa and Diff-Quik (Fig. 23.12b). Another option is silver-based triple stain that simultaneously allows visualization of *H. pylori* and the morphological changes in the mucosa (see Figs 23.9–23.11). Because this stain includes Alcian blue at pH 2.5, it makes detection of small foci of intestinal metaplasia easier (Fig. 23.13).

Endoscopic appearance
Hyperemia, erosions, ulcerations, hypertrophy, and atrophy may coexist in various combinations in the same stomach,

juxtaposed to one another and to apparently normal areas, and none of these features has been proven useful for predicting the presence or absence of chronic *H. pylori* gastritis. Although there is no distinct endoscopic pattern of chronic *H. pylori* gastritis, the pattern of follicular gastritis (Fig. 23.14) is almost invariably associated with this infection.

Chemical gastropathy

The collection of endoscopic and histological features caused by chemical injury to the gastric mucosa is known as chemical gastropathy. In clinical practice, it is found almost exclusively in patients who use aspirin and other nonsteroidal antiinflammatory drugs (NSAIDs), and rarely in patients who have ingested alcohol or chemicals accidentally or for suicidal purposes. Reactive gastropathy has been documented (endoscopically or histologically) in 10%–45% of long-term users of NSAIDs and may be the first clue of surreptitious NSAID use.

Endoscopic appearance
The mucosa of chronic NSAID users, unless they have gastric ulcers or erosions, has no distinctive appearance. Erosions due to NSAID use are typically found in the antrum, often on the tops of folds. The erosions are generally multiple, and are characterized by a central depression with or without a necrotic floor, a red rim, and prominent reaction in the surrounding mucosa. Most are small (2–4 mm), but they can be more than 1 cm in diameter. Figures 23.15–23.20 represent NSAID-associated lesions ranging from very superficial erosions to ulcers.

Histopathology
The histopathological diagnosis of chemical gastropathy remains a challenging problem. Several mucosal changes have been associated with reactive gastropathy; however, the specificity and predictive value of any of these features is low, with many patients with *H. pylori* infection having one or more of these histological features (Fig. 23.21). Superficial erosions without surrounding inflammation (Fig. 23.22) are almost always caused by chemical injury, whereas the etiology of multiple inflamed erosions (Fig. 23.23) is virtually impossible to determine. Thus, the pathologist can suspect chemical gastropathy, but a firm diagnosis can be made only when supportive clinical data are available and no confounding factors (e.g., *H. pylori* infection) are present.

Bile-reflux gastropathy
Postgastrectomy bile reflux may present with a syndrome characterized by burning midepigastric pain unresponsive to antacids and aggravated by eating and recumbency, sometimes accompanied by bilious vomiting, anemia, and weight

loss. Endoscopic confirmation of bile reflux with characteristic histopathological findings supports the diagnosis, and corrective surgery (e.g., creation of a 40- to 50-cm Roux-en-Y gastrojejunostomy) is successful in about one-half of all cases.

Endoscopic appearance

The gastric mucosa at the anastomotic site may have a polypoid appearance with congestion, edema, and friability (Fig. 23.24). Superficial erosions may also be present in more proximal areas of the gastric stump.

Histopathology

The most characteristic changes include evidence of epithelial regeneration, extreme foveolar hyperplasia, edema of the lamina propria, and expansion of the smooth muscle fibers into the upper third of the mucosa (Figs 23.25 and 23.26). The enhanced epithelial proliferation may cause the foveolar cells to have an increased nuclear–cytoplasmic ratio and mild to moderate architectural disarray. These findings (known to pathologists as "atypia") may be incorrectly interpreted as dysplasia or neoplasia.

Partial gastrectomy and carcinoma

The polypoid appearance of the distal portions of the gastric stump in postgastrectomy patients has been referred to as gastritis cystica polyposa. Several European and Japanese studies have reported a high prevalence of low-grade dysplasia or gastric adenocarcinoma, but these findings have not been confirmed in the United States.

Watermelon stomach

Watermelon stomach, or gastric antral vascular ectasia (GAVE) syndrome, is a rare condition of unknown etiology that is frequently associated with gastric atrophy and autoimmune and connective tissue disorders, particularly systemic sclerosis. More than 70% of reported cases have occurred in older women. Occult bleeding is seen at presentation in almost 90% of the cases, and melena or hematemesis in 60%. In most patients, the chronic blood loss causes iron deficiency anemia.

Endoscopic appearance

Watermelon stomach was so named because of the "longitudinal antral folds seen converging on the pylorus, containing visible and ectatic vessels resembling the stripes on a watermelon" (Fig. 23.27). In other metaphors, the prominent dilated vessels have been described as resembling "a large, flat mushroom" or a "honeycomb."

Histopathology

In the antrum, the lamina propria shows smooth muscle proliferation and fibrosis, and contains markedly dilated mucosal capillaries (Fig. 23.28). Fibrin thrombi are often found within the dilated capillaries (Fig. 23.29).

Management

Therapeutic endoscopy, with obliteration of the dilated vessels by argon plasma coagulation, is the accepted treatment of choice and has greatly reduced the need for antrectomy.

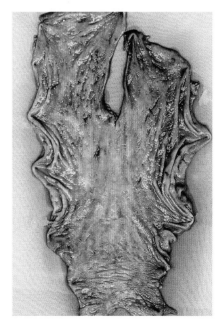

Figure 23.1 Total gastrectomy performed in a patient with end-stage autoimmune atrophic gastritis and multiple carcinoid tumors. The mucosa of the corpus is completely devoid of rugae, whereas the antrum maintains its normal anatomy.

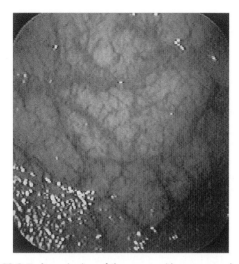

Figure 23.2 Endoscopic view of the corpus with severe atrophy. The mucosa appears thin and the underlying vasculature is prominent.

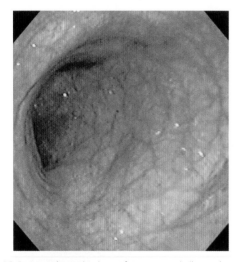

Figure 23.3 An endoscopic picture from a case similar to that depicted in Fig. 23.2 with clearly visible mucosal and submucosal vessels is seen in a patient with antral atrophy. The bluish discoloration in the upper left corner is the shade of the liver seen through the thin distended gastric wall.

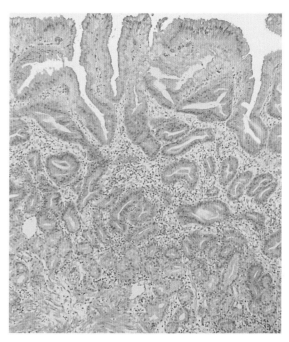

Figure 23.4 The mucosa of the corpus has completely lost its normal appearance. The normal tightly packed acid-secreting oxyntic glands have been progressively destroyed by the autoimmune inflammatory process and are replaced by mucus-secreting glands similar to those found in the distal antrum. The phenomenon is known as pyloric (or pseudopyloric) metaplasia.

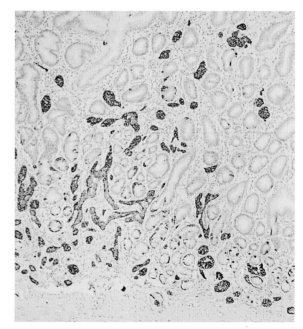

Figure 23.5 Chromogranin stain of the fundic mucosa shows severe enterochromaffin-like (ECL) cell hyperplasia and dysplasia. This is a consequence of the stimulus caused by the hypergastrinemia the patients develop in response to the low or absent acid content of the atrophic stomach. Both ECL cell hyperplasia and dysplasia are considered to be a precursor of carcinoid tumors, which frequently arise in the corpus of patients with autoimmune atrophic gastritis.

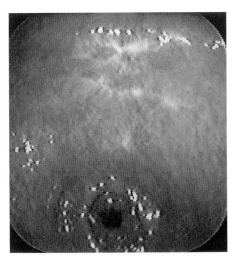

Figure 23.6 Intestinal metaplasia is usually difficult to diagnose endoscopically. Histopathological examination of biopsy specimens obtained from the flat yellowish areas visible in this antrum, originally interpreted as either metaplastic or fibrotic areas (scars), showed diffuse intestinal metaplasia.

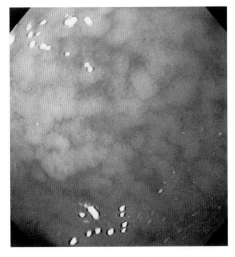

Figure 23.7 Large area of intestinal metaplasia in the antral mucosa. The appearance is characteristically pale and velvety.

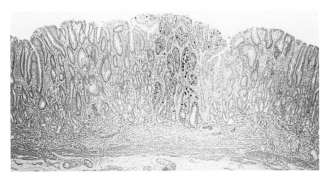

Figure 23.8 Antral mucosa with a small focus of intestinal metaplasia. Goblet cells are best visualized when Alcian blue at pH 2.5 is added to the traditional hematoxylin–eosin stain. Intestinal metaplasia is a marker for increased risk of dysplasia and adenocarcinoma. The larger the area of the gastric mucosa with atrophy (e.g., affected by metaplasia), the greater the risk for gastric cancer.

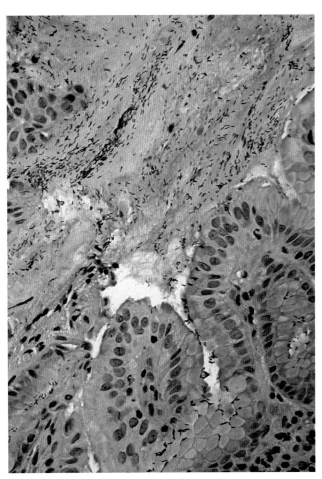

Figure 23.9 Gastric mucus with innumerable *Helicobacter pylori*. Organisms are seen both in the mucus and adhering to the antral mucosa.

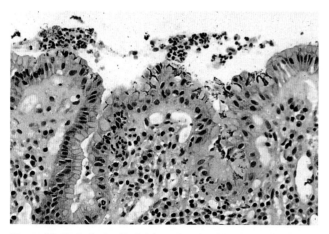

Figure 23.10 Surface epithelial damages caused by the adherence of *Helicobacter pylori*. Cells reduce or lose their apical mucin droplet, may take irregular cuboidal shapes, and occasionally drop out, leaving small gaps that give the gastric epithelium a ragged, uneven appearance.

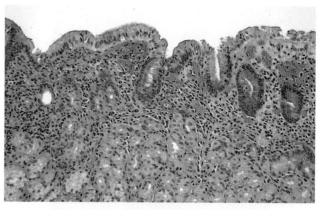

Figure 23.11 Chronic superficial gastritis in the corpus: a band of mononuclear cells separated the surface epithelium from the subjacent oxyntic glands. The surface epithelium is heavily infiltrated by neutrophils.

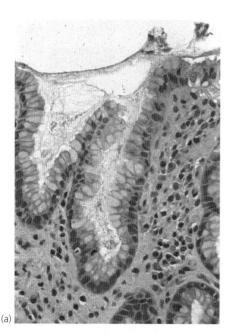

(a)

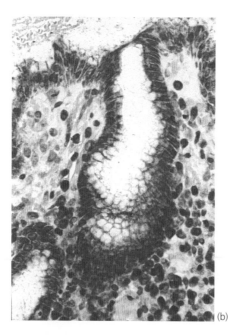

(b)

Figure 23.12 *Helicobacter pylori* can be visualized with the hematoxylin–eosin stain **(a)** as well as with inexpensive, although suboptimal, quick stains like the Giemsa **(b)**.

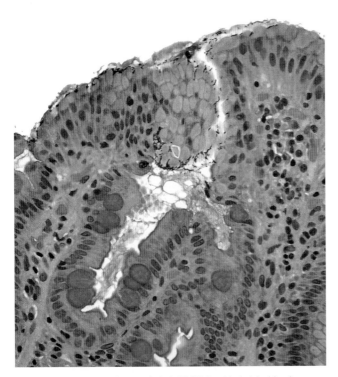

Figure 23.13 Intestinal metaplasia is highlighted in bright blue by an Alcian blue-containing silver-based triple stain for the detection of *Helicobacter pylori*. Organisms adhere to the native gastric mucosa only, apparently avoiding contact with metaplastic cells.

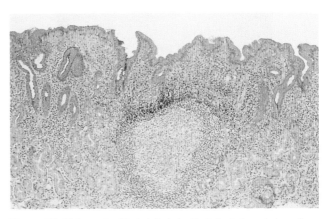

Figure 23.15 In most subjects infected with *Helicobater pylori*, small lymphoid follicles develop in the gastric mucosa. When their diameter is smaller than the mucosal thickness they are not visible endoscopically.

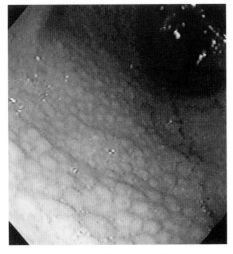

Figure 23.14 Innumerable small hemispherical elevations, many with a slightly depressed or umbilicated center, are characteristic of follicular gastritis.

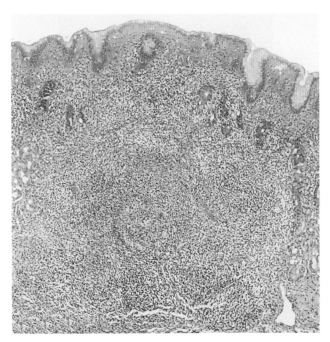

Figure 23.16 Larger lymphoid follicles increase the thickness of the mucosa and create endoscopically detectable elevations. When follicles are extremely numerous and most are large, the mucosal appearance is that of follicular gastritis.

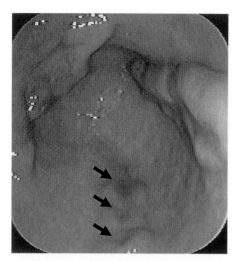

Figure 23.17 Superficial antral erosions (arrows) in a patient using nonsteroidal antiinflammatory drugs.

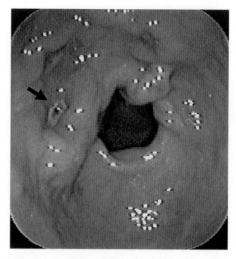

Figure 23.20 Nonsteroidal antiinflammatory drug-induced small ulcer.

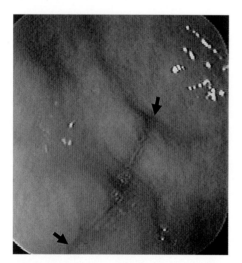

Figure 23.18 Characteristic of aspirin-induced linear erosion (extending between the two arrows).

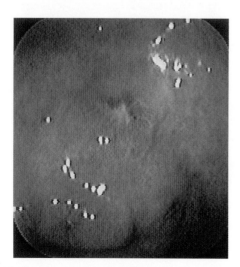

Figure 23.19 Large, deep erosion or superficial ulcer in a patient using nonsteroidal antiinflammatory drugs.

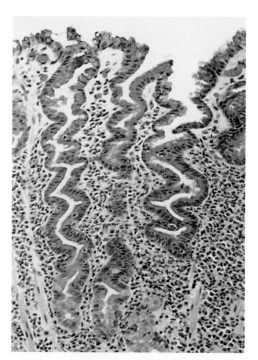

Figure 23.21 Foveolar hyperplasia is generally believed to be a characteristic histopathological finding in chemical gastropathy. This mucosal change, however, simply reflects increased epithelial turnover caused by superficial damage, and may occur in other conditions, including *Helicobater pylori* infection. In this patient with both *H. pylori* gastritis and a history of nonsteroidal antiinflammatory drug use, the etiology of the foveolar alterations cannot be determined.

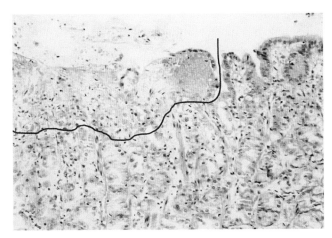

Figure 23.22 Superficial erosion of the oxyntic mucosa. The mucosa to the right and below the red line is completely normal and without inflammation. The affected portion shows hemorrhage, necrosis, and epithelial regeneration. This association of normal mucosa with an abrupt limited hemorrhagic and necrotic lesion is characteristic of chemical injury. The absence of inflammation all but excludes *Helicobater pylori* infection.

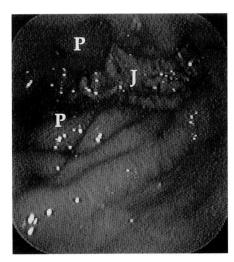

Figure 23.24 Polypoid appearance (*P*) of the gastric mucosa at the anastomotic site in a patient with Billroth II gastrojejunostomy. A portion of the jejunum (*J*) is visible, surrounded by thickened gastric mucosa.

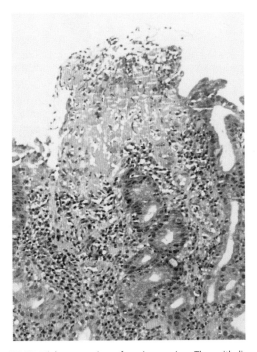

Figure 23.23 High-power view of a microerosion. The epithelium has disappeared and the uppermost part of the mucosa contains fibrin and inflammatory cells that are projected toward the lumen in a fashion that has been likened to a minuscule eruption.

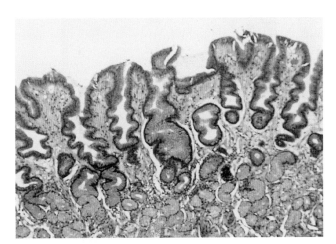

Figure 23.25 Foveolar hyperplasia without inflammation is probably caused by chemical injury.

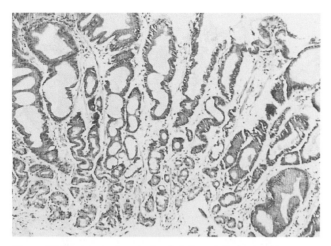

Figure 23.26 Extreme foveolar hyperplasia and dilation in a biopsy specimen from the gastric stoma in a patient with Billroth II gastrectomy. This degree of foveolar hyperplasia accounts for the juicy, polypoid aspect of the area immediately juxtaposed to the anastomotic site.

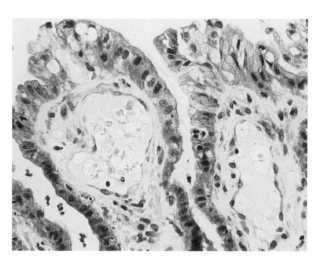

Figure 23.28 The antral mucosa shows innumerable dilated subepithelial capillaries.

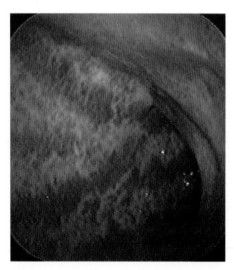

Figure 23.27 Hemorrhagic hyperemic streaks apparently converging toward the pylorus, in the antrum of a middle-aged woman with scleroderma and progressive anemia. The appearance of the streaks has been likened to the stripes of a watermelon, hence the term *watermelon stomach*.

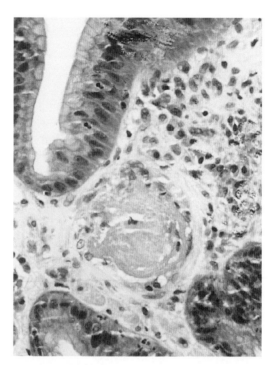

Figure 23.29 A characteristic – if not pathognomonic – finding in watermelon stomach is the presence of thrombi in the dilated superficial capillaries.

B STOMACH

24

Tumors of the stomach

Wai K. Leung, Enders K.W. Ng, Joseph J.Y. Sung

Gastric cancer is the second most common cause of death from cancer worldwide. According to data from the World Health Organization, it is estimated that more than 700 000 people died from this malignancy each year. There are considerable geographic differences in the incidence of gastric cancer. The highest rate is observed in eastern Asia, where the age-standardized rate in men is 46 per 100 000. The incidence rates in Japanese and Korean men are more than 60 per 100 000. Interestingly, there is a progressive decline in gastric cancer incidence in most countries in the past few decades (Fig. 24.1).

Adenocarcinomas comprise more than 90% of stomach cancers (Fig. 24.2) and the rest are predominantly lymphoma and stromal tumors. Detailed World Health Organization (WHO) classification of gastric tumors is presented in Table 24.1. Adenocarcinoma can be broadly categorized into intestinal and diffuse types, as proposed by Lauren (Acta Pathol Microbiol Scand 1965;64:31). Intestinal-type carcinoma is characterized by the presence of cohesive neoplastic cells forming glandular tubular structures, whereas diffuse-type cancer shows sheets of epithelial cells or cells scattered in a stromal matrix without evidence of gland formation (Fig. 24.3). Gastric carcinogenesis, particularly the intestinal type, is generally believed to be a multistep progression from chronic gastritis, which is usually triggered by chronic *Helicobacter pylori* infection, to atrophic gastritis, intestinal metaplasia, dysplasia, and carcinoma. Numerous genetic alterations have been demonstrated in this histological progression, including cyclooxygenase-2 overexpression, *p53* mutation, and microsatellite instability.

Radiological examination was once the investigation of choice for gastric diseases, but its role has been largely replaced by endoscopy. Diminished distensibility of the stomach on barium meal examination suggests a diffusely infiltrative cancer. In addition, the presence of an asymmet-

ric ulcer crater eccentrically located on an irregular mass with distortion or obliteration of normal mucosal fold strongly suggests malignant ulcer (Fig. 24.4). However, the definite diagnosis of malignancy is impossible without tumor biopsy obtained through endoscopic examination. Another advantage of endoscopy is the direct visualization of subtle mucosal changes found in early gastric cancer (Fig. 24.5). With the use of chromoendoscopy and magnifying endoscopes, the ability to detect early gastric cancer can be enhanced (Fig. 24.6).

The revised primary tumor node metastasis (TNM) staging of gastric cancer is given in Table 24.2. The T-staging remains unchanged (Fig. 24.7), but major modifications have been made in the classification of regional lymph nodes, which is now determined by the number instead of the anatomic location of the involved lymph nodes. Because the mainstay of treatment for gastric cancer is surgery, the importance of accurate preoperative staging cannot be overemphasized. The extent of surgical resection, especially the extent of lymph node dissection, is still a matter of debate. Because of the delay in presentation, not all gastric cancers could undergo curative resection.

Despite the advances in imaging techniques, no single imaging modality is sensitive or specific enough to detect local or distant metastasis. Approximately 10%–20% of patients being explored for potentially curative resection are found to have peritoneal seeding at the time of surgery. Because of the poor visualization of the stomach wall, computed tomography (CT) appears only to be useful in demonstrating local or distant invasion (Fig. 24.8). Even with the use of helical CT scan, about 25%–50% of tumor invasion into the colon or pancreas may be missed. On the other hand, the extent of local invasion, in particular the T-staging, is better delineated with the use of endoscopic ultrasound (EUS) (Fig. 24.9). The overall accuracy of EUS in T-staging was 78%. However, because of the poor penetration of high-frequency ultrasound, the role of EUS in assessing distant metastasis is limited. The use of EUS and CT scanning may be complementary in assessing local invasion and distant metastasis. Diagnostic accuracy can be further

Atlas of Gastroenterology, 4th edition. Edited by Tadataka Yamada, David H. Alpers, Anthony N. Kalloo, Neil Kaplowitz, Chung Owyang, and Don W. Powell. © 2009 Blackwell Publishing, ISBN: 978-1-4051-6909-7

improved by the use of preoperative laparoscopy that detects unexpected peritoneal and liver metastasis (Fig. 24.10), which is particularly useful in patients with locally advanced disease.

There is an increasing use of local therapy for early gastric cancer. In particular, endoscopic removal of tumors is favored by Japanese physicians for early gastric cancer, with low risk of lymph node and distant metastasis. Endoscopic mucosal resection (EMR) is currently the standard treatment for early gastric cancer in Japan (Fig. 24.11). Intestinal type mucosal cancer less than 2 cm in diameter is the best tumor type for EMR. Recently, more extensive endoscopic resection was introduced in Japan by the use of a new device called the insulation-tipped (IT) needle knife (Fig. 24.12). The procedure is usually called endoscopic submucosal dissection (ESD) to indicate the potential depth of resection. The advantage of this procedure over EMR is the provision of large en bloc specimen for histological staging and higher potential to prevent recurrent disease. Bleeding (7%) and perforation (4%) are more commonly encountered after this procedure than EMR.

Lymphoma accounts for about 10% of all gastric malignancies. The gastrointestinal tract is the most common extranodal site for non-Hodgkin lymphoma. The majority of gastric lymphomas are B-cell lymphomas, including high-grade lymphoma and low-grade mucosa-associated lymphoid tissue (MALT) lymphomas. MALT lymphoma is a special entity that is closely linked to *H. pylori* infection. Histologically, MALT lymphoma mimics that of normal MALT with marginal zone B-cell immunophenotypes (Fig. 24.13). The typical lymphoepithelial lesions are characterized by infiltration of the glandular epithelium by clusters of neoplastic lymphoid cells with associated destruction of gland architecture and morphological changes within the cells. Eradication of *H. pylori* alone has been shown to produce complete regression of low-grade MALT lymphoma. In this context, EUS may help to identify patients who would respond to antibacterial treatment; that is, patients with stage I_{E1} disease (confined to mucosa and submucosa) (Fig. 24.14).

Most gastric mesenchymal neoplasms are gastrointestinal stromal tumors (GIST) or smooth muscle types (Figs 24.15–20). Although the term GIST was originally reserved for tumors that were neither leiomyomata nor schwannomas, GIST has been loosely used to describe the majority of mesenchymal tumors. The cellular origin of GIST has been proposed to be the interstitial cell of Cajal, and most malignant GIST harbor mutations in the *c-kit* gene, which result in constitutive activation of the tyrosine kinase. In this context, immunoreactivity against c-KIT (CD117) was found to be present in 80%–100% of GIST (Fig. 24.16f). In general, tumors greater than 5 cm in size and with high mitotic counts (>10 mitoses/10 high-power field) are considered to be of higher malignant potential (Fig. 24.18).

Table 24.1 WHO histological classification of gastric tumors

Epithelial tumors	Nonepithelial tumors
Intraepithelial neoplasia or adenoma	Leiomyoma
Carcinoma	Schwannoma
Adenocarcinoma	Granular cell tumor
Intestinal type	Glomus tumor
Diffuse type	Leiomyosarcoma
Papillary adenocarcinoma	GI stromal tumor
Tubular adenocarcinoma	Benign
Mucinous adenocarcinoma	Uncertain malignant potential
Signet-ring cell carcinoma	Malignant
Adenosquamous carcinoma	Kaposi sarcoma
Squamous cell carcinoma	Others
Small cell carcinoma	Malignant lymphomas
Undifferentiated carcinoma	Marginal zone B-cell lymphoma of MALT type
Others	Mantle cell lymphoma
Carcinoid (well-differentiated endocrine neoplasm)	Diffuse large B-cell lymphoma
	Others
	Secondary tumors

GI, gastrointestinal; MALT, mucosa-associated lymphoid tissue; WHO, World Health Organization.

Table 24.2 The sixth edition of the UICC TNM classification of gastric carcinoma

(a) TNM classification

T: primary tumor

Tis	Carcinoma in situ; intraepithelial tumor without invasion of lamina propria
T1	Tumor invades lamina propria or submucosa
T2	Tumor invades muscularis propria or subserosa
T2a	Tumor invades muscularis propria
T2b	Tumor invades subserosa
T3	Tumor penetrates serosa (visceral peritoneum) without invasion of adjacent structures
T4	Tumor invades adjacent structures

N: regional lymph node

N0	No regional lymph node metastasis
N1	Metastasis in 1–6 regional lymph nodes
N2	Metastasis in 7–15 regional lymph nodes
N3	Metastasis in more than 15 regional lymph nodes

M: distant metastasis

M0	No distant metastasis
M1	Distant metastasis

(b) Stage grouping

Stage	T	N	M
0	Tis	N0	M0
IA	T1	N0	M0
IB	T1	N1	M0
	T2a/b	N0	M0
II	T1	N2	M0
	T2a/b	N1	M0
	T3	N0	M0
IIIA	T2a/b	N2	M0
	T3	N1	M0
	T4	N0	M0
IIIB	T3	N2	M0
IV	T4	N1–3	M0
	T1–3	N3	M0
	Any T	Any N	M1

TNM, primary tumor, regional nodes, metastasis; UICC, International Union Against Cancer.

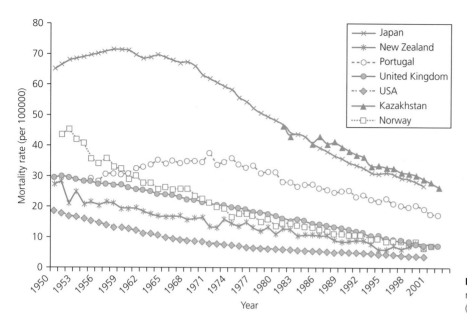

Figure 24.1 The age-adjusted mortality rates of gastric cancer in different countries (1950–2004).

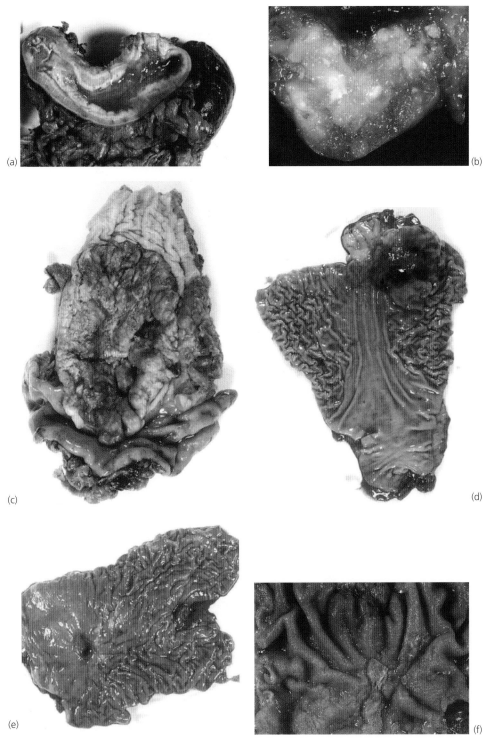

Figure 24.2 Macroscopic appearances of gastric adenocarcinoma. **(a)** Linitis plastica. The gastric wall is diffusely thickened and the spleen and omentum were removed en bloc in radical gastrectomy. **(b)** Mucoid carcinoma of stomach demonstrating multiple mucin pools. **(c)** An ulcerative tumor at the cardia. **(d)** A polypoid tumor at the cardia. **(e)** A malignant ulcer located in the lesser curve. **(f)** An early gastric cancer that resembles a benign ulcer. Courtesy of Dr K.F. To, Prince of Wales Hospital, Hong Kong.

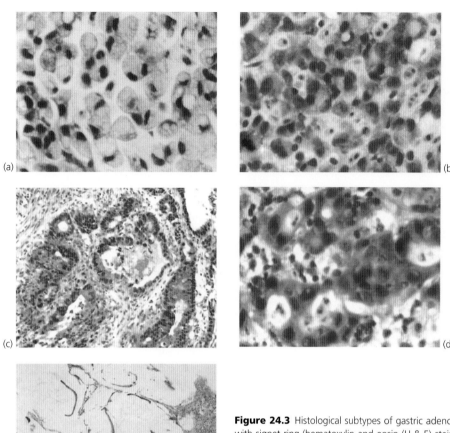

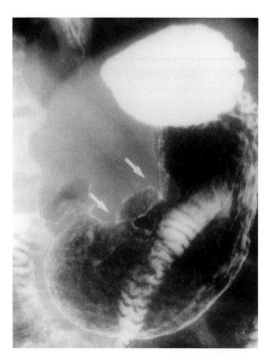

Figure 24.3 Histological subtypes of gastric adenocarcinoma. **(a)** Diffuse-type adenocarcinoma with signet ring (hematoxylin and eosin (H & E) stain; original magnification ×400). **(b)** Diffuse-type adenocarcinoma with discohesive sheets of carcinoma cells and moderate amount of pale eosinophilic cytoplasm (H & E stain; original magnification ×400). **(c)** Intestinal-type adenocarcinoma that was arranged in a tubular glandular pattern with invasion into the desmoplastic stroma (H & E section, ×200). **(d)** Intestinal-type adenocarcinoma with irregular fused small glandular pattern (H & E stain; original magnification ×400). **(e)** Mucinous adenocarcinoma (H & E stain; original magnification ×100). Courtesy of Dr K.F. To, Prince of Wales Hospital, Hong Kong.

Figure 24.4 Double-contrast barium meal examination demonstrating an ulcerative tumor in the angular incisura (arrows).

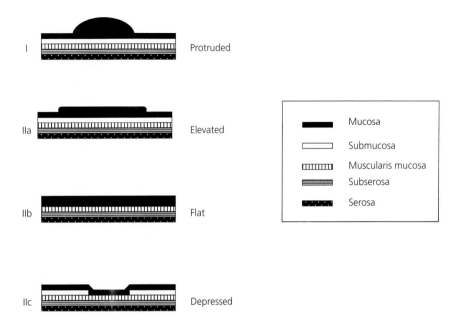

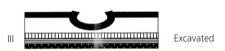

Figure 24.5 Classification of early gastric cancer. Type I is an exophytic lesion, type II is flat (or superficial), and type III is an ulcerated or depressed lesion. Type II is further divided into three subtypes depending on whether it is elevated (IIa), flat (IIb), or depressed (IIc).

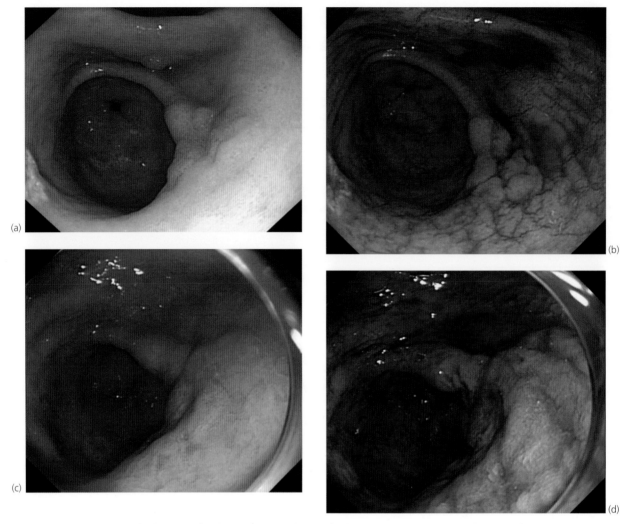

Figure 24.6 Chromoendoscopy for diagnosis of early gastric cancer. The use of indigocarmine can enhance the detection of early gastric cancer. **(a, b)** Type I protruded gastric cancer. **(c, d)** Type IIc depressed lesion.

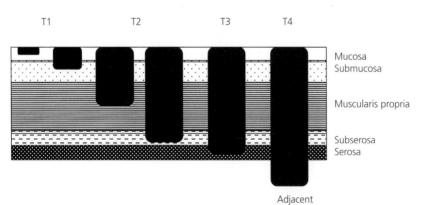

Figure 24.7 T-classification of gastric carcinoma. (Primary tumor node metastasis staging system.)

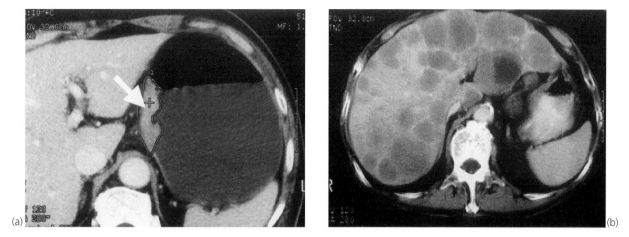

Figure 24.8 Computed tomography of gastric cancer. **(a)** Primary gastric carcinoma as illustrated by the arrow. **(b)** Multiple liver metastases from primary gastric carcinoma as shown by the hypodense lesions.

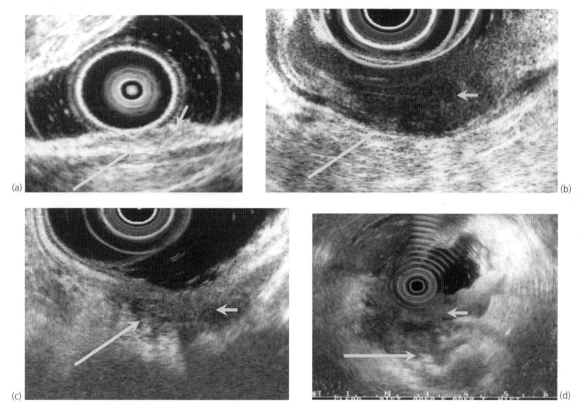

Figure 24.9 Preoperative staging of gastric carcinoma by endoscopic ultrasound. **(a)** Intramucosal early gastric cancer (Tis) with focal mucosal thickening (short arrow) and intact lamina propria (long arrow). **(b)** T2 gastric cancer (short arrow) invaded into the muscularis layer with intact serosa (long arrow). **(c)** Small gastric cancer (short arrow) invaded through the serosa (T3) (long arrow). **(d)** Large T4 gastric cancer (short arrow) invaded into the neck of pancreas (long arrow). Courtesy of Dr Y.T. Lee, Prince of Wales Hospital, Hong Kong.

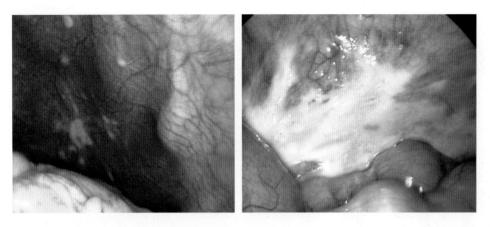

Figure 24.10 Laparoscopic views of peritoneal seeding from gastric adenocarcinoma. Courtesy of Dr Enders Ng, Prince of Wales Hospital, Hong Kong.

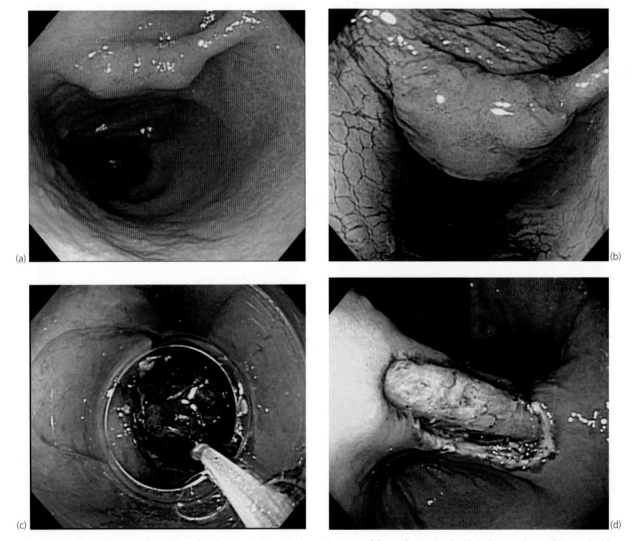

Figure 24.11 Endoscopic mucosal resection of early gastric cancer. Early gastric cancer **(a)** was first stained with indigocarmine and injected with normal saline to lift up the lesion **(c)**. The lesion was then sucked into the suction cap **(c)** and removed by EMR snare **(d)**.

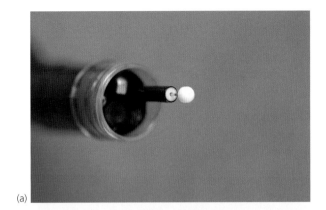

(a)

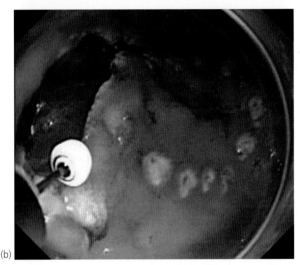

(b)

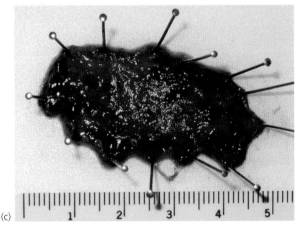

(c)

Figure 24.12 Endoscopic submucosal dissection of early gastric cancer.
(a) The insulation-tipped (IT) needle knife consists of a conventional
diathermic needle knife with a ceramic ball at the top to minimize the
risk of perforation. **(b)** The knife can be used in submucosal dissection
and complete en bloc resection of a larger lesion. **(c)** One-piece removal
of early gastric cancer.

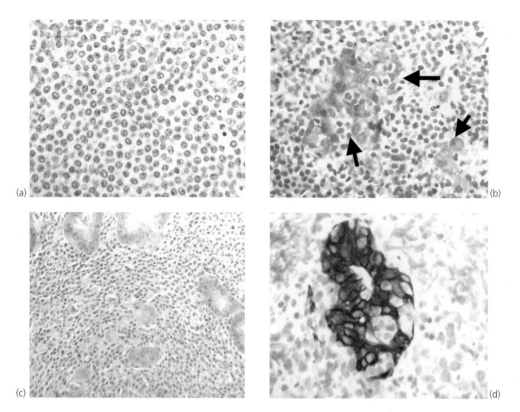

Figure 24.13 Gastric mucosa-associated lymphoid tissue (MALT) lymphoma. Characteristic features of low-grade MALT lymphoma: **(a)** centrocyte-like cells (H & E stain; original magnification ×200); **(c)** lymphoepithelial lesions (arrows) (H & E stain; original magnification ×200); **(c)** plasmacytic differentiation (H & E stain; original magnification ×100); and **(d)** lymphoepithelial lesions (immunostain for cytokeratin; original magnification ×200). Courtesy of Dr Wing Y. Chan, the Chinese University of Hong Kong, Prince of Wales Hospital, Hong Kong.

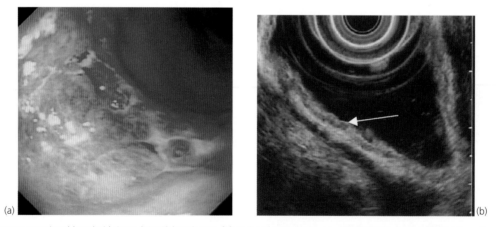

Figure 24.14 Mucosa-associated lymphoid tissue (MALT) lymphoma. **(a)** Endoscopic appearance of MALT lymphoma. **(b)** Thickened gastric mucosa without submucosa involvement (arrow) as shown by endoscopic ultrasonography (stage IE1).

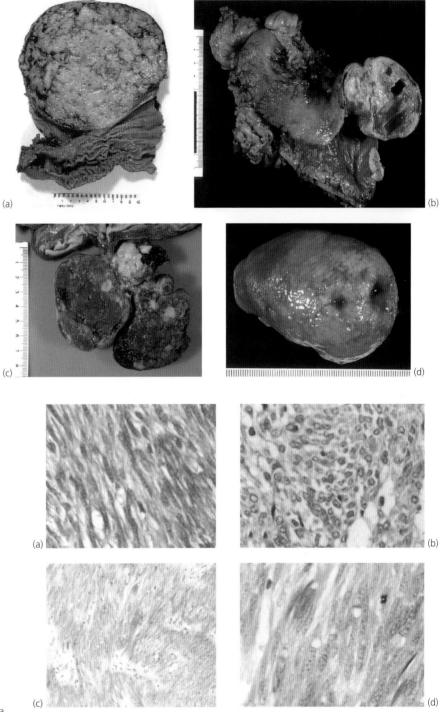

Figure 24.15 Gross appearances of gastric mesenchymal tumors. **(a)** A huge gastric stromal tumor arising from the gastric wall and protruding into the serosal surface. The tan-colored solid tumor was punctuated with areas of hemorrhage. **(b)** Another example of gastric stromal tumor that mainly protruded into the gastric lumen and exhibited cystic degeneration. **(c)** A gastric stromal tumor that was attached to the gastric wall by a narrow pedicle. **(d)** The surface of this tumor was covered by gastric mucosa with typical central umbilication. Courtesy of Dr K.F. To, Prince of Wales Hospital, Hong Kong.

Figure 24.16 Microscopic appearances of gastric stromal tumors. **(a–d)** Gastric stromal tumors have a wide range of histological and cytological patterns. **(a)** Fascicular pattern with spinal cell morphology (H & E stain; original magnification ×200). **(b)** Sheet-like pattern with epithelioid appearance (H & E stain; original magnification ×200). **(c)** Palisade pattern with resemblance to nerve sheet tumor (H & E stain; original magnification ×100). **(d)** Juxta-nuclear vacuolation suggestive of smooth muscle cells. **(e, f)** Strong immunoreactivity against CD34 **(e)** and CD117/c-KIT **(f)** in gastric stromal tumor. Courtesy of Dr K.F. To, Prince of Wales Hospital, Hong Kong.

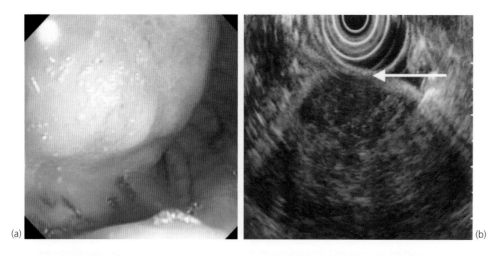

(a)

(b)

Figure 24.17 Gastric leiomyosarcoma. **(a)** Endoscopic examination showed a huge mass in the greater curve of the stomach with normal mucosa. **(b)** Endoscopic ultrasound examination (7.5 MHz, Olympus GF-UM240, Japan) revealed a 10-cm heterogeneous tumor arising from the muscularis layer with normal mucosa and submucosa (arrow). There were cystic changes within the parenchyma, whereas the pancreas was normal. Courtesy of Dr Y.T. Lee, Prince of Wales Hospital, Hong Kong.

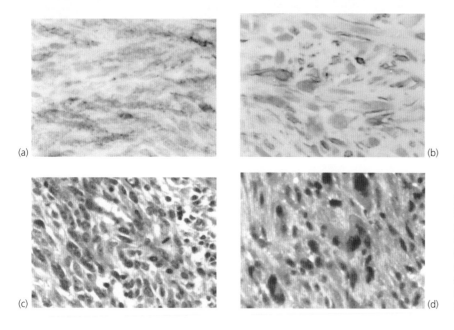

(a)

(b)

(c)

(d)

Figure 24.18 Smooth muscle tumor. **(a, b)** Smooth muscle origin was supported by the positive immunoreactivity against smooth muscle actin **(a)**, original magnification ×200, and desmin **(b)**, original magnification ×200. **(c, d)** Potential malignant smooth muscle tumor demonstrates cytological atypia and high mitotic activity. Courtesy of Dr K.F. To, Prince of Wales Hospital, Hong Kong.

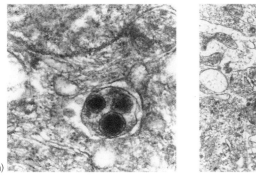

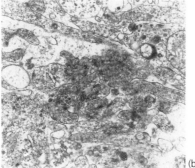

(a)

(b)

Figure 24.19 Gastrointestinal autonomic nerve tumor (GANT). The reconciliation of GANT relies on the typical ultrastructure appearances of interdigitating cell processes **(a)** and presence of neurosecretory granules **(b)**. Courtesy of Dr K.F. To, Prince of Wales Hospital, Hong Kong.

Figure 24.20 Gastric lipoma.
(a) Large submucosal mass at antrum with superficial ulceration on endoscopic examination.
(b) Endoscopic ultrasound examination (7.5 MHz, Olympus GF-UM240) showed a smooth regular hyperechoic mass (long arrow) situated in the submucosal layer with deep ulceration (short arrow). The muscularis and mucosal layers were normal. Courtesy of Dr Y.T. Lee, Prince of Wales Hospital, Hong Kong.

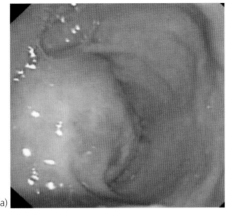
(a)

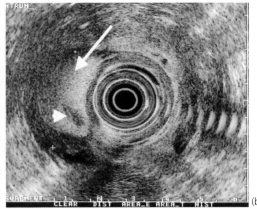
(b)

25

Surgery for peptic ulcer disease and postgastrectomy syndromes

Robert E. Glasgow, Sean J. Mulvihill

In the past, surgery for peptic ulcer disease was the most common indication for gastric surgery. However, the introduction of antisecretory agents, the development of endoscopic therapy for complications of ulcer disease, and the recognition of the importance of *Helicobacter pylori* in the pathogenesis of peptic ulcer disease have significantly changed the spectrum of gastric surgery. These improvements in medical management have dramatically reduced the frequency of hospitalizations and operations for uncomplicated ulcer disease. However, the incidence of complications of peptic ulcer disease is unchanged and, in this setting, surgical treatment is often necessary. Indications for surgical treatment include perforation, bleeding, intractability, and obstruction. Regardless of the indication for surgery, the fundamental goals of surgical therapy are to permit ulcer healing, prevent or treat ulcer complications, address the underlying ulcer diathesis, and to minimize postoperative digestive sequelae.

Surgery for peptic ulcer disease consists of three elements: primary management of the ulcer, vagotomy to decrease gastric acid secretion, and drainage of the stomach. In general, perforated duodenal ulcer is managed with oversew of the perforation and omental patch overlay (Graham patch) (Fig. 25.1). Bleeding duodenal ulcers are treated with ligation of the bleeding vessel, usually the gastroduodenal artery, through the ulcer bed (Fig. 25.2). Often, a vagotomy is performed to minimize the chance of ulcer recurrence. Three versions of vagotomy have been described: truncal, selective, and highly selective or parietal cell vagotomy (Fig. 25.3). When performing truncal or selective vagotomy,

gastric emptying is impaired because of a loss of coordination of the antral mill and pyloric sphincter mechanism. Therefore, a drainage procedure is indicated. Drainage options include antrectomy, pylorplasty, and gastrojejunostomy (Fig. 25.4). Surgical treatment of intractability and obstruction involves a combination of vagotomy and drainage.

The surgical treatment of gastric ulcers depends on their location and pathophysiology. A classification scheme for gastric ulcers is shown in Figure 25.5. When indicated, surgical treatment of gastric ulcers involves either wedge resection of the entire ulcer or formal gastric resection. This is shown in Figure 25.6. For ulcers associated with acid hypersecretion (Types 2 and 3), a vagotomy is included.

The changes in normal gastroduodenal anatomy and physiology resulting from gastric surgery are usually well-tolerated and have no clinically relevant sequelae. However, a small percentage of patients will develop a constellation of gastrointestinal symptoms resulting from their surgery. Collectively, these disorders of gastrointestinal function following gastric surgery are termed postgastrectomy syndromes (Fig. 25.7). Although some of these postgastrectomy disorders are mechanical in origin and require surgical intervention, the majority result from functional changes in normal physiology. In the latter group, remedial surgery is reserved for patients who fail conservative measures. Remedial operations for the common postgastrectomy syndromes are shown in Figure 25.8 (dumping syndrome), Figure 25.9 (postvagotomy diarrhea), Figure 25.10 (alkaline gastritis), Figure 25.11 (afferent limb syndrome), and Figure 25.12 (gastric stasis syndrome).

Atlas of Gastroenterology, 4th edition. Edited by Tadataka Yamada, David H. Alpers, Anthony N. Kalloo, Neil Kaplowitz, Chung Owyang, and Don W. Powell. © 2009 Blackwell Publishing, ISBN: 978-1-4051-6909-7

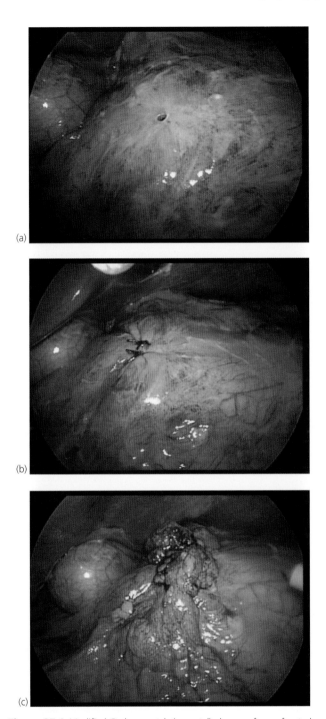

Figure 25.1 Modified Graham patch (omental) closure of a perforated duodenal ulcer. **(a)** Laparoscopic view of perforated anterior duodenal bulb ulcer. **(b)** Suture closure of the perforation. **(c)** Omental patch reinforcement of the perforation.

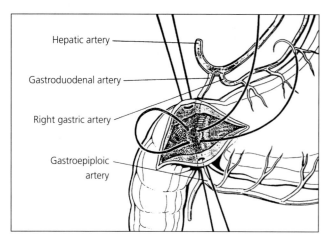

Figure 25.2 Suture closure of a posterior bleeding duodenal ulcer. Exposure is through a longitudinal gastroduodenotomy. The bleeding point within the ulcer is oversewn with monofilament sutures. Additional sutures are used above and below the ulcer to secure the gastroduodenal artery.

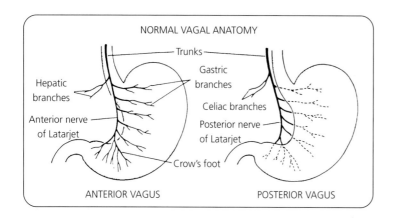

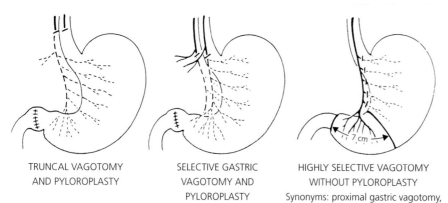

Figure 25.3 Normal vagal anatomy and types of vagotomy. Truncal and selective vagotomies are shown with a gastric drainage procedure (pyloroplasty). During truncal vagotomy, nerve trunks are divided above the celiac and hepatic branches. During selective vagotomy, the anterior and posterior nerves are divided distal to the celiac and hepatic branches, thus preserving extragastric innervation to the gastrointestinal tract. During highly selective vagotomy, individual branches of the anterior and posterior nerves of Latarjet to the body of the stomach are divided, sparing the branches to the antrum and pylorus ("Crow's foot"). Pyloroantral motor function is preserved and, therefore, a drainage procedure is not indicated.

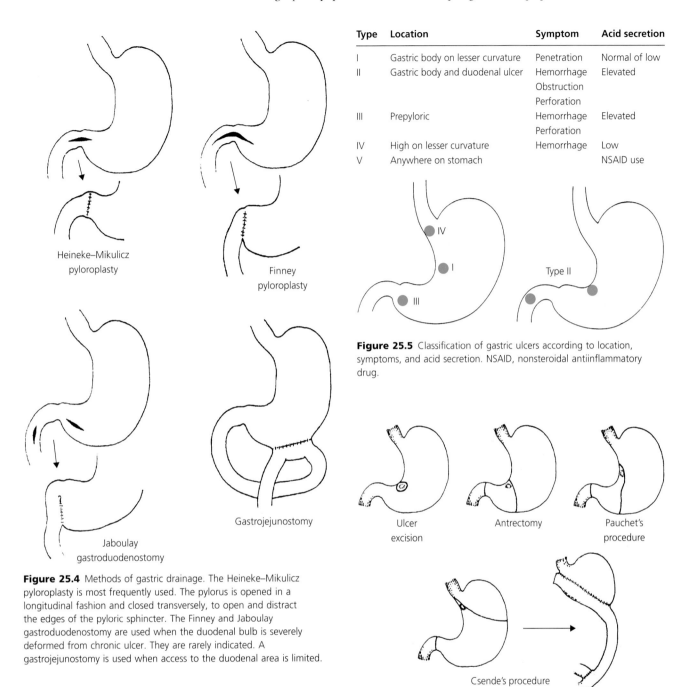

Type	Location	Symptom	Acid secretion
I	Gastric body on lesser curvature	Penetration	Normal of low
II	Gastric body and duodenal ulcer	Hemorrhage Obstruction Perforation	Elevated
III	Prepyloric	Hemorrhage Perforation	Elevated
IV	High on lesser curvature	Hemorrhage	Low
V	Anywhere on stomach		NSAID use

Heineke–Mikulicz
pyloroplasty

Finney
pyloroplasty

Type II

Figure 25.5 Classification of gastric ulcers according to location, symptoms, and acid secretion. NSAID, nonsteroidal antiinflammatory drug.

Jaboulay
gastroduodenostomy

Gastrojejunostomy

Ulcer
excision

Antrectomy

Pauchet's
procedure

Csende's procedure
for type IV gastric ulcer

Figure 25.4 Methods of gastric drainage. The Heineke–Mikulicz pyloroplasty is most frequently used. The pylorus is opened in a longitudinal fashion and closed transversely, to open and distract the edges of the pyloric sphincter. The Finney and Jaboulay gastroduodenostomy are used when the duodenal bulb is severely deformed from chronic ulcer. They are rarely indicated. A gastrojejunostomy is used when access to the duodenal area is limited.

Figure 25.6 Operations for benign gastric ulcer.

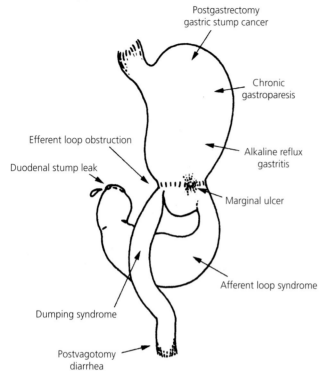

Figure 25.7 Postgastrectomy syndromes.

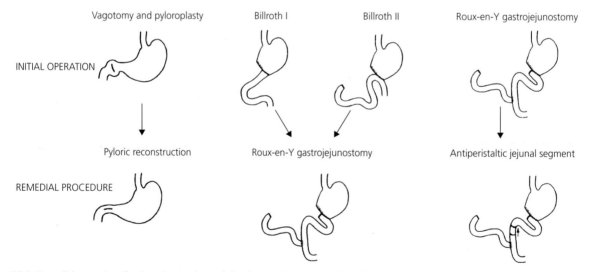

Figure 25.8 Remedial operations for dumping syndrome following gastric surgery. Although many options exist, for each initial operation, a reasonable remedial procedure is proposed.

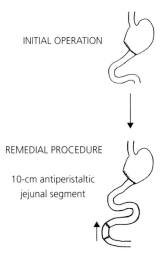

INITIAL OPERATION

REMEDIAL PROCEDURE

10-cm antiperistaltic
jejunal segment

Figure 25.9 Remedial operations for postvagotomy diarrhea includes construction of a 10 cm antiperistaltic jejunal segment located 100 cm from the ligament of Treitz.

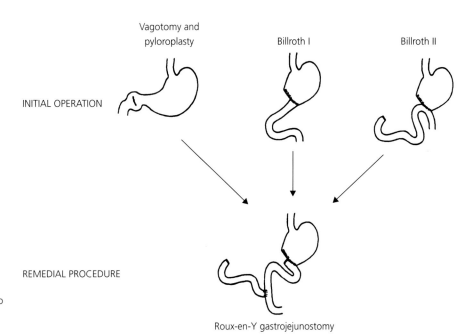

Vagotomy and
pyloroplasty

Billroth I

Billroth II

INITIAL OPERATION

REMEDIAL PROCEDURE

Figure 25.10 Remedial operation for alkaline reflux gastritis involves conversion to Roux-en-Y gastrojejunostomy, regardless of the initial operation.

Roux-en-Y gastrojejunostomy

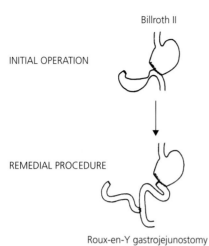

Figure 25.11 Remedial operations for afferent limb syndrome includes resection of the obstructed gastrojejunostomy with Roux-en-Y reconstruction.

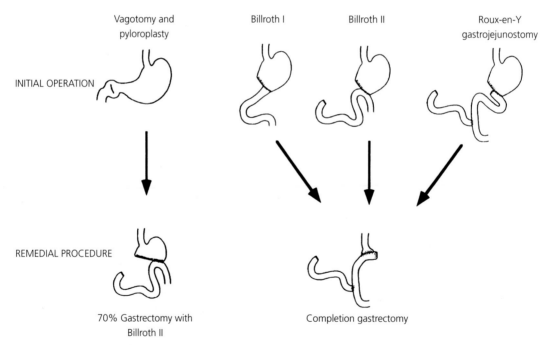

Figure 25.12 Remedial operations for gastric stasis syndrome following various gastric operations involve subtotal or total gastrectomy with gastrojejunostomy.

26

Miscellaneous diseases of the stomach

John C. Rabine, Timothy T. Nostrant

Hiatal hernias

Under normal circumstances, the stomach is held in position by the gastrophrenic, gastrohepatic, gastroduodenal, and gastrosplenic ligaments. Furthermore, the phrenoesophageal membrane helps to prevent herniation through the diaphragmatic hiatus. This membrane attaches near the squamocolumnar junction and extends approximately 1 cm above the junction. During swallowing and longitudinal esophageal muscle contraction, there is "physiological" herniation of the gastric cardia through the diaphragmatic hiatus. The phrenoesophageal membrane has a recoil action to pull the squamocolumnar junction back into its normal anatomical position. When these mechanisms are defective, true herniation can develop. The most common type of hernia is the sliding, or type I, hernia. This herniation is often transient and asymptomatic, but larger hernias are often nonreducing and predispose to gastroesophageal reflux (Fig. 24.1). Plain radiographs may suggest a hiatal hernia by demonstrating the presence of a large air bubble behind the cardiac silhouette. The cardia, identified by gastric folds, will be seen extending above the diaphragmatic impression, and the gastroesophageal junction is also displaced cephalad (Fig. 26.2).

Approximately 5% of hiatal hernias are types II, III and IV – the paraesophageal hernias. Unlike type I hernias, these hernias are associated with fundic herniation into the thoracic cavity (i.e., alongside the gastroesophageal junction); the gastroesophageal junction may or may not be displaced as well (Figs 26.3–26.5). Although relatively uncommon, these hernias are associated with severe complications, such as gastric volvulus and strangulation. In type II hernias there is a localized phrenoesophageal membrane defect allowing the gastric fundus to become the lead point of a herniation. The gastroesophageal junction is still in proper anatomic

attachment to preaortic fascia and the phrenoesophageal membrane. As more fundus herniates into the thoracic cavity, in part because of gastrocolic and gastrosplenic ligament laxity, gastric rotation can develop along the longitudinal axis of the stomach. This organoaxial volvulus results in the greater curve lying anterior to the lesser curve. Type II hernias can also result in a mesenteroaxial volvulus where rotation is along the transverse axis, but this is much less common. Type III hernias are a combination of types I and II; the fundus herniates through the hiatus, but stretching of the phrenoesophageal membrane results in displacement of the gastroesophageal junction above the diaphragm as well. Type IV hernias are rare and involve a massive hiatal defect that results in herniation of abdominal organs (colon, small bowel, spleen, and pancreas) into the thoracic cavity.

Gastric volvulus

A volvulus of the stomach occurs when one portion of the stomach twists around another. If the twist occurs around an imaginary line between the pylorus and the gastroesophageal junction, it is an organoaxial volvulus (Figs 26.6a and 26.7). Typically, the greater curve spins upward such that the stomach appears "upside-down" with the true posterior wall lying anteriorly. The antrum rotates anteriorly and superiorly while the fundus is displaced posteriorly and inferiorly. Alternatively, a mesenteroaxial volvulus develops when the distal stomach twists around an imaginary line between the center of the greater curve and the porta hepatis (see Figure 26.7a). This twisting resolves spontaneously in most patients (Fig. 26.7b). The antrum and distal body twist to the right (anteriorly and superiorly) such that the posterior wall again becomes anterior in placement.

Gastric bezoars

Bezoars are collections of foreign material that are retained most frequently within the stomach but have also been

Atlas of Gastroenterology, 4th edition. Edited by Tadataka Yamada, David H. Alpers, Anthony N. Kalloo, Neil Kaplowitz, Chung Owyang, and Don W. Powell. © 2009 Blackwell Publishing, ISBN: 978-1-4051-6909-7

found in the esophagus and rectum (Figs 26.8). Such matter may include plant and vegetable debris (phytobezoar), hair (trichobezoar), medications (pharmacobezoar), and persimmons (diospyrobezoar). Concretions are a type of bezoar that are typically very hard. Shellac, furniture polish, and concrete are classical components of such a bezoar, and surgery may be necessary to remove concretions; other therapies are generally ineffective. The formation of bezoars is likely multifactorial, and altered gastric motility and emptying are the primary etiologies. The size and digestibility of swallowed material are factors as well. Prior gastric surgery, whether pyloroplasty, antrectomy, or partial gastrectomy, clearly places patients at risk for phytobezoar or fungus ball formation. In addition to surgery, gastric stasis and bezoars have been linked to diabetic gastroparesis, mixed connective tissue disease, hypothyroidism, and myotonic dystrophy.

Heterotopic pancreas

Heterotopic pancreatic tissue, also termed a "pancreatic rest," can be found in the stomach, duodenum, or jejunum.

Typically, these rests are asymptomatic, but abdominal pain, nausea, vomiting, and rarely bleeding have been attributed to rests located in the stomach. These lesions typically appear as 2- to 4-cm submucosal masses in the prepyloric region, and it is not unusual that central umbilication is noted (Fig. 26.9). The nodules are firm and may have a yellow appearance. Endoscopic ultrasound will show a heterogenous submucosal mass with a pancreatic duct remnant.

Note

The views expressed in this article are those of the author and do not reflect the official policy or position of the U.S. Air Force, Department of Defense, or the U.S. Government.

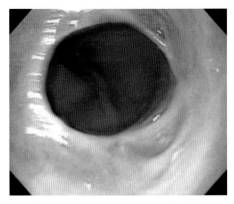

Figure 26.1 Endoscopic appearance of a large hiatal hernia with Schatzki ring.

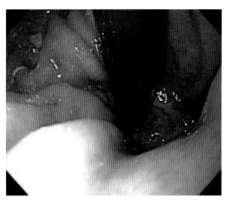

Figure 26.2 Endoscopic view of a type I hiatal hernia while in gastric retroflexion.

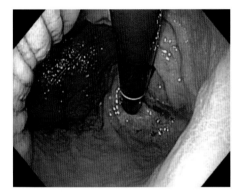

Figure 26.3 Endoscopic view of a paraesophageal hernia while in gastric retroflexion. The fundus is herniating into the thoracic cavity alongside a concomitant type I hernia.

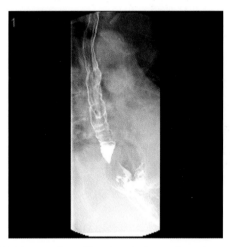

Figure 26.4 Paraesophageal hernia on barium radiograph.

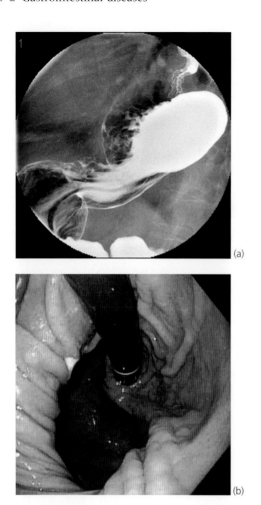

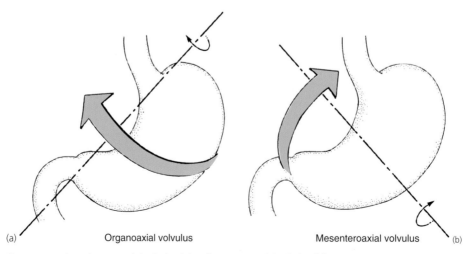

Figure 26.5 Type II paraesophageal hernia where the gastroesophageal junction remains below the diaphragm. **(a)** Barium radiograph demonstrating that the entire stomach has herniated into the chest, illustrating an "upside-down" appearance. **(b)** Endoscopic view of a paraesophageal hernia.

Figure 26.6 Schematic representation of organoaxial volvulus **(a)** and mesenteroaxial volvulus **(b)**.

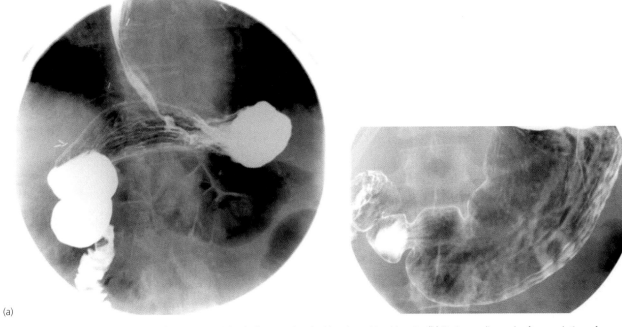

(a)

(b)

Figure 26.7 **(a)** Barium radiograph of an organoaxial volvulus associated with a large hiatal hernia. **(b)** Barium radiograph after resolution of organoaxial volvulus (same patient as in [a]).

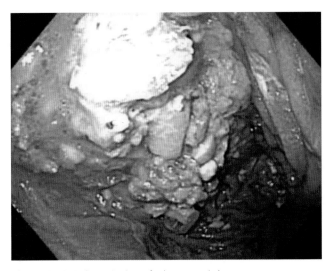

Figure 26.8 Endoscopic view of a large gastric bezoar.

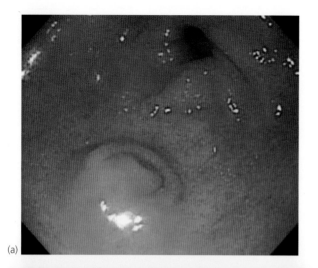

(a)

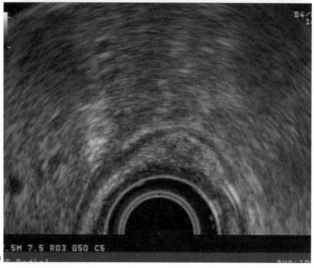

(b)

Figure 26.9 (a) Pancreatic rest identified in the antrum during upper endoscopy. **(b)** Endoscopic ultrasound view of a pancreatic rest.

27

Small intestine: anatomy and structural anomalies

Deborah C. Rubin, Jacob C. Langer

Embryology of the small intestine

The primitive human gut forms when the dorsal part of the yolk sac is incorporated into the embryo at 4 weeks' development, giving rise to the foregut, midgut, and hindgut. The foregut is the progenitor of the esophagus, stomach, duodenum up to the biliary duct ampulla, pharynx, respiratory tract, liver, pancreas, and biliary tract. The midgut gives rise to the duodenum distal to the common bile duct, jejunum, ileum, cecum, appendix, ascending colon, and one-half to two-thirds of the transverse colon. The rest of the colon and superior anal canal are derived from the hindgut.

The gut endoderm is the precursor of the gastrointestinal tract epithelium. Its endothelium arises from the ectoderm of the stomodeum and proctodeum as well as the endoderm. The splanchnic mesenchyme supplies the muscular and connective tissue components of the gastrointestinal tract. The midgut first freely communicates with the yolk sac and then narrows to be connected by the omphalomesenteric or vitelline duct. The primitive gut forms a U-shaped loop that grows so rapidly compared with the embryo that it herniates into the umbilical cord at the sixth week of gestation (Fig. 27.1). The proximal limb of the loop elongates into multiple intestinal loops, whereas the distal limb simply develops into the cecal diverticulum. The first stage of rotation is 90° counterclockwise around the superior mesenteric artery axis. At 10 weeks, the intestines return into the abdominal cavity and rotate a further 180° counterclockwise in the second stage. Finally, the cecum and appendix descend from the right upper quadrant to the right lower quadrant, and the proximal part of the colon elongates to form the hepatic flexure and ascending colon (third stage of rotation). Fixation occurs as the ascending colonic mesentery fuses with the parietal peritoneum and becomes fixed retroperitoneally. The mesentery of the small intestine attains a broad-based attachment to the posterior abdominal wall and extends from the duodenojejunal junction to the ileocecal region. The end result of this process is the normal location of the small and large intestines.

Congenital anomalies

A brief review of the main features of the common congenital anomalies is presented and illustrated with pictures of surgical specimens.

Meckel diverticulum

Meckel diverticulum is the most common congenital anomaly of the gastrointestinal tract. It results from failure of the vitelline duct to be completely resorbed (Fig. 27.2). Large autopsy series indicate a 2%–3% prevalence of Meckel diverticulum in the general population. Meckel diverticula are true diverticula, containing all layers of the bowel from serosa to mucosa. Heterotopic tissue is present approximately 50% of the time and includes gastric mucosa, pancreatic tissue and, less commonly, colonic mucosa, Brunner glands, and jejunal or hepatobiliary tissue. The presence of heterotopic mucosa correlates with increased risk for symptomatic, complicated Meckel diverticulum.

The complications of Meckel diverticulum include bleeding, intestinal obstruction, diverticulitis, perforation, and carcinoma. The frequency of specific complications varies between adult and pediatric patients. Among children, the most common complications are gastrointestinal bleeding and obstruction. For adults, intestinal obstruction is by far the most frequent complication and gastrointestinal bleeding is rare.

The diagnosis of Meckel diverticulum remains a challenge. Sodium pertechnetate technetium-99m radionuclide scanning is particularly useful in the care of children. This isotope is taken up into gastric mucosal cells and can help detect Meckel diverticula that contain ectopic gastric mucosa. Other examinations include enteroclysis and angiography, which may show the vitelline artery.

Atlas of Gastroenterology, 4th edition. Edited by Tadataka Yamada, David H. Alpers, Anthony N. Kalloo, Neil Kaplowitz, Chung Owyang, and Don W. Powell. © 2009 Blackwell Publishing, ISBN: 978-1-4051-6909-7

Management of complicated Meckel diverticulum is surgical. The management of asymptomatic Meckel diverticulum that is an incidental finding remains controversial, although prophylactic removal seems to be safe and produces low morbidity and mortality rates.

Duplications

Duplications of the gastrointestinal tract are rare congenital cystic anomalies attached to the intestinal mesenteric border (Fig. 27.3). Duplications may occur anywhere along the gastrointestinal tract, although those of small bowel origin are usually found in the ileum. Most duplications are diagnosed during infancy and early childhood, but duplications are occasionally newly discovered in adults. Symptoms in childhood include abdominal pain, obstructive symptoms, and hemorrhage. Adults frequently have no symptoms or have mild abdominal symptoms. Intussusception, gastrointestinal hemorrhage, or carcinoma occasionally develops in adults. Detection may be difficult. Small bowel follow-through shows a duplication only if the lumen of the normal intestine communicates with the duplication. Ultrasonography or computed tomographic scanning is valuable for detecting a cystic mass. Duplications are managed surgically.

Intestinal atresia and stenosis

Intestinal atresia is a condition in which segments of the lumen contain areas of total occlusion (Figs 27.4 and 27.5). Atresia is one of the common causes of intestinal obstruction among neonates. Atresia may be single or multiple and is found from the esophagus through to the rectum. The prevalence is from 1 in 3000–5000 live births. In type I atresia, a membranous septum or diaphragm of mucosa and submucosa obstructs the lumen, but the intestinal wall and mesentery are intact. Type II is characterized by two blind bowel ends connected by a fibrous cord, with intact mesentery in between (see Fig. 27.4). In type IIIa lesions (see Fig. 27.5), two blind bowel ends are separated by a mesenteric gap. Type IIIb is "apple peel" atresia, in which there is proximal atresia in the small intestine and absence of the distal superior mesenteric artery (less than 5% of all instances of atresia). In this case, the bowel distal to the atresia is foreshortened and coiled, and receives retrograde blood supply from the ileocolic, right colic, or inferior mesenteric artery. Type IV denotes multiple areas of atresia throughout the small bowel, which have the appearance of a string of sausages; the atresia may be type I, II, or IIIa.

Polyhydramnios is frequently detected in proximal gastrointestinal atresia, but amniotic fluid may be normal in distal atresia. Bilious vomiting soon after birth is a characteristic symptom of proximal atresia, whereas abdominal distention, later vomiting, and failure to pass meconium are found in distal atresia. Diagnosis may be made by means of prenatal ultrasonography followed by plain radiography, and cautious contrast radiography after birth and before surgical intervention.

Gastroschisis and omphalocele

Gastroschisis occurs when there is a small defect in the abdominal wall through which there is massive evisceration of the intestines (Fig. 27.6). The bowel has no membranous covering, has been exposed to amniotic fluid in utero, is thickened, and is covered with adhesions. Omphalocele occurs when the abdominal viscera herniate through the umbilical ring and persist outside the body covered by a membranous sac but not by skin (Fig. 27.7). Omphalocele is associated with a variety of other anomalies of chromosomal origin. The diagnosis of an abdominal wall defect is suggested by the presence of a high maternal serum α-fetoprotein level. Prenatal ultrasonography also is a sensitive method of prenatal diagnosis. Prenatal detection allows for obstetric planning so that the patient can be at a tertiary care facility for delivery. Treatment is surgical by means of primary closure, or use of a surgical silo or polymeric silicone sac.

Volvulus

Volvulus is abnormal twisting of the intestine around the axis of its own mesentery, resulting in obstruction of the more proximal bowel (Fig. 27.8). The twisting of the mesentery may involve the mesenteric vessels and make the involved loop particularly susceptible to strangulation and gangrene. In the United States, volvulus of the small intestine is usually caused by a preexisting defect such as an anomaly of rotation and fixation, postoperative adhesion, or congenital bands. Patients have symptoms of obstruction of the small intestine and an acute abdomen. The severity of pain may be out of proportion to the physical findings, which include abdominal distention, rebound tenderness, guarding and rigidity, and a palpable abdominal mass. The diagnosis is made with plain abdominal radiographs, which may demonstrate distended bowel with air–fluid levels consistent with obstruction or free air from a perforation. Barium studies can be useful in depicting disorders of rotation. A typical corkscrew-like appearance of barium in the distorted duodenum and jejunum also is diagnostic. Angiography may reveal twisting of the branches of the superior mesenteric artery. Rapid recognition of volvulus and prompt surgical intervention are the keys to decreasing the fatality rate associated with this condition.

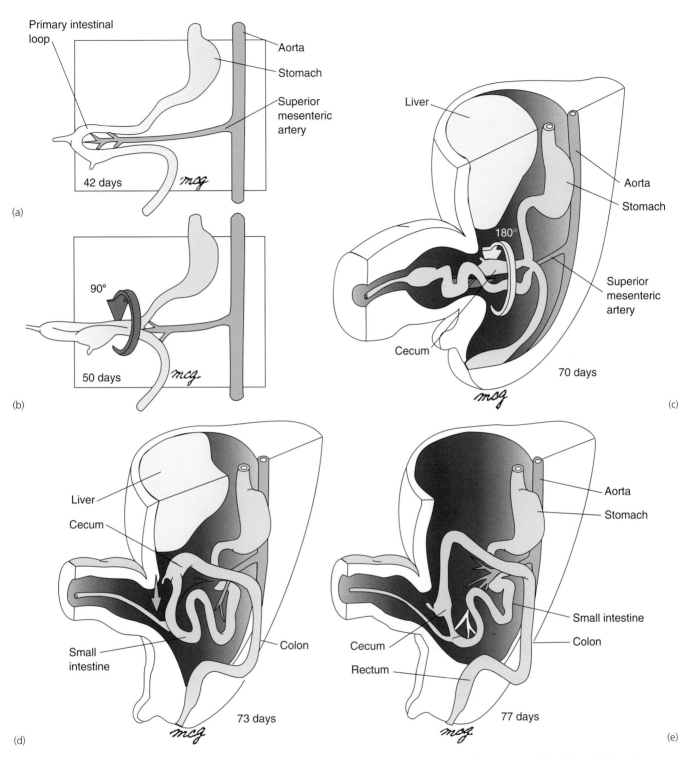

Figure 27.1 Herniation and rotation of the intestine. **(a, b)** At the end of the sixth week, the primary intestinal loop herniates into the umbilicus, rotating through 90° counterclockwise (in frontal view). **(c)** The small intestine elongates to form jejunoileal loops, the cecum and appendix grow, and at the end of the 10th week, the primary intestinal loop retracts into the abdominal cavity rotating an additional 180° counterclockwise. **(d, e)** During the 11th week, the retracting midgut completes this rotation as the cecum is positioned just inferior to the liver. The cecum is then displaced inferiorly, pulling down the proximal hindgut to form the ascending colon. The descending colon is simultaneously fixed on the left side of the posterior abdominal wall. The jejunum, ileum, and transverse and sigmoid colons remain suspended by mesentery.

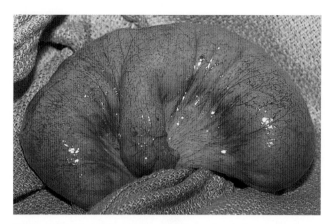

Figure 27.2 Meckel diverticulum. These true diverticula contain all layers of the intestinal wall. Ectopic gastric mucosa may appear as small, red nodules.

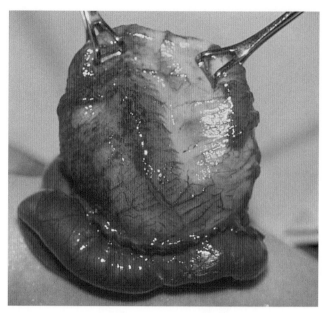

Figure 27.3 Jejunal duplication. Duplications are present on the mesenteric border and share a common blood supply with the adjacent bowel.

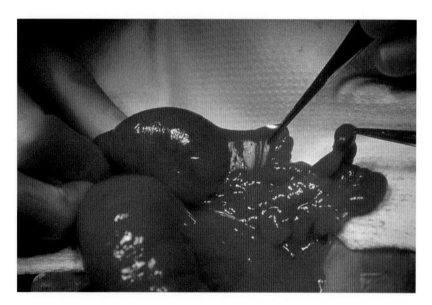

Figure 27.4 Jejunal atresia, type II. A cord-like fibrous segment connects the two ends of intestine.

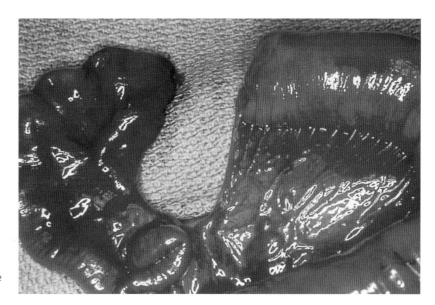

Figure 27.5 Atresia of the small intestine, type IIIa. There is complete separation of the blind ends of the small bowel and a mesenteric gap.

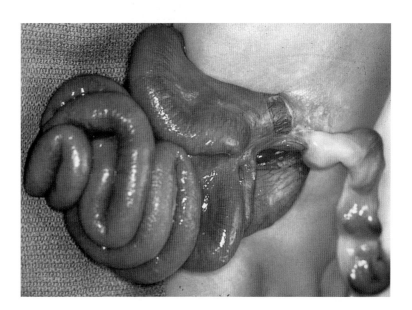

Figure 27.6 Gastroschisis. Multiple loops of exteriorized small intestine are depicted. The bowel is often dilated, edematous, and thickened, presumably because of direct exposure to amniotic fluid.

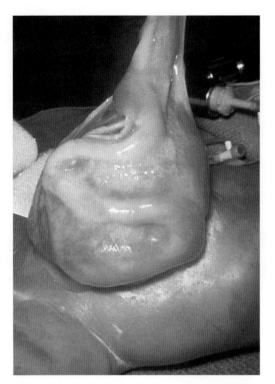

Figure 27.7 Omphalocele. Loops of intestine sit in a thin-walled sac composed of umbilical cord coverings.

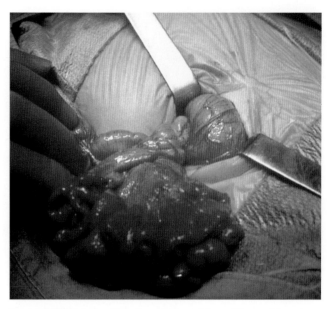

Figure 27.8 Volvulus. There is complete twisting of the small bowel around the axis of its mesentery. Although in this case the loops of the small intestine appear normal, ischemia or frank necrosis of the intestine may be present.

28

Dysmotility of the small intestine and colon

Michael Camilleri, Silvia Delgado-Aros

Motility of the digestive tract is the result of the myoelectric activity, contractile activity, tone, compliance, and transit. The correct function of all of these components of the motility of the small intestine ensures the appropriate absorption of the nutrients, propels the bolus through the intestine, and prevents bacterial overgrowth. Properly functioning colonic motility is particularly important to prevent diarrhea and constipation.

Motility is controlled by the enteric nervous system (ENS), which is modified by extrinsic nerves as well as gastrointestinal hormones. The effects of these neurons on the gut muscle partly rely on interstitial cells of Cajal (ICC). Dysfunctions in any of these components may cause intestinal or colonic dysmotility (Fig. 28.1).

Diseases that affect gastrointestinal smooth muscle include primary visceral myopathies, collagen diseases, muscular dystrophies, amyloidosis, and thyroid disease (Table 28.1). Enteric nerve dysfunction occurs in primary visceral neuropathies, Hirschsprung disease, diabetes mellitus, Chagas disease, ganglioneuromatosis, paraneoplastic visceral neuropathy, and Parkinson disease. Small intestine and colonic dysmotility may be also caused by drugs (such as phenothiazines, tricyclic antidepressants, ganglionic blockers, and narcotics) and occurs among patients with jejunoileal bypass and celiac disease. The effect of gastrointestinal hormones on the motility of the small and large intestine is manifested clinically by diarrhea in patients with carcinoid syndrome and irritable bowel syndrome. These syndromes are associated with elevated circulating serotonin levels and rapid intestinal transit that may partly reflect abnormal motor function or abnormal intestinal secretion.

Regardless of the underlying causes, patients with dysmotility of the small intestine and colon may have a wide range of clinical manifestations. Patients may be asymptomatic or, at the other end of the spectrum, they may present with chronic intestinal pseudoobstruction. Between the two

extremes, patients may have dyspeptic symptoms, including intermittent postprandial epigastric or periumbilical abdominal pain, bloating, nausea, vomiting, and diarrhea or constipation. Intestinal bacterial overgrowth occurs in severe cases of intestinal dysmotility and results in steatorrhea and sometimes diarrhea. Symptoms tend to occur in the postprandial period. Extraintestinal manifestations of the underlying disease may be detected among patients with the secondary causes of small intestine and colonic dysmotility.

Small intestine dysmotility seems to occur less frequently in comparison with colonic dysmotility. However, the lack of validated tests to evaluate small intestine motility makes it difficult to precisely estimate the prevalence. Novel techniques are being developed to improve measurements of the motor function of the small intestine that may help to diagnose and better estimate the prevalence of these dysfunctions. In contrast, constipation affects 12%–15% of the population and Hirschsprung disease; the prototypic congenital colonic dysmotility affects 1 in 5000 births. This chapter reviews primary and secondary causes of small intestine and colon motility diseases.

Primary causes

Visceral myopathies
Familial visceral myopathies
Familial visceral myopathies (FVMs) are a group of genetic diseases characterized by degeneration and fibrosis of the gastrointestinal smooth muscle and, in certain types, the urinary smooth muscle. There are at least three reported types of FVM based on gross lesions of the gastrointestinal tract and the pattern of inheritance (Table 28.2). Well-documented mitochondrial and gene alterations exist in type II FVM, also called mitochondrial neurogastrointestinal encephalomyopathy syndrome (MNGIE). On routine pathological examination, the histological findings in all three types of FVM are similar and are characterized by degenerated muscle cells and fibrosis. Recognition of milder lesions may be facilitated by use of trichrome stain (Fig. 28.2).

Atlas of Gastroenterology, 4th edition. Edited by Tadataka Yamada, David H. Alpers, Anthony N. Kalloo, Neil Kaplowitz, Chung Owyang, and Don W. Powell. © 2009 Blackwell Publishing, ISBN: 978-1-4051-6909-7

Intestinal manometric studies on patients with FVM reveal low-amplitude (usually <20 mmHg and on average <10 mmHg) intestinal contractions (Fig. 28.3). Recent advances in type II FVM or MNGIE warrant a more detailed discussion of this entity.

Type II familial visceral myopathies

This entity forms part of a heterogeneous group of disorders that result from structural, biochemical, or genetic derangements of mitochondria. Type II FVM has an autosomal recessive inheritance and it is characterized by gastrointestinal dysmotility, ophthalmoplegia, and peripheral neuropathy; on skeletal muscle biopsy, ragged red fibers demonstrated best on Gomori trichrome stain (Fig. 28.4). Additional clinical features include lactic acidosis, increased cerebrospinal fluid protein, and leukodystrophy, which is identified by magnetic resonance imaging of the brain. The ubiquity of mitochondria explains the association of neuromuscular, gastrointestinal, and other nonneuromuscular symptoms that are characteristic of this syndrome. Some patients have been found to have multiple mitochondrial DNA deletions in skeletal muscle. Mitochondrial DNA contains genes that encode polypeptides that are components of the cellular oxidative phosphorylation system. Nuclear genes, however, also encode for components of this system. It is believed that mutations of nuclear DNA genes that control the expression of the mitochondrial genomes are the underlying genetic defect of this syndrome. It was proposed that a unique gene located in the long arm of chromosome 22 (22q13.32qter), distal to locus D22S1161, is responsible for this syndrome.

Childhood visceral myopathies

Two distinct forms of childhood visceral myopathies (CVM) have been recognized (Table 28.3); the second is identified by the phenotype of megacystis-microcolon-intestinal hypoperistalsis. The two diseases differ from FVM in their clinical manifestations and modes of inheritance. Degeneration and fibrosis of gastrointestinal and urinary smooth muscle can be detected in both types of CVM and result in bowel dilation (Fig. 28.5), ureteropelvicaliectasis (Fig. 28.6), or megacystis, which results from bladder degeneration (Fig. 28.7).

Nonfamilial visceral myopathies

It is unclear whether cases of nonfamilial visceral myopathy among adults represent sporadic cases or unrecognized variants of FVM with a recessive pattern of inheritance. There is no histological difference between the familial and the nonfamilial forms of visceral myopathy, and both show low-amplitude contractions when investigated with intestinal manometry.

Visceral neuropathies

The ENS is a vast network of ganglionated plexuses located in the wall of the gastrointestinal tract, and it is in close contact with ICC. Normal migration, differentiation, and subsequent survival or maintenance of the precursor cells of the ENS derived from the neural crest has been demonstrated to be crucial for the normal function of the intestine. Different genetic defects in migration, differentiation, and maintenance of enteric neurons have been identified in several causes of gut dysmotility (Table 28.4). These include abnormalities of RET, the gene that encodes for the tyrosine kinase (Trk) receptor; the endothelin B system (which tends to retard development of neural elements, thereby facilitating colonization of the entire gut from the neural crest), Sox-10 (a transcription factor that enhances maturation of neural precursors), and c-Kit, which is a marker for ICCs. Disturbances in these mechanisms result in syndromic dysmotilities, such as Hirschsprung disease, Waardenburg syndrome (pigmentary defects, piebaldism, neural deafness, and megacolon), and idiopathic hypertrophic pyloric stenosis. Figure 28.8 demonstrates some of the mutations in the Trk receptor that have been reported in gut dysmotility associated with familial or sporadic medullary carcinoma of the thyroid, multiple endocrine neoplasia type 2A or B (Fig. 28.9), and Hirschsprung disease.

The effects of motor neurons on the gastrointestinal and colonic muscle cells are relayed, at least in part, via the ICCs, which are electrically coupled to the muscle (Figs 28.10 and 28.11). They have receptors for the inhibitory transmitters vasoactive intestinal peptide (VIP) and nitric oxide (NO), and for the excitatory tachykinin transmitters. The protooncogene c-kit encodes a transmembrane Trk receptor c-Kit. Activation of this receptor is responsible for the development of the ICCs. Disruption of ICCs by treatment of neonatal rats with antibodies to c-Kit receptor impairs excitatory and inhibitory transmission to the circular muscle of the small and large intestine. Because they generate physiological slow waves in the gastrointestinal tract, ICCs have also been recognized as the pacemaker cells of the gut. Slow waves are the rhythmic oscillations of the membrane potential that characterize the electrical activity of gut muscle. Slow waves are the rate-limiting step for contractile function in the smooth muscle cells. Contraction typically occurs when there is superimposition of spike bursts on the slow waves. The relevance of these functions of ICCs as neuromodulators and "pacemakers" of the gut is highlighted by the several examples of gut motility dysfunction associated with anomalous ICCs. A smaller number of ICCs were found in slow-transit constipation (Figs 28.12 and 28.13), and abnormal distribution of these cells has been found in Hirschsprung disease. Variants of enteric neuropathic dysmotility, such as hypoganglionosis, immature ganglia, neuronal intestinal dysplasia, and infantile pyloric stenosis, as well as in chronic and transient intestinal pseudoobstruction, also have been observed. A diminished number, altered networks, and altered ultrastructural features of gastric ICCs have been demonstrated in diabetic mice with gastroparesis (Fig. 28.14).

Visceral neuropathy may result in bowel dilation (Fig. 28.15), although this is generally less frequent or less severe than in visceral myopathy. In Hirschsprung disease, the aganglionic segment is permanently contracted, causing dilation proximal to it (Fig. 28.16). Intestinal manometry is characterized by normal-amplitude contractions with evidence of incoordination in, for example, the propagation of fasting migrating motor complexes (MMCs), or recurrence of MMC-like activity in the first postprandial hour.

Familial visceral neuropathies

Familial visceral neuropathies (FVNs) are a group of genetic diseases characterized by degeneration of the enteric nervous system. Two distinct phenotypes, I and II, have been distinguished, which are summarized in Table 28.5.

Hirschsprung disease (congenital megacolon)

Aganglionosis is caused by arrest of the caudal migration of cells from the neural crest, which is destined to develop as the gut's intramural plexuses. In Hirschsprung disease, the aganglionic segment always extends from the internal anal sphincter for a variable distance proximally; in most instances, it stays within the rectum and sigmoid colon ("classical type"), although involvement of very short segments and longer segments or the entire colon have also been described. The genetic disorders resulting in altered development of the neural crest in Hirschsprung disease have been discussed in detail above (see Table 28.4). The defect occurs once in every 5000 live births and is in some cases familial, with an overall incidence of 3.6% among siblings of index cases. Although most children have major manifestations before the second month of life, very short segment aganglionosis may not cause severe symptoms until after infancy. Mucosal suction biopsy can rule out the disease if submucosal ganglia are present. However, the absence of ganglion cells does not establish the diagnosis, and a deep or full-thickness biopsy from at least 3 cm proximal to the pectinate line should be obtained. Ganglia may be absent from the deep and superficial submucosal layers for even longer distances, and myenteric ganglia may also be absent in normal infants over that distance proximal to the internal sphincter. A very short aganglionic segment may be missed by biopsy and radiographs. In these cases, the absence of internal sphincter relaxation in response to rectal distention may help to confirm the diagnosis. However, distention of a balloon in a dilated rectum (that is, for chronic constipation or megarectum) may be associated with a false-positive result, because the intrarectal balloon may not sufficiently distend the rectum to elicit the reflex relaxation of the internal anal sphincter.

Idiopathic nonfamilial visceral neuropathies (chronic neuropathic intestinal pseudoobstruction of idiopathic variety)

Damage to the myenteric plexus can occur for a variety of different reasons, including chemical exposure, drug use, and viral infections. Patients with idiopathic nonfamilial visceral neuropathy may have dysmotility at any level of the gastrointestinal tract present with features of chronic intestinal pseudoobstruction, and a useful screening test is a solid-phase gastric emptying test. The intestine may be dilated but shows active, nonperistaltic contractions. Histological examination of the myenteric plexus shows a reduction in the total number of neurons; the remaining neurons may be enlarged with thick, clubbed processes. An increase in the number of Schwann cells and hypertrophy of the muscularis propria may also be observed. In patients with colonic inertia, the ICCs are reduced in number and are morphologically abnormal. The precise mechanism and neurotransmitter deficiencies of this disorder are unclear. Table 28.6 summarizes information from a number of studies in the literature regarding histological changes that have been found in patients with motility disorders, such as chronic intestinal pseudoobstruction or slow transit constipation, severe enough to warrant subtotal colectomy. Table 28.7 summarizes the literature pertaining to specific disorders of neurotransmitters in disease. In less severe cases, differentiation from constipation-predominant irritable bowel syndrome may be difficult, especially when the gut is not dilated. Features of intestinal manometry mimic those of familial and secondary neuropathies (Fig. 28.17). In slow-transit constipation, colonic manometry shows a reduction in high-amplitude peristaltic waves.

Secondary causes

Several systemic diseases may involve the digestive tract and result in intestinal dysmotility, although gastrointestinal manifestations rarely are the presenting feature. These secondary dysmotilities include diseases involving the intestinal smooth muscle, that is collagen diseases (such as scleroderma, dermatomyositis, systemic lupus erythematosus, and mixed connective tissue disease) (Fig. 28.18), muscular dystrophy, and amyloidosis. Secondary intestinal dysmotility may also occur in diseases with associated neurological derangement (diabetic neuropathy, Chagas disease, Parkinson disease, neurofibromatosis, and paraneoplastic visceral neuropathy), endocrine disorders (diabetes mellitus, thyroid and parathyroid disease), drug-induced conditions (by phenothiazines, tricyclic antidepressants, antiparkinsonian drugs, ganglionic blockers, and narcotics), and miscellaneous diseases (celiac disease, radiation enteritis, immunoproliferative disorders, jejunoileal bypass, and postgastrointestinal viral infection) (see Figs 28.17 and 28.19).

Table 28.1 Causes of gut dysmotility

Primary causes

Visceral myopathies
Familial visceral myopathies: type I, II (MNGIE), III
Childhood visceral myopathies: type I, II (megacystis-microcolon-
    intestinal hypoperistalsis)
Nonfamilial visceral myopathies

Visceral neuropathies
Familial visceral neuropathies: type I, II
Hirschsprung disease
Idiopathic nonfamilial visceral neuropathies

Secondary causes

Disease involving the intestinal smooth muscle
Collagen diseases (e.g., scleroderma, dermatomyositis, systemic lupus
    erythematosus, mixed connective tissue disease)
Muscular dystrophies (e.g., myotonic dystrophy, Duchenne muscular
    dystrophy)
Amyloidosis

Neurological diseases
Chagas disease, ganglioneuromatosis of the intestine, paraneoplastic
    neuropathy, Parkinson disease, spinal cord injury

Endocrine disorders
Diabetes mellitus, thyroid disease (i.e., hyperthyroidism,
    hypothyroidism), hypoparathyroidism

Pharmacological agents
Phenothiazines, tricyclic antidepressants, antiparkinsonian medications,
    ganglionic blockers, clonidine, narcotics (morphine and meperidine)

Miscellaneous intestinal disorders
Celiac disease
Radiation enteritis
Diffuse lymphoid infiltration of the small intestine
Jejunoileal bypass
Postgastrointestinal viral infection

MNGIE, mitochondrial neurogastrointestinal encephalomyopathy
syndrome.

Table 28.2 Classification of familial visceral myopathies

Characteristics	Type I	Type II (MNGIE)	Type III
Mode of transmission	Autosomal dominant	Autosomal recessive; isolated cases	Autosomal recessive
Gross lesions	Esophageal dilation, megaduodenum, redundant colon, and megacystis	Gastric dilation, slight dilation of the entire small intestine with numerous diverticula	Marked dilation of the entire digestive tract from the esophagus to the rectum
Microscopic changes	Degeneration and fibrosis of both muscle layers		
Clinical manifestations:			
Age at onset	After the first decade	Teens	Middle age
Percentage symptomatic	<50%	>75%	>75%
Symptoms of CIP	Variable severity	Severe plus pain	Classic CIP
Extra-GI manifestations	Megacystis, uterine inertia, and mydriasis	Ptosis and external ophthalmoplegia, muscle pain, peripheral neuropathy, and deafness	None observed
Treatment, prognosis	Prognosis good with or without surgery	No effective medical or surgical treatment; prognosis poor	No effective medical or surgical treatment; prognosis poor

CIP, chronic intestinal pseudoobstruction; GI, gastrointestinal; MNGIE, mitochondrial neurogastrointestinal encephalomyopathy syndrome.

Table 28.3 Classification of childhood visceral myopathies

Characteristics	Type I	Type II (megacystis-microcolon-intestinal hypoperistalsis)
Mode of transmission	Autosomal recessive (?)	Autosomal recessive (?)
Gross lesions	Dilation of entire GI tract	Short, malrotated small intestine and malfixation of microcolon
Microscopic changes	Degeneration and fibrosis of GI and urinary smooth muscle cells	Vacuolar degeneration of GI and urinary smooth muscle cells
Clinical manifestations:		
Age of onset	Infancy and young childhood	Infancy
Gender	Both	Predominantly female
Symptoms	Constipation, distention ± CIP	Obstipation, intestinal pseudoobstruction
Extra-GI manifestations	Megacystis and megaureters	Megacystis and megaureters
Treatment, prognosis	No effective medication; prognosis poor	No effective treatment; prognosis poor

CIP, chronic intestinal pseudoobstruction; GI, gastrointestinal.

Table 28.4 Genetic defects identified in different causes of gut dysmotility

Dysmotility: prevalence genetic defect	Phenotype	Associated non-GI disease	Dysmotility: prevalence in phenotype
RET/GDNF	Hirschsprung	None in humans	20%–50% *RET*, 5% *GDNF*
ET-3/ET-B	Hirschsprung or megacolon	Waardenburg-Shah	5%–10% Hirschsprung
SOX-10	Hirschsprung	Waardenburg-Shah	?
C-KIT	?CIP/Hirschsprung	None	?

CIP, chronic intestinal pseudoobstruction; GI, gastrointestinal.

Table 28.5 Classification of familial visceral neuropathies

Characteristics	Type I	Type II
Mode of transmission	Autosomal dominant	Autosomal recessive
Gross lesions	Dilation of lengths of small intestine, often distal small bowel; megacolon; gastroparesis in ~25% of patients	Hypertrophic pyloric stenosis, dilated short small intestine, malrotation of small intestine
Microscopic changes	Degeneration of argyrophilic neurons and decreased numbers of nerve fibers	Deficiency of argyrophilic neurons and increased neuroblasts
Clinical manifestations		
Age of onset	Any age	Infancy
Percentage symptomatic	>75%	100%
Symptoms	~67% CIP	All CIP
Extra-GI manifestations	None	± Malformation of CNS, patent ductus arteriosus
Treatment, prognosis	No effective medical or surgical treatment; prognosis fair	No effective medical or surgical treatment; prognosis poor

CIP, chronic intestinal pseudoobstruction; CNS, central nervous system; GI, gastrointestinal.

Table 28.6 Colonic neuropathy in slow transit constipation

Histological and immunohistochemical findings
Decreased number or abnormal appearance of silver staining neurons or axons
Increased number of variably sized nuclei within ganglia
Decreased colonic VIP nerves
Decreased neurofilament staining in myenteric plexus in 75% of patients
17/29 entire colon affected
12/29 segmental involvement
Increased number of PGP 9.5 reactive nerve fibers in muscularis layer of ascending and descending colon
Decreased total nerve density in myenteric plexus
Decreased VIP and increased NO positive neurons
Decreased substance P nerves in 7/10 patients
Decreased VIP nerves in 4/7 patients
Decreased substance P in mucosa and submucosa of rectal biopsies
Increased VIP, substance P and galanin in ascending colon
Increased VIP and galanin in transverse colon
Increased VIP and neuropeptide Y in descending colon myenteric plexus
Decreased VIP in submucosa
Decreased tachykinin (substance P) and enkephalin fibers in circular muscle
Decreased colonic total neuron density
Decreased VIP and NO neurons in myenteric plexus
Decreased VIP neurons in submucous plexus
Decreased enteroglucagon and 5-HT cells in mucosa
Decreased cell secretory indices of enteroglucagon and somatostatin cells
Decreased volume of interstitial cells of Cajal and neurons in circular muscle

5-HT, 5-hydroxytryptamine; NO, nitric oxide; PGP 9.5, protein gene product 9.5; VIP, vasoactive intestinal peptide.
From De Giorgio R, Camilleri M. Human enteric neuropathies: morphology and molecular pathology. Neurogastroenterol Motil 2004;16:515.

Table 28.7 Pathological features of enteric neuromuscular disease

Aganglionosis
Neuronal intranuclear inclusions and apoptosis
Neural degeneration
Intestinal neuronal dysplasia
Neuronal hyperplasia and ganglioneuromas
Mitochondrial dysfunction: syndromic and non-syndromic
Inflammatory neuropathies: cellular and humoral mechanisms
Neurotransmitter disorders
Interstitial cell pathology

From De Giorgio R, Camilleri M. Human enteric neuropathies: morphology and molecular pathology. Neurogastroenterol Motil 2004;16:515.

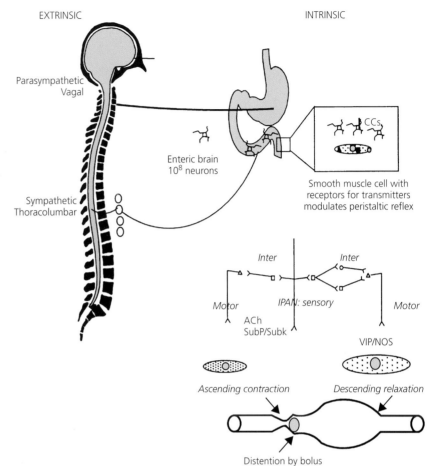

EXTRINSIC

INTRINSIC

Parasympathetic
Vagal

Sympathetic
Thoracolumbar

Enteric brain
10^8 neurons

CCs

Smooth muscle cell with
receptors for transmitters
modulates peristaltic reflex

Inter   Inter

Motor   IPAN: sensory   Motor

ACh
SubP/Subk

VIP/NOS

Ascending contraction   Descending relaxation

Distention by bolus

Figure 28.1 Extrinsic and enteric control of gut motility. The enteric nervous system (ENS) controls stereotypical motor functions, such as the migrating motor complex and the peristaltic reflex; enteric control is modulated by the extrinsic parasympathetic and sympathetic nerves, which respectively stimulate and inhibit nonsphincteric muscle. ACh, acetylcholine; ATP, adenosine triphosphate; CGRP, calcitonin gene-related peptide; ICCs, interstitial cells of Cajal; IPAN, intrinsic primary afferent neuron; NOS, nitric oxide synthase; PACAP, pituitary adenylate cyclase-activating polypeptide; SubP, substance P; VIP, vasoactive intestinal peptide.

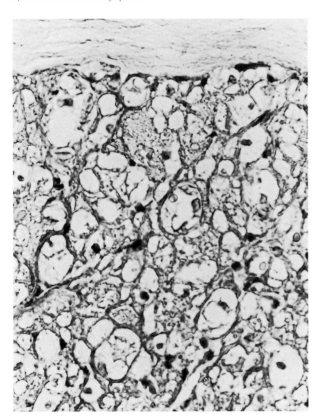

Figure 28.2 Characteristic vacuolar change with collagen fibers encircling spaces filled by fragmented muscle cells. This patient has familial visceral myopathy (trichrome stain; original magnification ×470).

1 min

30 mmHg

I

II

III

IV

V

Figure 28.3 Jejunal manometric record of a patient with type I familial visceral myopathy reveals weak contractions (amplitude <30 mmHg) of phase 3. Five tracings are shown and each is 5 cm apart. Phase 3 contractions were detected in only tracings I and II but not at other locations because of the weakness of contractions at these locations.

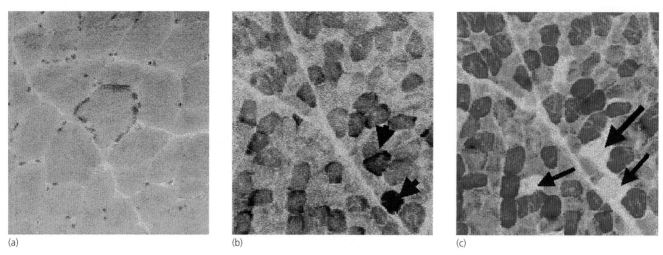

(a)

(b)

(c)

Figure 28.4 Histological and histochemical studies of skeletal muscle biopsy from a patient with mitochondrial myopathy. **(a)** Note the ragged red fibers characterized by the subsarcolemmal location of giant mitochondria in a few fibers, and the paucity of mitochondria in other fibers. **(b)** On histochemical analysis, a few fibers are succinate dehydrogenase positive (ragged blue appearance [arrowheads]) **(c)** The same fibers do not express cytochrome c oxidase (arrows), suggesting a defect in the respiratory enzyme chain that results in mitochondrial dysfunction and systemic acidosis.

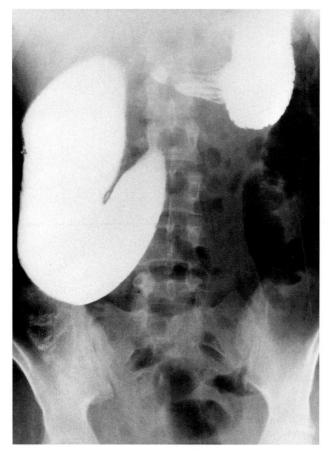

Figure 28.5 Upper gastrointestinal radiograph from a patient with type I familial visceral myopathy demonstrates severe megaduodenum.

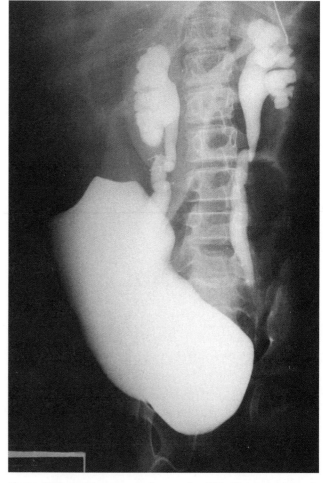

Figure 28.6 An intravenous pyelogram of a child with type I childhood visceral myopathy shows megacystis and bilateral ureteral pyelocaliectasis.

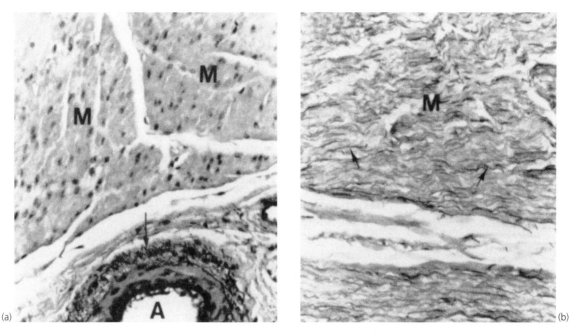

Figure 28.7 (a) Bladder muscularis from a control specimen demonstrates elastic fibers (arrow) in the adventitia of a small artery (A). No elastic fibers are present within muscle bundles (i.v.). **(b)** Bladder muscularis from a type I childhood visceral myopathy patient demonstrates numerous, parallel, coarse, wavy, elastic fibers (arrows) within muscle bundles (i.v.). (Verhoeff-van Gieson stain; original magnification ×325.)

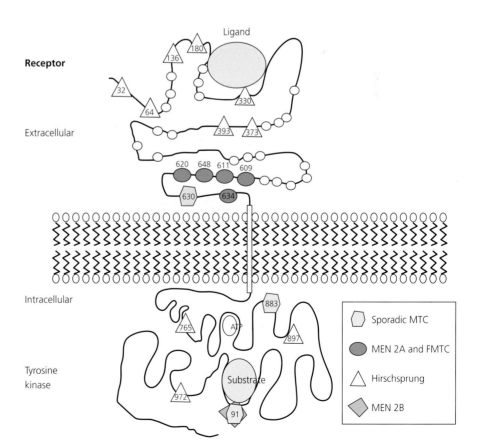

Figure 28.8 Tyrosine kinase receptor with examples of mutations associated with specific genetic disorders. ATP, adenosine triphosphate; [F] MTC, [familial] medullary carcinoma of the thyroid; MEN, multiple endocrine neoplasia.

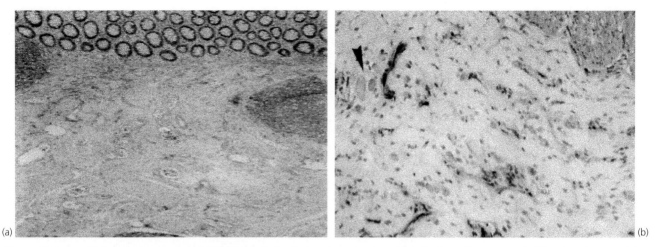

Figure 28.9 In multiple endocrine neoplasia (MEN) IIB, intestinal pathology shows transmural intestinal ganglioneuromatosis filling the submucosa **(a)**, and the myenteric plexus **(b)**. Note thick nerve trunks embedded with mature neurons (arrowhead).

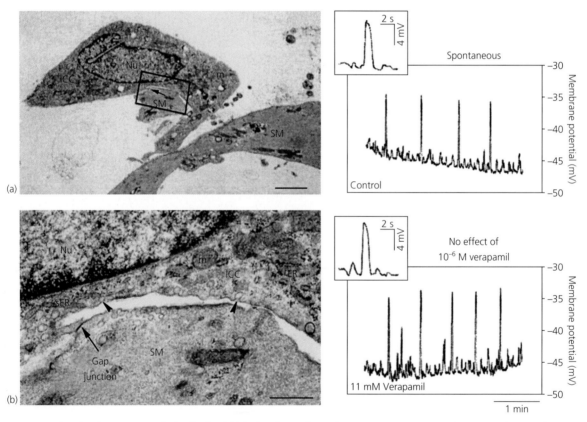

Figure 28.10 Gap junctions between interstitial cells of Cajal (ICCs) and smooth muscle cells; note spontaneous electrical oscillations of the resting membrane potential of ICCs **(a)** and lack of inhibition by the L-type calcium channel blocker, verapamil **(b)**. m, mitochondria; Nu, nucleus; RER, rough endoplasmic reticulum; SER, smooth endoplasmic reticulum; SM, smooth muscle.

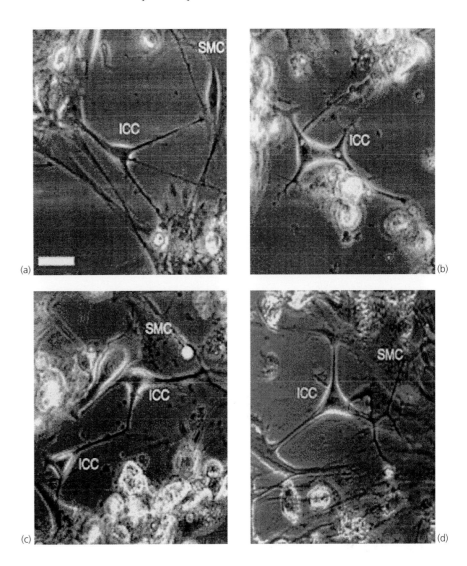

Figure 28.11 (a–d) In short-term culture, interstitial cells of Cajal (ICC) take a triangular shape, and have three to four branches that establish contact with cultured smooth muscle cells (SMC).

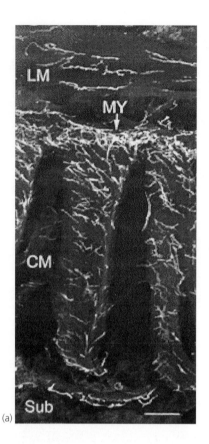

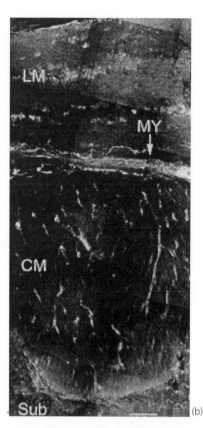

Figure 28.12 Distribution of interstitial cells of Cajal in whole transverse mounts of the sigmoid colon in a normal-appearing disease-control section of the sigmoid colon **(a)** and the sigmoid colon of a patient with slow-transit constipation **(c)**. CM, circular muscle; LM, longitudinal muscle; MY, myenteric plexus; Sub, submucosal plexus.

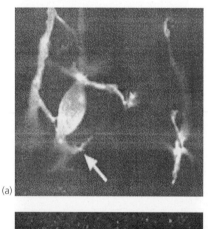

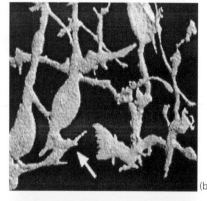

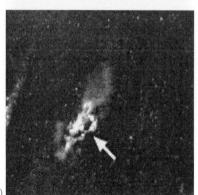

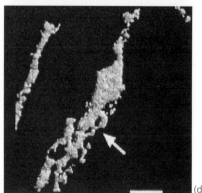

Figure 28.13 High-magnification confocal microscopy of the interstitial cells of Cajal (ICCs) from human sigmoid colon: **(a)** and **(c)** are single slices, **(b)** and **(d)** are reconstructions of 20 consecutive single slices, (a) and (b) are from healthy-appearing disease-control colons; note multiple fine processes and the network of interconnecting ICCs, and (c) and (d) are from a patient with slow-transit constipation. Note the irregular markings and loss of fine processes (bar = 10 µm).

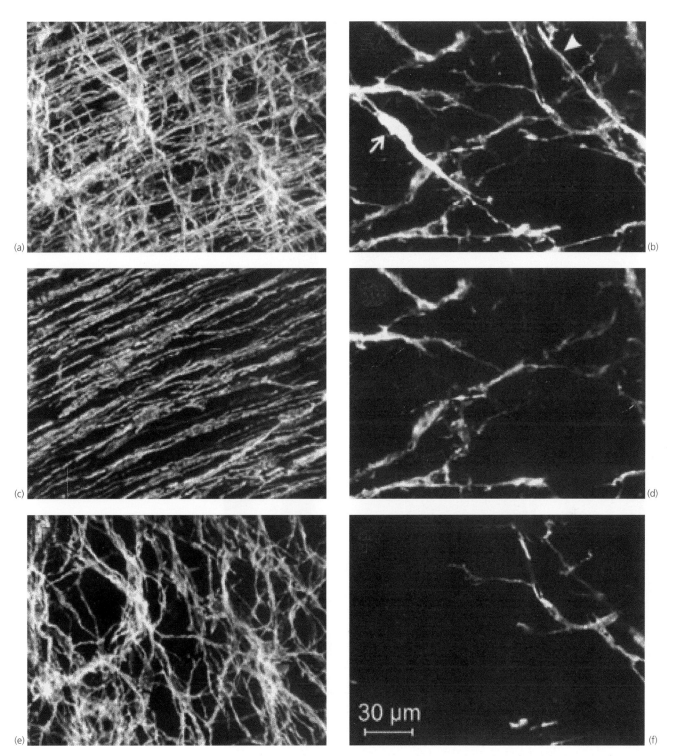

Figure 28.14 Effects of diabetes on gastric antral interstitial cells of Cajal (ICC) networks: Kit-like immunoreactivity in the proximal antrum of nondiabetic **(a, c, e)** and diabetic **(b, d, f)** mice. Confocal images representing the entire thickness of the tunica muscularis (a, b), the thickness of the circular muscle (c, d), and the myenteric region (e, f) are shown. Note the profound reduction in ICC number in the tunica muscularis of the diabetic animal. The arrow and arrowhead (b) indicate a cell body and process of an ICC, respectively. Scale bar applies to all panels.

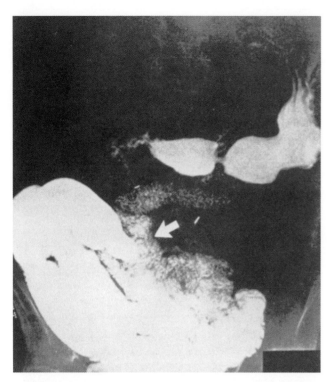

Figure 28.15 Small bowel radiograph from a patient with type I familial visceral neuropathy shows a normal stomach, duodenum, and proximal jejunum, but a dilated distal small bowel (arrow).

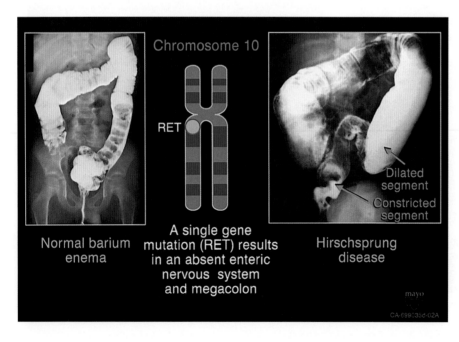

Figure 28.16 Barium enema in a normal child contrasted with megacolon and narrow segment of Hirschsprung disease.

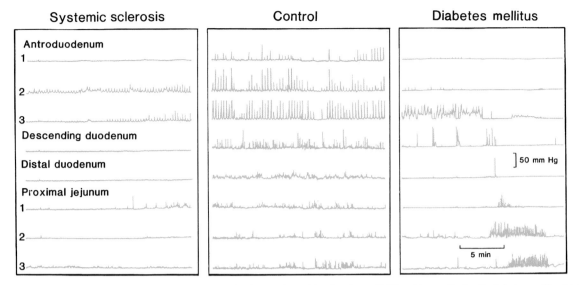

Figure 28.17 Altered postprandial intestinal manometric tracing in a patient with scleroderma **(left)** and in a patient with diabetes mellitus **(right)**. Note the low amplitude of contractions typical of a myopathic disorder in the **left panel**, and the normal amplitude but abnormal pattern typical of a neuropathic disorder in the **right panel**. The antral hypomotility, excessive pyloric tonic and phasic pressure activity, and the persistence of the migrating motor complex during the postprandial period are typical features of enteric nerve dysfunction.

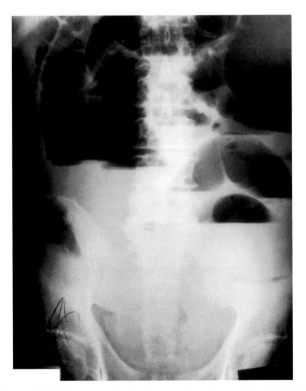

Figure 28.18 Plain abdominal radiograph of a patient with scleroderma and intestinal pseudoobstruction demonstrates dilated loops of small bowel with air–fluid levels.

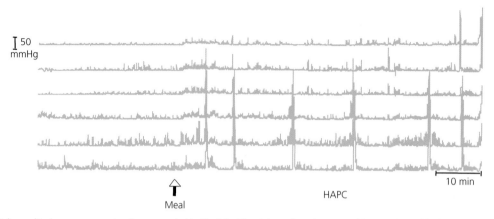

Figure 28.19 High-amplitude pressure contractions recorded in the left side of the colon after a meal in a patient with diarrhea caused by extrinsic neuropathy.

29

Bacterial, viral, and toxic causes of diarrhea, gastroenteritis, and anorectal infections

Gail A. Hecht, Jerrold R. Turner, Phillip I. Tarr

The spectrum of organisms that can infect and cause disease in the human colon includes bacteria, viruses, and protozoa. Reviewed in this chapter are the bacterial and viral pathogens of the large intestine. Although the symptoms associated with infection by enteric bacterial pathogens are essentially indistinguishable (including abdominal pain, diarrhea, and fever), the range of pathological appearances are somewhat more varied. For example, colonic biopsies of *Campylobacter* colitis often have features similar to those seen in inflammatory bowel disease, including crypt abscesses (Fig. 29.1), but typically lack changes associated with chronicity. Figures 29.2 and 29.3 portray the results of cholera infection and equipment used by patients to cope with the symptoms. Infection with enterohemorrhagic *Escherichia coli* (EHEC) typically induces histopathology that overlaps with ischemic colitis (Fig. 29.4). The colon can be quite severely affected, as demonstrated by contrast and computed tomography studies of affected children (Fig. 29.5), and of the colon at laparotomy because of severe abdominal pain (Fig. 29.6). Gastroenterologists need to be cognizant of the clinical progression of this infection, as patients can present at multiple different points during their illness, although it is most often the bloody diarrhea that prompts evaluation (Fig. 29.7). The histological features of colitis associated with enteroinvasive colitis and *Shigella* are typically identical (Fig. 29.8). This stems from the fact that the genes conferring the invasive phenotype are identical for these two pathogens. Despite these highlighted differences, colonic histology is usually not specific enough to conclusively determine the causative agent. The one exception to this statement is *Clostridium difficile*-associated pseudomembranous colitis. *C. dif-*

ficile holds the title of the number one cause of healthcare-associated diarrhea because hospitals and long-term care facilities serve as reservoirs, and establishment of infection in the colon by this spore-forming pathogen is dependent upon disruption of the resident colonic microflora by antibiotics (Fig. 29.9). Although the diagnosis of *C. difficile*-associated colitis is usually determined by assays that identify the presence of toxin A or B in the stool, the gross appearance of pseudomembranes seen at sigmoidoscopy, as are evident quite vividly following resection, (Fig. 29.10) and the characteristic histological volcano lesion (Fig. 29.11) are virtually pathognomonic for this infection. If a barium enema is performed, which is not recommended, then the presence of pseudomembranes may be demonstrated (Fig. 29.12).

Infections of the anus and rectum are most commonly seen in homosexual men and heterosexual women who engage in anoreceptive intercourse. Primary anorectal syphilis appears as a chancre of the squamous epithelial lining of the anal canal or rectum (Fig. 29.13). Condyloma lata represents the secondary phase of syphilis (Fig. 29.14). Biopsy of anorectal lesions from patients infected with *Treponema pallidum* may reveal spirochetes (Fig. 29.15). However, nonpathogenic spirochetes can also reside in the rectum, thus reducing the significance of this finding.

More commonly seen are condyloma acuminata (anal warts) caused by infection with human papillomavirus. These verrucous lesions are generally easy to differentiate from the flat, fleshy lesions of condyloma lata, but histology easily distinguishes between the two and is recommended to confirm the diagnosis (Fig. 29.16).

Atlas of Gastroenterology, 4th edition. Edited by Tadataka Yamada, David H. Alpers, Anthony N. Kalloo, Neil Kaplowitz, Chung Owyang, and Don W. Powell. © 2009 Blackwell Publishing, ISBN: 978-1-4051-6909-7

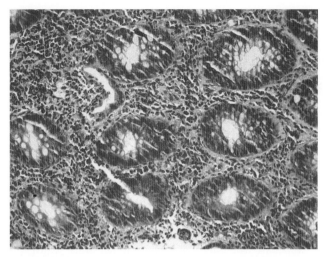

Figure 29.1 Photomicrograph of colonic mucosal biopsy from a patient with *Campylobacter jejuni* colitis. Note the presence of crypt abscesses, crypt destruction, and lamina propria infiltrates of neutrophils, eosinophils, and lymphocytes. These features can overlap with those present in inflammatory bowel disease. However, the uniform spacing and shape of the crypts, i.e., a lack of architectural distortion suggests that an alternative diagnosis, such as an infectious process, should be considered. Case courtesy of Dr Neal S. Goldstein, William Beaumont Hospital, Royal Oak, MI.

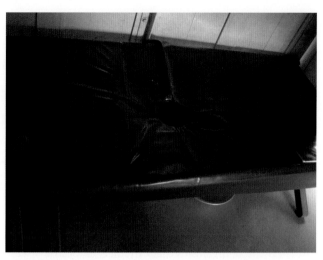

Figure 29.3 Cholera cot. Mattress covered with non-absorbable material to permit collection of high volume enteric effluent, as is produced during cholera infection. Photo courtesy of Matlab Hospital of the International Centre for Diarrhoeal Diseases Research, Bangladesh.

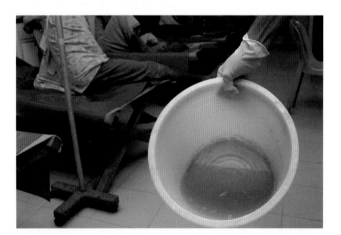

Figure 29.2 Classic rice water cholera stools. Liquid stool collected over one hour from an adult with *Vibrio cholerae*. In the five hours since this 54 kg man was admitted, he produced five liters of rice water stool. Photo courtesy of Matlab Hospital of the International Centre for Diarrhoeal Diseases Research, Bangladesh.

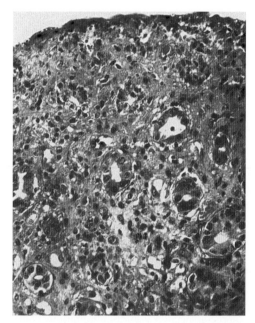

Figure 29.4 This colonic mucosal biopsy from a patient with *Escherichia coli* 0157:H7 colitis demonstrates superficial epithelial atrophy with crypt cell hyperplasia. These features overlap with those of ischemic colitis. Case courtesy of Dr Neal S. Goldstein, William Beaumont Hospital, Royal Oak, MI.

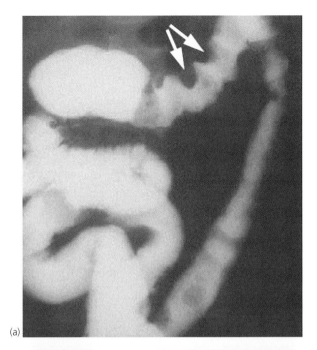

(a)

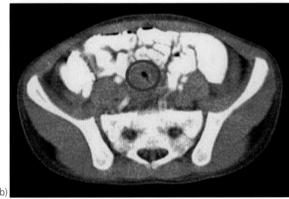

(b)

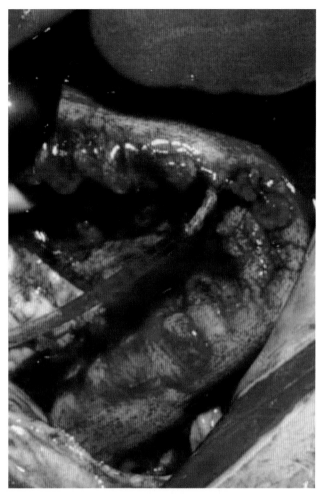

Figure 29.6 Colon of patient acutely infected with *Escherichia coli* O157:H7. Note marked hyperemia of serosal surface. Photograph courtesy of Dr David Tapper.

Figure 29.5 Radiographic features of *E coli* O157:H7 infection. **(a)** radiograph after barium enema with thumbprinting appearance of mucosa (arrows), suggesting colonic edema, in a patient who subsequently developed hemolytic-uremic syndrome (HUS). **(b)** CT of the pelvis of an eight-year-old boy on the eighth day of an *E. coli* O157:H7 infection. Note severely thickened colon (circled). This infection did not progress to HUS.

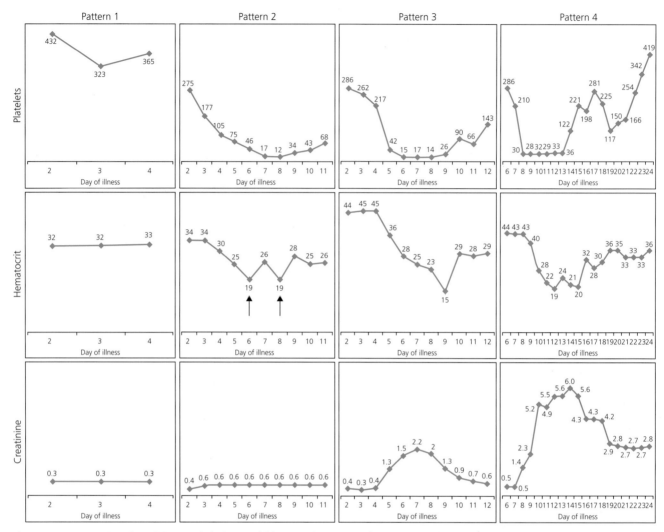

Figure 29.7 Progression of *E coli* O157:H7 infections in children. *E. coli* O157:H7 infections tend to follow a quite predictable pattern. We find that it is helpful to make clinical judgments based on stage of illness, in consideration of trends in laboratory tests.

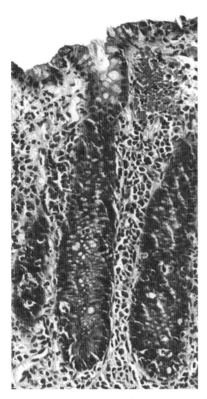

Figure 29.8 This colonic mucosal biopsy from a patient with enteroinvasive *Escherichia coli* colitis demonstrates pronounced infiltration of surface and crypt epithelium by neutrophils. The lamina propria also contains numerous neutrophils with admixed eosinophils and fewer lymphocytes and plasma cells. Some apoptotic epithelial cells can also be appreciated and can be present in even greater numbers in more severe cases. The clinical and pathological features can be indistinguishable from *Shigella* infection. The uniform spacing and shape of the crypts helps to exclude inflammatory bowel disease. Case courtesy Dr Neal S. Goldstein, William Beaumont Hospital, Royal Oak, MI.

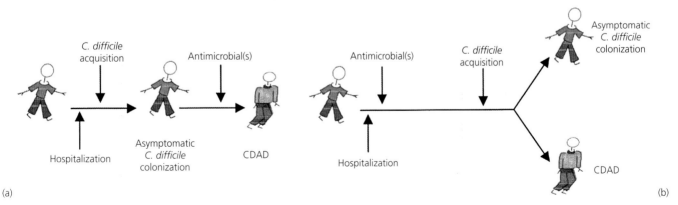

(a)

(b)

Figure 29.9 Hypotheses by which hospitalized patients acquire *Clostridium difficile* and the associated diarrhea. **(a)** depicts the initial hypothesis that hospitalized patients become colonized with *C. difficile* and upon exposure to antimicrobial agents develop the symptoms that typify this infection. More recently, a revised hypothesis has been put forth and is shown in **(b)**. In this case, the hospitalized patient may be exposed to *C. difficile* throughout the course of stay but is not susceptible to colonization until antibiotics are introduced. At that point, true acquisition of the organism occurs and host factors, such as the level of antibody production to the organism or its toxins, determines which patients will become colonized but remain asymptomatic and which will manifest the associated symptom of diarrhea. CDAD, *Clostridium difficile*-associated diarrhea.

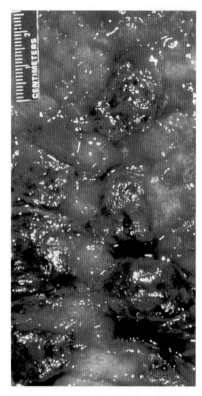

Figure 29.10 Gross appearance of *Clostridium difficile* pseudomembranous colitis. This photo shows the severe, nearly confluent, pale pseudomembranes that are typical of severe *C. difficile* pseudomembranous colitis. The pseudomembranes are composed of purulent debris and contrast sharply against the surrounding dark edematous mucosa.

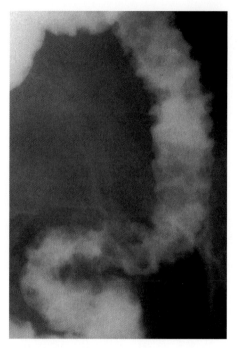

Figure 29.12 Radiograph of a barium enema performed on a patient with *Clostridium difficile*-induced pseudomembranous colitis. Note the presence of multiple filling defects within the colonic mucosa which represent pseudomembranes and mucosal edema.

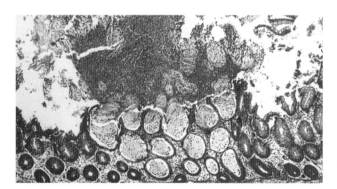

Figure 29.11 Histological appearance of *Clostridium difficile* pseudomembranous colitis. This photomicrograph shows a classic type II volcano-like eruption with a mushroom-shaped cloud of adherent inflammatory exudate.

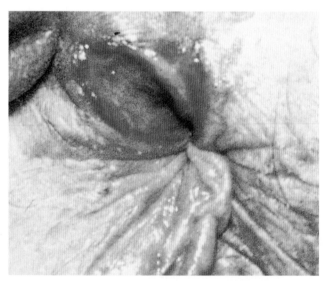

Figure 29.13 Primary syphilitic chancre of the anus. Such lesions occur in homosexual men and heterosexual women who engage in anoreceptive intercourse. Anorectal syphilitic chancres may be asymptomatic or painful, usually upon defecation.

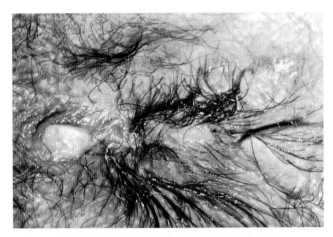

Figure 29.14 Condyloma lata of the anorectal area, shown here, represent the secondary stage of syphilis. Condyloma lata appear as smooth, moist, fleshy lesions which can secrete a discharge that is highly infectious. Condyloma lata are distinguishable from the verrucous anal warts or condyloma acuminata caused by infection with human papillomavirus.

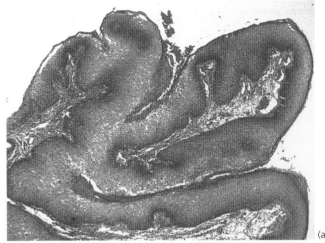

(a)

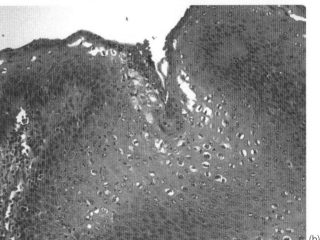

(b)

Figure 29.16 Condyloma acuminatum of the anal region. The low power view **(a)** shows the typical papillomatous growth pattern of this lesion. The higher magnification photomicrograph **(b)** demonstrates the typical vacuolization of koilocytotic human papillomavirus-infected squamous cells.

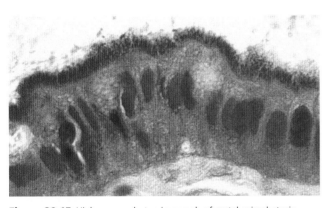

Figure 29.15 High-power photomicrograph of rectal spirochetosis showing the typical apical layer of spirochetes that stain dark blue on standard hematoxylin and eosin stain. The organisms are oriented parallel to the microvilli and, by electron microscopy, can be seen to interdigitate between the microvilli. Rectal spirochetes may represent *Treponema pallidum* or nonpathogenic organisms, diminishing the significance of such a finding.

30

Chronic infections of the small intestine

George T. Fantry, Lori E. Fantry, Stephen P. James, David H. Alpers

There are four chronic infections of the small intestine that occur in immunocompetent hosts: Whipple disease, tropical sprue, tuberculosis, and histoplasmosis. Other chronic infections of the small intestine are seen primarily among immunocompromised hosts and include mycotic infections such as aspergillosis, candidiasis, and mucormycosis, and *Mycobacterium avium* complex (MAC) occurring among patients with acquired immunodeficiency syndrome (AIDS). The last infection may mimic the histopathological findings of Whipple disease.

Whipple disease is a rare syndrome caused by infection with *Tropheryma whipplei*. The most important step in the evaluation of Whipple disease is to have a high degree of suspicion in the appropriate clinical setting. The challenge is to establish the correct diagnosis while avoiding the temptation to overdiagnose the disease. The diagnostic procedure of choice is endoscopic small intestine mucosal biopsy. The disease is usually diffuse but can be patchy; therefore, multiple (four to six) biopsy specimens should be obtained. The characteristic duodenal appearance consists of thickened mucosal folds coated with a yellow granular material or 1- to 2-mm yellow plaques that may be diffuse or patchy (Fig. 30.1).

The appearance with periodic acid–Schiff (PAS) staining often is sufficient to establish the diagnosis of Whipple disease for most patients (Figs 30.2–30.5); however, it can be confirmed with electron microscopic demonstration of the bacilli (Fig. 30.6). Occasional macrophages are found in the normal intestinal lamina propria. These macrophages usually stain faintly PAS positive, but the inclusions are not sickle shaped as in Whipple disease. There are three clinical entities in which the presence of numerous PAS-positive macrophages in the intestinal lamina propria may be misleading: AIDS with MAC infection, systemic histoplasmosis,

and macroglobulinemia. Macroglobulinemia can be differentiated from Whipple disease because of the faintly staining, homogeneously PAS-positive macrophages, and histoplasmosis can be differentiated by the large, PAS-positive, rounded, encapsulated *Histoplasma* organisms. More care must be taken in differentiating the histopathological findings in the intestinal mucosa of patients with Whipple disease from those in patients with AIDS and MAC infection. In MAC infection, the lamina propria is packed with macrophages containing MAC, which when stained with hematoxylin and eosin and PAS stain clearly resemble those seen in Whipple disease. However, MAC bacilli are acid fast, easily cultured, and have an electron microscopic appearance that is quite different from that of Whipple bacilli (Fig. 30.7). The diagnosis of MAC is easily established among persons with human immunodeficiency virus (HIV) infection. *T. whipplei* infection has not been reported among persons with HIV infection. Studies have suggested that the polymerase chain reaction may be a helpful confirmatory test for patients believed to have Whipple disease.

In very rare instances the diagnosis of Whipple disease has been established in the absence of intestinal involvement. In these cases the diagnosis was established with electron microscopic demonstration of bacilli in cerebrospinal fluid, brain biopsy specimens, or peripheral lymph nodes.

Considerable caution is required in the interpretation of gastric and rectal biopsy findings. PAS-positive macrophages frequently are present in the normal gastric and rectal mucosa, and in many diseases of the stomach and rectum. The stomach often contains faintly PAS-positive, lipid-containing macrophages (lipophages), whereas the rectal mucosa usually contains strongly PAS-positive muciphages and pigment-containing macrophages (Fig. 30.8). Electron microscopic demonstration of Whipple bacilli in these tissues usually is necessary to establish the diagnosis.

Barium studies of the small intestine usually are abnormal in Whipple disease and may reveal a characteristic but nonspecific finding of marked thickening of the mucosal folds (Fig. 30.9). These findings usually are more prominent in the duodenum and proximal jejunum and less prominent in the distal jejunum; the ileum is spared. In addition to marked thickening of the proximal small bowel, abdominal computed tomographic scanning often reveals marked mesenteric, paraaortic, and retroperitoneal adenopathy (Fig. 30.10).

Three specific chronic bacterial infections of the small intestine are caused by *Yersinia* (*Yersinia enterocolitica* and *Yersinia pseudotuberculosis*), *Mycobacterium tuberculosis*, and *Histoplasma capsulatum*. *Yersinia* penetrates the lamina propria and causes submucosal thickening that can mimic Crohn's disease (Fig. 30.11). Histologically, there are massively enlarged lymphoid follicles with prominent germinal centers (Fig. 30.12).

Intestinal tuberculosis is most common in patients with active pulmonary disease and is caused by swallowed organisms that cross the mucosa of the bowel segments rich in lymphoid tissue, i.e., the ileum and cecum. Figure 30.13 shows tuberculosis in the ileocecal region, where nearly all gastrointestinal infections occur. The tissue response can be either hypertrophic (Fig. 30.13b), ulcerative (Fig. 30.13c), or a combination of both. When tuberculosis becomes disseminated (miliary tuberculosis), tubercles are found on the serosal surface of the bowel (Fig. 30.14).

Histoplasmosis is originally a pulmonary infection that most often becomes generalized, as in immunocompromised patients. The causative organism can affect both the small or large intestine and the liver, although symptoms are most often attributed to small bowel disease (crampy abdominal pain, diarrhea, anemia, malabsorption). Figure 30.15a shows nodular ulcerated lesions. This ulceration is accompanied by intense mononuclear cell infiltration, possibly with granuloma formation (Fig. 30.15b), in those patients who are immunocompetent enough to mount a response. Oval yeast forms of 2–3 μm may be visualized in macrophages (Fig. 30.16).

Aspergillosis affects only severely immunocompromised patients, including those with AIDS, those undergoing organ transplantation or immunosuppressive chemotherapy, and premature infants. The small intestine is involved in about 5% of patients with disseminated aspergillosis. *Aspergillus* grows by branching and longitudinal extension of wide (2-5 μm) Y-shaped, branching, septate hyphae. Clinical disease is produced by vascular invasion and necrosis (Fig. 30.17).

Candida species are the fourth most common organisms isolated from the blood of hospitalized patients and are normal colonizers of the gastrointestinal tract. These organisms are commonly associated with esophageal disease in immunocompromised patients but rarely cause disease of the small intestine. Persons at highest risk include those with AIDS, chronic mucocutaneous candidiasis, or malignancies, and those taking immunosuppressive agents. The most common lesions associated with *Candida* are single or multiple ulcerations. Because *Candida* is a normal colonizer of the entire gastrointestinal tract, diagnosis requires biopsy evidence of invasion (Fig. 30.18).

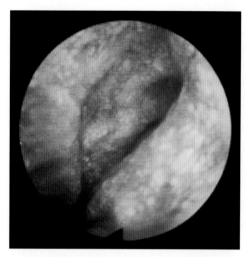

Figure 30.1 Characteristic duodenoscopic appearance of the duodenum of an untreated patient with Whipple disease. The folds are thickened and are covered with small yellowish-white plaques. This endoscopic appearance may be the first clue to the diagnosis.

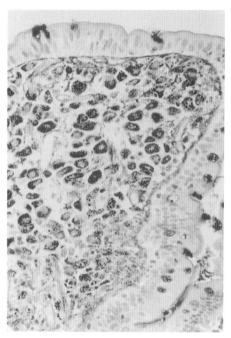

Figure 30.3 Periodic acid–Schiff and hematoxylin stain of the same villus as in Figure 30.2 shows prominence of the macrophages with this stain (original magnification ×200). Courtesy of Dr John E. Stone.

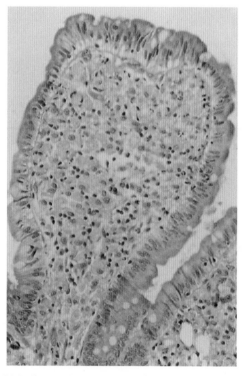

Figure 30.2 Characteristic appearance of a hematoxylin and eosin-stained intestinal villus in Whipple disease. The macrophages, although abundant throughout the lamina propria, are rather inapparent (original magnification ×200). Courtesy of Dr John E. Stone.

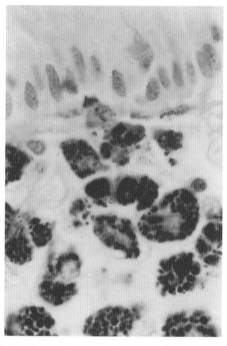

Figure 30.4 High-magnification (original magnification ×1000) photograph of macrophages stained with periodic acid–Schiff in the intestinal mucosa in Whipple disease. Note the characteristic rounded and sickle-shaped inclusions in the macrophages. This appearance alone is highly suggestive of the diagnosis.

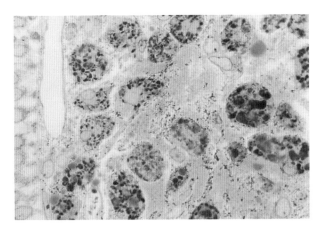

Figure 30.5 High-magnification (original magnification ×750) photograph of a toluidine blue-stained section of a plastic-embedded specimen of intestinal mucosa in Whipple disease. Characteristic macrophage inclusions and numerous extracellular bacilli are present throughout the lamina propria.

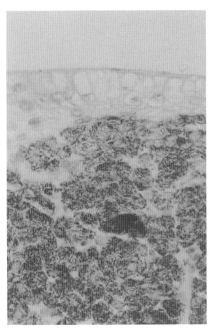

Figure 30.7 High-magnification (original magnification ×1000) photograph of an acid-fast stained intestinal villus in *Mycobacterium avium* complex infection in acquired immunodeficiency syndrome. Exclusively intracellular, very large bacilli are present. Whipple bacilli are much smaller, largely extracellular, and not acid fast. Courtesy of Dr Wilfred M. Weinstein.

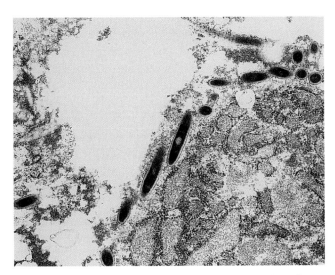

Figure 30.6 Electron micrograph of a duodenal biopsy specimen from a patient with Whipple disease shows the cytoplasm of a macrophage, with positive results at periodic acid–Schiff staining, and its surrounding extracellular space. Note the numerous bacilli with characteristic cell walls and pale central nuclei just outside the macrophage.

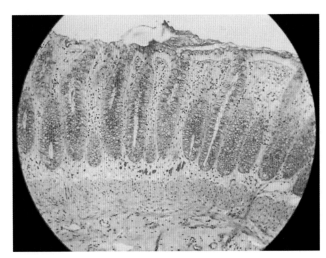

Figure 30.8 Periodic acid–Schiff and hematoxylin stain of a rectal biopsy specimen from a healthy person. Prominent macrophages are just below the crypts and above the muscularis mucosae. This finding is a frequent cause of confusion; however, the rectum and colon are very rarely involved in Whipple disease (original magnification ×100).

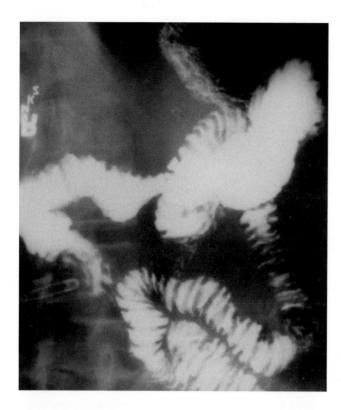

Figure 30.9 Radiograph shows coarsened folds in the duodenum and jejunum of an untreated patient with Whipple disease. Courtesy of Dr John E. Stone.

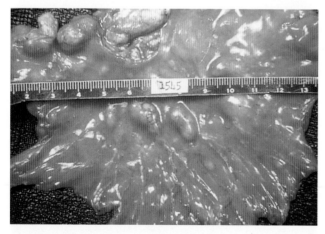

Figure 30.10 Autopsy image of the mesentery and nodes of a patient with Whipple disease shows marked thickening of the mesentery and a striking degree of adenopathy.

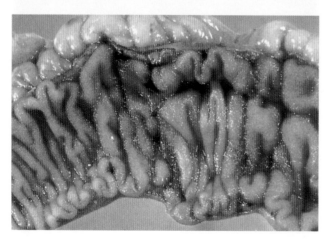

Figure 30.11 *Yersinia*. Gross appearance in a patient with culture-proven *Yersinia* infection. The mucosal folds are unduly prominent because of the granulomatous inflammation that extends into the submucosa.

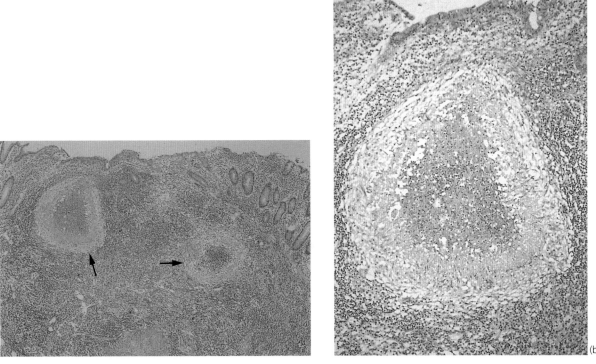

(a)

(b)

Figure 30.12 *Yersinia* enterocolitis. **(a)** and **(b)** demonstrate the presence of the prominent necrotizing granulomas that characterize *Yersinia* when it presents in a typical fashion. Two granulomas (arrows) are shown in (a). The overlying epithelium appears atrophic and ulcerated. (b) Higher magnification showing palisading histiocytes without foreign body giant cells. The entire granuloma is surrounded by a prominent cuff of lymphocytes.

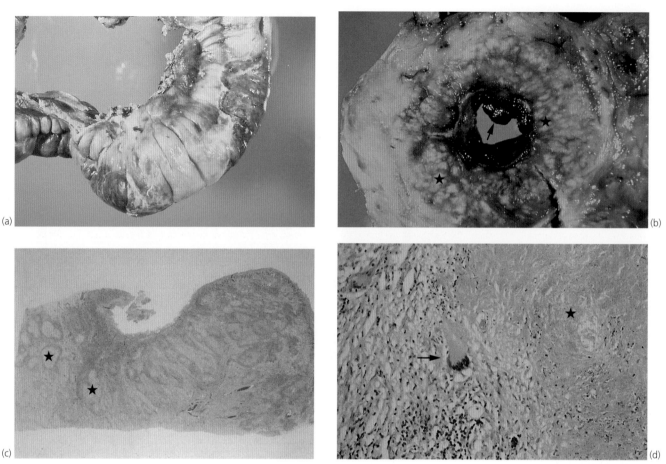

Figure 30.13 Ileocecal tuberculosis. **(a)** Gross photograph of the resection specimen demonstrating the presence of an ileocolectomy with transmural inflammation. It is difficult to delineate the exact ileocecal valve area. The serosal tissues are markedly congested and edematous and show fibrinous adhesions. **(b)** Cross-section through the specimen demonstrating transmural necrosis and replacement of the intestinal wall by numerous granulomas, several of which are indicated by stars. The intestinal lumen is severely compromised and narrowed. A hypertrophic lesion protrudes into the lumen (arrow). **(c)** Low-magnification photograph of the wall demonstrating the presence of the granulomas, some of which are indicated by stars. Granulomas appear centrally pale and are surrounded by a bluer rim. **(d)** Higher magnification photograph showing a portion of a granuloma with central caseous necrosis (star) and a surrounding giant cell (arrow).

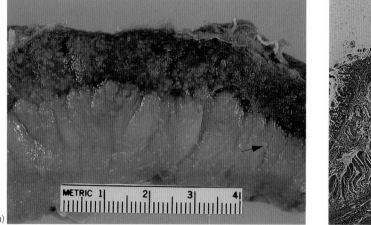

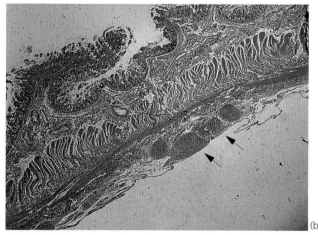

Figure 30.14 Miliary tuberculosis. Gross and microscopic features of miliary tuberculosis. **(a)** Gross resection specimen demonstrates numerous whitish nodules on the mucosal surface representing tubercles within the Peyer patches. The fat in the surrounding bowel also demonstrates large numbers of 1- to 2-mm whitish nodules, one of which is indicated by an arrow. Fine adhesions are also seen. **(b)** Histological section through several of the serosal tubercles (arrows). Mucosal and submucosal tubercles are not seen in this photograph.

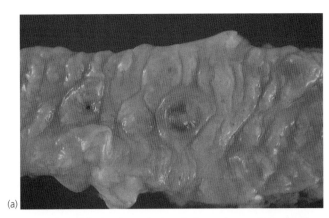

(a)

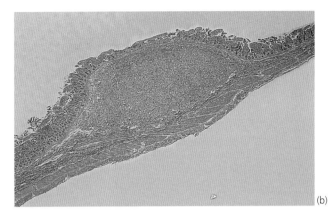

(b)

Figure 30.15 **(a)** Histoplasmosis. Intestinal resection specimen showing nodular ulcerated lesions located diffusely throughout the bowel wall, obliterating the normal mucosal fold pattern. **(b)** Histological section of the lesion shown in (a) indicating the presence of a submucosal granuloma.

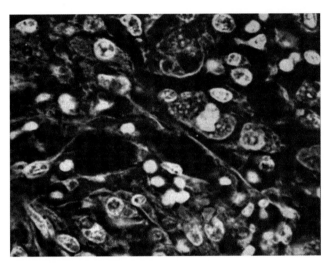

Figure 30.16 Light microscopic appearance of oval yeast forms of *Histoplasma capsulatum* within macrophages from a patient with disseminated histoplasmosis. High-power magnification.

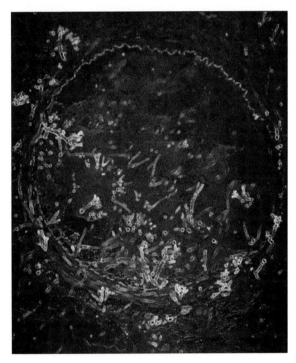

Figure 30.17 Light microscopic appearance of *Aspergillus* organisms showing vascular invasion.

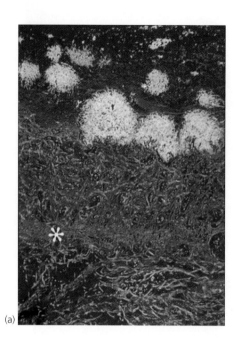

(a)

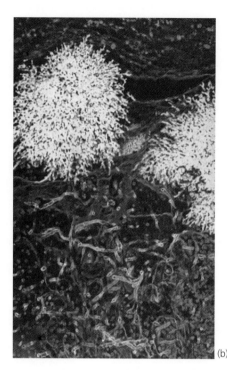

(b)

Figure 30.18 Light microscopic appearance of *Candida* organisms on the surface of infarcted bowel mucosa with *Aspergillus* hyphae in the underlying mucosa and submucosa. **(a)** Low magnification; **(b)** high magnification (Grocott–Gomori methenamine–silver stain).

31

Celiac disease

Peter H.R. Green, Anne R. Lee

Gluten and grains

Gluten is often used as the generic term for the storage protein in wheat, rye, and barley. The protein is found in the endosperm portion of the grain that is commonly used for flours and cereals (Fig. 31.1).

Definitions:

- Endosperm: The germ's food supply which, if the grain was allowed to grow, would provide essential energy to the young plant. As the largest portion of the kernel, the endosperm contains starchy carbohydrates, proteins, and small amounts of vitamins and minerals.
- Germ: The embryo, which, if fertilized by pollen, will sprout into a new plant. It contains B vitamins, vitamin E, antioxidants, phytonutrients, and unsaturated fats.
- Bran: The multilayered outer skin of the kernel that helps to protect the other two parts of the kernel from sunlight, pests, water, and disease. It contains important antioxidants, iron, zinc, copper, magnesium, B vitamins, fiber, and phytonutrients.

The taxonomy of the grasses (Family – Gramineae) is shown in Figure 31.2. One can see in the species of grains toxic to those with celiac disease (wheat, rye, and barley) that they have a close genetic relationship: all are members of the tribe Triticeae.

Oats are considered safe for most people with celiac disease, although the rare patient reacts with a celiac type lesion. Oats are a questionable grain for those with celiac disease because of the frequent cross contamination from wheat during the harvesting, milling, and processing. There are several companies that are beginning to grow, process, and mill uncontaminated oats.

Nutritional adequacy of the gluten-free diet

Table 31.1 outlines the fundamentals of a gluten-free diet and Table 31.2 outlines the gluten-free starch alternatives.

Atlas of Gastroenterology, 4th edition. Edited by Tadataka Yamada, David H. Alpers, Anthony N. Kalloo, Neil Kaplowitz, Chung Owyang, and Don W. Powell. © 2009 Blackwell Publishing, ISBN: 978-1-4051-6909-7

The grains that are the traditional cornerstone of the gluten-free diet – rice, corn, and potato – do not provide adequate amounts of nutrients [6]. As a result, patients are often vitamin deficient after about 10 years on the diet. This is partly accounted for by the fact that special dietary products are not required to be fortified or enriched as are their wheat-based counterparts. Grains such as quinoa, buckwheat, and millet (safe grains), however, provide texture, fiber, iron, B complex vitamins, and many minerals to gluten-free diets.

Clinical manifestations of celiac disease

There have been a decreasing number of patients presenting with diarrhea, or the classical presentation, over successive time periods. Figure 31.3 shows the number of individuals in each time period seen in a University Celiac Center since 1981.

The distribution of the major presentations is shown in Figure 31.4. This figure shows the distribution of modes of presentations of a group of patients diagnosed after the more frequent use of serological tests. Less than 50% of patients presented with diarrhea. Screening was the next most frequent mode of presentation, the screened groups were family members of individuals with celiac disease together with type I diabetics as well as Down syndrome. Incidental recognition at endoscopy refers to those who underwent endoscopy for a reason other than diarrhea, anemia, or the search for celiac disease.

Dermatitis herpetiformis

Dermatitis herpetiformis occurs in about 10% of those with celiac disease, and may be the only manifestation. Intensely itchy, usually blistering lesions can appear anywhere on the body (Figs 31.5 and 31.6). They are, however, frequently localized to the elbows, knees, buttocks, and scalp. The lesions may be symmetrical and tend to recur in the same location for any individual patient. The diagnosis is confirmed by the finding of granular deposits of immunoglobulin A (IgA) seen in the dermal papillae on direct immunofluorescence of biopsies taken about a millimeter from a lesion. Although dapsone given orally in a dosage of 50–100 mg once or twice daily may control outbreaks, the treatment is a gluten-free diet. Some patients are extremely sensitive to small amounts of ingested gluten. The lesions are considered to be caused by the reaction of antitissue transglutaminase antibodies generated in the intestine that react with tissue transglutaminase 3, present in skin.

Aphthous stomatitis

Aphthous stomatitis occurs more commonly in those with celiac disease compared with control populations. In addition they may be very gluten sensitive, responding to gluten withdrawal (Fig. 31.7).

Dental enamel defects

Dental enamel defects are imperfections in the enamel of the teeth. They are developmental and therefore symmetrical. They are a reflection on the health of a child, because adult enamel is formed by the age of 7 years. They occur more commonly in celiac disease (Fig. 31.8).

Endoscopic appearance of the duodenum in celiac disease

Typical appearances include reduced or absent folds and fissures (Fig. 31.9), scalloping and fissures (Figs 31.10 and 31.11), and nodularity (Fig. 31.12). Figures 31.12 and 31.13 show mucosal changes highlighted by the use of chromoendoscopy (indigo carmine). In Figure 31.13 the patchy nature of the villous atrophy is apparent. The endoscopic abnormalities are specific, but not sensitive for the detection of villous atrophy. If villous atrophy is suspected, biopsies should always be taken as celiac disease/villous atrophy occurs when the endoscopic appearance is entirely normal.

Pathological spectrum of celiac disease

Marsh initially created the concept of a spectrum of pathological changes in celiac disease (Figs 3.14, 3.15). Each grade may worsen or improve. It is difficult to diagnose celiac disease in the setting of a Marsh I lesion as there are many causes, including tropical sprue and *Helicobacter pylori*. Marsh II involves the presence of crypt hyperplasia with increased intraepithelial lymphocytosisn (Fig. 3.16). Marsh III includes

villous atrophy: IIIa partial villous atrophy, IIIb subtotal villous atrophy, IIIc total villous atrophy. Marsh IV is a less commonly encountered atrophic lesion. This is considered irreversible.

Marsh III lesions are shown in Figures 31.17–31.19, representing partial villous atrophy, subtotal villous atrophy and total villous atrophy. The pathological changes described are not specific for celiac disease.

Refractory celiac disease

Refractory celiac disease is considered to exist when an individual has persistent symptoms and villous atrophy, both without another apparent cause, despite at least 6 months of a strict gluten-free diet. Patients undergo extensive evaluation in order to exclude treatable causes of symptoms that include pancreatic insufficiency, bacterial overgrowth, and lymphoma. Persistent gluten ingestion is the most common cause; therefore, strict dietary counseling is imperative.

Patients are classified as having type I or type II refractory celiac disease, based on the characteristics of the intraepithelial lymphocytes. Normal intraepithelial lymphocytes have a normal complement of surface markers, including CD3$^+$, CD8$^+$. In the setting of active celiac disease or ongoing gluten ingestion the intraepithelial lymphocytes are normal (CD3$^+$, CD8$^+$). In addition, most patients with refractory disease have normal intraepithelial lymphocytes, CD3$^+$, CD8$^+$. When this finding is present, the patient is classified as having type I refractory celiac disease. This group is obviously difficult to distinguish from ongoing gluten ingestion. The antibodies may well be positive if there is gluten ingestion.

In type II refractory celiac disease the intraepithelial lymphocytes fail to express surface markers, although CD3 is present in the cell. Immunohistochemistry staining of the lymphocytes reveals the intraepithelial lymphocytes that stain for CD3, but not CD8 (CD3$^+$, CD8$^-$). In addition, the cells are clonally expanded. Refractory type II has a poor prognosis, with frequent progression to lymphoma. Figure 31.20 shows tissue from a patient with refractory celiac disease type II.

Table 31.1 Fundamentals of the gluten-free diet

Safe grains	Toxic grains
Amaranth	Wheat (includes spelt, kamut, semolina, triticale)
Millet	Rye
Quinoa	Barley (including malt)
Corn	
Sorghum	
Teff	
Oats	
Buckwheat	

Table 31.2 Gluten-free starch alternatives (flours used as a substitute for wheat flour)

Cereal grains (seeds of cultivated grasses): amaranth, buckwheat, corn (polenta), millet; quinoa, sorghum, teff; rice (white, brown, wild, basmati, jasmine); montina (Indian rice grass)

Tubers (swollen underground plant stem): arrowroot, jicama, taro; potato; white, sweet; tapioca (cassava, manioc, yucca)

Legumes (edible seeds from a pod): Beans including chickpea, lentil, kidney, navy, peas, soybean

Nuts (edible kernel of a hard shell): almonds, walnuts, chestnuts, hazelnuts, peanuts, cashews

Seeds: sunflower, flax, pumpkin

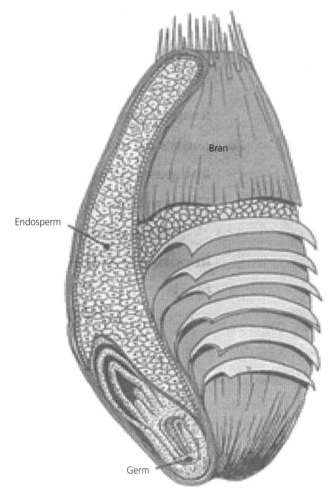

Figure 31.1 A whole kernel of wheat.

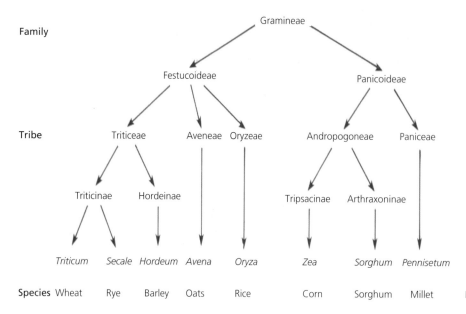

Figure 31.2 Taxonomy of the grasses.

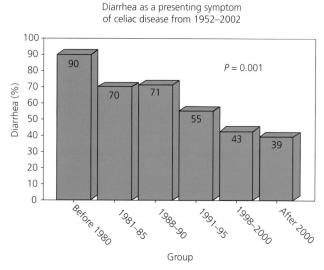

Figure 31.3 Percentage of patients presenting with diarrhea.

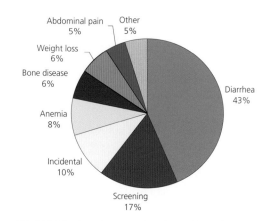

Figure 31.4 Distribution of presentations in a cohort of patients diagnosed after 1993.

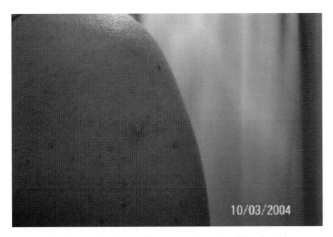

Figure 31.5 Dermatitis herpetiformis on the back of the shoulder.

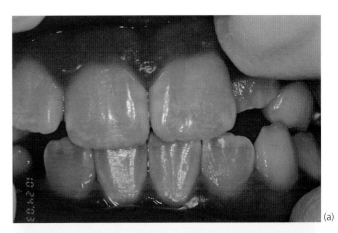

(a)

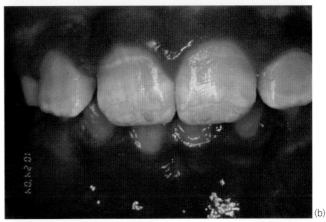

(b)

Figure 31.8 (a,b) Dental enamel defects.

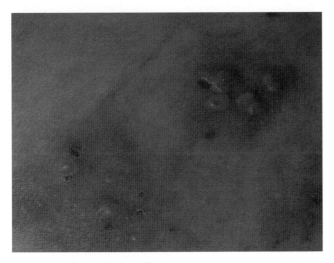

Figure 31.6 Dermatitis herpetiformis.

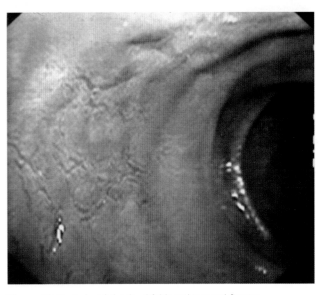

Figure 31.9 Reduced duodenal folds and mucosal fissures.

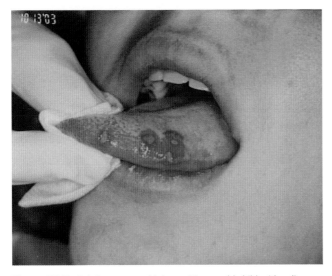

Figure 31.7 Aphthous stomatitis in an 11-year-old child with celiac disease.

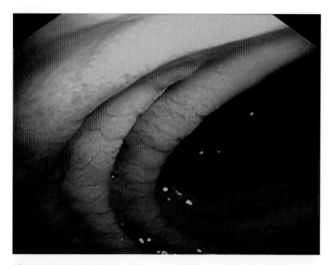

Figure 31.10 Scalloping and mucosal folds.

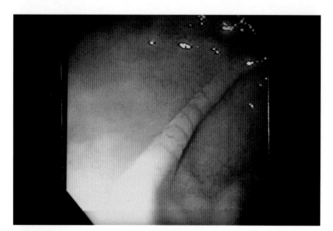

Figure 31.11 Scalloping of a duodenal fold.

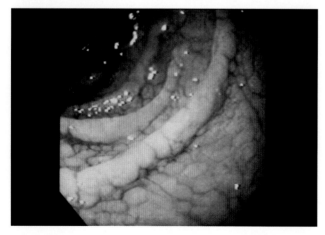

Figure 31.12 Nodularity of the duodenal mucosa. Appearance enhanced by the use of chromoendoscopy.

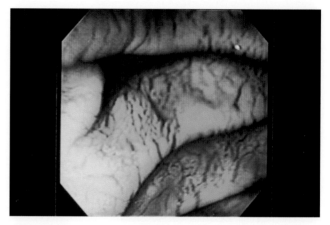

Figure 31.13 Patchy duodenal villous atrophy. Appearance enhanced by the use of chromoendoscopy.

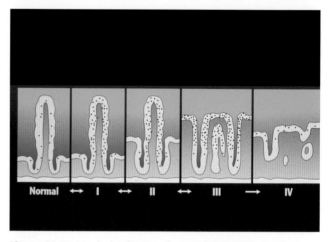

Figure 31.14 Marsh classification of mucosal abnormality in celiac disease. March 0 is normal with a crypt–villous ratio of 1:4. Marsh I consists of normal crypt/villous architecture together with an intraepithelial lymphocytosis (>20 lymphocytes per 100 epithelial cells). Marsh II has, in addition to an intraepithelial lymphocytosis, crypt hyperplasia. Marsh III lesions include villous atrophy together with crypt hyperplasia and an intraepithelial lymphocytosis. Marsh IV is a less commonly encountered lesion and can be irreversible.

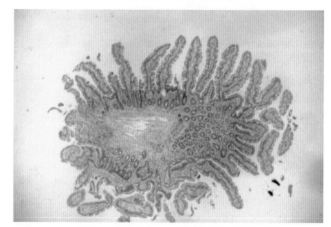

Figure 31.15 Normal duodenal biopsy. Long finger-like villi, no crypt hyperplasia, nor intraepithelial lymphocytosis. This is a Marsh 0 (normal) grade for an individual who had, or will develop celiac disease, the so-called latent celiac disease.

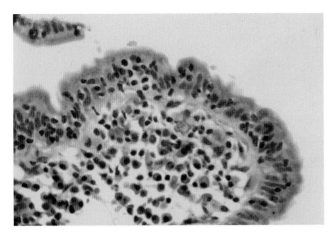

Figure 31.16 Epithelial changes in celiac disease. Intraepithelial lymphocytosis is demonstrated, present when there are greater than 25 lymphocytes per 100 epithelial cells. All celiac lesions, or Marsh types, will have an intraepithelial lymphocytosis. Also noted are distorted and abnormal epithelial cells.

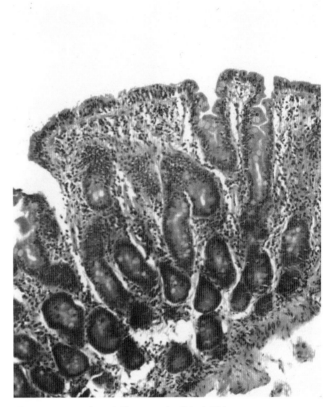

Figure 31.18 Subtotal villous atrophy (Marsh IIIb).

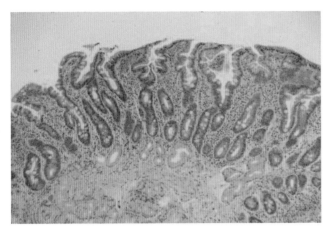

Figure 31.17 Partial villous atrophy (Marsh IIIa).

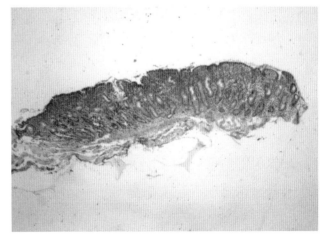

Figure 31.19 Total villous atrophy (Marsh IIIc).

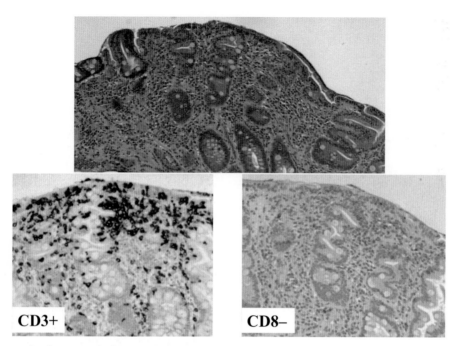

Figure 31.20 Refractory celiac disease. Total villous atrophy **(upper panel)** is shown, while immunohistological staining **(lower panels)** reveals the intraepithelial lymphocytes to be CD3+, CD8–.

32

Disorders of epithelial transport in the small intestine

Richard J. Grand, Mark L. Lloyd, Ward A. Olsen

Most inherited disorders of proteins involved in nutrient transport in the small intestine are rare. Two exceptions are lactase deficiency and cystic fibrosis. Lactase deficiency is normal among mammals and most humans after weaning from breastfeeding and is not, strictly speaking, a disease. Enzyme activities are regulated at the level of lactase mRNA transcription. However, the symptoms that arise from carbohydrate malabsorption must be differentiated from those caused by other intestinal disorders. The simplest screening test to identify lactose intolerance is withdrawal of dietary milk products. Should this maneuver produce confusing results, the next screening test can be breath hydrogen greater than 10 ppm over baseline after ingestion of a lactose load (Fig. 32.1).

Cystic fibrosis is the most commonly occurring lethal genetic disorder in the western continents. With modern treatment programs, more children are surviving to early adulthood and are experiencing symptoms involving extrapulmonary organs, including the intestine. Intestinal symptoms are caused by the presence of thick mucus produced by altered chloride secretion (Fig. 32.2) with prominent goblet cells and luminal retention of mucus (Fig. 32.3). These pathophysiological changes produce intestinal pseudoobstruction (Figs. 32.4 and 32.5) or actual mechanical obstructions. Colonic mucosa also shows the effects of abnormal mucus production (Fig. 32.6).

Much less common conditions include abetalipoproteinemia (Fig. 32.7) and sucrase-isomaltase deficiency. Of all the disorders of congenital carbohydrate absorption, the altered cellular events associated with sucrase-isomaltase deficiency have been best characterized. Studies have suggested that this condition may arise as a result of several different biosynthetic defects (Table 32.1).

The symptoms are characteristic of carbohydrate malabsorption. A presumptive diagnosis of sucrase deficiency can be made after a clinical response to sucrose exclusion from the diet. The diagnosis can be confirmed by means of breath hydrogen testing after administration of 2 g/kg body weight (maximum 25 g) oral sucrose (Fig. 32.8), or by means of mucosal disaccharidase assays that show low sucrase activity in biopsy specimens with normal mucosal histological features. Some patients with this condition lack any isomaltase activity. The associated decreased maltase activity is attributable to the fact that sucrase-isomaltase accounts for a substantial amount of normal maltose hydrolysis.

Two out of eight patients with sucrase-isomaltase deficiency in the series reported by Naim and colleagues (Naim HY, Roth J, Sterchi EE, et al. Sucrase–isomaltase deficiency in humans: different mutations disrupt intracellular transport, processing and function of an intestinal brush border enzyme. J Clin Invest 1988;82:667) showed exclusive synthesis of the high-mannose precursor and demonstrated accumulation of the protein in the Golgi apparatus at immunoelectron microscopic examination (Table 32.1). Other subjects had immunoreactive sucrase-isomaltase of a size that suggested that trimming reactions associated with the endoplasmic reticulum had failed to occur. A set of twins had identifiable sucrase-isomaltase in the brush border membrane that was catalytically inactive. These studies suggest that mutations leading to small changes in the primary structure of the sucrase-isomaltase gene product can have profound influences on the processing, intracellular transport, and function of the molecule. To date, no studies that have incorporated the technique of metabolic labeling have demonstrated complete absence of identifiable sucrase-isomaltase in this condition.

Atlas of Gastroenterology, 4th edition. Edited by Tadataka Yamada, David H. Alpers, Anthony N. Kalloo, Neil Kaplowitz, Chung Owyang, and Don W. Powell. © 2009 Blackwell Publishing, ISBN: 978-1-4051-6909-7

Table 32.1 Types of sucrase-isomaltase deficiency

	Type I	Type II	Type III
Forms of sucrase–isomaltase detected	High mannose (M_r = 212,000) +/– complex (M_r = 245 000) in reduced amounts	High mannose (M_r = 210 000) Sucrase (M_r = 45 000)	High mannose (M_r = 210 000) Complex (M_r = 245 000) Isomaltase (M_r = 151 000)
Immunolocalization defect	Not studied Incomplete trimming reaction in endoplasmic reticulum	Golgi Transport arrested in Golgi apparatus	Brush border Sucrase enzymatic active site altered

M_r, relative molecular mass.
Adapted from Naim HY, Roth J, Sterchi EE, et al. Sucrase-isomaltase deficiency in humans: different mutations disrupt intracellular transport, processing and function of an intestinal brush border enzyme. J Clin Invest 1988;82:667.

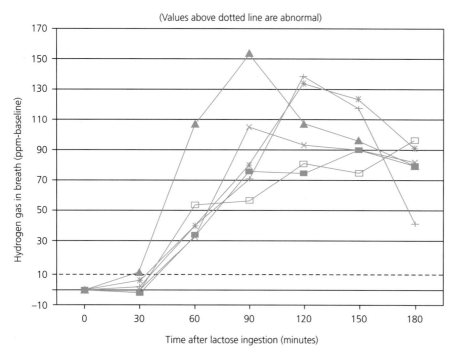

(Values above dotted line are abnormal)

Figure 32.1 Lactose breath hydrogen tests in four persons with lactose intolerance. Values above the dotted line are abnormal. After an overnight fast, a basal breath sample is obtained, and lactose (2 g/kg body weight) is administered in water. Breath is sampled every 30 min for 3 h and analyzed for hydrogen content in a dedicated gas chromatograph (in this study, a Quinton instrument [Quinton Instruments, Bothell, WA] was used). The peak in breath hydrogen occurs between 90 and 120 min in the subjects and remarkably similar curves are seen for all four subjects. It is customary to obtain a concomitant symptom chart to correlate breath hydrogen excretion with subjective symptoms.

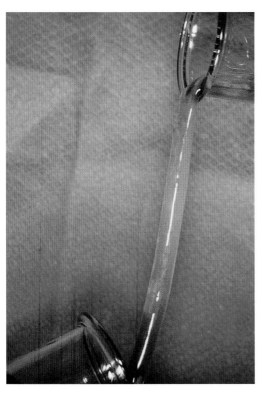

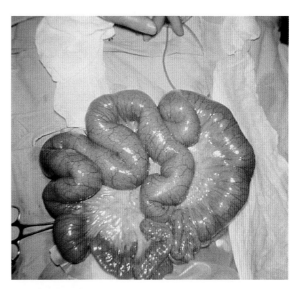

Figure 32.4 Photograph obtained at operation shows distal intestine of an adolescent patient with cystic fibrosis and distal intestinal obstruction. Terminal ileum is enlarged with impacted retained mucoid material, which failed to pass with nonoperative therapy. When surgical intervention is necessary, it is often sufficient to milk the retained intestinal contents distally. It is usually unnecessary to perform enterotomy or resection.

Figure 32.2 Duodenal mucus from a patient with cystic fibrosis obtained by means of intraduodenal intubation. Extremely viscid mucus retains its elastic properties even when poured from flask to flask.

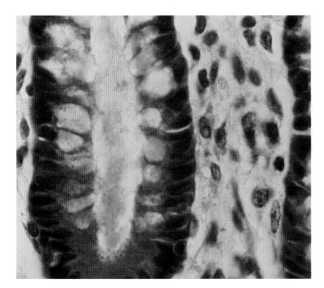

Figure 32.3 Ileal biopsy specimen from a patient with cystic fibrosis at operation for distal intestinal obstruction syndrome (periodic acid–Schiff stain). Prominent and enlarged goblet cells and retained mucus are present in the crypt lumen. This appearance is virtually pathognomonic of cystic fibrosis.

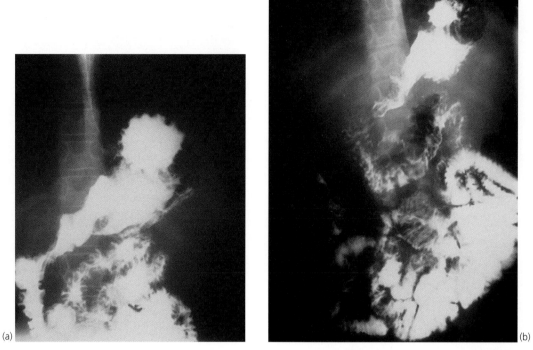

(a)

(b)

Figure 32.5 Upper gastrointestinal barium series with small bowel follow-through shows a 9-year-old patient with newly diagnosed cystic fibrosis. **(a)** The gastric and duodenal mucosa are nodular, thickened, and irregular. **(b)** The small intestine has a thickened, irregular mucosa with scattered nodularity.

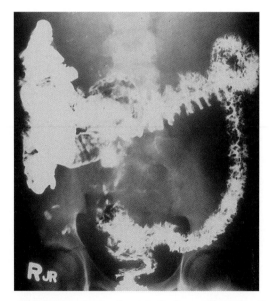

Figure 32.6 Barium enema radiograph of a 9-year-old patient with newly diagnosed cystic fibrosis. Spiculations, thickening, and irregularity of the mucosa are depicted. The nodularity is readily visible.

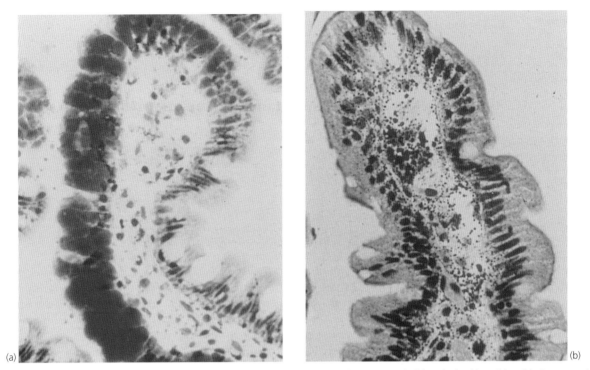

(a) (b)

Figure 32.7 Small intestine biopsy specimens after lipid feeding of a patient with abetalipoproteinemia **(a)** and a healthy subject **(b)**. Frozen sections were stained with Oil red O. Among patients with abetalipoproteinemia, lipid cannot be transported out of the enterocyte, and it accumulates intracellularly in large droplets, stained red here. Among healthy persons, lipid is transported into the lymphatic vessels, where it exists in small droplets.

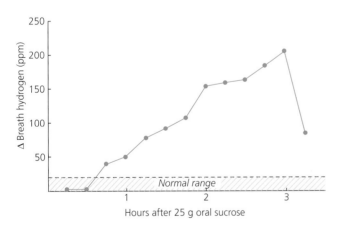

Figure 32.8 Breath hydrogen response to sucrose of a patient with sucrase–isomaltase deficiency. A marked increase in breath hydrogen level follows ingestion of 25 g of sucrose. The hydrogen production reflects colonic fermentation of the unabsorbed disaccharide.

33

Short bowel syndrome

Richard N. Fedorak, Leah M. Gramlich, Lana Bistritz

The term *short bowel syndrome* is used to refer to the clinical consequences and pathophysiological disorders associated with a malabsorptive state resulting from the removal of a large portion of the small and/or large intestine. The degree of nutrient and nonnutrient malabsorption that occurs in a patient with extensive intestinal resection is a consequence of a number of factors: the extent and site of the resected intestine; the presence or absence of an ileal cecal valve; the condition of the remaining intestine; and the degree of adaptation of the residual small intestine (Table 33.1). It is thus possible that the removal of similar lengths of small intestine might cause short bowel syndrome to develop in one person but not in another.

Diarrhea is inevitable for patients who have had extensive small intestinal resection and have developed short bowel syndrome. Diarrhea and fluid and electrolyte loss is multifactorial and often involves one or more of the following multiple causes: reduction of absorptive surface area, decreases in intestinal transit time, hormone-mediated intestinal hypersecretion, increases in the osmolality of intestinal contents, and bacterial overgrowth. Rational and judicious use of varying antidiarrheal therapies can significantly limit fluid and electrolyte losses and reduce or even eliminate the requirements for parenteral nutrition (Table 33.2).

In addition to the severe losses of fluid and electrolytes, micronutrient deficiencies (Fig. 33.1) and systemic complications such as gallstones (Fig. 33.2), enteric hyperoxaluria, renal calculi (Fig. 33.3; Table 33.3), and bacterial overgrowth are likely to occur. Almost all patients with short bowel syndrome at one time or another need parenteral nutrition or intravenous fluid and electrolyte therapy. Although the parenteral nutrition and electrolyte therapy may be tran-

sient, intermittent, or both, it is often life-sustaining therapy.

Tables 33.4–33.10 provide examples of total parenteral nutrition order forms, component composition, and suggested blood work and additive routines for the adult population. Tables 33.11–33.15 provide similar information for pediatric patients.

Once parenteral nutrition is initiated for short bowel syndrome patients it often becomes life sustaining, requiring lifetime home parenteral nutrition therapy. The complication rates of home parenteral nutrition therapy tend to be related to the central venous catheter (Table 33.16). Indeed, a minority of patients are susceptible to recurrent problems and many patients have very few complications. Quality of life for patients receiving home parenteral nutrition is generally reasonable and seems to plateau after 3–5 years (Table 33.17). The 1-year survival rate of patients receiving home parenteral nutrition is approximately 95% for the young Crohn's disease patient; however, this survival rate decreases dramatically in the elderly patient and over time (Table 33.18).

Intestinal transplantation has become a life-saving treatment that can be considered for patients with irreversible intestinal failure who cannot be maintained on parenteral nutrition. Figure 33.4 describes an algorithm for patients with intestinal failure and the management that should be considered in defining those individuals for intestinal transplantation. Figure 33.5 represents intestinal transplant graft and patient survival data by era of transplant from the intestinal transplant registry. Centers performing large numbers of intestinal transplants are reporting 1-year graft and patient survival rates of 90% and 70% respectively.

Atlas of Gastroenterology, 4th edition. Edited by Tadataka Yamada, David H. Alpers, Anthony N. Kalloo, Neil Kaplowitz, Chung Owyang, and Don W. Powell. © 2009 Blackwell Publishing, ISBN: 978-1-4051-6909-7

Table 33.1 Factors influencing short bowel syndrome

Extent of intestine removed
Site of intestine removed
Presence of an ileocecal valve
Extent of intestinal adaptation

Table 33.2 Antidiarrheal therapies

Drug	Dosage	Adverse effects	Comments
Opiate agonists			
Opium and belladonna suppository	One q12h PRN	Sedation, potentially addictive, nausea, dry mucous membranes	60–65 mg opium, 15–16 mg belladonna
Opium (Diban)	One q4h PRN	Sedation, nausea, potentially addictive	Capsule: 12 mg opium, 52 g hyoscyamine, 10 g atropine, 3 g scopolamine, 300 mg attapulgite, 71 mg pectin
Opium camphor (paregoric)	Varies depending on concentration	Sedation, nausea, potentially addictive	May not be generally available
Codeine	30–60 mg q4h PRN	Sedation, nausea, potentially addictive	Tablet: 15 or 30 mg; solution: 30 or 60 mg/mL
Diphenoxylate atropine sulfate (Lomotil, generics)	5 mg initially then 2.5 mg after each loose bowel movement to a maximum of 20 mg/day	Sedation, abdominal cramps, dry skin and mucous membranes (from atropine), some addiction potential	Capsule: 2.5 mg diphenoxylate, 0.025 mg atropine
Loperamide (Imodium, generics)	2 mg after each loose bowel movement to a maximum of 16 mg/day	Sedation, abdominal cramps	Capsule: 2 mg; solution: 2 mg/10 mL. After oral administration absorption is poor, ~40% excreted unabsorbed in feces
α_2-Adrenergic agonists			
Clonidine (Catapres, generics)	0.1–0.6 mg q12h	Centrally medicated sedation and hypotension	Tablets: 0.1 and 0.2 mg
Somatostatin			
Octreotide (Sandostatin)	50–500 µg q8–12h	Pain at injection site, diarrhea, abdominal pain	Ampules: 50, 100, and 500 µg; multidose vial: 200 and 1000 µg/mL
Sandostatin LAR depot	10–30 mg q4 weeks intragluteally	Pain at injection site, diarrhea, abdominal pain	Ampules: 10, 20, and 30 mg
Bulking agents			
Psyllium (Fibrepur, Metamucil, generics)	1 tsp (5–6 g) q12h	Inhaled psyllium powder may cause allergic reaction	Products in which psyllium has been mixed with laxatives need to be avoided
Cholestyramine resin (Questran, generics)	4 g q12h	Nausea, fat-soluble vitamin deficiency with long-term use, may bind other drugs in GI tract	One packet: 4 g; should not be taken dry, must be mixed with fluids; no oral drugs 1 h before or 4 h after

GI, gastrointestinal.

Table 33.3 Foods that contain high oxalate concentrations

Beets
Green beans
Spinach
Collard greens
Mustard greens
Turnip greens
Asparagus
Brussel sprouts
Cabbage
Carrots
Cranberries
Concord grapes
Oranges
Rhubarb
Tea
Cola
Chocolate
Celery
Peas
Tomatoes
Potatoes
Apples
Bananas
Cherries
Strawberries
Peaches
Pears
Plums

Table 33.4

Patient weight _____ kg

☐ Central administration　　☐ Peripheral administration

Components	Recommended requirements	24-hour intake (g)	Energy provided (kcal)	24-hour volume (mL)	Rate (mL/h)	Pharmacy use only
Amino acids (as 10%)	1–1.5 g/kg/24 h					
Dextrose (as D70W)	2–4 mg/kg/min					
Additional volume	150 mL minimum					
Total amino acid dextrose soln (mL)						
Lipid (as 20%)	1 g/kg/24 h					
Total fluid volume	30 mL/kg/24 h					
Total energy (kcal)	25–30 kcal/kg/24 h					

1. Volume for additives and/or free water.

Table 33.4 *Continued*

Additives[5]	Recommended requirements	Total 24-hour intake
Sodium (mmol)[1]	60–150 mmol/day	
Potassium (mmol)[1]	30–80 mmol/day	
Calcium (mmol)	5–15 mmol/day	
Magnesium (mmol)	4–8 mmol/day	
Phosphate (mmol)	15–30 mmol/day	
Acetate (mmol)	As required	
Multiple vitamin soln[3]	10 mL/day	
Vitamin K (mg)	10 mg/week	
Trace element soln[4]	1 mL/day	
Zinc (mg)	Additional as required	
Folic acid (mg)	Additional as required	
Ranitidine/famotidine (circle one)	As required	
Heparin (units)	As required	
Insulin, human regular (units) novolin/humulin (circle one)	As required	
Other (specify)		

1. Sodium and potassium will be added as chloride salts unless otherwise indicated.
2. Patient must reach glucose hemostasis for at least 48 hours.
3. See Table 3.
4. See Table 4.
5. See Table 2.

---

*Cycled administration (if appropriate).
Cycle over _____ hours at _____ mL/h Start time _____ Stop time _____ Decrease rate to _____ mL/h Start time _____
Stop time _____ Flush line per protocol, device dependent.

Duration of order: *Maximum 96 hours.*
Date ordered _____   Date to be reordered _____

Nutrition support service signature _____   Physician signature _____

Bag number				
Nursing initials				
Date				

Table 33.5 Additive equivalents for use in both adult and pediatric total parenteral nutrition solutions

Calcium gluconate: 1 mEq = 0.5 mmol Ca^{2+} = 216 mg Ca^{2+}
Potassium chloride: 1 mEq = 1 mmol K^+
Magnesium sulfate: 1 mEq = 0.5 mmol Mg^{2+} = 125 mg Mg^{2+}
Sodium acetate: 1 mEq = 1 mmol Na^+
Potassium acetate: 1 mEq = 1 mmol K^+
Potassium phosphate: 1 mL = 4.4 mmol K^+ and 3 mmol P
Sodium phosphate: 1 mL = 4 mmol Na^+ and 3 mmol P
1 g nitrogen = 6.25 g protein
1 g protein = 4 kcal
1 g fat = 9 kcal
1 g dextrose = 3.4 kcal
20% lipid: 1 mL = 2 kcal
Amino acid = 100 mOsm/g
Dextrose = 50 mOsm/g

Table 33.7 Intravenous trace element composition for use by both adults and children

Component	Amount per 1 mL
Zinc	5 mg
Copper	1 mg
Manganese	0.5 mg
Chromium	10 µg
Selenium	60 µg

Table 33.6 Intravenous multiple vitamins: 12-component composition for use by adults

Component	Amount per 10 mL
Vitamin A (IU)	3300
Vitamin B-1, thiamine (mg)	3.0
Vitamin B-2, riboflavin (mg)	3.6
Vitamin B-6, pyridoxine (mg)	4.0
Vitamin B-12, cyanocobalamin (µg)	5.0
Niacinamide (mg)	40
Vitamin C (mg)	100
Vitamin D (IU)	200
Vitamin E (IU)	10
D-panthenol (mg)	15
Biotin (µg)	60
Folic acid (mg)	0.4

Table 33.8 Suggested routine bloodwork for adults and children (6 months–14 years) on total parenteral nutrition

Initial: CBC, electrolytes, magnesium, phosphorus, calcium, albumin, PT (INR), PTT, creatinine, urea, glucose
Biweekly: CBC, sodium, potassium, CO_2, creatinine, urea, glucose
Weekly (as appropriate): alkaline phosphatase, albumin, ALT, bilirubin, magnesium, phosphorus, calcium, PT (INR), PTT
Others as needed: 24-h urine for electrolytes and nitrogen balance, cholesterol, triglycerides

ALT, alanine aminotransferase; CBC, complete blood count; INR, international normalized ratio; PT, prothrombin time; PTT, partial thromboplastin time.

Table 33.9 Suggested daily intravenous intake of vitamins for adults

Vitamin	RDA adult range
Ascorbic acid (mg)	45
Biotin (µg)	150–300[a]
Folacin (µg)	400
Niacin (mg)	12–20
Pantothenic acid (mg)	6–10[a]
Riboflavin (mg)	1.1–1.8
Thiamin (mg)	1.0–1.5
Vitamin A (IU)	4000–5000[b]
Vitamin B-8 (pyridoxine) (mg)	1.6–2.0
Vitamin B-12 (cyanocobalamin) (µg)	3
Vitamin D (IU)	400
Vitamin E (IU)	12–15

a Recommended daily allowance (RDA) not established; amount considered adequate in usual dietary intake.
b Assumes 50% intake as carotene, which is less available than vitamin A.
Results do not include requirements of pregnancy or lactation.

Table 33.10 Suggested daily intravenous intake of trace elements for adults

Trace element	Stable adult	Adult in acute catabolic state[a]	Stable adult with intestinal losses[a]
Zinc	2.5–4.0 mg	Additional 2.0 mg	Add 17.1 mg/kg of stool or ileostomy output
Copper	0.5–1.5 mg		
Manganese	0.15–0.8 mg		
Chromium	10–15 µg		
Selenium	40–80 µg		

a Frequent monitoring of blood levels for these patients is essential to provide proper dosage.

Table 33.11

Patient weight _____ kg   Height _____ cm

☐   Central administration   ☐   Peripheral administration (*Maximum 12.5% dextrose concentration*)

Components	24-hour intake (g)	Energy provided (kcal)	24-hour volume (mL)	Rate (mL/h)	Pharmacy use only
Amino acids (as 10%)					
Dextrose (as D70W)					
Additional volume					
Total amino acid-dextrose soln (mL)					
Lipid (as 20%)					
Total energy (kcal)					
Total volume					

1. Volume for additives and/or free water.

Additives[4]	Recommended requirements	Total 24-hour intake
Sodium (mmol)[1]	2–3 mmol/kg/day	
Potassium (mmol)[1]	1–3 mmol/kg/day	
Calcium (mmol)	0.5–1 mmol/kg/day	
Magnesium (mmol)	0.3–0.5 mmol/kg/day	
Phosphate (mmol)	0.5–1 mmol/kg/day	
Acetate (mmol)	For correction of acidemia	
Multiple vitamin soln, pediatric[2]	5 mL/day	
Trace element soln[3]	0.02 mL/kg to a maximum of 1 mL/day	
	Other (specify)	
Heparin (units)	As required	

1. Sodium and potassium will be added as chloride salts unless otherwise indicated.
2. See Table 9.
3. See Table 4.
4. See Table 2.

Duration of order: *Maximum 96 hours.*

Date ordered _____   Date to be reordered _____

Nutrition support service signature _____ Physician signature _____

Bag number				
Nursing initials				
Date				

Table 33.12 Intravenous multiple vitamin composition for use by children aged from 6 months to 14 years

Component	Amount per 5 mL
Vitamin A (IU)	2300
Vitamin B-1, thiamin (mg)	1.2
Vitamin B-2, riboflavin (mg)	1.4
Vitamin B-6, pyridoxine (mg)	1
Vitamin B-12, cyanocobalamin (μg)	1
Niacinamide (mg)	17
Vitamin C (mg)	80
Vitamin D (IU)	400
Vitamin E (IU)	7
D-panthenol (mg)	5
Biotin (μg)	20
Folic acid (mg)	0.14
Vitamin K (μg)	200

Table 33.13 Suggested protein, fat, and energy requirements for children

Age	Gender	Protein requirements (g/kg/day)	Fat requirements (g/kg/day)	Energy requirements[a]
0–2 months	Both	2.2	1–3 (initiate at 1 g/kg/d)	100–200 kcal/kg/day
3–4 months	Both	1.5		95–100 kcal/kg/day
6–8 months	Both	1.4		95–97 kcal/kg/day
9–11 months	Both	1.4		97–99 kcal/kg/day
1–3 years	Both	1.2		13.5 kcal/cm/day
4–6 years	Both	1.1	1–3 (initiate at 1 g/kg/d)	17 kcal/cm/day
7–9 years	M	1.0		17.5 kcal/cm/day
	F	1.0		15 kcal/cm/day
10–12 years	M	1.0		17.5 kcal/cm/day
	F	1.0		15.5 kcal/cm/day
13–15 years	M	1.0	2 (initiate at 1 g/kg/d)	17.5 kcal/cm/day
	F	0.9		14 kcal/cm/day
16–18 years	M	0.9		18.5 kcal/cm/day
	F	0.9		13 kcal/cm/day

a Actual energy requirements may vary by 20%–30% depending on stress and activity factors.

Table 33.14 Suggested daily intravenous intake of vitamins for children

Vitamin	Term infants and children (dose per day)
Lipid soluble	
A (µg)[a]	700
E (mg)[b]	7
K (µg)	200
D (µg)[c]	10
Water soluble	
Ascorbic acid (mg)	80
Biotin (µg)	20
Folate (µg)	140
Niacin (mg)	17
Pantothenate (mg)	5
Pyridoxine (mg)	1.0
Riboflavin (mg)	1.4
Thiamin (mg)	1.2
Vitamin B-12 (µg)	1.0

a 700 µg vitamin A = 2300 IU.

b 7 mg vitamin E (α-tocopherol) = 7 IU.

c 10 µg vitamin D = 400 IU.

Table 33.15 Suggested daily intravenous intake of trace elements in children

Element	Infants (µg/kg/day)		Children (µg/kg/day)
	Preterm	Term	
Zinc	400	250 < 3 months	50 (5000)[c]
		100 > 3 months	
Copper[a]	20	20	20 (300)
Chromium[b]	0.20	0.20	0.20 (5)
Manganese[a]	1.0	1.0	1.0 (50)
Selenium[b]	2.0	2.0	2.0 (30)
Molybdenum[a]	0.25	0.25	0.25 (5)
Iodide	1.0	1.0	1.0 (70)

a Omit for patients with obstructive jaundice.

b Omit for patients with renal dysfunction.

c Values in parentheses are maximum number of micrograms per day.

Table 33.16 Complications of home parenteral nutrition (episodes per catheter year unless indicated)

Study (author and publication year)	Catheter sepsis (95% CI)	Catheter sepsis (episodes per patient year) (95% CI)	Catheter occlusion (95% CI)	Central vein thrombosis (95% CI)	Liver/biliary problems (95% CI)	Metabolic bone disease (95% CI)	Other
Colomb, 2007	–	0.44 (0.40, 0.49)	–	–	0.09 (0.07, 0.11)[a]	–	–
Dray, 2007	–	–	–	–	Cholelithiasis 0.5 (0.35, 0.65)[a], biliary complications 0.77 (0.33, 1.51)[a]	–	–
Marra, 2007	0.85 (0.75, 0.96)	1.17 (1.03, 1.33)	–	0.06 (0.03, 0.09)	–	–	–
De Burgoa, 2006	–	1.41 (0.91, 2.08)[a]	0.17 (0.03, 0.49)[a]	–	–	–	–
Raman, 2006	–	–	–	–	–	0.81 (0.05. 0.13)[a]	–
Shirotani, 2006	0.30 (0.18, 0.47)	0.24 (0.14, 0.38)	0.03 (0.00, 0.09)	0.02 (0.00, 0.09)	–	–	–
Ugur, 2006	0.48 (0.42, 0.56)	–	–	0.02 (0.01, 0.04)	–	–	–
Hoda, 2005	0.13 (0.02, 0.41)	0.36 (0.21, 0.56)	0.24 (0.22, 0.26)	0.08 (0.02, 0.20)[a]	0.04 (0.00, 0.14)[a]	–	–
Ireton-Jones, 2005	–	–	–	–	–	–	–
Diamanti, 2003	–	–	–	–	0.125 (0.06, 0.20)[a]	–	–
Pironi, 2003	–	0.15 (0.09, 0.23)	–	0.04 (0.02, 0.09)[a]	0.15 (0.07, 0.26)	–	–
Bozzetti, 2002	0.22 (0.17, 0.28)	–	0.07 (0.04, 0.10)	0.00 (0.00, 0.02)	–	–	–
Moreau, 2002	0.17 (0.16, 0.17)	–	0.08 (0.08, 0.09)	–	–	–	–
Reimund, 2002	–	0.62 (0.42, 0.89)	–	–	–	–	–
Santarpia, 2002	–	1.96 (1.49, 2.52)	–	–	–	–	–
Scolapio, 2002	–	0.36 (0.25, 0.50)	–	–	–	–	–
Gambarara, 2001	–	0.21 (0.08, 0.32)	0.33 (0.20, 0.51)	0.02 (0.00, 0.10)[a]	–	–	–
Van Gossum, 2001	–	0.31 (0.24, 0.39)	–	0.09 (0.06, 0.14)[a]	–	–	–
Colomb, 2000	0.78 (0.67, 0.91)	0.70 (0.60. 0.82)	–	–	–	–	–
Terra, 2000	–	0.88 (0.47, 1.51)	–	–	–	–	–
Chan, 1999	–	–	–	–	0.20 (0.01, 0.05)[a]	–	–
Scolapio, 1999	0.07 (0.06, 0.09)	–	–	–	–	–	–
Tokars, 1999	0.36 (0.28, 0.46)	–	–	–	–	–	–
Nightingale, 1995	24 fungal infections; total number of lines not given	–	–	–	–	–	Four developed eye infections; two had recurrent infection
Buchman, 1994a	–	–	0.07 (0.06, 0.09)	0.02 (0.01, 0.03)	–	–	–
Buchman, 1994b	0.23 (0.2, 0.27); not possible to calculate rates for children	0.23 (0.2, 0.26)	–	–	–	–	–

Continued

Study (author and publication year)	Catheter sepsis (95% CI)	Catheter sepsis (episodes per patient year) (95% CI)	Catheter occlusion (95% CI)	Central vein thrombosis (95% CI)	Liver/biliary problems (95% CI)	Metabolic bone disease (95% CI)	Other
Dollery, 1994	–	–	–	16 episodes of major thrombosis in 12 of 34 patients	–	–	–
Buchman, 1993	–	–	–	–	–	–	Low plasma-free choline levels are prevalent, associated with elevated serum aminotransferases
Buchman, 1993	–	–	–	–	–	–	Fall in renal function of 3.5 ± 6.3%/year
Howard, 1993	–	–	–	–	–	–	Total complication rate is higher for those younger than 18 years
Johnston, 1993	0.16 (0.05, 0.47)	–	–	0.28 (0.06, 0.47)	–	–	–
King, 1993	0.54 (0.22, 1.11)	?	–	–	–	–	–
Pironi, 1993	0.12 (0.03, 0.3)	–	0.03 (0, 0.16)	0.09 (0.02, 0.26)	0.15 (0.05, 0.34)	–	–
Bisset, 1992	–	–	–	–	–	–	Sepsis 0.73
Burnes, 1992	0.27 (0.2, 0.35)	–	–	–	–	–	–
DePotter, 1992	0.40 (0.33, 0.49)	0.23	0.04 (0.02, 0.07)	–	0.03 (0.01, 0.05)	–	–
Herfindal, 1992	0.46 (0.3, 0.7)	0.14 (0.06, 0.29)	0.22 (0.12, 0.39)	–	0.42 (0.27, 0.63)	0.05 (0.01, 0.15)	Metabolic complications 0.61
Mukau, 1992	0.2 (0.1, 0.35)	?	–	0.07 (0.02, 0.17)	–	–	–
O'Hanrahan, 1992	0.47 (0.38, 0.58)	–	0.44 (0.36, 0.55)	0.06 (0.03, 0.11)	–	–	Metabolic complications 0.12 (0.08, 0.18)
Singer, 1991	A: 0.43 (0.05, 1.55); C: 0.2 (0.07, 1.43); H: 0.1 (0.04, 0.22)	–	A: 0.21 (0.05, 1.2); C: 0.03 (0, 0.18); H: 0.06 (0.02, 0.16)	–	–	–	Metabolic distribution: A: 0.43 (0.05, 1.55); C: 0.49 (0.28, 0.81); H: 0.17 (0.08, 0.3)
Beers, 1990	–	–	–	0.04 (0.02, 0.07)	–	–	–
Folders, 1990	–	–	–	–	–	90% (56%, 99%)	–
Galandiuk, 1990	0.27 (0.19, 0.38)	–	–	–	–	–	–
Hurley, 1990	0.30 (0.17, 0.49)	–	0.02 (0.06, 0.47)	–	–	–	Total complications: cancer 2.22 (1.4, 3.4), benign 0.89 (0.64, 1.2), $P < 0.01$

Continued

Study							
Schmidt-Sommerfeld, 1990	0.71 (0.5, 0.97)	—	0.29 (0.17, 0.47)	0.07 (0.02, 0.19)	—	—	—
Staun, 1994	—	—	—	—	—	4% decrease in bone mineral content/year	—
Manji, 1989	—	—	—	—	Symptomatic gallstones in 100%	—	—
Messing, 1989	0.38 (0.30, 0.48)	?	0.18	0.07	—	—	—
Gouttebel, 1987	0.70 (0.49, 0.97)	0.42 (0.26, 0.4)	—	—	—	—	—
Vargas, 1987	0.37 (0.29, 0.46)	0.20 (0.15, 0.28)	—	—	Any 0.06 (0.03, 0.1); severe 0.024 (0.008, 0.057)	—	—
Howard, 1986	0.37 (0.33, 0.42)	—	—	—	—	0.013 (0.005, 0.025)	—
Shike, 1986	—	—	—	—	15% (7%, 27%) liver problems	67% (35%, 90%)	—
Bowyer, 1985	—	—	—	—	3% (0.4%, 12%) deaths	—	—
Dudrick, 1984	0.39 (0.26, 0.54)	0.15 (0.08, 0.26)	0.1 (0.03, 0.24)	—	—	—	—
Robb, 1983	0.42 (0.25, 0.68)	—	—	—	—	—	—
Roslyn, 1983	—	—	—	—	Symptomatic gallstones in 23% (15%, 32%)	—	—
Steiger, 1983	—	—	—	—	—	—	Percent of hospitalized days: Crohn's, 24%; radiation enteritis, 13%
Weiss, 1982	0.2 (0.01, 1.11)	0.2 (0.01, 1.11)	—	—	—	—	—
Perl, 1981	—	—	—	—	—	—	Depression 80% (44, 98)
Shike, 1980	—	—	—	—	—	75% (48%, 93%)	—

a Episodes per patient year.
?, data in the study not sufficient for calculation of rates; 95% CI, 95% confidence interval; A, acquired immunodeficiency syndrome; C, cancer; H, home parenteral nutrition.

Table 33.17 Quality of life for patients receiving home parenteral nutrition

Study (author and publication year)	Whose values?	Instrument used	Profile or index	Index scores	Best QOL or outcome	Worst QOL or outcome	Comments
Chambers, 2006	Patient	SF-36, EQ5D	Index	QOL scores rose significantly within the first 6 months of HPN	Mental health, emotional role were same as normative data after 6 months of HPN	Body pain, general health, physical component did not significantly improve	All QOL scores at discharge were lower than normative data
Huisman-de Waal, 2006	Patient	Interviews	Profile	–	Psychosocial issues, physical problems, dependence, patient–care provider issues	One-third endorsed incapability due to physical limitations	Underlying theme expressed by respondents: loss, longing, and grief
Pironi, 2006	Patient	SF-36	Index	Physical functioning 2.3 and role 1.5; pain 1.0; health 1.2; vitality 0.5; social 0.9; emotional 0.7; mental 0.0	–	–	HPN subjects had poorer physical health scores compared with ITx
Gottrand, 2005	Patient, parent, sibling, doctor	Validated questionnaires; type dependent upon age	Index	No significant difference between QOL scores for all ages vs healthy children	Parents rated child's QOL higher vs doctors	Parents of HPN infants scored child's QOL lower than parents of healthy infants	Unlike adult HPN patients, pediatric QOL for HPN patients is not lower than their healthy counterparts
Orrevall, 2005	Patient, family	Semistructured interview	Profile	–	Acceptable: improved strength, activity, sense of relief, and security	Restrictive family life and social contacts	HPN benefits outweigh negative aspects
Persoon, 2005	Patient	Nonvalidated questionnaire and interview	Profile	–	–	Severe depression (65%) and fatigue (63%)	Low QOL associated with fatigue, sleeping disorders, anxiety, depression, and social impairment
Pironi, 2003	Patient	SF-36	Index	Only vitality and mental health scores were not significantly lower than those of the healthy population	Social functioning and emotional role better in women	Vitality scores lower for patients with motility disorder vs short bowel syndrome	–
Jeppesen, 1999	Patient	SIP and IBDQ	Index	HPN subjects scored worse than non-HPN subjects overall in both tests	–	–	The worse subgroup was those on HPN with a stoma

Continued

Study	Assessor	Instrument	Type	Score	Good QOL	Poor QOL	Comments
Carlson, 1995	Patient	Nonvalidated questionnaire	Index	0.64 (0–1 scale)[a]	–	–	QOL independent of variables tested; younger patients keen on intestinal transplantation
Richards, 1995	Patient	SF-36 and Euro QOL	Both	0.51	Age < 45 years	Age > 55 years, narcotic addiction	No significant difference between disease subgroups, stomas, recent hospitalization, and duration of HPN
Duclaux, 1993	Doctor	Nonvalidated simple questionnaire	Profile	–	–	–	QOL much improved at home; development and psychological well-being much improved
Pironi, 1993	Doctor	Functional assessment	Profile	–	–	–	Two-thirds in the upper two groups
Smith, 1993	Patient	Multiple validated instruments	Profile	–	Stable relationship	Long duration of HPN, poor income	Loss of friends, loss of employment, and depression were noted in two-thirds of families
O'Hanrahan, 1992	Doctor	Functional assessment	Profile	–	Crohn's disease	All other diagnostic groups	Same four-point scale used
Galandiuk, 1990	Patient plus doctor	QOL score, social activity score, psychological score	Index	Pre-HPN, 7.1; receiving HPN, 5.3[b]	–	–	Index scores were better when receiving HPN; pre-HPN QOL was significantly worse ($P < 0.01$); all patients in this study had Crohn's disease
Herfindal, 1989	Patient	Multiple validated instruments	Profile	–	Long duration (> 6 months)	Duration < 6 months	HPN patients had lower (worse) scores than renal transplant recipients and normal US population
Messing, 1989	Doctor	Functional assessment	–	–	Age < 65 years, benign	Age > 65 years, malignancy, pseudoobstruction	Simple four-stage rehabilitation profile; stage decided by physician, not the patient
Ladefoged, 1981	Patient	Nonvalidated questionnaire	Profile	–	Acceptable in two-thirds of cases	–	QOL parameters were independent of all variables, but not enough data to test

a Scale 0–1: 0 = death, 1 = best possible QOL.
b Scale 3–9: 9 = severe disablement, 3 = best possible QOL.
HPN, home parenteral nutrition; ITx, intestinal transplant; QOL, quality of life; SF, symptomatic function.

Table 33.18 Survival rates when receiving home parenteral nutrition

Study (author and publication year)	Benign underlying disease	Malignant underlying disease (including AIDS)
Colomb, 2007	2-year survival 97%, 5-year survival 89%, 10-year survival 81%	
Lloyd, 2006	1-year survival 86%; 3-year survival 77%; 5-year survival 73%; 10-year survival 71%	–
Ugur, 2006	–	Cancer: mean survival 1.0 year (0.2–2.4)
Gavazzi, 2005	5-year survival: radiation enteritis, 90%	–
Hoda, 2005	–	Cancer: median time to death 5 months (range 1–154 months)
Duerksen, 2004	–	Gastric or colon cancer: variable survival rate of 27–433 days; 67% survived for longer than 60 days
Vantini, 2004	1-year survival 95%; 4-year survival 79%; 6-year survival 66%. Survival better in patients with > 50 cm small bowel ($P < 0.05$) or in those starting HPN > age 45 ($P < 0.02$)	–
Pironi, 2003	1-year survival 97.3%; 3-year survival 82.6%; 5-year survival 67.8%	–
Scolapio, 2002	–	Cancer: 1-year survival 76%; 5-year survival 64%
Pasanisi, 2001	–	Cancer: survival ranged from 6 to 301 days, median of 74 days
Cavicchi, 2000	2-year survival 98%; 4-year survival 80%; 6-year survival 65%; 8-year survival 56%	–
Messing, 1999	2-year survival 86%; 5-year survival 75%	–
Scolapio, 1999	5-year survival: IBD, 92%; ischemic bowel, 60%; radiation enteritis, 54%; motility disorder, 48%	5-year survival: cancer, 38%
Van Gossum, 1999	~1-year survival: Crohn's, 96%; vascular disease, 87%; radiation enteritis, 79%	~1-year survival: AIDS, 66%; cancer, 26%
Howard, 1995	1-year survival (age 0–55 years) > 90%, 1-year survival (age > 55 years) ~ 65%	–
Messing, 1995	1-year survival 91%, 2-year survival 70%, 3-year survival 62%	–
Van Gossum, 1995	6-month mortality rates: Crohn's disease, 0%; vascular occlusion, 8%; miscellaneous, 13%; radiation enteritis, 7%	6-month mortality rates: cancer, 71%; AIDS, 88%
Howard, 1993	1-year survival: Crohn's disease, 95%; radiation enteritis, 76%	1-year survival: cancer, 30%
King, 1993	–	Gynecological malignancy: median survival 2 months (range 0–26)
Howard, 1991	1-year mortality rates: Crohn's disease, 5%; vascular occlusion, 20% (4% thereafter)	1-year mortality rates: cancer, 75%; AIDS, 93%; pseudoobstruction, 20%
August, 1991	–	Average months survived: ovarian cancer, 1.3; colon cancer, 3; appendiceal cancer, 6
Grabowski, 1989	Scleroderma: three of four died at 12, 14, and 17 months	–
Howard, 1986	50% survival at 36 months, 15% survival at year 8	50% survival at 6 months, 15% at 1 year, all dead by 23 months

AIDS, acquired immunodeficiency syndrome.

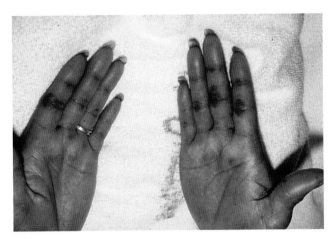

Figure 33.1 Acral skin lesions of a patient receiving home total parenteral nutrition without supplemental zinc.

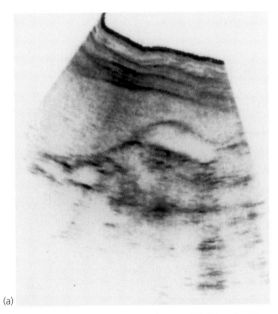

(a)

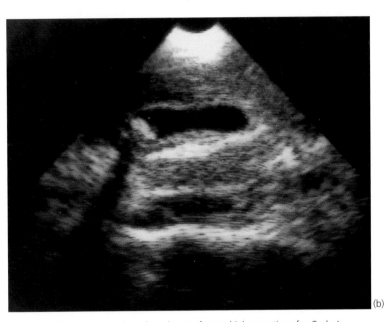

(b)

Figure 33.2 Ultrasound scans of the gallbladder of a 35-year-old woman with severe short bowel syndrome after multiple resections for Crohn's disease. **(a)** Ultrasound scan before home total parenteral nutrition (TPN) shows no stones. **(b)** Ultrasound scan after 2 years of home TPN demonstrates stones and sludge. The patient needed a cholecystectomy for symptomatic cholelithiasis.

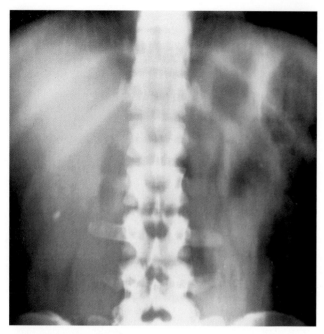

Figure 33.3 Nephrotomogram of a patient after resection of all but 100 cm of small intestine because of midgut volvulus with infarction showing bilateral renal calculi. The patient had hyperoxaluria (urinary oxalate excretion 70 mg/day). Analysis of a surgically extracted stone showed that it was composed of calcium oxalate.

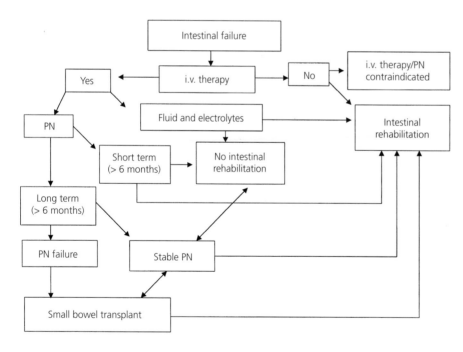

Figure 33.4 Algorithm for intestinal failure. i.v., intravenous; PN, parenteral nutrition.

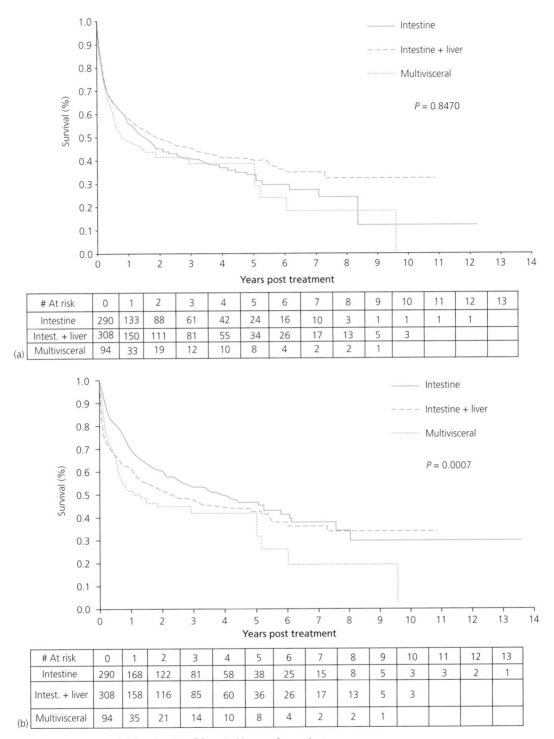

Figure 33.5 Intestinal transplant graft **(a)** and patient **(b)** survival by era of transplant.

34

Tumors of the small intestine

Robert S. Bresalier

Small intestinal tumors (tumors of the duodenum, jejunum, and ileum) are uncommon in comparison with those occurring elsewhere in the gastrointestinal tract. Although the small intestine is approximately 20 ft long, comprising 75% of the length of the gastrointestinal tract and 90% of its mucosal surface area, less than 2% of malignant gastrointestinal tumors are derived from this organ. Approximately 6000 new cases of small intestinal cancer are expected in the United States in 2008 (equally distributed between men and women), with 1100 estimated cancer deaths.

Primary small intestinal tumors are diverse in nature because they are derived from both epithelial and mesenchymal components of the small bowel (Table 34.1). The most frequent histological types of primary malignant tumors include adenocarcinomas, carcinoids, lymphomas, and sarcomas (most are now classified as gastrointestinal stromal tumors). Reports in the literature show that the relative frequency of these primary tumors is 24%–52% for adenocarcinoma, 17%–41% for malignant carcinoid, 12%–29% for lymphoma, and 11%–20% for sarcoma. In a review of the US National Cancer Data Base for the years 1985–1995, the relative frequency by histological type was 35.1% for adenocarcinoma, 27.6% for carcinoid, 20.8% for lymphoma, 10.1% for sarcoma, and 6.4% for other. This is similar to the histological distribution in other population-based studies. The pattern of distribution of tumors in the small intestine is dependent on histological type. In Western countries adenocarcinomas are most commonly found in the duodenum. In the setting of Crohn's disease, adenocarcinomas may occur distally in the ileum, reflecting the distribution of the underlying inflammatory bowel disease. Carcinoids and primary lymphomas occur predominantly in the ileum and jejunum. Sarcomas are found more evenly distributed throughout the small intestine. Metastases to the small bowel account for approximately 50% of all small bowel tumors. Metastases may arise from several sources including a variety of carcinomas and sarcomas.

Adenocarcinoma of the small intestine represents the most common primary malignancy of this organ in most series, but the overall incidence is low in comparison to malignancies of the colon. The incidence per million of small bowel adenocarcinoma ranges between 3.0 and 6.5 in population-based studies. Adenocarcinomas represent approximately 40% of primary small bowel tumors in most population-based studies (range 24%–42%), and between 20% and 69% in selected case studies. Small bowel adenocarcinoma accounts for approximately 2% of gastrointestinal tumors and 1% of gastrointestinal cancer deaths. In an analysis of the US National Cancer Data Base, a joint project of the American College of Surgeons Commission on Cancer and the American Cancer Society, there were 4995 small bowel adenocarcinomas reported between 1985 and 1995. Of these, 55% occurred in the duodenum, 18% in the jejunum, 13% in the ileum, and 14% in nonspecified sites. In total, 53% of those with small bowel adenocarcinomas were male and 47% were female. The overall 5-year survival rate was 30.5%, with a median survival of 19.7 months.

Adenocarcinomas arise from adenomas or dysplastic changes of the small intestine. Adenomas and adenocarcinomas of the small intestine, and especially of the duodenum and ampulla of Vater, are most frequently encountered in the setting of familial adenomatous polyposis (FAP). Duodenal adenomas have been reported in up to 90% of FAP patients but the potential for malignant degeneration and their natural history have not been studied in detail. Adenocarcinomas of the small bowel are also associated with hereditary nonpolyposis colorectal cancer (HNPCC), hamartomatous polyposis syndromes (especially the Peutz–Jeghers syndrome), Crohn's disease, bile diversion (previous cholecystectomy), and gluten-sensitive enteropathy. Other conditions that have been associated with adenocarcinoma of the small intestine include urinary diversion to the small bowel (ileal loop conduits), and long-standing ileostomies and ileal pouches in patients with inflammatory bowel diseases and FAP.

Atlas of Gastroenterology, 4th edition. Edited by Tadataka Yamada, David H. Alpers, Anthony N. Kalloo, Neil Kaplowitz, Chung Owyang, and Don W. Powell. © 2009 Blackwell Publishing, ISBN: 978-1-4051-6909-7

Adenomas in the small intestine display the same gross and microscopic features as those in the large intestine. They may be pedunculated or sessile. Tubular adenomas tend to be small, whereas those with villous architecture tend to be larger. The presence of multiple duodenal adenomas or adenomatous changes in the ampulla of Vater suggests the diagnosis of FAP. Small intestinal adenocarcinomas may appear grossly as flat, stenosing, ulcerative, infiltrating, or polypoid lesions. Most are moderately differentiated tumors with gland formation and variable degrees of mucin secretion. Adenocarcinomas invade the muscularis propria and bowel wall to invade veins, lymphatics, and nerves, and metastasize to regional lymph nodes and distant sites such as the liver and lungs. Tumors often invade adjacent structures and the retroperitoneum, including the pancreas.

The mean age of presentation for adenocarcinomas is approximately 65 years of age, with a wide range of age at presentation. Less than 1% of tumors occur before the age of 30 years and approximately 85% occur after the age of 50 years. Symptoms relate to tumor size, location, and blood supply. Small tumors are asymptomatic or may present with anemia secondary to chronic blood loss, but for the most part are indolent and difficult to diagnose. Abdominal pain and other obstructive symptoms such as nausea and vomiting are common late symptoms as tumors obstruct because of infiltration with lumenal narrowing or because of mass effect. Anorexia and weight loss are also common symptoms.

Endoscopy may be used to examine the duodenum when a lesion is suspected or in families with FAP. Small bowel follow-through (SBFT) has been reported to be 70%–80% accurate for detection of duodenal lesions. Barium studies, however, are not as accurate in detecting tumors that are more distal. Enteroclysis involves intubation of the duodenum and instillation of dilute barium into the small intestine. In a study comparing the sensitivity and tumor detection rate of enteroclysis and SBFT, SBFT had a sensitivity of 61% and enteroclysis had a sensitivity of 95%. Capsule endoscopy has emerged as a sensitive tool for detecting lesions throughout the small intestine and may be the preferred modality for detecting small mucosal lesions. Computed tomography (CT) is being used increasingly to demonstrate small bowel tumors and their complications. Endoscopic ultrasonography has emerged as an important tool for diagnosing and staging tumors of the gastrointestinal tract. A high-frequency transducer placed at the tip of the endoscope is used to obtain high-resolution transmural sonographic images of the intestinal wall and surrounding structures. Surgical resection is the treatment of choice for adenocarcinoma of the small intestine.

Carcinoid tumors (or argentaffinomas) belong to a family of rare neuroendocrine neoplasms that are also known as amine precursor uptake and decarboxylation tumors. This entire family of neoplasms has in common the ability to secrete amines and polypeptides, which produce the characteristic clinical syndromes with which they sometimes present. Over 40 different secretory products have been associated with carcinoid tumors. About 74% percent of carcinoid tumors occur in the gastrointestinal tract. The majority appear in the appendix, followed in frequency by the small bowel and rectum. Most of the clinically significant carcinoid tumors are located in the small bowel; 87% of small bowel tumors are in the ileum and 40% of these can be found within 2 ft of the ileocecal valve. Carcinoid tumors are malignant despite their sometimes indolent course. Small bowel carcinoids in particular are associated with local–regional spread or metastases at the time of diagnosis. The tumors are usually intramucosal and rarely ulcerate to the lumen of the bowel. Small bowel carcinoids spread locally through the muscularis propria toward the serosa. When serosal breach has occurred, an intense local fibroblastic reaction is commonly seen. The desmoplastic reaction is responsible for many of the clinical findings in patients with small bowel carcinoid.

Patients with small bowel carcinoids can present with nonspecific gastrointestinal symptoms, small bowel obstruction, intestinal ischemia, intussusception, gastrointestinal hemorrhage, hepatomegaly, or symptoms of the carcinoid syndrome. Many of the signs and symptoms of small bowel carcinoids are due to the intense desmoplastic reaction of the mesentery in proximity to the tumor. Fibrosis leads to partial small bowel obstruction, intermittent abdominal pain, and weight loss. Approximately 50% of patients with metastatic carcinoid initially present with intestinal obstruction requiring surgery. Patients with liver metastases from carcinoids may exhibit symptoms and signs of the carcinoid syndrome. Flushing of the face and neck may be episodic or permanent and is usually a deep red or purple color. Diarrhea manifests as intermittent episodes of explosive, watery diarrhea caused by intestinal hypermotility. Abdominal cramping may accompany the diarrhea episodes and is the third most common symptom of the syndrome. Dyspnea can be due to advanced carcinoid heart disease or less frequently to bronchoconstriction and asthma. About 65% of patients with carcinoid syndrome will present with a large liver or an abdominal mass, and 40% will have heart valve abnormalities that can be auscultated at presentation. Other less common signs include cyanosis, peripheral edema, arthritis, and pellagra.

Conventional barium studies of the small intestine may identify the primary lesion as a smooth, semilunar filling defect in the lumen. Scintigraphy has long been used for detecting neuroendocrine tumors. Octreotide-labeled scintigraphy is useful not only as a diagnostic modality but also to predict who will respond to octreotide therapy and to locate tumors before surgical debulking. Small bowel carcinoids have been detected endoscopically or by capsule endoscopy in the duodenum, proximal jejunum, and terminal ileum. The tumors generally appear as nodular, submucosal protuberances with a yellowish, shiny appearance. Duodenal carcinoids can also be diagnosed by endoscopic ultrasound.

Neoplasms of mesenchymal origin are uncommon in the gastrointestinal tract, accounting for less than 1% of all gastrointestinal malignancies. Given the uncertainty about the histogenesis and behavior of these tumors, the general term gastrointestinal stromal tumors (GISTs) was coined to describe the group. The majority of these tumors are now believed to share the same embryonic origin as Cajal cells. Malignant GISTs are gut-specific sarcomas and represent 11%–12.7% of all small bowel malignancies. GISTs of the small bowel occur most frequently in the jejunum, followed by the ileum and then the duodenum. GISTs mostly arise from the muscularis propria and generally tend to grow extramurally. Small bowel GISTs generally have a spindle cell-like appearance but infrequently can appear epithelioid.

Most GISTs contain gain-of-function mutations in the c-*kit* oncogene resulting in activation of the c-Kit tyrosine kinase. c-Kit activation is a crucial oncogenic mechanism in sporadic and familial GISTs. Mutations in c-*kit* are found in more than 90% of adult GISTs and predict response to therapy with tyrosine kinase inhibitors.

GISTs of the small bowel tend to invade locally and frequently present with peritoneal seeding or direct invasion to adjacent organs. The most useful indicators of survival and the risk of metastases are the size of the tumor at presentation and the mitotic index (the number of mitotic figures per 50 high-power fields). In addition, histological evidence of tumor invasion into the bowel lamina propria is a consistently poor prognostic indicator. More than 50% of patients with tumors larger than 5 cm will have either a palpable abdominal mass or gastrointestinal hemorrhage. Perhaps the greatest advance in the endoscopic diagnosis of submucosal gastrointestinal tumors is endoscopic ultrasound. GISTs appear as hypoechoic masses arising from the fourth echo layer (muscularis propria). Surgical resection is the treatment of choice for GISTs. A growing body of evidence indicates that imatinib and several newer tyrosine kinase inhibitors that target c-Kit and the platelet-derived growth factor receptor (PDGFR) are effective in the control of metastatic GISTs. The 1-year progression-free survival rate has increased from 10% with chemotherapy to 70% with imatinib. The response to targeted therapy may be monitored with computed tomography or [18]fluorodeoxyglucose positron emission tomography (FDG-PET).

Involvement of the intestine with lymphomatous neoplasms can occur in several settings. The following criteria should be met to designate a primary small bowel lymphoma:
• the absence of palpable peripheral lymphadenopathy
• a normal peripheral leukocyte count and differential
• no mediastinal lymphadenopathy on a chest radiograph
• involvement of only the organs of the gastrointestinal tract and proximal regional lymph nodes
• no involvement of the liver or spleen unless by direct extension from the primary gastrointestinal tumor.

Small bowel lymphomas represent 1%–10% of all extranodal lymphomas and 7%–25% of all small bowel tumors. Primary small bowel lymphomas (PSBL) occur most often in the ileum, followed by the jejunum and then the duodenum. They are generally localized to one segment of the bowel, except in the case of mantle cell lymphoma, otherwise known as multiple lymphoid polyposis.

The tumors have many different appearances. They may be large exophytic masses, polyp-like, ulcer-like, or appear as nodularity and inflammation. Tumor growth and extension is frequently intramural for a prolonged period of time before intralumenal ulceration or extralumenal invasion occurs. Involvement of regional lymph nodes is present in approximately 50% of patients with most types of PSBL. In contrast to PSBL, immunoproliferative small intestinal disease (IPSID) tends to be a very diffuse disease and most often involves the jejunum. Gross findings can range from thickened folds to discrete masses. Although the macroscopic appearance of IPSID is generally less impressive than that of PSBL, the disease affects a significant portion of the intestine in a contiguous fashion. The great majority of small bowel lymphomas are B-cell derived.

The symptoms of PSBL are usually nonspecific and may continue for 4–18 months before a diagnosis is rendered. Abdominal pain is reported in 65%–87% of patients with PSBL, and weight loss is seen in approximately 50%. The symptoms of IPSID differ from those of PSBL. Nearly all patients with IPSID will have diarrhea, weight loss, anorexia, and abdominal pain. Emesis and fever occur in 50% of patients. If a small bowel lymphoma is suspected, the diagnosis can be achieved by radiological, endoscopic, or surgical means. The mainstay of treatment for PSBL is surgical resection. PSBL that cannot be completely resected is usually treated by chemotherapy, sometimes with the addition of radiotherapy. IPSID is less amenable to surgical resection than PSBL because of the diffuse nature of the tumor and the low performance status of patients at the time of presentation.

Metastatic tumors represent the commonest tumors involving the small intestine in many series. Grossly, secondary tumors often present as submucosal nodules or plaques and may grow to form intramural masses, which cause obstruction, intussusception, or perforation. Tumors often present as stenotic or infiltrative lesions that simulate Crohn's disease. Metastases from melanoma as well as from carcinomas of the lung, testes, adrenal gland, ovary, stomach, large intestine, uterus, cervix, liver, and kidney to the small intestine have all been reported.

The benign tumors that are most often encountered clinically are adenoma, leiomyoma, Brunner gland hamartoma, and lipoma. Adenocarcinoma of the small intestine probably arises from adenoma. The incidence of periampullary adenocarcinoma is greatly increased among those with FAP.

The histological nature of a tumor of the small intestine is usually not apparent from the clinical features. Intermittent, partial obstruction of the small intestine is the most common way for both benign and malignant small bowel tumors to present themselves. Benign small bowel tumors are the most common cause of intussusception among adults. Occult blood loss and weight loss are each features in about 50% of cases of malignant tumors of the small intestine. Most patients with periampullary adenocarcinoma have jaundice. The diagnosis of a small bowel tumor is often not made before laparotomy.

Table 34.1 Classification of small intestinal tumors

Benign epithelial tumors
Brunner gland lesions[a]
Benign intestinal epithelial polyps: adenomas; hamartomas (Peutz–Jeghers syndrome, Cronkhite–Canada syndrome, juvenile polyposis, Cowden disease, Bannayan–Riley–Ruvalcaba syndrome)

Malignant epithelial lesions
Primary adenocarcinomas
Secondary carcinomas (metastases)
Carcinoid tumors (neuroendocrine tumors)

Lymphoproliferative disorders
B-cell: diffuse large cell lymphoma; small noncleaved cell lymphoma; MALT cell lymphoma; mantle cell lymphoma (multiple lymphomatous polyposis); immunoproliferative small intestinal disease
T-cell: enteropathy-associated T-cell lymphoma

Mesenchymal tumors[b]
Gastrointestinal stromal tumors (benign and malignant)
Fatty tumors (lipoma, liposarcoma)
Neural tumors (gut autonomic tumors, Schwannomas, neurofibromas, ganglioneuromas, granular cell tumors)
Paragangliomas
Smooth muscle tumors (leiomyoma, leiomyosarcoma)
Vascular tumors (hemangioma, angiosarcoma, lymphangioma, Kaposi sarcoma)

---

a→It is unclear whether these lesions should be classified as hyperplasias, neoplasias, hamartomas, or adenomatous proliferations.
b→Some mesenchymal tumors represent clear-cut diagnostic entities, whereas many are more difficult to classify into any specific cell lineage. The latter are designated as gastrointestinal stromal tumors.
This is a partial list of tumors found in the small intestine. Although the overall incidence of small intestinal tumors is low, a wide variety of benign and malignant lesions have been described in this organ.
MALT, mucosa associated lymphoid tissue.

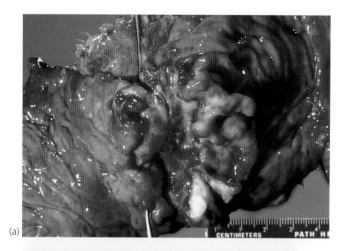

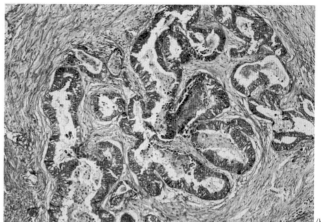

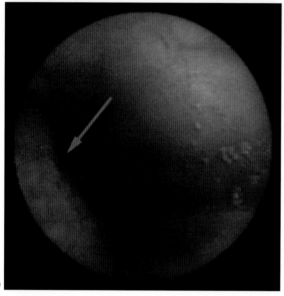

Figure 34.1 Small intestinal adenocarcinoma. **(a)** Gross specimen. Opened section of duodenum with stenosing, infiltrating lesion. **(b)** Histological section demonstrating typical gland formation in this moderately differentiated adenocarcinoma. **(c)** Small tumor (arrow) seen at capsule endoscopy demonstrating abnormal mucosal color, distortion of the villous pattern, and tumor bulge in the lumen. (a) Courtesy of Dr Chan Ma; (c) courtesy of Dr Peter E. Legnani.

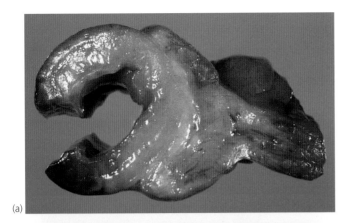

(a)

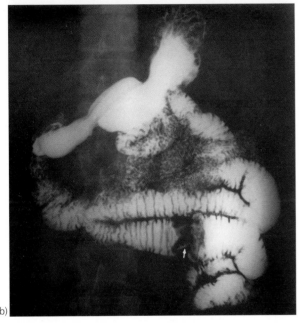

(b)

Figure 34.2 Small intestinal adenocarcinoma. Annular constricting lesion of the jejunum. **(a)** Gross specimen. Courtesy of Dr Chan Ma. **(b)** Upper gastrointestinal barium study demonstrating "apple core" lesion (arrow).

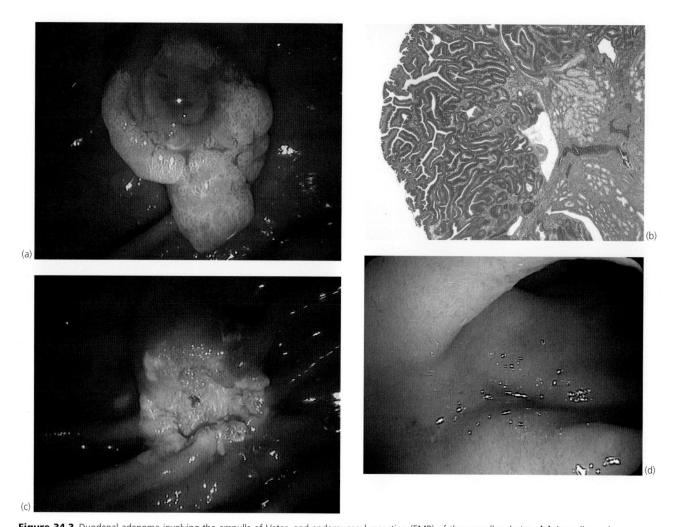

Figure 34.3 Duodenal adenoma involving the ampulla of Vater, and endomucosal resection (EMR) of the ampullary lesion. **(a)** Ampullary adenoma seen at endoscopy. **(b)** Histology showing branching dysplastic glands with crowding and hyperchromatic nuclei. Courtesy of Dr Norio Fukami and Dr T.T. Wu. **(c)** Polypectomy site after EMR of the lesion. **(d)** Healed EMR site. (c,d) Courtesy of Dr Norio Fukami.

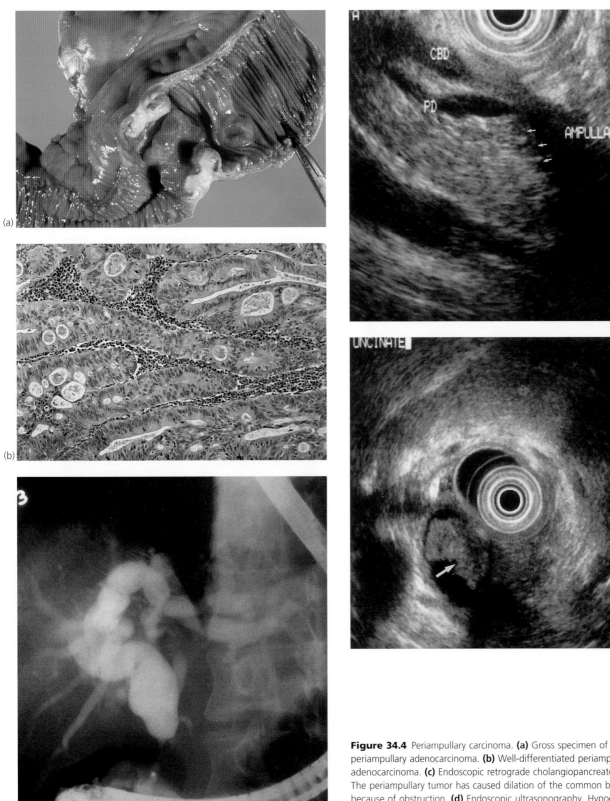

Figure 34.4 Periampullary carcinoma. **(a)** Gross specimen of periampullary adenocarcinoma. **(b)** Well-differentiated periampullary adenocarcinoma. **(c)** Endoscopic retrograde cholangiopancreatography. The periampullary tumor has caused dilation of the common bile duct because of obstruction. **(d)** Endoscopic ultrasonography. Hypoechoic lesion with frond-like extension into the parenchyma of the pancreas (arrows). **(e)** Pedunculated adenoma of the ampulla of Vater has prolapsed into the common bile duct (arrow). CBD, common bile duct; PD, pancreatic duct. (d,e) Courtesy of Dr Tamir Ben-Menachem.

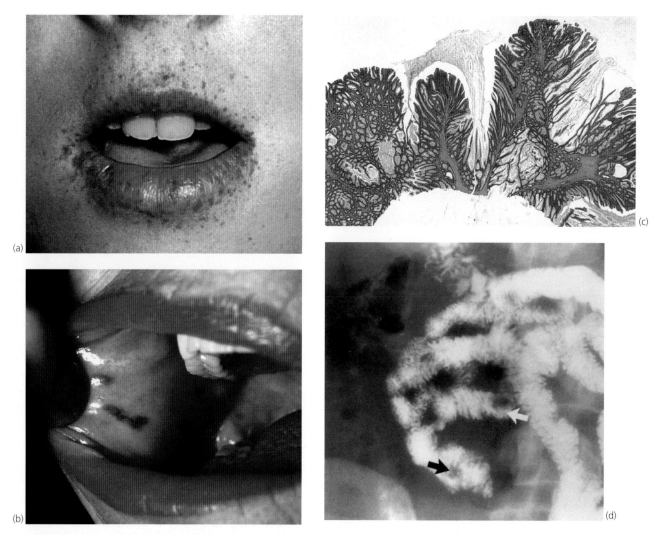

Figure 34.5 Peutz–Jeghers syndrome. **(a,b)** Characteristic buccal and perioral pigment spots characteristic of this syndrome. **(c)** Distinctive polyp with arborizing pattern of growth of the muscularis mucosae extending into the branching fronds of the polyp. **(d)** Small bowel follow-through demonstrating two polyps (arrows) in the midjejeunum. This image was supplied courtesy of M.L. Andres.

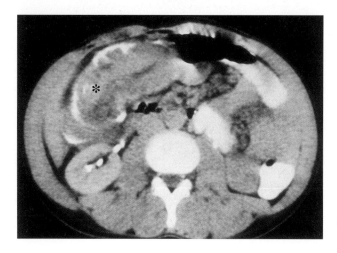

Figure 34.6 Computed tomography scan demonstrating intussusception in the terminal ileum caused by a small intestinal carcinoma (asterisk).

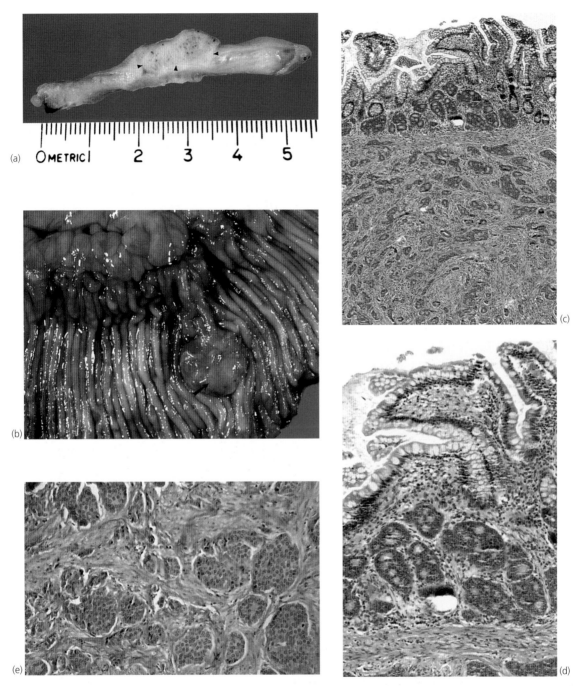

Figure 34.7 Carcinoid tumors of the small intestine. Carcinoid tumors develop deep in the mucosa and grow slowly, extending into the underlying submucosa and the overlying mucosa. They form firm intramural nodules that grossly appear tan or yellow. **(a)** Gross specimen of small intestinal carcinoid appearing as tan nodular tumor. **(b)** Small nodular carcinoid (arrow) can be distinguished in an unfixed opened specimen of this ileal resection. **(c–e)** Histological sections show small intestinal carcinoid tumors characterized by closely packed, round, regular, and monomorphous cell masses, buds, and islands. Lumina and rosette-like structures are present in (c) and (d); (c) demonstrates the desmoplastic reaction responsible for many of the clinical findings of small intestinal carcinoid tumors. Courtesy of Dr Raouf Nakhleh.

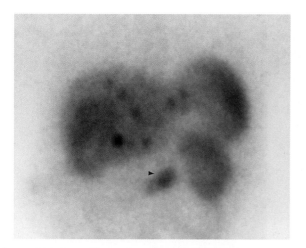

Figure 34.8 Octreotide scan demonstrating small intestinal carcinoid (arrow) and numerous hepatic metastases. Courtesy of Dr K. Karvelis.

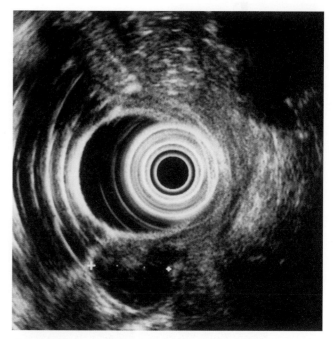

Figure 34.9 Carcinoid tumor. Endoscopic ultrasound demonstrating small noninvasive lesion arising in the third echo layer (submucosa) of the duodenum (marked by cursor +). Courtesy of Dr Tamir Ben-Menachem.

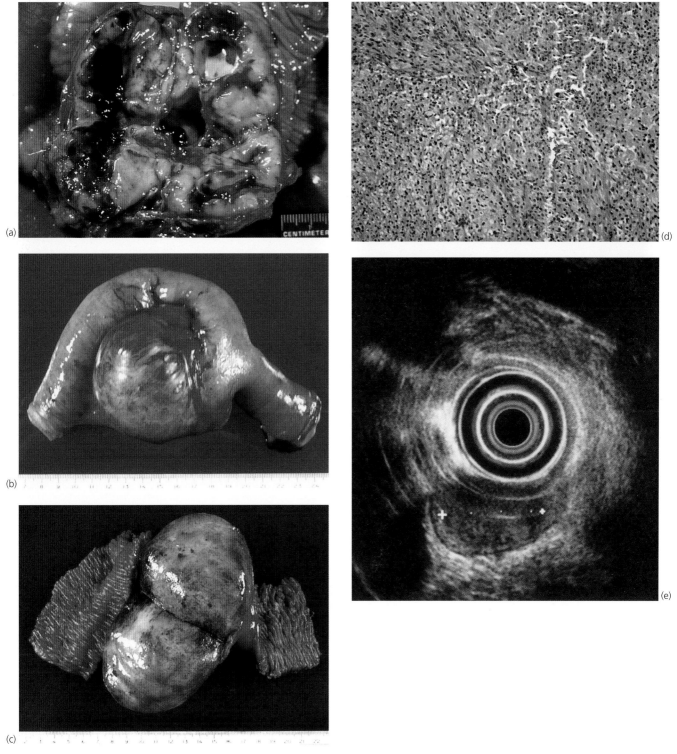

Figure 34.10 Gastrointestinal stromal cell tumor of the small intestine. **(a)** The cut surface of this tumor contains grossly evident areas of hemorrhage and necrosis. This particular lesion was designated a leiomyosarcoma. **(b)** Firm rubbery mass protruding from the wall of the small intestine. **(c)** The cut surface of the tumor depicted in (b); the fleshy tan-pink tumor has focal areas of hemorrhage. **(d)** Histological section demonstrating spindle cell appearance and several mitoses, which suggest malignancy. **(e)** Endoscopic ultrasound. Gastrointestinal stromal cell tumors arising from the fourth echo layer (muscularis propria) of the duodenum. (a) Courtesy of Dr Chan Ma; (c) courtesy of Dr Raouf Nakhleh; (e) courtesy of Dr Tamir Ben-Menachem.

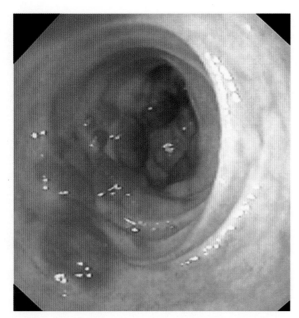

Figure 34.11 Kaposi sarcoma. Violaceous nodules in the duodenal mucosa seen at endoscopy in a patient with acquired immunodeficiency syndrome. Courtesy of Dr Tamir Ben-Menachem.

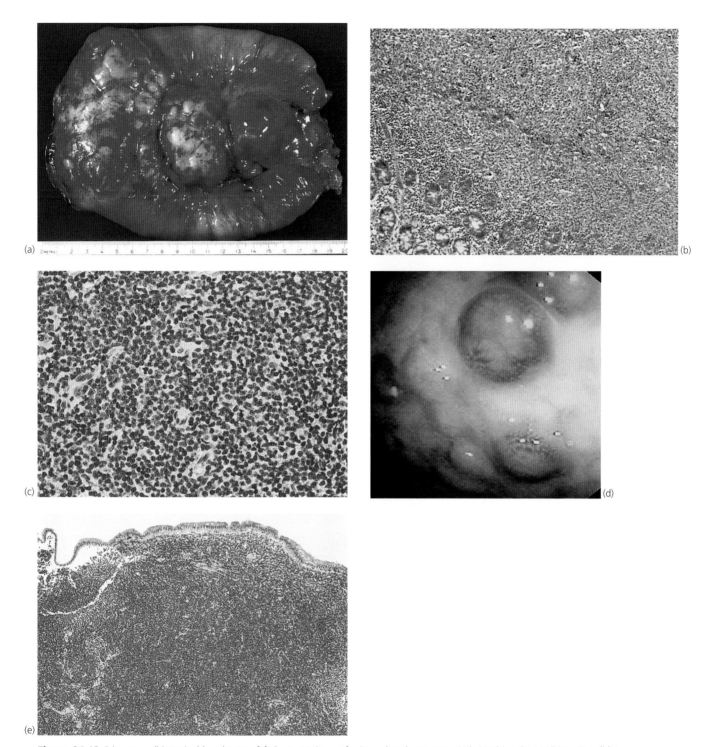

Figure 34.12 Primary small intestinal lymphomas. **(a)** Gross specimen of primary lymphoma extensively involving the small intestine. **(b)** Low-power photomicrographs of diffuse B-cell lymphoma of the small intestine. **(c)** High-power photomicrograph of intestinal B-cell lymphoma of the terminal ileum. **(d)** Mantle cell lymphomatous polyposis of the intestine seen endoscopically. The mucosa is studded with elevated polypoid nodules. **(e)** Low-power photomicrograph of polypoid lymphoma. (a) Courtesy of Dr Raouf Nakhleh.

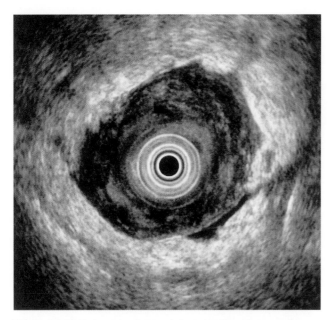

Figure 34.13 Endoscopic ultrasound demonstrating primary small bowel lymphoma of the duodenum. A characteristic irregular hypoechoic mass disrupts the architecture. All echo layers in the duodenum are obliterated, which suggests involvement of the entire duodenal wall. Courtesy of Dr Tamir Ben-Menachem.

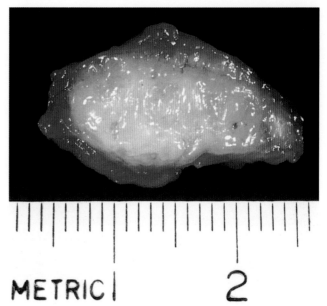

Figure 34.15 Gangliocytic paraganglioma of the duodenum. This is a rare submucosal polypoid tumor. Tumors contain proliferating neurites and Schwann cells, ganglion cells with Schwann cells, or proliferations of clear epithelioid cells resembling carcinoid tumors. Courtesy of Dr Raouf Nakhleh.

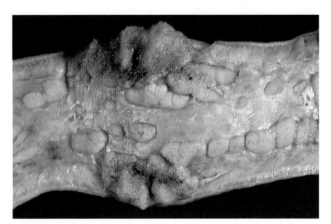

Figure 34.14 Fixed specimen of ileum demonstrating denuded and nodular mucosa characteristic of Crohn's disease, with small bowel lymphoma arising in this setting. Courtesy of Dr Raouf Nakhleh.

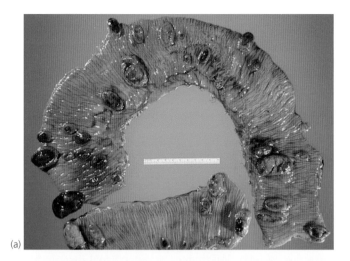

(a)

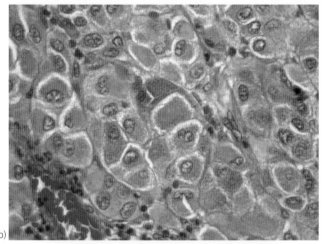

(b)

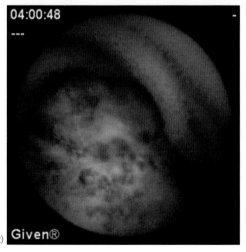

(c)

Figure 34.16 Metastatic melanoma. **(a)** Multiple submucosal metastases appear as plaques and nodules with a "target-like" appearance throughout this section of small intestine. **(b)** Pleomorphic pigmented neoplastic cells account for the black gross appearance seen in (a). **(c)** Pigmented metastatic lesion seen at capsule endoscopy. (b) Courtesy of Dr Chan Ma; (c) courtesy of Dr Alexander Dekovich.

35

Miscellaneous diseases of the small intestine

C. Prakash Gyawali, Marc S. Levin

Ulcers of the small intestine

There are many causes of ulcers of the small intestine (Table 35.1). Primary (idiopathic) small bowel ulcers are diagnosed when other identifiable causes of small bowel ulcers are eliminated. Seventy-five percent are located in the middle to distal ileum. Symptomatic complications include bleeding, perforation, and obstruction. The ulcers vary in size from 0.3 to 5 cm and usually have sharp, demarcated borders. The diagnosis sometimes is made with radiological studies, such as small bowel barium studies (Fig. 35.1) and enteroclysis, or small bowel enteroscopy, but most symptomatic idiopathic ulcers are first diagnosed at exploratory laparotomy. Therapy is dictated by the severity of complications. Perforation and bleeding usually necessitate surgical resection. Intraoperative enteroscopy may be a useful adjunct in the operative diagnosis.

Many medications have been known to cause ulcers and strictures of the small intestine (Table 35.2), and among them nonsteroidal antiinflammatory drugs (NSAIDs) are recognized as common causes. Although the exact pathogenesis is unknown, increased intestinal permeability is believed to increase susceptibility to lumenal macromolecules, bacteria, and toxins. NSAID-mediated cyclooxygenase inhibition is not believed to play an important role in the pathogenesis. NSAID-associated intestinal injury primarily affects the distal small intestine, which leads to diagnostic confusion with Crohn's disease. Therapy includes discontinuation of the offending agent whenever possible. Surgical intervention may be needed for symptomatic strictures or intestinal perforation. When an acceptable alternative medication is unavailable, use of prodrugs such as sulindac or nabumetone may lessen intestinal toxicity.

Other medications implicated as ulcerogens include enteric-coated potassium chloride, ferrous salts (Fig. 35.2),

digoxin, corticosteroids, cytarabine and other chemotherapeutic agents, and clofazimine. Parenteral gold therapy has been associated with enterocolitis characterized by edema and ulceration of the ileum. Ischemic damage can result from drugs that interfere with autonomic regulation of vascular supply to the bowel (see Table 35.2; Fig. 35.3), or with the coagulation process, resulting in intravascular thrombus formation (Fig. 35.4). On the other hand, anticoagulants can cause ulceration from intramucosal and transmural hematoma formation with mucosal pressure necrosis (Fig. 35.5). Drug smugglers sometimes ingest packets of illicit drugs for transport to avoid detection (body packer, Fig. 35.6), the rupture of which can result in overwhelming toxicity from the drug and often death of the smuggler.

Behçet syndrome is associated with intestinal ulceration among less than 1% of patients. These patients have multiple deep ulcers, often bleeding or penetrating, in the ileocecal region. Microthrombosis and vasculitis with intestinal ischemia can result in intestinal ulceration in systemic lupus erythematosus. Mesenteric vasculitis with small-bowel ischemia and stricture formation has been reported in rheumatoid arthritis, scleroderma, polyarteritis nodosa (Fig. 35.7), Henoch–Schönlein purpura, Wegener granulomatosis (Fig. 35.8), giant cell arteritis, Churg–Strauss syndrome, and Sézary syndrome. Spasm of the mesenteric arteries (see Fig. 35.3), sometimes induced by drugs such as ergot or cocaine, can cause mesenteric ischemia and result in ulceration if prolonged. Thrombosis of the mesenteric veins resulting from many conditions, including hypercoagulable states and collagen vascular diseases, can cause transmural hemorrhage, mucosal ulceration, or even perforation of the bowel (see Fig. 35.4). Angiodysplasia consists of ectatic submucosal blood vessels with a thin, overlying mucosal layer (Fig. 35.9), the erosion or rupture of which can result in ulceration and gastrointestinal bleeding. Radiation damage to the intestine can result in fibrosis of the submucosal layers and vascular insufficiency with the formation of intraepithelial telangiectasia (Fig. 35.10). Stricture formation can result in bowel obstruction, sometimes necessitating surgical intervention.

Atlas of Gastroenterology, 4th edition. Edited by Tadataka Yamada, David H. Alpers, Anthony N. Kalloo, Neil Kaplowitz, Chung Owyang, and Don W. Powell. © 2009 Blackwell Publishing, ISBN: 978-1-4051-6909-7

Chronic ulcerative jejunoileitis (CUJ) is a rare clinical syndrome. It occurs among patients with long-standing gluten-sensitive enteropathy in the sixth or seventh decade of life. It is characterized by malabsorption, abdominal pain, and multiple nonmalignant ulcers of the small intestine. Villous atrophy, which is believed to be related to infiltration by activated T cells, usually is present. Mucosal ulceration, crypt hyperplasia, and an inflammatory cell infiltrate also occur and result in malabsorption and protein-losing enteropathy. Other symptoms include midepigastric pain, weight loss, and complications of ulceration, including small bowel obstruction, bleeding, and perforation. The diagnosis should be considered in the care of patients with long-standing gluten-sensitive enteropathy with worsening malabsorption despite continued compliance with a gluten-free diet. Biopsies of the small intestine are essential to establish the diagnosis. Although oral steroids and surgical resection of severely affected bowel have been tried, no specific therapy has been shown to modulate the course of CUJ. Data suggest that CUJ may be an important risk factor for the development of enteropathy-associated T-cell lymphoma (Fig. 35.11).

Necrotizing enterocolitis

Acute jejunitis is largely a disease of nonindustrialized nations. Outbreaks are most frequent in communities in which protein deprivation and poor food hygiene are prevalent. *Clostridium perfringens* type C has been established as the causative organism. The illness is characterized by bloody diarrhea, fever, and abdominal pain. Nonocclusive small-intestinal ischemia results in necrosis of varying severity. Successful treatment involves early recognition, antibiotics, and surgical resection of severely affected bowel segments.

Neonatal necrotizing enterocolitis is a disorder of unknown causation. It affects premature infants and low-birth-weight neonates. It is characterized by focal or diffuse small intestine ulceration and necrosis (Fig. 35.12). Pathogenic etiological factors implicated include prematurity, intestinal ischemia, infectious agents, and initiation of enteral nutrition. There is a high prevalence among infants whose mothers used cocaine during pregnancy, suggesting a pathogenic role of hypoxic and ischemic injury. Although no organism has been consistently identified with neonatal necrotizing enterocolitis, a pathogenic role for bacteria is suggested by the occurrence of epidemics within intensive care units.

Protein-losing gastroenteropathy

The defining characteristic of protein-losing gastroenteropathy is hypoproteinemia resulting from gastric or intestinal loss of plasma proteins in abnormal amounts. A number of intestinal disorders have been implicated in the pathogenesis (Table 35.3; Figs 35.13 and 35.14; see Fig. 35.11). The diagnosis is established with documentation of excessive intestinal protein losses by means of measuring fecal α_1-antitrypsin clearance. There is no specific therapy for protein-losing gastroenteropathy, and management of the primary condition is the only effective remedy.

Table 35.1 Causes of small intestine ulceration

Infectious	Tuberculosis, typhoid, cytomegalovirus infection, syphilis, parasitic infestation, strongyloidosis hyperinfection, *Campylobacter* infection, yersiniosis
Toxic	Acute jejunitis (β-toxin-producing *Clostridium perfringens*), arsenic
Inflammatory	Crohn's disease, systemic lupus erythematosus with high serum antiphospholipid levels, diverticulitis
Mucosal lesions	Gluten-sensitive enteropathy (jejunoileitis)
Tumors:	
Primary	Malignant histiocytosis, lymphoma
Secondary	Adenocarcinoma, melanoma, Kaposi sarcoma
Vascular	Mesenteric insufficiency, giant cell arteritis, vasculitis, vascular abnormality, amyloidosis (ischemic lesion)
Metabolic	Uremia
Drugs	Potassium chloride, nonsteroidal antiinflammatory drugs, antimetabolites
Radiation	Therapeutic, accidental
Idiopathic	Primary ulcer, Behçet syndrome

Table 35.2 Drug-induced small bowel disease

Mechanism	Drugs implicated
Erosive damage:	Nonsteroidal antiinflammatory drugs, potassium chloride
Ischemic damage:	
Hypotension	Antihypertensives, diuretics
Direct vasoconstriction	Norepinephrine, dopamine, vasopressin
Decreased splanchnic blood flow	Digoxin
Increased sympathetic stimulation	Cocaine
Vasospasm	Ergot compounds
Arterial/venous thrombosis	Oral contraceptives
Hematoma formation	Anticoagulants
Motility disorders:	
Pseudoobstruction	Anticholinergics, phenothiazines, tricyclic antidepressants, opioids, verapamil, clonidine, cyclosporine
Neurotoxicity	Vincristine
Narcotic bowel syndrome	Narcotics
Malabsorption:	
Interference with intralumenal digestion	Tetracycline, cholestyramine, mineral oil, aluminum and magnesium hydroxide
Increased intestinal transit	Prokinetic agents, cathartics
Mucosal injury	Colchicine, neomycin, methotrexate, methyldopa, allopurinol, mefenamic acid
Direct inhibition of absorption	Sodium aminosalicylate, thiazide diuretics
Inhibition of epithelial cell turnover:	
Erosive enteritis	Methotrexate, 5-fluorouracil, actinomycin D, doxorubicin, cytosine arabinoside, bleomycin, vincristine, ara-C, interleukin-2

Table 35.3 Causes of protein-losing enteropathy

Increased interstitial pressure:
Congenital intestinal lymphangiectasia
Mesenteric lymphatic obstruction
  Tuberculosis
  Sarcoidosis
  Lymphoma
  Retroperitoneal fibrosis

Increased central venous pressure:
Constrictive pericarditis
Congestive heart failure

Ulcerative disease:
Erosive gastritis or enteritis
H. pylori associated gastritis
Neoplasia – carcinoma or lymphoma
Crohn's disease
Pseudomembranous enterocolitis
Acute graft-versus-host disease

Nonulcerative disease:
Giant hypertrophic gastropathy (Ménétrier disease)
Hypertrophic hypersecretory gastropathy
Viral enteritides
Bacterial overgrowth
Parasitic diseases (e.g., malaria, giardiasis, schistosomiasis, helminth infections)
Cystic fibrosis
Whipple disease
Allergic enteritis
Eosinophilic gastroenteritis
Gluten-sensitive enteropathy
Tropical sprue
Systemic lupus erythematosus

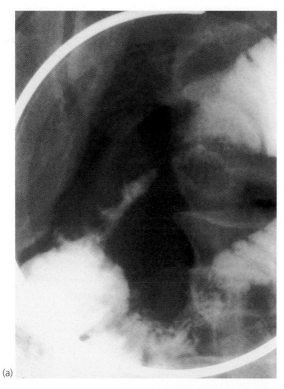

(a)

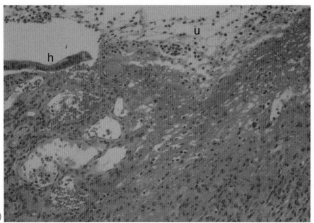

(b)

Figure 35.1 (a) Small bowel follow-through image of a patient who sought treatment with clinical features of obstruction of the small intestine shows intestinal spasm associated with ulceration and dilation of the proximal segment. The patient underwent exploratory laparotomy and resection of the affected bowel segment. Courtesy of Dr. Dennis Balfe. **(b)** Histopathological section of the resected segment of small bowel shows ulceration (u) with epithelialization of the healing edge (h). A nifedipine capsule was found in the vicinity of the ulcer at operation, raising the possibility of a causative association. Courtesy of Dr Paul Swanson.

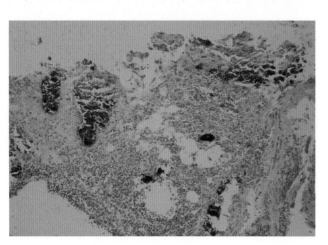

Figure 35.2 Prussian blue stain shows iron deposition in an ulcer of the terminal ileum. Iron tablets were thought to be the cause of small bowel ulceration and occult gastrointestinal bleeding in this patient. Courtesy of Dr Paul Swanson.

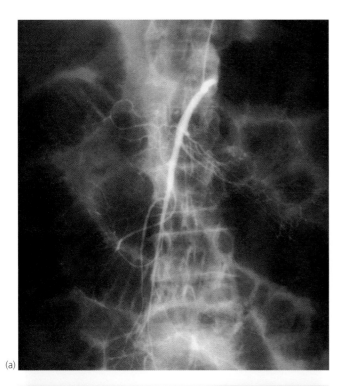

(a)

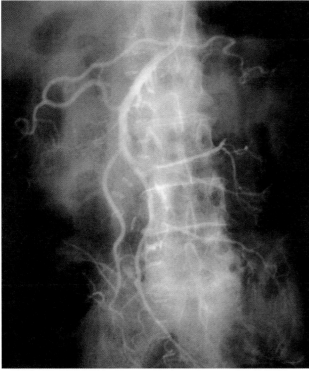

(b)

Figure 35.3 (a) Mesenteric arteriogram of a patient with abdominal pain and ileus shows spasm of the superior mesenteric circulation. Prolonged spasm of the mesenteric vessels can lead to vascular insufficiency and intestinal ulceration. **(b)** Repeat arteriography after intraarterial infusion of papaverine shows relief of the spasm and ileus and restoration of normal blood flow to the intestine. Courtesy of Dr Daniel Picus.

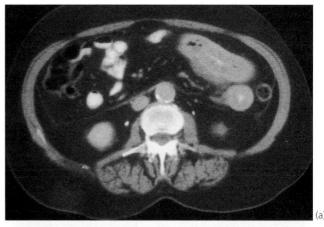

(a)

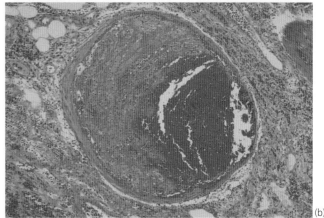

(b)

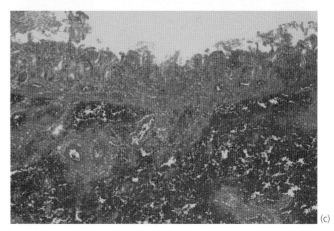

(c)

Figure 35.4 (a) Computed tomographic scan of a patient with superior mesenteric venous thrombosis shows a thickened loop of small bowel. This can cause mucosal sloughing with ulceration and intestinal perforation that necessitates exploratory laparotomy and bowel resection. Courtesy of Dr. Dennis Balfe. **(b)** Section through the superior mesenteric vein shows acute and organizing thrombus within the lumen. Courtesy of Dr. Paul Swanson. **(c)** Section through surgically resected segment of bowel shows transmural hemorrhage and acute inflammation with focal epithelial necrosis. Courtesy of Dr Paul Swanson.

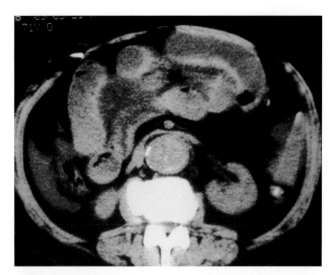

Figure 35.5 Abdominal computed tomographic scan of a patient who took an overdose of warfarin demonstrates bowel hemorrhage. The intestinal wall appears thickened because of the presence of intramural hematomas. Required therapeutic interventions included correction of coagulopathy and surgical resection of the affected bowel segments. Courtesy of Dr Dennis Balfe.

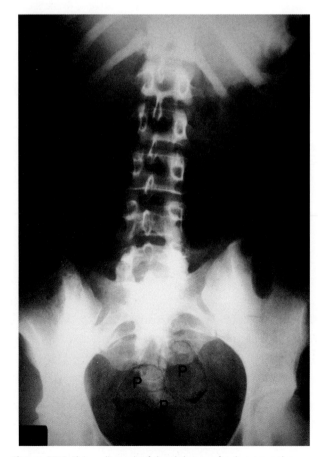

Figure 35.6 Plain radiograph of the abdomen of a drug smuggler shows multiple packets (P) of illicit drugs in the bowel lumen. Body-packer syndrome occurs when rupture of the drug-containing packets causes severe drug toxicity. Courtesy of Dr Dennis Balfe.

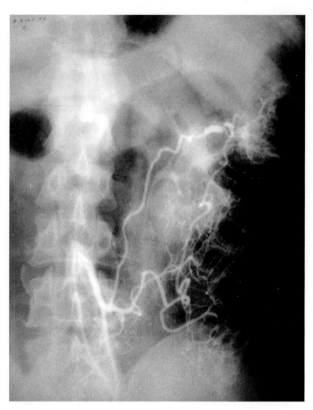

Figure 35.7 Mesenteric arteriogram of a patient with polyarteritis nodosa shows beaded appearance of the medium-sized arteries. Vasculitis of the arteries supplying the bowel can lead to intestinal ulceration. Angiography of other vessels, including the renal arteries, can show aneurysmal dilation. Courtesy of Dr Dennis Balfe.

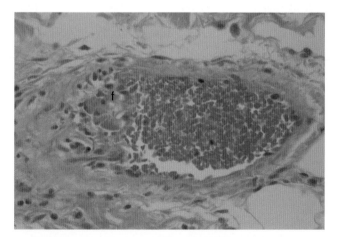

Figure 35.8 Section through a mesenteric artery shows evidence of vasculitis and fibrinoid necrosis (f) involving the arterial wall. This patient with Wegener granulomatosis had bowel ischemia, ulceration, and gastrointestinal bleeding that necessitated surgical resection of the affected bowel segment. Courtesy of Dr Paul Swanson.

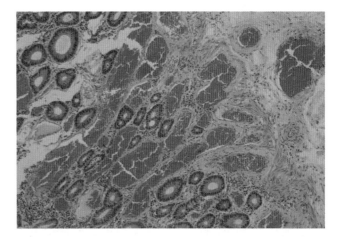

Figure 35.9 Section through angiodysplasia of the small intestine shows typical thickened and ectatic vasculature involving mucosa and submucosa (red). Rupture or erosion of the mucosa over areas of angiodysplasia can result in ulceration and gastrointestinal bleeding that can be difficult to localize. Intraoperative enteroscopy sometimes is necessary to identify the segment of bowel that needs surgical resection. Courtesy of Dr Paul Swanson.

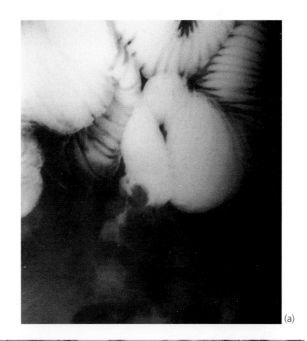

(a)

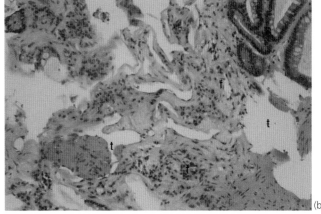

Figure 35.10 (a) Intestinal stricture with food impaction and dilation of proximal segment in a patient who had received radiation therapy for lymphoma. This patient had clinical features of small bowel obstruction and underwent surgical resection of the affected segment. Courtesy of Dr Dennis Balfe. **(b)** Histopathological section of the surgically resected segment shows fibrosis of the lamina propria (f) with mucosal telangiectasis (t), a common finding with radiation-induced intestinal injury. Courtesy of Dr Paul Swanson.

(b)

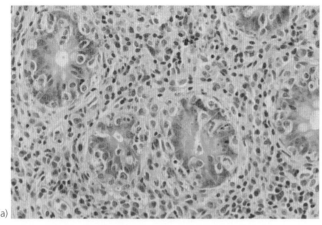

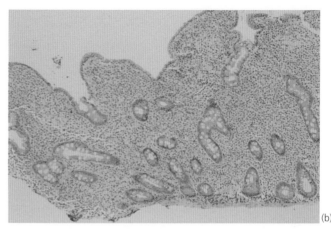

(a)

(b)

Figure 35.11 (a) Infiltration of a segment of small bowel with large atypical lymphoid cells consistent with enteropathy-associated T-cell lymphoma in a patient with refractory celiac disease. This condition can present with malabsorption, ulceration of the intestine, and protein-losing enteropathy. **(b)** Monotonous plasma cell infiltration of small-bowel mucosa in a patient with α-heavy-chain disease, which can also result in malabsorption and protein-losing enteropathy. Courtesy of Dr Paul Swanson.

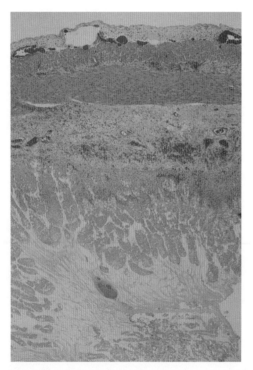

Figure 35.12 Section through a segment of bowel from a child with necrotizing enterocolitis shows submucosal hemorrhage, epithelial necrosis, and an acute inflammatory cell infiltrate. Courtesy of Dr Paul Swanson.

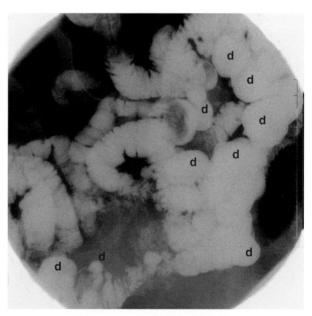

Figure 35.13 Images from small bowel follow-through series show multiple, large diverticula (d) of the small bowel. This patient had malabsorption caused by bacterial overgrowth. Treatment included long-term antibiotic therapy and correction of nutritional and vitamin deficiencies.

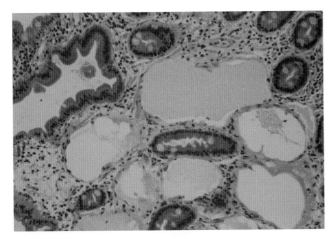

Figure 35.14 Intestinal lymphangiectasia can present as malabsorption and protein-losing enteropathy. Section shows lakes of ectatic lymphatic vessels within the lamina propria of the small intestine. Courtesy of Dr Paul Swanson.

36

Colon: anatomy and structural anomalies

Steven M. Cohn, Elisa H. Birnbaum

The gastroenterologist often encounters patients who have undergone previous surgical procedures involving the colon or rectum. An understanding of the postsurgical anatomy of the gastrointestinal tract often is crucial for effective treatment of these patients. Figures 36.1 and 36.2 illustrate the postsurgical anatomy that results from surgical procedures commonly performed on patients with inflammatory bowel disease or colorectal carcinoma.

Hirschsprung disease is rare among adults but must be considered in the evaluation of chronic constipation dating back to childhood. Hirschsprung disease can be a challenging diagnosis to establish for adult patients. It is a result of failure of neural crest cells (precursors of ganglion cells) to complete their caudal migration during normal colonic development. The aganglionic segment does not relax and causes functional obstruction. Anorectal manometry is often useful in the evaluation of suspected Hirschsprung disease. Figures 36.3 and 36.4 illustrate anorectal manometric findings for healthy adults and patients with Hirschsprung disease.

A normal sphincter profile (resting pressures 40–80 mmHg and squeeze pressures 80–160 mmHg) and an abnormal rectoanal inhibitory reflex typically occur among patients with Hirschsprung disease. The internal sphincter does not relax in response to rectal distention among patients with Hirschsprung disease, and an abnormal reflex during manometry aids in the diagnosis. However, the rectoanal inhibitory reflex may be normal among patients with short-segment Hirschsprung disease. These patients may have a short segment as the primary disease, or the short segment may be residual disease after surgical intervention. High anal resting pressures and impaired rectal emptying may occur.

Colonic volvulus is an infrequent cause of colonic obstruction. It may be difficult to diagnose without a high degree of suspicion. Volvulus is classified and managed according to its location in the colon. Figures 36.5 and 36.6 illustrate the radiographic findings for sigmoid volvulus and cecal volvulus. Sigmoid volvulus accounts for approximately 60% of all instances of volvulus in the United States. It usually occurs among elderly persons, patients in extended care facilities, or in patients with neuropsychiatric disorders. *Cecal volvulus* accounts for less than 20% of all cases of colonic volvulus and generally occurs among younger patients. It is believed to be caused by anomalous fixation of the right colon that leads to a freely mobile cecum. Other precipitating factors include adhesions from previous operations, pregnancy, and obstructing lesions of the left colon.

Atlas of Gastroenterology, 4th edition. Edited by Tadataka Yamada, David H. Alpers, Anthony N. Kalloo, Neil Kaplowitz, Chung Owyang, and Don W. Powell. © 2009 Blackwell Publishing, ISBN: 978-1-4051-6909-7

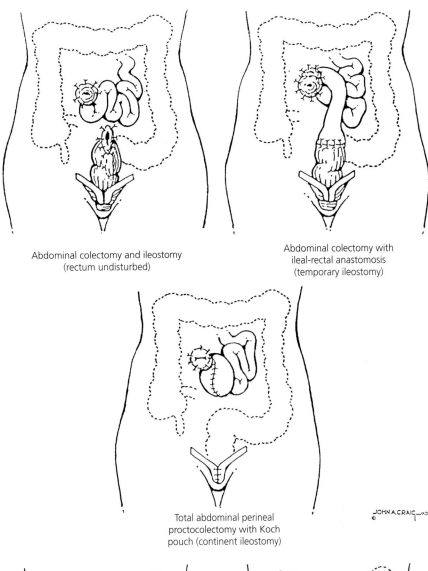

Abdominal colectomy and ileostomy
(rectum undisturbed)

Abdominal colectomy with
ileal-rectal anastomosis
(temporary ileostomy)

Total abdominal perineal
proctocolectomy with Koch
pouch (continent ileostomy)

JOHN A.CRAIG—MD

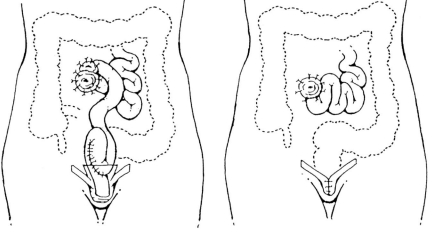

Total abdominal colectomy,
mucosal proctectomy, ileal
pouch anal anastomosis
(temporary ileostomy)

Total abdominal proctocoiectomy

Figure 36.1 Surgical options for ulcerative colitis. Abdominal colectomy with ileostomy usually is performed as an emergency procedure when the diagnosis is unclear. The rectum is removed at a later operation. Total abdominal colectomy with ileal–rectal anastomosis is rarely performed for ulcerative colitis. It is a more common surgical approach for Crohn's colitis. Total abdominal perineal proctocolectomy with Koch pouch is a continent ileostomy performed for the rare patient who has undergone removal of the rectum. Ileostomy requires intubation for passage of fecal contents. It is never performed as a primary procedure. In total abdominal colectomy with ileal pouch anal anastomosis, a continent anal reservoir allows normal evacuation of stool. The ileostomy is closed once healing is complete. Total abdominal proctocolectomy with permanent end ileostomy is performed on patients with inadequate anal sphincters.

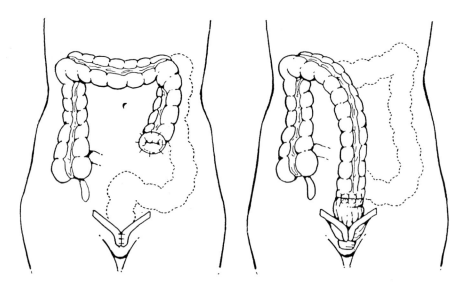

Abdominal perineal
proctosigmoidectomy with
permanent end colostomy

Low anterior resection
of rectosigmoid with
colorectal anastomosis

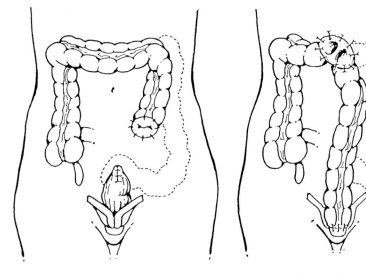

Hartmann resection

Low anterior resection
of rectosigmoid with
coloanal anastomosis
and protecting loop-
transverse colostomy

JOHN A. CRAIG—MD
©

Figure 36.2 Surgical options for
rectal cancer. Abdominal perineal
proctosigmoidectomy with permanent end
colostomy is performed on patients with
carcinoma in the lower third of the rectum.
Low anterior resection of the rectosigmoid
with colorectal anastomosis is performed for
lesions in the upper and some lesions in the
middle third of the rectum. Hartmann
resection is performed as an emergency
resection with an unprepared colon or
inadequate anal sphincter to allow
anastomosis without incontinence. Low
anterior resection of the rectosigmoid with
coloanal anastomosis and protecting loop-
transverse colostomy is performed on patients
with carcinoma in the lower third of the
rectum who have a spared functional anal
sphincter. The transverse colostomy is closed
electively after healing of the coloanal
anastomosis.

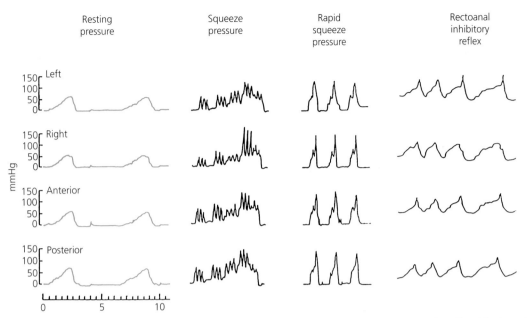

Figure 36.3 Normal anal manometric results with hydraulic capillary system. Resting pressures (normal 40–80 mmHg) are obtained as the catheter is pulled through the anal sphincter with the patient at rest. Squeeze pressures (normal 80–160 mmHg) are measured as the catheter is pulled through the anal sphincter in 0.5-cm increments with the patient squeezing. Rapid squeeze pressure (normal 80–160 mmHg) is determined as the catheter is removed quickly while the patient is generating maximal squeeze effort. The rectoanal inhibitory reflex is measured with a catheter placed within the sphincter zone. The rectal balloon is distended in 10-cm increments. A normal rectoanal inhibitory reflex is manifested by an increase over baseline, followed by involuntary relaxation below baseline, followed by return to baseline.

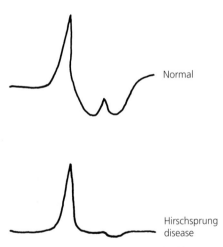

Figure 36.4 Rectoanal inhibitory reflex among healthy persons and those with Hirschsprung disease. Among healthy persons, sphincter presence increases over baseline, relaxes below baseline, and returns to baseline. Among persons with Hirschsprung disease, an increase over baseline occurs, but no relaxation of the internal anal sphincter is observed.

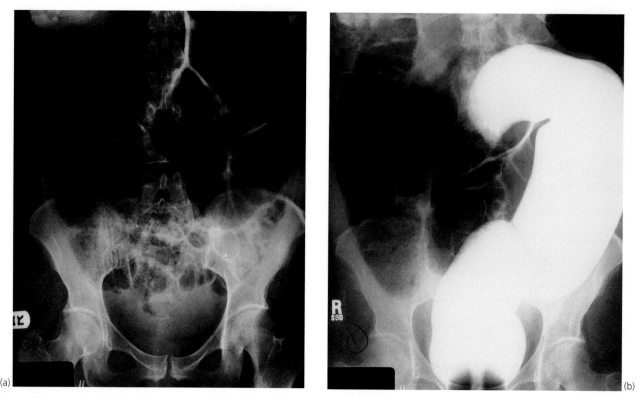

Figure 36.5 Sigmoid volvulus. **(a)** Gas-filled, dilated colon is evident on a plain radiograph of the abdomen. There is a paucity of gas in the rectum. **(b)** Hypaque enema image shows tapering of the column of contrast material at the site of torsion ("bird's beak sign") of the sigmoid colon.

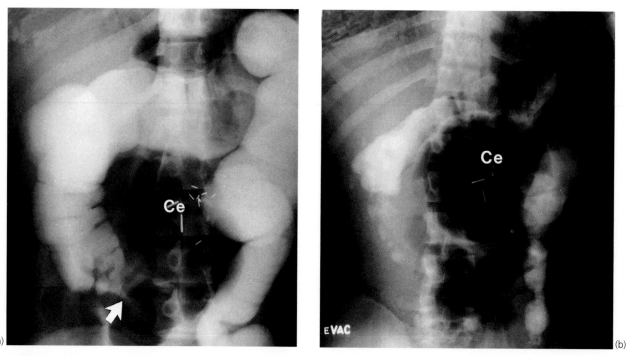

Figure 36.6 Cecal volvulus. **(a)** Hypaque enema image shows tapering of the column of contrast material at the site of torsion (arrow) and displacement of the cecum toward the epigastrium. **(b)** Postevacuation radiograph shows gas-filled, dilated cecum (Ce) in the epigastrium. There is a paucity of gas in the normal location of the cecum in the right lower quadrant of the abdomen.

37

Inflammatory bowel disease

William F. Stenson, William J. Tremaine, Russell D. Cohen

Pathology

Ulcerative colitis

The gross appearance of ulcerative colitis may be uniform involvement throughout the colon or a sharp demarcation between abnormal mucosa distally and normal mucosa proximally (Fig. 37.1). The appearance also may be diffusely abnormal, with a gradation from mild edema in the cecum to submucosal hemorrhage in the transverse colon to frank ulceration in the rectum. Sometimes the ulcerations can be seen only in histological sections but, in other cases, large distinct ulcerations may be seen in the gross specimen.

At histological examination, the inflammatory infiltrate in ulcerative colitis usually extends down to the muscularis mucosae. The inflammatory infiltrate includes both neutrophils, a sign of acute inflammation, and macrophages and lymphocytes, signs of more chronic inflammation. Crypt abscess (Fig. 37.2), a collection of neutrophils in a colonic crypt, is characteristic of ulcerative colitis but also is seen in other diseases, including Crohn's colitis. Crypt branching (Fig. 37.3) occurs in many patients with ulcerative colitis and persists even when the disease is inactive and the mucosal inflammation has resolved. Crypt branching is uncommon in other disease processes. Inflammatory polyps in ulcerative colitis may be filiform (Fig. 37.4), or they may be broad based and sessile. Often they are covered with a whitish cap of exudate (Fig. 37.5).

It is possible to screen for carcinoma in ulcerative colitis by identifying areas of dysplasia (Fig. 37.6). Dysplastic mucosa can be villiform owing to the proliferation of epithelial cells. At low-power microscopic examination, low-grade dysplasia is marked by enlarged goblet cells and atypical hyperchromatic nuclei, whereas high-grade dysplasia is characterized by more marked nuclear pleomorphism and pseudostratification of the nuclei. Under higher power magnification, low-grade dysplasia shows hyperchromatic cells with preservation of nuclear polarity, whereas high-grade dysplasia shows complete loss of nuclear polarity. Biopsy screening for dysplasia may reveal carcinoma in situ. Adenocarcinoma of the colon occurs with increased frequency in ulcerative colitis (Fig. 37.7) and Crohn's colitis. Adenocarcinoma of the small intestine occurs with increased frequency in Crohn's disease of the small intestine (Fig. 37.8).

The earliest pathological lesion in Crohn's disease is an aphthous ulcer. These small, sharply demarcated ulcers often occur over submucosal lymphoid aggregates. As the disease progresses, aphthoid ulcers can grow to form transverse or round ulcers (Fig. 37.9). Gross specimens in Crohn's disease may show intersecting longitudinal and transverse ulcerations resulting in a "cobblestone" appearance (Fig. 37.10). In ulcerative colitis, involvement of the colon is continuous, whereas in Crohn's disease of either the intestine or colon, involvement may be discontinuous, with areas of involvement interspersed with grossly normal areas (Fig. 37.11).

The inflammatory process in Crohn's disease often is transmural. In transmural inflammation, there are areas of clustering of inflammatory cells in all layers of the intestinal wall. Frequently, this transmural inflammation includes granulomas and lymphoid aggregates with germinal centers (Fig. 37.12). In some sections, granulomas are seen in both the submucosa and the serosa. Narrowing of the small intestine as a result of Crohn's disease can lead to obstruction (Fig. 37.13).

Extraintestinal manifestations

A common dermal manifestation of both ulcerative colitis and Crohn's colitis is pyoderma gangrenosum (Figs 37.14 and 37.15), marked by sharply defined areas of ulceration with serpiginous borders. Iritis is a potentially serious ophthalmological complication of ulcerative colitis and Crohn's disease. Iritis is accompanied by conjunctival injection (Fig. 37.16). Aphthous ulcers, which occur in the intestine and

Atlas of Gastroenterology, 4th edition. Edited by Tadataka Yamada, David H. Alpers, Anthony N. Kalloo, Neil Kaplowitz, Chung Owyang, and Don W. Powell. © 2009 Blackwell Publishing, ISBN: 978-1-4051-6909-7

colon in Crohn's disease, also can occur on the tongue, oral mucosa, or lips (Fig. 37.17).

Perianal Crohn's disease is marked by fistulae, bluish discoloration, edematous tags, and ulceration (Figs 37.18–37.20). Direct or "metastatic" extension to the external genitalia may involve painful swelling of the scrotum, penis, or labia (Fig. 37.21).

Radiology

Ulcerative colitis

Plain radiographs are helpful in establishing the diagnosis of toxic megacolon, which is characterized by dilation of a colonic segment, typically the transverse colon (Fig. 37.22). Double-contrast studies identify early changes in ulcerative colitis that would not be seen with full-column studies. Early changes in ulcerative colitis include mucosal edema, granularity, and loss of haustral markings (Fig. 37.23a). As the disease progresses, ulcerations develop with penetration of the mucosal layer (see Fig. 37.23b). Undermining of the mucosal layer gives the characteristic appearance of collar-button ulcers (Fig. 37.24).

Although ulcerative colitis tends to involve the left colon more than the right, the inflammatory process may affect the cecum and result in severe narrowing. The terminal ileum is affected among about 10% of patients with pancolitis. Involvement of the terminal ileum is manifested radiographically with thickening of the mucosal folds, spasm, and irritability. The ileocecal valve in ulcerative colitis tends to be gaping, as opposed to its position in Crohn's disease, in which it tends to be narrowed.

Crohn's disease

Crohn's disease can cause narrowing and obstruction of the duodenum (Fig. 37.25). Although isolated Crohn's disease in the duodenum can occur, disease usually is present elsewhere in the intestine as well.

One early radiographic finding in Crohn's disease is the presence of aphthous ulcers (Fig. 37.26). Another early radiographic finding in Crohn's disease is diffuse mucosal granularity. In the small bowel, this pattern is caused by widening and blunting of the villi with inflammatory infiltrate. As the inflammation progresses, there is thickening and distortion of the valvulae conniventes. Progression of the inflammatory process results in both transverse and longitudinal ulcers. These ulcers frequently cross each other in a grid pattern. The remaining islands of mucosa become thickened and have a cobblestone pattern on barium studies. Ulcers seen in cross-section have a collar-button appearance (Fig. 37.27).

Infiltration and thickening of the bowel wall produce the radiographic appearance of separation of loops of small bowel (Fig. 37.28). The loops of barium-filled intestine are pushed apart by a thickened edematous mesentery and matted mesenteric nodes. Narrowing of the intestinal lumen makes the loops appear farther apart. Severe inflammation results in a rigid segment of bowel with a narrowed lumen and total loss of mucosal detail. This constellation results in the "string sign" (Fig. 37.29) and is most commonly seen in the terminal ileum.

Terminal ileal involvement includes stricture (Figs 37.30 and 37.31), ulcers (see Fig. 37.31), and fissures (see Fig. 37.30). The standard surgical approach to Crohn's disease of the terminal ileum is resection of the affected segment with construction of an ileocolic anastomosis. Disease activity typically recurs on the ileal side of the anastomosis (Fig. 37.32). The terminal ileum or an ileocolic anastomosis can be depicted with oral barium examination (see Fig. 37.31), by means of enteroclysis (see Fig. 37.30), by computed tomographic enterography (Fig 37.33), by magnetic resonance enterographs (Fig 37.34), video wireless capsule endoscopy (Fig. 37.35), or by means of pneumocolon (oral administration of barium and insufflation of air into the colon).

Double tracking, which shows the presence of longitudinal extralumenal collections of barium paralleling the lumen, can be seen in diverticulitis as well as Crohn's disease. In Crohn's disease, this radiographic pattern reflects penetration of mucosa by ulcers and the development of a long intramural fistula.

Perianal Crohn's disease has a distinctive radiographic pattern of ulcers and deep lateral fissures. Extension of the ulcers results in branching sinus tracts and fistulae reaching to the skin.

Endoscopy

Ulcerative colitis

In quiescent ulcerative colitis, there is distortion of vascular markings without edema or erythema (Fig. 37.36). In mildly and moderately active disease, there is edema and erythema granularity and distortion of vascular markings (Figs 37.37 and 37.38).

In severe ulcerative colitis, the mucosa is friable, erythematous, and edematous with ulceration (Fig. 37.39). Although the severity of inflammation seen endoscopically may lessen as one moves proximally in the colon in ulcerative colitis, the degree of inflammation at a given level is uniform through the entire circumference of the colon. Thus, ulceration in ulcerative colitis always occurs in areas of diffuse edema and erythema. The mucosa surrounding ulcerations may become so edematous that the result is a coarsely nodular deformity (Fig. 37.40). The more proximally one moves, the less severe the endoscopic changes are likely to be. Sometimes there is sharp demarcation between normal and inflamed tissue (Fig. 37.41).

Pseudopolyps can occur in ulcerative colitis of any degree of activity (Figs 37.42–37.44; see Fig. 37.37).

Figure 37.45 shows sequential endoscopic studies of a patient with severe pancolitis. At the first colonoscopy (see Fig. 37.45a), there was almost universal ulceration with only a few islands of remaining mucosa. In Figure 37.45b, the mucosa is beginning to heal, and less ulcer and more epithelium are seen. In Figure 37.45c, there is further regression of ulcers with pseudopolyp formation. Full restoration of the epithelium with persistence of pseudopolyps is shown in Fig. 37.45d.

Dysplasia is most often found either when carcinoma is present in the colon or when the patient is at high risk for carcinoma. Dysplastic mucosa usually appears normal through an endoscope. When dysplasia is associated with a polypoid mass or other endoscopic abnormality, the lesion is called a *dysplasia-associated lesion or mass* (DALM) (Fig. 37.46). Identification of a DALM is an indication for resection because of the very high probability of an associated malignant tumor.

Ulcerative colitis can be treated surgically with total proctocolectomy and construction of an ileal pouch with an ileoanal anastomosis. Pouchitis (inflammation of the ileal pouch) occurs among some patients after this procedure. The endoscopic features of pouchitis include erythema, edema, mucous exudate, and superficial ulceration (Fig. 37.47).

Crohn's disease
Aphthous ulcers are the earliest endoscopic lesions in Crohn's disease (Figs 37.48 and 37.49) and are are surrounded by erythematous rings (Fig. 37.50). The mucosa between aphthous ulcers is endoscopically normal. As Crohn's disease progresses, small aphthoid ulcers grow to form deep excavated ulcers with distinct margins (Fig. 37.51). These ulcers may be rounded (Fig. 37.52) or linear

(Fig. 37.53). "Cobblestoning" is an endoscopic feature seen most often in Crohn's disease (Fig. 37.54). Cobblestoning is caused by the intersection of longitudinal and transverse ulcers in a grid pattern, with thickened erythematous mucosal bumps appearing between the ulcers. Severe Crohn's colitis can demonstrate diffuse ulceration in one portion of the colon (Fig. 37.55) and deep longitudinal ulcers in another portion (Fig. 37.56).

In some patients with involvement of the terminal ileum there is marked stenosis, and the colonoscope cannot be inserted into the ileum (Fig. 37.57). If the ileum can be entered, endoscopic examination reveals patterns similar to those in the involved part of the colon with longitudinal ulcers and cobblestoning (Fig. 37.58). This is differentiated from the endoscopic appearance of "backwash ileitis" in ulcerative colitis, in which there may be edema but no ulcers.

Crohn's disease of the cecum and terminal ileum often is managed with surgical resection of the affected segment and construction of an ileocolic anastomosis. Crohn's disease typically recurs on the ileal side of the anastomosis (Fig. 37.59). The endoscopic features of recurrent Crohn's disease are much the same as those of the initial presentation: ulcers, edema, erythema, and granularity.

Fistula formation is a common complication of Crohn's disease. Fistulae form between the affected segment of intestine and the skin, urinary bladder, vagina, or other segments of the intestine. Fistulae usually are easier to define with a barium enema or small bowel follow-through examination than with endoscopy. In some instances, however, fistulae can be easily appreciated with endoscopy (Fig. 35.60).

Successful medical therapy for active Crohn's disease results in healing of ulcers and loss of friability. In some cases, the endoscopic features revert to normal. In other cases, however, some superficial scarring, mucous exudate, and loss of vascular markings remain (Fig. 37.61).

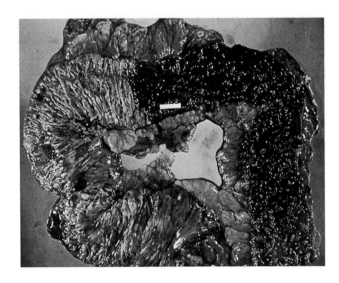

Figure 37.1 Colectomy specimen from a patient with ulcerative colitis demonstrates sharp demarcation in the midtransverse colon between involved and uninvolved mucosa. Courtesy of Dr Ira Kodner.

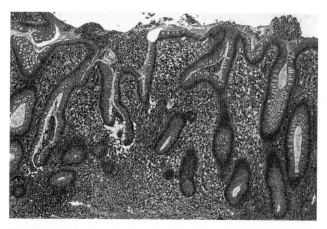

Figure 37.2 Histology of active ulcerative colitis, with distorted colonic crypts, inflammatory infiltrates, and crypt abscesses. Courtesy of Dr John Hart, Chicago, IL.

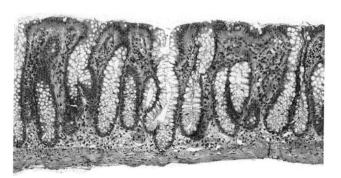

Figure 37.3 Histology of quiescent ulcerative colitis, with branched colonic crypts but no active inflammatory infiltrate. Courtesy of Dr John Hart, Chicago, IL.

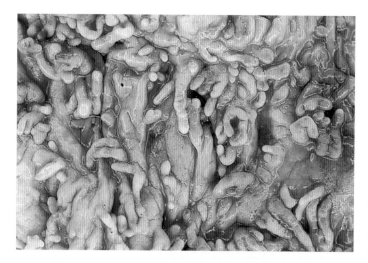

Figure 37.4 When inflammatory polyps assume the filiform appearance seen here, they are readily recognizable grossly; when smaller in numbers and rounded, they can be confused with adenomas or hyperplastic polyps.

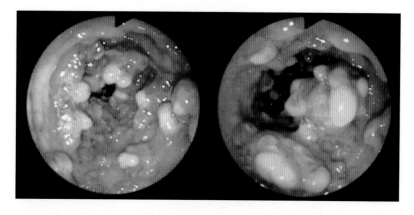

Figure 37.5 Multiple pseudopolyps in ulcerative colitis. Their surface is smooth and glistening. Detailed view of exudate creating whitish caps.

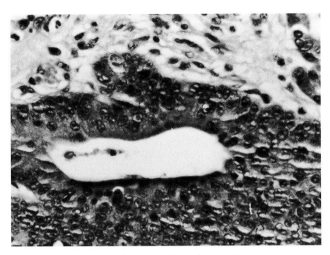

Figure 37.6 High-grade dysplasia with nuclear stratification, nuclear and cellular pleomorphism, and loss of nuclear polarity. Courtesy of Dr David Lacey.

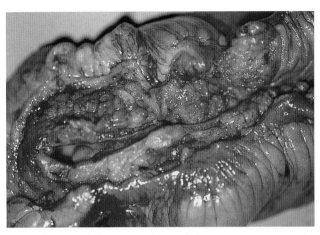

Figure 37.8 Gross specimen of Crohn's disease of the small intestine with adenocarcinoma. Courtesy of Dr Ira Kodner.

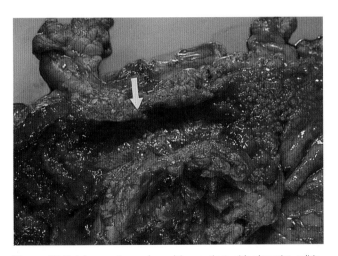

Figure 37.7 Adenocarcinoma (arrow) in a patient with ulcerative colitis. Courtesy of Dr Ira Kodner.

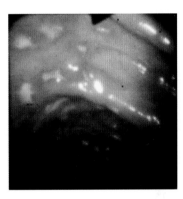

Figure 37.9 Crohn's colitis with discrete small, round ulcers separated by normal mucosa.

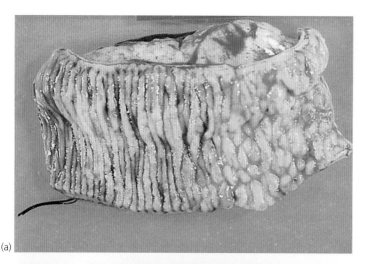

(a)

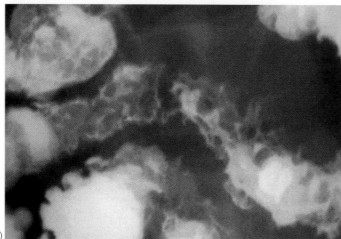

(b)

Figure 37.10 (a) One end of this ileal segment shows prominent cobblestoning, believed to result from the combined effect of multiple, small, longitudinal and transverse linear ulcers isolating areas of edematous mucosa. The mucosa is nearly normal at the other end, although variably severe and patchy involvement is present as pale areas of mucosal swelling and distortion. **(b)** Cobblestoning also can be detected radiographically, as in this case of Crohn's disease.

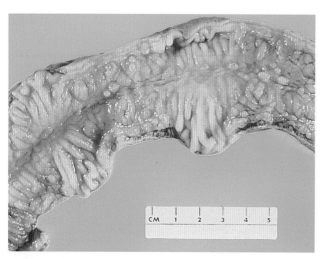

Figure 37.11 Skip areas in Crohn's disease of the jejunum are segments of involvement alternating with relatively normal segments. Courtesy of Dr Ira Kodner.

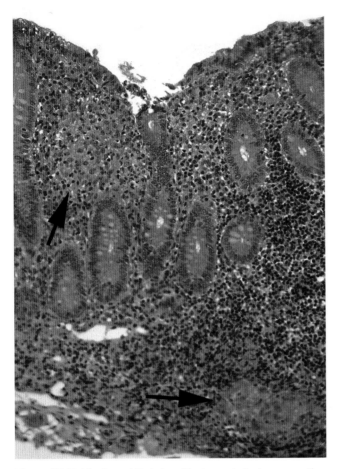

Figure 37.12 Histology of Crohn's colitis. Arrows indicate noncaseating granulomas. Courtesy of Dr John Hart, Chicago, IL.

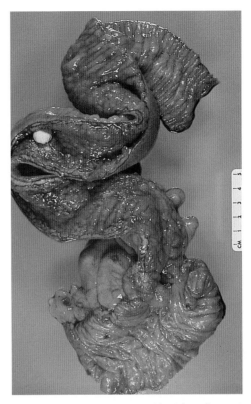

Figure 37.13 Ileal stricture in a patient with Crohn's disease. A pill is impacted in the lumen above a strictured area in the terminal ileum. An area of relatively normal cecum is at the bottom. Courtesy of Dr Ira Kodner.

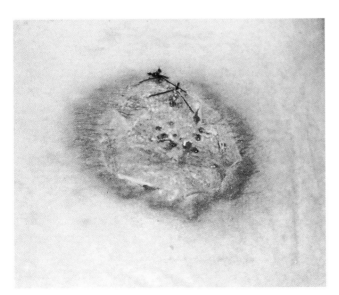

Figure 37.14 Pyoderma gangrenosum. Courtesy of Dr Ira Kodner.

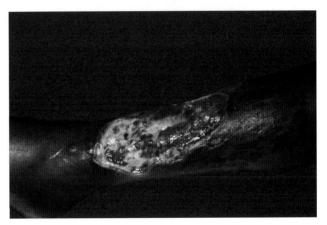

Figure 37.15 Severe pyoderma gangrenosum of the lower extremity. Note that the deep ulceration has reached the bone.

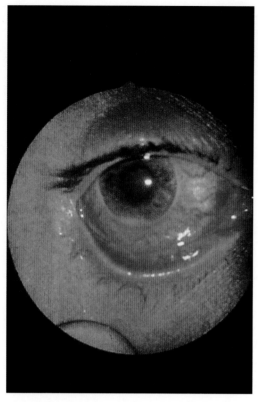

Figure 37.16 Marked conjunctival injection. A hypopyon also is present.

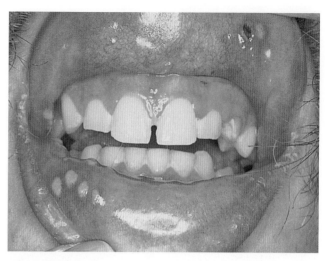

Figure 37.17 Aphthous ulcers. Courtesy of Dr Ira Kodner.

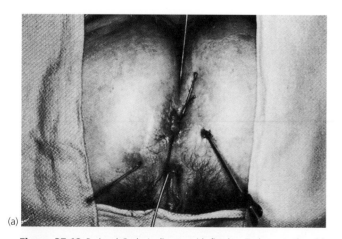

(a)

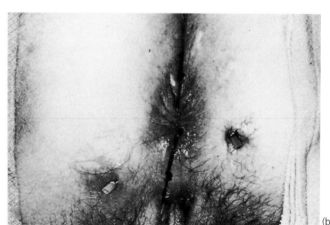

(b)

Figure 37.18 Perianal Crohn's disease with fistulae. Probes are placed intraoperatively to define fistulae **(a)**. Use of mushroom catheters and setons allows adequate drainage **(b)**. Courtesy of Dr Ira Kodner.

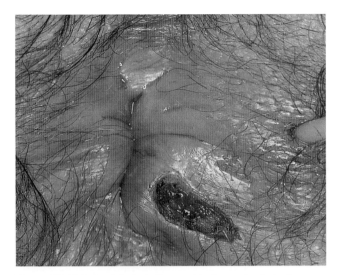

Figure 37.19 Perianal Crohn's disease with ulcer and catheter in a fistula. Courtesy of Dr Ira Kodner.

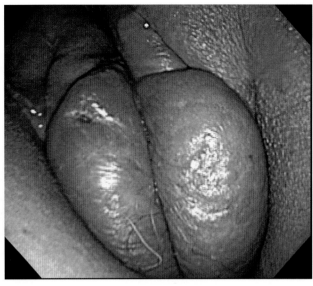

Figure 37.21 Chronic asymmetric labial swelling in a young woman with perianal Crohn's disease. Involvement of the genitals is typically by direct extension of fistulous tracts originating in the anorectum, but rarely can occur without any other obvious perineal or anorectal involvement, so-called "metastatic Crohn's disease."

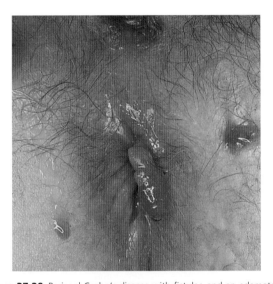

Figure 37.20 Perianal Crohn's disease with fistulae and an edematous tag. Courtesy of Dr Ira Kodner.

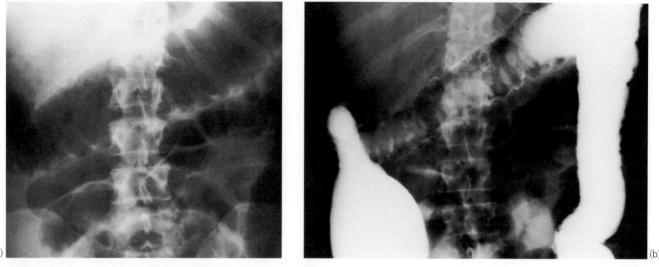

(a) (b)

Figure 37.22 Toxic megacolon. **(a)** Plain radiograph shows colonic dilation. **(b)** Contrast radiograph reveals large ulceration. Courtesy of Dr Dennis Balfe.

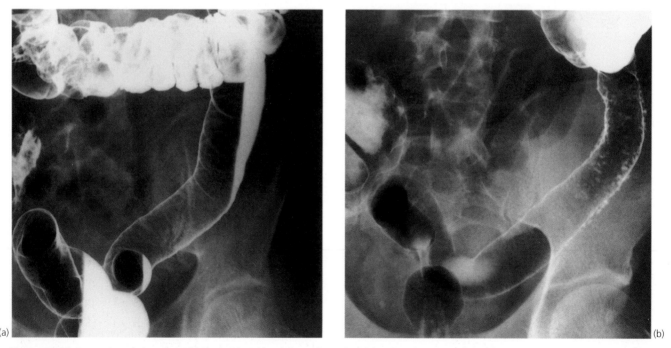

(a) (b)

Figure 37.23 Progression of ulcerative colitis in the sigmoid and descending colon. **(a)** Colon of a patient with mild ulcerative colitis. There is mucosal edema, granularity, and loss of haustral markings. **(b)** Two years later, there is shortening of the colon and mucosal ulcers. Numerous collar-button ulcers are present in the descending colon. Courtesy of Dr Dennis Balfe.

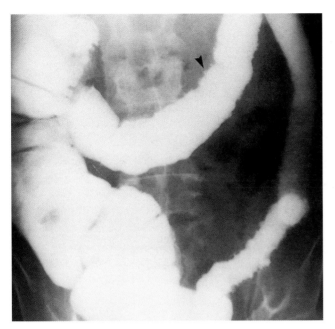

Figure 37.24 Ulcerative colitis extending to midtransverse colon with collar-button ulcerations in profile (arrowhead). Courtesy of Dr Dennis Balfe.

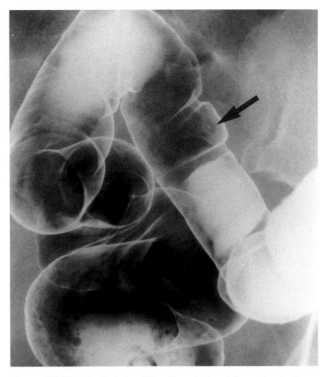

Figure 37.26 Early Crohn's colitis with a single aphthous ulcer in the sigmoid (arrow). Courtesy of Dr Dennis Balfe.

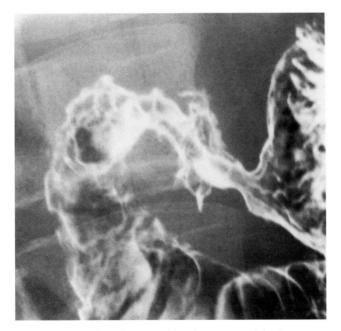

Figure 37.25 Crohn's disease involving the antrum and duodenum. Courtesy of Dr Dennis Balfe.

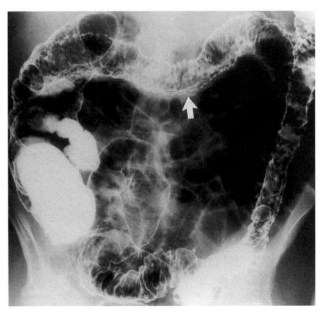

Figure 37.27 Severe Crohn's colitis involving the sigmoid, descending, transverse, and ascending colon. Numerous collar-button ulcerations are present (arrow). Courtesy of Dr Dennis Balfe.

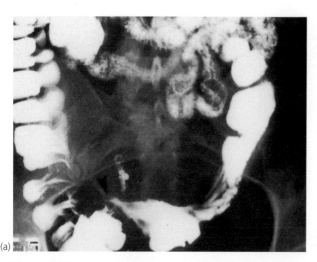
(a)

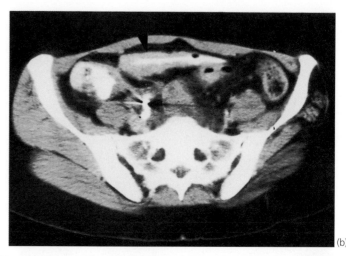
(b)

Figure 37.28 Crohn's disease of the terminal ileum (arrowhead) on small bowel follow-through image **(a)** and computed tomographic (CT) scan **(b)** of the same patient. Thickening of the intestinal wall is easily appreciated on the CT scan. On the small bowel follow-through image, wall thickening is indicated by the separation of the columns of barium. Courtesy of Dr Dennis Balfe.

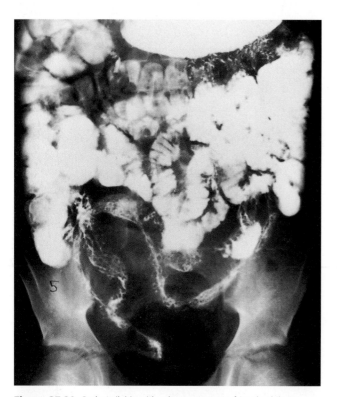

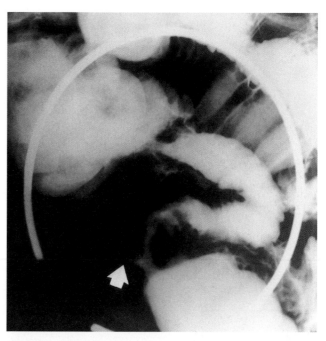

Figure 37.30 Crohn's disease of the terminal ileum. There is narrowing and ulceration of the terminal ileum with prestenotic dilation. There is also contrast material in a fissure (arrow). Courtesy of Dr Dennis Balfe.

Figure 37.29 Crohn's ileitis with a long segment of involved ileum. The barium columns are widely separated because of wall thickening. Courtesy of Dr Dennis Balfe.

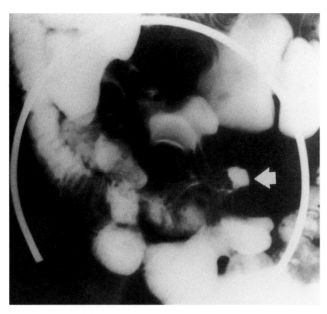

Figure 37.31 Crohn's disease of the terminal ileum with stricture and ulcer (arrow). Courtesy of Dr Dennis Balfe.

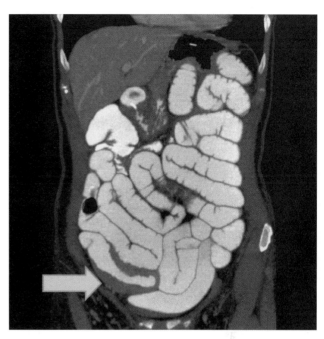

Figure 37.33 Computed tomographic enterography showing thickened terminal ileum (arrow) in a patient with Crohn's disease.

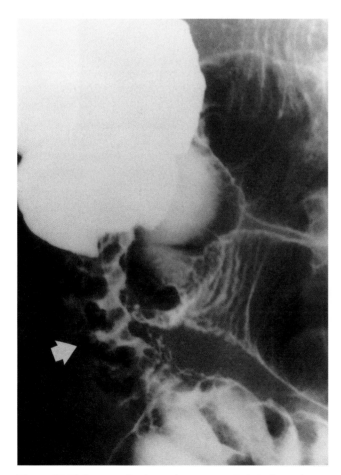

Figure 37.32 Pneumocolon image demonstrates Crohn's disease in a patient with an ileocolic anastomosis. There is active Crohn's disease with ulceration on the ileal side of the anastomosis (arrow). In a pneumocolon examination, barium is administered by mouth, and air is insufflated into the rectum. Courtesy of Dr Dennis Balfe.

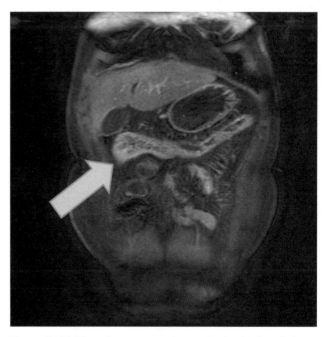

Figure 37.34 Magnetic resonance enterography showing long ileal stricture (arrow) in a patient with Crohn's disease. Courtesy of Dr David Rubin, Chicago, IL.

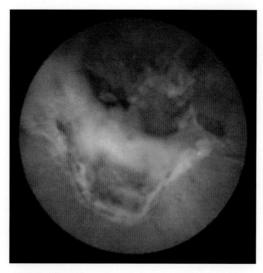

Figure 37.35 Wireless capsule endoscopy image of a small bowel stricture in a patient with Crohn's disease. Courtesy of Dr David Rubin, Chicago, IL.

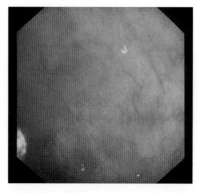

Figure 37.36 Quiescent (inactive) ulcerative colitis in a 39-year-old woman with ulcerative pancolitis for 11 years, now asymptomatic. There is distortion of the vascular markings but no granularity, edema, friability, mucous exudate, or ulcerations.

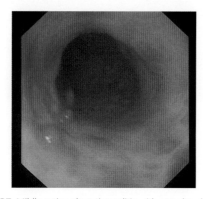

Figure 37.37 Mildly active ulcerative colitis with pseudopolyps. Same patient as in Fig. 37.36, 1 year after the endoscopic examination in Fig. 37.36, with a mild flare in symptoms. The disease is responding to prednisone 20 mg daily and mesalamine 4 g daily. There are two small pseudopolyps; the mucosa is mildly granular and erythematous; and the vascular markings are distorted.

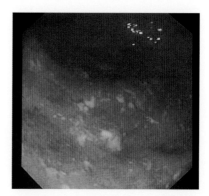

Figure 37.38 Moderately active ulcerative colitis in a 19-year-old woman with ulcerative pancolitis for 2 years. The patient has continuing symptoms despite oral mesalamine 4 g daily and prednisone 40 mg daily. Moderate granularity, edema, and mucus exudate is demonstrated.

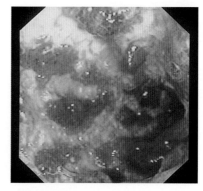

Figure 37.39 Severely active ulcerative colitis in a 54-year-old woman with left-sided ulcerative colitis for 7 years. There is marked ulceration. At least half of the surface area depicted is denuded by ulcers, and there are intervening areas of edematous granular mucosa.

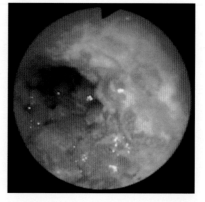

Figure 37.40 Coarsely nodular deformity of mucosal contour in ulcerative colitis. Mucosa is intensely erythematous and friable.

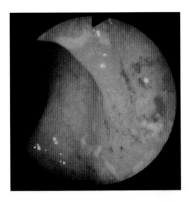

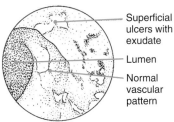

Superficial
ulcers with
exudate

Lumen

Normal
vascular
pattern

Figure 37.41 Sharp transition from normal to inflamed bowel is discernible at the rectosigmoid junction. Erythema and superficial ulceration of diseased mucosa contrast to the normal vascular pattern.

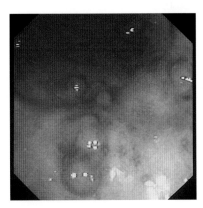

Figure 37.42 Mildly active ulcerative colitis with multiple pseudopolyps. This 54-year-old woman (same patient as in Fig. 37.39) about 1 year later after a course of topical 5-ASA (mesalamine) and prednisone 60 mg daily tapered and discontinued 9 months previously. There is mild granularity and erythema; the vascular markings are distorted, and multiple small pseudopolyps are present.

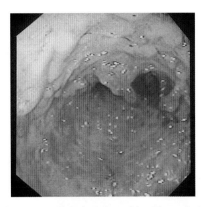

Figure 37.43 Long-standing ulcerative colitis with scarring and pseudopolyps. A 25-year-old man had a 9-year history of ulcerative colitis. The patient is now asymptomatic with azathioprine 150 mg daily and mesalamine 2.4 g daily. There is scarring and loss of the normal vascular markings. Two small pseudopolyps are present.

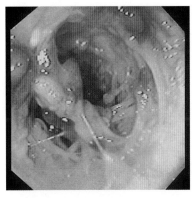

Figure 37.44 Ulcerative colitis with bridging pseudopolyps. A 25-year-old man has had ulcerative colitis for 9 years (same patient as in Fig. 37.43) and the disease is asymptomatic with azathioprine 150 mg daily and mesalamine 2.4 g daily. Endoscopic picture shows bridging pseudopolyps in the transverse colon.

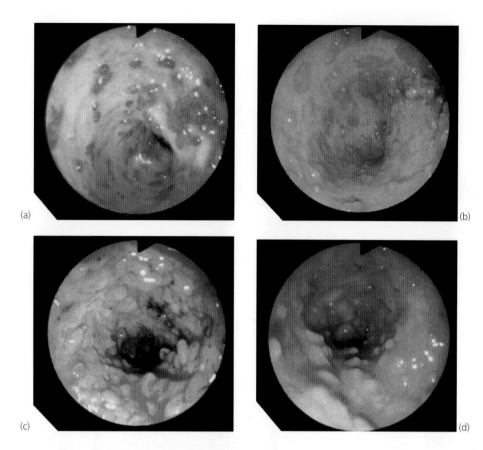

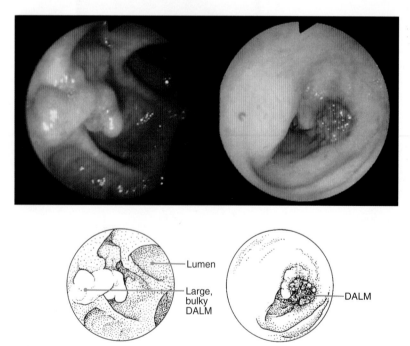

Figure 37.45 Sequential study of severe pancolitis. Massive ulceration of the colon was studied at intervals of 4–6 weeks after institution of medical therapy. **(a)** View of the proximal sigmoid shows extensive ulceration before therapy. Some islands of remaining mucosa are visible. **(b)** Regression of inflammation and early reepithelialization. **(c)** Ulcers are regressing with pseudopolypoid elevation of nonulcerated mucosal islands. **(d)** Full reepithelialization and pseudopolypoid transformation characterize healing.

Figure 37.46 Examples of dysplasia-associated lesions or masses (DALM) in long-standing, inactive ulcerative colitis.

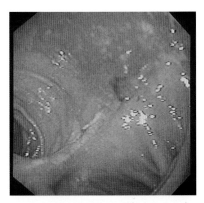

Figure 37.47 Mild to moderately active pouchitis. This 36-year-old woman has a history of ulcerative colitis for which she underwent colectomy with ileal J pouch–anal anastomosis 2 years previously. She had recurrent liquid stools and cramping discomfort relieved with bowel movements. Endoscopic image of the pouch, with views of the afferent limb of the neoterminal ileum in the left portion of the field and the blind end of the J pouch in the inferior aspect of the field, shows mucous exudate, superficial ulceration, and friability of the pouch mucosa but not of the mucosa in the neoterminal ileum.

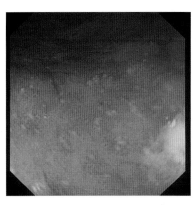

Figure 37.49 Crohn's disease involving the transverse colon with multiple aphthous ulcers. A 26-year-old woman with Crohn's disease for 2 years has persistent symptoms despite prednisone 25 mg daily and sulfasalazine 3 g daily. Endoscopic image shows multiple aphthous ulcers; edematous and erythematous mucosa with a loss of normal vascular markings; and mucous exudate.

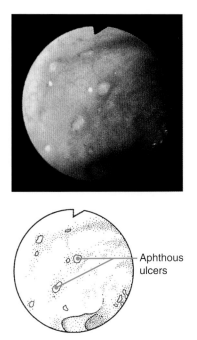

Figure 37.48 Colonoscopic appearance of aphthous ulceration.

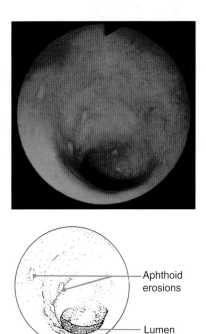

Figure 37.50 Characteristic superficial aphthoid erosions in Crohn's disease have erythematous rings.

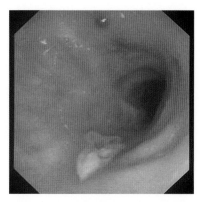

Figure 37.51 Crohn's disease of the colon with focal ulcer. A 24-year-old man with Crohn's disease for 2 years currently has minimal symptoms while taking metronidazole 250 mg three times daily and mesalamine 2.4 g daily. There is a focal ulcer in the distal sigmoid colon, mild inflammatory changes of the surrounding mucosa, distortion of the vascular markings, mild granularity, and erythema.

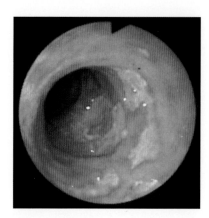

Figure 37.52 Multiple large, deep, excavated ulcers in severe ulcerating Crohn's disease show distinct margins. This patient has concomitant sclerosing cholangitis.

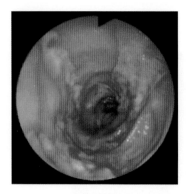

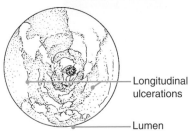

Longitudinal ulcerations

Lumen

Figure 37.53 Longitudinal alignment of ulceration causes a railroad-track appearance in Crohn's disease.

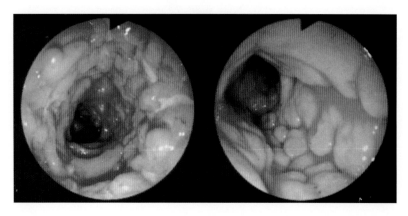

Figure 37.54 Active phase of Crohn's diseases shows cobblestoning caused by interconnecting ulcerations **(left)**. Area of cobblestoning after therapy **(right)**.

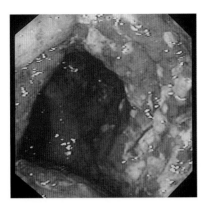

Figure 37.55 Severely active Crohn's disease of the colon. A 22-year-old man with a 1-year history of Crohn's disease has severe diarrhea, a 19-pound weight loss, and continuing symptoms despite prednisone 60 mg daily. Colonoscopic image shows severe ulceration in the transverse colon with markedly edematous, granular, and friable mucosa.

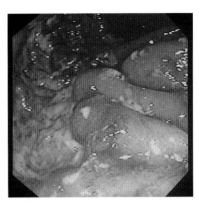

Figure 37.56 Severely active Crohn's disease of the colon (same patient as in Fig. 37.55). Deep rake ulcer in mid-descending colon with surrounding mucosal edema, granularity, and friability.

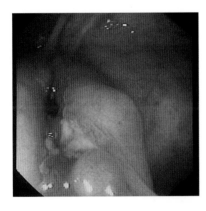

Figure 37.57 Crohn's disease with ulceration at the ileocecal valve. A 26-year-old woman with a history of Crohn's disease for 4 years has involvement of the terminal ileum. The disease was previously controlled with mesalamine 4 g daily, with worsening cramping abdominal pain in recent weeks. Colonoscopy revealed ulceration at the ileocecal valve with stenosis of the valve, which could not be intubated with a colonoscope. The colon otherwise appeared normal.

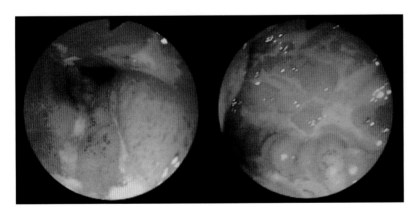

Figure 37.58 Diffuse, concentric involvement of the distal terminal ileum in Crohn's disease presents itself as swelling, erythema, punctiform bleeding, and ulceration **(left)**. Circumferential involvement of the distal terminal ileum with longitudinal ulcers and cobblestoning **(right)**.

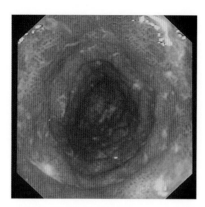

Figure 37.59 Crohn's disease involving the neoterminal ileum with multiple superficial ulcers. A 29-year-old woman with a history of Crohn's disease for 6 years had undergone resection of the terminal ileum and cecum with ileal-ascending colonic anastomosis. Symptoms of recurrent Crohn's disease (cramping abdominal pain and malaise) developed 4 months after resection. Colonoscopic image with visualization of the neoterminal ileum shows multiple focal superficial ulcers with edema, erythema, and granularity of the intervening mucosa.

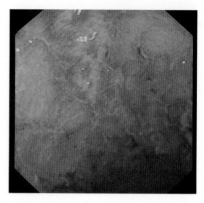

Figure 37.61 Mildly active Crohn's disease of the sigmoid colon in a 51-year-old man with a 4-year history of Crohn's colitis, now controlled with azathioprine 175 mg daily and metronidazole 250 mg twice daily. The mucosa shows superficial scarring, loss of normal vascular markings, and slight mucous exudate.

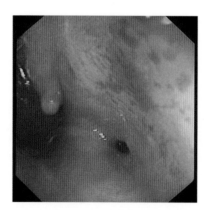

Figure 37.60 Crohn's disease – view of the rectum with rectovaginal fistula and prominent anal papilla. A 40-year-old woman has a 10-year history of Crohn's disease involving the colon. A symptomatic rectovaginal fistula developed with gas and stool passed per vagina. Retroflexed view of the rectum shows a central fistulous opening communicating with the vagina. The endoscope is in the left field of the photo, and a prominent anal papilla is present. The mucosa is granular, edematous, and friable.

38

Miscellaneous inflammatory and structural disorders of the colon

David H. Alpers, David H.B. Cort

A variety of structural and inflammatory conditions, apart from Crohn's disease and chronic ulcerative colitis, involve the colon. They have been divided into inflammatory conditions associated with motor disorders (including solitary rectal ulcer and colitis cystica profunda), inflammatory conditions associated with therapeutic interventions (including radiation-induced, drug-induced, and cathartic-induced inflammation as well as diversion colitis), and other disorders (including microscopic and collagenous colitis, nonspecific ulcers of the colon, endometriosis, and pneumatosis cystoides intestinalis). Figure 38.1 shows the endoscopic appearance of solitary rectal ulcer and Figure 38.2 demonstrates the characteristic histological finding of fibromuscular hyperplasia in the lamina propria. These ulcers are believed to recur from repeated prolapse associated with the failure of the levator ani muscles to relax during defecation. More specific ulcers in the ascending colon can look quite similar, although their cause is probably different (Fig. 38.3). Colitis cystica profunda is possibly related to the solitary rectal ulcer syndrome. Polypoid masses can occur in the presence (Fig. 38.4) and absence (Fig. 38.5) of surface ulceration. The characteristic histological features of submucosal mucin-filled cysts are shown in Figure 38.6. Inflammatory types of colitis other than idiopathic inflammatory bowel disease include Behçet disease (Fig. 38.7), radiation colitis (Figs 38.8–38.10), and diversion colitis (Fig. 38.11). Pneumatosis cystoides intestinalis is a benign condition with submucosal gas cysts (Figs 38.12 and 38.13).

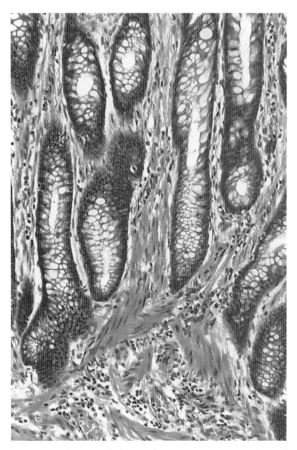

Figure 38.2 Solitary rectal ulcer syndrome. Biopsy specimen shows the characteristic appearance of fibroblasts (toward the 12 o'clock position) and muscle fibers (at the 6 o'clock position) within the lamina propria encircling crypts.

Figure 38.1 Solitary rectal ulcer. Well-demarcated margins and a clean ulcer base with mild adjacent inflammatory change are depicted.

Atlas of Gastroenterology, 4th edition. Edited by Tadataka Yamada, David H. Alpers, Anthony N. Kalloo, Neil Kaplowitz, Chung Owyang, and Don W. Powell. © 2009 Blackwell Publishing, ISBN: 978-1-4051-6909-7

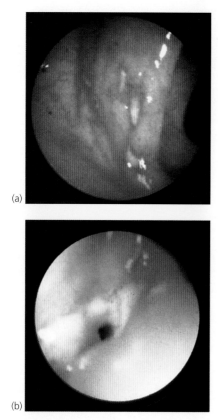

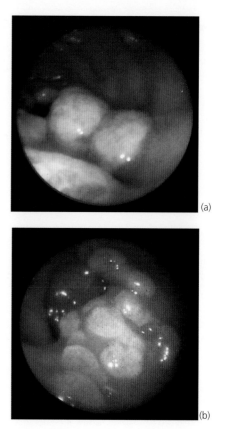

Figure 38.3 (a) Nonspecific colonic ulcers in the ascending colon. Three discrete ulcers were found in an 80-year-old man with a history of hematochezia. The cause of these ulcers is unknown. **(b)** Nonspecific colonic ulcer of the sigmoid with stricture. Deep ulceration in a patient with alcoholic pancreatitis and a pseudocyst was associated with stricture formation. There was no communication between the pancreatic pseudocyst and the stricture at operation, nor did the resected specimen show evidence of either inflammatory bowel disease or a malignant tumor. This was therefore considered to be nonspecific colonic ulceration.

Figure 38.4 Solitary rectal ulcer syndrome. **(a)** Ulcer stage with inflammatory polyps. Multiple 5- to 15-mm polypoid masses with ulcerated surfaces (composed of granulation tissue) are present rather than a discrete ulcer. **(b)** Ulcer stage with polypoid masses. Rather than multiple discrete inflammatory polyps as seen in (a), these appear together as one large (1.5 × 2.5 cm), relatively discrete mass with nodules, the surfaces of which are composed of granulation tissue. In this case, large-particle biopsy showed superficial ulceration and fibromuscular hyperplasia of the lamina propria and muscularis mucosae. No submucosal mucin-containing cysts were found, although the endoscopic appearance and the location (rectosigmoid) cannot be differentiated from those of colitis cystica profunda.

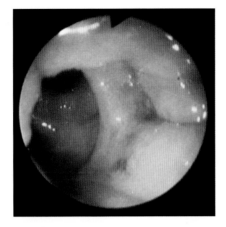
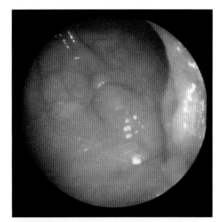
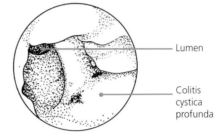

Lumen

Colitis
cystica
profunda

Figure 38.5 Multiple submucosal cysts in the rectum of a patient with colitis cystica profunda.

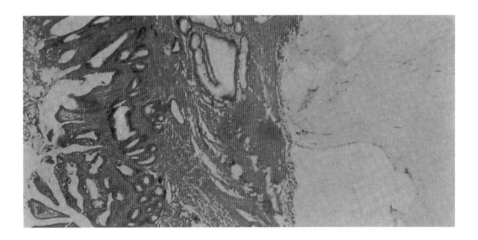

Figure 38.6 Submucosal mucin-filled cysts characteristic of colitis cystica profunda (H & E stain).

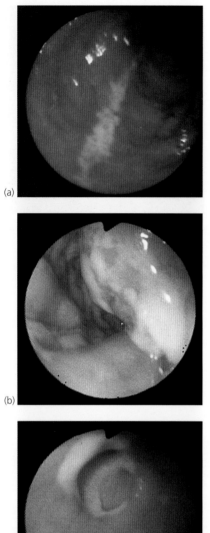

(a)

(b)

(c)

Figure 38.7 Behçet disease involving the colon. **(a)** A discrete, long, linear ulceration set in a background of nonspecific erythema. This was observed in a patient with oral and vaginal ulcerations and iritis, the clinical constellation of Behçet disease. **(b)** Discrete, deep ulceration of the sigmoid in a patient with clinical features favoring Behçet disease. The endoscopic appearance, however, does not allow differentiation from Crohn's disease, although colonic biopsies with evidence of vasculitis (lacking in this case) would have strongly favored Behçet disease. **(c)** Discrete, deep, punched-out ulcerations, not unlike those found in Crohn's colitis, are typical of colonic involvement in Behçet disease.

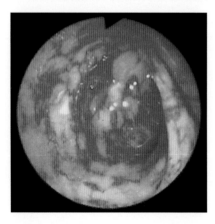

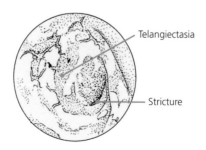

Figure 38.8 Chronic radiation-induced telangiectasia and stricture of the rectosigmoid colon.

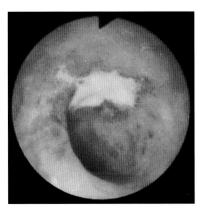

Figure 38.9 Chronic radiation-induced ulcer of the anterior wall of the rectum.

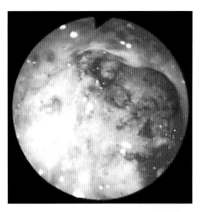

Figure 38.11 Characteristic diffuse mucosal inflammatory changes of diversion colitis. These findings are clinically indistinguishable from those of chronic idiopathic inflammatory bowel disease.

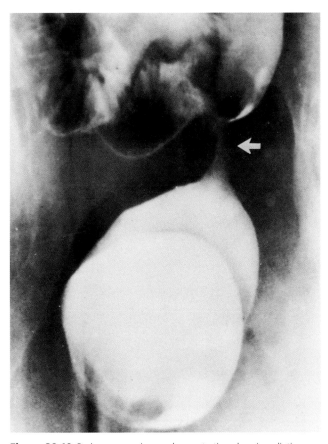

Figure 38.10 Barium enema image demonstrating chronic radiation-induced stricture of the rectosigmoid (arrow).

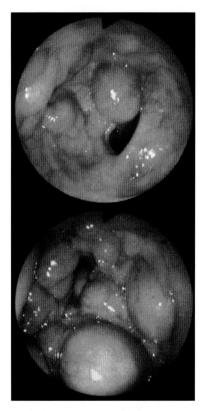

Figure 38.12 Multiple submucosal gas-filled cysts in pneumatosis cystoides intestinalis. There is partial lumenal obstruction by the cysts.

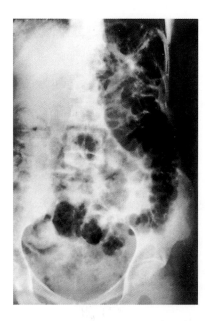

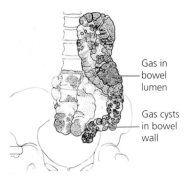

Gas in
bowel
lumen

Gas cysts
in bowel
wall

Figure 38.13 Plain abdominal radiograph
demonstrating gas-filled cysts in the wall of the sigmoid
colon.

39

Diverticular disease of the colon

Tonia M. Young-Fadok, Michael G. Sarr

Diverticular disease of the colon is an acquired condition. Diverticulosis, or the presence of diverticula, affects more than 30% of persons older than 60 years living in industrialized countries. The etiology of diverticular disease appears to be multifactorial. Most important are age-related changes in the structure of the colon wall that cause decreased tensile strength and chronic exposure to excessive intralumenal pressures (Fig. 39.1). Insufficient dietary fiber in the western diet has been implicated in the formation of diverticula, because African subjects with high-fiber diets rarely develop diverticula.

Diverticulosis primarily involves the sigmoid colon, although diverticula may develop in any segment of the intraperitoneal colon; in contrast, diverticula of the rectum are exceedingly uncommon. Diverticula are extralumenal structures composed of mucosa, submucosa, and serosa, but specifically lack the muscularis. They are, therefore, pseudo-diverticula, characteristic of the pulsion, acquired type (Fig. 39.2). Diverticula develop where the vasa recta penetrate the colon wall, and it is thought that these are points of weakness in the colonic wall. Indeed, close inspection of diverticula, seen at the time of endoscopy, frequently reveals one or more blood vessels entering the sac (Figs 39.3 and 39.4). As the site where the vasa recta pass through the colon wall is adjacent to the teniae, diverticulosis often appears to occur in longitudinal rows (Fig. 39.5). In extensive diverticulosis, this can present a "honeycomb" effect (Fig. 39.6).

The segment of colon affected by diverticulosis, usually the sigmoid, undergoes changes that are signaled by muscular thickening (myochosis), which leads to shortening of the bowel and decreased lumenal diameter. These changes may lead to a "concertina-like" or "picket fence" appearance radiographically (Fig. 39.7).

Many patients with diverticulosis are asymptomatic. Approximately 15%–25% of patients have intermittent abdominal pain and irregular bowel habits. Such symptomatic, uncomplicated disease may have an as yet undefined relationship to irritable bowel syndrome (IBS). Like IBS, uncomplicated diverticular disease is generally managed with increased dietary fiber. A high-fiber diet often ameliorates abdominal symptoms and may offer protection from the development and progression of diverticular disease.

Approximately 30% of patients with diverticulosis develop inflammation (diverticulitis) or bleeding, but rarely both. Diverticulitis is an inflammatory, peridiverticular process that begins with microperforation of a diverticulum, typically filled with inspissated stool. Diverticulitis manifests classically with lower abdominal pain, frequently left-sided, tenderness, fever, and leukocytosis. The diagnosis of acute diverticulitis is often made on the basis of clinical presentation. Additional evaluation beyond plain abdominal radiography (to rule out free air) should proceed if there is diagnostic doubt or if a secondary complication is suspected (i.e., perforation, fistula, abscess, stricture, or obstruction). Further evaluation is also indicated in the patient whose disease is severe enough to merit hospitalization, because documentation of the diagnosis is a necessary part of subsequent surgical decision making. The use of a barium enema examination to diagnose acute diverticulitis is contraindicated because of the complications associated with extralumenal spillage of barium. The most widely used investigation is computed tomography (CT) (Figs 39.8 and 39.9), which allows confirmation of the diagnosis and also stages the extent of extralumenal inflammation. In the absence of ready access to CT facilities, water-soluble contrast enema may be useful (Fig. 39.10). CT colonography or "virtual colonoscopy" has the ability to image diverticula, but its role in the management of acute disease is not yet defined (Fig. 39.11a–c).

Management of acute diverticulitis includes bowel rest, correction of fluid and electrolyte abnormalities, and broad-spectrum intravenous antibiotics effective against aerobic and anaerobic organisms. Most patients respond to this

Atlas of Gastroenterology, 4th edition. Edited by Tadataka Yamada, David H. Alpers, Anthony N. Kalloo, Neil Kaplowitz, Chung Owyang, and Don W. Powell. © 2009 Blackwell Publishing, ISBN: 978-1-4051-6909-7

medical management. After resolution of symptoms, a high-fiber diet may protect this subset of patients from recurrent attacks.

Elective operative intervention is reserved for patients with complicated diverticulitis (fistula [Fig. 39.12], abscess, and stricture), those with recurrent attacks, and when evaluation cannot exclude the possibility of an underlying carcinoma (Fig. 39.13). Elective surgical intervention is also indicated in the immunocompromised patient after just a single episode of diverticulitis. The management of young patients is more controversial; traditionally, operation has been offered after a single episode of diverticulitis but with improved diagnostic modalities it may be reasonable to base the need for operation on the severity of the disease rather than the age of the patient. Emergent operation is indicated for patients with free perforation or acute diverticulitis, which does not respond promptly to medical therapy.

For patients with a contained abscess (usually within the body of the colonic mesentery itself), CT-guided drainage (Fig. 39.14) may allow for postponement of surgical intervention until sepsis is controlled, the inflammatory process has subsided, and the bowel can be mechanically prepared for a one-stage resection of the affected colon with a primary colorectostomy. More urgent operations on an unprepared colon usually require a two-stage procedure: resection of the sigmoid colon and a diverting descending colostomy (Hartmann procedure). Formal resection of the diseased colonic segment, rather than proximal colonic diversion using colostomy and drainage, should be the aim of surgical management for perforated diverticulitis because the affected bowel is a source of continuing sepsis that can lead to increased morbidity and mortality. Recurrent diverticulitis after appropriate resection of the entire sigmoid colon is uncommon.

The laparoscopic approach is increasingly being used for surgical intervention. Most experience has been gained in the elective setting, for example elective sigmoid resection and closure of colostomy after a Hartmann procedure. Laparoscopic techniques in the acute setting may be appropriate in skilled hands for Hinchey stages I and II, but generally not for stages III and IV because of the difficulty of ensuring complete clearance of all loculated pockets of purulence or stool. When resection with anastomosis is performed, an intracorporeal anastomosis is necessary (Fig. 39.15a,b) because the distal margin of resection should be in the proximal rectum below the point where the teniae coalesce, to minimize the risk of recurrence.

Diverticular bleeding occurs much less frequently than acute diverticulitis. The true cause of erosion of the vasa recta at the neck of a diverticulum is unknown. The typical presentation involves an elderly patient with massive, painless bleeding that stops and starts abruptly and spontaneously. After initiating resuscitation, the site and source of bleeding should be sought. The timing and order of the diagnostic tests, including mesenteric angiography, red blood cell–tagged bleeding scintigraphy, and colonoscopy, depend on the clinical situation and the available facilities at the physician's institution. Mesenteric angiography is highly sensitive if performed when the rate of bleeding is greater than $0.5 \ mL \ min^{-1}$ (Fig. 39.16a,b). Extravasation of intravenous contrast into a diverticulum is pathognomonic of diverticular bleeding. The radiographic pattern is different from that of bleeding angiectasis. Angiography has the additional benefit of allowing therapeutic infusion of vasopressin in an attempt to halt the bleeding. Red blood cell–tagged scintiscans (Fig. 39.17) may be helpful to determine whether bleeding is ongoing but are often unreliable for localizing the precise site of bleeding, particularly in patients with chronic bleeding.

When significant bleeding persists, operative intervention is indicated. When the site of bleeding is known, segmental colonic resection is possible and is associated with low morbidity, mortality, and recurrence rates. When the site is unknown, intraoperative colonoscopy may be helpful. If the site cannot be identified, abdominal colectomy is usually indicated to deal effectively with the problem. This approach, however, is associated with increased morbidity among older patients, emphasizing the need to identify a site, whenever possible, to allow for the directed segmental resection.

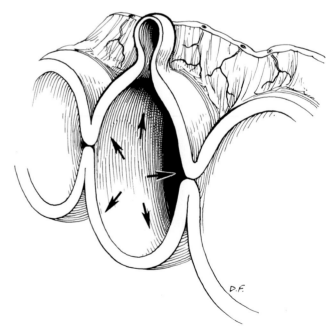

Figure 39.1 The concept of Painter and Burkitt of segmentation causing formation of pulsion diverticula.

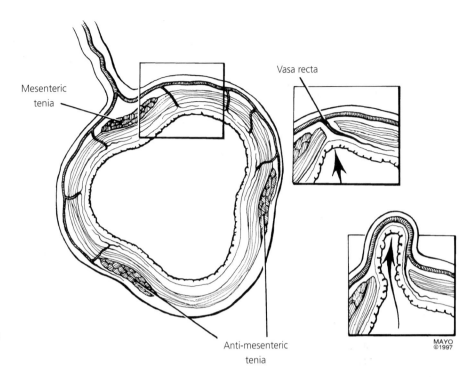

Figure 39.2 Cross-section of the sigmoid colon. The main illustration indicates the points of penetration of the vasa recti around the bowel circumference. Insets: the development of a diverticulum at one such point of weakness.

Mesenteric tenia

Vasa recta

Anti-mesenteric tenia

MAYO ©1997

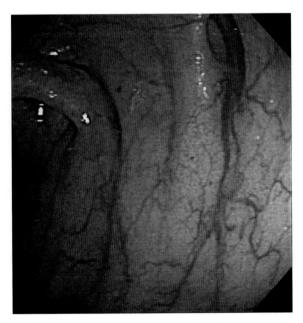

Figure 39.3 Appearance at colonoscopy showing blood vessels entering the mouth of the diverticulum.

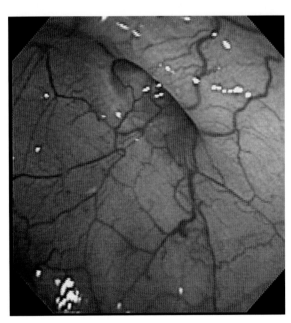

Figure 39.4 Appearance at colonoscopy showing blood vessels entering the mouth of the diverticulum.

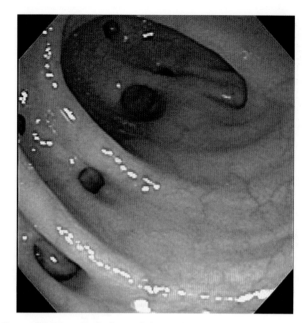

Figure 39.5 Longitudinal row of diverticula.

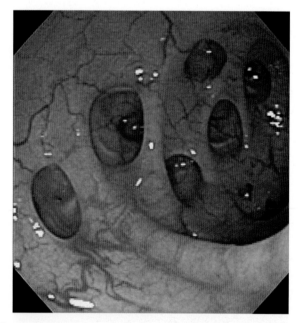

Figure 39.6 Multiple longitudinal rows of diverticula creating a "honeycomb" appearance.

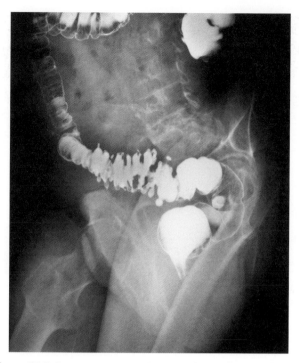

Figure 39.7 Contrast enema revealing picket fence appearance of the sigmoid colon, associated with symptoms of obstruction.

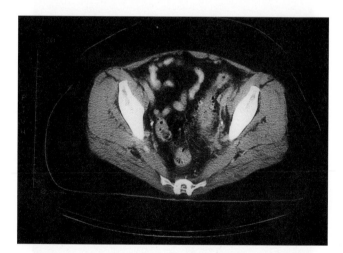

Figure 39.8 Computed tomography with oral and intravenous contrast in a 59-year-old woman with increasing abdominal pain for 3 weeks. Mild changes of diverticulitis are seen with narrowing of the colonic lumen, bowel wall thickening in the midsigmoid, tissue stranding in pericolic pelvic fat, and diverticula. There is no pericolic fluid collection.

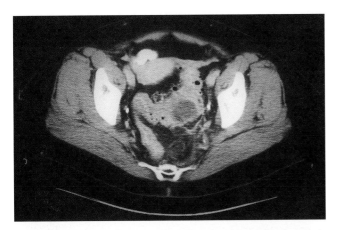

Figure 39.9 Computed tomography with oral and intravenous contrast in a 60-year-old woman with a 2-week history of crampy lower abdominal pain, fever, and chills showing a low-density mass adjacent to the sigmoid in the left pelvis. The central, low-density region within the mass, the pockets of surrounding gas, and inflammatory changes in pericolic tissues are consistent with diverticular disease.

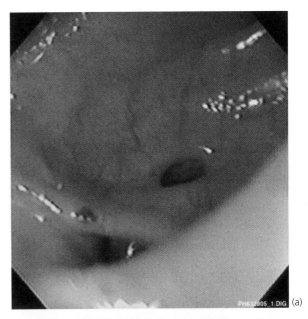

(a)

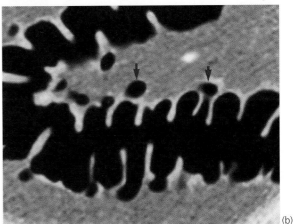

(b)

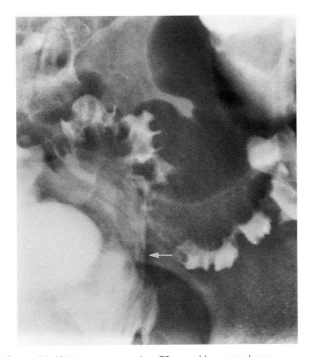

Figure 39.10 Hypaque enema in a 79-year-old woman shows nonanatomic distribution of contrast (arrow) around the rectum, demonstrating perforation.

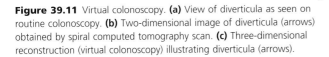

Figure 39.11 Virtual colonoscopy. **(a)** View of diverticula as seen on routine colonoscopy. **(b)** Two-dimensional image of diverticula (arrows) obtained by spiral computed tomography scan. **(c)** Three-dimensional reconstruction (virtual colonoscopy) illustrating diverticula (arrows).

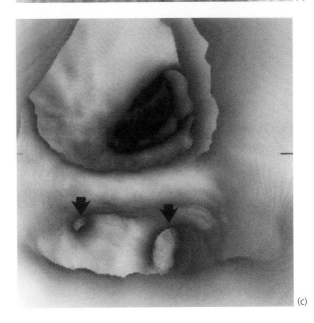

(c)

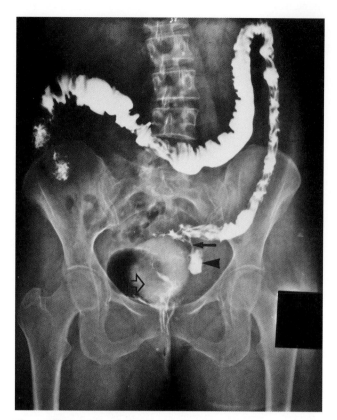

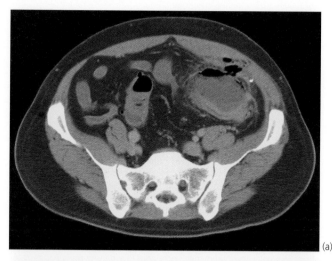

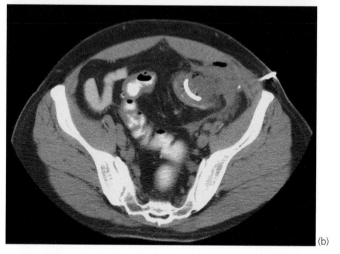

(a)

(b)

Figure 39.12 Barium enema in a 54-year-old woman with pneumaturia and left lower quadrant pain. A fistulous tract (arrow) arises in the midsigmoid passing into an abscess cavity (arrowhead) and then into the bladder, where contrast is also seen (open arrow).

Figure 39.14 Computed tomographic scan in a 43-year-old man. **(a)** Large pericolic abscess. **(b)** Following placement of a pigtail catheter to drain the abscess.

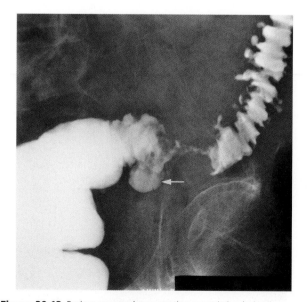

Figure 39.13 Barium enema demonstrating constricting lesion in sigmoid colon in a region of diverticulosis. There is also a 3-cm localized collection of barium (arrow) off the lateral colonic wall consistent with an abscess cavity. The most likely radiological diagnosis is diverticulitis but carcinoma cannot be excluded.

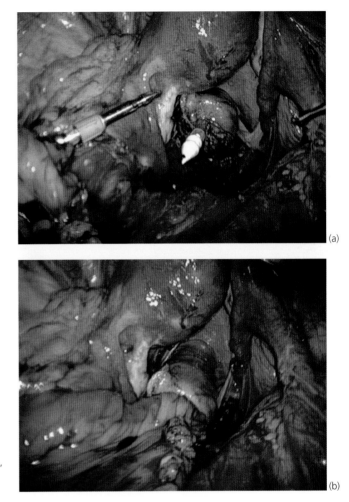

(a)

(b)

Figure 39.15 A 53-year-old woman undergoing elective laparoscopic sigmoid resection. **(a)** The distal resection margin is in the proximal rectum, just below the sacral promontory. **(b)** The completed anastomosis employing the circular stapler.

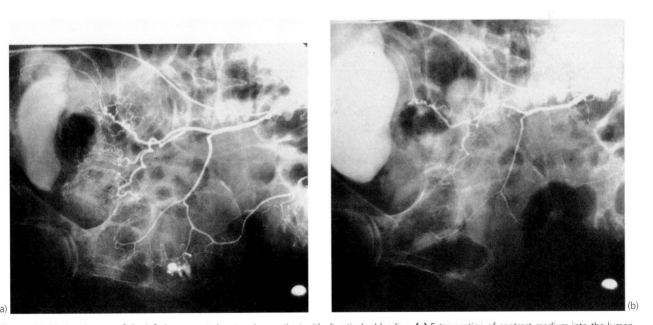

(a)

(b)

Figure 39.16 Arteriogram of the inferior mesenteric artery in a patient with diverticular bleeding. **(a)** Extravasation of contrast medium into the lumen of the descending colon. **(b)** Arteriogram of the same patient after infusion of vasopressin. Note the markedly reduced flow in the left colonic and sigmoidal branches.

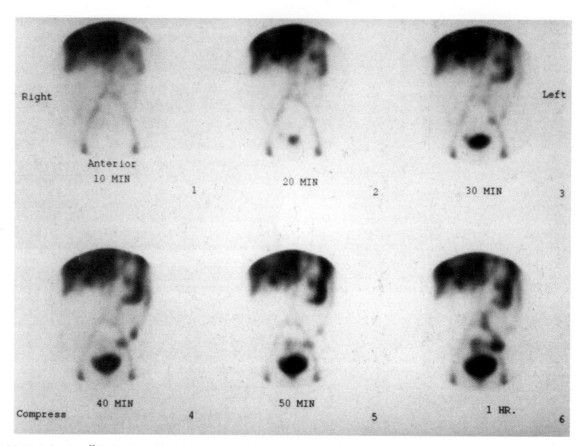

Figure 39.17 Technetium ^{99m}Tc-labeled red blood cell scan for evaluation of lower gastrointestinal bleeding in a 63-year-old woman with a 24-h history of bright red blood per rectum. Increased activity in the distal transverse colon near the splenic flexure progresses toward the descending colon and sigmoid colon by termination of the examination at 1 h. Findings are consistent with a bleeding source in the distal transverse colon near the splenic flexure.

40

Neoplastic and nonneoplastic polyps of the colon and rectum

Graeme P. Young, Finlay A. Macrae, Anthony C. Thomas

Overview

Colorectal polyps may be classified in various ways. On the basis of location they may be mucosal (such as an adenoma) or submucosal (such as a lipoma). Mucosal lesions are by far the most common and are further subdivided into neoplastic and nonneoplastic lesions. Neoplastic polyps are of greatest clinical significance because of their premalignant nature and their potential to progress to carcinoma. Nonneoplastic polyps have minimal or no premalignant potential. Submucosal lesions are rare and their clinical significance depends on the underlying cause. A series of figures (photomicrographs, endoscopic and macroscopic photographs, radiological studies) are presented in Figures 40.1–40.85 as examples of the different types of polyps. In addition, some figures depict endoscopic therapy.

Polyps are generally asymptomatic and are usually detected in the context of screening or serendipitous diagnostic investigation. If the possibility of polyps is high, the definitive diagnostic procedure is colonoscopy, often coupled with polypectomy and histological examination to ascertain the true nature of the tissue. Endoscopic polypectomy provides adequate management of most adenomatous polyps unless they are very large. Many sessile polyps can now be removed, sometimes requiring a submucosal injection of saline (a "saline lift") followed by snare polypectomy. However, some malignant polyps may necessitate surgical resection if removal is incomplete, clearance is not certain, and histology is poorly differentiated. Because polyps are most often seen at endoscopy, many of the photographs presented here have been obtained at endoscopy. Selected radiographs are also presented because polyps are occasionally diagnosed in this way.

Atlas of Gastroenterology, 4th edition. Edited by Tadataka Yamada, David H. Alpers, Anthony N. Kalloo, Neil Kaplowitz, Chung Owyang, and Don W. Powell. © 2009 Blackwell Publishing, ISBN: 978-1-4051-6909-7

The potential for malignancy now or in the future depends on the size of the adenomatous polyp, the number of such polyps, histological features such as degree of dysplasia, and architectural type such as degree of villous change. Adenomatous polyps larger than 1 cm in diameter, those with a large villous architectural component, or those with severe dysplasia carry a higher risk for malignancy. Persons with more than two adenomas of any size or with certain types of serrated adenomas are also at increased risk. The natural history of the progression of adenomatous polyps has been deduced from observational studies and remains largely speculative. It appears that most adenomas take 2–10 years to progress to frank malignant tumors. Exceptions include adenomas in hereditary nonpolyposis colorectal cancer (HNPCC) and perhaps some flat adenomas outside of this setting.

Because histopathological examination is the crucial issue for any polyp, examples of the histopathological features of the various types of polyps are provided. Figures are grouped and generally follow the following sequence: tubular adenomas (Figs 40.1–40.8), tubulovillous adenomas (Figs 40.9–40.15), villous adenomas (Figs 40.18–40.22), serrated adenomas (Figs 40.23–40.25), examples of polypectomy (Figs 40.26–40.39), malignant polyps (Figs 40.16 and 40.17, and 40.40–40.43), familial adenomatous polyposis (Figs 40.44–40.50), other polyposis syndromes (Figs 40.51–40.55), lymphoid accumulations (Figs 40.56–40.59), hyperplastic polyps (Figs 40.60–40.63), inflammatory polyps (Figs 40.64–40.66), submucosal lesions (Figs 40.67–40.77), and miscellaneous (Figs 40.78–40.95).

Epidemiological association of adenomas and cancer

Autopsy studies show that the prevalence of adenomas varies widely among countries and parallels the frequency of colorectal cancer in that country (Table 40.1), confirming the close association of adenomas with colorectal carcinomas. Most studies show prevalence rates that are 30% higher in men than in women.

Anatomic distribution

Colonoscopic studies and some autopsy studies show that colorectal adenomas are more common in the distal colon and rectum, similar to the distribution of colorectal cancer (Table 40.2). Distribution, however, relates to size. Small adenomas are more uniformly distributed throughout the entire colon, whereas large adenomas (>1 cm) show a distal predominance.

Association of adenomas with other diseases

Associations between colonic polyps and other diseases are summarized in Table 40.3. None of the conditions with a strong association is common. In a prospective study of acromegalic patients, nearly 50% had adenomas, especially when older.

Table 40.1 Prevalence of colorectal neoplasia in men in various regions around the world

Population	Cancer incidence (per 100 000 per year)	Adenoma prevalence (%, ~ age 50 years)
Hawaiian Japanese	34	65
New Orleans, white	28	40
New Orleans, African American	26	30
Sweden (Trelleborg)	17	30
Japan (Akita)	16	30
Spain (Barcelona)	13	20
Brazil	12	15
Sweden (Bolinas)	10	10
Japan (Miyagi)	8	10
Colombia (Cali)	5	5
Costa Rica	3	5
Iran	<2	<5
Bolivia	<2	<5

Table 40.2 Anatomic distribution of colorectal adenomas

Examination	Ascending colon (%)	Transverse colon (%)	Descending colon (%)	Sigmoid colon (%)	Rectum (%)
Colonoscopy	10	10	30	45	5
Autopsy (all adenomas)	30	20	15	15	20
Autopsy (adenomas > 1 cm)	15	15	25	35	10

From: Cronstedt J, et al. Geographic differences in the prevalence and distribution of large-bowel polyps: colonoscopic findings. Endoscopy 1987;19:110. Jass JR. Subsite distribution and incidence of colorectal cancer in New Zealand 1974–1983. Dis Colon Rectum 1991;34:56. Vukasin AP, et al. Increasing incidence of cecal and sigmoid carcinoma: data from the Connecticut Tumor Registry. Cancer 1990;66:2442. Luk GD. Epidemiology and etiology of colorectal neoplasia. Curr Opin Gastroenterol 1992;8:19.

Table 40.3 Confirmed, postulated, and unconfirmed disease associations with colorectal polyps (excluding familial syndromes) and their strengths of association

Disease	Polyp type	Strength of association
Ureterosigmoidostomy	Adenoma/carcinoma	Strong
	Juvenile	
	Inflammatory	
Acromegaly	Adenoma/carcinoma	Strong
Streptococcus bovis infections	Adenoma/carcinoma	Strong
Breast cancer	Adenoma	Weak
Atherosclerosis	Adenoma	Weak
Cirrhosis	Adenoma	Weak
Skin tags	Adenoma	Very weak
Cholecystectomy	Adenoma	Very weak
Diverticula (colon)	Adenoma	Very weak
Lymphoid follicles	Adenoma	Very weak

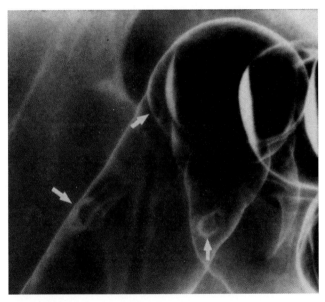

Figure 40.1 Double-contrast radiographic appearance of three small sessile polyps (arrows) ranging in size from 0.5 to 0.8 cm, which were subsequently found to be tubular adenomas. The distinction between adenomas, which have malignant potential, and mucosal or hyperplastic polyps, which have no malignant potential, cannot be made at radiography or endoscopy. Biopsy (or polypectomy) and histological examination must be performed. Whenever possible, all polyps should be removed and retrieved for examination because they will not all be the same.

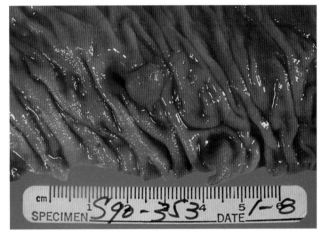

Figure 40.2 Typical macroscopic appearance of a 1-cm pedunculated tubular adenoma. Dark red coloration and the fine granular surface are depicted. The surfaces of tubular adenomas are typically fine and granular, as shown here, or lobulated. However, a definitive diagnosis can be made only by means of histopathological study.

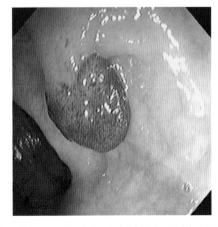

Figure 40.3 Colonoscopic photograph of an 8-mm tubular adenoma on a moderate-sized stalk.

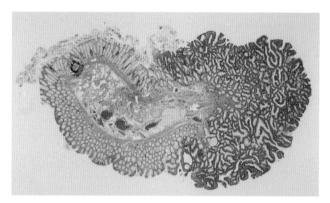

Figure 40.4 Low-power photomicrograph of a section of a small tubular adenoma with a long stalk (H & E stain). The adenoma comprises closely packed glands imparting a tubular appearance and shows few goblet cells. There is no complexity of glandular architecture and, at higher power, the columnar cells had basal nuclei and a moderate amount of cytoplasm. These findings are characteristic of low-grade (mild) dysplasia. The diathermy burn is at the base of the stalk, well clear of the adenoma.

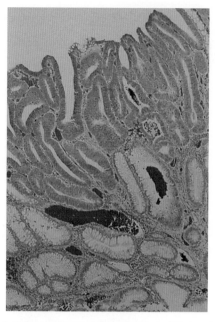

Figure 40.6 Higher-power view of another part of the specimen in Figure 40.5 shows closely packed epithelial tubules, pseudostratification, scant cytoplasm, and enlarged and elongated hyperchromatic nuclei in the dysplastic area.

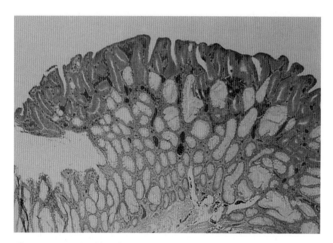

Figure 40.5 Histological appearance of a small tubular adenoma with mild dysplasia.

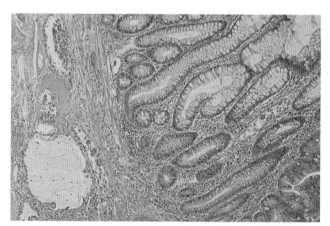

Figure 40.7 Medium-power photomicrograph of a section of part of a tubular adenoma (lower right) with "misplaced" mucin (lower left) within the submucosa deep to the muscularis mucosae (H & E stain). These appearances can be misinterpreted as invasive carcinoma, but note the absence of epithelium and the presence of lamina propria around the mucin pool indicating that this is not true invasion. Similarly, "misplaced" glands surrounded by lamina propria should not be interpreted as invasive carcinoma. Nonneoplastic mucosa is seen adjacent to the adenoma (top right).

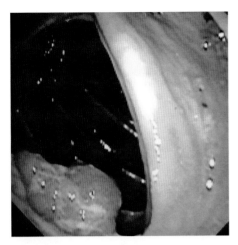

Figure 40.8 Colonoscopic photograph of a large adenoma in the ascending colon of a patient with hereditary nonpolyposis colorectal cancer.

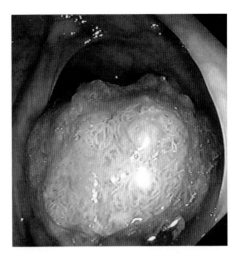

Figure 40.11 Colonoscopic photograph of a moderately large tubulovillous adenomatous polyp. Courtesy of Dr Michael Bourke.

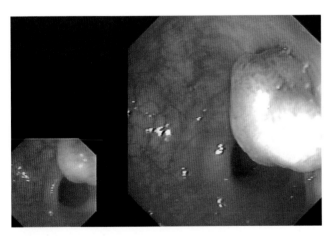

Figure 40.9 Endoscopic photograph showing semisessile sigmoid 1.5-cm tubulovillous adenoma partly obscured by a sigmoid fold in a patient without symptoms but at risk for hereditary nonpolyposis colorectal cancer.

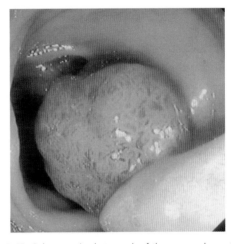

Figure 40.12 Colonoscopic photograph of the same polyp as in Figure 40.11 from a different perspective and showing its thick stalk.

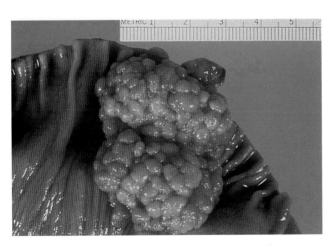

Figure 40.10 Macroscopic appearance of a tubulovillous adenoma.

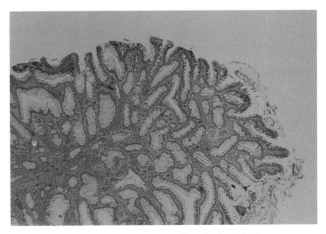

Figure 40.13 Histological appearance of a mixed tubulovillous adenoma. Image shows predominant epithelial tubules, villous projections at the surface, and the eosinophilic core of the polyp (lower left corner).

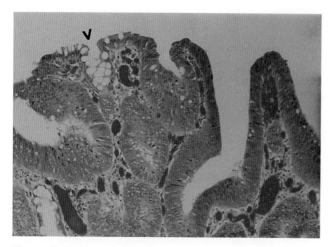

Figure 40.14 Histopathological appearance of a tubulovillous adenoma with high-grade dysplasia. There is marked variation in the cellular appearance of the dysplastic superficial cells with loss of basal polarity of nuclei and an increased nuclear-to-cytoplasmic ratio. Focal persistence of normal mucosa is present (arrowhead).

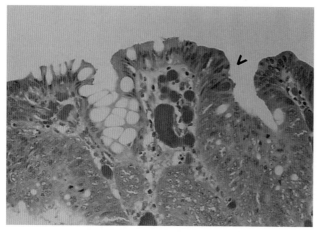

Figure 40.15 Higher-power view of tubulovillous adenoma in Figure 40.14 shows marked variation in nuclear and cytoplasmic appearance (arrowhead), pleomorphic hyperchromatic nuclei, crowding of the glands, and frequent mitotic figures.

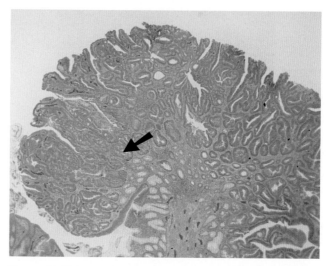

Figure 40.16 Low- to medium-power photomicrograph of a section of a portion of a 20-mm sigmoid polyp showing a tubulovillous adenoma with focal intramucosal carcinoma (arrow) (H & E stain). Note the complex glandular architecture with back-to-back arrangement and budding of glands. There is no submucosal invasion and the diathermy margin passed through normal epithelium (not apparent in this section).

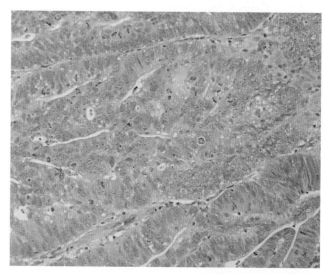

Figure 40.17 High-power photomicrograph of the same area of intramucosal carcinoma depicted in Figure 40.16 showing more clearly the complex glandular architecture with crowding and distortion of crypts. In addition there is high-grade cytological atypia with a high nuclear-to-cytoplasmic ratio, prominent nucleoli, some stratification, and conspicuous mitotic figures. Despite the lack of an obvious desmoplastic response, the constellation of these features is often regarded as intramucosal carcinoma rather than merely high-grade dysplasia. Because the resection margin was well clear of neoplasia and there was no invasion of vessels in the stalk, polypectomy alone was considered adequate in this case.

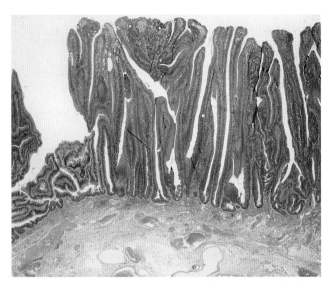

Figure 40.18 Medium-power photomicrograph of a section of a villous adenoma (H & E stain). Note the frond-like projections and relative lack of glandular architecture when compared with tubular adenomas.

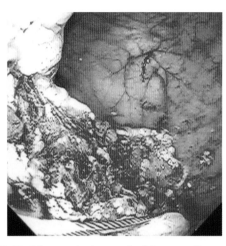

Figure 40.20 Colonoscopic photograph of the same villous adenoma as in Figure 40.19 after submucosal saline injection to lift the adenoma followed by polypectomy. The submucosal injection elevates the base and makes polypectomy a little easier and more likely to remove the base of the adenoma.

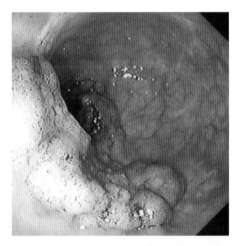

Figure 40.19 Colonoscopic photograph of an extensive, almost circumferential villous adenoma in the rectum that extended for 8 cm. This patient was not an ideal candidate for surgery and agreed to undergo attempted endoscopic removal.

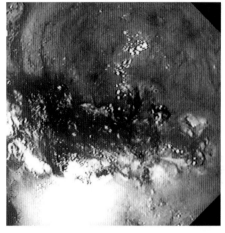

Figure 40.21 Colonoscopic photograph of the same villous adenoma as in Figure 40.20 after polypectomy followed by destruction of residual adenoma at the margins by argon plasma coagulation. Close follow-up is required to check for recurrence because total destruction cannot be guaranteed.

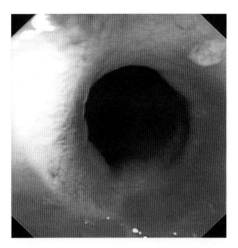

Figure 40.22 Colonoscopic photograph of the rectum of the same patient as in Figure 40.21, 14 months later. There is scarring but no residual tumor on biopsy of the pale area. The yellow patch is fecal material.

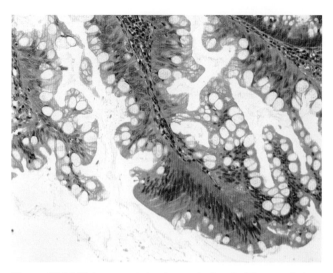

Figure 40.24 High-power photomicrograph of part of the same lesion depicted in Figure 40.23 showing more clearly the intermingling of the two components. The serrated surface typical of a hyperplastic polyp can be clearly seen, but the surface epithelium is also hyperchromatic and stratified with, in some foci, a high nuclear-to-cytoplasmic ratio indicative of dysplasia.

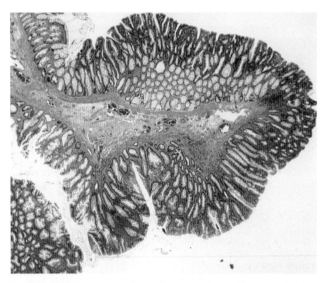

Figure 40.23 Low-power photomicrograph of a section of a typical serrated adenoma (H & E stain). Note the intermingling of the dysplastic component (imparting an appearance similar to that of a tubular adenoma) with the hyperplastic component characterized by the typical surface serrations. Some use the term "combined" or "mixed" when the adenomatous component lies adjacent to the hyperplastic component, reserving the term "serrated adenoma" for when the two components are intimately intermingled, as in this case.

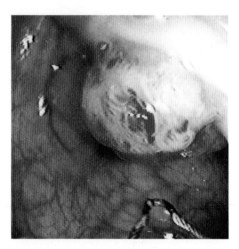

Figure 40.25 Colonoscopic photograph of a large serrated adenoma about to be removed from a patient with hyperplastic polyposis.

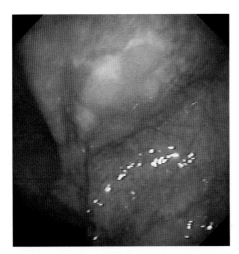

Figure 40.26 Endoscopic photograph shows a 1-cm flat, multilobulated polyp adjacent to the cecal sling fold. The polyp is pale pink whereas the surrounding mucosa is brown because of melanosis. Adenomas do not take up melanin and stand out in melanosis coli.

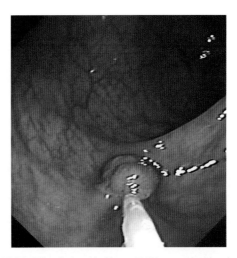

Figure 40.28 Polyp depicted in Figure 40.27 grasped with colonoscopic snare before electrocauterization. The colonoscope has been rotated to allow better apposition of the snare to the polyp base to optimize clearance. Better clearance and safety could be facilitated by submucosal injection of up to 10 mL of saline (not shown).

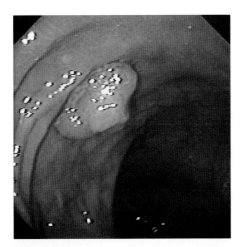

Figure 40.27 Colonoscopic photograph shows a semisessile, 1.4-cm polyp in the proximal rectum. Some irregularity of the surface and possible ulceration are evident by scalloping of the surface on the upper aspect.

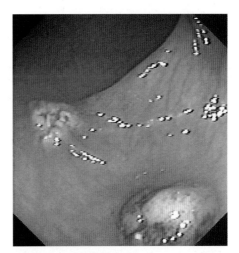

Figure 40.29 Clean polypectomy base interpreted by endoscopist as complete polypectomy of polyp depicted in Figure 40.27. The separated free-lying polyp is present in the foreground.

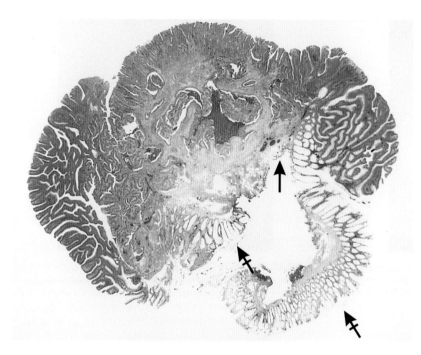

Figure 40.30 Histopathological examination of the polyp depicted in Figure 40.27 shows centrally placed, invasive, moderately differentiated adenocarcinoma arising in a sessile, moderately dysplastic tubulovillous adenoma. The malignant glands and surrounding desmoplastic stroma are approximately 600 μm from the closest point of the diathermized deep margin (arrow). Because of the closeness, this represents a relative indication to proceed to surgical resection. Crossed arrows point to the cuff of normal rectal mucosa included in the polypectomy specimen. The subsequent low anterior resection specimen did not contain any residual malignant tissue or lymph node metastases.

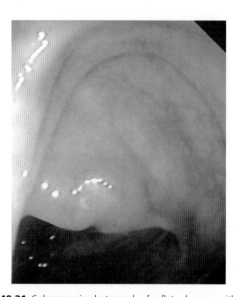

Figure 40.31 Colonoscopic photograph of a flat adenoma with slight central depression on the edge of a fold in the sigmoid colon. These are likely to show high-grade dysplasia. Flat adenomas are recognized more commonly in Japan, although one study has shown that they may be as common in Western countries such as the United Kingdom. Courtesy of Dr Michael Bourke.

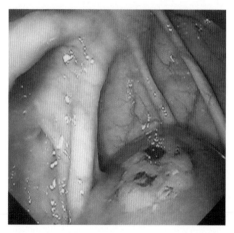

Figure 40.32 Colonoscopic photograph of a flat adenoma in the cecum that has been lifted by a submucosal injection of indigo carmine to facilitate colonoscopic removal. The wall of the cecum is thin and presents a higher risk of perforation than elsewhere in the colon. Courtesy of Dr Michael Bourke.

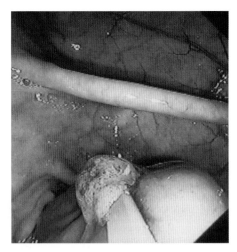

Figure 40.33 Colonoscopic photograph of the same lesion as in Figure 40.32 after application of the snare for polypectomy. Courtesy of Dr Michael Bourke.

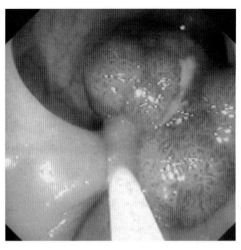

Figure 40.35 Colonoscopic photograph of a large, multilobulated tubulovillous adenoma showing the diathermy loop secured to the stalk a good distance below the adenoma tissue. Histopathology confirmed total removal with a 4-mm margin. Such polyps have a chance of containing a focus of carcinoma and complete removal at the first attempt is desirable. Courtesy of Dr Michael Bourke.

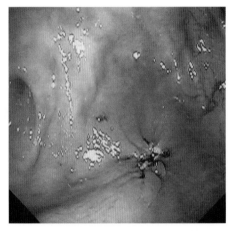

Figure 40.34 Colonoscopic photograph of the same lesion as in Figure 40.33 after snare polypectomy. Note the clean base and how the saline–indigo carmine lift helps ensure complete removal with less chance of perforation. Courtesy of Dr Michael Bourke.

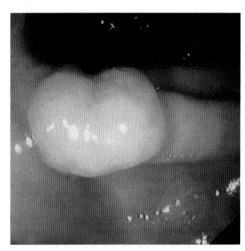

Figure 40.36 Colonoscopic photograph of a sessile polyp on a fold. Saline injection prior to polypectomy is desirable to aid complete removal and lessen the chance of perforation. Courtesy of Dr Michael Bourke.

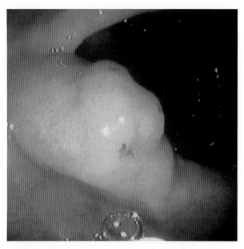

Figure 40.37 Colonoscopic photograph of the same sessile polyp as in Figure 40.36 after saline injection. Courtesy of Dr Michael Bourke.

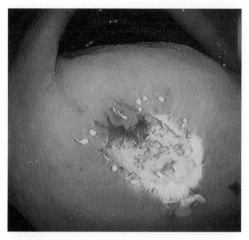

Figure 40.39 Colonoscopic photograph of the same sessile polyp as in Figure 40.38 after polypectomy. There is no obvious residual material. Note the bulge on the fold remaining from the saline injection into the submucosa. Courtesy of Dr Michael Bourke.

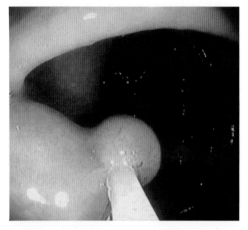

Figure 40.38 Colonoscopic photograph of the same sessile polyp as in Figure 40.37 after saline injection and subsequent snaring. In this situation it may be difficult to ensure that all of the adenoma is included because there is no discrete stalk; histopathological examination and possible early follow-up examination within 1 year are required to ensure the adequacy of removal. Courtesy of Dr Michael Bourke.

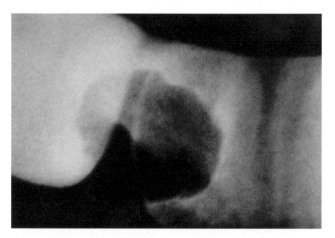

Figure 40.40 Radiographic appearance of a 2-cm sessile polyp with a somewhat lobulated surface. This was subsequently found to be tubulovillous adenoma with early invasive carcinoma. The carcinomatous invasion cannot be determined with radiography alone, or with endoscopy or biopsy. Large polyps must be removed in toto so that the degree of carcinomatous invasion, if any, can be determined. The drawing in of a haustral fold suggests malignant tethering.

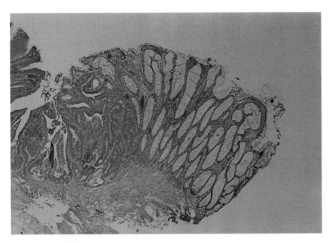

Figure 40.41 Histological appearance of a tubulovillous adenoma with severe dysplasia and invasion into and through the muscularis mucosae, typical of a malignant polyp. There is marked cell crowding with hyperchromatic, elongated nuclei, marked loss of basal polarity, an increased nucleus-to-cytoplasm ratio, and architectural distortion in the malignant focus. A lesion such as this highlights the inadequacy of biopsying such lesions because the carcinoma can easily be missed. All large polyps should be removed in toto and subjected to careful histological study.

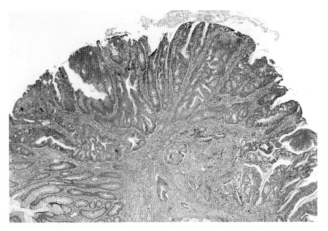

Figure 40.43 Medium-power photomicrograph of a section of an adenomatous polyp with a focus of invasive carcinoma in the submucosa of the stalk (H & E stain). In contrast to "misplaced" glands, note the lack of surrounding lamina propria and early desmoplastic response indicating true invasion.

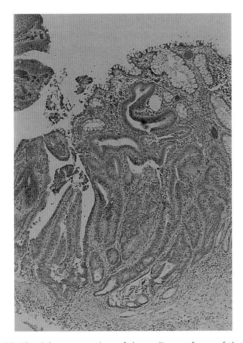

Figure 40.42 Higher-power view of the malignant focus of the adenoma in Figure 40.41 showing cytological detail with invasion into the muscularis mucosae.

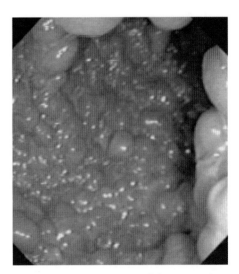

Figure 40.44 Colonoscopic photograph of the rectum of a teenage boy undergoing his first sigmoidoscopic surveillance for familial adenomatous polyposis. Many adenomas are apparent up to 10 mm in size. These extended well into the transverse colon and became sparse in the cecum. Residual fecal material accentuates the polyps.

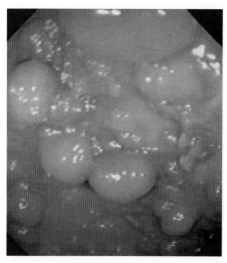

Figure 40.45 A close-up colonoscopic view of the same polyps from the patient shown in Figure 40.44.

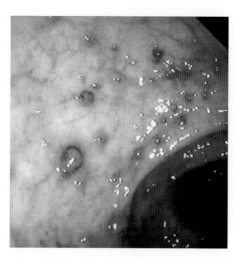

Figure 40.47 Colonoscopic photograph of scattered small polyps in the rectum of a patient with familial adenomatous polyposis who has undergone colectomy and ileorectal anastomosis.

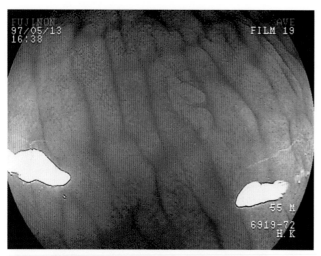

Figure 40.46 Magnifying colonoscopic view of a cluster of aberrant crypts with histopathological features of dysplasia. These are the earliest stage of adenoma formation. *APC* or *Ras* mutations (or both) may already be established in these lesions.

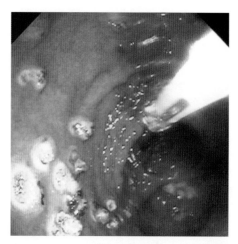

Figure 40.48 Colonoscopic photograph of the same patient shown in Figure 40.47 after destruction of the polyps by argon plasma coagulation.

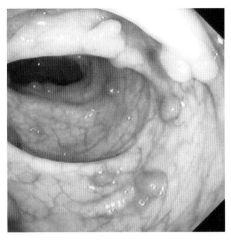

Figure 40.49 Colonoscopic photograph of sparse rectal polyps found at the first sigmoidoscopic examination of a patient in a family with attenuated (also termed "atypical") familial adenomatous polyposis. Note the dramatic difference in density of the polyps compared with that shown in Figure 40.44.

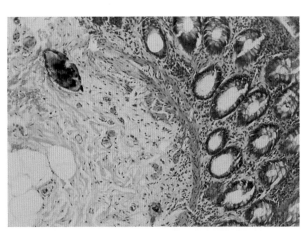

Figure 40.51 Typical histological appearance of an inflammatory polyp. The colonic glands are preserved and there is an increase of inflammatory cells in the lamina propria. This specimen was a result of schistosomiasis. A *Schistosoma haematobium* ovum, partially calcified, is lodged in the submucosa. Other inflammatory polyps, such as those found in inflammatory bowel disease, show similar histological features.

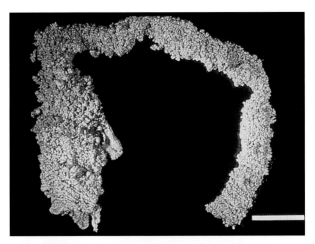

Figure 40.50 Colon resection specimen from a patient with familial adenomatous polyposis. The normal mucosa seems to be almost completely replaced by adenomas.

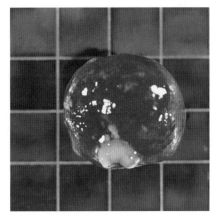

Figure 40.52 Macroscopic appearance of a juvenile polyp with a cherry-red, smooth, congested surface and a short, shiny mucosal stalk.

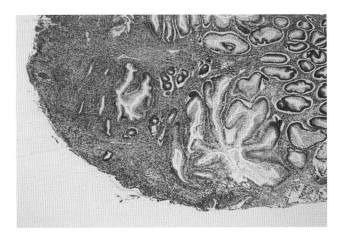

Figure 40.53 Histological features of the juvenile polyp from Figure 40.52 include cystically dilated glands without mucosal hyperplasia and an edematous, mildly inflamed lamina propria. The surface erosion is common with inflammatory exudate. The cystic dilation seen here is not as marked as usual.

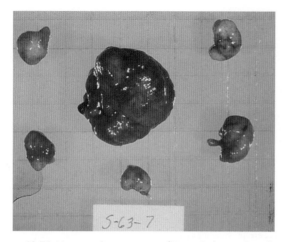

Figure 40.54 Macroscopic appearance of Peutz–Jeghers polyps: five small (0.3- to 0.8-cm) polyps and a 2.5-cm lobulated polyp. The polyps had a short stalk.

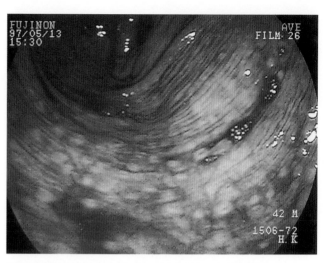

Figure 40.56 Colonoscopic photograph of lymphoid follicles highlighted by methylene blue dye. The methylene blue dye acts as a background against which the small follicles are raised above it like islands.

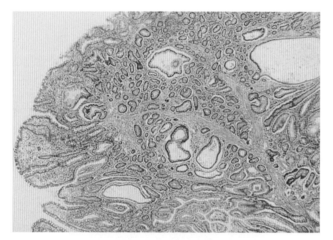

Figure 40.55 Histological features of Peutz–Jeghers polyps include atypical branching of the muscularis separating and surrounding islands of variably sized glands lined by normal colonic epithelium.

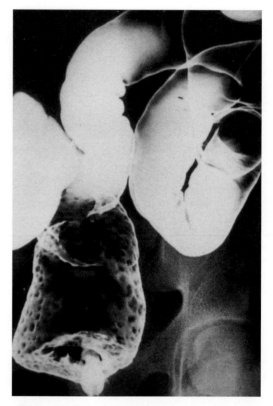

Figure 40.57 Large lymphoid polyps in the rectum typical of nodular lymphoid hyperplasia. Biopsy must be performed to differentiate this condition from multiple adenomas and lymphomas.

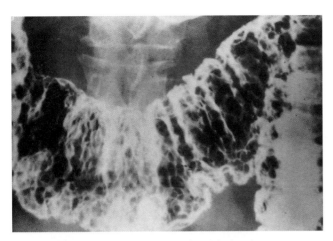

Figure 40.58 Radiological appearance of nodular lymphoma. Differentiation from lymphoid hyperplasia is difficult at radiology and biopsy is essential.

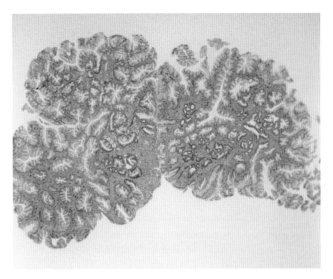

Figure 40.60 Low-power photomicrograph of an H & E-stained section of a hyperplastic polyp showing the typical serrated appearance of the surface epithelium and foci of hyperchromatic glandular epithelium within the crypts deeper in the lamina propria.

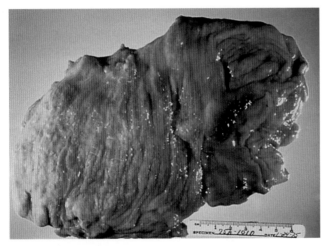

Figure 40.59 Macroscopic appearance of lymphosarcoma that appeared as multiple minute polyps, which suggest diffuse nodular lymphoid hyperplasia (which is benign).

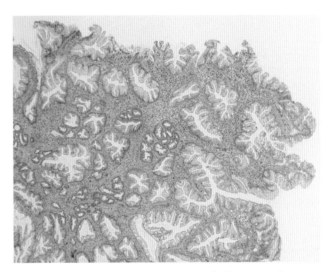

Figure 40.61 Medium-power photomicrograph of a section of a hyperplastic polyp showing the typical serrated appearance of the surface epithelium and the hyperchromatic glandular epithelium of the crypts deeper in the lamina propria (H & E stain).

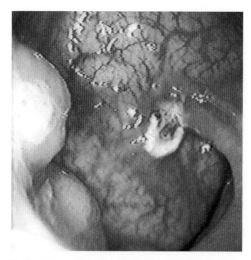

Figure 40.62 Colonoscopic photograph of hyperplastic polyps in the left colon of a patient with hyperplastic polyposis. These polyps are not distinguishable from adenomas without histological examination, preferably performed after polypectomy.

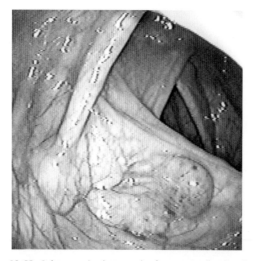

Figure 40.63 Colonoscopic photograph of sparse small polyps from the right side of the colon in the same patient as in Figure 40.62 with hyperplastic polyposis.

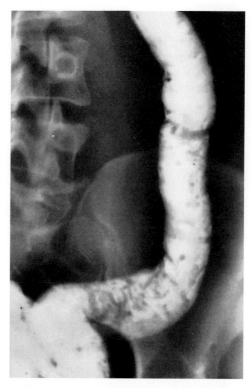

Figure 40.64 Radiological appearance of multiple inflammatory polyps ("pseudopolyps") in the descending colon of a patient with ulcerative colitis. Colonoscopy and biopsy are necessary for proper characterization of the lesions. During colonoscopy, the endoscopist should perform a biopsy on atypical polyps and suspicious plaque-like areas because these may show dysplasia. Dysplastic lesions, and not the inflammatory pseudopolyps, are the premalignant lesions.

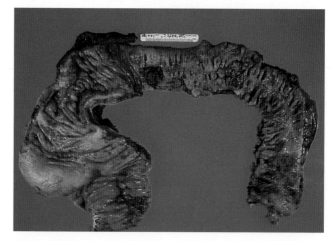

Figure 40.65 Total colon resection specimen from a 49-year-old man with a 20-year history of ulcerative colitis. In addition to the diffuse inflammatory mucosal changes and multiple inflammatory (pseudo) polyps, at least three distinct tumors, located 8, 15, and 25 cm distal to the ileocecal valve, are present.

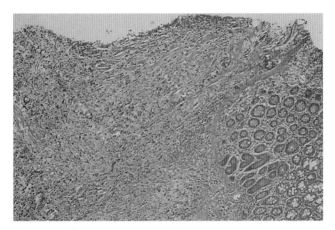

Figure 40.66 Microscopic section of the most proximal tumor from Figure 40.65 shows the abrupt change from fairly normal lining mucosa to invasive, pleomorphic, poorly differentiated carcinoma typical of ulcerative colitis.

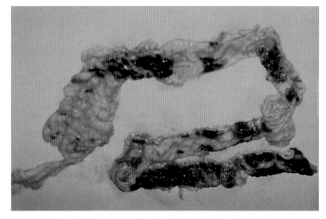

Figure 40.67 Colon resection specimen of pneumatosis cystoides intestinalis. Extensive pneumatosis and necrosis are depicted. The glistening, translucent, air-filled blebs vary in size. This case was caused by necrotizing enterocolitis, hence the poor state of the colon. Most cases of pneumatosis are idiopathic and asymptomatic.

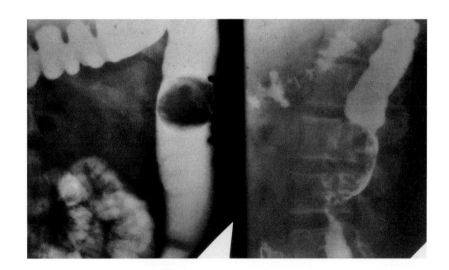

Figure 40.68 Characteristic radiographic appearance of a lipoma. The submucosal nature is suggested on the postevacuation radiograph (the image on the **right**) by the round, smooth, radiolucent appearance.

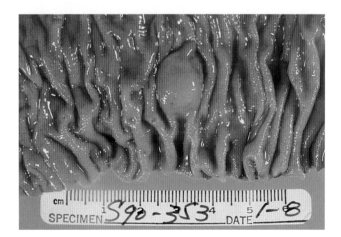

Figure 40.69 Macroscopic appearance of a 1 × 1.3-cm lipoma shows a normal smooth mucosal surface over the submucosal lipoma with a translucent yellowish color.

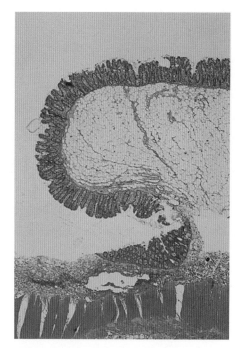

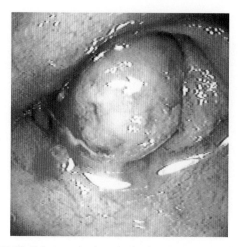

Figure 40.72 Colonoscopic photograph of an asymptomatic ileal carcinoid tumor (1.5 cm) found at surveillance colonoscopy for hereditary nonpolyposis colon cancer.

Figure 40.70 Histological section of the lipoma from Figure 40.69 shows well-defined areas of mature, well-vascularized adipose tissue expanding the submucosal space and forming a sessile polyp covered by normal mucosa.

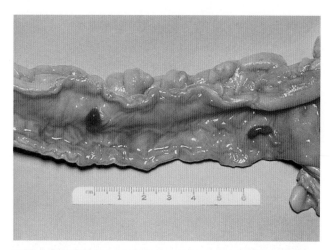

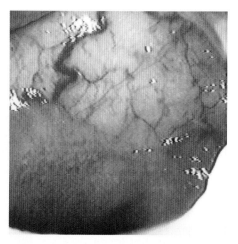

Figure 40.73 Colonoscopic photograph of the base adjacent to the carcinoid tumor shown in Figure 40.72 depicting the "feeding" vessel characteristic of larger carcinoids.

Figure 40.71 Macroscopic appearance of hemangiomas (blue rubber bleb nevus syndrome). Two hemangiomas, one 0.5 × 0.5 cm, the other 1.0 × 0.3 cm, are depicted. The hemangiomas are cherry-red, vascular-appearing polypoid lesions. Biopsy of these and other vascular-appearing lesions may be hazardous.

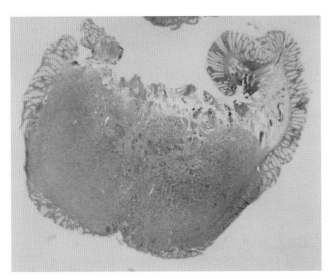

Figure 40.74 Low-power photomicrograph of a section from a biopsy of a 13-mm rectal polyp removed by loop diathermy and found to be a carcinoid (H & E stain). Note that although there is mucosal involvement and focal ulceration, the bulk of the lesion lies within the submucosa. Higher-power views showed the typical nests of small uniform cells having a stippled nuclear chromatin pattern characteristic of a carcinoid tumor. The tumor extends to the cauterized margin and complete removal cannot be guaranteed.

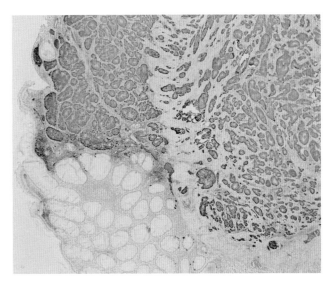

Figure 40.75 Medium-power photomicrograph of an immunoperoxidase-stained section of the same lesion shown in Figure 40.74 using antibodies to the neuroendocrine marker chromogranin, with diaminobenzidine as the chromogen (brown reaction). Note the small rosettes and solid nests typical of a carcinoid tumor involving the mucosa and underlying submucosa. Adjacent mucosa shows only an occasional positively staining cell in keeping with the more normal distribution of neuroendocrine cells within the mucosa.

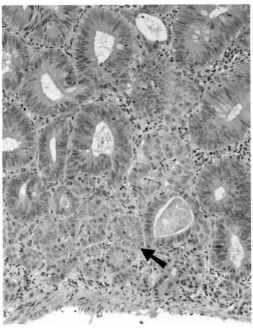

Figure 40.76 High-power photomicrograph of a section from a biopsy of a most unusual cecal polyp (H & E stain). This polyp was sessile and had an atypical appearance on endoscopy; hence, polypectomy was not attempted. Microscopic examination revealed the typical features of a tubular adenoma with low-grade dysplasia (upper half of photograph), but also showed small rosettes of rounded, uniform cells with eosinophilic cytoplasm adjacent to the muscularis mucosae suggestive of a neuroendocrine tumor (arrow).

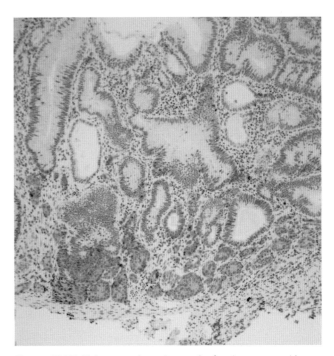

Figure 40.77 High-power photomicrograph of an immunoperoxidase-stained section of the same lesion shown in Figure 40.76 using antibodies to the neuroendocrine marker chromogranin, with diaminobenzidine as the chromogen (brown reaction). In comparison with the tubular adenoma component, the small rosettes of cells noted in the section stain intensely brown (H & E stain), confirming that this is a composite tubular adenoma–carcinoid tumor. Co-occurrence of these two pathologies is rare. Provided excision is complete, and there is nothing to suggest more extensive infiltration by the carcinoid, polypectomy alone should be adequate because small benign carcinoids are not uncommon in the cecum.

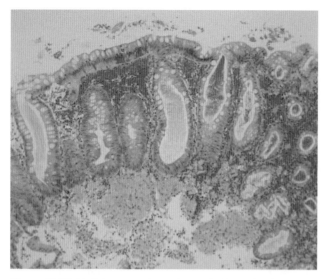

Figure 40.78 Medium-power photomicrograph of a section from a biopsy from an unusual rectal polypoid lesion caused by amyloidosis in a patient presenting with rectal bleeding (H & E stain). Note the pale-staining eosinophilic amyloid deposition, particularly at the base of the crypts, in contrast to the extravasation of red cells in the more superficial lamina propria.

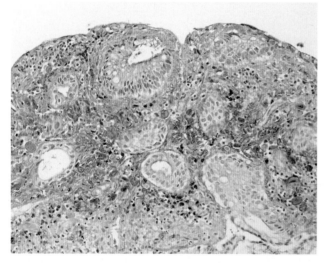

Figure 40.79 Corresponding photomicrograph of an immunoperoxidase-stained section of the biopsy shown in Figure 40.78 using antibodies to amyloid P protein, with diaminobenzidine as the chromogen (brown reaction). Note the widespread deposition of amyloid throughout the lamina propria, which was previously masked in the section by the red cell extravasation.

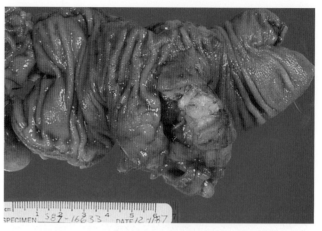

Figure 40.80 A firm, submucosal, ill-defined mass in the wall of the cecum of a 44-year-old woman with endometriosis appearing as a polypoid lesion at colonoscopy. The mass has been cut open for frozen-section studies.

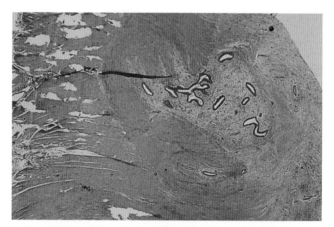

Figure 40.81 Histological section of the endometriosis depicted in Figure 40.80 shows islands of endometrial tissue (glands lined by benign columnar epithelium and surrounded by spindle cell stroma) in the submucosa and muscularis of the colonic wall.

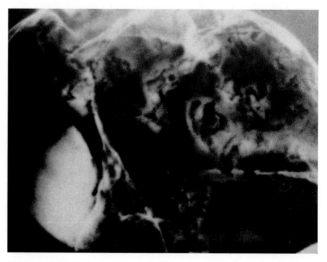

Figure 40.82 Radiographic artifact mimicking polyps caused by mucoid fecal material. Thorough colonic cleansing is important for radiographic and endoscopic studies.

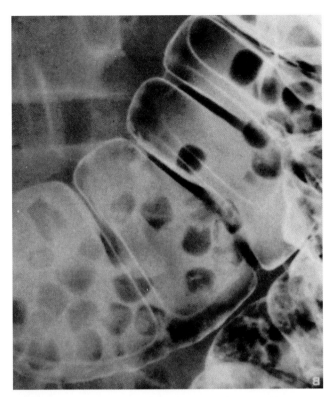

Figure 40.83 Radiographic artifact mimicking polyps caused by undigested kernels of corn. Undigested food remnants, especially corn and peas, often produce this artifact.

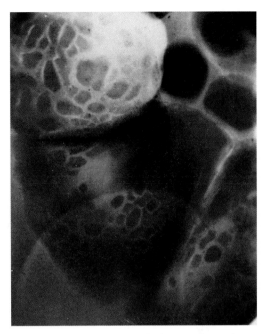

Figure 40.85 Radiographic appearance of cecal urticaria. The papular appearance of the urticarial lesions is depicted. These lesions often respond to antihistamine or corticosteroid therapy. They can be misdiagnosed as multiple polyps.

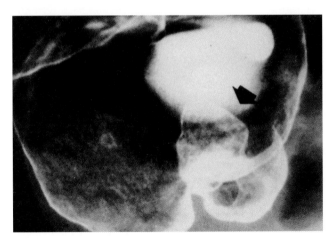

Figure 40.84 The appendiceal stump often mimics a polyp at radiological and endoscopic examinations. A history of appendectomy within the previous few years should alert the clinician to this artifact.

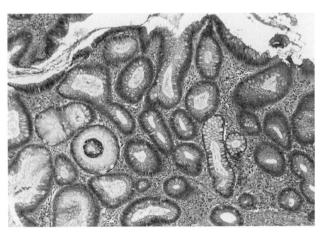

Figure 40.86 Histological appearance of a tubular adenoma with low-grade dysplasia. Architectural organization includes orderly, closely packed epithelial tubules. Cells have a normal nuclear-to-cytoplasmic ratio, nuclei have a predominantly basal orientation, and goblet cells are present.

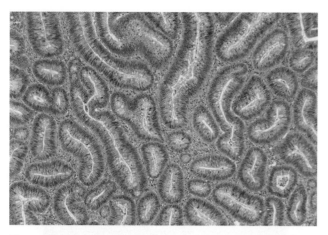

Figure 40.87 Histological appearance of a tubular adenoma with low-grade dysplasia but slightly more architectural distortion than in Figure 40.86. There is also more cellular crowding, variation in nuclei, and occasional loss of basal polarity with an increased nuclear-to-cytoplasmic ratio. No goblet cells are seen. In the three-tier system of grading dysplasia, this could be classed as moderate in grade.

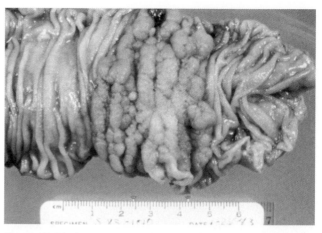

Figure 40.89 This cecal villous adenoma is virtually circumferential, with submucosal carcinomatous invasion. The lesion is sessile in nature and has a cauliflower appearance with a shaggy, frond-like, friable surface.

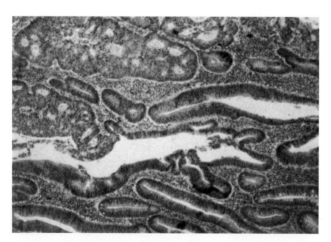

Figure 40.88 Histological appearance of a tubulovillous adenoma with severe dysplasia and contiguous carcinoma. Note the hyperchromatic elongated nuclei with loss of basal polarity and the increased nuclear-to-cytoplasmic ratio. There is a sharp and drastic transition between these adenomatous features and carcinoma.

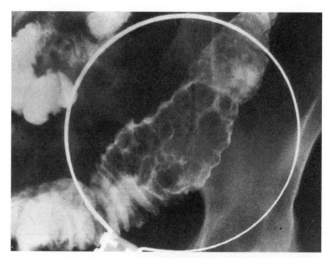

Figure 40.90 A very large, multilobulated, polypoid mass is demonstrated in the colon by radiography. Note the shaggy-appearing mucosal surface. The mass was subsequently found to be a large, sessile, villous adenoma that was virtually circumferential, similar to the lesion in Figure 40.89.

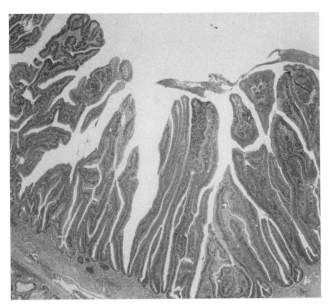

Figure 40.91 Histological section of a villous adenoma with typical frond-like appearance. Note the more marked architectural disturbance than is seen with tubular adenomas. The nuclear-to-cytoplasmic ratio is increased, and nuclei are not always basally situated.

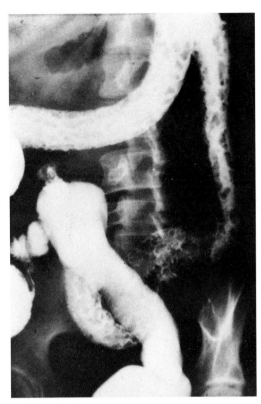

Figure 40.93 Multiple inflammatory polyps are present throughout the colon in a patient with ulcerative colitis. Colonoscopy and biopsy are necessary for proper identification of the lesions.

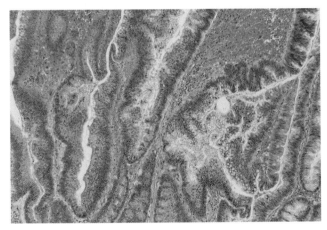

Figure 40.92 Section of a tubulovillous adenoma showing high-grade dysplasia. Note the substantial architectural disturbance and pallisading of nuclei.

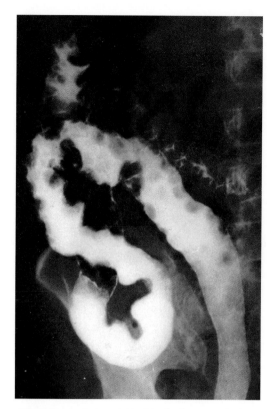

Figure 40.94 Pneumatosis cystoides intestinalis seen on barium-enhanced radiography. The intramural gas-filled cysts could have been identifiable on a plain abdominal radiograph.

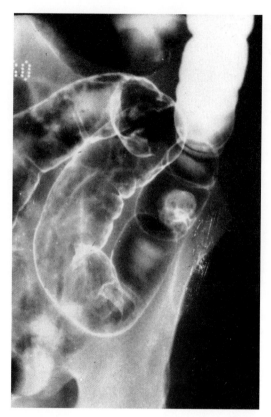

Figure 40.95 A pedunculated polyp demonstrated by double-contrast radiography. Note the lobulated appearance of the polyp surface. The mass was subsequently found at polypectomy to be a tubulovillous adenoma.

Polyposis syndromes

Randall W. Burt, Russell F. Jacoby

The gastrointestinal polyposis syndromes are a set of uncommon diseases considered together because they each express multiple polypoid lesions of the gut. A number of separate syndromes can be defined in terms of pathological and clinical characteristics. Genetic advances have allowed an even more precise definition and categorization of these conditions. The syndromes are important because they each exhibit benign and malignant complications. They are sufficiently common that all gastroenterologists and gastrointestinal surgeons will deal with them. Furthermore, because intestinal issues are central to the diagnosis and management of patients with polyposis, gastroenterologists are often the primary care physicians of polyposis patients and families. The conditions are summarized in Tables 41.1 and 41.2.

Atlas of Gastroenterology, 4th edition. Edited by Tadataka Yamada, David H. Alpers, Anthony N. Kalloo, Neil Kaplowitz, Chung Owyang, and Don W. Powell. © 2009 Blackwell Publishing, ISBN: 978-1-4051-6909-7

Table 41.1 Distinguishing features of the polyposis syndromes

Syndrome	Gene (frequency mutation found)	CRC risk (mean age of diagnosis)	Polyp histology	Polyp distribution	Mean age of GI symptom onset	Most prominent extraintestinal features Benign	Malignant
Familial adenomatous polyposis[a]	APC (70%–90%)	100% (39 years); AFAP, 69% (58 years)	Adenomatous, except stomach: fundic gland polyps	Stomach: 23%–100%; duodenum: 50%–90%; jejunum: 50%; ileum: 20%; colon: 100%	33 years	Desmoid tumors, epidermoid cysts, fibromas, osteomas, CHRPE, adrenal adenomas, dental abnormalities, nasal angiofibromas	Duodenal or periampullary: 3%–5%; rare pancreatic, biliary, thyroid, gastric, CNS, hepatoblastoma, small bowel
MYH-associated polyposis	MYH (recessive inheritance, 16%–40% if 15–100 adenomas)	93-fold increased risk (61 years)	Adenomatous	Possible gastric, duodenal; colon usually	Not determined	None known	None known
Peutz–Jeghers syndrome	STK11 (LKB1) (50%–60%)	39% (46 years)	Peutz–Jeghers	Stomach: 24%; small bowel: 96%; colon: 27%; rectum: 24%	22–26 years	Orocutaneous melanin pigment spots	Pancreatic: 36%; gastric: 29%; small bowel: 13%; breast: 54%; ovarian: 21%; uterine: 9%; lung: 15%; testes: 9%; cervix: 10%
Juvenile polyposis	SMAD4 (DPC4), BMPR1A, ENG (53%)	9%–68% (34 years)	Juvenile	Stomach: 14%; duodenum: 7%; small bowel: 7%; colon: 98%	18.5 years	Macrocephaly, hypertelorism, 20% congenital abnormalities in sporadic type	Stomach and duodenum combined up to 21%; pancreatic increased
Cowden syndrome[b]	PTEN (80%–90%)	Little, if any	Juvenile, lipomas, inflammatory, ganglioneuromas, lymphoid hyperplasia	Esophagus: 66%; stomach: 75%; duodenum: 37%; colon: 66%	Not determined	Facial trichilemmomas, oral papillomas, multinodular goiter, fibrocyctic breast disease	Thyroid: 3%–10%; breast: 25%–50%; uterine: 2%–5%
Hereditary mixed polyposis syndrome	Locus on chromosome 6	Increased, but uncertain (47 years)	Atypical juvenile, adenomatous, hyperplastic	Primarily colon	40 years	None known	None known
Gorlin syndrome	PTCH	Not known	Hamartoma	Only gastric reported	Not determined	Mandibular bone cysts, pits of palms and soles, macrocephaly	Basal cell carcinoma

a Includes Gardner syndrome, two-thirds of Turcot syndrome cases, and attenuated familial adenomatous polyposis (AFAP).

b Includes Bannayan–Riley–Ruvalcaba syndrome and Lhermitte–Duclos disease.

CHRPE, congenital hypertrophy of the retinal pigment epithelium; CNS, central nervous system; CRC, colorectal cancer; GI, gastrointestinal.

Table 41.2 Additional conditions that exhibit gastrointestinal polyposis

Category	Condition	Cause	Histology of polyps	GI areas affected	Other disease manifestations	
					Benign	Malignant
Syndromes in which polyps contain neural elements	Neurofibromatosis type I (NF1)	Mutations of *NF1* gene, autosomal dominantly inherited	Neurofibromas and ganglioneuromas	Small bowel > stomach > colon	Café au lait spots; cutaneous neurofibromas	Ampullary carcinoid, pheochromocytoma, GISTs
	Multiple endocrine neoplasia type IIB (MEN2B)	Mutation at codon 918 of *RET* protooncogene, autosomal dominantly inherited	Ganglioneuromas	Lips to anus, but most common in colon and rectum	Pheochromocytoma; parathyroid adenoma	Medullary thyroid carcinoma
Syndromes of uncertain etiology	Cronkhite–Canada syndrome	Possibly infectious	Juvenile polyps	Stomach to anus	Skin hyperpigmentation, hair loss, nail atrophy, hypogeusia	12%–15% colon cancer
	Hyperplastic polyposis	Possibly inherited	Hyperplastic	Colon	None known	Colon cancer risk probably increased
Conditions with inflammatory polyps	Inflammatory bowel disease	Crohn's disease and ulcerative colitis	Pseudopolyps	Colon	As in inflammatory bowel disease	
	Devon polyposis	Inherited	Fibroid polyps	Ileum, stomach	None known	
	Cap polyposis	Unknown, possibly internal prolapse	Similar to solitary rectal ulcer	Rectosigmoid	Rectal bleeding	None
Polyposis conditions arising from lymphoid tissue	Nodular lymphoid hyperplasia	Isolated > immunodeficiency > lymphoma	Hyperplasia of lymphoid nodules	Small bowel, stomach, colon	Related to underlying disease	
	Multiple lymphomatous polyposis	A type of mantle cell lymphoma	Multiple malignant lymphomatous polyps	Small bowel and colon > stomach	None known	
	Immunoproliferative small intestinal disease (a MALT lymphoma)	Most cases from *Campylobacter jejuni* infection	Plasma cell proliferation	Small bowel	Malabsorption, progression to lymphoplasmacytic and immunoblastic lymphoma if not treated in early stages	
Miscellaneous noninherited polyposis conditions	Leiomyomatosis	Not known	Leiomyoma	Colon, other	None known	
	Lipomatous polyposis	Not known	Lipoma	Colon, other	None known	
	Multiple lymphangiomas	Not known	Lymphangioma	Colon	None known	
	Pneumatosis cystoides intestinalis	Not known	Inflammatory and air spaces	Colon and other GI locations	None known	

GI, gastrointestinal; GISTs, gastrointestinal stromal tumors; MALT, mucosa-associated lymphoid tissue.

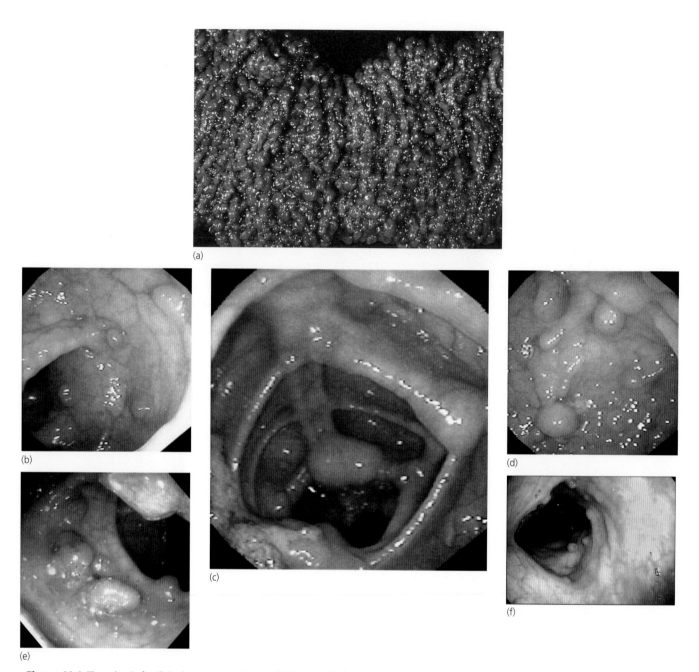

Figure 41.1 The colon in familial adenomatous polyposis. **(a)** Section of colon exhibiting fully developed familial adenomatous polyposis. **(b–f)** Colonoscopic views of patients with familial adenomatous polyposis. (a) Courtesy of Robert Flinner, MD, Salt Lake City, UT; (b–d) courtesy of Dr Robert Kiyomura; (e) courtesy of Dr Robert J. Pagano; (f) courtesy of Dr James DiSario.

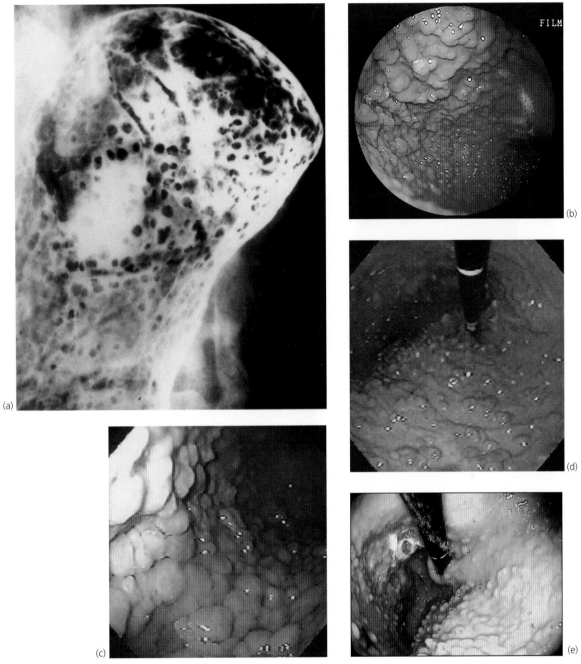

Figure 41.2 Fundic gland polyps of familial adenomatous polyposis. **(a)** Upper gastrointestinal radiograph of the proximal stomach showing numerous small polyps. **(b–e)** Endoscopic photographs of the proximal stomach demonstrating the typical pattern of numerous fundic gland polyps. (a) Courtesy of Dr Kyosuke Ushio. (*Continued on next page.*)

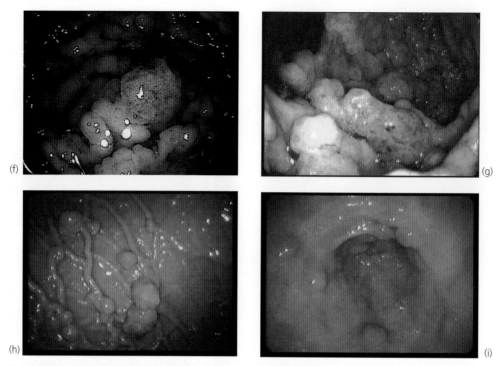

(f)

(g)

(h)

(i)

Figure 41.2 *Continued* **(f–h)** Endoscopic photographs of the proximal stomach demonstrating the typical pattern of numerous fundic gland polyps. **(i)** Endoscopic photograph of antral adenomas. (h,i) courtesy of Dr James DiSario.

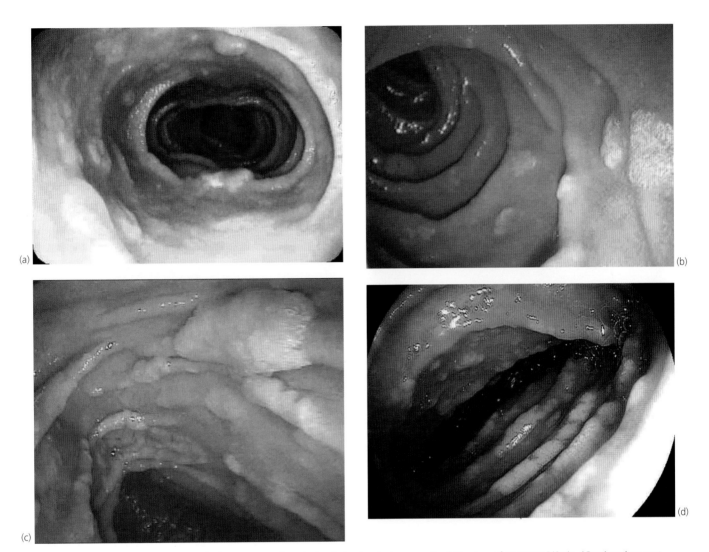

Figure 41.3 Duodenal polyps in familial adenomatous polyposis: **(a–d)** duodenal adenomas; (b–d) Courtesy of Dr James DiSario. (*Continued on next page.*)

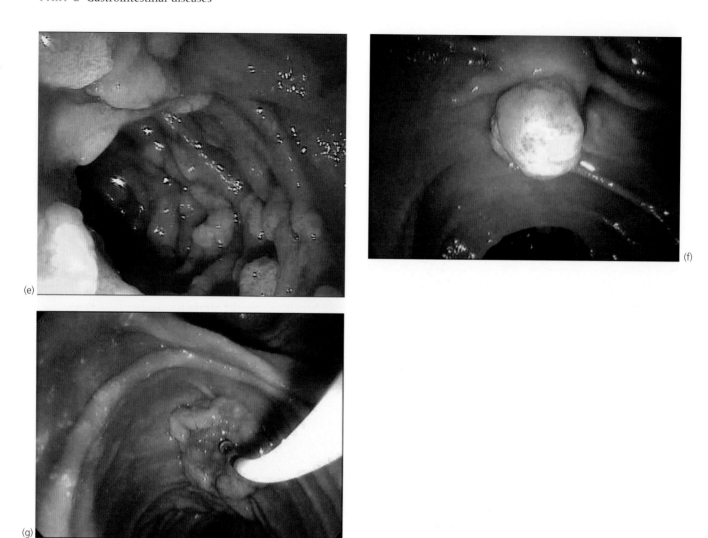

Figure 41.3 *Continued* **(e)** Duodenal adenomas; **(f)** ampullary adenoma; **(g)** ampullary mass. **(e–g)** Courtesy of Dr James DiSario.

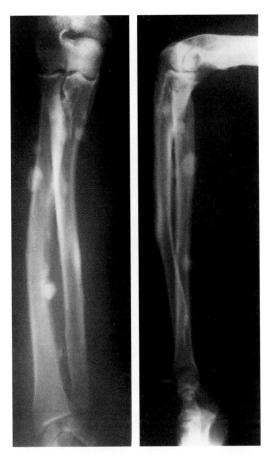

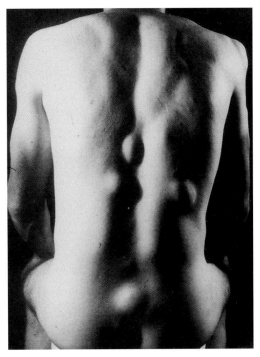

Figure 41.5 Epidermoid cysts on a patient with Gardner syndrome. These may occur anywhere on the cutaneous surface. They often occur before puberty and may grow to several centimeters in diameter.

Figure 41.4 Osteomas of Gardner syndrome. In this syndrome osteomas may form on any bone of the body. They occur most commonly at the angle of the mandible and elsewhere on the skull but they may also be observed on long bones, as seen on the forearm and leg in these radiographs.

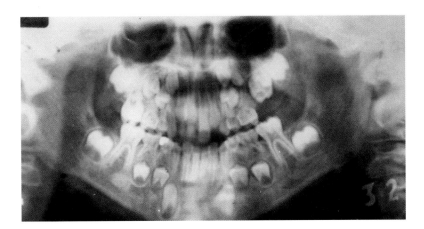

Figure 41.6 Dental abnormalities in a patient with Gardner syndrome. Opacities of the mandible as well as supernumerary teeth are evident in this panoramic radiograph of the maxilla and mandible.

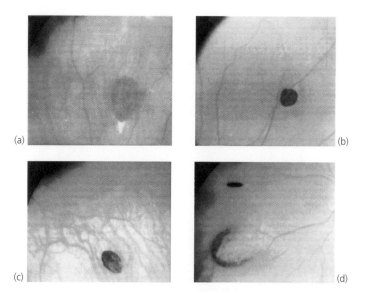

Figure 41.7 Congenital hypertrophy of the retinal pigment epithelium. **(a–d)** Several sizes and hues of the retinal pigment are observed in pedigrees with adenomatous polyposis who exhibit *APC* mutations distal to exon 9. Although such lesions are common, the presence of bilateral or more than four retinal lesions is specific for familial adenomatous polyposis.

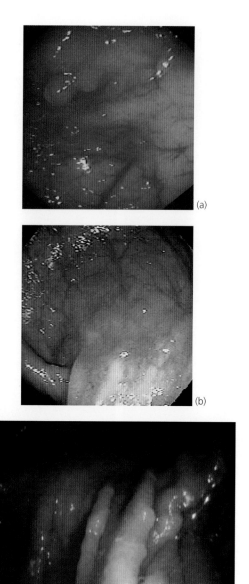

Figure 41.8 (a–c) Small, more subtle colonic adenomas of attenuated adenomatous polyposis coli. (a,b) Courtesy of Dr James DiSario.

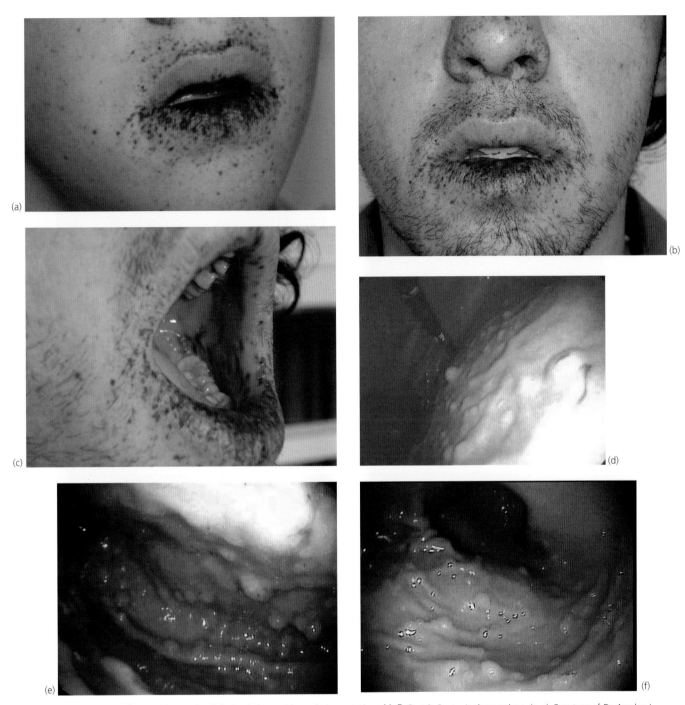

Figure 41.9 Peutz–Jeghers syndrome. **(a–c)** Perioral, lip, and buccal pigmentation. **(d–f)** Gastric Peutz–Jeghers polyps. (a–c) Courtesy of Dr Asadur J. Tchekmedyian. (*Continued on next page.*)

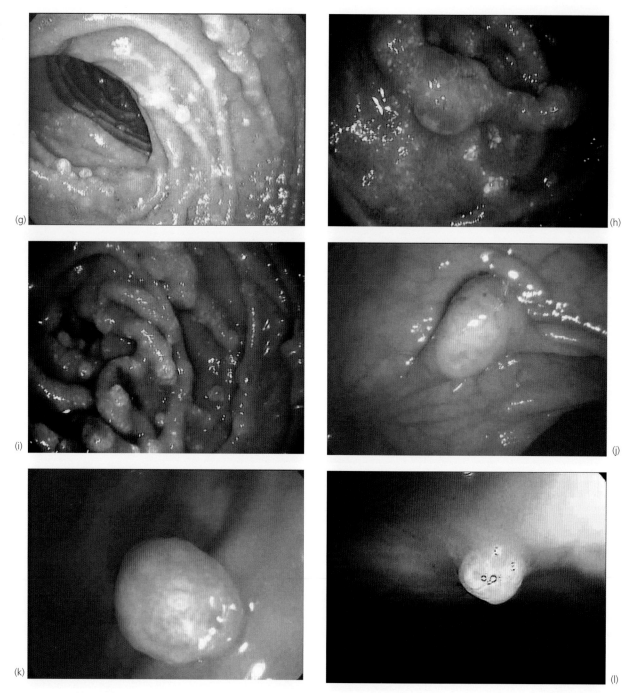

Figure 41.9 *Continued* **(g–i)** Duodenal Peutz–Jeghers polyps. **(j–l)** Colonic Peutz–Jeghers polyps.

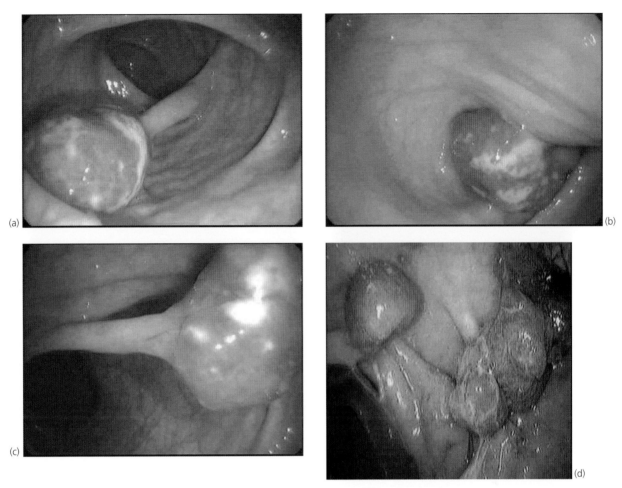

(a)

(b)

(c)

(d)

Figure 41.10 Juvenile polyposis syndrome. **(a–d)** Colonic juvenile polyps in patients with juvenile polyposis.

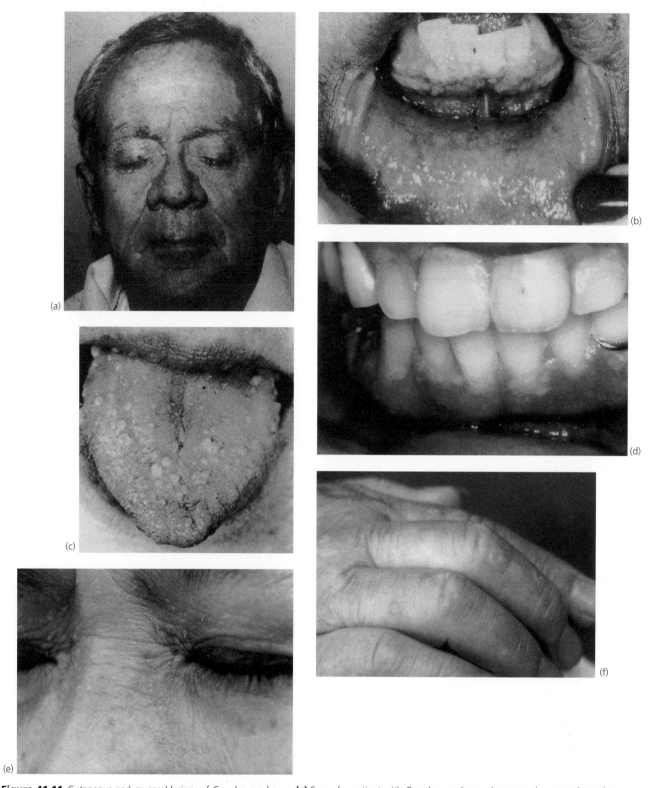

Figure 41.11 Cutaneous and mucosal lesions of Cowden syndrome. **(a)** Face of a patient with Cowden syndrome demonstrating central papules. **(b)** Labial mucosa and gingiva showing cobblestone papules. **(c)** Tongue with typical papules. **(d)** Fibromas on the gingiva. **(e)** Trichilemmomas of the face. **(f)** Hyperkeratosis of the digits. (d–f) courtesy of Dr Kyosuke Ushio. (*Continued on next page.*)

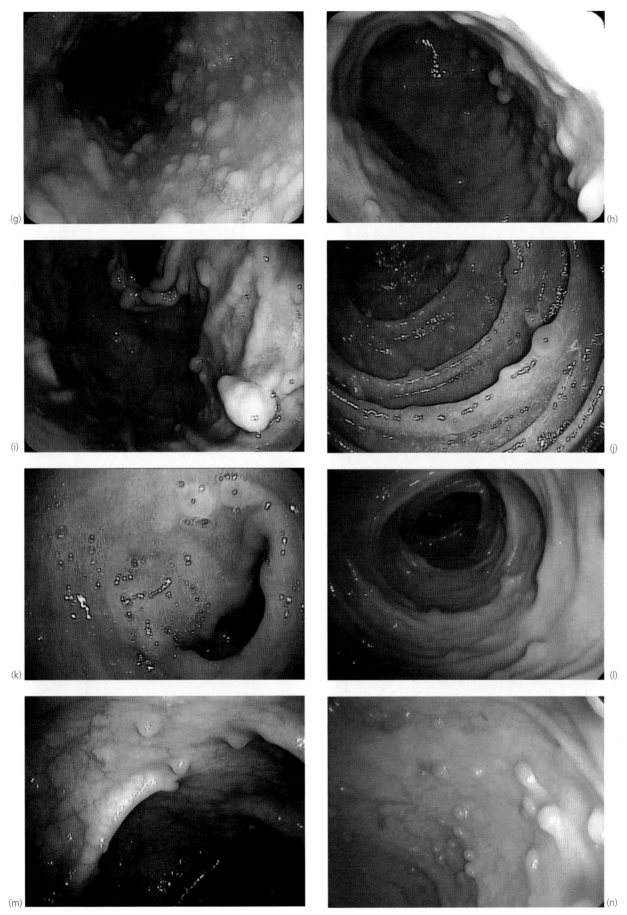

Figure 41.11 *Continued* **(g)** Endoscopic photograph of the esophageal lesions, glycogenic acanthosis. **(h,i)** Gastric polyps in Cowden syndrome, which are hamartomas. **(j)** Duodenal hamartomatous polyps in Cowden syndrome in the second part of the duodenum. **(k)** Duodenal hamartomatous polyps in Cowden syndrome in the bulb of the duodenum. **(l–n)** Colonic hamartomatous polyps of Cowden syndrome.

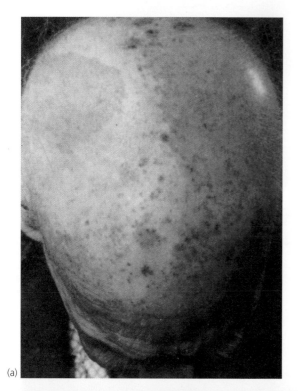

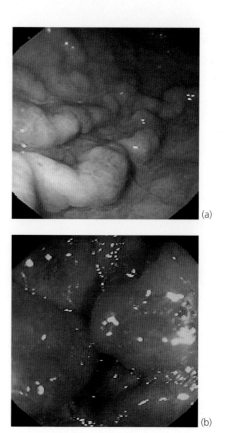

Figure 41.13 Endoscopic views of a patient with Cronkhite–Canada syndrome. The patient presented with dysgeusia, alopecia, onychodystrophy, and diarrhea. **(a)** Stomach. **(b)** Colon: the largest polyp is a pedunculated adenomatous polyp; all other polyps shown exhibited histology typical of Cronkhite–Canada lesions. Courtesy of Dr Edward L. Krawitt.

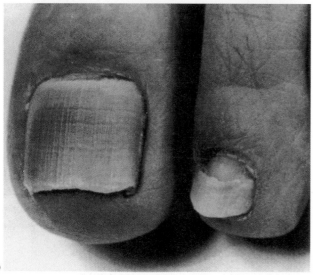

Figure 41.12 Cronkhite–Canada syndrome. **(a)** Scalp showing almost total alopecia. **(b)** Onychodystrophy of toenails with lines of separation from the normal nail.

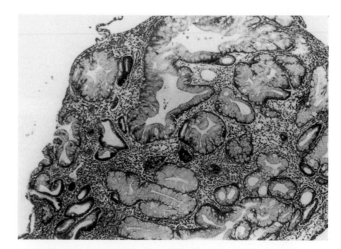

Figure 41.14 Polyp from a patient with Cronkhite–Canada syndrome. The polyp demonstrates cystically dilated glands with abundant generous, edematous, and inflamed lamina propria. The polyps of Cronkhite–Canada syndrome are very similar to those of juvenile polyposis. Intervening mucosa in Cronkhite–Canada syndrome, however, is abnormal, with edema and inflammation of the lamina propria.

42

Malignant tumors of the colon

David H. Alpers, Francis M. Giardiello

Colorectal adenocarcinoma is a major human health problem worldwide affecting approximately one million individuals per year and causing 500 000 deaths annually. Over the past two decades, a significant basic science and clinical research effort has focused on colorectal cancer. These investigations have resulted in a series of seminal discoveries in the pathogenesis of colorectal cancer. In some individuals with these tumors, germline mutations are the readily identifiable cause; however, in most, the development of this malignancy appears to be a complex interaction between the host genome and environmental factors. Advances in knowledge of colorectal cancer have resulted in improvements in surgical/endoscopic techniques, epidemiology, screening, and surveillance of high-risk groups. Moreover, in the past decade several new chemotherapeutic agents have been released that have been developed from basic scientific understanding of tumor biology. Despite these advances, surgery still remains the treatment that offers the greatest hope for cure. Because colorectal cancer usually arises over a prolonged period and is accessible to screening techniques, secondary prevention remains the best modality to decrease death from this malignancy.

Illustrations of the epidemiological features of colorectal cancer are shown in Figures 42.1–42.3 and Table 42.1. A model of the genetic events involved in the production of colorectal cancer is illustrated in Figures 42.4 and 42.5.

The value of fecal occult blood testing for colorectal cancer screening has been demonstrated by many investigators. Results from major studies are documented in Tables 42.2–42.8. The accuracy of screening an average risk population for colorectal neoplasia with standard fecal occult blood testing compared with DNA stool testing is shown in Table 42.9. Table 42.10 presents data from one study reporting the highest rates of sensitivity and specificity for detection of colorectal adenomas during screening of average risk persons

with virtual colonoscopy in comparison to optical colonoscopy. An algorithm for the screening of colorectal cancer is shown in Figure 42.6. Family history is important in deciding who is at increased risk for colorectal cancer; these risk estimates are shown in Figure 42.7 and Table 42.11. Genetic testing is commonly used to define colorectal cancer risk. Table 42.12 gives the common clinical indications for genetic testing.

Knowledge of pathological stage of colorectal cancer is important in patient management and prognosis. Figure 42.8 illustrates the Dukes–Turnbull classification system and the correlation with tumor, node, and metastasis (TNM) stages. Table 42.13 and Figures 42.9 and 42.10 describe the TNM staging system and associated rates of survival and the clinical outcome of patients presenting with colorectal cancer. The distribution of another colon tumor (carcinoid) at the time of presentation is shown in Table 42.14.

Illustrations of the pathological features of colon cancer are provided in Figures 42.11–42.33. Most lesions are moderately or well-differentiated adenocarcinoma. Relatively few pathological features are effective predictors of the invasive and metastatic potential of a colon cancer. However, less well-differentiated, poorly differentiated, and signet cell tumors are associated with an adverse prognostic outcome.

A spectrum of cellular atypia or architectural dysplasia can occur within adenomatous polyps. Cells within a small adenoma can look almost normal and tend to progress to greater degrees of cellular atypia as the polyp size grows. Foci of high-grade dysplasia may be found in adenomas, which are sometimes termed "carcinoma in situ." Carcinoma in situ is a confusing misnomer; in this situation the pathologist is describing dysplastic cells confined by the muscularis mucosa and, consequently, the lesion by definition is not cancer. Foci of cancer may be confined to the polyp itself (Fig. 42.17) and can be cured by endoscopic polypectomy. A well-differentiated variant of colon cancer that is associated with a poor clinical outcome is the mucin-producing colon cancer (Fig. 42.18). The production of large amounts of mucin correlates with an increased ability to metastasize in animal models of the disease.

Atlas of Gastroenterology, 4th edition. Edited by Tadataka Yamada, David H. Alpers, Anthony N. Kalloo, Neil Kaplowitz, Chung Owyang, and Don W. Powell. © 2009 Blackwell Publishing, ISBN: 978-1-4051-6909-7

Instructive clinical cases are highlighted in Figures 42.19 and 42.20. In Figure 42.19, an asymptomatic 42-year-old man had occult fecal bleeding detected by guaiac testing. A barium enema examination was interpreted as negative; however, a large mass was detected in the sigmoid by means of colonoscopy. In Figure 42.20, a 52-year-old man with episodes of hematochezia was observed for a year before a barium enema and rigid sigmoidoscopy were performed, which were negative. Additional examination by colonoscopy found cancer of the sigmoid and further workup revealed metastatic disease. These cases highlight the limitations of the barium enema, especially for detecting rectal and sigmoid lesions, and the difficulty in obtaining an adequate examination by rigid sigmoidoscopy.

Adenocarcinoma is usually diagnosed by lower colonoscopy and confirmed by mucosal biopsy. This tumor may appear plaque-like (Fig. 42.22) or as a lesion that obstructs the lumen (Figs 42.23 and 42.24). The tumor may appear as a stricture with normal overlying mucosa (Fig. 42.23a), with exophytic growth (Fig. 42.23b), or as an annular mass (Fig. 42.23c). Often synchronous lesions are found (Fig. 42.24). Malignant strictures in the colon occasionally result from metastases from adjacent tissues such as the cervix (Fig. 42.25). Malignant lymphoma occurs as either polypoid or ulcerating lesions (Fig. 42.26) but does not usually occlude the lumen.

Strictures from adenocarcinoma can arise in areas of diverticular disease and the malignancy may not be suspected without biopsy (Fig. 42.27). Carcinoma that perforates can produce a localized inflammatory response and present in a similar way to diverticulitis (Fig. 42.28).

Usually the definitive management of colorectal cancer is surgical resection. The affected colorectum should be removed en bloc with associated lymph node drainage (Fig. 42.29). Reanastomosis of large bowel segments has been simplified with gastrointestinal and triangulation anastomosis staplers (Figs 42.30–42.32). In rectal cancer the location of the tumor determines whether an anal sphincter-preserving operation can be carried out. The rectal tumor is localized by the number of centimeters it is from the anal verge. Because the surgical anal canal length is variable, ranging from 2 to 7 cm depending on body habitus and gender (Fig. 42.33), a tumor with a lower margin 8 cm from the anal verge may fall within the middle one-third of the surgical canal in a thin woman but the lower one-third in a muscular man.

Table 42.1 Age-specific incidence rates per 100 000 population for cancers of the colon and rectum

Age (years)	Men	Women
0–4	0.0	0.0
5–9	0.0	0.0
10–14	0.0	0.0
15–19	0.2	0.1
20–24	0.4	0.4
25–29	1.2	1.1
30–34	2.5	2.4
35–39	5.9	5.9
40–44	12.3	11.9
45–49	27.7	24.6
50–54	57.2	46.3
55–59	102.6	76.7
60–64	164.9	105.7
65–69	243.9	155.5
70–74	320.5	226.9
75–79	411.3	293.6
80–84	463.5	365.5
85+	497.6	391.5

From Eddy DM. Screening for colorectal cancer. Ann Intern Med 1990;113:373.

Table 42.2 Bleeding from colorectal cancers

Location of cancer	Mean blood loss (^{51}Cr-labeled erythrocytes)	Positive Hemoccult II test[a]	
		Nonrehydrated	Rehydrated
Cecum, ascending colon ($n = 10$)	9.3 mL/day	83%	96%
Transverse and descending colon ($n = 5$)	1.5 mL/day	54%	54%
Sigmoid colon ($n = 3$)	1.9 mL/day	64%	97%
Rectum ($n = 18$)	1.8 mL/day	69%	93%
Total sample		69%	91%

a Hemoccult II tests performed with and without rehydration; Hemoccult II test considered positive if any of six tests are positive in a 3-day test period.

Data from Macrae FA, St John DG. Relationship between patterns of bleeding and Hemoccult sensitivity in patients with colorectal cancers or adenomas. Gastroenterology 1982;82:891.

Table 42.3 False-negative Hemoccult II tests correlated with duration of testing in patient with known colorectal carcinoma

	Duration of testing (days)									
	1	2	3	4	5	6	7	8	9	10
Unrehydrated Hemoccult false-negative rate	181/359 (50%)	117/313 (37%)	84/267 (31%)	56/222 (25%)	41/177 (23%)	28/136 (21%)	18/100 (18%)	10/68 (15%)	5/39 (13%)	2/15 (13%)
Rehydrated Hemoccult false-negative rate	80/359 (22%)	39/313 (12%)	23/267 (9%)	15/222 (7%)	9/177 (5%)	7/136 (5%)	5/100 (5%)	3/68 (4%)	2/39 (5%)	1/15 (7%)

Results are the proportion and percentage of tests in which patients with known colorectal cancers had falsely negative Hemoccult II tests. This demonstrates that 50% of cancers are missed by performing a single (unrehydrated) test; the false-negative rate decreases to 31% after 3 days of testing and is reduced to 13% with 10 days of testing. When the rehydrated test is used the false-negative rate is only 9% with 3 days of testing, but the prohibitive rate of false positives produced makes rehydration a maneuver of questionable value.

From Macrae FA, St John DG. Relationship between patterns of bleeding and Hemoccult sensitivity in patients with colorectal cancers or adenomas. Gastroenterology 1982;82:891.

Table 42.4 Relation between fecal hemoglobin concentration and Hemoccult II tests in patients with colorectal cancers

Stool hemoglobin concentration (mg Hb/g stool)	Proportion of positive tests	
	HO	HO(R)
0–2	86/766 (11%)	212/758 (28%)
2–6	127/314 (40%)	213/304 (70%)
6–10	50/80 (63%)	75/80 (94%)
10–15	50/64 (78%)	60/64 (94%)
15–20	11/18 (61%)	14/18 (78%)
>20	30/58 (52%)	56/58 (97%)

HO, Hemoccult II developed without rehydration; HO(R), Hemoccult II developed with preliminary rehydration.

From Macrae FA, St John DG. Relationship between patterns of bleeding and Hemoccult sensitivity in patients with colorectal cancers or adenomas. Gastroenterology 1982;82:891.

Table 42.5 A combination strategy for fecal occult blood screening

Test	Positive tests[a]	True-positive tests[b]	False-positive tests[c]	True-negative tests[d]	False-negative tests[e]	Sensitivity	Specificity	Positive predictive value
Hemoccult II	2.5% (n = 198)	0.6% (n = 46)	1.9%	96.4%	1.2% (n = 96)	32.4%	98.1%	23.2%
Hemoccult SENSA	13.6% (n = 1073)	1.3% (n = 99)	12.3%	85.9%	0.5% (n = 40)	71.2%	87.5%	9.2%
HemeSelect	5.9% (n = 440)	1.2% (n = 90)	4.7%	93.5%	0.6%	67.2%	95.2%	20.5%
Sequential strategy[f]	3.0% (n = 23)	0.92% (n = 72)	2.1%	96.2%	0.8% (n = 62)	53.7%	97.9%	30.9%

Approximately 8000 patients were screened, although not all with every fecal occult blood test. Patients with positive tests were evaluated by colonoscopy and followed further in a health maintenance organization, with chart follow-up of the screened population.

a Percent of asymptomatic, screened patients with positive test.

b Percent of all screened patients with a cancer or polyp ≥1 cm and a positive test.

c Percent of all screened patients with a positive test but no cancer or polyp ≥1 cm.

d Percent of all screened patients with a negative test and no cancer or polyp ≥1 cm.

e Percent of all screened patients with a cancer or polyp ≥1 cm who had a negative test.

f Stool screened first with Hemoccult SENSA, with only positive stools rescreened with HemeSelect; positive test indicates both tests positive.

From Boland CR. Malignant tumors of the colon. In: Yamada T, Alpers DH, Owyang C (eds). Textbook of Gastroenterology, 2nd edn. Philadelphia, PA: Lippincott Williams & Wilkins, 1999.

Table 42.6 Development of colorectal neoplasms in 20 000 patients during first year after screening

Patient group	Carcinomas		Adenomas	
	Number	Rate per 1000	Number	Rate per 1000
Positive screening Hemoccult test (n = 77/3613)	13	3.6	42[a]	7.9
Negative screening Hemoccult test (n = 3536/3613)	1	0.3		
Offered Hemoccult test (refused or no response) (n = 6143)	8	1.3	3	0.5
Control group (not screened) (n = 10 272)	10	1.0	5	0.5

a In 29 patients.

From Hardcastle JD, Farrands PA, Balfour TW. Controlled trial of faecal occult blood testing in the detection of colorectal cancer. Lancet 1983;2:1.

Table 42.7 Pathological stage of cancers in 20 525 patients followed for 2 years after randomization to screening or no screening

Stage	Test group			Control group (10 272)
	Responders (3613)[a]	Nonresponders (6640)[b]	Overall (10 253)	
A	12 (60%)	2 (14%)	14 (43%)	0
B	4 (20%)	7 (50%)	11 (33%)	8 (47%)
C	2 (10%)	1 (7%)	3 (9%)	6 (35%)
D	2 (10%)	4 (29%)	6 (15%)	3 (18%)
Total	20	14	34	17

a Responders: patients who completed the Hemoccult II fecal screening test.

b Nonresponders: patients randomized to be screened but who did not respond to request.

Data from Hardcastle JD, Farrands PA, Balfour TW. Controlled trial of faecal occult blood testing in the detection of colorectal cancer. Lancet 1983;2:1.

Table 42.8 Distribution of colorectal cancer patients by pathological stage

Stage[a]	Estimated distribution[b]	Detection by screening[c]
A	10%	60%
B	50% (±10%)	20%
B1	15%	
B2	35%	
C	25%	10%
C1	13%	
C2	13%	
D	15%	10%

a Pathological stage varies by investigator.

b These are estimates drawn from several reported studies that used differing methods to recruit and exclude patients.

c In several large studies, 65%–90% of cancers were stage A or B when detected by screening.

Data from Boland CR. Diagnosis and management of primary and metastatic colorectal cancers. Semin Gastrointest Dis 1992;3:33; in several large studies, 65%–90% of cancers were stage A or B when detected by screening. Permission pending from WB Saunders and Co.

Table 42.9 Most advanced finding at colonoscopy and results of fecal DNA panel and occult blood test in subgroups

Most advanced finding at colonoscopy	Positive fecal DNA panel		Positive occult blood test[a]	
	Number/total number	% (95% CI)	Number/total number	% (95% CI)
Colorectal cancer	16/31	51.5 (34.8, 68.0)	4/31	12.9 (5.1, 28.9)
Colorectal cancer and high-grade dysplasia	29/71	40.8 (30.2, 52.5)	10/71	14.1 (7.8, 24.6)
Advanced adenoma[b]	61/403	15.1 (12.0, 19.0)	43/403	10.7 (8.0, 14.1)
Adenoma < 1 cm	23/286	8.0 (5.9, 12.7)	15/286	5.2 (3.5, 9.2)
No polyps on colonoscopy	79/1423	5.6 (4.5, 6.9)	68/1423	4.8 (3.9, 58)

a Occult blood testing by Hemoccult II cards.

b Advanced adenoma is defined as a polyp with high-grade dysplasia or villous adenoma or equal to or greater than 1 cm in size.

CI, confidence interval.

Data from Imperiale TF, Ransohoff DF, Itzkowitz SH, et al., N Engl J Med 2004;351:26.

Table 42.10 Per-patient sensitivity and specificity of virtual colonoscopy detection of colorectal polyps by size calculated by metaanalysis of 33 studies comprising 6393 patients

Variable	Size of polyp		
	<6 mm	6–9 mm	>9 mm
Sensitivity (%)	48 (25–70)	70 (55–84)	85 (79–91)
Specificity (%)	92 (89–96)	93 (91–95)	97 (96–97)

Parentheses are the 95% confidence intervals.

Data from Mulhall BP, Veerappan GR, Jackson JL, et al., Ann Intern Med 2005;142:635.

Table 42.11 Lifetime risk of colorectal cancer according to family history of colorectal cancer with reference to the general population

Category	Lifetime risk of colorectal cancer (%)
General population	6
First-degree relative with CRC over 59 years	11
First-degree relative with CRC between 45 and 59 years	14
First-degree relative with CRC under 45 years	23
Two first-degree relatives with CRC	26

CRC, colorectal cancer.
From Johns LE, Houlston RS. A systematic review and meta-analysis of familial colorectal cancer risk. Am J Gastroenterol 2001;96:2992.

Table 42.12 Common indications for genetic testing for inherited syndromes causing colorectal cancer and associated genetic tests

Indications	Disorder suspected	Genetic testing[a]
Revised Bethesda criteria: colorectal cancer (CRC) diagnosed at less than 50 years old; presence of synchronous, metachronous CRC or other hereditary nonpolyposis colorectal cancer (HNPCC)-associated tumors, regardless of age; CRC with MSI-H[b] histology diagnosed at less than 60 years old; CRC diagnosed in one or more first-degree relative with an HNPCC-related tumor, with one cancer diagnosed under 50 years old; CRC diagnosed in two or more first- or second-degree relatives with HNPCC-related tumors, regardless of age	HNPCC	MSI/IHC testing[c]; *MLH1, MSH2, MSH6*
Sebaceous adenoma, carcinoma, epithelioma	Muir–Torre syndrome	*MSH2* (primarily), *MLH1, MSH6*
100 or more adenomatous polyps with/without family history of polyposis	Familial adenomatous polyposis	*APC*
100 or more adenomatous polyps without family history of polyposis	Familial adenomatous polyposis	*APC*
	MYH-associated polyposis	*MYH*
10 or more adenomatous polyps	Attenuated familial adenomatous polyposis	*APC*
	MYH-associated polyposis	*MYH*
5 or more juvenile polyps	Juvenile polyposis	*SMAD4/MADH4, BMPR1A*
Trichilemmomas, pedigree with breast cancer, thyroid cancer, gastrointestinal hamartomatous polyps	Cowden syndrome	*PTEN*
Macrocephaly, penile pigmentation, gastrointestinal hamartomatous polyps	Bannayan–Riley–Ruvalcaba syndrome	*PTEN*
Labial pigmentation and gastrointestinal Peutz–Jeghers polyps	Peutz–Jeghers syndrome	*STK11/LKB1*

a Genetic tests are in italics.
b Microsatellite instability, high frequency.
c Microsatellite instability testing and immunohistochemistry testing.

Table 42.13 American Joint Commission on Cancer (AJCC) and the Union Internationale Contre Le Cancer (UICC) staging and corresponding 5-year survival rates

Stage	T, primary tumor	N, lymph nodes	M, metastatic disease	5-year survival (%)
Stage 0	Tis	N0	M0	
Stage I	T1–T2	N0	M0	93.2
Stage IIA	T3	N0	M0	84.7
Stage IIB	T4	N0	M0	74.2
Stage IIIA	T1–T2	N1	M0	83.4
Stage IIIB	T3–T4	N1	M0	64.1
Stage IIIC	Any T	N2	M0	44.3
Stage IV	Any T	Any N	M1	8.1

T stage (T0): no evidence of primary tumor. Tis – in situ adenocarcinoma (high-grade dysplasia, carcinoma in situ); tumor confined to the mucosa, not breaching mucularis mucosae. T1 – tumor invades submucosa but not into the mucularis propria. T2 – tumor invades into but not through the muscularis propria. T3 – cancer invades through muscularis propria into subserosa or nonperitonealized extramural tissues. T4 – cancer directly invades other organs or structures (T4a) or perforates visceral peritoneum (T4b).

N stage (Nx): lymph nodes cannot be assessed. N0 – no lymph node involvement. N1 – metastasis in one to three regional lymph nodes. N2 – metastasis in four of more regional lymph nodes. Of note, prognosis correlates with the number of lymph nodes inspected in the pathological resection specimen. Consequently the AJCC–UICC mandates that a minimum of seven lymph nodes should be inspected. M stage (Mx): distant metastasis cannot be assessed. M0 – no distant metastasis. M1 – presence of distant metastasis. Involvement of nonregional lymph nodes including common iliac, external iliac, paraaortic, supraclavicular is considered distant metastasis.

Table 42.14 Distribution of 3000 gastrointestinal carcinoid tumors

Organ	Percentage of total	Percentage with metastasis
Stomach	3	18
Duodenum	1	16
Jejunum	2	35
Ileum	28	35
Appendix	47	3
Colon	2	60
Rectum	17	12

Data from Orloff MJ. Carcinoid tumors of the rectum. Cancer 1971;28:175.

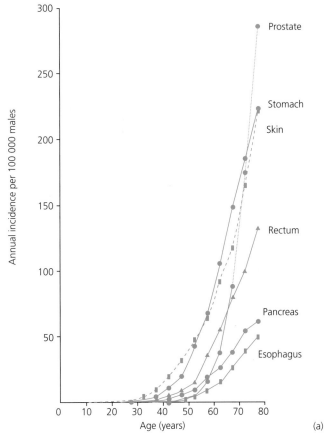

TOTAL	<15	15–24	25–34	35–44	45–54	55–64	65–74
306.7	12.4	36.3	118.9	200.9	407.9	789.6	1344.0

(a)

(b)

Figure 42.1 The relation between cancer incidence and age. **(a)** Site-specific increases in cancer incidence with advancing age. **(b)** Crude age-specific total cancer incidence per 100 000 population for all sites.

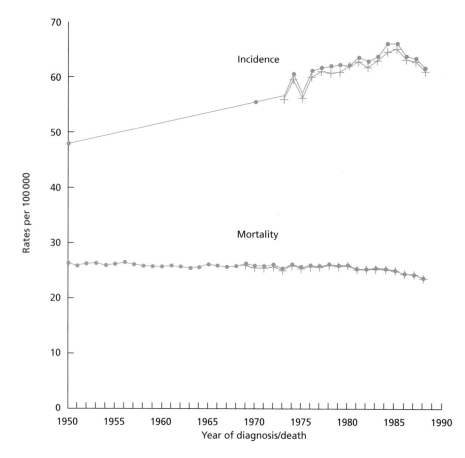

Figure 42.2 Incidence of colorectal cancer from five geographic regions of the United States from 1950 to 1988 **(top)** and mortality rates for the entire United States during that time **(bottom)**. Both curves are age-adjusted to a 1970 standard population.

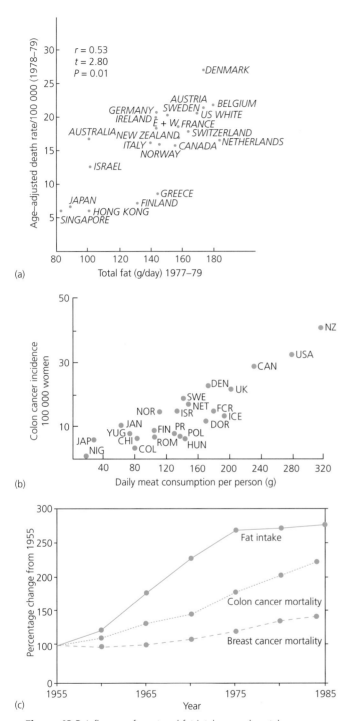

Figure 42.3 Influence of meat and fat intake on colorectal cancer incidence. **(a)** Correlation between incidence of colon cancer and per capita fat consumption. **(b)** Correlation between incidence of colon cancer and per capita meat consumption. **(c)** Correlation between changing fat intake and age-adjusted mortality from cancer of the colon and breast from 1955 to 1985 in Japan, a period when fat intake increased by 180%.

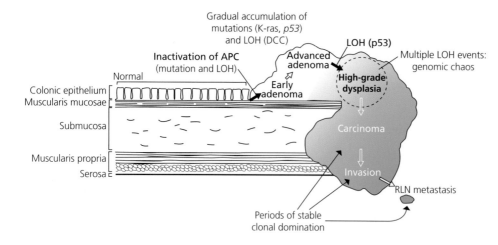

Figure 42.4 A proposed model of genetic events through which normal colorectal epithelium develops into neoplasia. This involves the inactivation of the *APC* gene followed by the accumulation of other events that can include mutations in the genes for K-ras and p53 or loss of heterozygosity (LOH) at tumor suppressor gene loci. RLN, regional lymph nodes.

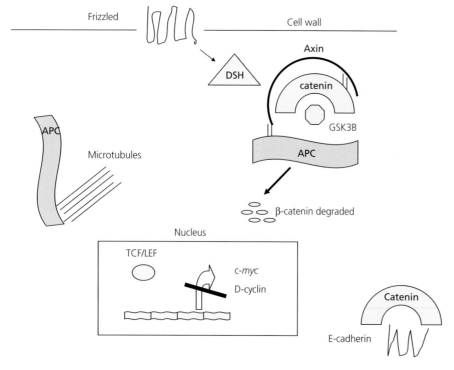

Figure 42.5 The Wnt pathway. The *APC* gene product is involved in the Wnt signaling pathway. Normally, β-catenin is found in the cytoplasm of the cell and is degraded by phosphorylation. Phosphorylation of β-catenin is facilitated by the *APC* gene product–axin complex. Also, the *APC* gene product binds to microtubules and stabilizes growth. If the *APC* gene product is nonfunctional (i.e., there is mutation of the *APC* gene), β-catenin is not degraded but instead is translocated to the nucleus where it stimulates transcription, including that of oncogenes such as c-*myc* and cyclin D1, via the TCF4/LEF complex. Activation of the Wnt pathway can also occur through ligand stimulation of Frizzled, which stimulates the protein Disheveled (DSH), disrupting the APC–axin–β-catenin complex. GSK3B, glycogen synthase kinase-3-beta.

Symptom assessment

Risk assessment

Screening

Diagnosis

Surveillance

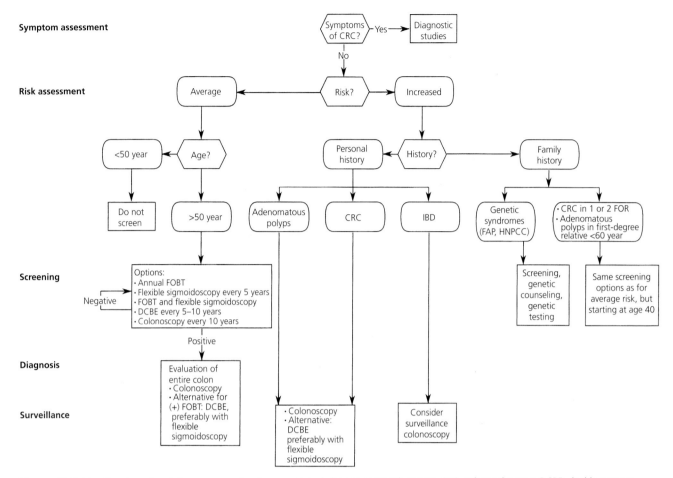

Figure 42.6 Algorithm for colorectal cancer screening for average and above average risk groups. CRC, colorectal cancer; DCBE, double contrast barium enema; FAP, familial adenomatous polyposis; FOR, first order relatives; FOBT, fecal occult blood test; HNPCC, hereditary nonpolyposis colorectal cancer; IBD, inflammatory bowel disease.

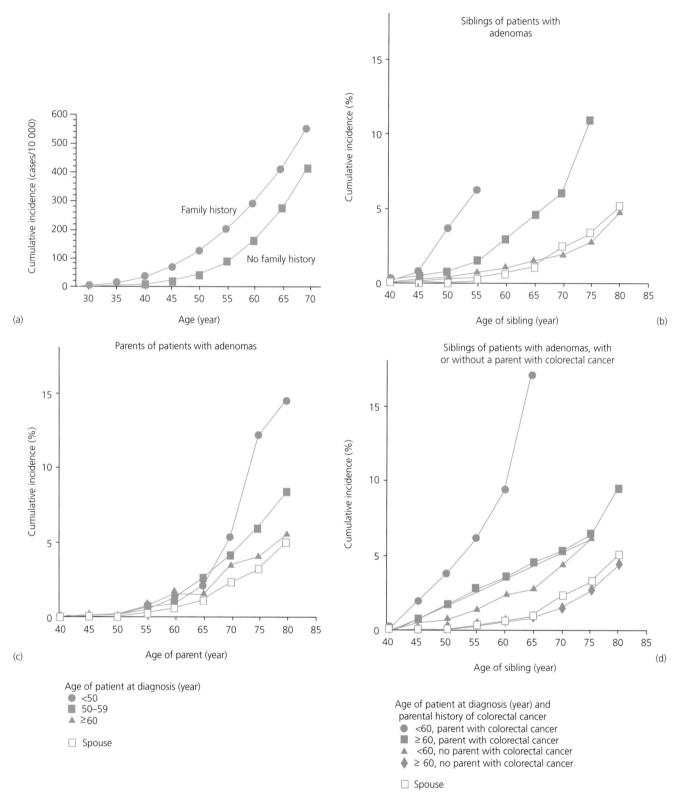

Figure 42.7 (a) The influence of family history of colorectal cancer in siblings and the age at diagnosis on the cumulative incidence of colorectal cancer. **(b)** The influence of a history of colorectal cancer in siblings and the age at diagnosis on the cumulative incidence of colorectal adenoma. **(c)** The influence of a history of colorectal cancer in parents and the age at diagnosis on the cumulative incidence of colorectal adenoma. **(d)** The influence of the combined history of colorectal cancer in a parent and sibling and the age at diagnosis on the cumulative incidence of colorectal adenoma.

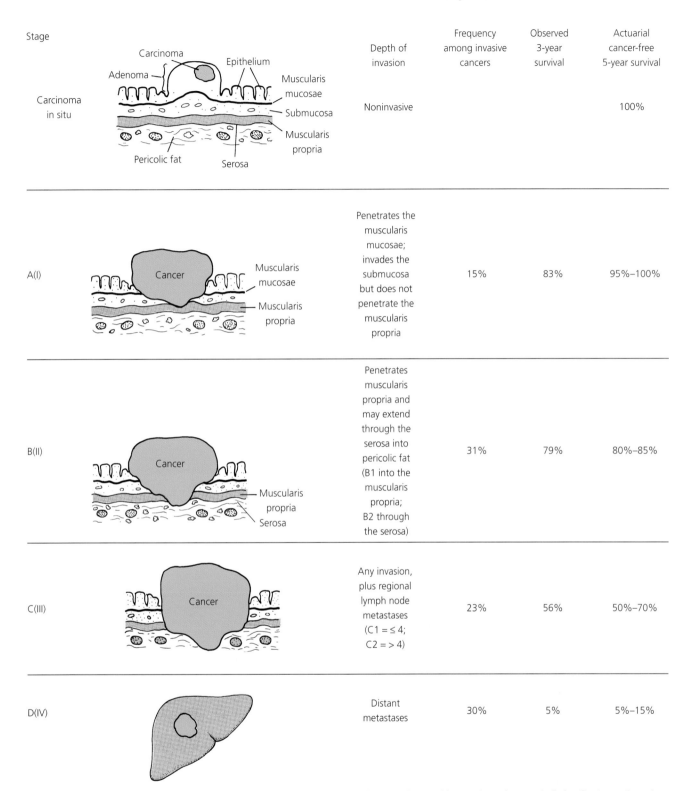

Stage		Depth of invasion	Frequency among invasive cancers	Observed 3-year survival	Actuarial cancer-free 5-year survival
Carcinoma in situ		Noninvasive			100%
A(I)		Penetrates the muscularis mucosae; invades the submucosa but does not penetrate the muscularis propria	15%	83%	95%–100%
B(II)		Penetrates muscularis propria and may extend through the serosa into pericolic fat (B1 into the muscularis propria; B2 through the serosa)	31%	79%	80%–85%
C(III)		Any invasion, plus regional lymph node metastases (C1 = ≤ 4; C2 = > 4)	23%	56%	50%–70%
D(IV)		Distant metastases	30%	5%	5%–15%

Figure 42.8 Numerous classification systems have been proposed for colorectal cancer. Illustrated here is the Dukes–Turnbull classification A through D accompanied by the tumor, node, metastasis (TNM) stage in parentheses. The observed 3-year survivals and actuarial cancer-free 5-year survivals are estimated for each stage. The actuarial survival estimates reflect excessive disease-related mortality from the cancer, and the crude survival rates are considerably lower because of comorbidity.

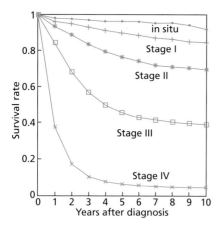

Figure 42.9 Relative rates of survival for patients with colon cancer by stage of disease from a database of more than 110 000 patients using the tumor, node, metastasis (TNM) staging system.

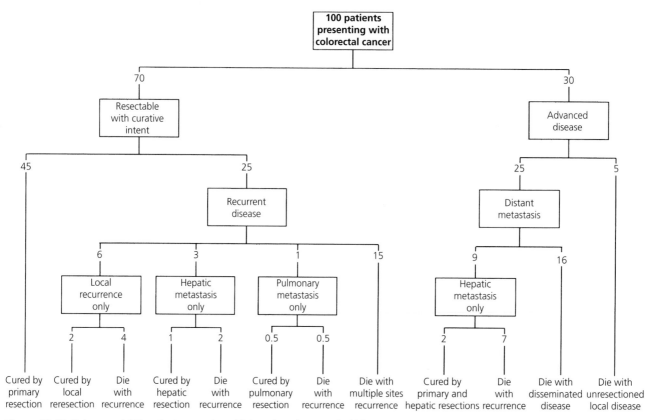

Figure 42.10 Outcomes of 100 patients presenting with large bowel cancer of which 70% appeared to be resectable for cure: 64% of this group were cured by primary resection but the other 36% experienced recurrent disease. A total of 55% either presented with advanced disease (30%) or developed postoperative recurrence (25%); about 11% of this group may be cured by additional surgery.

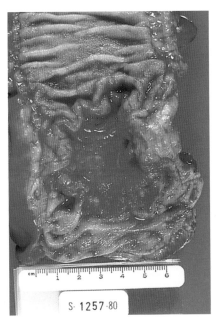

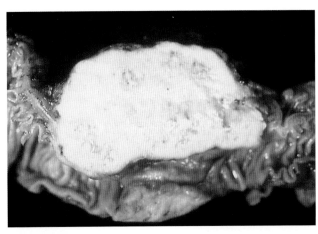

Figure 42.13 Cross-section of a bulky cancer from the ascending colon that invades the serosa to the subserosal percolic fat layer but without lymph node involvement, making it a TNM stage IIA cancer.

Figure 42.11 En face view of carcinoma of the colon. The features include heaped-up edges and the ulcerated center of the lesion.

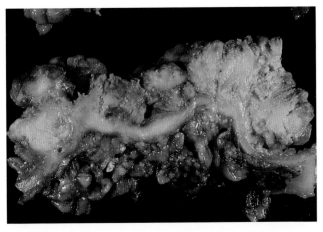

Figure 42.12 Cross-section of polypoid colon cancer. This lesion is a TNM stage I neoplasm because it does not invade the muscularis propria. Although a bulky intralumenal lesion, the patient's prognosis is excellent due to limited bowel wall invasion and absence of positive lymph nodes.

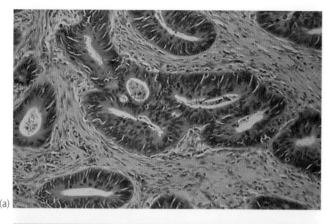

(a)

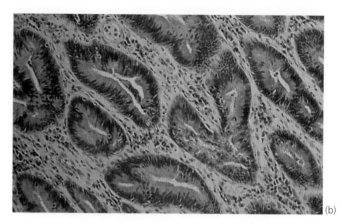

(b)

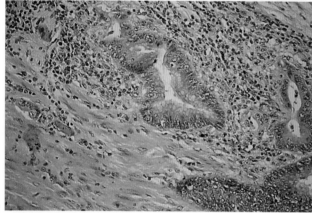

(c)

Figure 42.14 Histopathological features of well-differentiated carcinoma. **(a)** High-power microscopic view of a well-differentiated carcinoma of the colon shows typical, darkly stained glands within a poorly stained stroma. The nuclear-to-cytoplasmic ratio is high, and the nuclei palisade away from the basal lamina. **(b)** Microscopic field from a benign adenomatous polyp demonstrates similarities to a malignant neoplasm. However, the smaller nuclei with basal orientation are more characteristic of a benign lesion. **(c)** Well-differentiated adenocarcinoma invading into the muscularis propria.

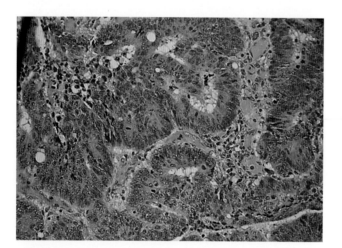

Figure 42.15 Less well-differentiated adenocarcinoma in which formation of the characteristic glands is less evident and nuclei are larger and more irregular. A poorly differentiated adenocarcinoma may consist of sheets of such cells and confers a poorer prognosis.

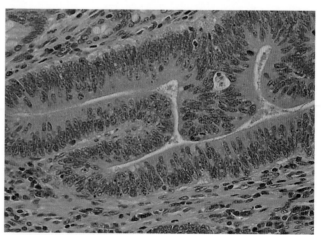

Figure 42.16 High-grade dysplasia in an adenomatous polyp. The nuclei are large with poorly condensed chromatin and the nuclei palisade up from the basal lamina. This lesion occurring in the confines of an adenomatous polyp is not capable of invasion or metastasis.

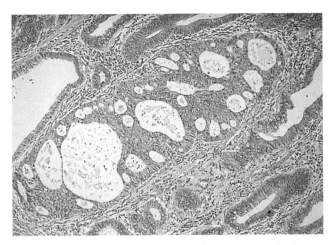

Figure 42.17 Histopathological appearance of carcinoma in situ in a polyp.

(a) 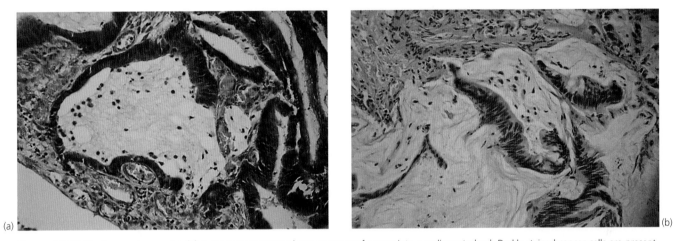 (b)

Figure 42.18 Mucinous colon cancer. **(a)** Some tumors secrete large amounts of mucus into a malignant gland. Darkly stained cancer cells are present and the nuclei are suspended in the central pool of mucin. **(b)** Liver metastasis of mucinous cancer with nests of cells secreting large pools of mucin.

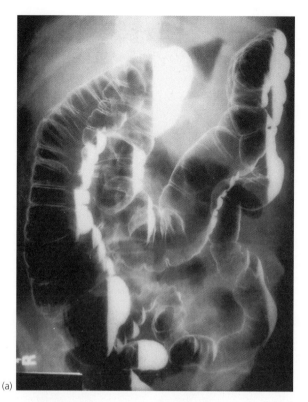

(a)

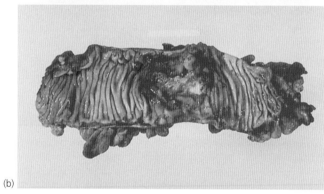

(b)

Figure 42.19 Large colon cancer, missed on initial diagnostic testing, resected for cure. A 42-year-old asymptomatic man had occult fecal bleeding detected at routine examination by stool guaiac testing. **(a)** Air contrast barium enema study interpreted as normal. On review, a constricting lesion was found in the midsigmoid colon. **(b)** A 4.5 × 6-cm ulcerative mass in the sigmoid colon noted on histopathlogical review to be a mucin-producing adenocarcinoma. The patient had no lymph node involvement and was disease free 3 years after surgery.

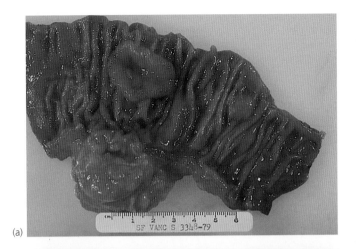

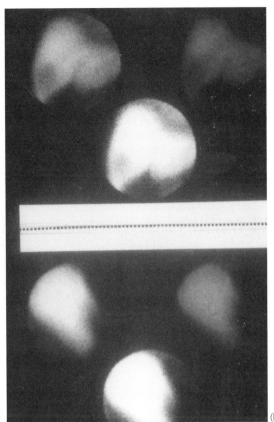

(a)

(b)

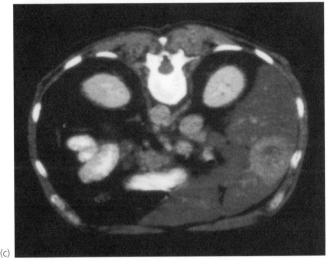

(c)

Figure 42.20 Metastatic colon cancer not detected on multiple diagnostic testing. A 55-year-old man had hematochezia and a 1-year history of guaiac-positive stools attributed to alcohol misuse and salicylate use. A single-contrast barium enema was read as normal, and no lesion was seen on rigid sigmoidoscopy. **(a)** A 3 × 4-cm elevated cancer in the sigmoid colon. The lesion was recognized on retrospective review of the barium enema. **(b)** Area of decreased uptake in the right lobe of the liver on a radionuclide scan. **(c)** Metastatic lesion in the liver on computed tomography scanning. The patient died of metastatic disease within 6 months of diagnosis. Although the primary lesion was smaller than that described in Figure 42.19, this was an aggressive TMN stage IV lesion.

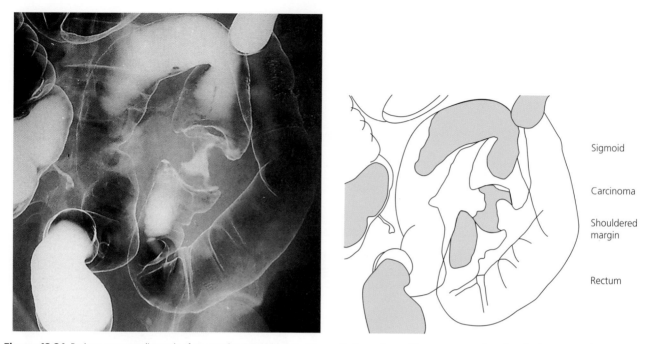

Figure 42.21 Barium enema radiograph of an annular sigmoid colon cancer with the radiographic appearance often described as an "apple core lesion."

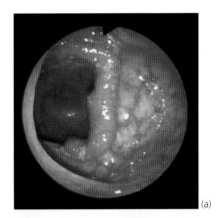

(a)

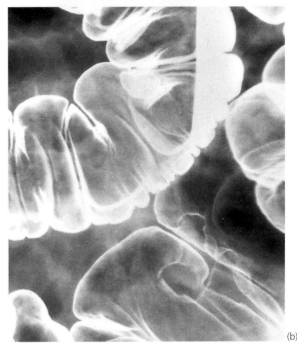

(b)

Figure 42.22 (a) Adenocarcinoma, plaque-like mass. The lesion, located proximal to the cecum (on the posterior wall at the 3 o'clock position), appears as a slightly raised, discrete mass with central depressions. **(b)** Radiographic appearance of plaque-like adenocarcinoma. The lesion (left lower quadrant) has raised margins around a central depression giving the appearance of a saddle.

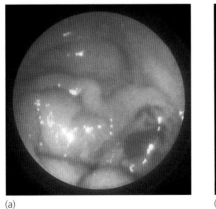

(a)

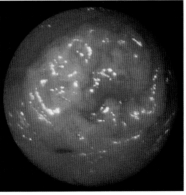

(b)

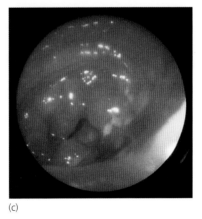

(c)

Figure 42.23 (a) Adenocarcinoma, stricture. Folds radiate to a pinpoint narrowing. The intact overlying mucosa suggests an infiltrating rather than an exophytic growth pattern. Biopsies of the mouth of the stricture revealed normal histology, but brush cytology findings were abnormal, emphasizing the usefulness of this technique in diagnosing these types of lesions. **(b)** Adenocarcinoma, stricture. A mass effect is apparent, suggesting that this lesion may have an exophytic growth pattern. Generally, the mucosa is intact, as in (a), except for a small rim at the mouth of the stricture. **(c)** Adenocarcinoma, annular mass. In this case the stricture is entirely the result of tumor, which has broken through at the point of lumenal narrowing.

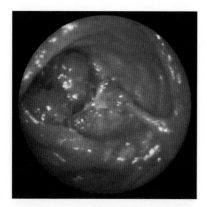

Figure 42.24 Adenocarcinoma, sigmoid with synchronous (sentinel) adenoma. A cancer with an ulcerated mass appearance was found at the splenic flexure (in the distance at the 3 o'clock position). Just distal to this in the proximal descending colon, a pedunculated polyp is present as a sentinel neoplasm. The possibility that other adenomas or even cancers are present in this colon emphasizes the need to perform colonoscopy at the time of diagnosis to clear the colon of other lesions that could alter patient management.

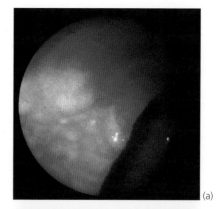
(a)

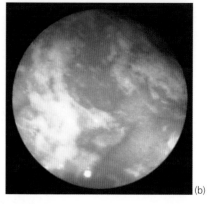
(b)

Figure 42.26 (a) Lymphoma. Multiple polyps in the cecum of a patient with abdominal lymphoma always suggests involvement of this segment, even when the patient is asymptomatic. **(b)** Lymphoma simulating ulcerative colitis. Ulcerations and friability in this patient with watery diarrhea caused this appearance, which was initially mistaken for inflammatory bowel disease. Biopsies, however, showed poorly differentiated lymphoma.

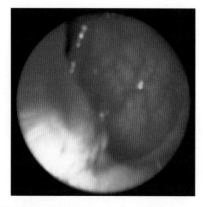

Figure 42.25 Metastatic carcinoma to the colon from a cervical primary lesion. Local spread produced a mass and lumenal narrowing at the rectosigmoid junction. Biopsies showed squamous carcinoma similar to that found in the original cervical carcinoma.

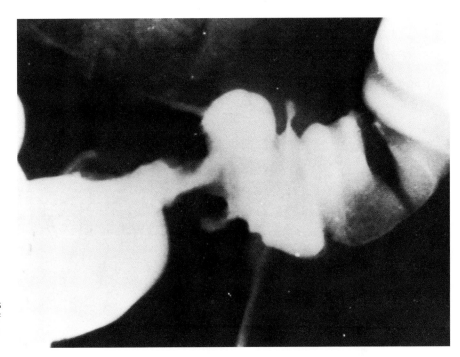

Figure 42.27 Carcinoma of the sigmoid with diverticular disease. Diverticular outpouchings are noted in the setting of an annular lesion constricting the colon lumen as noted in the center of the picture. Because of the relative frequency of both conditions, this is commonly seen.

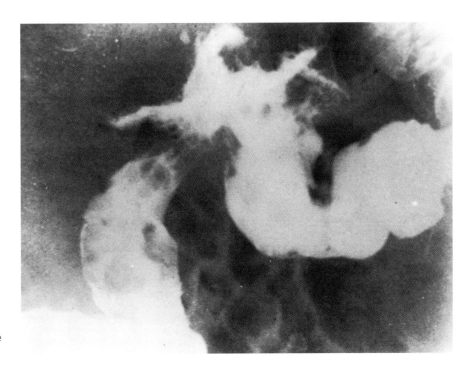

Figure 42.28 Perforated carcinoma may be indistinguishable from diverticulitis.

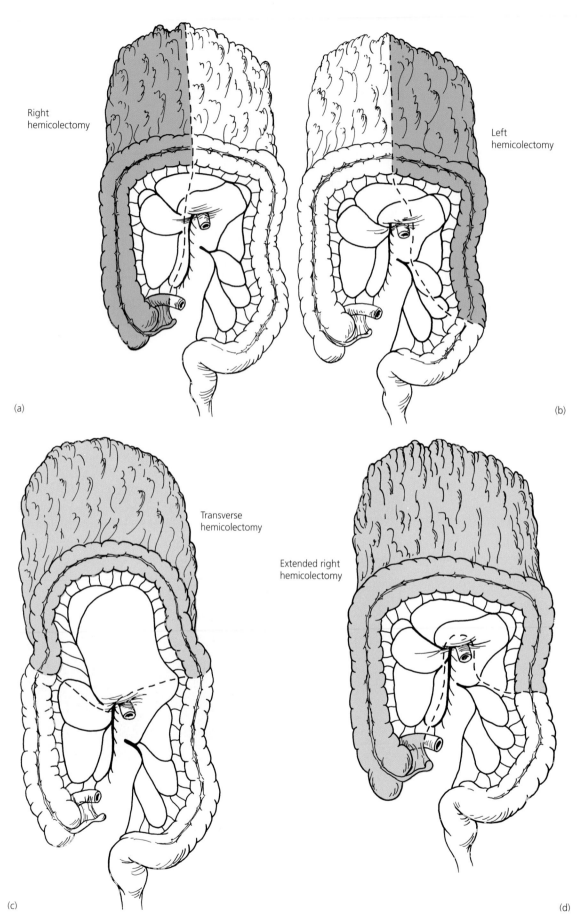

Figure 42.29 (a–e) Oncological colon resections. (*Continued on next page.*)

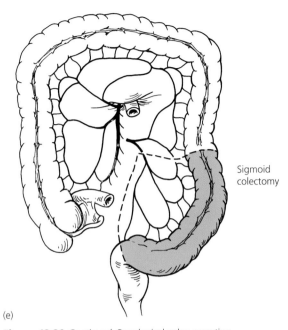

(e)

Figure 42.29 *Continued* Oncological colon resection.

Sigmoid
colectomy

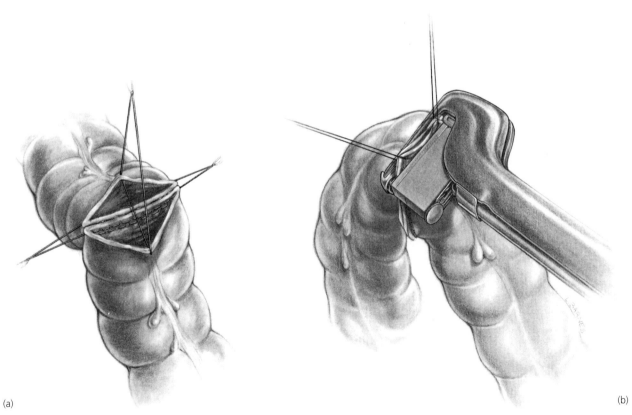

(a)

(b)

Figure 42.30 Triangulation anastomosis by means of inversion of the posterior (mesenteric) wall **(a)** and eversion of the anterior walls **(b)**.

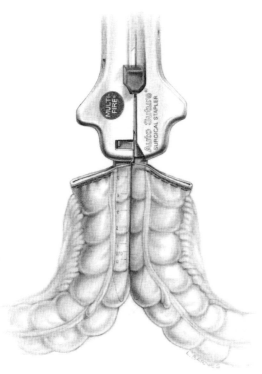

Figure 42.31 Functional end-to-end anastomosis by means of the closed technique after construction of two enterotomies for insertion of the separate limbs of the gastrointestinal anastomosis stapler.

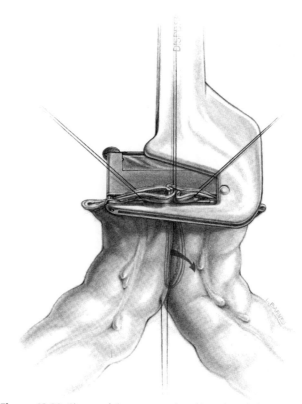

Figure 42.32 Closure of the enterotomies with a triangulation anastomosis stapler.

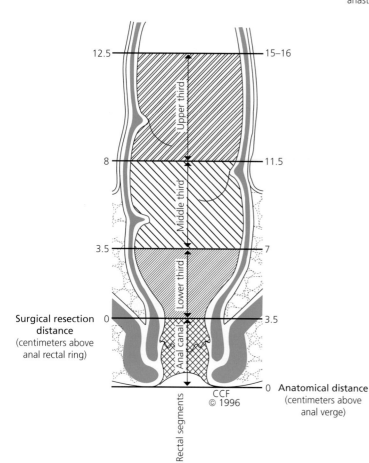

Figure 42.33 Surgical and purely anatomical regions of the rectum as related to the anal sphincters and pelvic floor.

43

Anorectal diseases

Adil E. Bharucha, Arnold Wald

This chapter provides a visual review of anorectal anatomy, functions, and pathologies. We begin with a coronal section of the anorectum which highlights the orientation of the anal sphincters and pelvic floor muscles (Fig. 43.1). Common instruments for anorectal examinations more frequently used by a colorectal surgeon than a gastroenterologist are shown in Figure 43.2. The equipment used for rigid procto-sigmoidoscopy is shown in Figure 43.2a. Because symptomatic internal hemorrhoids are one of the most common lesions seen by the practicing gastroenterologist, we have elected to show a photograph of the simplest, most widely used instrument for management of internal hemorrhoids, the Barron-type rubber band ligator with its ancillary equipment (see Fig. 43.2c).

Hemorrhoids are the most common anal lesions seen in practice; therefore, pictures of external and different degrees of internal hemorrhoids are critical to any atlas on anal disorders (Figs 43.3–43.8). Hemorrhoids may be treated using a variety of nonsurgical techniques. One modality is banding using a ligator device attached to the tip of an endoscope (Fig. 43.9). Examples of an anorectal abscess, the classification of anorectal fistulae, rectal prolapse, solitary rectal ulcer, and chronic anal fissure, are shown in Figures 43.10–43.14. These important lesions are all best diagnosed by means of simple inspection. Figures 43.15 and 43.16 depict normal anorectal and pelvic floor motion during defecation and when subjects squeeze (i.e., contract) their pelvic floor muscles. Figures 43.17–43.27 illustrate the techniques for digital rectal examination and encapsulate the pathophysiology of fecal incontinence. Figures 43.28–43.30 summarize the cardinal clinical features of syndromes associated with functional anorectal pain. Finally, we show examples of carcinoma of the anus (Figs 43.31–43.32). One fairly subtle lesion is Bowen disease (cutaneous squamous cell carcinoma in situ), which may be confused with the anal lesions of dermatitis and psoriasis.

Atlas of Gastroenterology, 4th edition. Edited by Tadataka Yamada, David H. Alpers, Anthony N. Kalloo, Neil Kaplowitz, Chung Owyang, and Don W. Powell. © 2009 Blackwell Publishing, ISBN: 978-1-4051-6909-7

Table 43.1 Manometric patterns of fecal incontinence

| | IAS weakness | EAS trauma | Neurogenic | |
			Peripheral	Central
Resting P	↓	NI	NI	NI
Squeeze P	NI	↓	↓	↓
PRM	NI	NI	↓	↓
Sensation	NI	NI	NI	↓

Internal and anal sphincter (IAS, EAS) dysfunctions manifest as
reduced anal resting and squeeze pressures (P), respectively.
Peripheral neurogenic injury may result in external sphincter weakness
and, if the sacral roots are affected, also cause puborectalis (PRM)
weakness. Central neurogenic injury also affects rectal sensation.

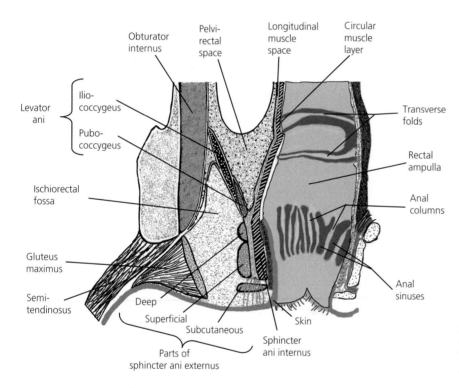

Figure 43.1 Diagram of a coronal section of
the rectum, anal canal, and adjacent structures.
The pelvic barrier includes the anal sphincters
and pelvic floor muscles.

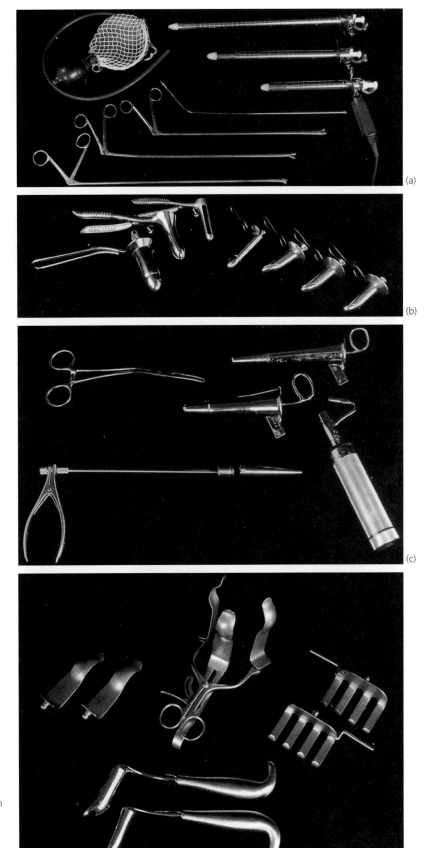

Figure 43.2 Instruments for anorectal examinations. **(a)** Equipment necessary for performance of rigid proctosigmoidoscopy – air insufflator, interchangeable proctoscopes with light source, suction wand, and assorted biopsy forceps. **(b)** Instruments for anorectal examination that require an external light source. **Left to right:** Fansler proctoscope, Pratt rectal speculum, Sims rectal speculum, Buie-Hirschman anoscope, and Hirschman anoscopes (small, medium, and large). Disposable anoscopes are also commonly used (not shown). **(c)** Instruments for rubber-band ligation of internal hemorrhoids. Barron-type ligator with grasping forceps, and device for loading bands **(left)**. Welch-Allyn self-illuminated anoscope with large and small specula **(right)**. **(d)** Anal retractors. **Top to bottom:** Parks' anal retractor with interchangeable blades, Ferguson-Moon anal retractor, and Hill-Ferguson anal retractor.

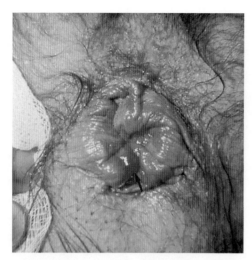

Figure 43.3 First-degree (nonprolapsing) internal hemorrhoid (arrow) and external hemorrhoids.

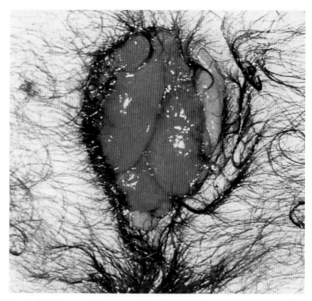

Figure 43.5 Second-degree internal hemorrhoids. These hemorrhoids prolapse but are spontaneously reducible.

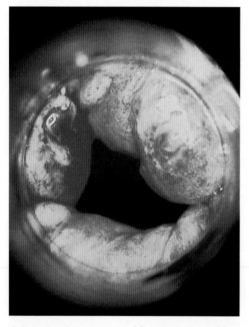

Figure 43.4 Anoscopic appearance of first-degree internal hemorrhoids.

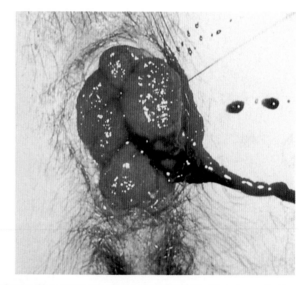

Figure 43.6 Third-degree internal hemorrhoids. These hemorrhoids prolapse and require manual reduction. Spontaneous bleeding is apparent.

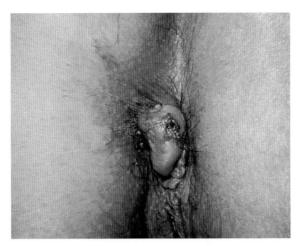

Figure 43.7 Thrombosed external hemorrhoid with cutaneous ulceration and superficial necrosis.

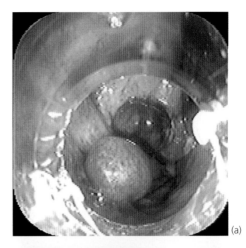

(a)

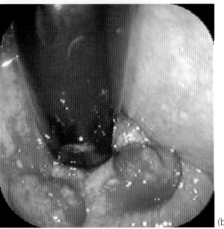

(b)

Figure 43.9 **(a)** A view through the endoscope after placing bands on two separate internal hemorrhoids using a multibanding ligator device attached to the instrument tip. **(b)** A retroflexed endoscopic view of banded internal hemorrhoids.

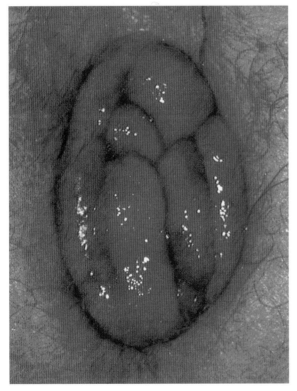

Figure 43.8 Fourth-degree (nonreducible) internal hemorrhoids.

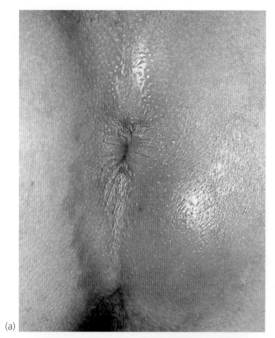

(a)

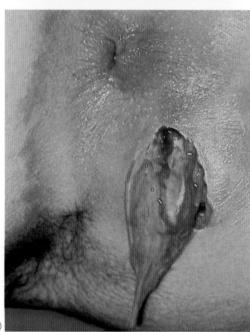

(b)

Figure 43.10 Anorectal abscess. **(a)** A ripe ischiorectal abscess in the left posterior quadrant. **(b)** The same abscess expressing pus immediately after incision.

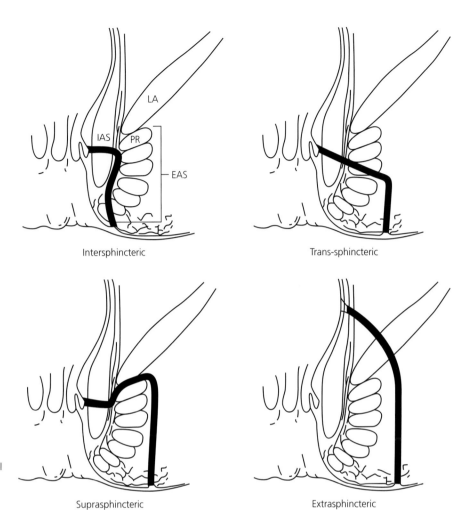

Intersphincteric

Trans-sphincteric

Suprasphincteric

Extrasphincteric

Figure 43.11 Classic location of several fistulas and their relationship to pelvic musculature depicted schematically. Anorectal anatomy: PR, puborectalis; LA, levator ani; IAS, internal anal sphincter; EAS, external anal sphincter.

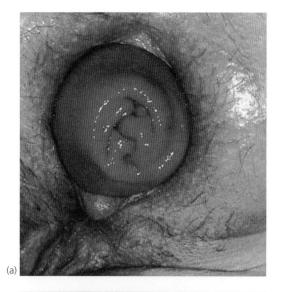

(a)

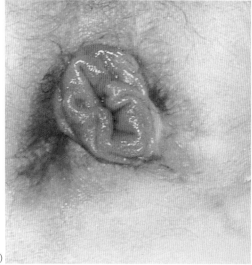

(b)

Figure 43.12 Rectal prolapse. **(a)** Complete rectal prolapse.
(b) Incomplete rectal prolapse.

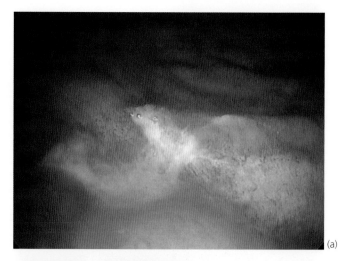

(a)

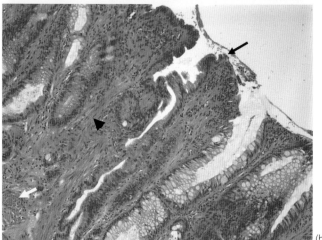

(b)

Figure 43.13 Solitary rectal ulcer. **(a)** Gross and **(b)** microscopic
appearance. Observe the hyperplastic mucosa with a surface erosion
(black arrow), vascular congestion (white arrow), and hyperplastic muscle
fibers between the crypts (black arrowhead). (a) and (b) courtesy of Dr
Deepak Gopal, University of Wisconsin School of Medicine and Public
Health and Dr Thomas Smyrk, Department of Pathology, College of
Medicine, Mayo Clinic, Rochester, MN respectively.

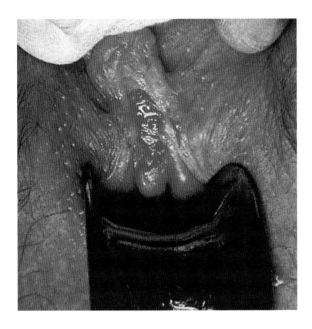

Figure 43.14 Typical appearance of a chronic anal fissure triad consisting of a sentinel pile **(top)**, the fissure itself, and a hypertrophic papilla.

Rest   **Defecation**

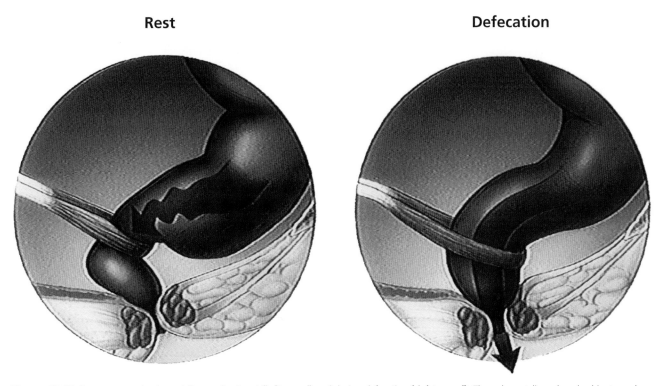

Figure 43.15 Anorectum and puborectalis muscle at rest **(left panel)** and during defecation **(right panel)**. The puborectalis and anal sphincters relax allowing opening of the anal canal and perineal descent during defecation.

Rest   Evacuation   Rest   Squeeze

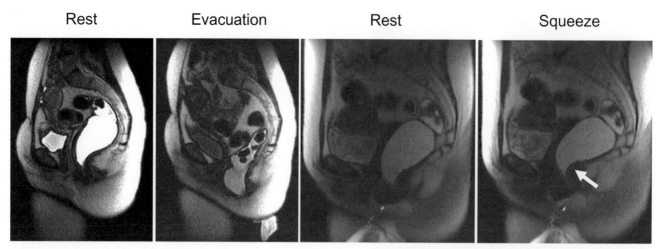

Figure 43.16 Left panel – sagittal dynamic magnetic resonance imaging images of normal puborectalis relaxation, perineal descent (2.6 cm), and opening of the anal canal during rectal evacuation in an asymptomatic subject. Right pane – during squeeze, the anal canal was elevated upward and anteriorly by pelvic floor contraction. Observe increased indentation (white arrow), reflecting contraction of the puborectalis muscle on the posterior rectal wall during squeeze (i.e., contraction of pelvic floor muscles).

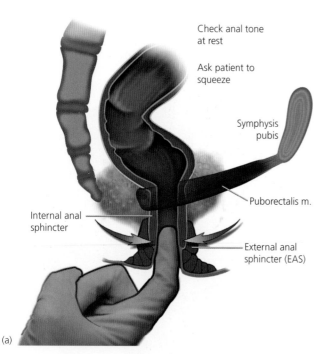

(a)

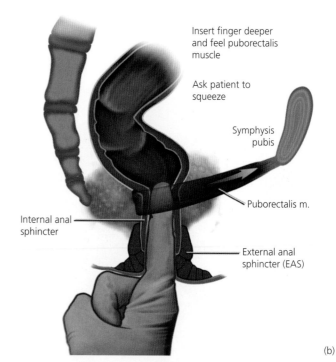

(b)

Figure 43.17 Digital examination of the anorectum of an adult with fecal incontinence. **(a)** When patient is asked to squeeze, the strength and duration of the contraction of the external anal sphincter (arrows) may be assessed after resting tone has been assessed. **(b)** The examining finger is then advanced and oriented posteriorly to assess the puborectalis muscle. When the patient is asked to squeeze, the contraction of the puborectalis muscle is felt as an anterior and upward tug as the muscle shortens (arrow). Simultaneously, the external anal sphincter contracts to increase the pressure in the anal canal. Courtesy of Dr Arnold Wald and Jerry Schoendorf, MAMS.

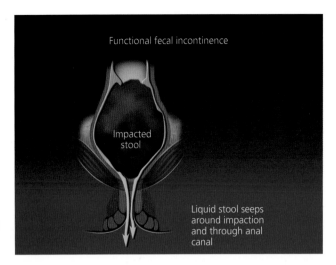

Figure 43.18 In functional fecal incontinence, impacted stool in the rectum reflexively inhibits the tone of the internal anal sphincter which is responsible for most of the resting tone in the anal canal. This allows liquid stool to seep around the impaction and escape through the anal canal. Courtesy of Dr Arnold Wald and Jerry Schoendorf, MAMS.

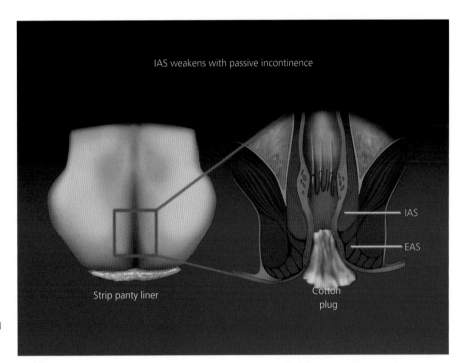

Figure 43.19 In patients with fecal seepage associated with a weakened internal anal sphincter, the placement of a cotton plug in the anal canal creates a physical and absorbent barrier to the passage of gas or mucus to effectively ameliorate the problem. IAS, internal anal sphincter; EAS, external anal sphincter. Courtesy of Dr Arnold Wald and Jerry Schoendorf, MAMS.

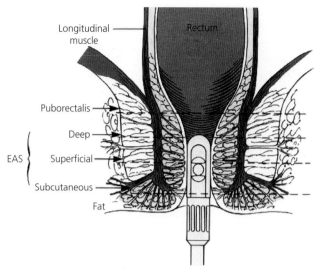

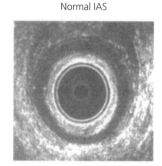
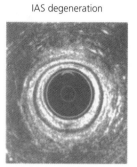

Figure 43.20 Illustration of a 360-degree anal sonographic probe shown in relationship to relevant anorectal anatomy. This technique is very reliable, although operator dependent, for evaluation of the internal anal sphincter but is less reliable for external anal sphincter and puborectalis muscle anatomy when assessing for structural causes of fecal incontinence. EAS, external anal sphincter. Courtesy of Dr Arnold Wald and Jerry Schoendorf, MAMS.

Figure 43.21 Axial sonographic views of the sphincter muscles of the anal canal. In the left panel is a structurally intact, concentric hypoechogenic internal anal sphincter (IAS). The right panel illustrates a structurally intact but very thin internal anal sphincter associated with low resting anal canal pressures, characteristic of some patients with passive incontinence. Lateral to the internal anal sphincter is a concentric ring of mixed echogenicity representing the external anal sphincter. Courtesy of Dr Arnold Wald and Jerry Schoendorf, MAMS.

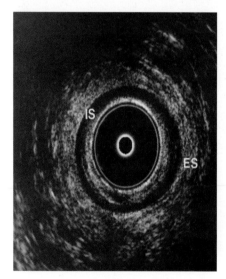
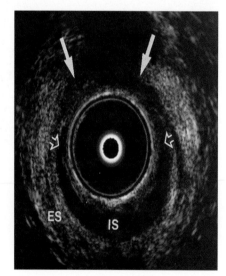

Normal

Sphincter disruption

Figure 43.22 (Left panel) Axial views of the anal canal illustrating normal internal anal sphincter (IS) and external anal sphincter (ES). **(Right panel)** There is anterior disruption of both the IS (short arrows) and ES (long arrows) characteristic of traumatic tear during childbirth.

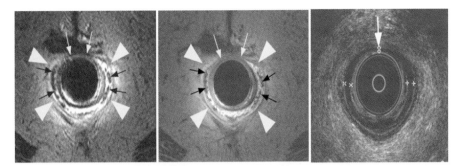

Figure 43.23 Endoanal fast spin-echo T2-weighted **(left panel)** and spin-echo T1-weighted **(center panel)** magnetic resenance (MR) images demonstrate marked atrophy of the external anal sphincter (arrowheads) in a 75-year-old incontinent patient, making the internal anal longitudinal muscle prominent (black arrows). Corresponding endoanal ultrasound images **(right panel)** identified patchy thinning of the internal sphincter also seen on the MR images (white arrows), but not external sphincter atrophy.

Figure 43.24 Endoanal and dynamic magnetic resonance (MR) proctogram in a 70-year-old female with urinary and fecal incontinence. Endoanal MR images show partial tear and atrophy of the right puborectalis **(upper panel, arrow)**. Dynamic rest and squeeze images **(lower panel)** show lift of the levator posteriorly, but little anterior or upward movement of the anorectal junction, consistent with puborectalis injury. Observe a cystocele (white arrowhead) and a small rectal intussusception (white arrow) during defecation.

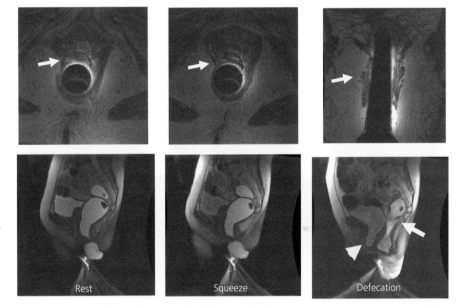

Figure 43.25 Illustration of a sacral nerve stimulator shown with relevant anatomy. A permanent electrical stimulator electrode is placed into a sacral nerve root via one of the sacral foramina. The nerve is selected as the one which produces optimal stimulation of the external anal sphincter. Shown here is the electrode in place and connected to a permanently implanted pulse generator which delivers a continuous stimulation.

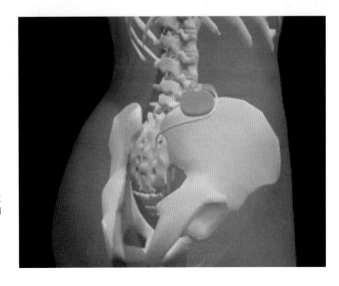

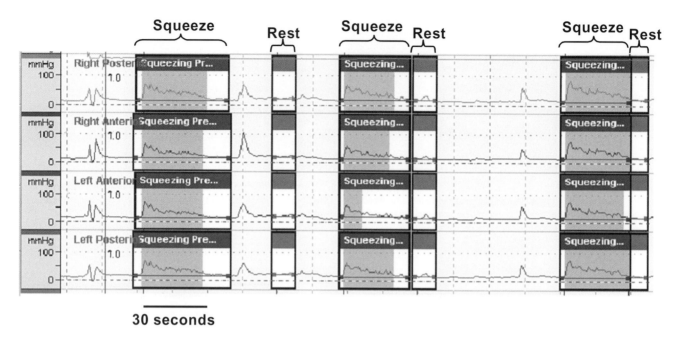

30 seconds

Figure 43.26 Anal sphincter pressures assessed on three separate occasions by four circumferentially oriented transducers stationed at 1 cm from the anal verge; transducers were located in separate quadrants. The maximum squeeze pressure is the highest pressure recorded by all four transducers during one of three maneuvers; the average squeeze pressure is calculated by averaging pressures across all four maneuvers. In this example, resting and squeeze pressures were comparable in all four quadrants.

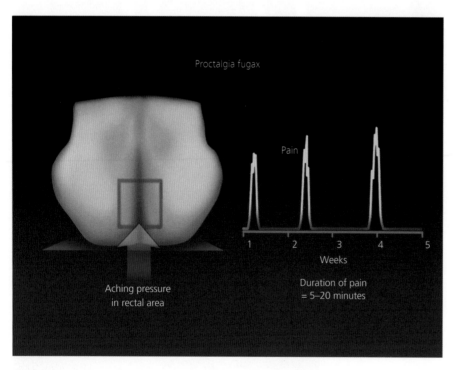

Figure 43.27 Characteristic location and pain pattern in proctalgia fugax. Typically, patients are asymptomatic between discrete episodes of rectal pain which last less than 60 min before disappearing completely. Courtesy of Dr Arnold Wald and Jerry Schoendorf, MAMS.

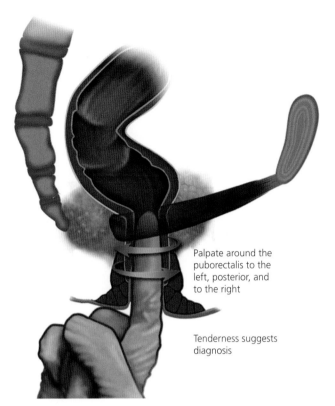

Palpate around the
puborectalis to the
left, posterior, and
to the right

Tenderness suggests
diagnosis

Figure 43.28 Illustration of the digital examination in patients with
chronic proctalgia syndrome. There is often palpable tenderness of the
puborectalis/levator muscles as the examining finger moves posteriorly to
anteriorly. Tenderness is often asymmetric and most commonly found on
the left side. Courtesy of Dr Arnold Wald and Jerry Schoendorf, MAMS.

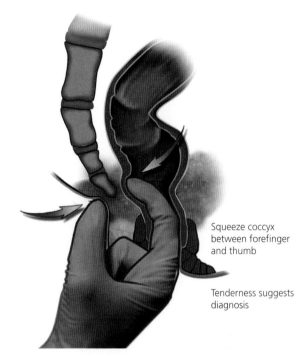

Squeeze coccyx
between forefinger
and thumb

Tenderness suggests
diagnosis

Figure 43.29 Anorectal examination in patients with coccygodynia. The
key to the diagnosis is the reproduction of the pain when the coccyx is
manipulated between the examining finger and the thumb. Courtesy of
Dr Arnold Wald and Jerry Schoendorf, MAMS.

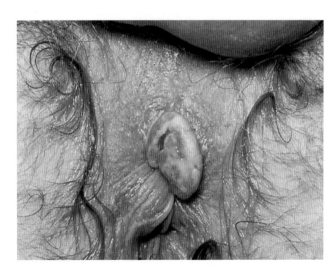

Figure 43.30 Squamous cell carcinoma of the anus. Courtesy of
Dr Karen Guice.

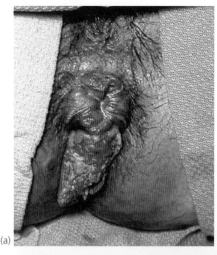

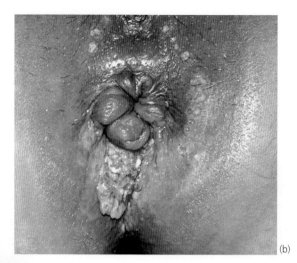

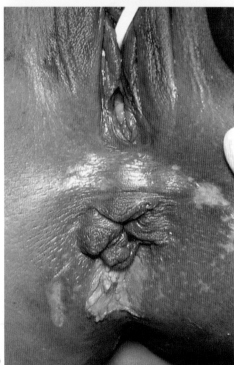

Figure 43.31 Large perianal squamous cell carcinoma just posterior to the anus. **(a)** Bulky tumor at the time of initial diagnosis. **(b)** The same tumor 3 weeks later, after partial treatment with radiation therapy and chemotherapy. **(c)** Complete disappearance of tumor 3 months after diagnosis and a full course of radiation therapy and chemotherapy. Courtesy of Dr Karen Guice.

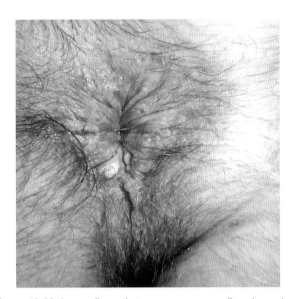

Figure 43.32 Bowen disease (cutaneous squamous cell carcinoma in situ) of the anus. The lesion has a scaly, plaque-like appearance. Courtesy of Dr Richard Burney.

44

Pancreas: anatomy and structural anomalies

David G. Heidt, Michael W. Mulholland, Diane M. Simeone

Knowledge of the anatomic and structural relations of the pancreas has become increasingly important with the advent of cross-sectional imaging, innovations in endoscopy, and the introduction of methods for percutaneous biopsy of the gland. The central location of the gland in the upper retroperitoneum complicates the medical and surgical management of pancreatic disease.

Pancreatic development begins during the fourth week of gestation from two primordial anlagen associated with the duodenum (Fig. 44.1). The dorsal pancreatic bud, destined to form a portion of the pancreatic head and all of the body and tail of the pancreas, enlarges more rapidly and extends into the dorsal mesentery. The ventral pancreatic bud, the source of the uncinate process and a portion of the pancreatic head, develops in association with the hepatic rudiment and biliary ductal structures. Rotation of the ventral pancreatic bud to the left of the duodenum brings it below the dorsal bud. Fusion occurs in the seventh week of gestation. In most instances, fusion of the ventral duct with the dorsal duct results in formation of a single pancreatic duct that empties through the ventral ductal segment (Fig. 44.2). Failure of ductal fusion results in formation of the congenital anomaly pancreas divisum (Figs 44.3 and 44.4).

The pancreas is an elongated organ (12–20 cm in length in adults) that lies transversely in the upper retroperitoneum. The gland may be divided arbitrarily into head, uncinate process, neck, body, and tail (Fig. 44.5). The head of the pancreas lies on the right in the concavity of the duodenal sweep. The head of the gland also is related to the gastroepiploic foramen, the right kidney, the inferior vena cava, and the right portion of the transverse mesocolon (Figs 44.6 and 44.7). The distal common bile duct traverses the head of the pancreas before entering the duodenum.

The neck of the pancreas is bordered inferiorly by both the transverse mesocolon and the root of the mesentery of the small intestine. Posteriorly, the neck of the pancreas is associated with the confluence of the superior mesenteric and splenic veins, which, together, form the portal vein (Fig. 44.8). The body and tail of the pancreas are related, along the superior border, to the splenic artery and vein (Fig. 44.9). The transverse mesocolon is attached to the inferior border of the tail of the gland; the stomach contacts the anterior surface. The tail of the pancreas extends to the left in the leaves of the splenorenal ligament to the hilum of the spleen. Some of these anatomic relations, as seen with cross-sectional imaging, are shown in Figure 44.10. The arterial blood supply of the pancreas is derived from both the celiac axis and the superior mesenteric artery. Venous drainage is entirely portal.

The pancreas is a mixed endocrine and exocrine gland (Fig. 44.11). The exocrine pancreas is organized in lobular units composed of ductules and acini. Acinar cells are pyramidal and have a highly basophilic cytoplasm. Numerous zymogen granules are visualized by means of electron microscopic examination of the cellular apex. Centroacinar cells (which express the surface marker Hes-1, a Notch pathway signaling molecule) and ductal cells (which express cytokeratin-19) are more columnar. The acini rest on a thin basal lamina penetrated by numerous blood vessels and nerve fibers. Centroacinar cells have been recently implicated as a possible cell of origin in pancreatic ductal carcinoma.

The endocrine pancreas is composed of approximately 1 million islets of Langerhans. The islets contain endocrine cells that stain positively for insulin (75%–80%), glucagon (10%–20%), and somatostatin (5%). Pancreatic polypeptide and several other enteric peptides are also expressed within cells of the pancreatic islets.

Atlas of Gastroenterology, 4th edition. Edited by Tadataka Yamada, David H. Alpers, Anthony N. Kalloo, Neil Kaplowitz, Chung Owyang, and Don W. Powell. © 2009 Blackwell Publishing, ISBN: 978-1-4051-6909-7

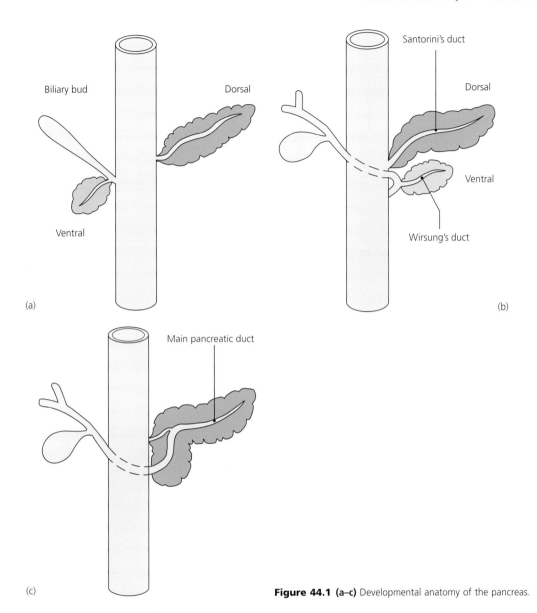

Figure 44.1 (a–c) Developmental anatomy of the pancreas.

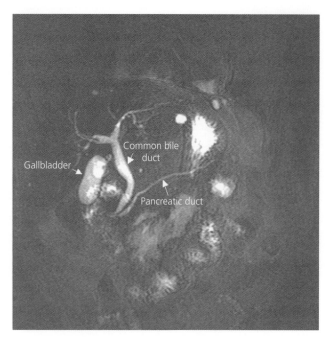

Figure 44.2 Magnetic resonance cholangiopancreatography demonstrates standard pancreatic ductal anatomy, with a single main pancreatic duct emptying through the ventral segment.

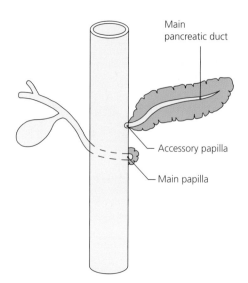

Figure 44.3 Failure of fusion of ventral and dorsal pancreatic buds results in pancreas divisum.

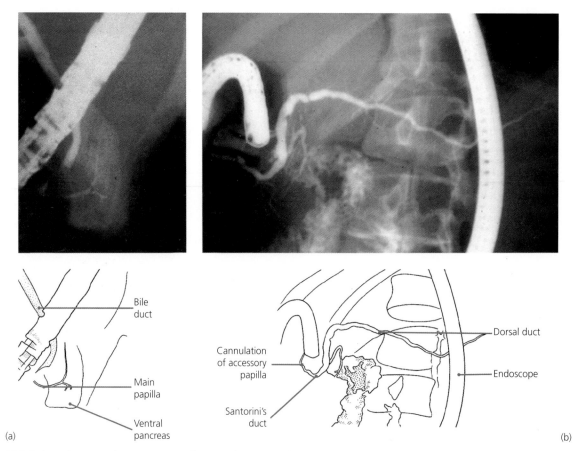

Figure 44.4 Endoscopic retrograde pancreatogram illustrates the congenital anomaly pancreas divisum. The dorsal pancreatic duct is filled through the accessory pancreatic duct **(a)**. The ventral pancreatic duct **(b)** fills through the major papilla. The two ductal systems do not communicate.

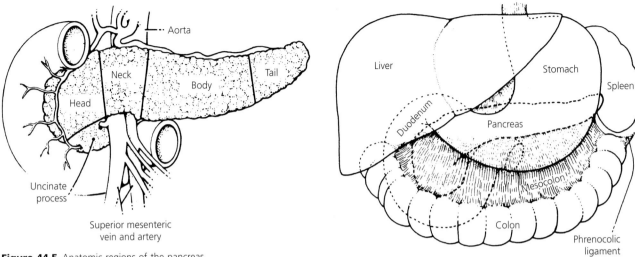

Figure 44.5 Anatomic regions of the pancreas.

Figure 44.6 Anterior relations of the pancreas.

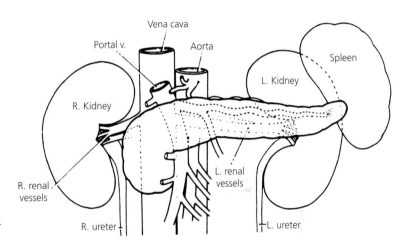

Figure 44.7 Anatomic relations posterior to the pancreas.
L., left; R., right; v., vein.

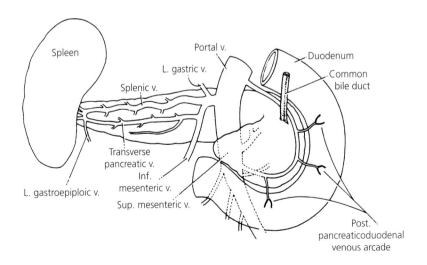

Figure 44.8 Posterior view of the pancreas
demonstrates relations to portal venous tributaries. Inf.,
inferior; L., left; Post, posterior; Sup., superior; v., vein.

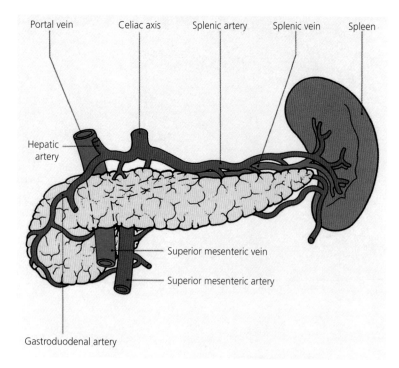

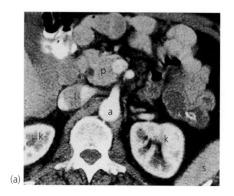

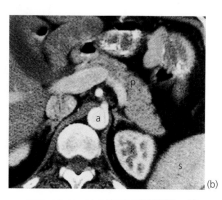

Figure 44.9 Arterial supply to the pancreas.

Figure 44.10 Computed tomographic scan of the abdomen demonstrates the relation of the head **(a)** and body and tail **(b)** of the pancreas to surrounding structures. a, aorta; l, inferior vena cava; k, kidney; p, pancreas; s, spleen.

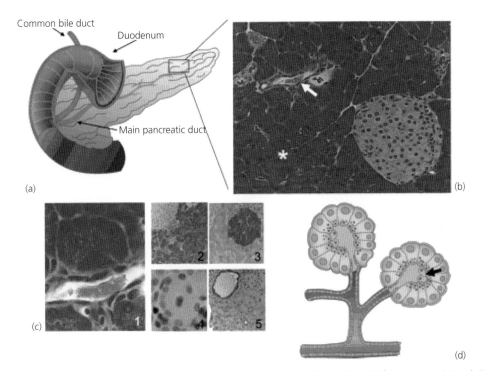

(a)

(b)

(c)

(d)

Figure 44.11 Anatomy of the pancreas. **(a)** Gross anatomy of the pancreas demonstrating its close anatomical relationship with the duodenum and common bile duct. **(b)** The major components of the pancreatic parenchyma on a histological level. At the lower right is an islet of Langherhans, the endocrine portion of the pancreas, which is principally involved in regulating glucose homeostasis. The asterisk is placed among acini, which are involved in secreting various digestive enzymes (zymogens) into the ducts (indicated by the solid arrow). **(c)** Photomicrographs of hematoxylin and eosin- and immunohistochemical-stained sections of pancreatic tissue, demonstrating the various cell types. **(Panel 1)** An acinar unit in relationship to the duct. **(Panel 2)** Acinar units visualized with an antibody to amylase are seen as brown owing to diaminobenzidine staining. **(Panel 3)** Islet of Langerhans shown stained with an antibody to insulin. **(Panel 4)** A centroacinar cell showing robust Hes1 staining. **(Panel 5)** Ductal cells (seen in cross-section) are stained with an antibody to cytokeratin-19. **(d)** Representation of an acinar unit showing the relationship to the pancreatic ducts. Also depicted are centroacinar cells (arrow), which sit at the junction of the ducts and acini.

45

Acute pancreatitis

Anil B. Nagar, Stephen J. Pandol

Acute pancreatitis is an acute inflammatory process of the pancreas. This inflammation may be mild with minimal abnormalities or severe, with pancreatic necrosis or fluid collections observed on imaging studies. Severe pancreatitis can also result in the systemic inflammatory response and dysfunction of organ systems (i.e. acute respiratory distress syndrome). The two most common etiologies, alcohol misuse and gallstones, together account for 60%–80% of acute pancreatitis (Table 45.1). Approximately 10% of cases are idiopathic, despite extensive diagnostic evaluation. Two histological forms of acute pancreatitis are recognized: acute interstitial and acute necrotic/hemorrhagic. Microscopically, acute interstitial pancreatitis demonstrates interstitial edema, infiltration of neutrophils and focal areas of fat necrosis in the pancreas and peripancreatic fat. In the more severe form, necrosis involves the acinar and ductal tissue as well as may involve the islets of Langerhans along with diffuse hemorrhage into the gland. Arterial and venous thrombosis often accompany pancreatic necrosis. In the life-threatening complication of infected necrosis, Gram stains of pancreatic aspirates can usually demonstrate the infectious pathogens. Although histological examination of pancreatic tissue is rarely available, classification systems have been developed to determine severity of disease using clinical observations, laboratory tests, specific serum inflammatory markers and imaging studies (Table 45.2).

The specific mechanisms whereby gallstones and alcohol abuse cause pancreatitis are yet unknown. Intracellular activation of pancreatic enzymes is an important early event in acute pancreatitis; along with inhibition of secretion. The resulting cell injury leads to activation of inflammatory cell signaling via NF-κB (nuclear factor- κB) and AP-1 (activated protein-1). This results in production of multiple inflammatory cytokines, such as TNF-α (tumor necrosis factor-α) platelet activating factor, interleukin-6 and macrophage migration inhibitory factor, among others. These inflammatory mediators have multiple targets, including vascular endothelium, recruitment of and activation of inflammatory cells, and damage to remote organs such as the lungs. The vascular response and injury are important in acute pancreatitis, with vasospasm described early in the course of pancreatitis associated with necrosis. In addition to inflammatory and vascular factors, neural pathways also play an important role in inflammation, particularly the formation of edema. Both substance P and calcitonin gene-related peptide are released from neural endings within the pancreas and mediate the neurovascular inflammatory response. The pathway of cell death influences the severity of acute pancreatitis. Cell death can occur by necrosis and apoptosis. Apoptosis is an ordered process that is mediated by a family of proteases called capsases; however, the level of intracellular ATP appears to be important in determining necrosis. Understanding the regulation and interaction between inflammation and necrosis is important because inflammation and its mediators precede necrosis, and attenuation of the inflammatory response may decrease that amount of necrosis.

In addition to gallstone disease and alcohol abuse, there are many less common causes of acute pancreatitis. The identification of the underlying etiology is important in prevention of recurrent attacks. Microlithiasis or crystals in the bile can cause acute recurrent pancreatitis in the absence of gallstones. Microlithiasis can be identified on transabdominal ultrasound or endoscopic ultrasound as amorphous nonshadowing layering or bright echogenic crystals. Microscopic examination of bile demonstrates birefringent cholesterol crystals or reddish brown calcium bilirubinate granules. Treatment is usually cholecystectomy with biliary sphincterotomy reserved for patients who cannot undergo surgery.

Pancreas divisum results from congenital partial or absent fusion between the duct of Wirsung and the duct of Santorini, resulting in the dorsal duct draining most of the pancreas through the minor papilla of the duct of Santorini. Some patients with pancreas divisum experience recurrent attacks of acute pancreatitis, which might be secondary to obstruction to the flow of pancreatic secretions at the duct

Atlas of Gastroenterology, 4th edition. Edited by Tadataka Yamada, David H. Alpers, Anthony N. Kalloo, Neil Kaplowitz, Chung Owyang, and Don W. Powell. © 2009 Blackwell Publishing, ISBN: 978-1-4051-6909-7

of Santorini or at a diminutive orifice of the minor papilla. Diagnosis of pancreas divisum can be made by endoscopic retrograde cholangiopancreatography (ERCP), magnetic resonance cholangiopancreatography (MRCP) or endoscopic ultrasound (EUS). In complete pancreas divisum, injection of the major ampulla demonstrates a short duct of Wirsung that terminates in the pancreatic head. To demonstrate filling of the pancreatic duct in the body and tail, the minor ampulla must be cannulated and injected with contrast. Careful examination of the ERCP images is required to distinguish pancreas divisum from duct obstruction caused by benign or malignant disease involving the main pancreatic duct. When treatment of pancreas divisum is undertaken, it can consist of careful sphincterotomy of the intraduodenal portion of the minor papilla with short-term stenting to prevent obstruction to the minor ampulla as a result of edema. Patients with chronic pancreatitis and persistent abdominal pain are less likely to respond to endoscopic therapy. Sphincter of Oddi dysfunction is another cause of pancreatitis. Obstruction to the flow at the sphincter of Oddi can be a result of stenosis or spasm, both of which may be associated with acute pancreatitis. Pancreatic sphincter hypertension can be diagnosed by sphincter of Oddi manometry performed during ERCP; a pressure greater than 40 mmHg is considered abnormal. Surgical or endoscopic ablation of the sphincter in these patients may prevent attacks of acute pancreatitis. Metabolic causes of acute pancreatitis include hypertryglyceridemia and hypercalcemia.

Lymphoplasmacytic sclerosing pancreatitis or autoimmune pancreatitis is rare and usually presents with subacute symptoms and obstructive jaundice. Acute pancreatitis is an unusual presentation. Imaging of the pancreas usually demonstrates a diffusely enlarged "sausage-shaped" pancreas or a focal pancreatic mass. A diffusely narrowed irregular pancreatic duct is usually demonstrated by ERCP. Common bile duct involvement is also described with intrapancreatic strictures or hepatic hilar strictures simulating malignancy. Endoscopic ultrasound examination may demonstrate an enlarged hypoechogenic pancreas and provide the opportunity to perform a Tru-Cut biopsy for histological diagnosis. Histology demonstrates lymphoplasmacytic infiltrate around small pancreatic ducts and venules, with a positive stain for IgG_4 immunocytochemistry. The most characteristic laboratory abnormality is an elevation of serum IgG_4 levels. Autoimmune pancreatitis must be differentiated from malignancy whenever possible; a helpful feature can be the response of autoimmune pancreatitis to systemic corticosteroids, with resolution of strictures and masses.

ERCP is a recognized cause of acute pancreatitis with a reported incidence of about 5%. Avoiding ERCP by using less invasive tests, such as MRCP and EUS as the preferred diagnostic approaches, will avoid post-ERCP pancreatitis. For patients at highest risk for pancreatitis (e.g. sphincter of Oddi dysfunction), the use of temporary pancreatic duct stenting has been demonstrated to reduce the risk of post-ERCP pancreatitis.

Pancreatic duct disruption secondary to trauma is a common cause of acute pancreatitis in children. The mid-pancreatic duct, as it crosses the vertebral column, is particularly susceptible to blunt trauma. In patients at risk for this complication, ERCP, MR or CT scanning can demonstrate duct disruption. Pancreatic duct disruption can also be seen in severe acute pancreatitis not associated with abdominal trauma.

The diagnosis of acute pancreatitis is based on the presence of acute abdominal pain and biochemical evidence of pancreatic injury. Abdominal pain is present in more than 95% of patients and is usually severe mid abdominal pain and may radiate to the back, accompanied by nausea, vomiting and fever. A small percent of patients do not complain of pain and the diagnosis of acute pancreatitis may be missed on presentation. These patients may present with acute respiratory changes or changes in mental status. Depending on the severity and presence of distal organ failure, patients can develop tachycardia, hypotension, confusion, reduced urine output, and hypoxemia. In addition to tenderness, examination of the abdomen of patients with severe pancreatitis may demonstrate abdominal rebound and guarding, reduced or absent bowel sounds, ascites, and rarely flank ecchymosis (Grey Turner's sign), or periumbilical ecchymosis (Cullen's sign). Periumbilical ecchymosis has been described in other causes of hemoperitoneum. Severe pancreatic necrosis may be accompanied by subcutaneous fat necrosis, resulting in panniculitis.

The serum amylase and lipase levels are elevated in acute pancreatitis. Serum amylase and lipase levels rise within the first hours after the onset of pancreatitis. Elevation of one or both of the pancreatic enzymes can be observed in non-pancreatic diseases, including renal failure, intestinal ischemia and perforation, acute cholecystitis, ruptured ectopic pregnancy, and certain neoplasms. Lactescent sera can cause falsely lower amylase levels, which are resolved by dilution of the sample. Liver tests are important in differentiating biliary from non-biliary pancreatitis and in identifying those patients that may benefit from early ERCP and biliary sphincterotomy. The alanine aminotransferase (ALT) is the single most sensitive liver test of acute biliary obstruction. Rapid rise and fall in transaminase and very high (>1000) levels are also very suggestive of biliary pancreatitis. Persistent elevation of the alkaline phosphatase and bilirubin are suggestive of a retained common bile duct stone and persistent biliary obstruction. Biliary tract imaging by ultrasound, MRCP or EUS is helpful in confirming retained stones in this setting (Table 45.3).

In patients with acute and severe abdominal pain, plain films of the abdomen and chest should be taken to exclude intestinal perforation. Chest radiographic findings include pleural effusions (most commonly on the left, occasionally bilateral, and rarely right sided), atelectasis, and adult respiratory distress syndrome. The inflammatory exudates in acute pancreatitis can spread anteriorly and inferiorly to involve the transverse mesocolon, resulting in spasm of the transverse colon, which is observed as the "colon cut-off" sign. This finding is not specific for acute pancreatitis and may be seen in ischemic colitis or mechanical obstruction. Other findings on abdominal plain films include localized dilation of small bowel (sentinel loop) or generalized ileus.

Imaging studies establish the diagnosis of acute pancreatitis, provide prognostic information, document presence or absence of biliary obstruction, and assess possible complications. Abdominal ultrasound examination is helpful in documenting cholelithiasis (>95% sensitive for gallbladder stones) and biliary obstruction. It is less sensitive for biliary sludge (microlithiasis) and choledocholithiasis. The inflamed pancreas is often not well-visualized secondary to overlying bowel gas. Ultrasound findings of acute inflammation include enlargement of the gland, loss of normal internal echo's, and hypoechogenicity secondary to increased water in the parenchyma.

Although the diagnosis of acute pancreatitis is made based on an elevated serum amylase and lipase, the level of elevation does not predict severity. Multiple biological markers and scoring systems have been proposed to predict severity, but the contrast enhanced dynamic CT scan remains the most widely used diagnostic technique (Table 45.4). CT scanning is helpful in establishing the diagnosis of acute pancreatitis (edema and inflammatory stranding around the gland), predicting the degree of necrosis (lack of contrast enhancement of >30% of the pancreas), and imaging of pancreatic and peripancreatic fluid collections. Development of necrosis may take 48 h and CT scanning for documentation of necrosis should be performed after adequate fluid resuscitation and preferably 24–48 h after the onset of pancreatitis. The severity of changes by dynamic CT scan correlates with morbidity and mortality in acute pancreatitis (Table 44.5). In management and follow-up of local complications of acute pancreatitis (Table 45.6), CT scanning and other imaging procedures are useful. Unlike ultrasonography, overlying bowel gas does not interfere with CT images. CT scanning is useful in the follow up of peripancreatic fluid collections and pseudocysts. However, CT scanning cannot differentiate sterile from infected necrosis. The diagnosis requires percutaneous aspiration for gram stain and culture of the necrotic area under CT or ultrasound guidance. The presence of air within a fluid collection suggests infection. Magnetic resonance imaging (MRI) may be used in acute pancreatitis. Changes in acute pancreatitis seen through the use of MRI include edema, enlargement of the organ, and lack of tissue enhancement with intravenous gadolinium in the presence of necrosis. It is an attractive alternative to CT scanning because it does not require iodine-containing intravenous contrast and can provide an MRCP image at the

same setting; this is a sensitive test to detect choledocholithiasis and is especially useful when there is a need to avoid ERCP. In patients with necrotizing pancreatitis, MRI can also document pancreatic duct disruption. EUS is A useful test in acute pancreatitis is EUS, which may be helpful in detecting biliary sludge and choledocholithiasis not seen on abdominal ultrasound imaging and can be used to identify patients who may benefit from ERCP. In women who are pregnant, EUS can also be used prior to ERCP to potentially obviate the need for ERCP and its use of X-rays. It can also aid in the diagnosis of pancreatic divisum and endoscopic drainage of pancreatic pseudocysts. The choice of imaging test depends on the question that needs to be answered at the time of the patient's presentation. If the diagnosis is uncertain a CT scan is helpful to confirm pancreatitis or demonstrate an alternative diagnosis such as perforation or ischemia. Ultrasound is helpful if biliary pancreatitis is suspected, as it detects gallstones and identifies patients with biliary dilation. In patients with chronic pancreatitis or a suspected pancreatic mass, CT scanning is preferred. If severe acute pancreatitis is suspected, dynamic contrast enhanced CT scanning can document necrosis and identify patients who may have pancreatic abscess and those who may benefit from prophylactic antibiotics.

It is important to define the severity of pancreatitis, as this allows identification of a subset of patients who will require careful monitoring and interventions. Severe pancreatitis is defined as the occurrence of local or systemic complications or death. Complications have been defined in the 1992 Atlanta conference and the Multiple Organ Dysfunction Syndrome classification. Laboratory tests, clinical and physiological assessment, and imaging tests have all been used to predict severity of pancreatitis (see Table 45.2). Pancreatitis may be classified as mild or severe to assist the clinician in management decisions (Table 45.7).

Complications of acute pancreatitis may be local or systemic. Local complications include fluid collections, necrosis, vascular complications, and obstruction of the duodenum, biliary tract or colon. Systemic complications include organ failure manifesting as respiratory insufficiency, circulatory shock, DIC (disseminated intravascular coagulation), renal failure, and a sepsis-like picture. The syndrome of multiple organ dysfunction may occur. Fat necrosis is seen in a minority of patients.

An acute fluid collection is the most common local complication. These occur early in the course of the disease, do not have a defined wall, and usually resolve spontaneously. Early intervention, such as percutaneous drainage, is only necessary if the collection becomes infected or causes intestinal obstruction. Once fluid collections persist for longer than 4 weeks and develop a wall of granulation tissue and fibrosis, they are referred to as pseudocysts. Most pseudocysts do not require any intervention unless they are increasing in size or causing symptoms. Pseudocyst drainage can be accomplished endoscopically, surgically, and percutaneously. The endoscopic approach is preferable because of its less invasive nature, high success, and low complication rates. Surgical cystgastrostomy should be considered in complicated multilocular collections and in those collections that cannot be differentiated from cystic neoplasms, so that a surgical biopsy may be obtained at the time of drainage. Endoscopic drainage can be transpapillary or transmural. Endoscopic ultrasound can assist with endoscopic pseudocyst drainage by identifying the best site for drainage, avoiding major blood vessels and providing the ability to obtain cyst contents for analysis and cytology. Communicating pseudocysts in the pancreatic head are best drained by the transpapillary approach. The transduodenal and transgastric approach can be used for pseudocysts close to the duodenum or stomach walls.

Dynamic contrast-enhanced CT scanning is used to document pancreatic necrosis, which appears as a well-demarcated area of nonenhanced pancreatic tissue. Organ failure (i.e. pulmonary, renal and cardiovascular) is more common in patients with an estimated necrosis of >50% of the gland. Necrotic tissue is at risk for infection from bowel flora that gets translocated across the intestinal lumen and then seeds the pancreatic necrosis directly or indirectly (via lymphatics and bacteremia). Infected necrosis is a leading cause of death in acute pancreatitis and usually occurs late in the presentation (second week), although early infected necrosis has been reported. The standard diagnostic modality used to document infected necrosis is CT-guided fine needle aspiration of infected tissue. Based on past studies, prophylactic antibiotics are often used to prevent the development of infected necrosis. However, recent clinical data suggest that antibiotic prophylaxis may not be effective (see below). Once infected necrosis develops, surgery with debridement is necessary. Sterile pancreatic necrosis may resolve, develop into organized pancreatic necrosis after a few weeks or may cause persistent organ dysfunction and systemic inflammatory response, requiring surgical drainage. Pancreatic abscess can sometimes complicate acute pancreatitis. Due to their walled-off nature they can be drained and seldom require surgery. Other uncommon local complications of acute pancreatitis include pancreatic ascites and fistula formation. Disruptions of the pancreatic duct can be treated either by endoscopic stenting of the pancreatic duct, by keeping the patient nil per os (NPO, nothing by mouth) and providing total parenteral nutrition, or by inhibiting pancreatic secretions with octreotide. Endoscopic therapy appears to be the most effective.

Vascular complications are not uncommon in acute pancreatitis, and include splenic vein thrombosis leading to development of gastric varices. This can be managed by splenectomy. Pseudocysts can erode into a major artery, with bleeding into the pseudocyst and formation of a pseudoaneurysm. These patients can present with circulatory collapse, and CT scanning confirms the diagnosis. Angiography with embolism of the involved artery is usually effective.

Aggressive fluid replacement and the monitoring and management of systemic complications are mainstays of therapy. Hypocalcemia is frequently seen in the acute setting. Replacement is only necessary in symptomatic patients or those with a low ionized calcium level in the serum. Pharmacological therapies for inhibition of enzyme activation and immune-modulating agents that reduce the inflammatory cytokine response have not clearly demonstrated benefit in human acute pancreatitis. There is increasing evidence that enteral feeding is associated with less infectious complications than parenteral nutrition. Enteral nutrition also has the theoretical advantage of preserving gut integrity and thereby reducing bacterial translocation, which may play an important role in infected pancreatic necrosis and the systemic inflammatory response. Patients with severe acute pancreatitis should be initiated on a semielemental diet, using enteral (i.e., jejunal) administration early (within 48 h) in the course of their disease. Patients with mild to moderate pancreatitis do not benefit form early enteral feeding and these patients can be kept NPO until resolution of their symptoms. Because infected necrosis is associated with a poor prognosis, strategies have been developed to prevent necrosis from becoming infected, including the use of prophylactic antibiotics and selective gut decontamination. The clinical data is mixed about the benefit of the use of prophylactic antibiotics. A recent metaanalysis of six controlled studies suggested no reduction in infectious complications or benefit in mortality for patients with severe acute pancreatitis. Thus, it is unclear which, if any, patient with severe acute pancreatitis should be given prophylactic antibiotics. If a decision is made to use prophylactic antibiotics, they should be started within 48 h, in patients with >30% pancreatic necrosis on CT scan, and continued for 2 weeks. The most effective antibiotic in this setting is Imipenem.

Gallstones are among the most common cause of acute pancreatitis. Patients are usually treated conservatively. Clinical studies have demonstrated the benefit and safety of early ERCP in patients with severe acute biliary pancreatitis. Emergent ERCP with biliary sphincterotomy and bile duct stone extraction is reserved for patients with persistent biliary obstruction or cholangitis. Occasionally, an impacted stone is seen at the ampulla; this can usually be dislodged by a cannula. If sphincterotomy is difficult or contraindicated (e.g. in DIC), a temporary plastic biliary stent or nasobiliary drain can be placed to secure immediate bile duct drainage. If liver tests normalize, it is not necessary to proceed with ERCP prior to cholecystectomy.

After an episode of acute pancreatitis, there is usually complete recovery of pancreatic morphology and function. Prevention of additional episodes is dependent on identifying and treating the underlying etiology of the initial attack.

Table 45.1 Etiology of acute pancreatitis

Common etiologies
Gallstones and microlithiasis
Alcohol misuse

Less common etiologies
Structural/obstruction of PD (pancreas divisum, sphincter of Oddi dysfunction)
Hypertryglyceridemia
Medications
Trauma
ERCP
Viral (mumps and Coxsackie B)
Ascaris lumbricoides
Inflammatory bowel disease (structural and medications)
Idiopathic

Uncommon etiologies
Autoimmune
Hypercalcemia
Genetic (CFTR mutations, cationic trypsinogen mutations)
Postoperative
Infectious (*Salmonella*, *Campylobacter*)
Tumors
Ischemia
Toxins (mushroom poisoning, scorpion venom)
Other (coronary bypass, peritoneal dialysis, peptic ulcer)

CFTR, cystic fibrosis transmembrane regulator; ERCP, endoscopic retrograde cholangiopancreatography; PD, pancreatic duct.

Table 45.2 Indicators used to assess severity of disease in acute pancreatitis

Clinical
Shock, respiratory failure, distended, tender and silent abdomen
Hematocrit >44
Pleural effusion

Scoring systems
Ranson criteria
Modified Glasgow Score
APACHE II with obesity

Serum markers
C-reactive protein
Interleukin-6
Procalcitonin (PCT)
Granulocyte colony-stimulating factor (G-CSF)
Urinary trypsinogen activated peptide (TAP)
Serum amyloid A
Urinary trypsinogen-2

Imaging
Dynamic contrast-enhanced CT scan
Magnetic resonance imaging (MRI)

APACHE, Acute Physiology and Chronic Health Evaluation; CT, computed tomography.

Table 45.3 Laboratory findings and imaging in biliary versus alcoholic pancreatitis

Test	Biliary pancreatitis	Alcoholic pancreatitis
Amylase	Usually > 1000 IU	Usually < 500 IU
AST, ALT	Acute elevation with rapid resolution	Minimal elevation that does not fluctuate
Alkaline phosphatase and bilirubin	Increased	Not usually elevated
Ultrasound	Gallstones, dilated common bile duct	Changes of chronic pancreatitis
CT scan	Gallstones, dilated common bile duct	Pancreatic calcification, dilated pancreatic duct with stones

ALT, alanine aminotransferase; AST, aspartate aminotransferase; CT, computed tomography.

Table 45.4 CT grading of acute pancreatitis according to Balthazar et al. 1990

	Score
Staging	
A. Normal	0
B. Focal or diffuse enlargement of gland	1
C. As B plus involvement of peripancreatic fat	2
D. Single, ill-defined fluid collection	3
E. Two or more ill-defined fluid collections and/or intrapancreatic gas	4
Degree of necrosis (%)	
0	0
<33 of pancreas	2
33–<50 of pancreas	4
≥50 of pancreas	6
Maximum	10

Staging score + degree of necrosis score = CT severity index.
Data from: Balthazar EJ, Robinson DL, Megibow AJ, et al. Acute pancreatitis: value of CT scan in establishing prognosis. Radiology 1990;174:331.

Table 45.5 Computed tomography severity index (CTSI) correlates with mortality in acute pancreatitis

CTSI	Morbidity (%)	Mortality (%)
0–3	8	3
4–6	35	6
7–10	92	17

Table 45.6 Selected local complications of acute pancreatitis

Complication	Imaging	Management
Acute fluid collection	CT scan	Conservative management
Pancreatic abscess	CT scan with needle aspiration for determining infection	Transcutaneous drainage or surgery
Pancreatic necrosis	CT scan with needle aspiration for determining infection	Antibiotics with surgery for infected necrosis
Pseudocyst	CT scan or ultrasound	Conservative management, endoscopic or surgical drainage if indicated
Pancreatic fistula	ERCP, CT scan, MRCP	PD stenting, somatostatin (Octreotide), surgery
Splenic vein thrombosis	Contrast CT, MRA	Splenectomy for bleeding gastric or esophageal varices
Pseudoaneurysm formation	Contrast CT, angiography MRA	Angiographic embolism of feeding artery

CT, computed tomography; ERCP, endoscopic retrograde cholangiopancreatography; MRA, magnetic resonance angiography; PD, pancreatic duct.

Table 45.7 Classification of mild and severe pancreatitis

Model	Mild pancreatitis	Severe pancreatitis
Clinical		
Hematocrit (%)	Normal	>44
Physical examination	Abdominal pain without organ dysfunction	Peritonitis, shock, hypoxemia, renal failure
Scoring system		
Ranson	0–1	>3
APACHE-O	1–6	>8
Modified Glasgow Score	0	>2
Serum markers		
CRP at 48 h	25–100 mg/L	150 mg/L
IL-6	Normal	2.7 pg/mL
UTAP	<15	37 nmol/L
Imaging studies		
CTSI	1–3	>6
MRSI	1–3	>6

APACHE-O, Acute Physiology and Chronic Health Enquiry with Obesity; CRP, C-reactive protein; CTSI, computed tomography severity index; IL-6, interleukin-6; MRSI, magnetic resonance severity index; UTAP, urinary trypsin activation peptide.

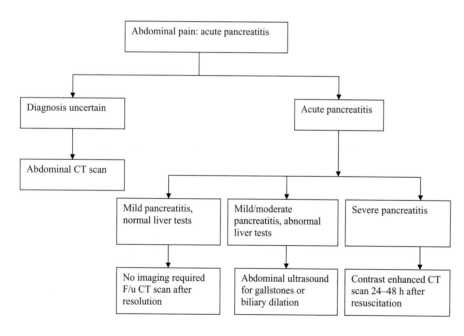

Figure 45.1 Algorithm showing an approach to imaging in acute pancreatitis. CT, computed tomography; F/u, follow up.

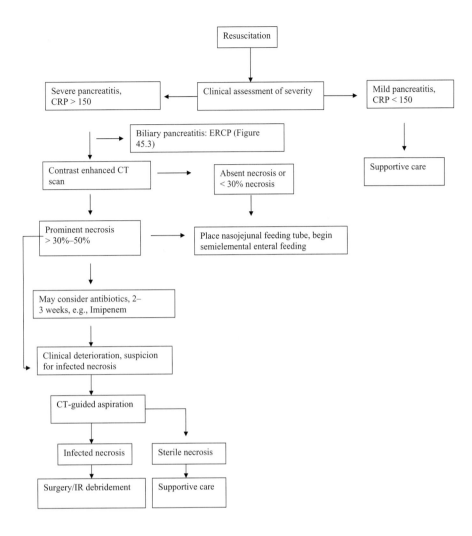

Figure 45.2 Algorithm showing an approach to management in acute pancreatitis. CRP, C-reactive peptide; CT, computed tomography; ERCP, endoscopic retrograde cholangiopancreatography; IR, Interventional radiology.

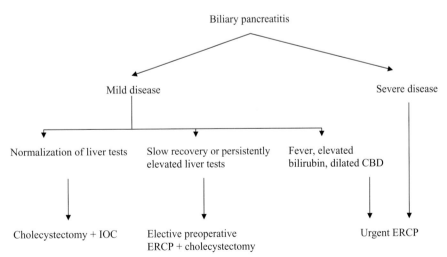

Figure 45.3 Approach to endoscopic retrograde cholangiopancreatography (ERCP) in acute biliary pancreatitis. CBD, common bile duct; IOC, intraoperative cholangiogram.

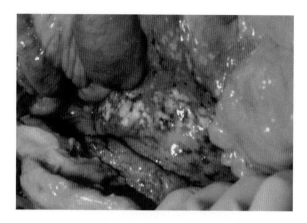

Figure 45.4 Gross specimen of acute hemorrhagic pancreatitis. White chalky fat necrosis and hemorrhage is seen. Courtesy of Robert Homer, MD, Yale University.

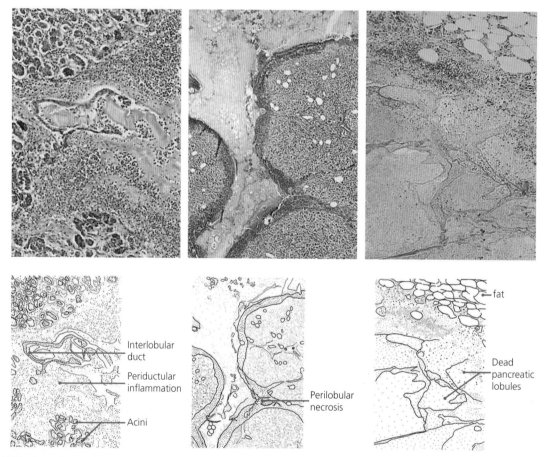

Figure 45.5 Histology of acute pancreatitis.

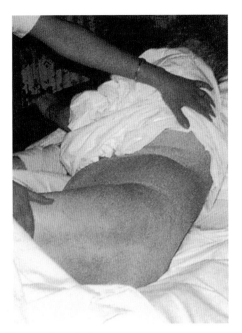

Figure 45.6 Grey Turner's sign.

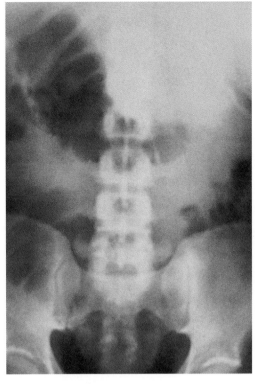

Figure 45.8 Colon cut-off sign.

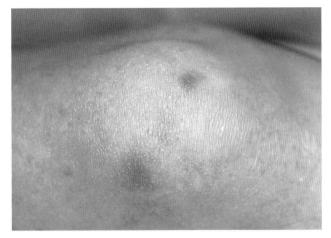

Figure 45.7 Panniculitis.

Figure 45.9 **(a)** Ultrasound image of a normal pancreas (arrows). **(b)** Transabdominal ultrasound image of acute pancreatitis. The pancreas is enlarged, hypoechoic, and heterogeneous (arrows). The splenic vein is shown by the arrowhead. L, liver; PC, portal confluence. Images courtesy of Carl Reading and Mark Topazian, Mayo College of Medicine.

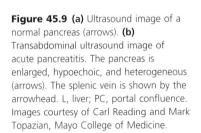

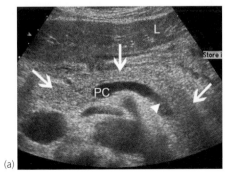

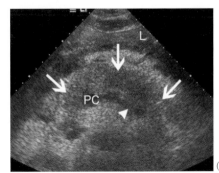

(a)

(b)

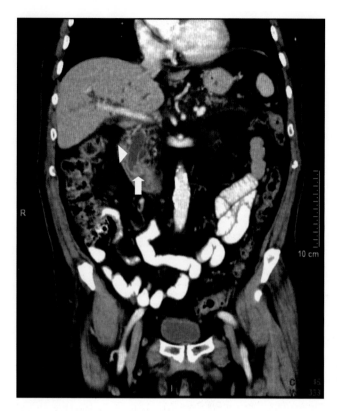

Figure 45.10 Impacted common bile duct (CBD) stone: computed tomography scan in cross-section demonstrating a dilated CBD (arrowhead) with a stone impacted in the distal CBD (arrow) leading to dilation of the ducts above. The pancreas is not seen in this cross-section.

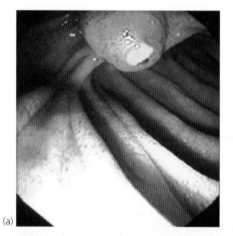

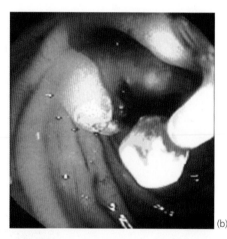

(a)

(b)

Figure 45.11 (a, b) Impacted stone: endoscopic view of a bulging papilla due to an impacted stone, which was removed following sphincterotomy using a needle knife (8B). Courtesy of Mark Topazian, Mayo Clinic.

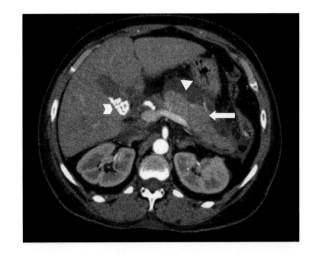

Figure 45.12 Computed tomography scan with intravenous contrast demonstrating moderate acute pancreatitis. The pancreas (arrow) is edematous, but enhances throughout, demonstrating absence of necrosis. There is peripancreatic fluid and stranding (arrowhead). Gallstones are present in the gallbladder (double arrowhead).

Figure 45.13 Computed tomography scan of pancreas in minimal necrosis. **(a)** Without contrast. **(b)** With intravenous contrast. The absence of contrast enhancement within part of the pancreas indicates necrosis (arrow). Fluid is seen around the pancreas tail (arrowhead).

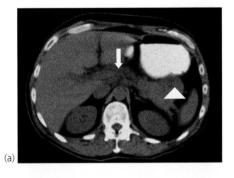

(a)

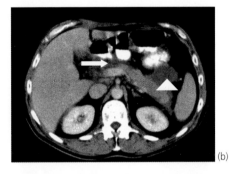

(b)

Figure 45.14 Contrast-enhanced computed tomography scans of the pancreas. **(a)** Day 1. Most of the pancreas demonstrates enhancement (arrow); contrast is seen in the aorta (arrowhead). **(b)** forty-eight hours later, there is absence of contrast enhancement with complete necrosis of the pancreas (arrow); contrast is seen in the aorta (arrowhead). Courtesy of Harold Schwartz.

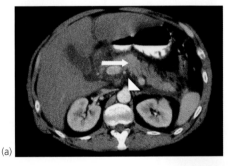

(a)

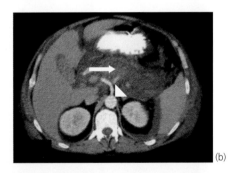

(b)

Figure 45.15 Magnetic resonance image with T1-weighted sections demonstrating peripancreatic fluid collections (arrowhead) and decreased parenchymal enhancement in acute pancreatitis, indicative of pancreatic necrosis (arrow). Courtesy of M. Arvanitakis.

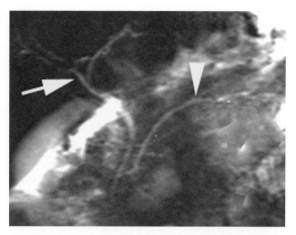

Figure 45.16 Magnetic resonance cholangiopancreatography in acute pancreatitis demonstrating a normal appearing common bile duct (arrow) and pancreatic duct (arrowhead). Courtesy of M. Arvanitakis.

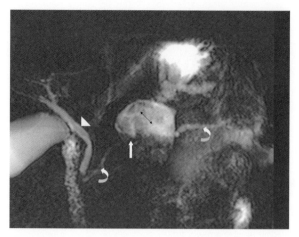

Figure 45.17 T2 heavily weighted coronal magnetic resonance imaging section following secretin injection demonstrating disruption of the main pancreatic duct (arrow) in setting of acute pancreatitis. The common bile duct (arrowhead) and pancreatic duct (curved arrow) are visualized. A fluid collection is seen at the site of pancreatic duct disruption (double arrow). Courtesy of M. Arvanitakis.

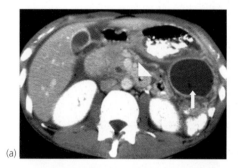

(a)

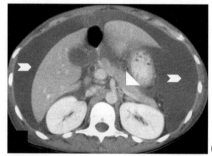

(b)

Figure 45.18 Contrast computed tomography scan of pancreas. **(a)** Pseudocyst is seen near the tail of pancreas (arrow), the pancreas is seen (arrowhead). **(b)** Ascites is observed (double arrowheads) with resolution of pseudocyst following the rare complication of pseudocyst rupture. Pancreas is also seen (arrowhead). Courtesy of Carolyn Taylor.

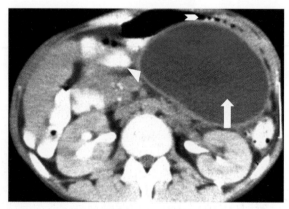

Figure 45.19 Contrast computed tomography of pancreas demonstrating a large pseudocyst (arrow) with thick walls (arrowhead), compressing the stomach (double arrowhead).

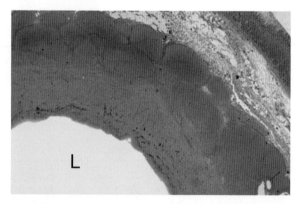

Figure 45.20 Histology of pseudocyst showing nonepithelial lining. The cyst is enclosed in a fibrous connective tissue from the inflammatory reaction. L, cyst lumen.

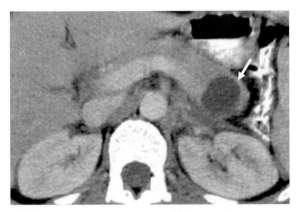

Figure 45.21 Contrast computed tomography (CT) of pancreas showing a cystic lesion in the tail (arrow). A CT scan may not differentiate a pseudocyst from a cystic neoplasm. Courtesy of Howard Taubin.

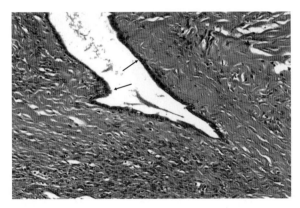

Figure 45.22 Histology of this cystic lesion demonstrated the columnar epithelial lining (arrows) of a cystadenoma.

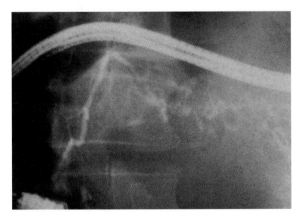

Figure 45.23 Endoscopic retrograde cholangiopancreatography of pancreatic duct trauma.

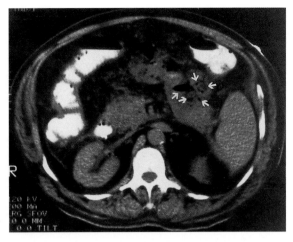

Figure 45.24 Computed tomography of pancreatic abscess. Air is noted in an area of pancreatic fluid collection (arrows).

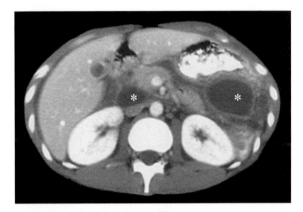

Figure 45.25 Contrast computed tomography scan demonstrating multiple fluid collections (*) complicating acute pancreatitis. The collections appear to be organizing into pseudocysts and would usually resolve spontaneously.

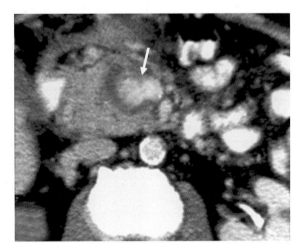

Figure 45.26 Contrast computed tomography demonstrating extravasation of intravenous contrast (arrow) into a pseudoaneurysm of the splenic artery. The patient was successfully treated by angiographic embolization of the feeding vessel. Courtesy of Caroline Taylor, Yale University.

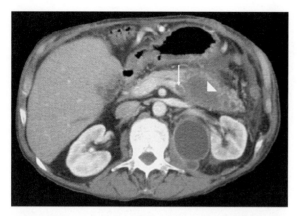

Figure 45.27 Contrast computed tomography scan of abdomen demonstrating splenic vein thrombosis (filling defect within the splenic vein indicated by arrow). Note the adjacent inflammation of the pancreatic tail (arrowhead). Courtesy of Caroline Taylor, Yale University.

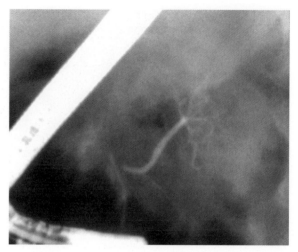

Figure 45.28 Endoscopic retrograde cholangiopancreatography image in pancreas divisum. Injection of the major ampulla results in filling of the duct of Wirsung, which terminates in the pancreas head with arborization and does not fill the dorsal pancreatic duct. Injection of the minor ampulla would have filled the dorsal pancreatic duct in the body and tail.

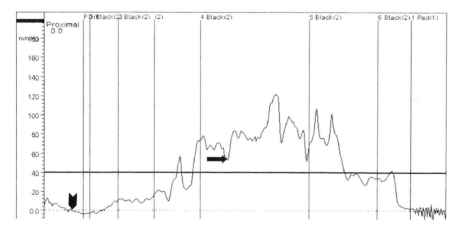

Figure 45.29 Sphincter of Oddi manometry tracing of the pancreatic duct sphincter demonstrating an elevated basal pancreatic sphincter pressure (arrow) measured on pulling back the proximal manometric catheter through the sphincter. The baseline duodenal pressure (double arrowhead) is zero reference. A pressure of greater than 40 mmHg is considered elevated. Marks are 1 mm apart and indicate depth of insertion. Courtesy of Dr Priya Jamidar and Sue Lynn, Yale University.

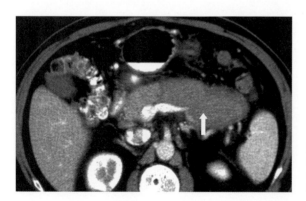

Figure 45.30 Contrast computed tomography of autoimmune pancreatitis demonstrating diffuse pancreatic enlargement involving the body and tail (arrow) without evidence of peripancreatic inflammation. Courtesy of Jeff Lee and David Carr-Locke.

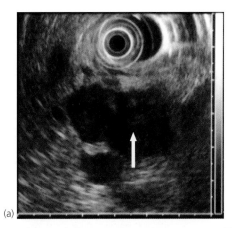
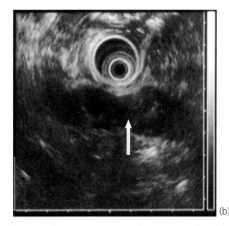

(a) (b)

Figure 45.31 Endoscopic ultrasound of pancreas in autoimmune pancreatitis **(a)** Diffuse hypoechoic mass in the pancreatic head (arrow). **(b)** Diffuse lobular hypoechoic body of the pancreas (arrow). Courtesy of Mark Topazian, Mayo Clinic.

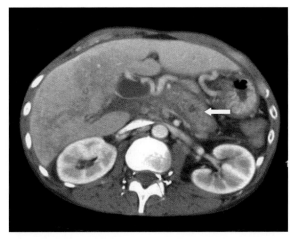

Figure 45.32 Contrast-enhanced computed tomography scan of pancreas in pancreatic lymphoma. The pancreas is diffusely enlarged in the body and tail (arrow). Although rare, it should be differentiated from autoimmune pancreatitis.

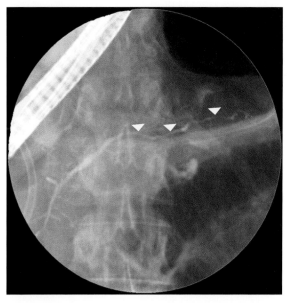

Figure 45.33 Endoscopic retrograde pancreatography in autoimmune pancreatitis. Injection of the pancreatic duct demonstrates a diffusely irregularly narrowed main pancreatic duct (arrowheads). Courtesy of Mark Topazian, Mayo Clinic.

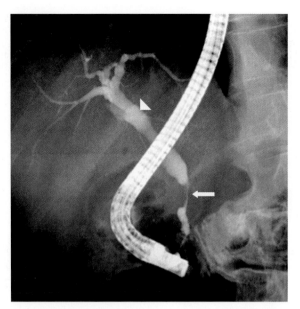

Figure 45.34 Endoscopic retrograde cholangiopancreatography in a patient with autoimmune pancreatitis. Injection of the common bile duct (CBD) demonstrating a distal CBD stricture (arrow), which simulates malignancy. The CBD is dilated above the stricture (arrowhead). Courtesy of Mark Topazian, Mayo Clinic.

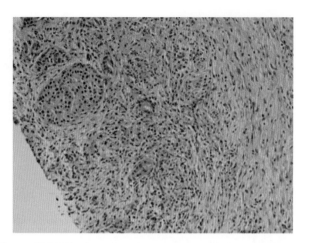

Figure 45.36 Histology of autoimmune pancreatitis demonstrating lymphoplasmacytic infiltrate, around ductules with fibrosis. Courtesy of Mark Topazian, Mayo Clinic.

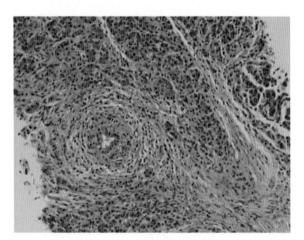

Figure 45.35 Histology of autoimmune pancreatitis demonstrating a periductular lymphoplasmacytic infiltrate involving the perivenular areas and small ducts. Courtesy of Mark Topazian, Mayo Clinic.

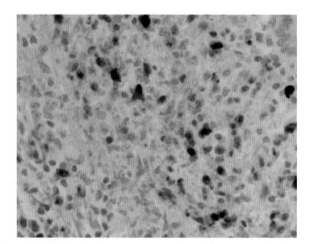

Figure 45.37 Histology of autoimmune pancreatitis demonstrating a lymphoplasmacytic infiltrate that stains for IgG4. Courtesy of Mark Topazian, Mayo Clinic.

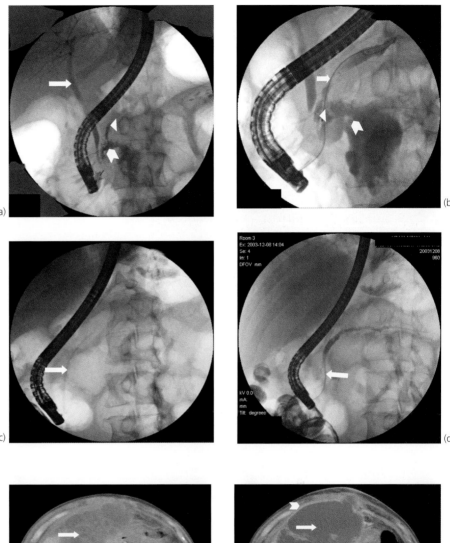

Figure 45.38 Pancreatic duct disruption following rupture of a pseudocyst. This was successfully managed endoscopically with endoscopic retrograde cholangiopancreatography and pancreatic duct stenting. **(a)** Injection of the ampulla demonstrates a normal appearing common bile duct (arrow) and disruption of the pancreatic duct in the head (double arrowhead). The pancreatic duct is seen distal to the disruption (arrowhead). **(b)** A 0.35 wire (arrow) is placed across the disruption. Pancreatic duct (arrowhead) and leak (double arrowhead) are seen. **(c)** Pancreatic duct stent (arrow) is placed across the duct disruption. **(d)** Follow-up 6 weeks later demonstrates healing of the pancreatic duct disruption (arrow).

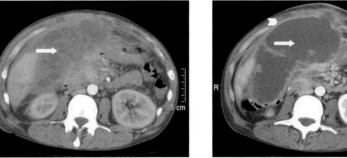

Figure 45.39 A computed tomography scan demonstrating progression of an acute fluid collection that complicated acute pancreatitis. **(a)** Edema, stranding, and multiple small fluid collections. Multiple fluid collections are seen (arrow). **(b)** Organization and development of a large pancreatic pseudocyst (arrow) with formation of a thick wall (arrowhead).

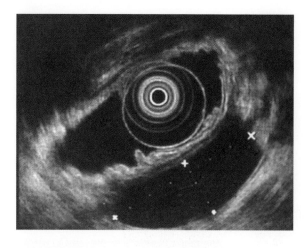

Figure 45.40 Endoscopic ultrasound (EUS) of a pseudocyst. The ultrasound probe is seen in the water-filled stomach. The pseudocyst is noted adjacent to the stomach (walls marked). An EUS is helpful prior to endoscopic drainage of a pseudocyst to measure the distance between bowel wall and pseudocyst and to avoid large blood vessels at the drainage site. Courtesy of Mark Topazian, Mayo Clinic.

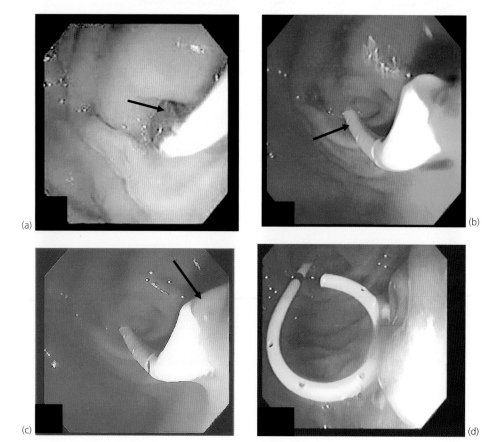

Figure 45.41 Endoscopic drainage of infected pseudocyst using the transgastric approach. Endoscopic views. **(a)** Dilation of the initial needle tract with a 6-mm balloon (arrow). **(b)** Deployment of a 10 F double pigtail stent (arrow). **(c)** Purulent material is seen draining out of the stent (arrow). **(d)** Pigtail stent is completely deployed (arrow). Multiple stents are necessary to adequately drain a pseudocyst endoscopically.

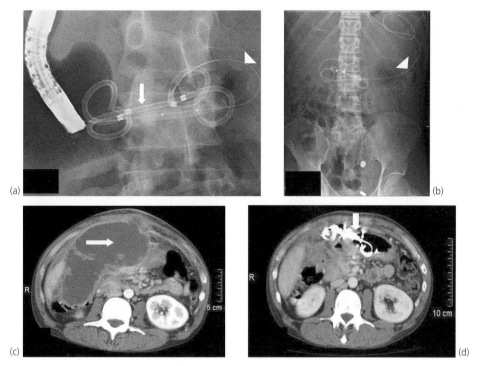

Figure 45.42 Endoscopic drainage of infected pseudocyst. Fluoroscopic views. **(a)** Multiple transgastric double pigtail stents (arrow) are placed along with a nasocystic drain (arrowhead). **(b)** Nasocystic drain (arrowhead) noted in the stomach; this is placed to enable lavage of the infected cavity following drainage. **(c)** A computed tomography (CT) scan demonstrating a large pseudocyst (arrow). **(d)** A CT scan in the same patient following endoscopic drainage, demonstrating drainage stents (arrow) and resolution of the fluid collection.

46

Chronic pancreatitis

Chung Owyang, Cyrus Piraka

Chronic pancreatitis is defined as an inflammatory disease of the pancreas characterized by persistent and often progressive lesions resulting in functional impairment and structural alterations. Alcohol misuse in Western societies (70%–80%) and malnutrition worldwide represent the leading causes of chronic pancreatitis. Metabolic and mechanical disturbances and hereditary disposition have also been implicated (Fig. 46.1).

Pain is the most important symptom of chronic pancreatitis. Possible causes include inflammation of the pancreas, increased intrapancreatic pressure, neural inflammation, and extrapancreatic causes such as common bile duct stenosis and duodenal stenosis. Clinical and experimental evidence suggests that pain may be related to increased intraductal pressure caused by continued pancreatic secretion in the face of ductal obstruction due to strictures, intraductal stones (Fig. 46.2), or destruction of pancreatic ducts (Fig. 46.3). Intrapancreatic neural inflammation is another factor that may play an important role in the genesis of pain in chronic pancreatitis. Morphological studies indicate that there is an alteration in the perineurial sheath that ordinarily shields nerves from surrounding connective tissue (Fig. 46.4). The damaged perineurium allows penetration of biologically active materials from the surrounding extracellular matrix, and pain may result from continual stimulation of the sensory nerves by noxious substances. Malabsorption is a serious problem in chronic pancreatitis. Malabsorption, however, occurs only after the capacity for enzyme secretion is reduced by more than 90% (Fig. 46.5). In chronic pancreatitis caused by alcoholism, it usually takes 10–20 years for severe pancreatic insufficiency and steatorrhea to develop.

The multiple tests available for the diagnosis of chronic pancreatitis can be separated into chemical measurements of pancreatic function and radiological procedures that provide information on pancreatic structure. Among the pancreatic function tests, the direct stimulatory tests with secretin or cholecystokinin (CCK) are the most sensitive and specific for evaluation of pancreatic function.

Pancreatic structural changes such as calcification, masses, ductal irregularities, enlargements, and cysts may be detected with various radiological and ultrasonic techniques. The demonstration of diffuse, speckled calcification of the pancreas on a plain radiograph of the abdomen is diagnostic of chronic pancreatitis (Fig. 46.6). Although the sensitivity of this finding is limited (30%–40%), plain radiography of the abdomen should be the first diagnostic test used to establish the diagnosis of chronic pancreatitis, because a positive finding obviates the need for additional testing.

The development over the past 15 years of ultrasound, computed tomographic (CT) scanning, and endoscopic retrograde cholangiopancreatography (ERCP) has made it possible to assess routinely the gross structure of the pancreas. These tests all have excellent specificity and reasonably good sensitivity. Ultrasound is the simplest and least expensive of the three imaging techniques. Characteristic findings include calcification, dilation of the pancreatic duct, and pancreatic enlargement (Fig. 46.7). The reported sensitivity of ultrasound scanning for chronic pancreatitis is about 70% and the specificity is 90%. CT scanning is 10%–20% more sensitive than ultrasound scanning in the diagnosis of chronic pancreatitis. The most helpful diagnostic findings on CT scans include ductal dilation, calcification (Fig. 46.8), and cystic lesions. Less helpful diagnostic findings include enlargement or atrophy of the pancreas and heterogeneous density of the parenchyma. ERCP is considered to be the most sensitive and specific test for the diagnosis of chronic pancreatitis. In minimal pancreatitis, the changes are limited to the branches and fine ducts, which show dilation and irregularity (Fig. 46.9). Moderate pancreatitis is characterized by the additional finding of minor irregularity of the main pancreatic duct. Advanced pancreatitis has the additional findings of cystic dilation of the main pancreatic duct and pancreatic atrophy (Fig. 46.10). Pancreatic divisum results from failure of the ducts of the embryonic dorsal and

Atlas of Gastroenterology, 4th edition. Edited by Tadataka Yamada, David H. Alpers, Anthony N. Kalloo, Neil Kaplowitz, Chung Owyang, and Don W. Powell. © 2009 Blackwell Publishing, ISBN: 978-1-4051-6909-7

ventral pancreas to fuse. Characteristic findings of the ductal anatomy can be observed during ERCP (Fig. 46.11). In patients with autoimmune pancreatitis, ERCP usually shows segmental or diffuse narrowing of the main pancreatic duct and stenosis of the common bile duct, mainly in the intrapancreatic area, resulting in dilation of the proximal biliary tract (Fig. 46.12).

Endoscopic ultrasound (EUS) has emerged as a means of obtaining detailed images of the pancreas (Figs 46.13 and 46.14). Several reports suggest that this technique is equivalent to ERCP; both tests exhibit sensitivities and specificities of more than 80% in moderate and severe chronic pancreatitis. However, the role of EUS in the diagnosis of mild chronic pancreatitis remains to be determined. The diagnosis of chronic pancreatitis by EUS is based on abnormalities in the pancreatic duct and parenchyma. Most reports used nine features, of which a minimum of three must be present. Parenchymal abnormalities include hyperechoic foci, hyperechoic strands, glandular lobularity, and cysts. Ductal findings may include duct dilation (Fig 46.15), irregularity, hyperechoic ductal margins, dilated side branches, and stones. Unlike ERCP, EUS has no risk for inducing pancreatitis. EUS-guided fine-needle aspiration can differentiate chronic pancreatitis from malignancy. ERCP and EUS are costly, invasive procedures that should be used only when less invasive procedures fail to substantiate the diagnosis of chronic pancreatitis.

Pancreatic pseudocyst is the most common complication of chronic pancreatitis; it occurs in as many as 25% of cases in some series. It represents a collection of pancreatic juice outside the normal boundaries of the ductal system, which is enclosed by a fibrous tissue membrane (Fig. 46.16). Abdominal ultrasound is most frequently used in the diagnosis and management of pseudocyst (Fig. 46.17). CT scanning has emerged as the single most accurate method of diagnosing pancreatic pseudocyst (Fig. 46.18). In addition to having a high accuracy rate, CT scanning provides structural details, such as the size of the common duct or pancreatic duct, that have important bearing on the choice of operative approach. Pancreatic pseudocyst may also be seen on EUS (Fig. 46.19). ERCP may demonstrate the anatomic relation between a pseudocyst and the main pancreatic duct (Fig. 46.20); however, not all gastroenterologists and surgeons have found routine preoperative ERCP desirable, for fear of secondary infection.

Treatment of pseudocyst includes excision and internal or external drainage. Pseudocysts that are more than 6 weeks old usually have a mature cyst wall that permits internal drainage in which the cyst is anastomosed to the stomach (cystogastrostomy), duodenum (cystoduodenostomy), or jejunum (cystojejunostomy). Endoscopic drainage can also be performed for the treatment of pseudocysts in chronic pancreatitis. A pseudocyst that indents to the stomach or duodenum can be punctured transendoscopically using elec-

trocautery or lasers to create a fistulous tract between the pseudocyst and the stomach (Figs 46.21 and 46.22).

Splenic venous thrombosis occurs among at least 20% of patients with chronic pancreatitis. It is usually caused by compression and fibrosis due to pancreatitis. Splenic venous thrombosis may cause gastric varices (Fig. 46.23) and at times either esophageal or colonic varices. The most important symptom of splenic venous thrombosis is bleeding from varices. The diagnosis can be made by means of CT scanning with bolus injection, which demonstrates varices around the stomach and in proximity to the spleen (Fig. 46.24). The treatment of choice is splenectomy, which decreases venous outflow through the varices, thereby reducing pressure.

Medical treatment of chronic pancreatitis is aimed mainly at the control of pain and correction of malabsorption with adequate pancreatic enzyme replacement. Control of pain includes avoidance of alcohol, use of analgesics, and celiac plexus block. Celiac plexus block can be done percutaneously (Figs 46.25 and 46.26) and should be considered only for patients with refractory pain that does not respond to medical therapy. The outcome of celiac block is, however, not as good in pancreatitis as in pancreatic cancer. This may reflect the fact that pain from chronic pancreatitis usually has a "central" component, which means that specialized nociceptive impulses are not needed to experience pain and so a nerve block is not expected to have a significant beneficial effect.

An increase in intrapancreatic pressure is believed to play an important role in the pathogenesis of pain in chronic pancreatitis. Hence, strategies to reduce intrapancreatic pressure have been designed to combat pain in chronic pancreatitis. These include endoscopic stenting in patients with an isolated stricture of the main pancreatic duct (Figs 46.27 and 46.28), pancreatic enzyme replacement, and surgical decompression. A number of studies show that oral pancreatic enzymes may reduce pain in some patients with chronic pancreatitis. The mechanism appears to involve a process termed "negative feedback inhibition," i.e., intraduodenal administration of trypsin or chymotrypsin is capable of inhibiting the release of CCK and pancreatic enzyme secretion. It is therefore conceivable that, in patients with chronic pancreatitis, decreased enzyme secretion may result in hyperstimulation of the pancreas, producing pain. Effective enzyme replacement therapy might reduce stimulation of the pancreas, decrease intraductal pressure, and diminish pain.

After all medical measures have failed to relieve pain, surgery should be considered. The type of surgery is selected according to the perceived mechanism for the pain. Patients who have ductal dilation have a 60%–70% chance of obtaining pain relief with either a partial resection with pancreaticojejunostomy or a lateral pancreaticojejunostomy (modified Puestow) (Fig. 46.29). The modified Puestow pancreaticojejunostomy is particularly suitable for patients who have ductal obstruction and dilation. It is a safe and effective operation with a morbidity of less than 5%, mortality of less than 2%, and effective pain relief of about 60%. On the other hand, for patients with moderate to severe parenchymal disease and no ductal dilation, partial pancreatic resection should be considered. A 95% distal resection is recommended for patients with diffuse parenchymal disease, whereas local resection of the major site of involvement may be sufficient for those with regional parenchymal disease. Overall, 50% of these patients have had satisfactory results.

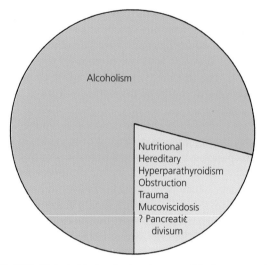

Figure 46.1 Etiological factors in chronic pancreatitis. Factors associated with or known to cause chronic pancreatitis are shown. Alcoholism accounts for 70%–80% of cases in Western societies.

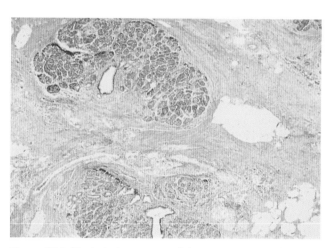

Figure 46.3 Histological appearance of chronic pancreatitis. Bands of fibrous tissue have replaced the acini, and the ducts have been destroyed (H & E stain). Courtesy of Dr Henry Appelman.

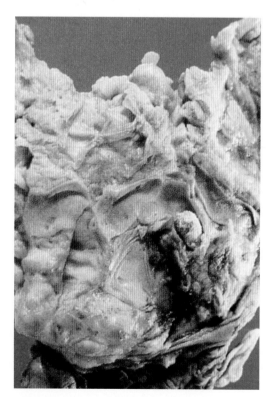

Figure 46.2 Surgical specimen of pancreas from a patient with advanced chronic pancreatitis. A pancreatic stone in the main pancreatic duct is causing obstruction.

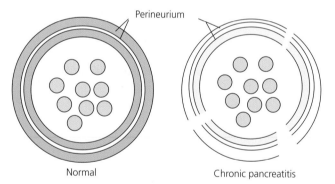

Figure 46.4 Diagram of damage to the perineurium that occurs in chronic pancreatitis. Intact perineurium normally provides a barrier, whereas damaged perineurium allows penetration of biologically active materials from the surrounding extracellular matrix.

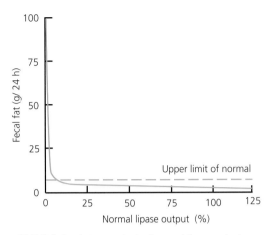

Figure 46.5 Relation between steatorrhea and lipase output. Steatorrhea does not occur until lipase output is reduced to less than 10% of normal.

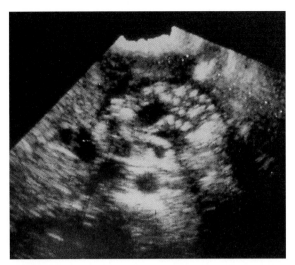

Figure 46.7 Transverse sonogram of a patient with chronic pancreatitis demonstrates a pancreas that is densely echogenic because of a combination of multiple calculi within the ducts and pancreatic fibrosis.

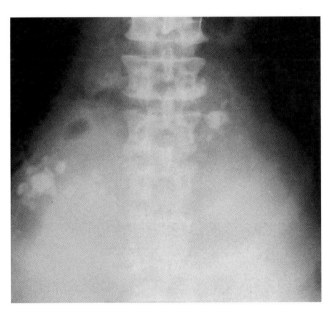

Figure 46.6 Plain abdominal radiograph demonstrates extensive calcification in the duct system of a patient with chronic calcific pancreatitis due to alcoholism.

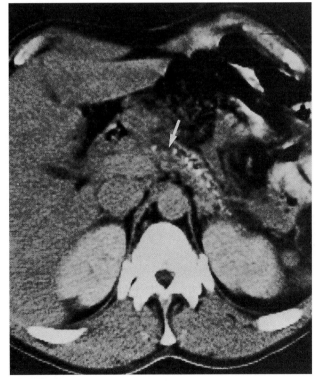

Figure 46.8 Chronic pancreatitis. Computed tomography scan shows pancreatic atrophy along with multiple intraductal calculi and dilation of the pancreatic duct (arrow).

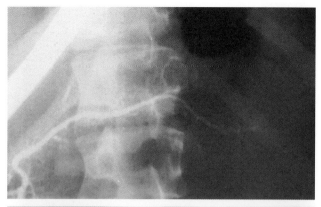

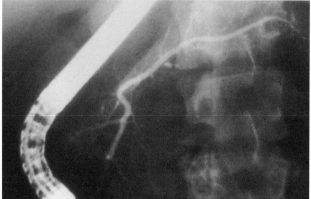

Figure 46.9 Endoscopic retrograde cholangiopancreatogram shows mild chronic pancreatitis. The main duct is of normal caliber, but the side branches are irregular. Courtesy of Jeffrey L. Barnett, MD.

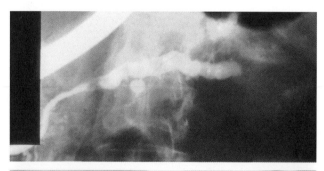

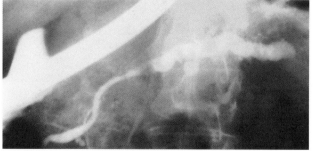

Figure 46.10 Endoscopic retrograde cholangiopancreatogram shows severe chronic pancreatitis. There is gross irregularity of the side branches and irregular dilation of the pancreatic duct. Courtesy of Jeffrey L. Barnett, MD.

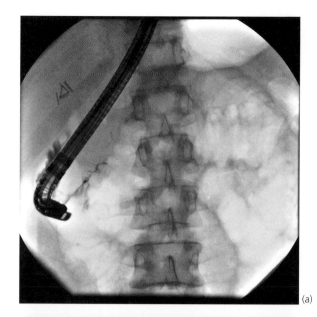

(a)

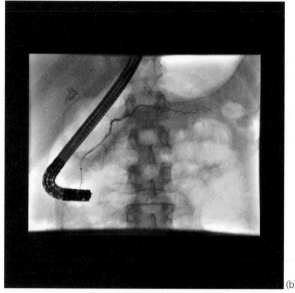

(b)

Figure 46.11 Pancreatogram in a patient with pancreas divisum.
(a) Ventral: contrast injection into the ventral duct reveals filling only in the head of the pancreas; contrast did not flow into the main pancreatic duct despite adequate injection to produce acinarization. **(b)** Dorsal: injection into the minor papilla reveals patency of the duct of Santorini and communication and filling of the main pancreatic duct without filling of the duct of Wirsung. This confirms the diagnosis of pancreas divisum.

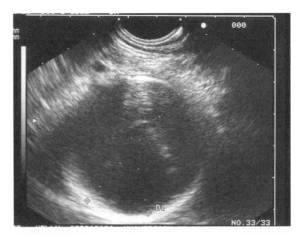

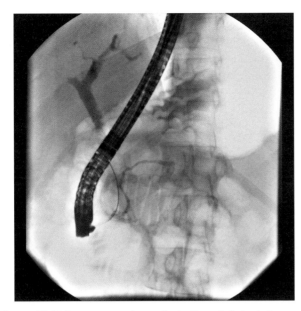

Figure 46.12 Pancreatogram in a patient with partially treated autoimmune pancreatitis.

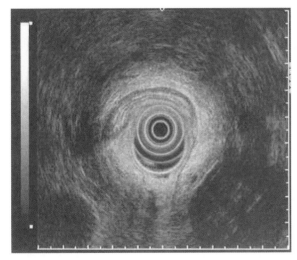

Figure 46.13 Endoscopic ultrasound showing mild chronic pancreatitis. Characteristic features include hyperechoic pancreatic duct margins and irregular contour of the pancreatic duct.

Figure 46.14 Endoscopic ultrasound showing a large pseudocyst (4.4 × 4.6 cm) with a calcified rim from a patient with chronic pancreatitis.

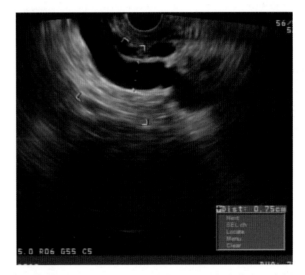

Figure 46.15 Endoscopic ultrasound showing marked dilation of the main pancreatic duct in a patient with chronic pancreatitis. A dilated side branch is also visible. The duct measures 7.5 mm in diameter.

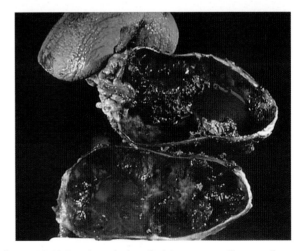

Figure 46.16 Pseudocyst in the tail of the pancreas. Courtesy of Dr Henry Appelman.

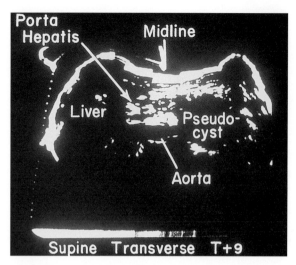

Figure 46.17 Transverse sonogram of a patient with chronic pancreatitis shows a large pseudocyst in the body and tail of the pancreas.

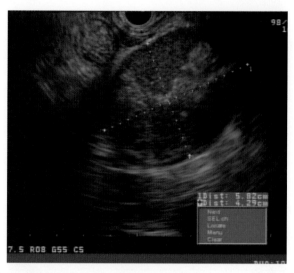

Figure 46.19 Linear endoscopic ultrasound image showing a 5.8 × 4.3-cm pseudocyst, also seen on computed tomography scanning (not shown). On endosonography, a moderate amount of internal debris is visible and the walls of the pseudocyst are thickened.

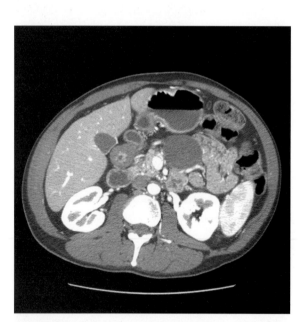

Figure 46.18 Computed tomography scan showing an atrophic pancreas and a pseudocyst in a patient with heavy alcohol use. Parenchymal atrophy is most visible on the head of this image.

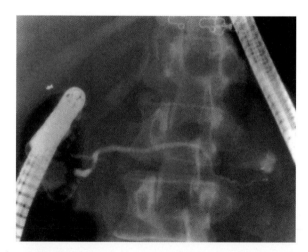

Figure 46.20 Endoscopic retrograde cholangiopancreatogram demonstrates extravasation of contrast material from the pancreatic duct into a pseudocyst.

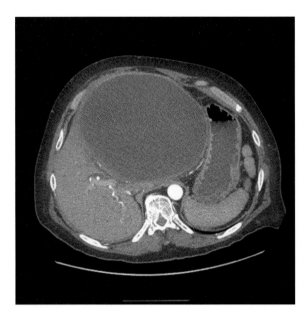

Figure 46.21 Large pancreatic pseudocyst measuring 20 × 17 cm following an episode of acute pancreatitis in a patient with alcoholism. The wall of the pseudocyst is thick and in close proximity to the wall of the stomach. This image is from a computed tomography angiogram that was carried out to rule out associated pseudoaneurysm prior to planned endoscopic cyst gastrostomy. The patient was symptomatic with abdominal pain, nausea, and early satiety.

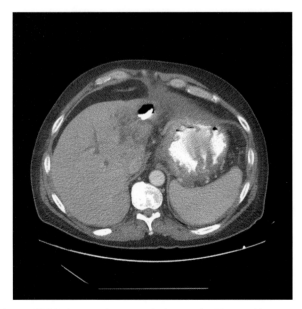

Figure 46.22 Computed tomography image of a 54-year-old man 4 weeks after successful single-step endoscopic ultrasound-guided pseudocyst gastrostomy. Visible in the anterior abdomen is a pocket of air with internal pigtails of the cyst gastrostomy stent. The pseudocyst has completely collapsed at this point.

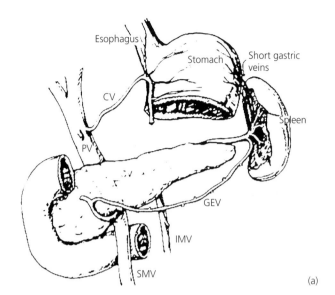

(a)

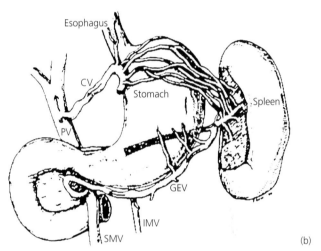

(b)

Figure 46.23 (a) Normal venous anatomy. The splenic vein is posterior to the pancreas. **(b)** Splenic venous thrombosis. Reversed direction of flow is shown (arrow). Left-sided portal hypertension leads to gastric varices and dilation of the short gastric veins, gastroepiploic vein (GEV), and coronary vein (CV). The portal vein (PV) is patent. IMV, inferior mesenteric vein; SMV, superior mesenteric vein.

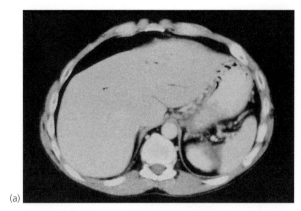

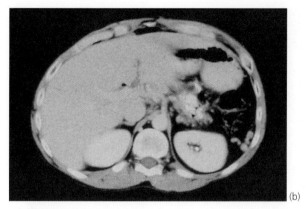

Figure 46.24 Computed tomographic scan shows splenic venous thrombosis. **(a)** Varices of short gastric veins next to the enlarged spleen. Varices are also present next to the lesser curve of the stomach. **(b)** Calcifications in the pancreas and varices (lower right corner).

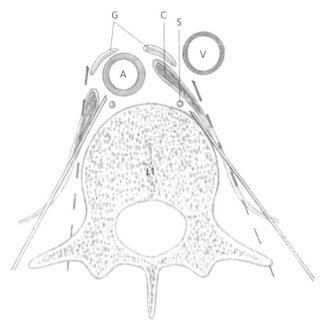

Figure 46.25 Diagram (transverse section) of needle position using classic and transcrural approaches to the celiac plexus. A, aorta; C, right diaphragmatic crus; G, celiac ganglia; L1, vertebral body of first lumbar vertebra (upper part); S, splanchnic nerve(s); V, vena cava.

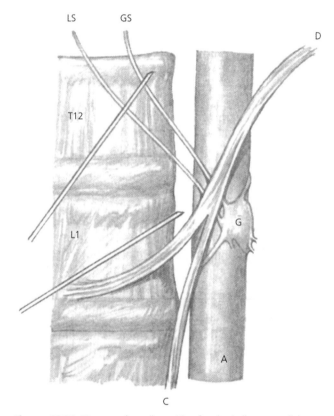

Figure 46.26 Diagram of needle position for classic (lower needle) celiac plexus block and splanchnic (upper needle) nerve block. A, aorta; C, right crus; D, diaphragma; G, celiac ganglia; GS, greater splanchnic nerve; L1, vertebral body of first lumbar vertebra; LS, lesser splanchnic nerve; T12, vertebral body of twelfth thoracic vertebra.

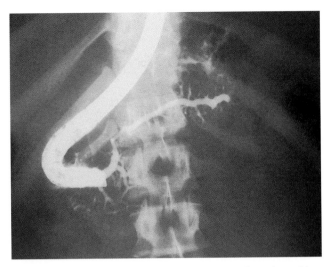

Figure 46.27 Endoscopic retrograde cholangiogram of a patient with chronic pancreatitis shows a stricture in the proximal pancreatic duct.

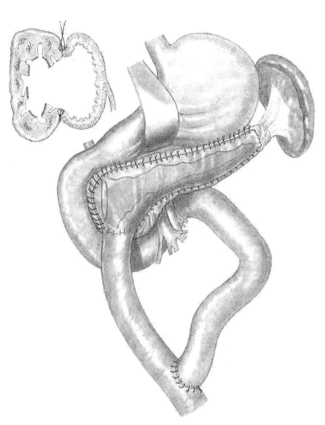

Figure 46.29 The lateral pancreaticojejunostomy is performed by anastomosing the jejunum to the anterior capsule of the pancreas. Nonabsorbable suture material is used to make this anastomosis. It can be carried out in a continuous or interrupted manner. The jejunojejunostomy is made approximately 40 cm distal to the pancreaticojejunostomy.

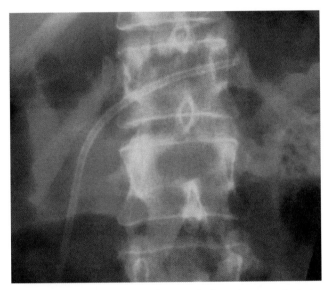

Figure 46.28 Endoscopic stent placement in the main pancreatic duct to facilitate pancreatic drainage.

47

Nonendocrine tumors of the pancreas

James J. Farrell, Howard A. Reber

Nonendocrine tumors of the pancreas include multiple pathological entities, such as ductal adenocarcinoma, mucinous cystadenoma, serous cystadenoma, intraductal papillary mucinous neoplasia (IPMN), solid and papillary epithelial neoplasms of the pancreas (SPENP), giant cell tumors, and acinar cell tumors. By far the most important of these, and the main focus of this chapter, is adenocarcinoma of the pancreas.

Adenocarcinoma of the pancreas

Adenocarcinoma of the pancreas is the fourth leading cause of cancer death in the United States, with approximately 31 000 new cases diagnosed each year. At diagnosis, the majority of patients have advanced disease, and only 15%–20% of patients are candidates for potentially curative surgical resection. The overall 5-year survival rate for pancreatic adenocarcinoma remains dismal at 3%. However, recent series demonstrate operative mortality rates less than 2% and 5-year survival rates after resection of 17%–20%. Patients whose tumors are resected with clean surgical margins and without microscopic nodal metastases have 5-year survival rates as high as 25%, and those with well-differentiated tumors may have a 5-year survival rate as high as 50%. These figures emphasize the important role of surgical resection as the only therapy with the potential to cure this aggressive disease.

Ductal adenocarcinoma makes up more than 90% of all malignant exocrine pancreatic tumors. Most of these neoplasms (67%) occur in the head of the gland, where they often obstruct the intrapancreatic portion of the common bile duct, as well as the pancreatic duct. More advanced tumors may invade or compress the duodenum, causing

bleeding or duodenal obstruction. Tumors of the head of the pancreas are usually at least 2 cm in diameter when they are first diagnosed, and most tumors that are resected have a median diameter of 2.5–3.5 cm. The rest occur in the body or tail, or diffusely throughout the pancreas. Because they are anatomically distant from the common bile duct, tumors of the body and tail produce fewer early symptoms and commonly are larger (5–7 cm) and more advanced when discovered. Advanced body and tail tumors may produce abdominal or back pain as a result of malignant infiltration of retroperitoneal structures and nerves. Although nearly all body and tail pancreatic adenocarcinomas are unresectable by the time of diagnosis, resectable body tumors have a similar prognosis to resectable head tumors.

Several notable pathological characteristics of pancreatic ductal adenocarcinomas deserve mention. These tumors are usually associated with an intense desmoplastic reaction, producing a rock-hard mass that is capable of compressing nearby structures. These tumors also demonstrate a unique tendency to aggressively infiltrate lymphatic and perineural spaces. By the time adenocarcinomas of the head of the pancreas are discovered, 70%–80% of them have metastasized to regional lymph nodes, which worsens the prognosis but does not preclude a cure.

Although distant metastases (e.g., to the lung) may occur, pancreatic cancer typically infiltrates locally into the adjacent structures, such as the stomach, duodenum, colon, transverse mesocolon, portal and superior mesenteric veins, or celiac or superior mesenteric arteries. The liver is the most common site of intraabdominal metastasis, and peritoneal seeding of the tumor can also occur. In patients without distant spread, vascular invasion by tumor is the most common reason for unresectability.

Patients with pancreatic cancer usually present with complaints such as weight loss, abdominal pain, back pain, and jaundice. The classical presentation of "painless" jaundice is actually uncommon. Pancreatic cancer can also manifest clinically as new-onset diabetes mellitus or, if pancreatic duct obstruction is present, as pancreatic exocrine insufficiency with malabsorption and steatorrhea. Light-colored

Atlas of Gastroenterology, 4th edition. Edited by Tadataka Yamada, David H. Alpers, Anthony N. Kalloo, Neil Kaplowitz, Chung Owyang, and Don W. Powell. © 2009 Blackwell Publishing, ISBN: 978-1-4051-6909-7

acholic stools are associated with biliary obstruction and are accompanied by jaundice and biliuria. Hepatomegaly, a palpable abdominal mass, or ascites usually reflect advanced unresectable disease. The classical Courvoisier gallbladder is actually palpable in only one-half of jaundiced patients with pancreatic cancer. Dermal lichenification or excoriation can be seen in those patients with intense pruritus associated with obstructive jaundice.

When the patient's history and physical examination suggest the diagnosis of pancreatic cancer, the workup should strive to achieve two main goals: to establish the diagnosis with a high degree of certainty (usually without a tissue diagnosis), and to determine if the patient is an appropriate candidate for surgical resection. The evaluation should be as cost and time efficient as possible to formulate an appropriate treatment plan. Transcutaneous ultrasound can be used to show large tumors and associated common bile or pancreatic duct dilation but usually provides limited information about resectability. The best overall test for the diagnosis and staging of pancreatic cancer is the dynamic helical contrast-enhanced computed tomographic (CT) scan of the abdomen. It provides extraordinary detail about the nature of the primary tumor, the adjacent vascular anatomy, and the presence of metastases (e.g., liver). Helical CT scans are better than conventional CT scans at both tumor detection and identification of metastatic disease. Pancreatic adenocarcinomas are seen on CT as hypodense, nonenhancing areas of the pancreas because they are less well perfused with blood compared with the surrounding normal parenchyma. An experienced gastrointestinal radiologist can accurately predict resectability from a helical CT scan in 80% of patients. However, the study has its greatest sensitivity in the assessment of masses at least 2 cm in diameter. For smaller lesions, or in patients with a negative or equivocal CT scan, endoscopic ultrasound (EUS) may be indicated.

Tumors as small as 1 cm can be demonstrated by EUS. Its sensitivity for tumor detection may be as high as 99% and it is also an accurate technique for local staging (70%). Other findings visible on EUS include a dilated common bile duct or a distended main pancreatic duct or side branch duct. For evaluating vascular involvement, EUS may be particularly useful; vascular involvement can manifest as abnormal vessel contour, loss of normal vessel-parenchymal interface, visible tumor within the vessel lumen, or nearby dilated peripancreatic venous collaterals. When tissue for diagnosis is desired, EUS allows for sampling of the tumor or nearby lymph nodes using fine-needle aspiration (EUS-FNA) with minimal morbidity (1%–2%). It is important to emphasize, however, that a negative FNA result never rules out the presence of malignancy.

With advances in other imaging techniques (e.g., CT, magnetic resonance imaging [MRI], EUS), endoscopic retrograde cholangiopancreatography (ERCP) is used less com-

monly for the diagnosis of pancreatic cancer. However, it does demonstrate certain typical abnormalities. The classical double-duct sign can be seen on ERCP when pancreatic cancer obstructs and dilates both the common bile and pancreatic ducts in the head of the pancreas. In tumors of the body or tail of the gland, the pancreatic duct may be narrowed or obstructed. The use of ERCP also enables the collection of cytology brushings from pancreatic or common bile ductal strictures, which prove the diagnosis of malignancy in 40%–60% of cases. The most valued use of ERCP is as a therapeutic modality. Intraductal stents can be placed to relieve biliary obstruction preoperatively, or as palliation in those patients who are not surgical candidates. For patients whose clinical presentation suggests pancreatic cancer (e.g., pain, jaundice, weight loss), and with a CT scan that demonstrates a mass in the head of the pancreas, ERCP is unnecessary. If a CT scan does not show a mass or raise questions about the diagnosis, ERCP or EUS examination should be performed, depending on the expertise available.

Additional techniques for the diagnosis and staging of pancreatic cancer include MRI with angiography (MRA) or cholangiopancreatography (MRCP), percutaneous transhepatic cholangiography (PTC), CT-guided FNA, and angiography. Excellent detail of the vascular and biliary anatomy can be seen using MRA and MRCP. For the patient with proximal common bile duct obstruction (e.g., Klatskin tumor), PTC is most useful, whereas ERCP is preferred for those with evidence of periampullary disease. Angiography has largely been replaced by helical CT and MRA, which provide high resolution vascular detail.

The only potentially curative therapy for pancreatic adenocarcinoma is surgical resection in patients with disease localized to the pancreas and adjacent lymph nodes, and without distant metastases or involvement of nearby vascular structures. Neither advanced age nor large tumor size are contraindications to resection. At specialized high-volume pancreatic surgery centers, perioperative mortality rates for pancreaticoduodenectomy have been lowered from about 20% two decades ago to the current level of less than 2%. For tumors of the head of the pancreas, Whipple resection with pylorus preservation provides adequate tumor extirpation and it has become the standard operation in most centers. Tumors of the body and tail of the pancreas require distal pancreatectomy and splenectomy.

Surgical resection begins with meticulous examination of the peritoneal cavity and its contents. Areas suspicious for metastatic disease are biopsied and sent for frozen-section analysis. In the absence of distant metastases, resectability usually depends on whether the tumor has invaded any major blood vessels. Assessment of vascular involvement requires mobilization of the tumor from surrounding structures. Involvement of the superior mesenteric, celiac, or hepatic arteries precludes resection. In most cases, so too does invasion of the superior mesenteric or portal vein. If the vessels appear to be free of tumor, the resection proceeds. It is unusual for vascular involvement to be found at the time of operation if it was not already suspected on the basis of helical CT or EUS examination performed preoperatively. It is more common (10%–15% of cases) to find small hepatic or peritoneal metastases that were not evident from the preoperative studies.

For this reason, some surgeons prefer to begin with operative laparoscopy, which permits examination of the liver and peritoneal surfaces and biopsy of any suspicious lesions. If metastatic tumor is found, laparotomy may be avoided. In some cases, palliative gastric and biliary bypasses may even be completed laparoscopically. Laparoscopy may also be appropriate for patients with a high likelihood of unresectability (unconfirmed by preoperative studies), for patients with body or tail masses (all of whom have a lower chance of having resectable disease), and for patients with pancreatic masses and ascites (likely the result of unrecognized peritoneal tumor implants). The major drawbacks of laparoscopy are the additional time and expense required for the procedure and the inability to determine the presence of vascular invasion. The latter often requires more extensive dissection and the tactile sensation only afforded by laparotomy.

Despite being undertaken only in those patients with apparently curable disease, resection of pancreatic cancer is not curative in the majority of cases, and postoperative 5-year survival is 17%–20%. However, there is evidence that survival is improved with the addition of adjuvant chemotherapy (European Study Group for Pancreatic Cancer 1 [ESPAC-l] Trial). Other factors that favorably affect prognosis include absence of lymph node involvement, clear surgical resection margins, small tumor size, and well-differentiated tumor grade. The prognosis for patients with unresectable disease remains poor, with median survival for only 6 months after diagnosis. For these patients, palliation is the main goal, and it can be achieved through surgical or nonsurgical means. Biliary bypass using choledochojejunostomy or cholecystojejunostomy effectively relieves jaundice, as do endoscopically placed bile duct stents. Duodenal obstruction occurs in the minority of patients, often as a near-terminal event. Surgical bypass (gastrojejunostomy) is the preferred therapy but endoscopically placed duodenal stents represent an alternative that may work well in some patients. Cholecystojejunostomy and gastrojejunostomy also can be performed laparoscopically, which minimizes postoperative morbidity. If a patient develops pancreatic exocrine insufficiency, enzyme replacement is useful to palliate steatorrhea and malabsorption. Palliative chemotherapy is also an option and gemcitabine, in particular, has been associated with decreased pain and improved quality of life in some patients. The most effective treatment of these patients requires carefully orchestrated efforts from a multidisciplinary team of surgeons, gastroenterologists, and oncologists.

Less common pancreatic neoplasms

Mucinous cystic neoplasms are large (often >5 cm), bulky, unilobular or multilobulated cysts containing mucin that comprise 1%–2% of exocrine pancreatic tumors. These tumors exhibit a marked female predominance (female–male ratio of 6:1) and have a peak age of occurrence between the fifth and seventh decades. The cysts are lined with a mucinous columnar epithelium that forms papillary projections, which may contain foci of dysplastic cells or invasive carcinoma. Radiographic studies reveal calcification within the cysts in about 10% of cases; calcification almost never occurs in pseudocysts. Mucinous cystadenomas are premalignant and should be resected. These tumors have a better prognosis than pancreatic adenocarcinoma; the 5-year survival probability after a curative resection of a mucinous cystadenocarcinoma is at least 50%.

Serous cystic neoplasms are typically large, encapsulated, multiloculated cystic tumors filled with watery fluid. They usually have a characteristic honeycomb appearance and the individual cysts are usually smaller than the individual cysts in mucinous cystic neoplasms. They account for about 1% of neoplastic pancreatic lesions and usually occur in elderly females in the sixth and seventh decades of life. These microcystic adenomas are usually asymptomatic and are often discovered incidentally on ultrasound examination or CT scans performed for another reason. Although uncommon, malignant transformation of serous lesions does occur, and these tumors should be resected if it can be accomplished safely. These fluid-filled neoplasms, as well as the mucinous cystic tumors just discussed, should not be confused with pseudocysts, which can be treated with internal or external drainage procedures.

SPENPs are rare neoplasms that are most common in adolescent girls and young women, usually occur in the pancreatic body or tail, can become large enough to produce vague abdominal discomfort, and have a characteristic appearance on CT scan. SPENPs have a favorable prognosis, and most patients are cured by resection. Nevertheless, some may recur locally, and liver metastasis has been reported.

IPMN is an increasingly recognized disease, often associated with repeated episodes of pancreatic inflammation. Intraductal tumor growth or secretion of mucus from these lesions can cause obstruction of the pancreatic duct and obstructive chronic pancreatitis. CT scans reveal a dilated pancreatic duct, and EUS can demonstrate dilated main and side branch pancreatic ducts. ERCP can confirm the ductal dilation as well as intraductal tumor and mucus, which appear as filling defects. A glob of mucus emanating from the gaping orifice of the papilla of Vater is characteristically seen at the time of ERCP. Approximately half the lesions show papillary malignant changes, but even these tumors have a better prognosis than the usual ductal adenocarcinoma. Surgical resection is required to remove any premalignant or malignant disease that may be present and also to relieve the episodes of pancreatitis. This may require total pancreatectomy because the entire pancreatic duct may be affected.

Other less common nonendocrine tumors of the pancreas include giant cell tumors, which are rare tumors characterized by bizarre giant and sarcomatoid cells supported by minimal fibrous tissue. Giant cell tumors have a poor prog-

nosis, even worse than ductal adenocarcinoma. Acinar cell carcinomas are uncommon and characterized by acinar arrangement of cells with little surrounding fibrous stroma. Zymogen granules are present and may be identified by electron microscopy. These tumors are most commonly seen in the elderly and they can be associated with elevated serum lipase levels, nonsuppurative panniculitis of the extremities and bone marrow, subcutaneous nodules, and polyarthritis.

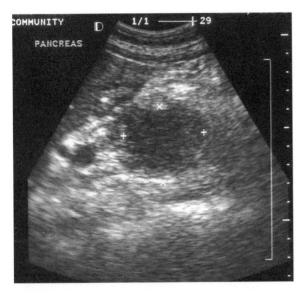

Figure 47.1 Transabdominal ultrasound in a patient showing a hypoechoic mass in the head of the pancreas.

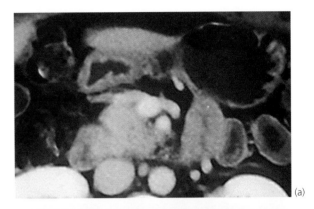

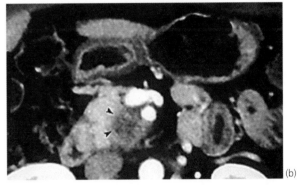

Figure 47.2 (a) On a conventional computed tomography (CT) scan, the primary tumor in the uncinate process of the pancreas is not seen. **(b)** The helical (spiral) CT scan performed 4 days later reveals the tumor (arrowheads). Courtesy of David Lu, UCLA Department of Radiology, Los Angeles.

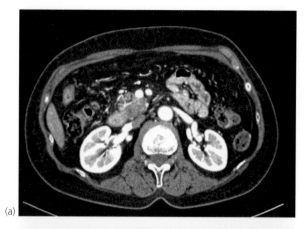

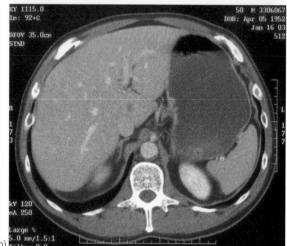

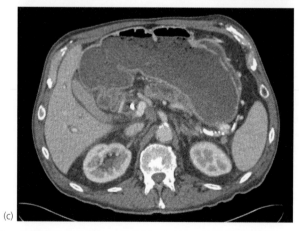

Figure 47.3 Computed tomography provides evidence of surgical unresectability. **(a)** Pancreatic head mass with superior mesenteric vein involvement. **(b)** Hypointense liver lesion suggestive of metastasis. **(c)** Celiac lymph node metastasis.

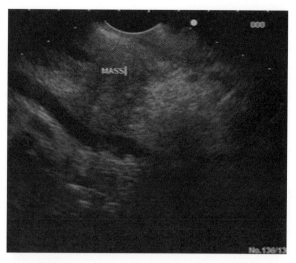

Figure 47.4 Endoscopic ultrasonogram showing a hypoechoic pancreatic head mass involving the portal vein

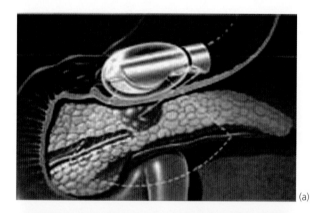

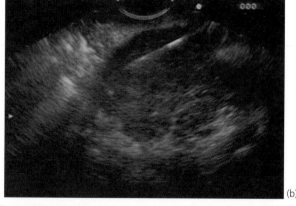

Figure 47.5 (a) Endoscopic ultrasound and fine-needle aspiration (FNA) demonstrating a linear echoendoscope biopsying the pancreas transgastrically. **(b)** Endoscopic ultrasound and FNA of a 2.5-cm localized hypoechoic mass in the head of the pancreas. The FNA needle is seen in the top right corner. Cytological analysis of the aspirated specimen revealed adenocarcinoma.

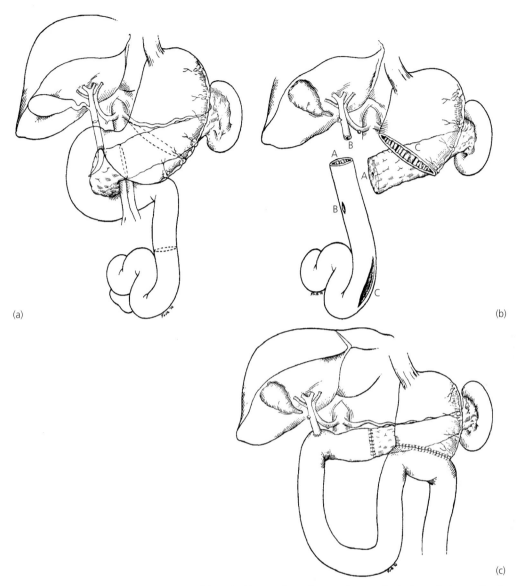

(a)

(b)

(c)

Figure 47.6 The standard Whipple pancreaticoduodenectomy. **(a)** Dashed lines indicate the resection margins in the typical operation for a tumor in the head of the pancreas. **(b)** The specimen has been resected. A, B, and C represent the sites for subsequent anastomoses between the bowel and the pancreas, bile duct, and stomach. **(c)** The completed anastomoses are shown.

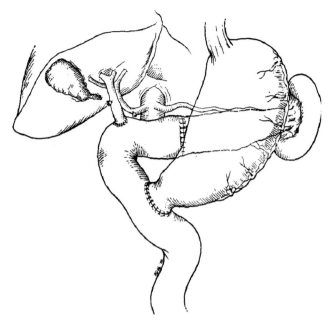

Figure 47.7 The pylorus-preserving modification of the standard Whipple pancreaticoduodenectomy is shown. The entire stomach, the pylorus, and several centimeters of the duodenum are retained.

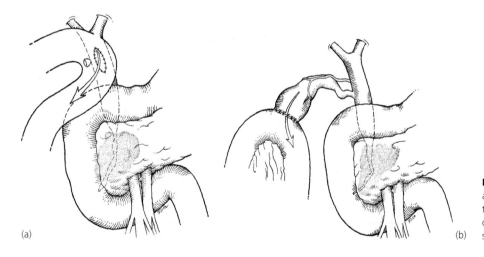

(a)

(b)

Figure 47.8 (a) Choledochojejunostomy and **(b)** Cholecystojejunostomy. Each of these operations effectively relieves biliary obstruction by diverting the bile into the small intestine proximal to the tumor.

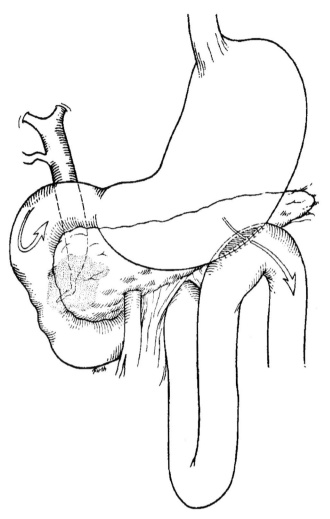

Figure 47.9 Gastrojejunostomy. The stomach can now empty into the small intestine directly when the tumor obstructs the duodenum.

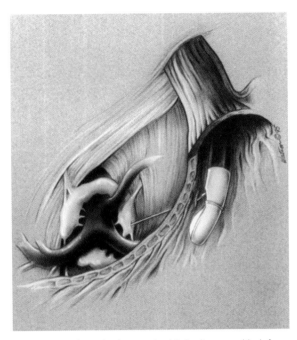

Figure 47.10 Endoscopic ultrasound-guided celiac nerve block for palliation of pain.

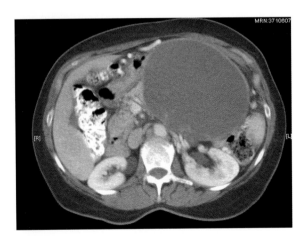

Figure 47.11 Computed tomography scan of a patient with a malignant mucinous cystadenocarcinoma, which was resected.

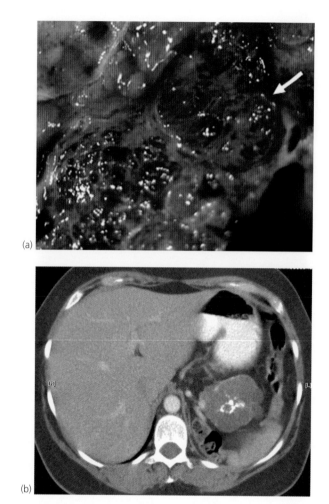

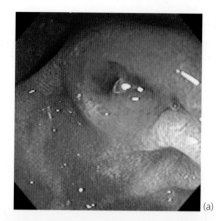

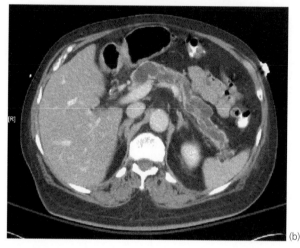

Figure 47.12 (a) Surgical resection of a serous cystadenoma with the honeycomb appearance. **(b)** Computed tomography scan of a patient with a benign serous cystadenoma with the characteristic central calcification.

Figure 47.13 Main-duct intraductal papillary mucinous neoplasm (IPMN). **(a)** Endoscopic image of mucin extruding from the ampulla in a main-duct IPMN. **(b)** Computed tomography imaging revealing a diffusely dilated main pancreatic duct in main-duct IPMN.

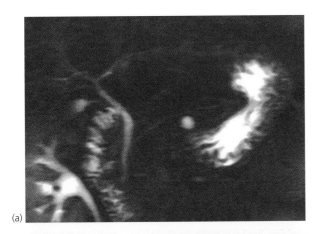

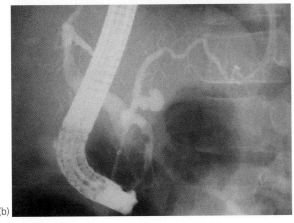

Figure 47.14 Branch duct intraductal papillary mucinous neoplasm.
(a) Magnetic resonance cholangiopancreatogram showing a normal
pancreatic duct with an associated pancreatic body cyst. **(b)** Endoscopic
retrograde cholangiopancreatogram showing a pancreatogram
that includes opacification of a side-branch cyst.

48

Endocrine neoplasms of the pancreas

Robert T. Jensen, Jeffrey A. Norton

Endocrine tumors of the pancreas are classified according to the type of clinical syndrome they cause. The seven generally accepted pancreatic endocrine tumor (PET) syndromes include gastrinoma that causes Zollinger–Ellison syndrome, insulinoma, glucagonoma, vasoactive intestinal peptide-secreting tumor (VIPoma) that causes the Verner–Morrison syndrome (also called pancreatic cholera or the WDHA syndrome [watery diarrhea, hypokalemia, and achlorhydria]), somatostatinoma, growth hormone releasing factor-secreting tumor (GRFoma), and nonfunctional tumors. Other syndromes that should be included in this category are adrenocorticotropic hormone-secreting tumors (ACTHomas) and PET-secreting factors that cause hypercalcemia (such as parathyroid hormone-related peptide [PTHrP]), PETs causing the carcinoid syndrome, PETs secreting renin (one case), and PETs secreting luteinizing hormone that causes masculinizing effects; these syndromes are much more uncommon and not as well characterized as the seven well-established PETs. Some have proposed that PETs secreting neurotensin (neurotensinomas), PETs secreting calcitonin, and PETs secreting ghrelin, a 28-amino-acid growth hormone secretogogue, also be included. At present there is no general agreement that these are distinct clinical syndromes and, therefore, are not included as a specific PET syndrome. In all cases, except nonfunctional tumors, the ectopic hormone release is associated with a distinct clinical syndrome. With nonfunctional tumors, the clinical symptoms and signs are entirely due to the presence of the tumor itself (e.g., hepatomegaly, weight loss, abdominal mass) and not to the ectopically released peptides. Not all nonfunctional tumors are truly nonfunctional in that many release pancreatic polypeptide-producing tumors (PPomas); some release neurotensin and almost all release chromogranin A. However, none of these secreted peptides is associated with specific clinical symptoms. All of these PETs share a number of common features, including various aspects of their natural history, pathology, medical treatment options, approaches to tumor localization, surgical options, and treatment options when the tumor is metastatic.

Even although these tumors are generally slow growing, recent studies show a subset demonstrate aggressive growth. Therefore, effective therapy requires both treatment of the effects of the ectopic hormone overproduction and treatment directed at the tumor itself. With each of these tumors, surgical resection is the treatment of choice. However, similar to carcinoids, liver metastases are already present in the majority of tumors at the time of diagnosis, except for insulinomas and gastrinomas. Almost all PETs, except insulinoma, possess high densities of somatostatin receptors. Their presence is now used for novel localization methods using radiolabeled somatostatin analogues (see section on tumor localization) and for treatment with somatostatin analogues. With each of the symptomatic PETs except for insulinomas, the long-acting somatostatin analogues, such as octreotide or lanreotide, are frequently used to control medically the clinical syndrome resulting from the ectopic hormone release. With this increased ability to control the symptoms caused by hormone overproduction, the prognosis will be increasingly determined in the future by the natural history of the tumor itself.

Clinical manifestations, pathogenesis, differential diagnosis, and diagnosis

Because these PET syndromes are uncommon, the proper diagnosis requires a continual awareness of the presenting manifestations of these tumor syndromes as well as an awareness that these syndromes can initially present with symptoms that are similar to other much more common conditions. In most patients, except those with nonfunctional tumors, the early symptoms are caused by the actions of the ectopically released hormone, whereas late in the course of the disease, symptoms owing to metastatic spread of the tumor itself (pain, bleeding, cachexia) may become increasingly important. The general approach to the

Atlas of Gastroenterology, 4th edition. Edited by Tadataka Yamada, David H. Alpers, Anthony N. Kalloo, Neil Kaplowitz, Chung Owyang, and Don W. Powell. © 2009 Blackwell Publishing, ISBN: 978-1-4051-6909-7

diagnosis and treatment of all PET syndromes except insulinomas is shown diagrammatically in Figure 48.1. In general, for these syndromes inappropriate hormonal hyperfunction, such as increased stool output, acid output, effects on blood glucose, and so on, needs to be demonstrated at the same time as an inappropriately elevated plasma hormone concentration is shown. After diagnosis it is important to establish whether the PET is occurring alone (sporadic tumor) or is part of an inherited disorder. The most common inherited disorder associated with PETs is multiple endocrine neoplasia-type 1 (MEN1) (nonfunctional > gastrinomas > insulinomas > GRFomas, VIPomas, and glucagonomas), but PETs can also occur with von Recklinghausen disease (duodenal somatostatinomas), von Hippel–Lindau syndrome (usually nonfunctional) and tuberous sclerosis. It is important to establish if an inherited syndrome is present because its presence affects the treatment approach and may determine the need for family studies. This should be followed by imaging studies to both localize the primary tumor and to assess the tumor extent (see Fig. 48.1). All of these investigations should be carried out preferably by a group with considerable experience with PETs because interpretation of these tests requires considerable expertise, and procedures such as sampling for hormone gradients, somatostatin receptor scintigraphy with SPECT imaging or intraoperative ultrasound are not frequently performed in many centers and their interpretation as well as performance may require considerable experience (see Fig. 48.1).

The approach and treatment of a patient with possible insulinoma is summarized in Figure 48.2. This is the typical approach when plasma insulin is measured by radioimmunoassay. Increasingly, plasma insulin is being measured in many centers by insulin-specific immunoradiometric assays (IRMAs) or immunochemoluminescent assays, which have no cross-reactivity with proinsulin and give lower values and can effect the approach (Fig. 48.2). The essential point in the diagnosis is to demonstrate hypoglycemia in the presence of an inappropriately elevated insulin or proinsulin level. Important tests used to differentiate a patient with hypoglycemia due to an insulinoma from a patient with hypoglycemia due to the surreptitious use of either insulin or sulfonylureas are shown in Table 48.1. With the availability of human insulin and its low antigenicity, the traditional method of demonstrating antiinsulin antibodies for the diagnosis of surreptitious use of insulin will not generally be useful, thus compounding the difficulty of this diagnostic problem. If suppressed plasma C-peptide levels can be established when the patient is hypoglycemic, this will add diagnostic verification (see Table 48.1). It is also important to remember that free C-peptide should be measured because proinsulin bound to antiinsulin antibodies may cause false elevations of the C-peptide level. After diagnosis, tumor localization (Fig. 48.2) is essential and is discussed in the following section.

In Figure 48.3 the approach to a patient suspected of having a VIPoma is outlined. Both patients with Zollinger–Ellison syndrome and VIPoma can present with secretory diarrhea. These two syndromes can be differentiated by measuring plasma VIP levels, which are normal in patients with gastrinomas and elevated in patients with VIPomas; by measuring gastrin, which is elevated in Zollinger–Ellison syndrome and normal to minimally elevated in patients with VIPomas; measuring gastric acid secretion, which is elevated in Zollinger–Ellison syndrome and normal to low in patients with VIPomas, or by measuring stool output during nasogastric aspiration or omeprazole treatment because increased stool output persists only in patients with VIPomas. In most series, more than 50% of all patients with VIPomas have metastatic, nonresectable disease at the time of diagnosis, and thus prolonged symptomatic treatment of the secretory diarrhea with a long-acting somatostatin analogue, such as octreotide or lanreotide, is required. If tumor progression occurs then treatment with chemotherapy, as outlined in Figure 48.4, may be required.

Tumor localization

As indicated in Figures 48.1–48.3, all patients with PET syndromes require imaging studies to assess both the extent of tumor and the possible location of the primary tumor. The best initial screening imaging test is somatostatin receptor scintigraphy (SRS) using ^{111}In-labeled octreotide (see Figs 48.1–48.3). Except in patients with insulinomas, the ability of SRS to localize these tumors is based on the fact that all PETs except insulinomas have a high density of somatostatin receptors. For all PETs except insulinomas, SRS has higher sensitivity than conventional imaging studies (CT scan, MRI, angiography, ultrasound) for detecting metastatic disease to the liver and for detecting distant metastases. SRS also allows screening of all body regions with one study and detects the primary tumor with greater sensitivity than other imaging methods. Because insulinomas frequently possess a low density of somatostatin receptors subtype 2 and 5, which are needed to bind radiolabeled octreotide with high affinity when SRS is performed, either CT or MRI scanning is recommended to detect liver metastases in the 5%–15% with malignant disease (see Fig. 48.2). Endoscopic ultrasound is recommended as the initial study to localize insulinomas because insulinomas are almost invariably intrapancreatic in location and are small (<1 cm). If endoscopic ultrasound is negative, selective intraarterial injection of calcium with hepatic venous sampling for insulin gradients is particularly helpful for regional localization of the tumor (see Fig. 48.2). Recent studies in Europe report that positron emission tomographic imaging with ^{11}C-5-hydroxytryptophan (^{11}C-5-HTP) or ^{68}Ga somatostatin analogues in patients with PETs may have greater sensitivity than SRS for both identifying the primary tumor and also for identifying metastatic sites in the liver and extrahepatically. These methods are under investigation in the United States but are not established or approved here.

In other PETs except insulinomas, for SRS to have maximal sensitivity it is essential that SPECT (single photon emission computed tomography) imaging be used to analyze the results. If extensive metastatic disease to the liver is present, the diagnosis should be confirmed by biopsy. If metastatic disease is not present on SRS and no primary tumor is seen, additional imaging studies should be undertaken (see Fig. 48.1). SRS only detects 50%–80% of primary PETs, primarily depending on their size. If SRS is negative, endoscopic ultrasound and angiography with determination of hormonal gradients after calcium (VIPoma, glucagonoma) or secretin (gastrinoma) should be performed to further localize the tumor.

A typical result determining an insulinoma's location by hormonal sampling is shown in Figure 48.4. In this patient a marked increase in insulin release occurs with injection of calcium into the gastroduodenal artery, supplying the head of the pancreas. Subsequently, an insulinoma was found in the pancreatic head. The ability of endoscopic ultrasound to localize a PET in a patient with the MEN1 syndrome is shown in Figure 48.5. In this patient, a 3.5-cm tumor was localized in the pancreatic body with two adjacent lymph nodes, each of which were subsequently removed at surgery. At surgery all patients should have intraoperative ultrasound performed because small lesions missed by palpation can be detected see (Figs 48.1–48.3).

Metastatic glucagonoma to the liver as well as metastatic disease with other PETs is frequently localized by CT scanning, especially if combined with intravenous contrast medium (Fig. 48.6). A number of recent studies show that PETs can also be detected by MRI; results from a patient with primary VIPoma in the pancreatic tail are shown in Figures 48.7 and 48.8, and from a patient with metastatic glucagonoma of the liver in Figure 48.9. With MRI, variations of the magnetic field and imaging sequence allow the same tumor to appear dark on one scan (T1 weighted) and bright (T2 weighted) on another scan sequence (Figs 48.7–48.9). MRI scans have the additional advantage that no ionizing radiation is involved. Glucagonomas are hypervascular tumors, as are other PETs, and are well seen on angiography, as is demonstrated in Figure 48.10 for a patient with metastatic glucagonoma of the liver. In some cases, small metastases in the liver and small primary tumors can be seen on angiography when SRS is negative; therefore, it is recommended by some that angiography should be performed on a patient with a PET with a negative SRS, prior to surgery (see Figs 48.1–48.3).

SRS is particularly sensitive for detecting hepatic metastases and, in one recent comparative study, it was equal in sensitivity to all conventional imaging studies combined (ultrasound, CT scan, MRI, selective angiography). Figure 48.11 demonstrates greater sensitivity with SRS than MRI in a patient with a metastatic PET to the liver with a serum chromogranin A level of 5200 ng/mL (nl < 50). An additional left lobe liver metastasis is seen on the SRS that is not seen on the MRI. Increasingly, bone metastases are being diagnosed late in the disease course in patients with malignant PETs and their detection is essential for determining appropriate therapy. For detection of bone metastases, SRS is superior to bone scanning and has the advantage over MRI that distant metastases to ribs and nonspinous areas can easily be detected and, therefore, is the recommended method. Figure 48.12 shows results of these three methods and the greater sensitivity of somatostatin receptor scintigraphy for detecting bone metastases in a patient with a malignant PET releasing ACTH and causing Cushing syndrome.

In Figure 48.13 the increased sensitivity of positron emission tomography over SRS or conventional imaging (CT scan) is shown in a patient with a malignant PET with ultrasound-proven liver metastases, but with an unknown primary tumor location. Both the CT (top panel) and the SRS (middle panel) images show the liver metastases, but the location of the primary tumor is not seen on the CT and is suggested in the pancreatic area on the SRS. The positron emission tomographic scan after administration of ^{11}C-5-hydroxytryptophan clearly shows both a pancreatic tail tumor and the presence of liver metastases. Although not generally available at present in the United States, a number of studies from Europe have demonstrated the increased sensitivity of positron emission tomography using ^{11}C-5-HTP or ^{68}Ga-labeled somatostatin analogues.

In Figure 38.14 the approach to a patient with a metastatic PET syndrome is outlined. Whereas in patients with insulinoma only 5%–15% of the tumors are found to be malignant, in older studies more than 50% of patients with the other PETs had metastatic disease at the time of diagnosis. In a small percentage of cases (<5%–20%), it may be possible to resect the tumor either because it is localized to regional lymph nodes or to only one lobe of the liver. It has been recommended that surgical resection should be considered in these cases (see Fig. 48.14). However, in the majority of cases the tumor is not resectable, and in these cases, if the tumor is functional, a long-acting somatostatin analogue such as lanreotide or octreotide should be used to control the symptoms (see Fig. 48.14). Progressive disease occurs in >60% of patients with liver metastases. Among patients with symptomatic tumors, chemotherapy with dacarbazine (DTIC) should be considered to treat patients with malignant glucagonoma, and streptozotocin and doxorubicin should be considered for patients with other PETs. Recent studies show that treatment with long-acting somatostatin analogues, either alone or in combination with α-interferon, may not only control the hormone excess state but also decrease tumor growth rate. At present, it is not established that the direct antitumor growth effects of somatostatin analogues or interferon increase survival rates, although this is being investigated in a number of large trials. Chemoembolization of a symptomatic tumor may also help control symptoms (see Fig. 38.14). More than 80% of patients with nonfunctional tumors at presentation have metastatic disease to the liver. If progression occurs or symptoms develop because of the tumor itself, treatment with somatostatin analogues (±α-interferon) or chemother-

apy with streptozotocin and doxorubicin is recommended by various groups. Recent studies from Europe demonstrate that treatment of advanced metastatic PETs with radiolabeled somatostatin analogues ([111]indium, [90]yttrium, [177]lutetium) can result in tumor shrinkage as well as stabilization in progressive cases. This treatment is being investigated now in a number of centers. At present, this form of treatment is not approved in the United States and therefore is not listed on the figure as an option generally available.

Table 48.1 Results of laboratory tests used to distinguish factitious hypoglycemia from hypoglycemia caused by insulinoma

Laboratory test	Insulin	Sulfonylureas	Insulinoma
Plasma insulin	Normal or elevated	Normal or elevated	Normal or elevated
Plasma proinsulin	Normal or decreased	Normal	Increased >85%
Plasma C-peptide	Decreased	Normal or elevated	Normal or elevated
Plasma antibodies to insulin	Present	Not present	Not present
Plasma or urine sulfonylureas detected	Not present	Present	Not present

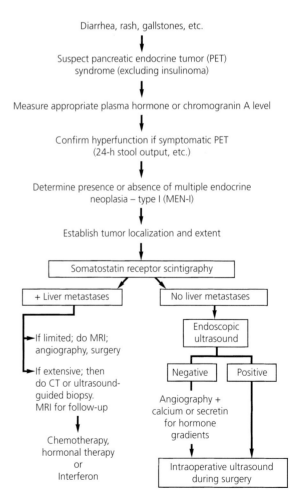

Figure 48.1 The general approach to diagnosis and treatment of all pancreatic endocrine tumor (PET) syndromes except insulinomas. Insulinomas are considered separately because they differ from all of the other PETs in frequency being missed (30%–50%) with somatostatin receptor scintigraphy (SRS) and being primarily nonmalignant (>90% are benign). SRS is shown to be the initial localization study because it is the most sensitive and allows imaging of the entire body. Other imaging studies detect few patients with liver metastases if the SRS is negative; however, endoscopic ultrasound or angiography with venous sampling for hormonal gradients can detect primary tumors in >20% of patients not seen on SRS. Recent studies show that positron emission tomographic imaging, with ^{11}C-5-hydroxytryptophan or ^{68}Ga somatostatin analogues, may have greater sensitivity than SRS but is not available in the United States (see Fig. 48.13). CT, computed tomography; MRI, magnetic resonance imaging.

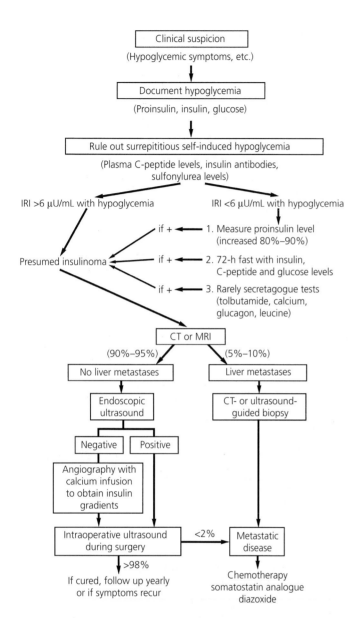

Figure 48.2 Algorithm for the diagnosis and treatment of a patient with insulinoma. After documentation of the hypoglycemia, it is important to rule out self-induced hypoglycemia either owing to surreptitious use of insulin or sulfonylureas. If plasma insulin-like immunoreactivity (IRI) assessed by radioimmunoassay exceeds 6 µU/mL and hypoglycemia is present, the proinsulin level is elevated and a presumed diagnosis of insulinoma can be made. The diagnosis is generally confirmed by a 72-h fast performed under supervised conditions with regular assessment of blood glucose, insulin, proinsulin and C-peptide. Secretagogue provocative tests (tolbutamide, calcium, glucagon, or leucine) are rarely needed. Insulinomas are usually benign (90%–95% of cases) and the malignant cases can be detected by computed tomography (CT) or magnetic resonance imaging (MRI) for liver metastases. Endoscopic ultrasound is more sensitive than other imaging studies, detecting insulinomas in 80%–95% of cases. If endoscopic ultrasound does not localize the insulinoma, selective intraarterial injection of calcium with sampling of hepatic veins for insulin concentrations should be done to localize the insulinoma to the appropriate pancreatic area. Intraoperative ultrasound should be routinely used during surgery. Many centers are increasing the use of insulin-specific assays, which result in lower insulin levels, such that as many as 30%–60% of patients with insulinomas have plasma insulin levels of <6 µU/mL during a fast. Using insulin, proinsulin, and C-peptide specific assays, the most sensitive criterion (100%) for diagnosis of insulinoma is an elevated proinsulin when the glucose is <45 mg%. Vezzosi, D. Europ J Endocrinol 2007;157:75.

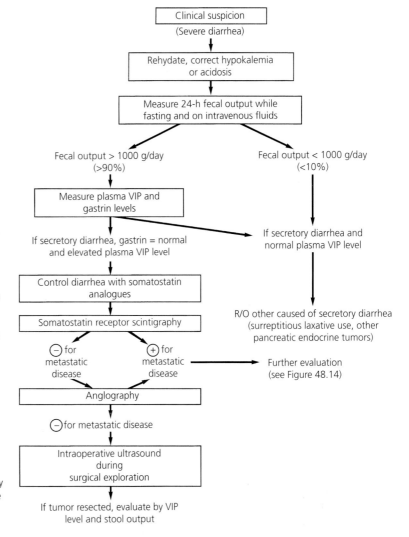

Figure 48.3 Algorithm summarizing the approach and treatment of a patient with suspected VIPoma syndrome. It is important to measure 24-h fecal output while keeping the patient completely fasted and rehydrated after correction of electrolyte or acid–base imbalance by intravenous fluids. Greater than 80% of patients with VIPomas have ≥3000 g/day of stool output, and it has been reported that no patients with VIPoma have daily stool output <700 g/day. Angiography is recommended if somatostatin receptor scintigraphy (SRS) is negative prior to surgery because it can detect small liver metastases not seen on SRS. Intraoperative ultrasound should be used because recent studies with other pancreatic endocrine tumors demonstrate that some small tumors are only localized with this procedure. If metastatic disease is present and nonresectable, or if no tumor is found, postoperative treatment with long-acting somatostatin analogues (octreotide, lanreotide) should be continued, adjusting the dosage to control symptoms. If metastatic disease is present and there is progressive disease, or symptoms are not controlled with octreotide, chemotherapy should be considered, as outlined in Figure 48.14. R/O, rule out; VIP, vasoactive intestinal peptide; VIPoma, vasoactive intestinal peptide-secreting tumor.

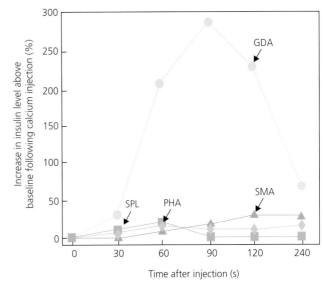

Figure 48.4 Localization of an insulinoma by selective intraarterial injection of calcium with hepatic venous insulin sampling. Calcium (0.025 mEq Ca/kg normally, or 0.01 mEq Ca/kg in obese patients) was injected selectively into the gastroduodenal artery (GDA), superior mesenteric artery (SMA), splenic artery (SPL), or proper hepatic artery (PHA) and hepatic venous blood was sampled for insulin concentration prior to injection and 30, 60, 90, 120, and 210 s post injection. A 275% increase over the preinjection value was seen with the gastroduodenal artery injection, which is consistent with a 0.9-cm insulinoma located in the pancreatic head area at surgery.

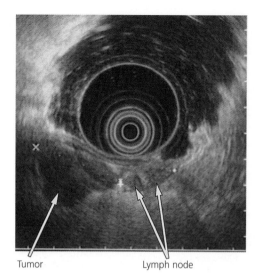

Tumor   Lymph node

Figure 48.5 Endoscopic ultrasound image in a patient with multiple endocrine neoplasia type 1 (MEN1). A 3-cm tumor was found in the pancreatic body (labeled tumor) and two adjacent enlarged lymph nodes. At surgery a 3.5-cm pancreatic endocrine tumor with two lymph nodes containing metastases were found.

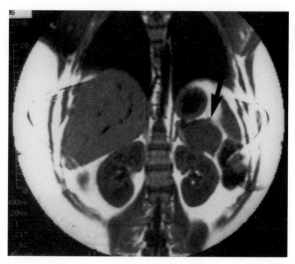

Figure 48.7 Magnetic resonance imaging scan of a patient with a large 5-cm VIPoma located in the tail of the pancreas (arrow). This scan represents a sagittal view of a T1-weighted sequence. The tumor is posterior to the stomach, medial to the spleen, and anterior to the kidney. The tumor appears dark on a T1-weighted sequence.

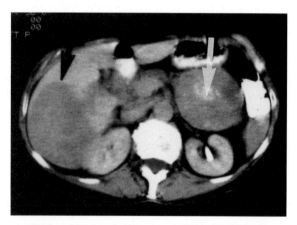

Figure 48.6 Computed tomogram in a patient with metastatic glucagonoma obtained with both intravenous and oral contrast media. This patient had a 7-cm glucagonoma in the pancreatic tail (white arrow) and a large 10-cm metastatic deposit in the right lobe of the liver (black arrow).

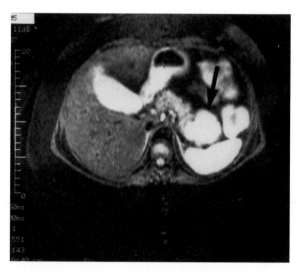

Figure 48.8 Cross-sectional magnetic resonance image of a patient with a VIPoma. This is the same patient seen in Figure 48.7. The tumor is a large VIPoma (arrow) located in the tail of the pancreas. The tumor appears bright (white) on this T2-weighted short inversion time inversion recovery (STIR) sequence and is easier to see than on the T1-weighted STIR image (Fig. 48.7). The gallbladder, stomach, spleen, and colon also appear bright.

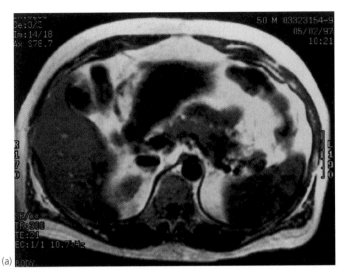 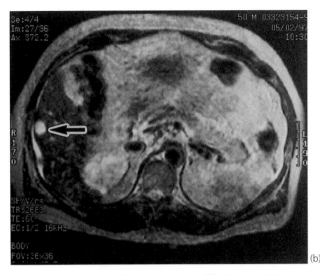

(a)   (b)

Figure 48.9 Magnetic resonance imaging scan of a patient with metastatic glucagonoma of the liver. **(a)** T1-weighted image. **(b)** T2-weighted image. The metastasis is shown by the arrow. This case demonstrates that pancreatic endocrine tumor liver metastases are much better seen on the T2-weighted image.

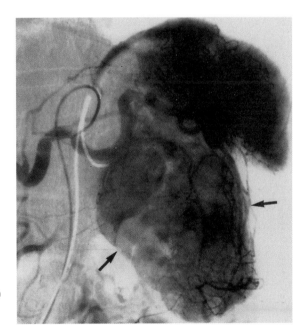

Figure 48.10 Selective abdominal angiogram in a patient with metastatic glucagonoma demonstrating the primary glucagonoma. The splenic artery injection demonstrates a large 8-cm hypervascular primary tumor in the tail of the pancreas (arrows) next to the spleen. This is the same patient as shown in Figure 48.6.

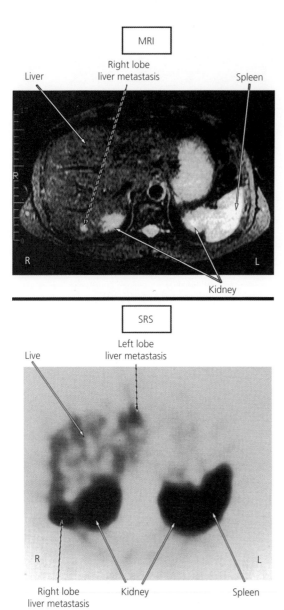

Figure 48.11 An example of the greater sensitivity of somatostatin receptor scintigraphy (SRS) than magnetic resonance imaging (MRI) for identifying bilateral liver metastases in a patient with a malignant pancreatic endocrine tumor metastatic to the liver. The top panel is an MRI image showing one metastasis in the right lobe of the liver. No left lobe metastases were observed. The bottom panel is a single photon emission computed tomography image of the SRS showing a left lobe liver metastasis and a right lobe liver metastasis. L, left; R, right.

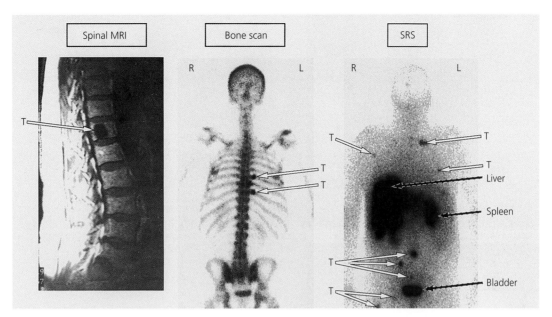

Figure 48.12 Detection of bone metastases in a patient with a malignant pancreatic endocrine tumor secreting adrenocorticotrophic hormone and with liver metastases. The magnetic resonance image (MRI) **(left)** shows a single metastasis (T) in a thoracic vertebral body. The bone scan **(middle)** shows two new left rib metastases, whereas the somatostatin receptor scintigraphy (SRS) **(right)** shows new metastases to the left and right ribs, left scapula, thoracic and lumbar spine, right sacroiliac joint, and right femoral head. The extensive liver metastases are also seen on the SRS. Recent studies demonstrate the SRS is the best overall method to detect bone metastases in malignant pancreatic endocrine tumors.

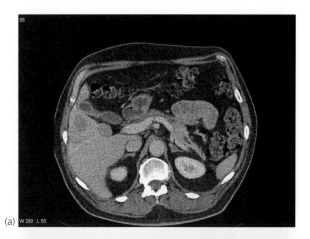

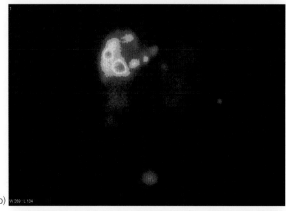

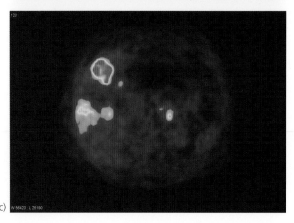

Figure 48.13 Increased sensitivity of positron emission tomography **(c)** compared with computed tomography (CT) **(a)** and somatostatin receptor scintigraphy (SRS) **(b)** in a patient with a malignant pancreatic endocrine tumor (PET). The CT image (a) of a patient with malignant PET shows liver metastases but no primary tumor. The SRS (anterior view) (b) confirms the liver metastases and raises the question of a possible pancreatic primary tumor. Positron emission tomographic scanning after administration of ^{11}C-5-hydroxytryptophan (c) clearly shows both a pancreatic tail tumor and the liver metastases. Images courtesy of Prof. Anders Sundin, Department of Radiology, Uppsala University Hospital, Uppsala, Sweden.

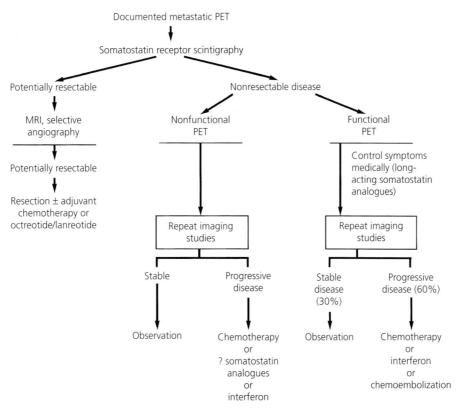

Figure 48.14 Algorithm of the treatment of a patient with a metastatic pancreatic endocrine tumor (PET). For all PETs, except metastatic insulinoma, recent studies demonstrate somatostatin receptor scintigraphy (SRS) should be the initial tumor localization method because of its greater sensitivity and ability to give a complete body scan. If surgical resection is feasible without a high morbidity, this should be considered by a surgeon who is experienced in the surgical treatment of such tumors. Additional imaging with magnetic resonance imaging (MRI) and selective angiography are helpful in better defining the location of the liver metastases and detecting possible small lesions not seen on the SRS. If the tumor is not resectable in a patient with a functioning pancreatic endocrine tumor, symptoms should be controlled with a long-acting somatostatin analogue (octreotide or lanreotide). If symptoms are not controlled or there is progressive disease, chemotherapy, interferon, or chemoembolization should be considered. Dacarbazine is recommended for patients with metastatic glucagonomas and streptozotocin or chlorozotocin with fluorouracil is advised for patients with the other functional pancreatic endocrine tumor syndromes or with nonfunctional tumors. Treatment of advanced PETs with radiolabeled somatostatin analogues ([111]indium, [90]yttrium, [177]lutetium) is being investigated in a number of centers and shows promising results. At present, this form of treatment is not approved in the United States and therefore is not listed on the figure as an option generally available.

49

Hereditary diseases of the pancreas

Carlos G. Micames, Jonathan A. Cohn

Cystic fibrosis (CF) is the most common inherited disease of the exocrine pancreas. It is an autosomal recessive disease caused by loss-of-function mutations of the CF gene. Typical features of CF include lung disease, pancreatic insufficiency, male infertility and excessive salt secretion by the sweat glands. The CF gene encodes the CF transmembrane conductance regulator (CFTR), a protein which functions as a cyclic adenosine monophosphate (cAMP)-dependent anion channel and as an ion transport regulator in many epithelial tissues.

The molecular pathogenesis of CF can be understood using the CFTR structural model shown in Figure 49.1. The CFTR occurs at the luminal surface of the polarized epithelial cells that line many gastrointestinal tissues. In the pancreas and liver, CFTRs occur at the apical plasma membrane of duct cells (Fig. 49.2). During normal pancreatic secretion, CFTRs contribute to the secretion of fluid and bicarbonate by duct cells (Fig. 49.3).

Early features of CF pancreatic disease include blockage of the smaller ducts with eosinophilic plugs owing to insufficient dilution and alkalinization of the pancreatic juice. Pancreatic insufficiency occurs in approximately 85% of CF individuals and is usually recognized by one year of age. The CF pancreas is typically atrophic with prominent lobulation and progressive cystic changes, fibrosis, and fatty replacement (Fig. 49.4). Similar changes occur at the microscopic level in patients with CF who have pancreatic insufficiency (Fig. 49.5).

Other gastrointestinal organs are also greatly affected by CF. In the liver, steatosis is common and 2%–5% of individuals develop multilobular biliary cirrhosis (Fig. 49.6). In the intestine, meconium ileus and distal intestinal obstruction syndrome (DIOS) are distinctive clinical presentations

seen in patients with CF. In both conditions, the terminal ileum is blocked by impacted mucofecal material. The typical CT findings of DIOS are shown in Fig. 49.7. In patients with CF who do not have overt intestinal obstruction, the ileal mucosa is often partially coated with concretions consisting of inspissated mucofecal material (Fig. 49.8).

Most mortality and morbidity of patients with CF is due to lung disease. Aggressive nutritional support is important for delaying the progression of lung disease in patients with CF. Many individuals with CF are malnourished and poor pulmonary function correlates closely with having a low body mass index (BMI) (Fig. 49.9). It is difficult to achieve target BMI values in most individuals with CF. Clinical management usually includes pancreatic enzyme replacement therapy, a high-fat (high-calorie) diet, and vitamin supplements formulated specifically for individuals with CF.

A second common inherited disease of the exocrine pancreas is hereditary pancreatitis (HP). This is an autosomal dominant disease caused by mutations of the PRSS1 gene. This gene encodes cationic trypsinogen, the principal trypsin proenzyme in human pancreatic juice. The most common HP-causing mutation is R122H. The molecular pathogenesis of HP due to this PRSS1 mutation can be understood using the trypsinogen structural model shown in Fig. 49.10. The CT findings in HP resemble those of other forms of chronic pancreatitis (Fig. 49.11). As HP causes recurrent and progressive pancreatic injury, it gradually leads to pancreatic exocrine insufficiency, diabetes mellitus, and pancreatic cancer over a period of decades (Fig. 49.12).

Other inherited diseases of the exocrine pancreas are rare. Among these, the most common is Shwachman–Diamond syndrome (SDS), an autosomal recessive condition caused by mutations of the SBDS gene. Patients with SDS usually develop pancreatic insufficiency by the age of one year. Common additional findings include neutropenia, and growth or skeletal abnormalities. Pancreatic insufficiency in SDS results from defective development of the pancreatic acini. Typical histopathological features in the pancreas include fatty replacement of the acini with relative sparing of the pancreatic ducts and islets (Fig. 49.13).

Atlas of Gastroenterology, 4th edition. Edited by Tadataka Yamada, David H. Alpers, Anthony N. Kalloo, Neil Kaplowitz, Chung Owyang, and Don W. Powell. © 2009 Blackwell Publishing, ISBN: 978-1-4051-6909-7

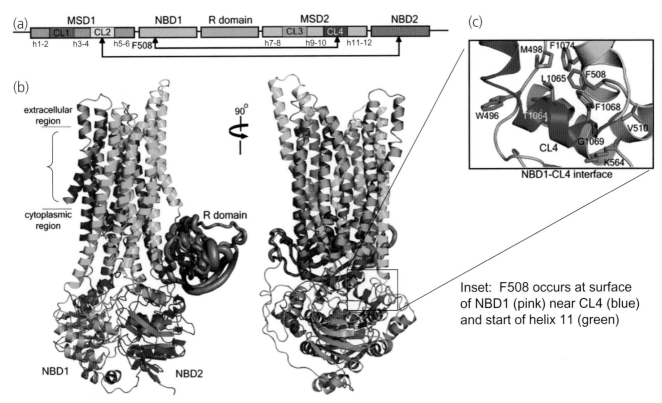

Figure 49.1 A proposed structure for cystic fibrosis transmembrane conductance regulator (CFTR). This model builds on the crystal structures of one cytoplasmic domain (NBD1) of CFTR and of a bacterial transporter related to CFTR (Sav1866). **(a)** CFTR contains two membrane spanning domains (MSD1 and MSD2 in dark and light green), two nucleotide binding domains (NBD1 and NBD2 in light and dark pink), and a regulatory domain (R domain, in gray). Each MSD contains six transmembrane helices (h1–h6, h7–h12) and two cytoplasmic loops (CL1–2, CL3–4). Together, the 12 helices (h1–h12) surround an aqueous pore which forms a channel through the lipid bilayer and allows anions to passively flow through the cell membrane. Channel gating is controlled by the impact of nucleotides and cAMP-dependent signaling on the cytoplasmic NBD1, NBD2, and R domains. **(b)** This model highlights how cytoplasmic regulatory events are thought to control the structure and ion channel function of the MSD domains through NBD/CL interactions. The most common CF-causing *CFTR* mutation results in deletion of the phenylalanine normally in position 508 in the NBD1 domain of CFTR (delta F508). CFTR molecules with this mutation misfold and exhibit reduced function because of defective intracellular trafficking, instability at the cell surface, and defective ion channel gating. Based on crystallography data for NBD1 and on modeling studies for full-length CFTR, F508 occurs on the surface of NBD1 in a region where NBD1 normally interacts with the CL4 loop near the base of helix 11 **(c)**. This region contains a hydrophobic pocket where F508 probably interacts with L1065, F1068, and F1074 in CL4. Even though the deletion of F508 has little impact on the intrinsic structure of NBD1 (comparing crystal structures for the mutant and normal forms of NBD1), this mutation may cause misfolding and malfunction of full-length CFTR by disrupting the NBD1/CL4 interface. Adapted from Serohijos AW, Hegedus T, Aleksandrov AA, et al. Phenylalanine-508 mediates a cytoplasmic-membrane domain contact in the CFTR 3D structure crucial to assembly and channel function.

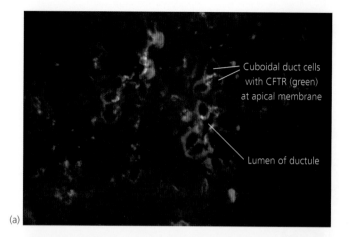

Cuboidal duct cells
with CFTR (green)
at apical membrane

Lumen of ductule

(a)

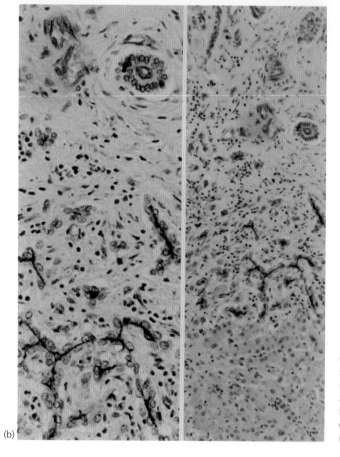

(b)

Figure 49.2 Localization of cystic fibrosis transmembrane conductance regulator (CFTR) protein in human pancreas and liver.
(a) Double-label immuofluorescence staining of CFTR (green) and of the sodium/potassium ATPase (orange) in human pancreas. Small pancreatic ducts are surrounded by cuboidal epithelial cells which express CFTR at the apical plasma membrane and the sodium–potassium ATPase at the basolateral plasma membrane. **(b)** Immunoperoxidase staining of CFTR (brown signal) in human liver. CFTR occurs on the lumenal surface of intrahepatic bile ducts.

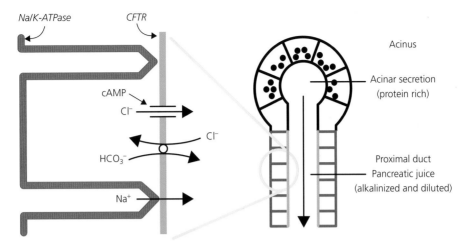

Figure 49.3 Proposed role of cystic fibrosis transmembrane conductance regulator (CFTR) during pancreatic exocrine secretion. As pancreatic juice flows through the intralobular duct, the protein-rich acinar secretions are diluted and alkalinized by the duct epithelial cells. CFTR functions at the apical plasma membrane of these cells to promote the cAMP-mediated secretion of fluid at bicarbonate into the lumen.

When CFTR function at this site is reduced (e.g., in CF), inadequate dilution and alkalinization of the pancreatic juice may promote the formation of protein plugs (possibly by affecting solubility or viscosity) and thereby contribute to the ductal obstruction and progressive pancreatic insufficiency that occur in CF.

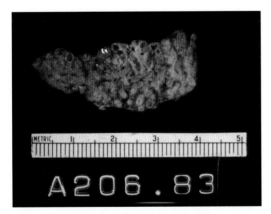

Figure 49.4 A pathological specimen of pancreas from a patient with cystic fibrosis with severe pancreatic insufficiency. This atrophic gland is fibrotic and shows prominent lobulation with cystic changes. Courtesy of Dr Peter Durie, Hospital for Sick Children, Toronto.

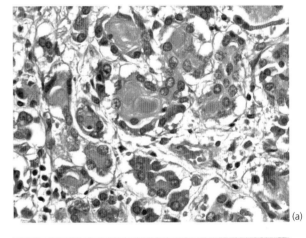

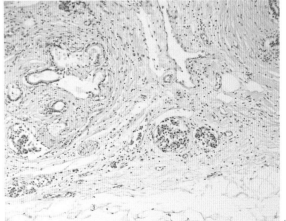

Figure 49.5 Photomicrographs of the pancreas from patients with cystic fibrosis. **(a)** Early findings include acinar atrophy and ductular plugging with insipissated eosinophilic concretions. Courtesy of Dr David Myerholz and Dr Marcus Nashelsky, University of Iowa Medical Center. **(b)** Typical pancreatic findings with exocrine insufficiency include prominent fibrosis and fatty infiltration with relative preservation of the islets. Courtesy of Dr Alan Proia, Duke University Medical Center.

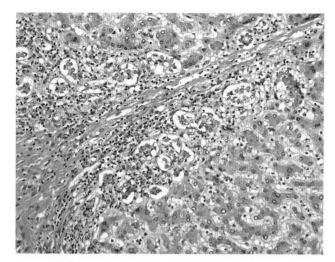

Figure 49.6 Photomicrographs of the liver from patients with cystic fibrosis showing focal biliary cirrhosis. Typical findings include focal portal and periportal fibrosis, ductular proliferation and periductular inflammation. Steatosis and ductal plugging also are common. Courtesy of Dr David Meyerholz and Dr Marcus Nashelsky.

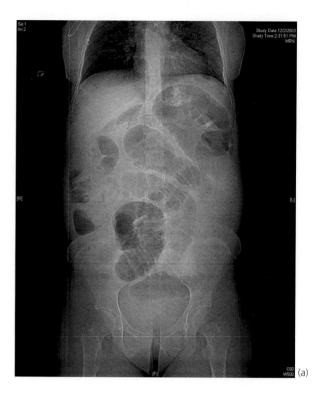

(a)

Distended small bowel with thickened bowel wall and fecal material containing small gas bubbles

Terminal ileum containing solid stool

Colon containing contrast; the lumen is not distended and the bowel wall thickness is normal

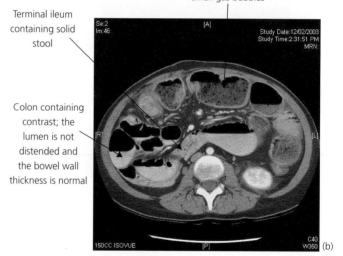

(b)

Figure 49.7 (a) Abdominal imaging of an adult with cystic fibrosis with distal intestinal obstruction syndrome. **(b)** The terminal ileum is filled with solid stool. Proximal to this obstruction, the small bowel is distended (note thickened bowel wall and gas bubbles in fecal material). Distal to the transition point, the colon contains contrast and is not distended.

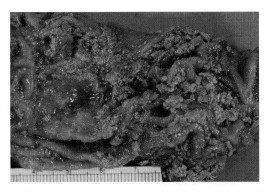

Figure 49.8 A pathological specimen of ileum from an adult with cystic fibrosis (CF) who had severe CF lung disease but who did not have overt intestinal disease. Much of the mucosal surface is covered with concretions consisting of inspissate mucofecal material. Courtesy of Dr Peter Durie.

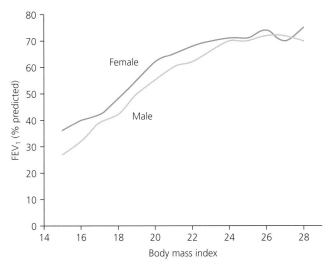

Figure 49.9 Relationship between nutritional status and lung function in adults with cystic fibrosis (CF). For patients with CF at age 20–40 years, lung function drops sharply as the body mass index falls below 22. Data like this provide the rationale for providing patients with CF with aggressive nutritional support. FEV$_1$, forced expiratory volume in 1 s.

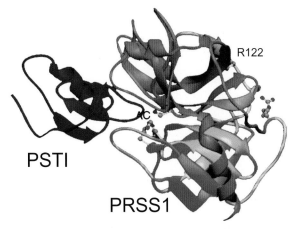

Figure 49.10 The structure of cationic trypsinogen (PRSS1) and of pancreatic secretory trypsin inhibitor (PSTI). PSTI blocks tryptic proteolysis by binding to the catalytic site of trypsinogen (AC), as shown. Mutations of the *PRSS1* and *PSTI* genes can each lead to hereditary forms of pancreatitis. The most common cause of hereditary pancreatitis is the *PRSS1* R122H mutation. R122 occurs at the trypsinogen surface as shown. If active trypsin accumulates in the pancreatic parenchyma, this potentially could cause an uncontrolled proteolytic chain reaction because additional activated trypsin can be produced by the action of trypsin on trypsinogen. To prevent this, trypsinogen normally contains an inactivating cleavage site at an accessible site on its surface (R122). Once trypsinogen is digested at R122 (e.g., by trypsin), trypsinogen can no longer be activated. In hereditary pancreatitis, the R122H mutation prevents digestion of trypsinogen at R122 and this allows active trypsin to accumulate in an uncontrolled manner. Thus, excessive activation of trypsin is thought to be the primary event causing pancreatic injury in many patients with hereditary pancreatitis.

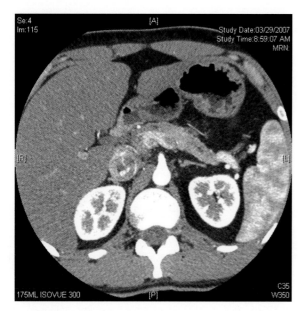

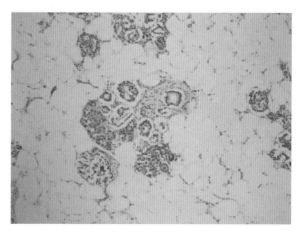

Figure 49.13 A histological section of pancreas from a patient with Shwachman–Diamond syndrome. Typical exocrine gland features include fatty replacement of acini with sparing of ducts. Many islets are preserved but have distorted architecture. Courtesy of Dr Peter Durie.

Figure 49.11 Computed tomography scan for an adult with hereditary pancreatitis. The pancreas shows changes consistent with chronic pancreatitis including mild atrophy and multiple punctate parenchymal calcifications (especially in the pancreatic head).

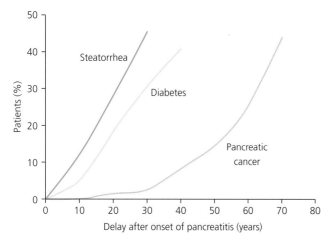

Figure 49.12 Steatorrhea, diabetes mellitus, and pancreatic cancer are common complications of hereditary pancreatitis in patients who are followed for decades. Steatorrhea and diabetes mellitus often occur two to four decades after the onset of pancreatitis, while pancreatic cancer is usually delayed by an additional two to three decades.

50

Gallbladder and biliary tract: anatomy and structural anomalies

Theodore H. Welling, Diane M. Simeone

Anatomy

The gallbladder lies in a depression along the inferior surface of the liver in a plane dividing the liver into its anatomic right and left lobes. The gallbladder is intimately attached to the liver by loose connective tissue that contains small veins and lymphatic vessels. The rest of the gallbladder, which is not in direct contact with the liver, is covered with peritoneum reflected from the liver and is in contact with the duodenum and hepatic flexure of the colon (Fig. 50.1). The gallbladder is divided into four anatomic areas: fundus, body, infundibulum, and neck. The neck tapers into the cystic duct, which joins the common hepatic duct to become the common bile duct. Although the cystic duct typically joins the common hepatic duct directly, it may join the extrahepatic biliary tract anywhere from the right hepatic duct down to the level of the ampulla (Figs 50.2 and 50.3). The blood supply to the gallbladder and cystic duct is usually from a single artery arising from the right hepatic artery, although variations in this configuration are common (Fig. 50.4). The gallbladder is innervated by branches of both the sympathetic and parasympathetic nervous systems (Fig. 50.5), which play a role in modulating gallbladder contractility. The gallbladder has five layers: epithelium, lamina propria, muscularis, perimuscular connective tissue, and serosa. The gallbladder mucosa is lined with columnar epithelial cells that are covered with abundant microvilli and joined by tight junctions.

Bile drains from the liver into the right and left hepatic ducts, which *usually* join outside the liver to form the common hepatic duct. The cystic duct then joins the common hepatic duct to become the common bile duct. The common bile duct lies anterior to the portal vein and to the right of the hepatic artery. The common bile duct is divided into four segments: supraduodenal, retroduodenal, pancreatic, and intraduodenal. The intraduodenal common bile duct joins the main pancreatic duct to form the ampulla of Vater, which empties into the lumen of the duodenum. The intraduodenal common bile duct and ampulla of Vater are surrounded by a sheath of smooth muscle fibers referred to as the sphincter of Oddi (Fig. 50.6). Regulation of bile flow is controlled primarily by the sphincter of Oddi.

Embryology

The biliary tract is first apparent during the fifth week of gestation and develops as a ventral sacculation in the distal foregut (Fig. 50.7). This sacculation grows into the ventral mesentery, which divides into two buds: the cranial bud develops into the liver and intrahepatic bile ducts, and the caudal bud develops into the gallbladder and cystic duct (Fig. 50.8). Another small bud arises from the inferior aspect of the caudal bud and ultimately develops into the ventral pancreas (Fig. 50.9). The ventral pancreatic bud rotates 180° from right to left, fusing with the dorsal pancreatic bud to form the complete pancreas. Because the lower end of the common bile duct is attached to the ventral pancreatic bud, it also rotates and fuses with the duodenum along its posteromedial wall (Fig. 50.10). Variations in this developmental process give rise to structural anomalies in the biliary tract (Fig. 50.11). In addition, viral etiologies along with host response may result in various forms of atresia (Fig. 50.12). Type II and type III choledochal cysts are likely secondary to variations in development (Fig. 50.13) whereas type I choledochal cysts are related to an aberrant junction of the pancreatic and biliary ducts such that a common channel of more than 20 mm (normal <10 mm) exists, resulting in reflux of pancreatic juice into the biliary epithelium, leading to gradual inflammation and ectasia.

Atlas of Gastroenterology, 4th edition. Edited by Tadataka Yamada, David H. Alpers, Anthony N. Kalloo, Neil Kaplowitz, Chung Owyang, and Don W. Powell. © 2009 Blackwell Publishing, ISBN: 978-1-4051-6909-7

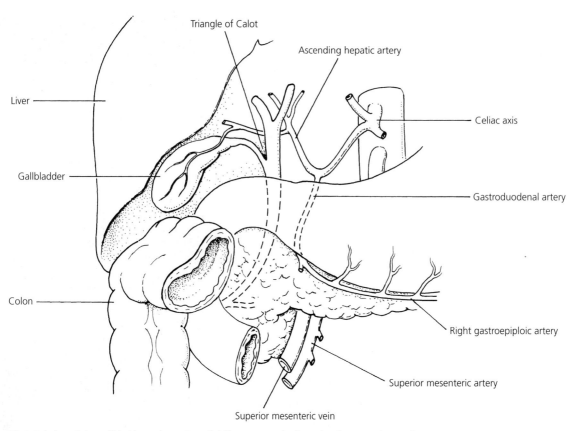

Figure 50.1 Relation of the gallbladder and extrahepatic biliary tract to the liver, duodenum, colon, and pancreas.

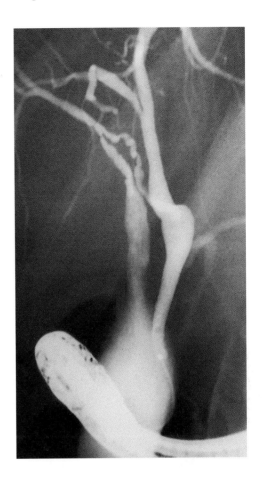

Figure 50.2 Endoscopic retrograde cholangiopancreatogram demonstrates an anomalous junction of the cystic duct with an accessory right hepatic duct.

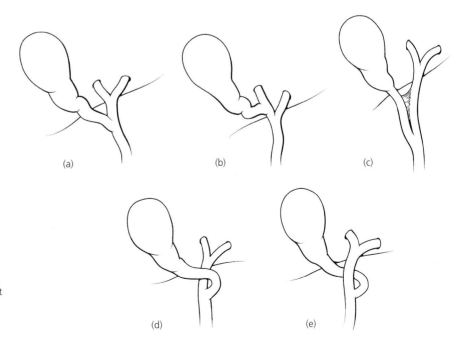

Figure 50.3 Variations in cystic duct anatomy. **(a)** Cystic duct joins common hepatic duct directly (most common). **(b)** Cystic duct joins the right hepatic duct. **(c)** Low junction of cystic duct with common hepatic duct. **(d)** Anterior spiral of cystic duct before joining common hepatic duct. **(e)** Posterior spiral of cystic duct before joining common hepatic duct.

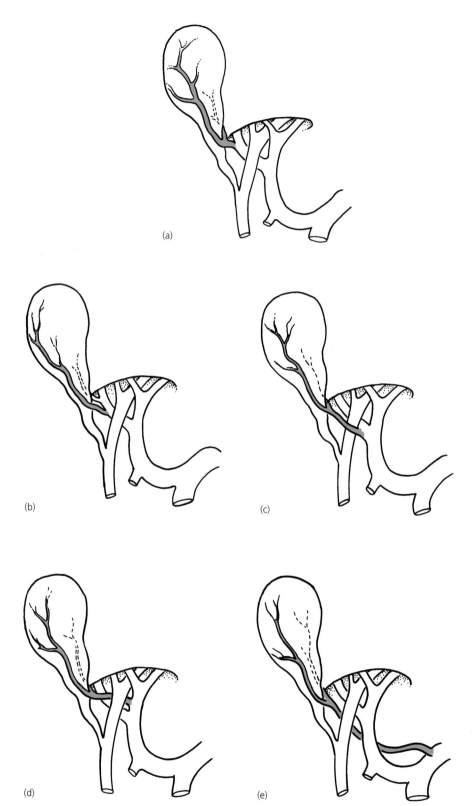

Figure 50.4 Common variations in the origin of the cystic artery. It originates most commonly from the right hepatic artery, traverses the triangle of Calot, and on reaching the gallbladder divides into two main branches **(a)**. Occasionally the two branches come off the right hepatic artery independently **(b)**. The cystic artery may cross the hepatic duct anteriorly **(c)**, come off the left hepatic artery **(d)**, or, more rarely, come directly from the celiac axis **(e)**.

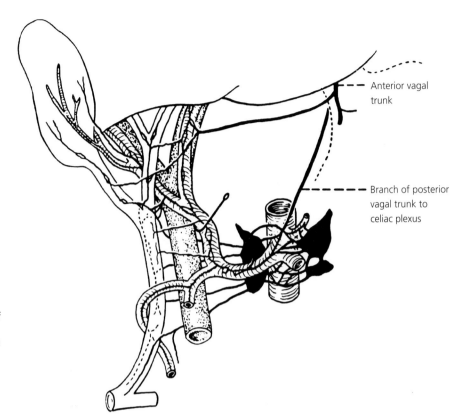

Anterior vagal trunk

Branch of posterior vagal trunk to celiac plexus

Figure 50.5 Schematic of the innervation of the gallbladder and extrahepatic biliary tract. The nerves originate both from vagi and from the celiac axis. They reach the biliary tract traveling along the walls of the hepatic artery, except for direct branches of the anterior vagus that cross through the gastrohepatic ligament.

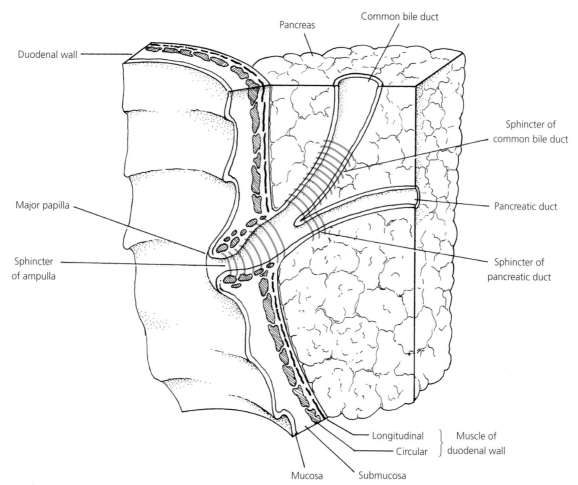

Figure 50.6 Muscular apparatus at the terminal end of the common bile duct. The bile duct is closely associated with the pancreatic duct and they both enter the medial wall of the duodenum tangentially. Each duct has its own sphincter, which is poorly developed in the pancreatic duct.

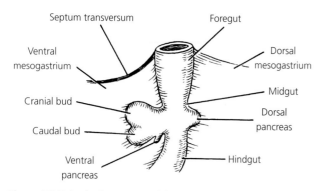

Figure 50.7 At the 3-mm stage of the embryo, the ventral bud enters the mesogastrium and soon divides into a cranial and a caudal bud. A smaller caudal bud represents the origin of the ventral pancreas.

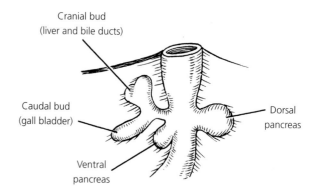

Figure 50.8 As the embryo reaches 5 mm, the cranial bud (which will form the liver and intrahepatic biliary tract) moves toward the septum transversum, pulling the caudal bud (gallbladder and extrahepatic bile ducts).

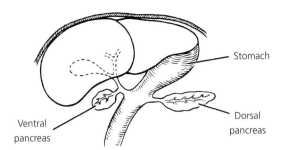

Stomach

Ventral pancreas

Dorsal pancreas

Figure 50.9 When the embryo reaches 7 mm, the right and left lobes of the liver occupy the position under the septum transversum. The ventral pancreas and the extrahepatic biliary tract are visible. As the ventral pancreas rotates to reach the dorsal pancreas, it pulls the lower end of the common bile duct with it.

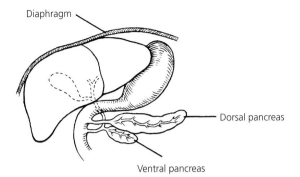

Diaphragm

Dorsal pancreas

Ventral pancreas

Figure 50.10 At the 12-mm stage, the ventral pancreas has rotated and the normal anatomic relations of the bile ducts and gastrointestinal tract have taken place.

Figure 50.11 (a) Two gallbladders. **(b)** Bilobed gallbladder. **(c)** Diverticulum at the neck. **(d)** Septated gallbladder. All are anatomic variations that relate to the embryological development of the biliary tract.

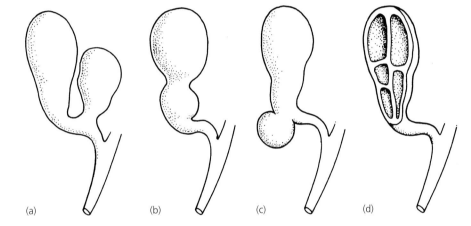

(a)   (b)   (c)   (d)

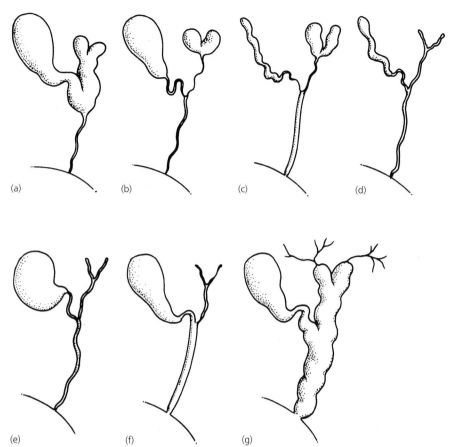

(a)   (b)   (c)   (d)

(e)   (f)   (g)

Figure 50.12 (a–g) Different forms of biliary atresia. Biliary atresia may be partial, affecting the intrahepatic or extrahepatic portions of the biliary tract, or may be a complete process.

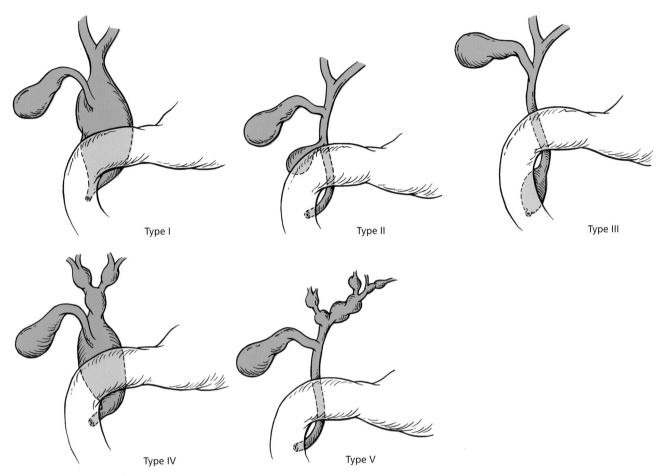

Figure 50.13 Classification of choledochal cysts.

51 Gallstones

Cynthia W. Ko, Sum P. Lee

Cholelithiasis and its complications are the most common diseases of the biliary tract. The prevalence of gallstones varies greatly among ethnic and national groups. In the United States, more than 20 million persons harbor gallstones. Cholesterol stones predominate in Western societies. During the last two decades, important advances have been made in understanding the pathogenesis and treatment of gallstones.

Classification of gallstones

Gallstones are classified by content as cholesterol or pigment stones. In Western countries about 80% of stones are cholesterol stones. About 5% of cholesterol gallstones are composed of pure cholesterol. This type of stone often occurs singly (cholesterol solitaire) (Fig. 51.1a). The very pure cholesterol monohydrate crystalline structure is well appreciated in the fractured surface (Fig. 51.1b). This subgroup of cholesterol gallstones is characterized by an excellent response to oral bile acid therapy or lithotripsy. The long-term recurrence rate of these single cholesterol stones after medical treatment is surprisingly low – about 10% over 15 years.

More commonly, cholesterol gallstones contain other constituents, including proteins and calcium salts of bilirubin or carbonate. Although sometimes called mixed stones, they are still classified as cholesterol stones because cholesterol is the predominant component (more than 70% by weight). These stones are typically multiple and faceted (Fig. 51.2). The fractured surface shows a pigmented center and concentric "growth" rings, suggesting that the chemical composition of bile may have varied during the development of these stones. Sometimes smaller stones aggregate to form a larger concretion. Figure 51.3 shows a large cholesterol gallstone, the surface of which has a mulberry appearance composed of small subunits. In contrast, pigment gallstones are either dark brown or black, small, and amorphous (Fig. 51.4).

Atlas of Gastroenterology, 4th edition. Edited by Tadataka Yamada, David H. Alpers, Anthony N. Kalloo, Neil Kaplowitz, Chung Owyang, and Don W. Powell. © 2009 Blackwell Publishing, ISBN: 978-1-4051-6909-7

Pathogenesis of cholesterol gallstones

Applying the principles of physical chemistry has significantly advanced the basic scientific and clinical understanding of gallstone pathogenesis. The principal site for cholesterol synthesis and metabolism in the body is the liver (Fig. 51.5). Cholesterol is insoluble in water and bile. Cholesterol is initially secreted into bile with phospholipids as unilamellar vesicles measuring 40–75 nm. If bile salt concentrations are low, the cholesterol in bile is predominantly carried in the vesicular form. With the addition of bile salts, mixed micelles form. Mixed micelles contain bile salts, lecithin, and cholesterol. In these mixed micelles, cholesterol is solubilized by the bile salts and phospholipids. Mixed micelles are high in buoyant density (>1.15 g/mL) and measure about 25 Å. Gallstones are formed from "supersaturated" or "lithogenic" bile, which implies that the cholesterol content in bile has exceeded the cholesterol-carrying capacity of other biliary lipids. Implicit within this lithogenic bile hypothesis are two principles. First, the initial abnormality in gallstone formation comes from the liver, which secretes abnormal bile. Second, cholesterol supersaturation is a prerequisite factor for gallstone formation and differentiates persons who form gallstones from those who do not. The cholesterol saturation index (CSI), the ratio of the actual amount of cholesterol in a given bile sample to the maximal cholesterol-carrying capacity of that sample determined in vitro, allows quantification of bile lithogenicity. Bile that has a CSI of more than 1 is considered supersaturated.

A crucial step in cholesterol gallstone formation is nucleation, which is the formation of solid cholesterol crystals from lithogenic bile. The propensity of a bile sample to nucleate is a much better predictor of the gallstone-forming risk than the degree of supersaturation. Figure 51.6 provides a schematic summary of the physical and chemical events involving biliary lipids in nucleation. It is believed that aggregation and fusion of vesicles precede nucleation. Fused vesicles can be seen at transmission electron microscopic examination as large lipid aggregates (Fig. 51.7) or at polarizing microscopic examination as lipid crystals. When cholesterol monohydrate crystals form, they are derived almost exclusively from vesicular cholesterol. Factors in addition to cholesterol supersaturation are important in nucleation. Biliary proteins may have a crucial role in promoting or inhibiting nucleation.

Diagnosis of gallstones

Examination of bile with a polarizing microscope is a useful way of diagnosing gallstone disease. Macroscopic concretions of more than 2 mm often are not found in the gallbladder. Smaller cholesterol crystals may be found, and their presence in bile is referred to as biliary sludge, microcrystalline disease, or microlithiasis. Biliary sludge may be a precursor to gallstones in certain situations. Sludge is composed of cholesterol monohydrate crystals, calcium bilirubinate, and calcium carbonate granules in bile high in mucus content (Figs 51.8–51.11). Similar to patients with gallstones, most patients with sludge have no symptoms. However, patients may have typical biliary pain or complications such as pancreatitis. Biliary sludge may be detected by means of ultrasound scanning. On scans it appears as low-level echoes that layer in the dependent portion of the gallbladder without acoustic shadowing (Fig. 51.12).

Gallstones are usually diagnosed with ultrasonography, appearing as high-amplitude, mobile echoes with postacoustic shadowing (Fig. 51.13). If choledocholithiasis is suspected, percutaneous transhepatic, endoscopic retrograde (Fig. 51.14), or magnetic resonance cholangiography (Fig. 51.15) may be used. Endoscopic ultrasound is also highly sensitive for detecting choledocholithiasis. Oral cholecystography is used infrequently (Fig. 51.16). Acute cholecystitis with obstruction of the cystic duct by stone or inflammatory edema can be diagnosed using hepatobiliary scintigraphy with high sensitivity (Figs 51.17 and 51.18). Ultrasonographic features suggestive of cholecystitis include thickening of the gallbladder wall, the presence of pericholecystic fluid, and air in the gallbladder wall (Fig. 51.19).

Worldwide, a common biliary tract problem is recurrent pyogenic cholangitis (also known as Oriental cholangiohepatitis). This syndrome is characterized by intrahepatic stone formation with recurrent abdominal pain, fever, and jaundice. This syndrome often preferentially involves the left intrahepatic ducts (Fig. 51.20). Management of these patients is difficult and often involves a combination of surgical and radiological techniques.

Management of gallstones

It is estimated that 60%–80% of all gallstones are asymptomatic at a given time. When gallstones do form, the risk factors for developing symptoms are unknown. However, the rate at which stones give rise to symptoms and complications is relatively small. More than 90% of complications, such as cholecystitis, cholangitis, and pancreatitis, are preceded by attacks of pain. Therefore, for most people with asymptomatic gallstones, watchful waiting is appropriate (Fig. 51.21). Once symptoms or complications develop, treatment should be considered. Because biliary sludge can cause symptoms or complications, treatment of sludge should be considered in situations similar to those for gallstones.

Surgery is the definitive curative method for treatment of gallstones. The advent of laparoscopic cholecystectomy and its widespread acceptance has revolutionized surgical treatment of gallstones. Laparoscopic cholecystectomy is now regarded as the treatment of choice for symptomatic gallstones. For patients unable or unwilling to undergo surgery, nonsurgical methods such as oral bile acid therapy are available (Table 51.1).

Table 51.1 Therapeutic options for symptomatic gallbladder stones

Therapy	Candidates	Stone clearance (%)	Mortality (%)	Disadvantages
Laparoscopic cholecystectomy	No previous abdominal surgery, normal gallbladder wall	100	<1	Invasive, requires general anesthesia, possible bile duct injury
Oral bile acids	Patent cystic duct, functioning gallbladder, floating radiolucent stones < 5 mm in diameter	80–90 (well selected)	0	Delayed stone clearance, possible stone recurrence
ESWL with oral bile acids	Patent cystic duct, functioning gallbladder, solitary radiolucent stones up to 20 mm in diameter	70–90	<0.1	Post-ESWL biliary pain and acute pancreatitis (3%–5%), delayed stone clearance, possible stone recurrence
Contact dissolution with MTBE	Radiolucent stones, GB attached to liver, patent cystic duct	50–90	Limited experience	Invasive, bile leakage (5%), leakage of MTBE (erosive duodenitis, hemolysis, pathologic somnolence), stone recurrence

ESWL, extracorporeal shock wave lithotripsy; GB, gallbladder; MTBE, methyl tert-butyl ether.

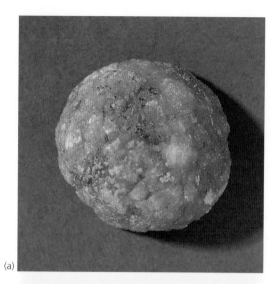

(a)

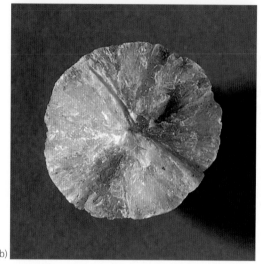

(b)

Figure 51.1 (a) Pure, usually solitary, cholesterol gallstone (cholesterol solitaire). **(b)** Almost 99% of this stone is cholesterol monohydrate. The crystalline structure arrangement can be seen in the fractured surface.

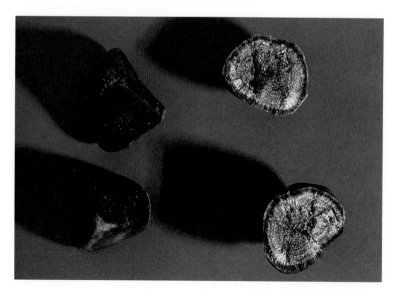

Figure 51.2 Mixed cholesterol gallstones. Usually multiple and faceted, the fractured surface shows a pigment center and concentric "growth" rings. These stones are at least 70% cholesterol by weight and thus are classified as a form of cholesterol gallstones. When multiple stones are present in the gallbladder they are usually identical in chemical composition.

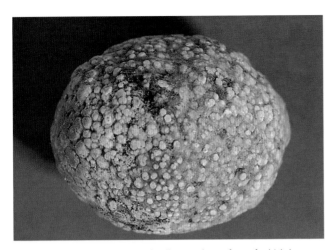

Figure 51.3 A large cholesterol gallstone, the surface of which has a mulberry appearance with multiple small subunits.

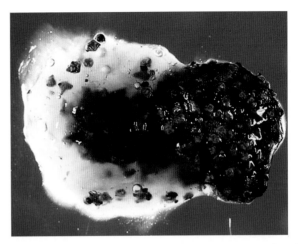

Figure 51.4 Pigment stones are either dark brown or black, small, and multiple. These pigment stones are embedded in a mucus gel.

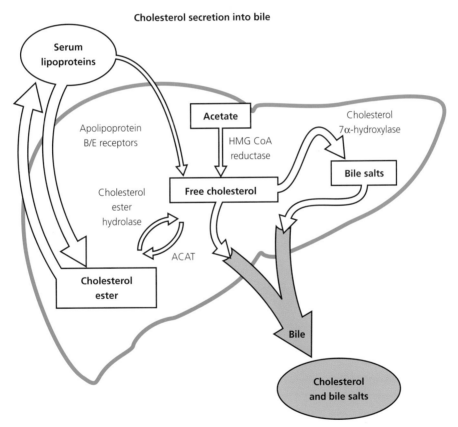

Figure 51.5 Schematic representation of cholesterol and bile acid metabolism in the liver. The liver is the major site for cholesterol synthesis and metabolism in the liver. The free pool of cholesterol in the liver is derived from de novo cholesterol synthesis or uptake from plasma lipoproteins. Cholesterol synthesis from acetate is regulated by hydroxymethylglutaryl coenzyme A (HMG CoA) reductase. Cholesterol may be esterified by acyl:cholesterol:lecithin transferase (ACAT) for storage in the cholesterol ester pool in the body. Cholesterol may be eliminated from the body by secretion into bile or transformation into bile acids by the rate-limiting enzyme 7α-hydroxylase.

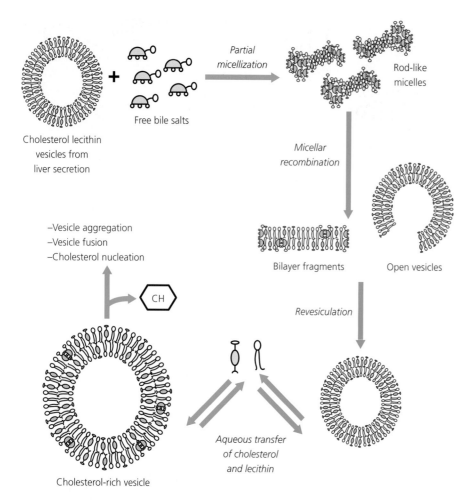

Figure 51.6 Schematic representation of cholesterol nucleation. In bile, cholesterol exists in two soluble forms, vesicles and mixed micelles. These forms are in dynamic equilibrium depending on the total bile salt and lipid concentration. With concentration, vesicles are depleted of phospholipid and enriched in cholesterol, resulting in a tendency for vesicles to aggregate and fuse. Pronucleators may also cause vesicular fusion. The fused vesicles lead to formation of multilamellar liposomes or liquid crystals. Cholesterol separates from the liquid to the solid crystalline form during nucleation. Whether vesicles can nucleate into solid cholesterol crystals is unclear.

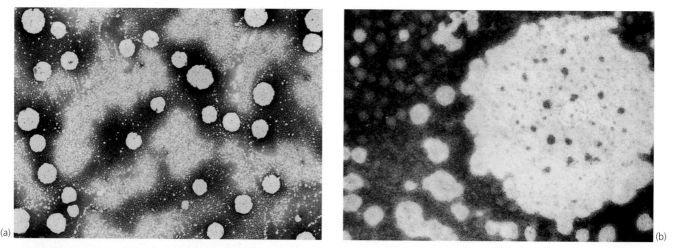

Figure 51.7 Transmission electron microscopy shows vesicular cholesterol and vesicular fusion. **(a)** Monodispersed cholesterol–lecithin vesicles of approximately 600 Å in mean hydrodynamic radius. **(b)** Vesicular fusion into large lipid aggregates, also known as multilamellar vesicles. At polarized microscopic examination they appear as liquid crystals.

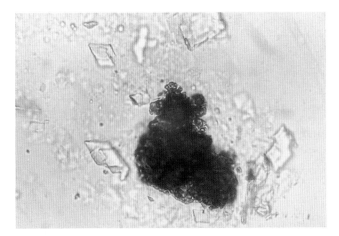

Figure 51.8 Phase-contrast photomicrograph of gallbladder sludge. A central dark calcium bilirubinate granule is surrounded by cholesterol monohydrate crystals. The crystals are typically rhomboidal with a notch. All are embedded within amorphous strands of mucus.

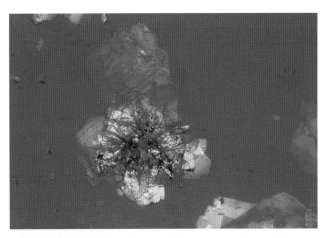

Figure 51.9 Polarizing photomicrograph of gallbladder sludge. A clump of cholesterol monohydrate crystals surrounds a pigmented center of calcium bilirubinate. These crystal aggregates have been referred to as biliary sludge.

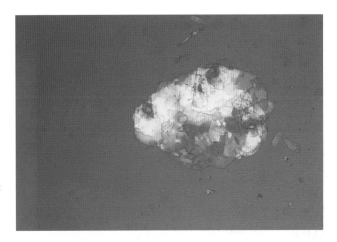

Figure 51.10 Polarizing photomicrograph of gallbladder sludge. Adherent cholesterol monohydrate crystals form a small oval structure. This is probably a cholesterol gallstone in its embryonic stage. This miniature gallstone will grow with further precipitation of cholesterol.

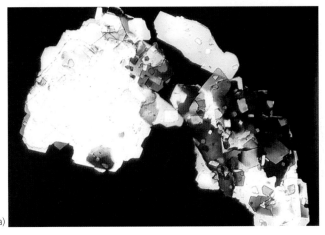

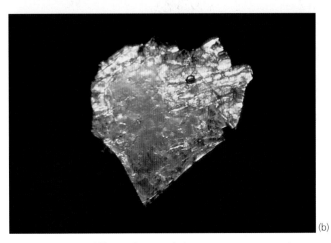

(a)   (b)

Figure 51.11 (a,b) Polarizing photomicrographs of gallbladder sludge. Crystals can be present in different shapes and sizes. In contrast to smooth, rounded cholesterol gallstones, crystals in sludge often have sharp, irregular edges. It is conceivable that such crystals can damage the mucosa of the bile ducts or the sphincter of Oddi, causing inflammation and symptoms.

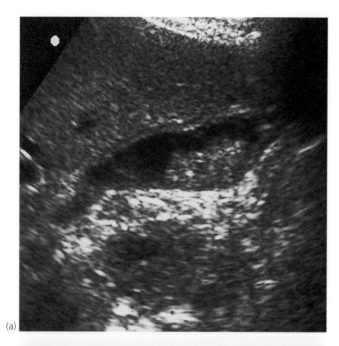

(a)

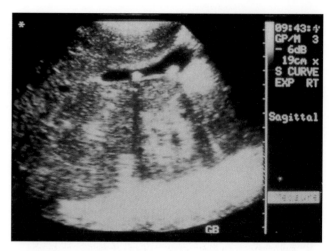

Figure 51.13 Ultrasound scan of gallstones. The stones generate high-amplitude echoes and are large and dense enough to produce substantial acoustic impedance in the path of the ultrasound beam. This produces a void behind the stone, which is known as the postacoustic shadow.

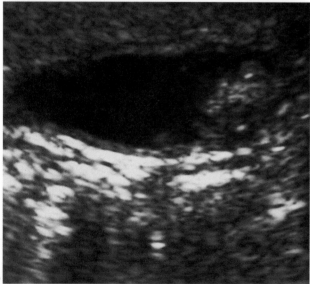

(b)

Figure 51.12 Ultrasound scan of gallbladder sludge. **(a)** The particulate matter within the gallbladder generates low-amplitude echoes without postacoustic shadowing. **(b)** With positioning changes the material forms progressive layers in the most dependent part of the gallbladder. The high-amplitude echoes contained within the sludge may represent small early gallstones.

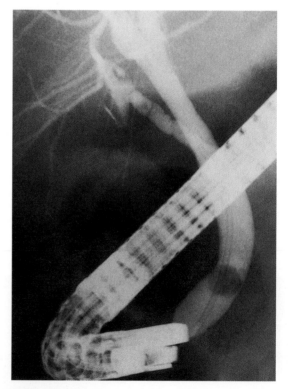

Figure 51.14 Endoscopic retrograde cholangiogram shows a stone within the common bile duct. There is also a small stone or debris within the cystic duct. Courtesy of Dr Scott Schulte.

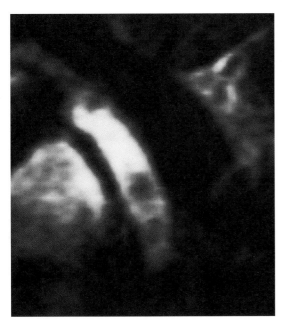

Figure 51.15 Magnetic resonance cholangiogram shows two stones within the common bile duct. The gallbladder is adjacent to the common bile duct. Courtesy of Dr Scott Schulte.

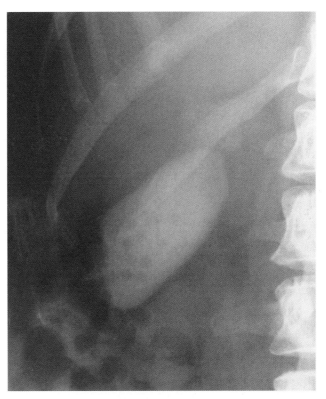

Figure 51.16 Oral cholecystogram shows several small stones within an opacified gallbladder.

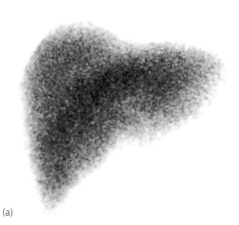

(a)

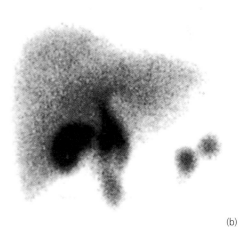

(b)

Figure 51.17 Technetium 99m iminodiacetic acid scintigraphy, normal study. **(a)** Homogeneous hepatic uptake occurs within 5 min. **(b)** Fifteen minutes after radionuclide administration, the gallbladder, common bile duct, and a portion of small bowel are visible. Courtesy of Dr Arnold Jacobson.

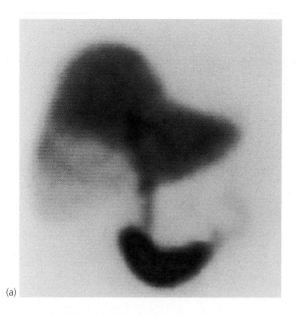

(a)

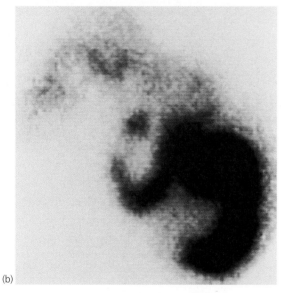

(b)

Figure 51.18 Technetium 99m iminodiacetic acid scintigraphy, abnormal study. **(a)** The 5-min scan demonstrates normal liver uptake. **(b)** Morphine (0.04 mg/kg intravenously) has been given to enhance gallbladder filling. Inability to visualize the gallbladder by 90 min after radionuclide administration if adequate images of the liver, common duct, and small bowel have been obtained is consistent with the diagnosis of acute cholecystitis. A rim sign, a region of increased activity in the liver adjacent to the gallbladder fossa, is present and represents transmural inflammation of the gallbladder. Courtesy of Dr Arnold Jacobson.

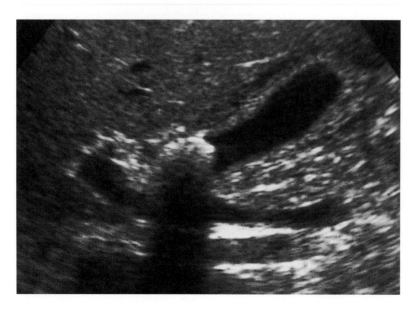

Figure 51.19 Ultrasound scan shows acute cholecystitis. A large gallstone is impacted within the neck of the gallbladder. Other findings that suggest acute cholecystitis include a thickened gallbladder wall and a small amount of pericholecystic fluid.

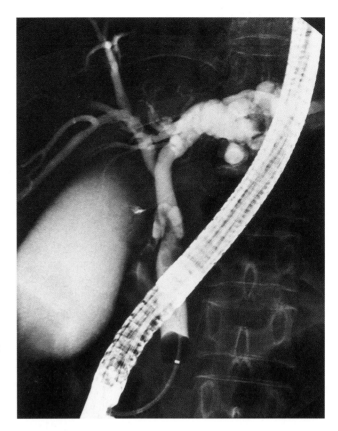

Figure 51.20 Cholangiogram showing findings characteristic of recurrent pyogenic cholangitis. The left intrahepatic duct is preferentially involved, with dilation and intraductal filling defects characteristic of intrahepatic stones. The right intrahepatic ducts show characteristic changes of pruning and decreased arborization. A balloon catheter is used to obtain the occlusion cholangiogram. Courtesy of Dr Charles Rohrmann.

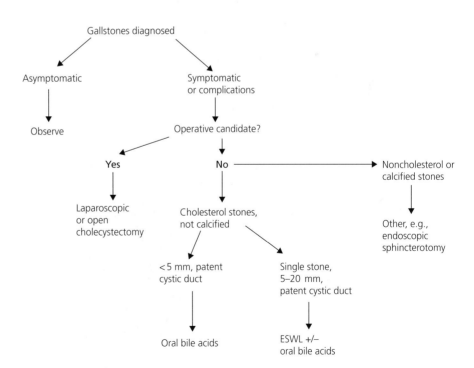

Figure 51.21 Algorithm for management of biliary sludge and gallstones. ESWL, extracorporeal shock wave lithotripsy.

52

Primary sclerosing cholangitis and other cholangiopathies

Russell H. Wiesner, Kymberly D.S. Watt

Primary sclerosing cholangitis (PSC) is a chronic cholestatic liver disease characterized by inflammation and fibrosis of the intra- and extrahepatic bile ducts. Disease progression often results in biliary cirrhosis and hepatic failure. The only successful treatment has been liver transplantation. The etiology and etiopathogenesis remain poorly understood.

The diagnosis of PSC is made by cholangiography (Fig. 52.1). Intrahepatic duct involvement is nearly universal with extrahepatic duct sparing occurring in 20% of cases. Segmental bile duct fibrosis with subsequent saccular dilation with normal intervening areas results in the characteristic beaded pattern frequently noted on the cholangiogram. The use of abdominal computed tomography or magnetic resonance cholangiopancreatography for accurate detection of suspected PSC has been increasingly useful (Fig. 52.2a,b). Liver biopsy is required for staging disease severity of PSC; histological findings include periductal fibrosis with inflammation, bile duct proliferation, and ductopenia (Fig. 52.3a,b). Fibroobliterative cholangiopathy (Fig. 52.4) is considered the most diagnostic finding on liver biopsy but is present in only about 10% of biopsies obtained in PSC patients. Explant findings often reveal liver fibrotic reactions surrounding the large bile ducts (Fig. 52.5).

The recognition of elevated serum hepatic biochemistries consistent with cholestasis in a male patient with concurrent inflammatory bowel disease (IBD) is strongly suggestive of PSC. IBD, most commonly chronic ulcerative colitis, occurs in 70%–80% of patients with PSC. In those PSC patients who undergo proctocolectomy, the formation of peristomal varices with severe bleeding can be a major complication and a cause of significant morbidity (Fig. 52.6). In such cases a surgical portocaval shunt or a transjugular intrahepatic portal shunt (TIPS) procedure has been effective. In addition, pouchitis following proctocolectomy seems to be more frequent and more severe in PSC patients than in patients with ulcerative colitis alone (Fig. 52.7).

The differential diagnosis of PSC includes biliary obstruction from choledocholithiasis, stricture, or malignancy,

primary biliary cirrhosis, autoimmune pancreatitis, recurrent pyogenic cholangitis, fungal cholangitis, acquired immunodeficiency syndrome cholangiopathy, choledochal cysts, cystic fibrosis, primary portal hypertension, intrahepatic hepatocellular carcinoma, and eosinophilic cholangitis.

Metabolic bone disease, most commonly osteoporosis, is seen in relation to PSC patients (Fig. 52.8). Approximately 50% of patients have osteopenia, whereas osteoporosis develops in less than 10% of cases. Initial treatment with calcium and weight-bearing activity is essential. Oral replacement therapy with vitamin D is indicated if measured serum levels are reduced. The use of bisphosphonates has been proven to be effective in preventing bone mineral loss. When present, steatorrhea may be caused by impaired small intestinal bile acid delivery, celiac disease, or exocrine pancreatic insufficiency. Malabsorption of fat-soluble vitamins A, D, E, and K is common in patients with advanced PSC and usually responds to oral replacement therapy.

Bacterial cholangitis is most commonly associated with a previous history of biliary tract surgery, bile duct calculi, or dominant stricture. Therapy includes empiric broad-spectrum intravenous antibiotics and biliary decompression when clinically indicated. Dominant strictures occur in 15%–20% of PSC patients (Fig. 52.9a,b). Clinical manifestations include progressive jaundice, symptoms of bacterial cholangitis, and dark urine. Diagnosis and therapy include endoscopic or radiological approaches to dilate the dominant stricture and often provide significant and clinical improvement. Of note, there appears to be an increased incidence of gallbladder cancer associated with gallstones in patients with PSC.

The most serious complication of PSC is the development of cholangiocarcinoma. Primary anatomic sites of involvement include the hilum (75% of cases), intrahepatic ducts (16%), and the gallbladder (8%). Risk factors include advanced age, long duration of IBD, advanced hepatic disease, cigarette smoking, colorectal neoplasia, or carcinoma. Confirming the diagnosis of cholangiocarcinoma in PSC is challenging. The distinction between benign and malignant biliary strictures with cross-sectional imaging and cholangiography can be helpful in making the diagnosis (Fig. 52.10a,b). Serum tumor markers, including carbohy-

Atlas of Gastroenterology, 4th edition. Edited by Tadataka Yamada, David H. Alpers, Anthony N. Kalloo, Neil Kaplowitz, Chung Owyang, and Don W. Powell. © 2009 Blackwell Publishing, ISBN: 978-1-4051-6909-7

drate antigen 19-9 and carcinoembryonic antigen, remain insensitive for detecting early stage disease. Rarely, bile duct dysplasia or carcinoma can be diagnosed on liver biopsy (Fig. 52.11). At least one report has suggested that positron emission tomography (PET) scanning can be helpful in diagnosing cholangiocarcinoma in the presence of PSC (Fig. 52.12). The use of biliary cytology, digital image analysis, and fluorescence in situ hybridization (FISH) studies can also be useful in diagnosing cholangiocarcinoma in patients with PSC (Figs 52.13 and 52.14a,b). Some studies also suggest that the use of cholangioscopy can be helpful in distinguishing between malignant and benign dominant bile duct strictures in patients with PSC (Fig. 52.15a,b).

Finally, the only known successful therapy for PSC is liver transplantation; PSC is the fourth most common indication for liver transplantation in the United States. Survival rates ranging between 90% and 95% at 1 year and 83% and 88% at 5 years have been reported. Long-term graft survival is affected by a higher incidence of rejection in hepatic artery thrombosis. An increasing body of evidence suggests that PSC can recur after liver transplantation in up to 30% of cases (Fig. 52.16). To date, there is no recognized effective medical therapy that appears to alter disease progression. Multiple therapies studied include antifibrotic agents, anticupric agents, and immunosuppressive agents, all of which have been proven unsuccessful in preventing disease progression. Three randomized, placebo-controlled trials with ursodeoxycholic acid (UDCA) have also failed to show significant improvements in histology and survival. Of note, secondary causes of sclerosing cholangitis often reveal radiological and histological findings that are similar to those of PSC (Fig. 52.17).

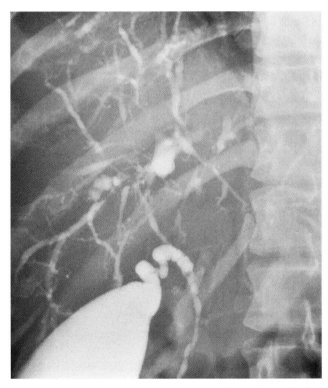

Figure 52.1 Cholangiogram showing beading and irregularity of both the intra- and extrahepatic biliary tract, typical of primary sclerosing cholangitis.

Figure 52.2 **(a)** Typical changes of primary sclerosing cholangitis on magnetic resonance cholangiography: diffuse changes throughout the intra- and extrahepatic bile ducts are seen without evidence of a dominant stricture or filling defect. **(b)** Images of primary sclerosing cholangitis seen on the corresponding endoscopic retrograde cholangiogram. As is seen, magnetic resonance cholangiography gives a better visualization of the peripheral branches of the biliary tree, not seen on this particular endoscopic retrograde cholangiogram.

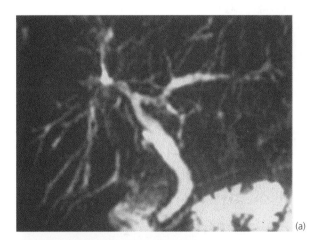

(a)

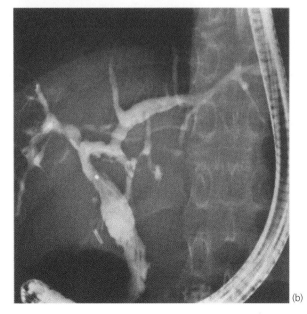

(b)

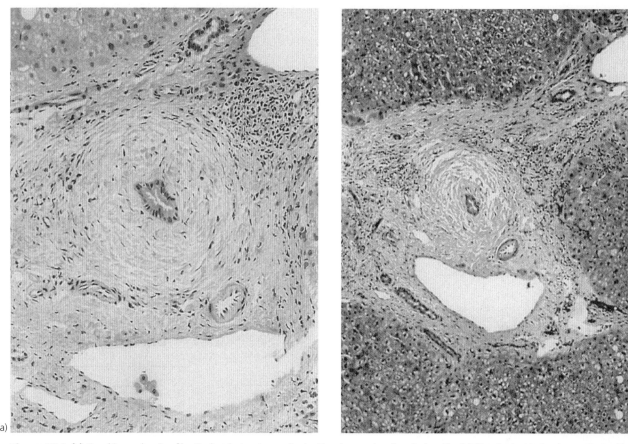

(a)   (b)

Figure 52.3 (a) Liver biopsy showing fibrotic duct lesions in a patient with primary sclerosing cholangitis. **(b)** Fibrotic duct lesion in a patient with primary sclerosing cholangitis. Tissue sample was stained with Mason trichrome.

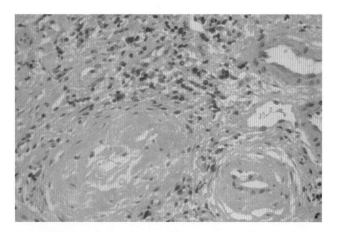

Figure 52.4 Liver biopsy showing obliterative duct lesion with only the ghost of a previous bile duct remaining.

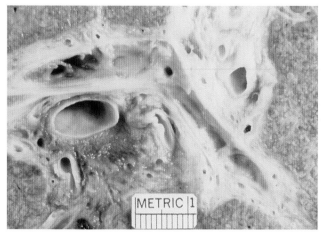

Figure 52.5 Explant liver with intense fibrosis surrounding the biliary tract, which is typical of primary sclerosing cholangitis.

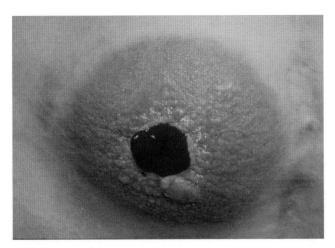

Figure 52.6 Abdominal photograph of a severe abdominal peristomal varix in a patient with primary sclerosing cholangitis with a history of chronic ulcerative colitis who underwent total proctocolectomy and ileostomy.

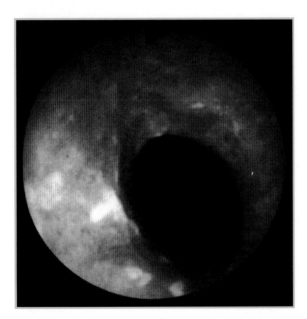

Figure 52.7 Pouchitis in a patient who has undergone proctocolectomy and ileorectal pouch anastomosis. This is seen more frequently and is more severe in patients with primary sclerosing cholangitis than in patients with ulcerative colitis alone.

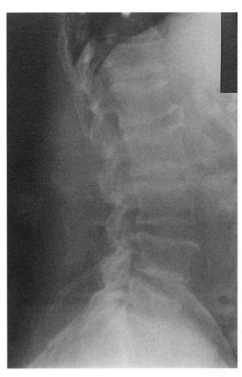

Figure 52.8 Spine radiograph of a patient with severe osteoporosis, a finding seen in 25% of patients with primary sclerosing cholangitis who undergo liver transplantation. Because of available therapies at this time, early diagnosis is important.

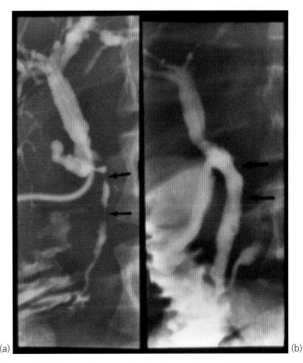

(a)　　　　(b)

Figure 52.9 Cholangiogram of a dominant stricture of the common hepatic bile duct before **(a)** and after **(b)** dilation.

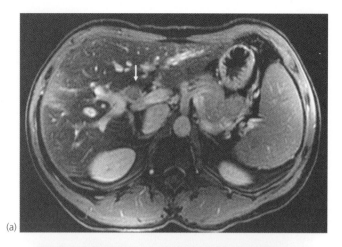

(a)

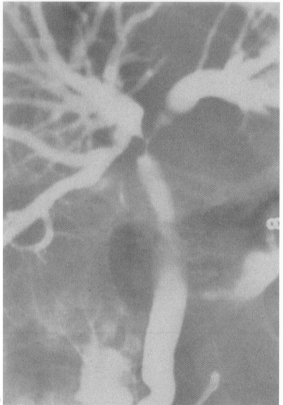

(b)

Figure 52.10 (a) Magnetic resonance cholangiogram showing a dominant stricture of the right hepatic duct with a tumor mass (arrow) in a patient with primary sclerosing cholangitis. **(b)** Cholangiogram of a hilar lesion typical of cholangiocarcinoma in a patient with long-standing chronic ulcerative colitis.

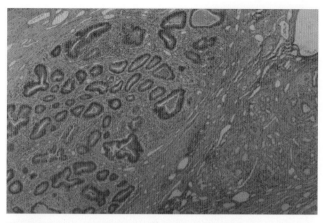

Figure 52.11 Liver biopsy showing severe dysplasia and bile duct carcinoma in a patient with primary sclerosing cholangitis.

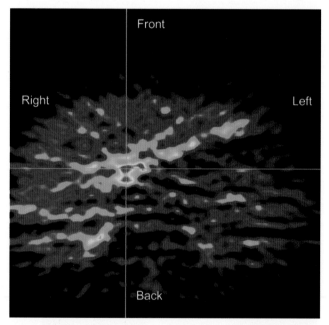

Figure 52.12 A positron emission tomography study demonstrating a perihilar irregularity in a patient with primary sclerosing cholangitis, which represented an infiltrating cholangiocarcinoma.

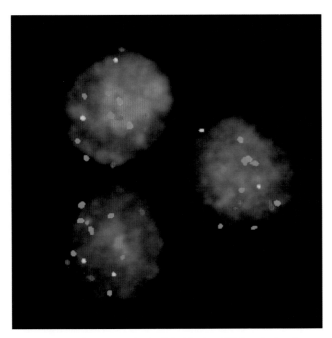

Figure 52.13 Fluorescence in situ hybridization (FISH) study showing cysts positive for polysomy with two or more copies for two or more of the four probes utilized. This is typical of malignant cells.

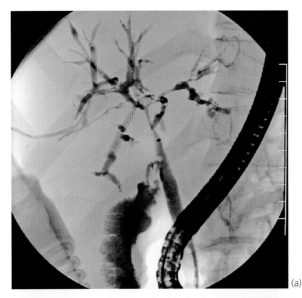

(a)

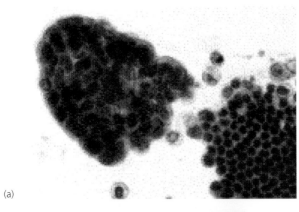

(a)

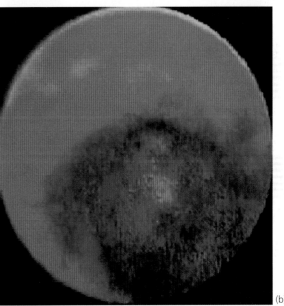

(b)

Figure 52.15 **(a)** Cholangiogram in a patient with cholangiocarcinoma showing bilateral intrahepatic ductal dilation and irregularity along with a high-grade irregular stricture of the proximal extrahepatic bile duct. **(b)** Cholangioscopy showing an intraductal polypoid mass in the stenotic segment of the cholangiogram noted above.

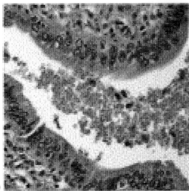

(b)

Figure 52.14 **(a)** Cytological specimen from a patient with primary sclerosing cholangitis showing low-grade dysplasia. **(b)** Epithelium from the resected main bile duct from the same patient, again showing low-grade dysplasia.

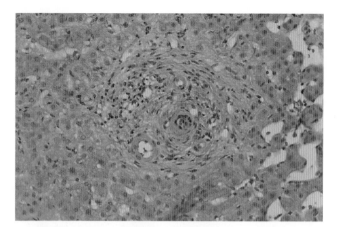

Figure 52.16 Liver biopsy that shows early recurrence of primary sclerosing cholangitis in a patient who underwent liver transplantation for primary sclerosing cholangitis 5 years previously. An early fibrotic obliterative duct lesion is present.

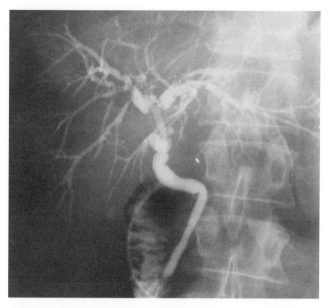

Figure 52.17 Patient with acquired immune deficiency syndrome cholangiopathy who had a positive culture for cytomegalovirus and *Cryptosporidium*: the findings are indistinguishable from cholangiographic findings in primary sclerosing cholangitis.

53

Cystic diseases of the liver and biliary tract

Albert J. Chang, Jung W. Suh, Shelly C. Lu

Biliary cysts are cystic dilations that occur anywhere in the biliary system. They mainly afflict children and young adults. Most biliary cysts are congenital. Todani and colleagues have proposed the most useful classification of biliary cysts. The most common are type I common bile duct cysts or choledochal cysts. Type II are diverticulum cysts that are found anywhere in the extrahepatic ducts; type III are choledochocele cysts; type IV are multiple cysts in the intrahepatic and extrahepatic ducts; type V are intrahepatic bile duct cysts (single or multiple); and type VI are isolated cystic duct dilations.

The clinical presentation of biliary cysts depends on the patient's age. In infancy, jaundice with or without acholic stools is the most common finding. Vomiting, failure to thrive, and hepatomegaly are often found. The classic clinical triad (pain, jaundice, and a palpable abdominal mass) has been reported in 11%–63% of large series. In patients older than 2 years of age the most common presentation is chronic and intermittent pain. Intermittent jaundice and recurrent cholangitis can also occur. The classic clinical triad, cirrhosis, and portal hypertension are less often encountered than in the infantile form. Recurrent pancreatitis has been reported only in older patients. Patients may present with carcinoma of the biliary tract, the most feared complication of biliary cysts (Fig. 53.1).

Diagnosis of biliary cysts requires a high index of suspicion. Percutaneous transhepatic cholangiography (PTC) and endoscopic retrograde cholangiopancreatography (ERCP) provide the most detailed examinations (Figs 53.2, 53.3a, 53.4, 53.5a, and 53.7a). In infants, hepatobiliary scintigraphy and ultrasonography provide a sound basis for diagnosis (Figs 53.3b and 53.6). Ultrasonography is an excellent screening tool but provides little anatomical or functional information. Hepatobiliary scintigraphy provides information about excretory patterns (Fig. 53.3b) and is excellent for postoperative patient follow-up. Computed tomography

(CT) is superior to ultrasonography in older patients (Figs 53.3c and 53.7b). Magnetic resonance cholangiopancreatography (MRCP) is an attractive alternative to ERCP or PTC (Fig. 53.8).

The presence of an anomalous pancreaticobiliary ductal union occurs commonly in cases of choledochal cysts (Figs 53.4a,b). In many patients with choledochal cysts, the common bile duct enters the pancreatic duct at a right angle, abnormally far from the ampulla of Vater. This abnormal anatomy impairs normal sphincteric function at the pancreaticobiliary junction, which may lead to reflux of pancreatic juice into the bile duct causing injury and cystic malformation.

Cholangiography best diagnoses choledochoceles (Fig. 53.5a). Typically, the distal common bile duct appears "clubbed." Emptying of contrast material is often delayed. Choledochoceles are easily distinguished from duodenal diverticuli and duodenal duplication cysts by filling during cholangiography but not during upper gastrointestinal contrast studies (Fig. 53.5b). Sarris and Tsang proposed a further anatomic classification of choledochoceles (Fig. 53.9), which is useful for therapeutic implications. Thus, excision of the duodenal lumenal portion of the cyst, leaving the medial portion containing the ampulla intact, is the preferred treatment for types IIIA1 and IIIA2 cysts. Transduodenal sphincteroplasty and ERCP with papillotomy have been advocated for type IIIA3 cysts. Type IIIB cysts should be treated by excision and sphincteroplasty.

Type V intrahepatic bile duct cysts represent Caroli disease (Fig. 53.7). There is a simple type and a periportal fibrosis type. The periportal fibrosis type is also known as Caroli syndrome. In addition to intrahepatic cystic dilation, congenital hepatic fibrosis, cirrhosis, portal hypertension, and esophageal varices are frequently seen. Intrahepatic bile duct cysts are often associated with the renal abnormalities of autosomal recessive polycystic kidney disease.

Congenital hepatic fibrosis refers to a unique congenital liver histology characterized by bland portal fibrosis, hyperproliferation of interlobular bile ducts within the portal areas with variable shapes and sizes of bile ducts, and preservation of normal lobular architecture (Fig. 53.10).

Atlas of Gastroenterology, 4th edition. Edited by Tadataka Yamada, David H. Alpers, Anthony N. Kalloo, Neil Kaplowitz, Chung Owyang, and Don W. Powell. © 2009 Blackwell Publishing, ISBN: 978-1-4051-6909-7

The treatment of choice is total cyst excision in patients with choledochal cysts and diverticulum cysts. The malignant potential of choledochoceles depends on the type of epithelium that lines the cysts. Carcinoma has been reported only in choledochoceles that were lined by biliary or undifferentiated epithelium internally. Thus, some advocate complete excision of the choledochocele if the choledochocele is lined by biliary or undifferentiated epithelium, with sphincteroplasty for those lined by duodenal epithelium.

Intrahepatic cyst (i.e., types IVA, V) treatment depends on the degree of involvement. When segmental cystic disease is confined to one lobe (more often the left lobe), lobectomy is usually curative. If both lobes are involved, some have advocated establishing a permanent-access hepaticojejunostomy after partial hepatectomy to allow easy biliary tree access. Ultimately, if attacks of cholangitis are frequent and quality of life poor, hepatic transplantation may be a therapeutic option. Cholecystectomy should be performed at the time of cyst excision because the gallbladder is predisposed to malignant change in patients with biliary cysts. If definitive surgical procedure is successful, the prognosis is generally excellent.

Biliary cysts are distinct from polycystic liver disease (PCLD), which is a rare hepatobiliary fibropolycystic disorder characterized by the progressive development of fluid-filled biliary epithelial cysts in the liver. The most common form of PCLD coexists with autosomal dominant polycystic kidney disease (ADPKD); however, PCLD can occur without renal involvement (Fig. 53.11). The hepatic cysts are rarely detected before puberty, but approximately 80% of patients with renal cysts have liver cysts by the fifth decade of life. They are more prevalent and prominent in women, and increase dramatically in number and size through the childbearing years.

Most patients with PCLD are asymptomatic. The cysts range in size from less than 1 mm to more than 10 cm and may be diffuse or involve only one lobe. The most common presenting symptom is abdominal pain, with or without distention. Complications of PCLD include hepatic cyst hemorrhage, rupture, or infection.

Abdominal ultrasound and CT scanning are excellent in the detection of hepatic cysts. MRCP can also be a useful modality for better visualizing intrahepatic ductal dilations and distinguishing PCLD from other lesions such as biliary hamartomas and Caroli disease.

There is no effective medical therapy for PCLD. Surgical fenestration of hepatic cysts, involving the deroofing of as many cysts as possible, can be performed through open laparotomy or by laparoscopy. Patients with severely symptomatic PCLD and significant comorbid conditions or diffuse liver involvement by small cysts may benefit from orthotopic liver transplantation.

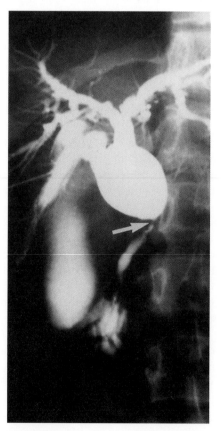

Figure 53.1 Choledochal cyst with cholangiocarcinoma. Cystic dilation of the common bile duct with irregularities in the wall (arrow) consistent with cholangiocarcinoma. Courtesy of Dr Randall Radin, Department of Radiology, LAC/USC Medical Center.

Figure 53.2 Choledochal cyst – type IA. Mild stenosis (arrow) of the common bile duct immediately distal to the cyst contributes to the slight intrahepatic ductal distention.

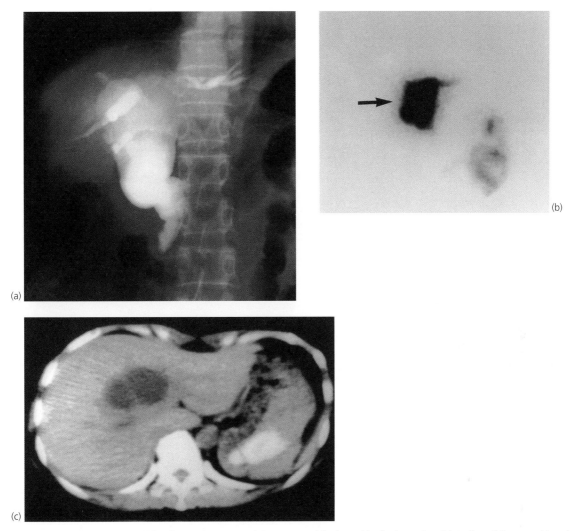

Figure 53.3 Choledochal cyst – type IC. **(a)** Diffuse enlargement of the common bile duct with distal tapering. **(b)** Radionuclide scan with activity predominantly in the cyst (arrow) and left hepatic duct. Bowel activity indicates patency of the common bile duct. **(c)** Computed tomographic scan at the level of the cephalic portion of the cyst shows slight extension of the dilation into both the right and left hepatic ducts.

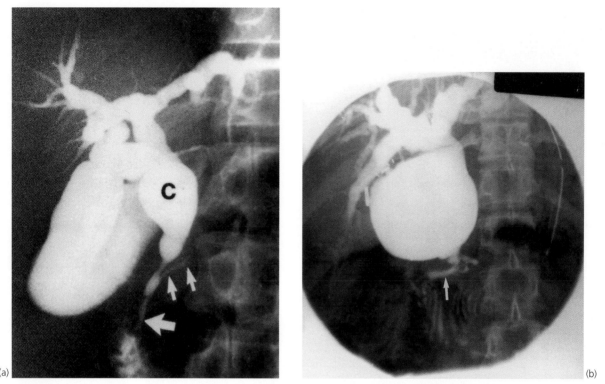

(a)   (b)

Figure 53.4 Choledochal cyst – anomalous ductal relationship. **(a)** Cystic enlargement of the common bile duct (C) with associated dilation of the common hepatic and intrahepatic ducts. The abnormal junction of the pancreatic (small arrows) and common bile ducts and the long common channel (large arrow) are displayed. **(b)** A large cyst involves the common hepatic and common bile ducts accompanied by intrahepatic ductal dilation. A long common channel (arrow) results from the abnormally high junction with the pancreatic duct.

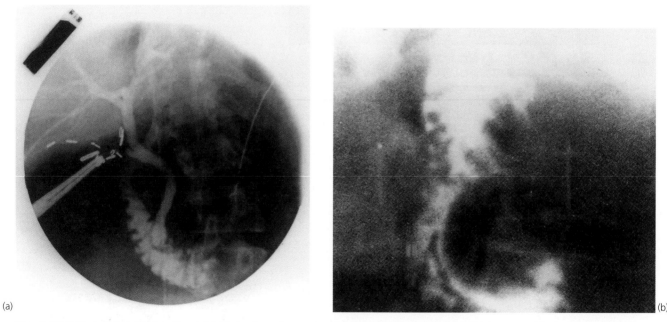

(a)   (b)

Figure 53.5 Choledochocele – type III cyst. **(a)** Cholangiography reveals a club-shaped enlargement of the distal common bile duct bulging into the duodenum. **(b)** Upper gastrointestinal series reveals a smoothly rounded filling defect in the second portion of the duodenum.

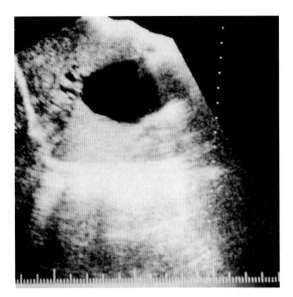

Figure 53.6 Choledochal cyst – sonographic findings. The anechoic mass with enhanced through-transmission is characteristic of a cystic structure. Note one and possibly two ducts entering the cephalic aspect of the cyst. Absence of dilation of the bile ducts proximal to the cystic mass is typical for most type I cysts.

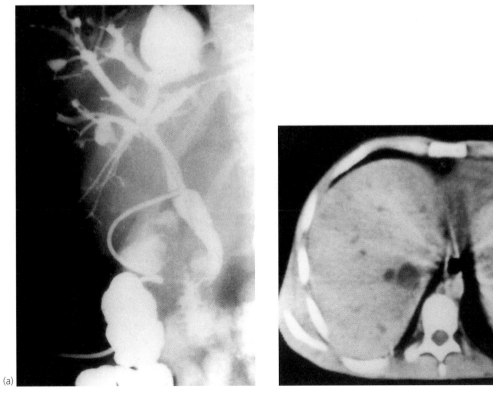

(a)

(b)

Figure 53.7 Caroli disease – type V cyst. **(a)** T-tube cholangiography demonstrates cystic dilation of multiple intrahepatic bile ducts representing type V biliary cysts. **(b)** Computed tomographic scan of the same patient showing several of the intrahepatic cysts.

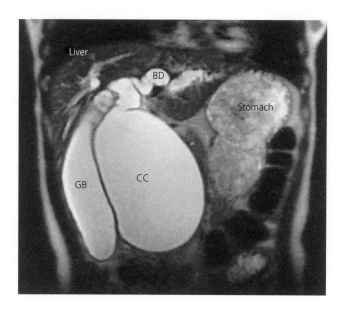

Figure 53.8 Magnetic resonance cholangiopancreatography (MRCP) of a choledochal cyst. Coronal T2-weighted fast spin-echo MRCP performed on a 16-year-old female patient presenting with right upper quadrant pain, jaundice, and amylasemia shows a very dilated segment of the common bile duct compatible with a choledochal cyst distal to the origin of the cystic duct. The intrahepatic ducts are normal in size and shape. BD, bile duct; CC, choledochocele; GB, gallbladder. Courtesy of Dr Fergus Coakley, Department of Radiology, UCSF.

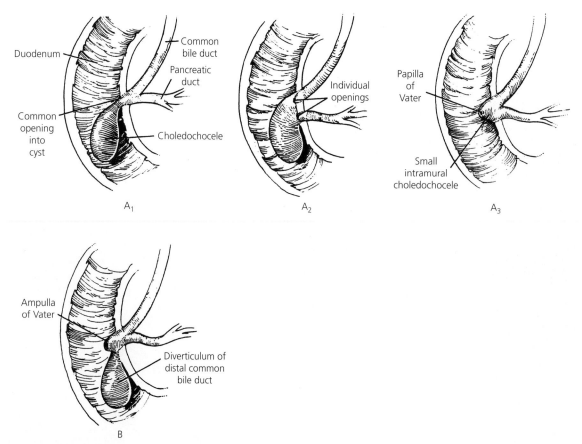

Figure 53.9 Proposed subclassification of choledochoceles (type III biliary cysts). In type A the ampulla opens into the choledochocele, which in turn communicates with the duodenum by way of another small opening. Type A is subclassified into A$_1$, in which the pancreatic and common bile duct share a common opening into the cyst (33% of cases); A$_2$, in which the openings are distinct (4% of cases); and A$_3$, in which the choledochocele is small and entirely intramural (25% of cases). In type B the ampulla opens directly into the duodenum with the choledochocele communicating with the distal common bile duct (21% of cases).

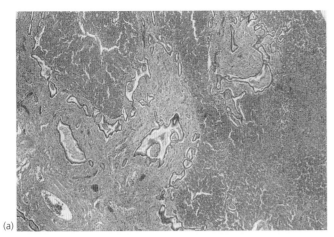

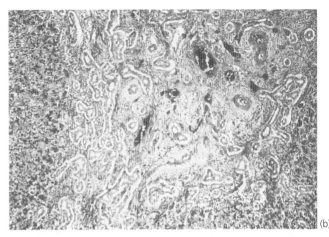

(a)

(b)

Figure 53.10 Congenital hepatic fibrosis. A 27-year-old woman presented with periodic right upper quadrant discomfort and persistent, mildly elevated alkaline phosphatase levels. A liver biopsy was performed. **(a)** The liver parenchyma is normal but the portal areas show prominent portal fibrosis without inflammation. The interlobular bile ducts are numerous and dilated and some contained inspissated bile (hematoxylin and eosin, low power). **(b)** Marked portal fibrosis as demonstrated by trichrome staining. Note the sharp demarcation of the fibrotic area from the parenchyma (trichrome stain, high power). Courtesy of Dr Gary Kanel, Department of Clinical Pathology, Keck School of Medicine, University of Southern California.

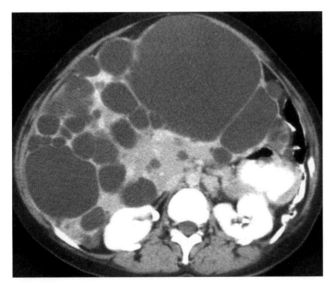

Figure 53.11 Polycystic liver disease. Small and large cysts fill the liver of a patient without polycystic kidneys. Courtesy of Dr Randall Radin, Department of Radiology, LAC+USC Medical Center.

54

Tumors of the biliary tract

Joseph J.Y. Sung, Yuk Tong Lee

Tumor of the bile ducts

Bile duct cancer, or cholangiocarcinoma, is rare in the Western world but is relatively common in Asia. Chronic inflammation and bile stasis are considered to be important in the development of the disease. Risk factors include chronic infestation by liver flukes; chronic suppurative cholangitis (recurrent pyogenic cholangitis); inflammatory bowel disease associated with sclerosing cholangitis; congenital bile duct disorders (choledochal cyst and Caroli disease); and use of Thorotrast, a radiological contrast medium, in the 1930s and 1940s. Evidence of old or current infestation by *Clonorchis* (*Clonorchis sinensis*) and *Opisthorchis* (*Opisthorchis viverrini*) has been associated with cholangiocarcinoma in China and southeast Asia. The leaf-shaped adult worms live and proliferate in the intrahepatic biliary tract and cause chronic inflammation, ductal proliferation, and mucin secretion of the biliary epithelium (Fig. 54.1). Cholangiocarcinoma is also associated with hepatolithiasis and strictures of the bile duct (Fig. 54.2).

At macroscopic examination, cholangiocarcinoma is a solid, grayish-white tumor with a nodular, sclerosing, or diffuse infiltrative appearance. The distribution of extrahepatic bile duct cancer is 49% in the upper third, 25% in the middle third, 19% in the lower third, and diffuse among 7% of patients according to Tompkins and colleagues. Cholangiocarcinoma originating from the hilum of the liver is called Klatskin tumor. These tumors are usually small and can be missed, even during an operation, and they remain localized at the confluence of the right and left hepatic ducts. Bismuth and colleagues classified these tumors according to extent of involvement and communication between the right and left ductal system as follows:

Type I: unobstructed primary confluence (tumor in the main hepatic duct)

Type II: obstruction limited to primary confluence (tumor at the confluence)

Type III: obstruction of the primary confluence with extension to either the right (IIIa) or left (IIIb) secondary confluence

Type IV: tumor growth along both hepatic ducts causing multiple segmental obstructions.

Most Klatskin tumors present themselves in a type II or type III distribution. This classification reflects increasing difficulty in treatment options as the tumor grows into segmental bile ducts.

At microscopic examination most bile duct cancers are adenocarcinoma. They are usually differentiated tubular adenocarcinoma with abundant fibrous stroma and variable mucin-secreting ability (Fig. 54.3). The tumor penetrates lymphatic vessels and regional lymph nodes, portal vessels, and adjacent neural tissues. Despite advances in biliary imaging, the treatment results of cholangiocarcinoma have not improved substantially.

Tumor of the gallbladder

Tumor of the gallbladder is the most common biliary tract cancer in the Western world. Gallbladder cancer occurs more frequently among women. Gallbladder stones, found among 75% of patients, are considered an important risk factor for gallbladder cancer. It is hypothesized that gallstones cause chronic trauma to and inflammation of the gallbladder mucosa, which induce dysplastic changes and carcinogenesis. Porcelain gallbladder is also associated with a high risk of infiltrative carcinoma of the gallbladder; some experts advocate prophylactic cholecystectomy for such patients. There appears to be a high incidence of an anomalous junction between the cystic duct and common bile duct among patients with gallbladder cancer. The malignant potential of benign lesions such as adenoma (gallbladder polyp) and adenomyoma is unconfirmed. No clear adenoma-

Atlas of Gastroenterology, 4th edition. Edited by Tadataka Yamada, David H. Alpers, Anthony N. Kalloo, Neil Kaplowitz, Chung Owyang, and Don W. Powell. © 2009 Blackwell Publishing, ISBN: 978-1-4051-6909-7

to-carcinoma sequence has been demonstrated as it has with colonic cancer.

At macroscopic examination the tumor is seen to produce diffuse thickening of the gallbladder wall. Fungating growth in the gallbladder lumen and infiltration of surrounding structures are commonly found. Most gallbladder cancers are mucin-secreting adenocarcinoma. Gallbladder cancer spreads by means of direct local invasion of the liver, duodenum, and colon. The common hepatic duct is often invaded by cancer that arises from the neck of the gallbladder or the Hartmann pouch and which mimics cholangiocarcinoma in clinical presentation. A presumptive diagnosis of chronic cholecystitis is often made at laparotomy. Only about 20% of patients with gallbladder cancer have a correct preoperative diagnosis. In total, 80% of tumors are considered unresectable at surgical exploration. The overall 5-year survival rate remains less than 5%. Benign tumors of the gallbladder are not uncommon. They are often detected incidentally during ultrasound examination of the abdomen for other reasons. In general, follow-up ultrasonography within 3–6 months is recommended for gallbladder polyps. If no enlargement is detected, cholecystectomy is unnecessary.

Periampullary tumors

Tumors of the papilla and ampulla of Vater are grouped together as periampullary tumors. The cause of periampullary cancer is unclear. The tumors appear as papillary growths in the periampullary region, which makes identification of the opening of the ampulla difficult (Fig. 54.4). Similar to other biliary tract cancers, periampullary cancers are adenocarcinoma. Periampullary tumor is considered a separate entity from carcinoma of the pancreas, with a much better prognosis. Because of the early presentation, most periampullary tumors are resectable and the postoperative survival rate is very high.

Clinical features

Patients with biliary tract cancers usually have vague symptoms such as anorexia, malaise, weight loss, and pain. Cholangiocarcinoma and gallbladder cancer cause jaundice when the confluence of the common hepatic duct or the common bile duct is obstructed. Intermittent jaundice is an early sign of periampullary cancer. In complete biliary obstruction, urine turns dark and stool turns pale. Unlike choledocholithiasis or benign biliary strictures, cholangitis is an uncommon presenting feature of cholangiocarcinoma. Sepsis of the biliary tract usually occurs only after endoscopic or radiological intervention. Cholangitis is distinctly more common with periampullary cancer. Periampullary cancer occasion-

ally ulcerates and causes frank gastrointestinal bleeding or iron-deficiency anemia. A mass can be palpated in the right upper quadrant in some cases of gallbladder cancer.

Diagnosis

An initial ultrasound or computed tomographic (CT) scan provides valuable information about the level of obstruction and invasion of adjacent structures. In cholangiocarcinoma, dilated intrahepatic ducts proximal to the tumor and a normal or collapsed gallbladder are usually seen (Figs 54.5 and 54.6). Segmental or lobar atrophy of the liver resulting from portal vein or bile duct occlusion is an important finding on CT scans, because it might affect decisions about surgical resection and biliary drainage. A complex mass shadow in the region of the gallbladder or an intralumenal mass with thickened wall is highly suggestive of gallbladder cancer (Fig. 54.7). A low-density area of the liver adjacent to the tumor may imply local invasion. Periampullary cancers are usually too small to be detected with ultrasonography or CT scanning. Dilation of the common bile duct that extends to the most distal end and distention of the gallbladder suggest periampullary tumor. Endoscopic ultrasonography (EUS) is considered to be the most sensitive test in detecting small periampullary tumor (Fig. 54.8).

Cholangiography is the most accurate method for delineating the extent of tumor involvement and defining segmental ducts. The choice of cholangiography lies between magnetic resonance cholangiopancreatography (MRCP), percutaneous transhepatic cholangiography (PTC), and endoscopic retrograde cholangiopancreatography (ERCP). MRCP is the preferred choice for diagnosis (Fig. 54.9). PTC and ERCP should be considered as therapeutic procedures. A cholangiogram that shows dilated intrahepatic ducts with a normal common bile duct suggests cholangiocarcinoma (Figs 54.10 and 54.11). Gallbladder cancer may cause extrinsic compression or direct invasion into the common bile duct (Fig. 54.12). Patients with periampullary tumors have a distended gallbladder and dilated ductal system up to the level of the distal common bile duct.

A definitive diagnosis of biliary cancer rests on histological or cytological proof of malignant growth. Fine-needle aspiration cytological examination guided by ultrasound or CT scanning often confirms the diagnosis of gallbladder cancer. Unfortunately, a mass is seldom detected in bile duct cancer, making direct aspiration difficult. Brush cytological specimens can be obtained at ERCP or PTC (Fig. 54.13). The sensitivity of brush cytological examination ranges from 35% to 70%, depending on the type and location of tumor, method of brushing, and experience of the cytologist. On the other hand, endoscopic biopsy of the ampulla provides good tissue samples for histological diagnosis. Biopsy after endoscopic sphincterotomy may further improve the diagnostic yield. EUS-guided fine-needle aspiration is shown to have high sensitivity and accuracy in differentiating benign from malignant disease, and has a significant impact on patient management.

Angiography is important in assessing the resectability of a tumor. It shows a nonvascular mass in the biliary tract that is nonspecific for the diagnosis. The main purpose of angiography is to exclude invasion of the blood vessels and major arterial anatomic variants.

Treatment

The two objectives in the treatment of patients with biliary tract cancer are to cure the patient of the tumor or to relieve bile duct obstruction by means of establishing biliary–enteric drainage. Resection of the proximal bile duct (with or without hepatic resection) and reconstruction by means of hepaticojejunostomy is the standard procedure for the management of cholangiocarcinoma. Patients with complete resection of tumor and histologically verified tumor-free margins have a satisfactory chance of survival. Cholangiocarcinoma is not considered suitable for transplantation at most centers. Most cases of resectable gallbladder cancer are found incidentally at cholecystectomy. In confirmed cases of gallbladder cancer, cholecystectomy with resection of the liver and dissection of lymph nodes and hepatoduodenal ligament is recommended. In these cases, survival is good. The Whipple procedure is widely accepted as therapy for periampullary cancer, although some surgeons claim that local resection is sufficient. The outcome among these patients is the best among all tumors of the biliary tract.

Palliative treatment is aimed at relieving the obstruction of bile flow to preserve liver function and metabolism. It can be achieved with endoscopic–radiological drainage of the bile ducts or surgical biliary–enteric bypass. Successful endoscopic insertion of a biliary endoprosthesis can be achieved in 80%–90% of cases (Fig. 54.14) and results in normalization of bilirubin levels in the blood. Endoscopic stenting results in lower immediate mortality and morbidity rates and shorter hospital stays, and thus is less expensive. However, the long-term results of surgical bypass are better than those of endoscopic drainage. The latter is associated with recurrent cholangitis in subsequent months. For proximal bile duct obstruction, the success of endoscopic stenting is reduced, and higher procedural complication rates and lower rates of resolution of jaundice occur. Percutaneous drainage is a better option. The plastic stents in current use tend to clog as a result of bacterial colonization and sludge formation on the stent.

Self-expanding metallic stents have been developed to avoid early clogging of endoprostheses. The Wallstent endoprosthesis (Schneider, Minneapolis, MN), which opens to a much larger diameter in the bile duct than a plastic stent, allows good drainage of bile (Fig. 54.15). The metal mesh of this stent also facilitates drainage of segmental bile ducts in proximal cholangiocarcinoma. Tumor ingrowth may still cause obstruction to bile flow within a period of 6–9 months (Fig. 54.16). The obstruction can be relieved by insertion of a plastic stent into the metal stent to resume bile drainage. A metal stent designed to drain tumor involving bifurcation of the bile duct has been developed (Fig. 54.17). There is little evidence to support the use of radiation therapy and chemotherapy in the palliation of biliary tract cancers.

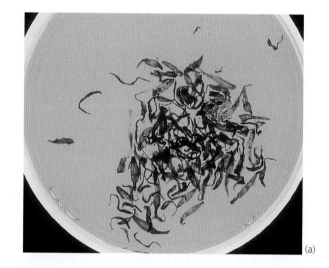
(a)

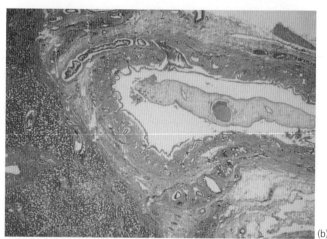
(b)

Figure 54.1 *Clonorchis sinensis* infestation. **(a)** Liver flukes extracted from the bile of a patient with cholangiocarcinoma. **(b)** Liver fluke in the bile duct causing chronic inflammation and ductal injury.

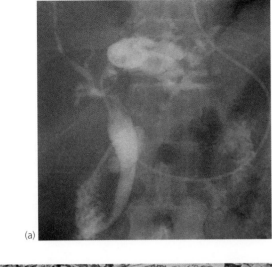

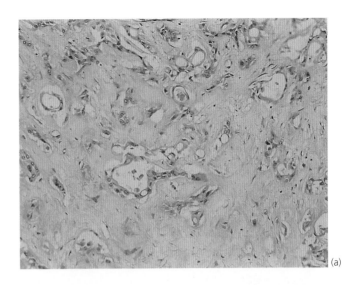

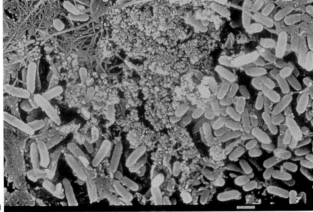

Figure 54.2 Intrahepatic pigment stones. **(a)** Intrahepatic ductal dilation and stone impaction in the left hepatic duct of a patient with bile duct cancer. **(b)** Bacteria inside the pigment stones.

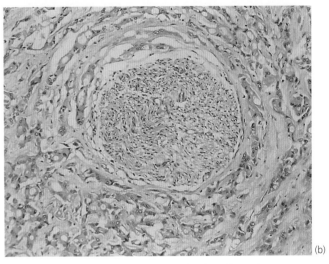

Figure 54.3 Cholangiocarcinoma. **(a)** Cholangiocarcinoma is adenocarcinoma with abundant fibrosis. **(b)** Perineural infiltration by cholangiocarcinoma.

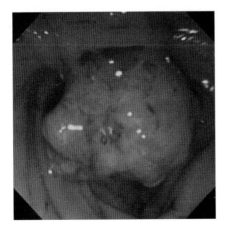

Figure 54.4 Periampullary cancer. Papillary growth of periampullary cancer obscures the opening of the ampulla.

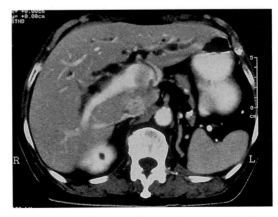

Figure 54.5 Computed tomographic scan demonstrates intrahepatic ductal dilation with tumor invasion in the portal vein.

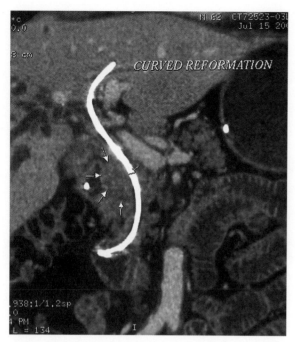

Figure 54.6 Curved reformation computed tomographic scan image shows a circumferential but eccentric tumor at the upper common bile duct that has invaded the adjacent pancreas and duodenal wall (arrows). Despite the insertion of the biliary stent, the right intrahepatic ductal system is not decompressed suggesting segmental infiltration.

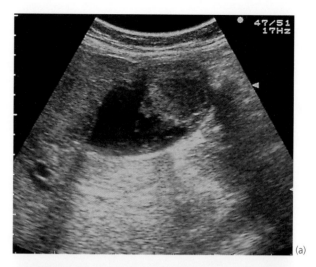
(a)

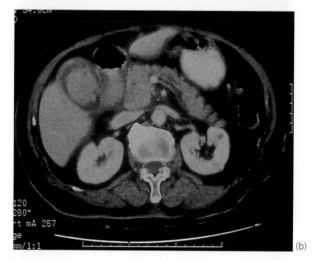
(b)

Figure 54.7 Cancer of the gallbladder. **(a)** Ultrasound scan shows a complex mass in the gallbladder. **(b)** Computed tomographic scan shows tumor filling the lumen of the gallbladder.

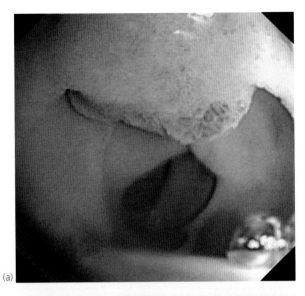

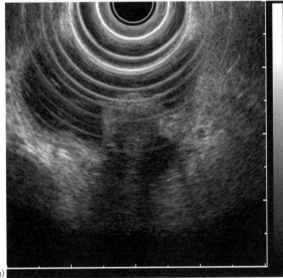

Figure 54.8 (a) Endoscopic view shows mild bulging of the papilla. **(b)** Endoscopic ultrasonography showing a small ampullary tumor under the surface.

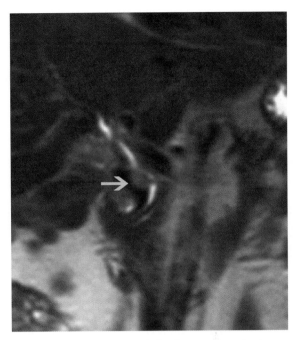

Figure 54.9 Magnetic resonance cholangiopancreatography shows a mid common bile duct stricture (arrow) due to tumor.

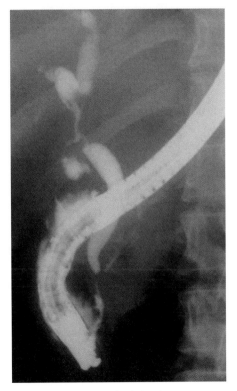

Figure 54.10 Endoscopic retrograde cholangiopancreatogram shows a stricture at the common hepatic duct and a normal-sized common bile duct.

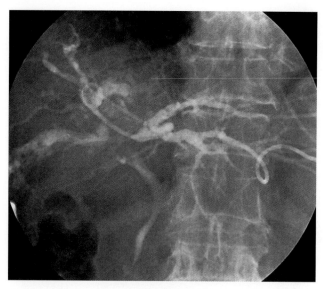

Figure 54.11 Percutaneous transhepatic cholangiogram shows a bile duct cancer at the confluence causing proximal ductal obstruction. A pigtail catheter is inserted for drainage.

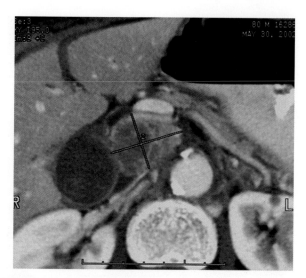

Figure 54.12 Computed tomography shows a tumor arising from the neck of the gallbladder that has invaded the common bile duct.

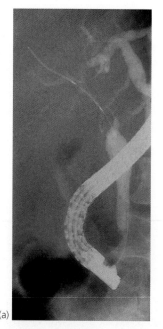

(a)

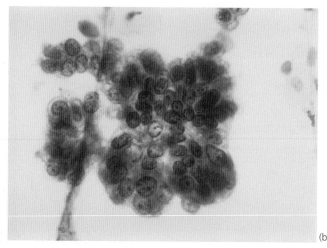

(b)

Figure 54.13 Brush cytological examination. **(a)** A cytological brush is inserted through the endoscope into the proximal biliary tract. **(b)** The presence of malignant cells confirms the diagnosis of bile duct cancer.

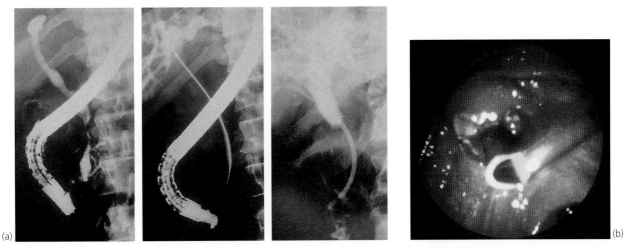

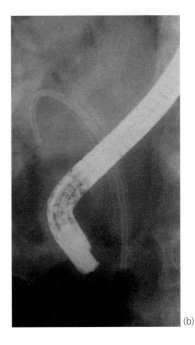

Figure 54.14 Endoscopic stenting. **(a)** Endoscopic insertion of a polyethylene stent to manage distal bile duct cancer. **(b)** Good drainage of bile after stenting.

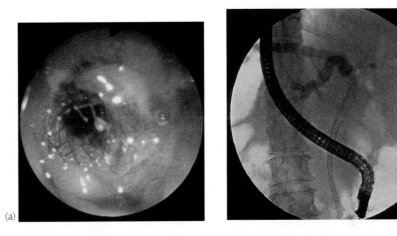

Figure 54.15 Wallstent endoprosthesis for drainage of bile duct cancer. **(a)** Endoscopic view shows mesh wire extending into the duodenum. **(b)** The metallic stent opens the lumen in instances of biliary stricture.

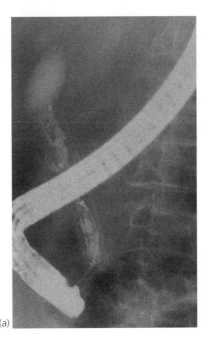

Figure 54.16 Blockage of a Wallstent endoprosthesis. **(a)** Tumor ingrowth in a Wallstent causing recurrent biliary obstruction. **(b)** A plastic stent is inserted inside the Wallstent to resume the drainage of bile.

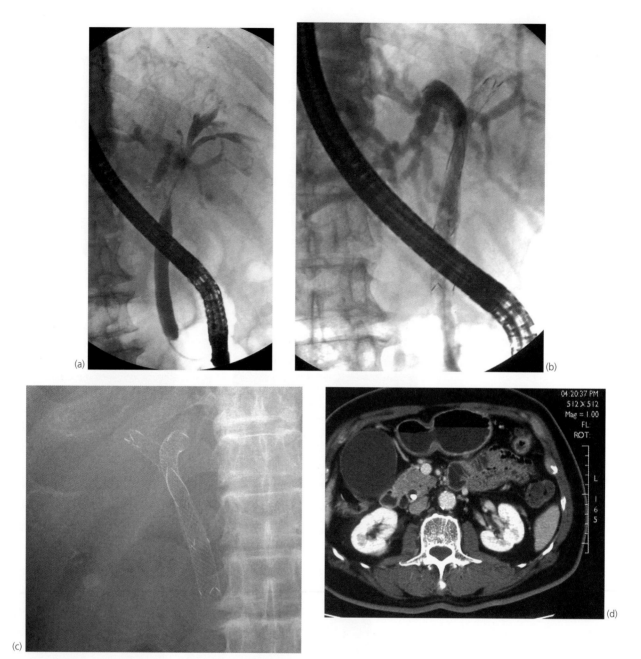

Figure 54.17 Metallic stent for malignant stricture at bifurcation of the bile duct. The larger (common bile duct) stent has a space in the midportion that allows a smaller (intrahepatic) stent to go through. **(a)** Cholangiogram showing a stricture at the common hepatic duct and intrahepatic branches. **(b)** Self-expanding metallic stents were inserted to bypass the strictures. **(c)** Two metallic stents, one draining the left hepatic duct and one draining the right hepatic ducts, are shown on this abdominal film. **(d)** Computed tomography of the abdomen shows a tumor arising from the head of both the body and tail of the pancreas.

55

Liver: anatomy, microscopic structure, and cell types

Gary C. Kanel

Embryology

The hepatic primordium anlage first appears towards the end of the third week of gestation and is seen as a hollow midline outgrowth stalk (hepatic diverticulum). By the fourth week the diverticulum enlarges by proliferation of the endodermal cell strands (hepatoblasts) and projects cranially into the mesoderm of the septum transversum, eventually giving rise to the hepatic parenchyma and intrahepatic duct structures.

The vascular network is originally derived from the development of both the vitelline and umbilical veins. The hepatic cords and vessels anastomose, forming the hepatic sinusoids. By week 5 most of the major vessels are identified, including the right and left umbilical veins, the transverse portal sinus, and the ductus venosus. The portal vein develops from the vitelline vein and then subdivides into the right and left branches.

The biliary apparatus develops from membranous infoldings occurring between the junctional complexes of adjacent hepatoblasts and appears initially as intercellular spaces with no distinct wall. A ductal plate develops from the hepatoblasts immediately adjacent to the portal mesenchyme, eventually forming an anastomosing network of portal duct structures.

Gross anatomy

The liver extends from the right lateral aspect of the abdomen 15–20 cm transversely towards the xiphoid. The weight of the adult liver varies from 1200 to 1800 g, depending on the overall body size. Anatomically it has four lobes: right, left, caudate, and quadrate. The right and left lobes are divided

by a line extending from the inferior vena cava superiorly to the middle of the gallbladder fossa inferiorly. A total of eight functional segments are present, each demarcated by their vascular and biliary drainage.

The portal vein is formed through the merger of the superior mesenteric and splenic veins. The hepatic vein is composed of three major tributaries (right, middle, and left), while the hepatic artery ascends along the hepatoduodenal ligament and eventually divides into the right and left main branches.

The biliary drainage of the right lobe is derived from anterior and posterior segmental branches that merge to form the right hepatic duct. Lateral and medial segmental branches merge to form the left hepatic duct, which drains the left lobe.

Microanatomy

The portal tract contains one to two interlobular bile ducts that are usually seen adjacent to the hepatic arterioles, the latter responsible for their blood supply. The portal venule is a single vascular structure. The fibrous tissue, which supports the major portal components, varies in amount depending on the distance of the portal tract from the hepatic hilum. The hepatic lobules are composed predominantly of liver cell cords one cell thick. The adjacent sinusoids are lined by both endothelial and Kupffer cells, whereas the perisinusoidal space, located between the endothelial cells and hepatocytes, contains stellate cells and collagen fibers.

The hepatocytes average from 25 to 40 μm in diameter and are polyhedral and multifaceted. The cells have three distinct cell boundaries: sinusoidal, lateral (intercellular), and canalicular membranes. The liver cell nucleus is centrally located within the hepatocyte and measures approximately 10 μm in diameter.

The liver cell cytoplasm contains numerous functionally important organelles. The superstructure is maintained by the cytoskeleton of the hepatocyte, which includes three major subdivisions: microfilaments, microtubules, and

Atlas of Gastroenterology, 4th edition. Edited by Tadataka Yamada, David H. Alpers, Anthony N. Kalloo, Neil Kaplowitz, Chung Owyang, and Don W. Powell. © 2009 Blackwell Publishing, ISBN: 978-1-4051-6909-7

intermediate filaments. The numerous mitochondria maintain critical functions such as oxidative phosphorylation and fatty acid oxidation and also contain components that are essential for the urea and citric acid cycles. The endoplasmic reticulum (ER) is composed of a convoluted network of cisternae, saccules, tubules, and vesicles and is divided into two components, the rough ER and the smooth ER. The Golgi apparatus is composed of highly polarized parallel flattened dilated saccules or vesicles. Lysosomes appear as electron-dense pleomorphic single membrane-bound vesicles containing various enzymes such as acid phosphatase, esterases, proteases, and lipases.

The Kupffer cells are sinusoidal lining cells that function as tissue macrophages. The endothelial cells are flattened elongated sinusoidal cells. Numerous cytoplasmic projections and clustered fenestrae or gaps that range in size from 0.1 to 0.2 μm are present. The stellate cells are located within the perisinusoidal liver cell recesses along the space of Disse and often contain variably sized lipid droplets that carry a high concentration of vitamin A (retinol palmitate). The space of Disse lies between the hepatocytes and the endothelial cells.

The stroma overall supports the basic hepatic architectural arrangement and is composed of five basic types of collagen. Types I and III represent more than 95% of the total collagen, type I representing mature collagen strands and type III representing new collagen (reticulin fibers).

The biliary tract can be divided into its structural components, the smallest of which are the biliary canaliculi, which are located along the intercellular spaces between hepatocytes and are lined by microvilli. The canaliculi that enter the portal tracts, labeled the terminal ductules or ducts of Hering, are derived from hepatocytes located at the limiting plate and communicate with the interlobular bile ducts. The interlobular bile ducts within the smaller portal structures are lined by a single layer of cuboidal cells, whereas the larger interlobar and septal ducts have a fibrous wall and are lined by a single layer of cuboidal to columnar epithelium. These lead into the segmental ducts, eventually forming the major hilar ducts that ultimately branch into the main right and left hepatic ducts.

The major blood vessels that supply the liver are the portal vein and the hepatic artery. The portal vein sequentially develops interlobar, segmental, and interlobular veins, and preterminal branches. The terminal portal venules are seen in the smaller triangular portal tracts. The hepatic artery branches accompany the portal vein and divide within the smaller portal tracts into the periportal plexus and the peribiliary plexus, which supply blood to the accompanying interlobular bile ducts through small capillaries that are layered around the ducts.

The hepatic acinus can be divided into three segments: simple, complex, and acinar agglomerate. The simple acinus is the smallest functional parenchymal unit and centers on a portal tract. The acinus is divided into three zones (zones of Rappaport): periportal (zone 1), which includes the limiting plate; midzone (zone 2); and perivenular (zone 3), with the terminal hepatic venule at its outer lateral margin. The complex acinus is derived from three adjacent simple acini fed by a preterminal portal vein and arterial branch. The acinar agglomerate is composed of approximately four complex acini and is fed by a portal venous branch.

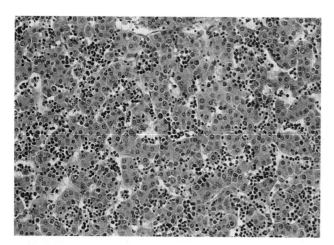

Figure 55.1 Embryonic development of the hepatic lobule. Extramedullary hematopoiesis is prominent in the hepatic lobules, begins at approximately 6 weeks, and is most active during the sixth and seventh months of gestation.

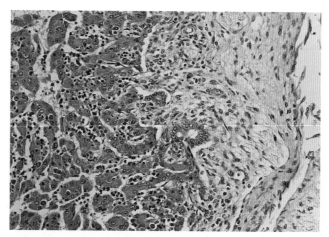

Figure 55.2 Embryonic development of the duct plate. Duct plates form by invasion of hepatoblasts into the portal mesenchyme.

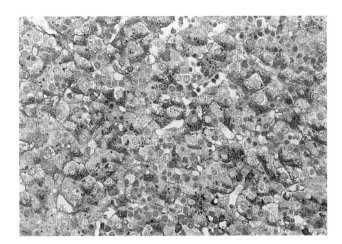

Figure 55.3 α-Fetoprotein during embryonic development. This protein, which is present at high concentration at birth, is initially identified in the liver at 1 month of gestation.

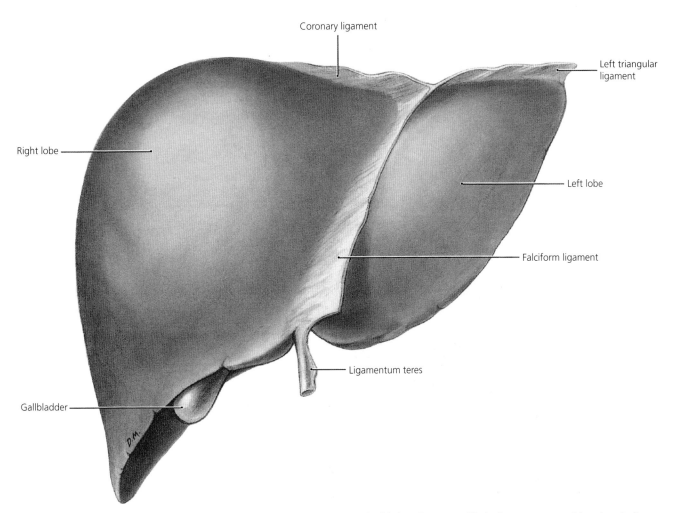

Figure 55.4 Anterior surface of the liver. The right and left lobes are divided by the falciform ligament, with the ligamentum teres lying along its free edge.

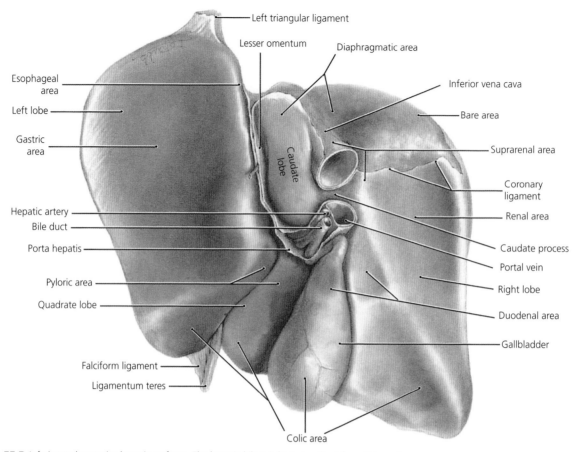

Figure 55.5 Inferior and posterior hepatic surfaces. The hepatic hilum is best visualized from this angle.

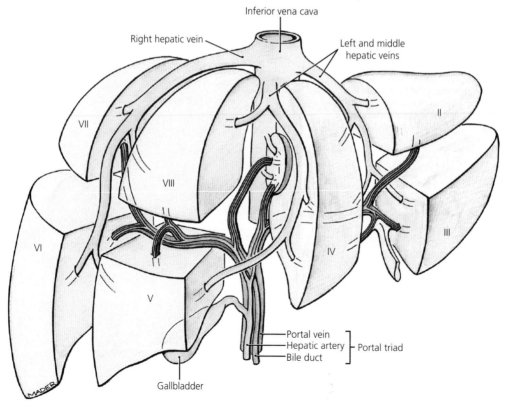

Figure 55.6 Segmental and vascular hepatic components. The eight functional components are demarcated by their vascular supply and biliary drainage.

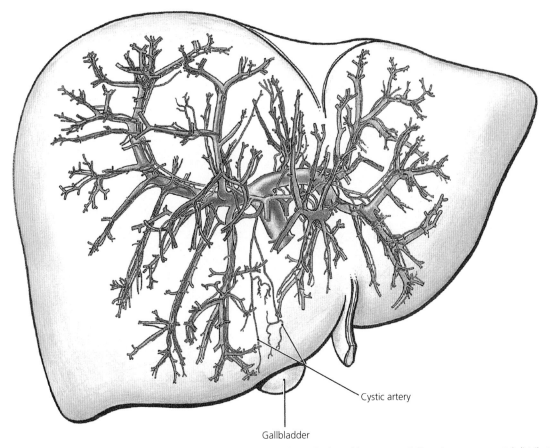

Cystic artery

Gallbladder

Figure 55.7 Intrahepatic network of the portal vein, hepatic artery, and bile duct. The branching patterns follow along a segmental distribution.

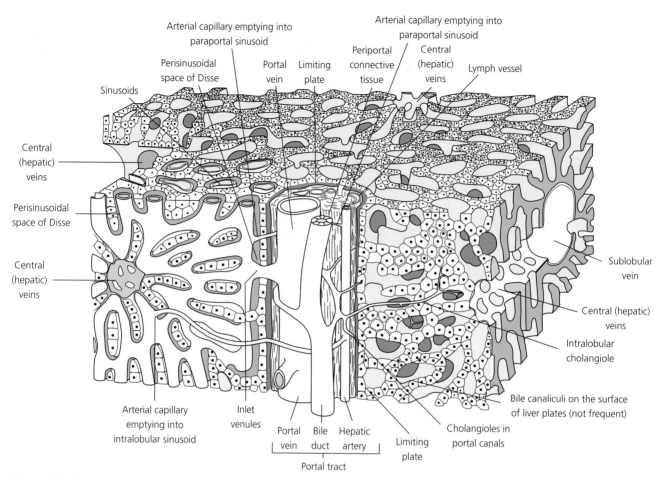

Figure 55.8 The structure of the normal liver.

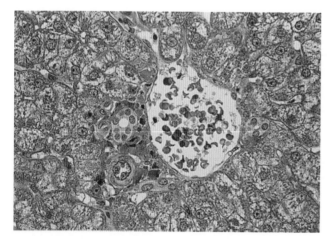

Figure 55.9 Portal tract (Masson trichrome stain). The major components include the hepatic arteriole, portal venule (large vessel), and bile ductule (cuboidal epithelium). There is a normal amount of collagen seen in this portal tract.

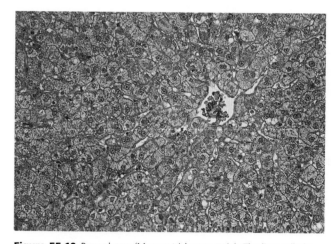

Figure 55.10 Parenchyma (Masson trichrome stain). The liver cell plates are one cell thick and are divided by sinusoids lined by Kupffer and endothelial cells, with vascular outflow via the terminal hepatic venule. No sinusoidal collagen deposition is appreciated on light microscopy in the normal liver.

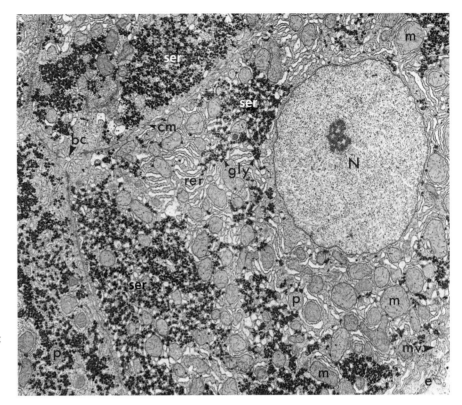

Figure 55.11 Hepatocyte (electron microscopic image). The hepatocyte is composed of a single nucleus (N). The cytoplasm demonstrates many mitochondria (m), rough (rer) and smooth (ser) endoplasmic reticulum, glycogen (gly), and peroxisomes (p). Also seen are the cell membrane (cm), a bile canaliculus (bc), endothelium (e), and microvilli (mv).

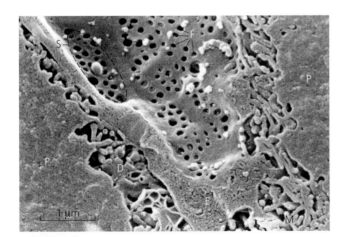

Figure 55.12 Scanning electron micrograph of the hepatic sinusoid. Numerous fenestrae (F), which are grouped into sieve plates (S), are demonstrated. D, space of Disse; E, endothelial cell; M, microvilli; P, parenchymal cell.

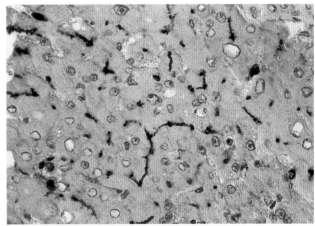

Figure 55.13 Biliary canaliculi (immunoperoxidase stain). Polyclonal carcinoembryonic antigen stains biliary glycoprotein and is useful in demonstrating the biliary canalicular network.

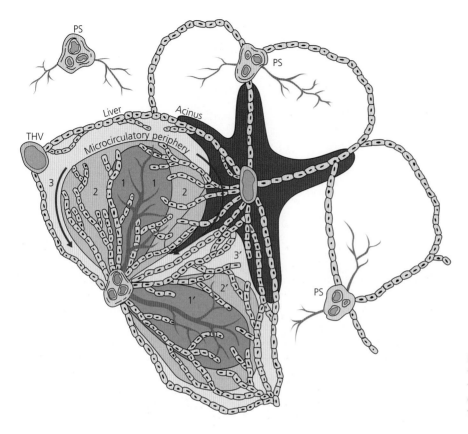

Figure 55.14 The simple liver acinus. The three hepatic zones and their relationship to the microcirculatory blood supply are demonstrated. PS, portal structures; THV, terminal hepatic venule.

56

Acute viral hepatitis

Marc G. Ghany, T. Jake Liang

Acute viral hepatitis is a syndrome characterized by a constellation of clinical, biochemical, and pathological features following primary infection of the liver by viruses that cause injury to hepatocytes. Five hepatotrophic viruses, hepatitis A, B, C, D, and E viruses, account for over 90% of cases. The hepatotrophic viruses are found worldwide (see Figs 56.1–56.5); the prevalence varies greatly from region to region and their individual distribution is partly dependent on their mode of transmission. Hepatitis A virus (HAV) and hepatitis E virus (HEV) are transmitted enterically, whereas hepatitis B, C, and D viruses (HBV, HCV, and HDV) are transmitted via percutaneous/permucosal routes. The liver is the primary site of infection and replication of hepatotrophic viruses. Four (HAV, HCV, HDV, and HEV) are single-stranded RNA viruses; HBV is a partially double-stranded DNA virus.

The genomic organization of HAV is shown in Figure 56.6. The replication process of HAV has been inferred from studies of other picornaviruses. Entry of the virus into the host is mediated by a cell surface receptor, which has been proposed to be a mucin-like class 1 integral membrane glycoprotein. Viral entry is followed by uncoating and initiation of viral protein synthesis. Viral RNA synthesis proceeds from negative to positive strand and occurs in the cytoplasm. Viral assembly follows a sequence similar to that of picornaviruses in a cellular membrane compartment.

The infectious HBV virion (Dane particle) has a 42-nm spherical, double-shelled structure consisting of a lipid envelope containing the hepatitis B surface antigen (HBsAg), which surrounds an inner nucleocapsid. The hepatitis B core antigen (HBcAg) complexes with the viral-encoded polymerase and viral DNA genome to form the nucleocapsid. The genome of the hepatitis B virus is a partially double-stranded circular DNA of approximately 3.2 kilobase pairs (kbp). The viral genome encodes four overlapping open reading frames (ORF) from which four mRNA transcripts are derived, coding for seven viral proteins (see Fig. 56.7 for details). HBV replicates through a RNA intermediate and this process is summarized in Figure 56.8.

HCV has a positive-sense, single-stranded RNA genome of approximately 9.6 kb in length with a single large ORF and highly conserved untranslated regions (UTR) at the 5' and 3' ends. The genomic organization is summarized in Figure 56.9. HCV replicates in the cytoplasm, presumably in a membrane-associated compartment. The replication process is illustrated in Figure 56.10.

HDV requires coinfection with HBV for replication. Delta antigen is the inner ribonucleoprotein component of a subviral particle that is enveloped by HBsAg. The ribonucleoprotein complex consists of small (SHDAg) and large (LHDAg) delta antigens and a single-stranded circular RNA genome of 1.7 kb in length that has extensive self-complementarity, allowing it to form a rod-like structure (Fig. 56.11). The antigenome is synthesized from the genomic RNA and is the template for synthesis of HDV mRNA, which encodes the delta antigens. The antigenome also serves as the template for genome synthesis. The HDV genome utilizes host RNA polymerase II to carry out RNA-directed RNA synthesis, which is dependent on the small delta antigen. Both genomic and antigenomic RNAs possess ribozyme activity, which catalyzes RNA self-cleavage and self-ligation. Transcription and replication are integrated into a single process using a double rolling-circle mechanism. After entry into cells, the HDV genome serves as a template for replication, resulting in the production of multimeric antigenomes. Nascent antigenomes, through their intrinsic ribozyme activity, form circular monomeric RNAs, which in turn serve as templates for the production of HDV genomes. Alternatively, the elongating product can be cleaved and released as polyadenylated mRNA, which then directs delta antigen synthesis. HDV assembly begins with the association of the delta antigens with the newly synthesized genome to yield a ribonucleoprotein complex (RNP). The RNP is transported from the nucleus to the cytoplasm, presumably mediated by the nucleocytoplasmic shuttling function of delta antigens.

Atlas of Gastroenterology, 4th edition. Edited by Tadataka Yamada, David H. Alpers, Anthony N. Kalloo, Neil Kaplowitz, Chung Owyang, and Don W. Powell. © 2009 Blackwell Publishing, ISBN: 978-1-4051-6909-7

The LHDAg of the RNP interacts with HBsAg to facilitate assembly, whereas the SHDAg is copackaged but not required for particle formation.

The HEV genome is a single-stranded, positive-sense RNA of approximately 7.5 kb. The genome is organized into three overlapping ORF flanked by noncoding regions (Fig. 56.12). Replication of HEV has not been characterized. The mechanisms of viral attachment, entry, and uncoating are unknown.

During primary infection, the initial pathway of the antiviral immune response is largely unknown. Initial viral infection is associated with activation of innate immunity in the liver. Recognition of infected hepatocytes by resident natural killer (NK) and natural killer T (NKT) cells leads to activation of these cells and induction of antiviral cytokines including interferons. This phase of innate immunity leads to the initial control of viral replication. As this antiviral response is likely to be associated with a noncytopathic mechanism, little or no hepatocellular injury is evident. The innate immunity also plays a critical role in the activation of adaptive immunity including humoral and cellular responses. Induction of a humoral immune response with production of neutralizing antibodies prevents viral spread and leads to subsequent elimination of circulating viruses. For HBV, the antibody response to the envelope proteins is a T cell-dependent process (Fig. 56.13).

The other limb of the immune response, cell-mediated immunity (CMI), is critical for the long-term control of viral infections including hepatitis virus infections. In acute HBV infection, individuals can mount a vigorous, multispecific, and polyclonal cellular immune response to HBV. In contrast, chronically infected patients have a weak or barely detectable anti-HBV response. This is true for both CD4 and CD8 responses. During acute hepatitis B, a vigorous human leukocyte antigen (HLA) class II-restricted CD4$^+$ helper T cell response to multiple epitopes of HBc/eAg predominates in virtually all patients. By helping B cells to produce neutralizing antienvelope antibodies and activating HBV-specific cytotoxic T lymphocytes (CTLs), this CD4$^+$ T helper population may direct the initial antiviral response.

In most viral infections, the activation of virus-specific CD8+ CTLs is critical for viral clearance. Patients acutely infected with HBV develop a strong polyclonal HLA class I-restricted CTL response that is directed against multiple epitopes in all viral proteins. This response appears to persist for many years after recovery from acute HBV infection.

The molecular and cellular mechanisms of viral clearance and hepatocellular injury have been elucidated for HBV infection (see Fig. 56.13). CD8+ HLA class I-restricted HBsAg-specific CTLs target the liver through interaction between the HBV-specific T-cell receptors and the antigen-presenting HLA class I molecules on the hepatocytes and cause scattered apoptosis of hepatocytes. By secreting cytokines, including interferons, the CTLs recruit a variety of antigen-nonspecific inflammatory cells into the liver, resulting in more extensive necroinflammatory injury of the liver. The predominant infiltrating effector cells are the macrophages, which probably mediate most of the hepatocellular injury. The CTLs, although not primarily responsible for the majority of hepatocellular injury, initiate the cascade of immunological events leading to hepatitis. They also play a role in elimination of infected hepatocytes through noncytolytic inhibition of HBV gene expression and viral replication. The detection of virus-specific CD4 and CD8 cells in the peripheral blood and liver of chronically infected individuals suggests a pathogenic relationship between the indolent cellular immune response and necroinflammatory liver disease associated with chronic hepatitis. Therefore, the CMI is a double-edged sword: vigorous response leads to viral clearance, whereas ineffective response results in chronic hepatocellular injury.

Following infection, the hepatotrophic viruses give rise to similar clinical, biochemical, and pathological features. Serological testing is the only reliable way to determine the infecting agent (see Figs 56.14–56.19). The incubation period differs for each virus, ranging from 2 weeks to 6 months. The clinical course ranges from an asymptomatic illness to fulminant hepatitis and is typified by three phases, prodromal, symptomatic, and convalescent, lasting from 6 weeks to 6 months. Approximately 20% of cases present with jaundice. The primary biochemical abnormality is an acute rise in serum alanine and asparate aminotransferases, markers of hepatocellular necrosis, to greater than 2.5 times the upper limit of normal and more commonly to greater than 10 times the upper limit of normal. The basic pathological lesion is an acute inflammation of the entire liver. The severity can range from mild, involving a few hepatocytes, to moderate, to massive necrosis, involving almost all hepatocytes (see Figs 56.20–56.22). The classic pathological features of acute viral hepatitis are swollen hepatocytes, apoptotic hepatocytes (acidophil bodies), and the presence of inflammatory cells within the hepatic lobule, predominantly lymphocytes and macrophages, which result in distortion of the normal liver architecture.

HAV and HEV do not lead to chronic infection, and development of antibody protects against reinfection for HAV. HBV, HCV, and HDV have the propensity to cause chronic infection and are associated with an increased risk of hepatocellular carcinoma. Effective and safe vaccines exist for the prevention of infection with HAV and HBV and are recommended in the pre- and postexposure setting and for persons with non-A non-B (NANB)-related chronic liver disease. Institution of risk-behavior modifications is the only effective way to prevent HDV superinfection in persons with chronic hepatitis B. No vaccine exists for HCV and strategies for preventing infection include screening of blood donors and risk-behavior modification. Improving hygiene and providing safe drinking water should lower the risk of HEV infection.

Treatment is supportive with the aim being to maintain adequate nutrition and hydration and to monitor for the development of fulminant hepatitis. Antiviral therapy is rarely indicated, especially for HAV and HEV, in which the course is benign and recovery the rule. Most adults with acute HBV infection recover spontaneously and, given the low response rate of current regimens, specific antiviral treatment is not currently advised. Household and sexual contacts of persons with acute HBV infection should receive hepatitis B immune globulin (HBIG) and HBV vaccine. Based on data indicating a high response rate to interferon therapy, it may be reasonable to treat patients with acute hepatitis C.

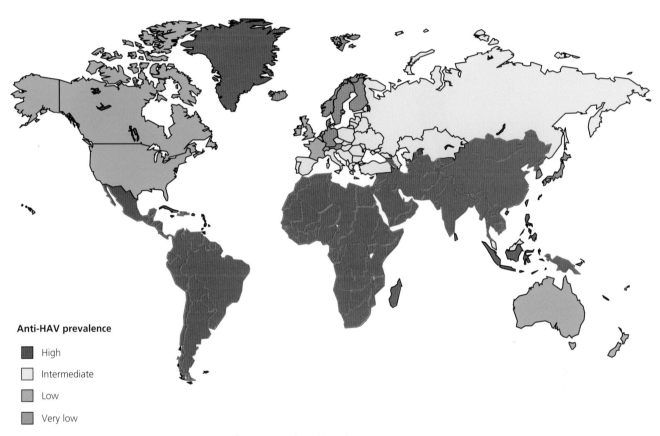

Anti-HAV prevalence

- High
- Intermediate
- Low
- Very low

Figure 56.1 Worldwide prevalence of hepatitis A infection. HAV, hepatitis A virus.

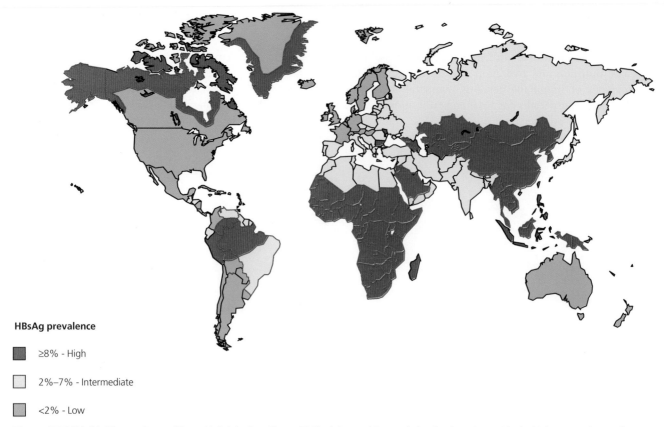

HBsAg prevalence

■ ≥8% - High

□ 2%–7% - Intermediate

■ <2% - Low

Figure 56.2 Worldwide prevalence of hepatitis B infection. Almost 50% of the world's population live in regions with the highest prevalence of hepatitis B virus infection, where 8%–20% of the population are hepatitis B surface antigen (HBsAg) positive. Another 40% of the global population live in areas with an intermediate prevalence, where 2%–7% of the population are positive for HBsAg.

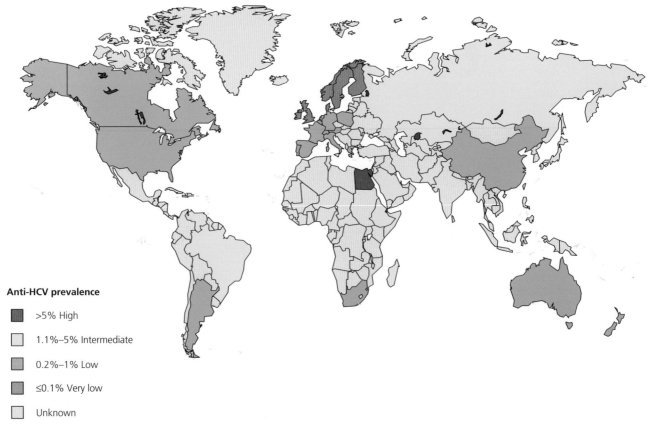

Anti-HCV prevalence

■ >5% High

□ 1.1%–5% Intermediate

■ 0.2%–1% Low

■ ≤0.1% Very low

□ Unknown

Figure 56.3 Worldwide prevalence of hepatitis C infection. Worldwide, the prevalence of anti-hepatitis C virus (HCV) is fairly consistent, ranging from 0.5% to 2%. Note areas of high prevalence in Egypt and Japan compared with the low prevalence in Northern Europe.

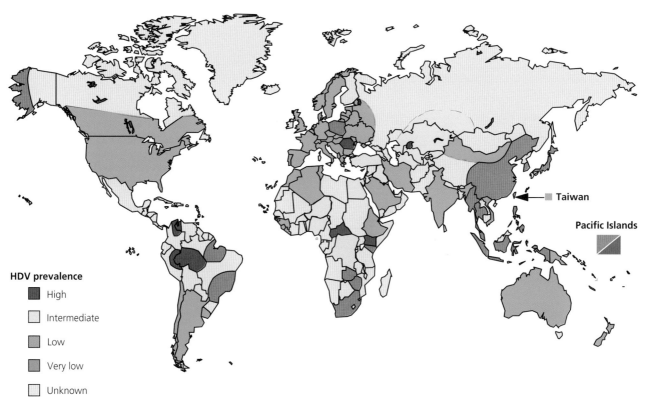

HDV prevalence

- High
- Intermediate
- Low
- Very low
- Unknown

Taiwan

Pacific Islands

Figure 56.4 Worldwide prevalence of hepatitis D infection. The prevalence of hepatitis D virus (HDV) mimics that of hepatitis B virus (HBV) because of its dependency on HBV for its life cycle. However, areas of discordance exist, such as China, where the rate of HDV infection is low but the rate of HBV infection is high. The reasons for this finding are not known.

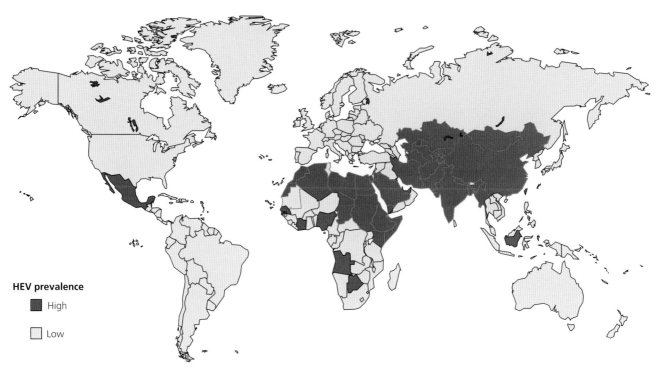

HEV prevalence

- High
- Low

Figure 56.5 Worldwide prevalence of hepatitis E infection. The prevalence of anti-hepatitis E virus (HEV) in the colored red areas is estimated to range from 2.5% to 25%. In the remaining areas, the prevalence of anti-HEV is estimated to range from 0% to 2.5%.

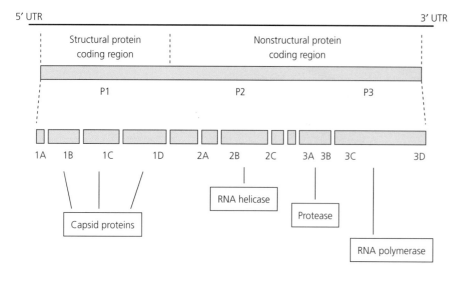

Figure 56.6 Structure of the hepatitis A virus and genetic organization. The top line represents the hepatitis A virus RNA genome. The hepatitis A virus has a linear, positive-sense, single-stranded RNA genome of approximately 7.5 kb. Translation of the genome yields a single polyprotein that can be divided into three main functional domains (P1, P2, and P3) from which the individual viral proteins are cleaved. P1 encodes the viral capsid proteins while P2 and P3 encode the nonstructural proteins. The lower diagram illustrates the three regions of the polyprotein and the individual protein products. Four capsid proteins designated 1A–1D are encoded in P1, with the P2 and P3 regions encoding proteins 2A–2C and 3A–3D respectively. UTR, untranslated region.

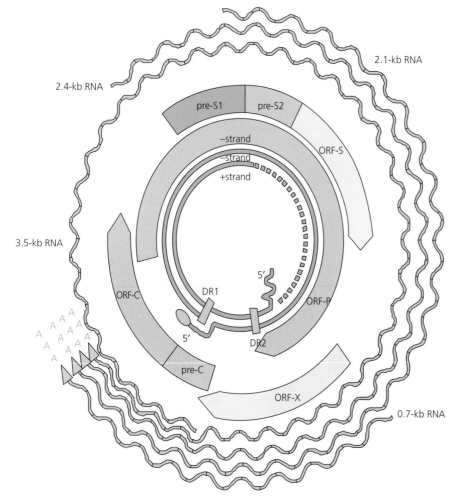

Figure 56.7 Genomic structure and organization of hepatitis B virus. The hepatitis B virus open reading frames (ORF) pre-C and C (precore and core proteins), P (polymerase protein), pre-S1, pre-S2, and S (L, M, and S surface envelope proteins), and X protein are shown. The viral genome structure is composed of the full-length (–)-DNA strand and the variable-length (+)-DNA strand (solid followed by dashed line). The polymerase protein is covalently attached to the 5' end of the (–) strand and a capped oligoribonucleotide (angulated line) to the (+) strand. Direct repeats (DR) 1 and 2 (small rectangular boxes) are shown on the genome. The outer lines represent the four transcripts all terminating at a common polyadenylation site. The S open reading frame encodes the viral surface envelope protein, hepatitis B surface antigen (HBsAg), and comprises the pre-S1, pre-S2, and S regions. The core gene consists of precore and core regions; separate initiation codons give rise to the hepatitis B e antigen and the viral nucleocapsid (HBcAg). The polymerase open reading frame P encodes the polymerase protein, which is involved in encapsidation and initiation of negative strand synthesis, possesses reverse transcriptase activity and catalyzes genome synthesis, and possesses RNAse H activity, which degrades pregenomic RNA and facilitates replication. The HBX protein is translated off the X transcript and is a viral protein with pleotrophic functions that plays an integral role in the viral life cycle.

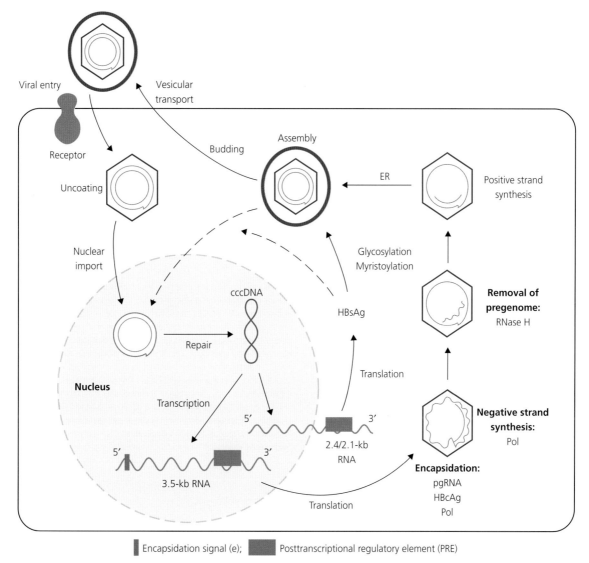

Encapsidation signal (e); Posttranscriptional regulatory element (PRE)

Figure 56.8 Replication of hepatitis B virus. Infectious virions probably attach to hepatocytes via the pre-S1 domain of the L protein. On entering, the nucleocapsid is delivered to the nucleus and the viral genome is repaired to the covalently closed circular form (cccDNA). Viral transcripts are translated in the cytoplasm, and the core and polymerase proteins interact with the genomic-length RNA to form the nucleocapsids. Reverse transcription occurs and the mature virions are assembled in the endoplasmic reticulum (ER), where they acquire the surface proteins. The virion is then secreted via vesicular transport. The encapsidation signal and posttranscriptional regulatory element on the hepatitis B virus transcripts are shown as rectangular boxes.

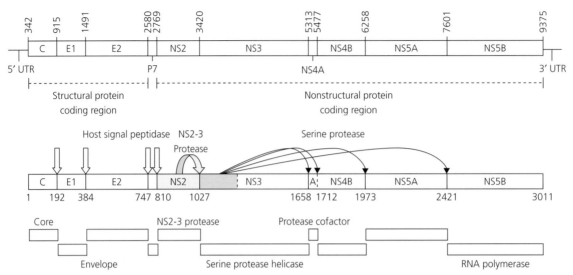

Figure 56.9 Genomic organization of hepatitis C virus (HCV). The 5' and 3' untranslated regions (UTR) flanking a polyprotein open reading frame are shown at the top. Numbering refers to the nucleotide positions of genes, based on the sequence of an HCV genotype 1a infectious clone. The HCV polyprotein of approximately 3000 amino acids is processed co- and posttranslationally by cellular and viral proteases to produce the individual gene products. Cellular proteases in the endoplasmic reticulum catalyze the cleavage of the structural proteins, whereas viral-encoded proteases cleave the nonstructural proteins. The middle panel shows HCV polyprotein processing with the cleavage sites of host signal peptidase (open arrows), NS2-3 protease (green arrow), and NS3 serine protease (thin arrows). Numbering denotes amino acid position upstream of cleavage sites. The processed HCV proteins are shown at the bottom. The highly conserved core protein is the putative viral nucleocapsid and encompasses the first 191 amino acids of the polyprotein. E1 and E2 are envelope glycoproteins with C-terminal hydrophobic transmembrane domains. The NS2 region encodes a metalloproteinase. The NS2-3 protease mediates autocatalytic cleavage between NS2 and NS3. The NS3 region encodes a multifunctional protein with an N-terminal serine protease and a C-terminal RNA helicase and nucleotide triphosphatase (NTPase). The NS3 protease, distinct from NS2-3 protease activity, is involved in processing the downstream polyprotein. NS4A interacts with and acts as a cofactor for the NS3 protease. The function of NS4B is unknown. NS5A may play a role in sensitivity to interferon. NS5B is the RNA-dependent RNA polymerase that mediates viral replication.

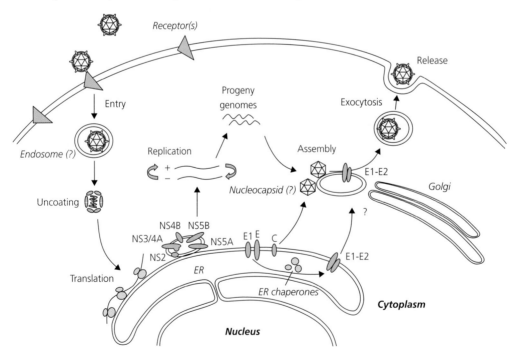

Figure 56.10 Replication of hepatitis C virus (HCV). The virion attaches and enters the susceptible cell via pathways that are not yet completely defined. The viral genome is then directed to a membranous component in the perinuclear endoplasmic reticulum (ER) region and serves as a template for hepatitis C virus protein synthesis. The nonstructural proteins form a replication complex with the genomic RNA and direct RNA replication (to negative and then positive strands). The structural proteins, which are retained in the ER, interact with the progeny genomes and assemble into virions. The virions are then secreted via an unknown exocytotic pathway, probably not passing through the Golgi compartment.

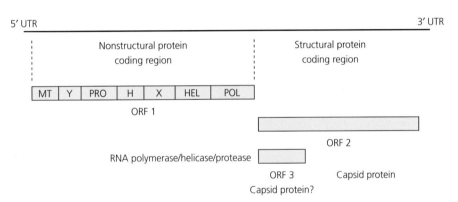

Figure 56.11 Genomic organization of hepatitis D virus (HDV). The RNA genome has a rod-like structure and contains an RNA editing and a self-cleavage site (circle). The antigenome is synthesized from the genomic RNA and is the template for hepatitis D virus mRNA encoding the delta antigens. The antigenome also serves as the template for genome synthesis. The estimated copy numbers of the RNA species in the infected liver are shown below.

Figure 56.12 Genomic organization of hepatitis E virus. The genome is organized into three overlapping open reading frames (ORFs) flanked by 5′ and 3′ noncoding regions and a 3′ polyadenylation signal. ORF 1 appears to encode the nonstructural gene products: MT (methyltransferase), X and Y (unknown functions), Pro (protease), Hel (helicase), H (proline-rich hinge region), and Pol (RNA-dependent RNA polymerase). ORF 2 codes for the capsid, and ORF 3 codes for a protein with possible nucleocapsid function. UTR, untranslated region.

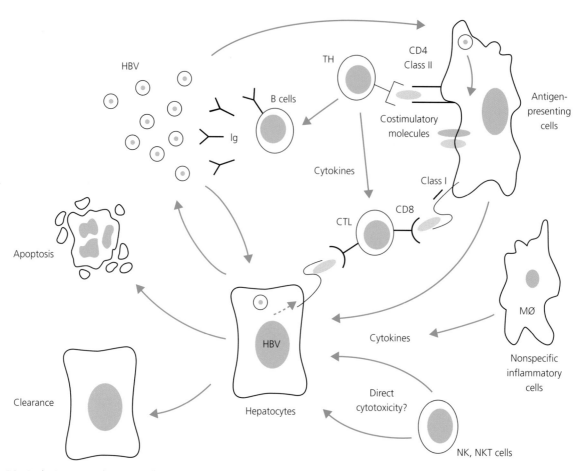

Figure 56.13 The immunopathogenesis of hepatitis B (see text for details). CTL, cytotoxic T lymphocyte; HBV, hepatitis B virus; NK, natural killer cell; NKT, natural killer T cell; TH, thymocyte.

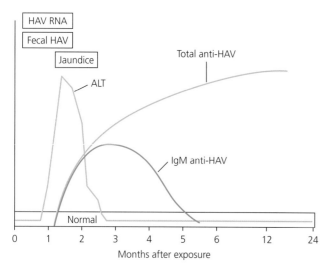

Figure 56.14 Serological course of acute hepatitis A. Hepatitis A virus (HAV) can be detected in stool before the onset of clinical symptoms by electron microscopy and polymerase chain reaction assays. Persons are therefore infectious during the incubation period. Levels of virus fall and become almost undetectable with the onset of symptoms and the peak of the alanine aminotransferase (ALT) level. Antibody to HAV (anti-HAV) first becomes detectable during this period. The initial antibody response is IgM anti-HAV; levels usually peak at 3 months following acute exposure and rapidly decline to undetectable by month 5 or 6. Occasionally IgM anti-HAV may remain detectable for up to 1 year or longer. IgG anti-HAV is also present at low levels during acute infection but levels rise as IgM anti-HAV levels begin to fall. IgG anti-HAV persists for life and confers protection against reinfection. Thus, diagnosis of acute hepatitis A rests on the demonstration of IgM anti-HAV in serum. IgG anti-HAV is a marker of past infection. One caveat: commercial assays for total anti-HAV measure both IgM and IgG and therefore are not helpful in diagnosing acute infection.

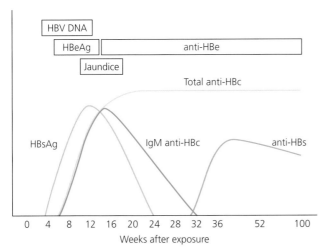

Figure 56.15 Serological course of acute hepatitis B. Diagnostic tests are available for most of the hepatitis B virus (HBV) antigens and corresponding antibodies. The presence or absence of each of these antigens and antibodies serologically defines the stage of illness as acute, chronic, or recovered. Detection of hepatitis B surface antigen (HBsAg) in serum is the serological hallmark of HBV infection. It usually appears in serum 1–10 weeks after acute exposure and 2–6 weeks before the onset of symptoms. It is detectable in both acute and chronic sera. Hepatitis B e antigen (HBeAg) is the next viral antigen to appear in serum soon after HBsAg. Its presence correlates with other markers of viral replication such as HBV DNA and it is a useful marker of infectivity. Hepatitis B core antigen (HBcAg) is not detectable in serum but can be demonstrated in liver tissue. With the onset of symptoms, HBeAg and HBV DNA levels may become undetectable and the level of HBsAg also begins to decline. HBsAg may persist in the convalescent phase but should disappear by 6 months. Antibody against HBcAg, anti-HBc, appears before the onset of symptoms. IgM anti-HBc is usually the first to appear and the titer peaks with the onset of symptoms but declines to undetectable levels within 6 months. IgG anti-HBc is also present during acute infection but, unlike IgM anti-HBc, remains elevated lifelong and is a marker of past infection. Thus, diagnosis of acute HBV infection is made by the demonstration of HBsAg and IgM anti-HBc in serum. During the convalescent phase, HBsAg disappears and antibodies to HBsAg, anti-HBs, appear. Therefore, loss of HBsAg and HBeAg and development of anti-HBs indicates recovery from acute infection and immunity against reinfection. Rarely, all markers of HBV infection, HBsAg, HBeAg, and HBV DNA, are cleared from serum before the development of anti-HBs. If testing is performed during this period, IgM anti-HBc may be the only marker to indicate HBV infection and this "serologically silent" period is referred to as the window period.

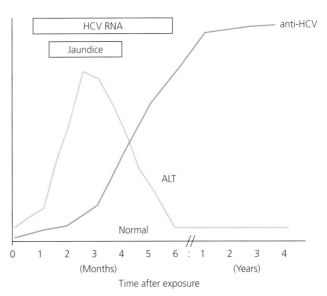

Figure 56.16 Serological course of acute hepatitis C virus (HCV) infection. Following exposure to HCV, the virus can be detected within 2 weeks in serum and liver using sensitive polymerase chain reaction assays. An antibody response can be demonstrated as early as week 4 but more commonly by week 12, coinciding with the onset of clinical symptoms. Anti-HCV usually persists for life but may disappear in up to 25% of persons who recover spontaneously. Anti-HCV does not confer immunity against reinfection. ALT, alanine aminotransferase.

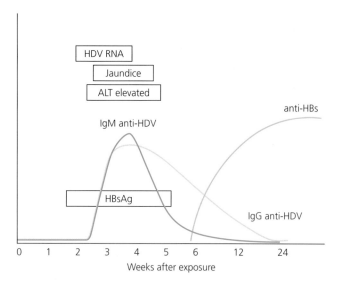

Figure 56.17 Serological course of hepatitis D virus (HDV) coinfection. Acute HDV infection occurs in two settings: simultaneously with acute hepatitis B virus (HBV) infection (coinfection) or following exposure in a patient with chronic HBV infection (superinfection). The serological course is different in each instance. In acute coinfection, markers of HBV are usually evident before HDV is detected. HDVAg and HDV RNA can be detected in serum before the peak in alanine aminotransferase (ALT) level; however, these are research tests and are not commercially available. IgM anti-HDV can be detected by week 4 following exposure but is often weak and may disappear before the development of IgG anti-HDV. IgG anti-HDV is usually delayed for several weeks following exposure and in some cases is only present transiently during convalescence. Therefore, both acute and convalescent sera should be tested for anti-HDV. Following recovery, levels of anti-HDV may decline to undetectable and no serological markers of HDV may remain. Thus, some cases may be diagnosed as acute HBV infection alone. The presence of IgM anti-HBc, which is associated with acute HBV infection, is an important marker for distinguishing HDV coinfection from superinfection. Thus, the diagnosis of HDV coinfection is determined by the presence of IgM anti-HDV, hepatitis B surface antigen (HBsAg), and IgM anti-HBc.

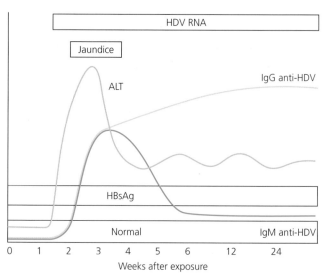

Figure 56.18 Serological course of hepatitis D virus (HDV) superinfection. The incubation period of HDV superinfection is usually shorter than for coinfection. HDV RNA and HDVAg are present during the incubation period and symptomatic phase. The titer of hepatitis B surface antigen (HBsAg) usually falls when HDVAg appears in serum. Most cases of HDV superinfection result in chronic infection and HDV RNA and HDVAg persist in serum. In contrast to HDV coinfection, IgM and IgG anti-HDV are both present during the symptomatic phase of infection and persist indefinitely. IgM anti-HBc is usually absent or present in low titer. Thus, diagnosis of acute HDV superinfection rests on the detection of anti-HDV and HBsAg and the absence of IgM anti-HBc.

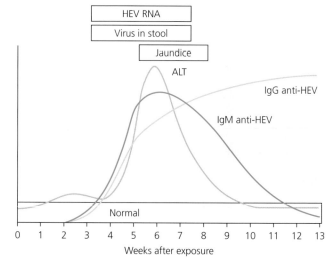

Figure 56.19 Serological course of hepatitis E virus (HEV) infection. Following acute exposure to the virus, viral excretion is detectable within 2 weeks in serum and stool. Similar to hepatitis A virus (HAV) infection, virus levels are highest during the incubation phase and begin to decline with the onset of symptoms. Both IgM and IgG antibodies are elicited during acute infection. IgM anti-HEV is detectable within 2 weeks of exposure and peaks with the onset of symptoms and alanine aminotransferase (ALT) levels. It disappears rapidly over 4–5 months. IgG anti-HEV is present during the acute illness and remains elevated for several years and then levels begin to decline. Current assays for anti-HEV vary widely in their sensitivity and false negatives can result in diagnostic error.

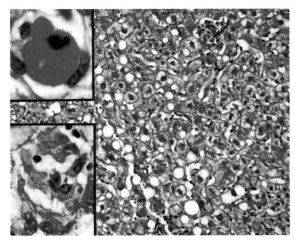

Figure 56.20 Acute viral hepatitis. The biopsy demonstrates typical features of acute viral hepatitis with a mild inflammatory infiltrate, ballooning degeneration, scattered acidophil bodies, and mild lobular disarray. **Upper left** insert shows a high-power view of an acidophil body with densely eosinophilic, irregularly shaped cytoplasm and a pyknotic nucleus. **Lower left** insert shows a high-power view of the inflammatory infiltrate. There are lymphocytes, pigmented macrophages, and occasional plasma cells. Mild steatosis is present (hematoxylin and eosin stain).

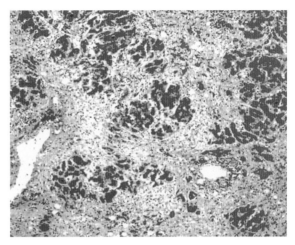

Figure 56.22 Acute viral hepatitis with submassive necrosis. There is almost complete involvement of the acini with extensive loss of parenchyma. Islands of hepatocytes are seen, separated by reticulin and inflammatory cells that form bridges (hematoxylin and eosin stain).

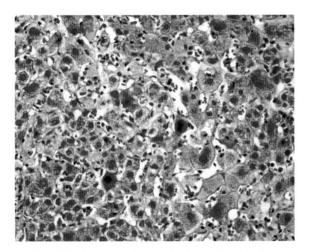

Figure 56.21 Acute viral hepatitis, moderate severity. Note the ballooned hepatocytes together with scattered acidophil bodies (towards the center of biopsy specimen). There is a moderate inflammatory infiltrate (hematoxylin and eosin stain).

57 Chronic hepatitis B viral infection

Robert G. Gish

Hepatitis B viral (HBV) infection remains one of the most common chronic infections in the world. HBV accounts for one of the most devastating and common cancers in the world, hepatocellular carcinoma. The lifetime risk of death caused by HBV is approximately 30% in individuals who are chronically infected. Unfortunately, most patients with chronic hepatitis B remain undiagnosed because of the lack of population screening. If a diagnosis of chronic HBV infection is made, often little intervention takes place because of the lack of symptoms in most patients and a lack of knowledge of the rapidly evolving therapies available for HBV infection. It is important for all practitioners to understand that HBV infection is suppressible and controllable in many patients. Viral suppression can markedly improve long-term outcomes and decrease the rate of death, cirrhosis, and liver cancer. Understanding all aspects of HBV disease is essential to the management of this complex problem. The physician managing HBV infection must be a liver specialist, virologist, radiologist, clinician, pathologist, and oncologist combined. Each practitioner must understand the natural history of the various forms of chronic hepatitis B infection and recognize the multiple ways in which a patient may present. Each patient group with chronic HBV infection is quite heterogeneous in the initial presentation and clinical course. Each patient needs to be monitored for changes in liver enzymes, liver function tests, and serological status and viral replication at least every 6 months. This monitoring process allows interventions to take place for those patients who have ongoing replication and those who clinically manifest with progressive liver disease. Ultrasound testing every 6 months for patients with cirrhosis or for those who have carried HBV infection for more than 40–50 years will identify many patients who develop hepatocellular carcinoma. Liver biopsy should be considered in all patients with elevated liver enzymes if therapy is not recommended. Understanding the

scoring system for liver fibrosis and inflammation, and applying this system to the liver biopsy for each patient is important. This information can be used to counsel patients about the chances of developing cirrhosis, the current evidence for the presence of cirrhosis, the risk of liver cancer, and the possibility of identifying additional diagnoses.

A 26-year-old man who had a history of more than 50 sexual partners presented with elevated liver enzymes that normalized after 1 month of follow-up. The serum liver enzyme levels were markedly elevated again 3 months later. The patient underwent a liver biopsy and had active liver disease with positive core and surface antigen immunoperoxidase stains as well as grade 3 inflammation and stage 3 fibrosis (Fig. 57.1a–d). The patient was treated with interferon therapy but could not tolerate the severe fatigue associated with the treatment. Interferon treatment was subsequently discontinued. The patient's liver tests normalized for 4 months and serum levels of HBV DNA were 2000 IU/mL. After this 4-month interval there was a sudden increase in liver enzymes and the serum level of HBV DNA increased to more than 10 million IU/mL. Entecavir (0.5 mg orally per day) was initiated. There was a subsequent rapid decrease in liver enzyme levels and the serum HBV DNA became unmeasurable after 2 months of therapy. The patient's serum became negative for hepatitis B early antigen (HBeAg) and positive for anti-HBe at month 11. The serum levels of liver enzymes were normal and HBV DNA was negative 1 year after entecavir therapy was stopped. Table 57.1 outlines the suggested patient groups for observation or treatment.

A 35-year-old Romanian woman who was infected with HBV and hepatitis D virus (HDV) presented with jaundice, ascites, and encephalopathy. She rapidly developed coma within the ensuing 6 weeks and underwent a liver transplant. A liver biopsy was performed 6 months before her clinical presentation with rapidly progressive liver disease. The patient died of recurrent HDV infection and liver failure after the liver transplant despite hepatitis B immunoglobulin therapy and adequate serum levels of immunoglobulin. Liver tissue photomicrographs are shown in Fig. 57.2a–c and

Atlas of Gastroenterology, 4th edition. Edited by Tadataka Yamada, David H. Alpers, Anthony N. Kalloo, Neil Kaplowitz, Chung Owyang, and Don W. Powell. © 2009 Blackwell Publishing, ISBN: 978-1-4051-6909-7

demonstrate hematoxylin and eosin, trichrome, and delta antigen staining respectively.

A 23-year-old woman with chronic HBV infection after a liver transplant developed a rapidly progressive liver disease, jaundice, and liver dysfunction. Liver biopsy results indicated fibrosing cholestatic hepatitis (Fig. 57.3a,b) and positive in situ HBV DNA stain throughout the liver tissue. The clinical course in this patient was modified by the addition of nucleoside analogues. Her jaundice, ascites, and abnormal coagulation tests corrected to normal within 3 months of initiating antiviral therapy. She remains well 8 years later and a liver biopsy shows early cirrhosis but no evidence of progression by physical examination or by liver synthetic abnormalities.

A 45-year-old man presented with chronic HBV infection and cirrhosis, and waited 2 years before undergoing a liver transplant. The patient had a known hepatoma at the time of transplant that was single and less than 5 cm, without evidence of vascular invasion by computed tomography. After the liver transplant, the explant and tumor (Fig. 57.4a) were examined microscopically in detail by the pathologist and were found to have vascular invasion (Fig. 57.4b). The patient died 1 year later of brain metastasis. The finding of vascular invasion often portends a poor prognosis and signifies that the patient may have stage 4 disease (disseminated cancer).

Fortunately, the incidence of acute HBV infection has been decreasing in the United States during the last two decades. With the introduction of neonatal vaccination and screening of pregnant mothers throughout the world, there is a clear expectation that not only will early deaths due to hepatocellular carcinoma decline but also that the incidence of end-stage liver disease caused by HBV will also decrease. The mandate for occupational safety, vaccination of adolescents, and education of individuals involved in high-risk activities are also very important public health policies.

Table 57.1 Management of chronic hepatitis B virus (HBV) infection

| HBV DNA level | ALT activity | |
	≤17–25 U/L[a]	>17–25 U/L
<~10^4 copies/mL; <2000 IU/mL for HBeAg(–); <20 000 IU/mL for HBeAg(+)	Observe[b]	Perform biopsy[c]
>~10^4 copies/mL; >2000 IU/mL for HBeAg(–); >20 000 IU/mL for HBeAg(+)	Perform biopsy and treat if active HBV infection	Treat: HBeAg(+): ≥6 months after eAg seroconversion; HBeAg(–): prolonged treatment (≥24 months) beyond NAT negative[d]. Consider biopsy or use noninvasive fibrosis testing

a Upper limit of normal for a person with a normal body mass index.
b Treat any patient with cirrhosis who is NAT positive, refer to specialist.
c Rule out fatty liver and other causes of chronic liver disease.
d Consider 3–5 years.
ALT, alanine aminotransferase; HBeAg, hepatitis B early antigen; NAT, nucleic acid testing, such as polymerase chain reaction, branched DNA, transcription-mediated amplification.
From Gish RG. Current treatment and future directions in the management of chronic hepatitis B viral infection. Clin Liver Dis 2005;9:541.

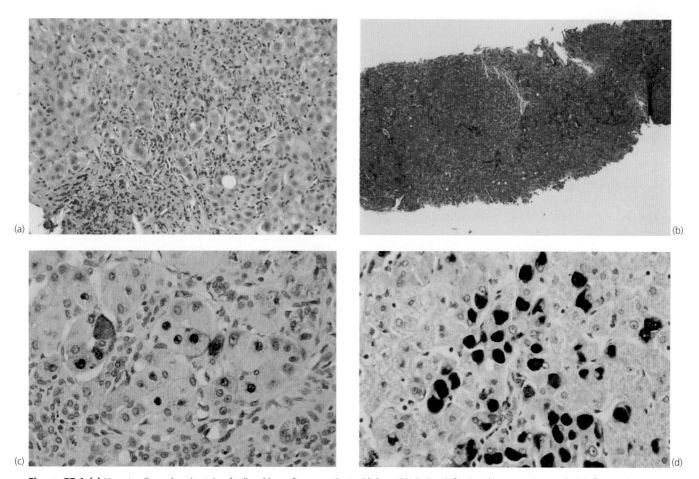

Figure 57.1 (a) Hematoxylin and eosin stain of a liver biopsy from a patient with hepatitis B virus infection demonstrating grade 3 inflammation. **(b)** Trichrome staining demonstrating stage 3 fibrosis. **(c)** Immunoperoxidase staining for hepatitis B core antigen. **(d)** Immunoperoxidase staining for hepatitis B surface antigen.

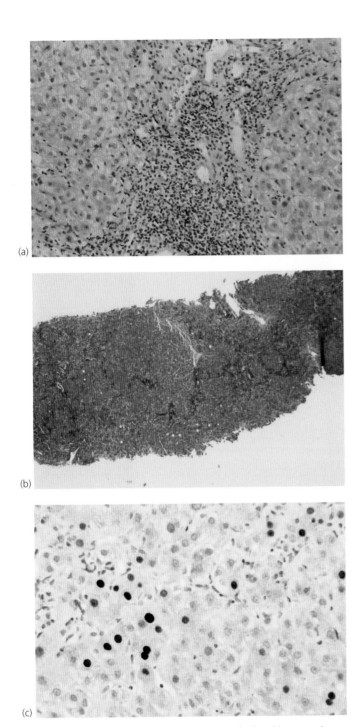

Figure 57.2 **(a)** Hematoxylin and eosin stain of a liver biopsy specimen demonstrating grade 3 inflammation. **(b)** Trichrome staining demonstrating stage 3 fibrosis. **(c)** Immunoperoxidase staining for hepatitis delta antigen.

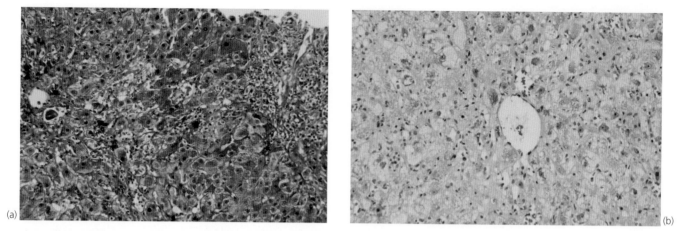

Figure 57.3 (a) Fibrosing cholestatic hepatitis (trichrome stain). **(b)** Fibrosing cholestatic hepatitis (hematoxylin and eosin stain).

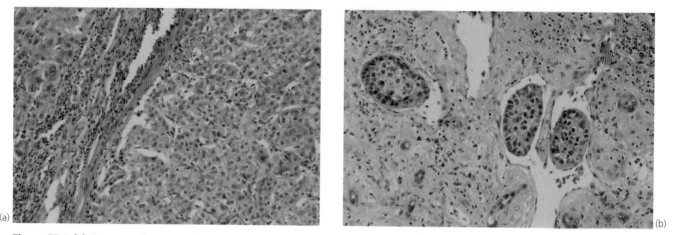

Figure 57.4 (a) Liver cancer (hepatoma, hepatocellular carcinoma). **(b)** Liver cancer invading a blood vessel.

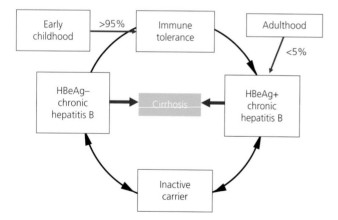

Figure 57.5 Natural history of chronic hepatitis B. Courtesy of W. Ray Kim, MD.

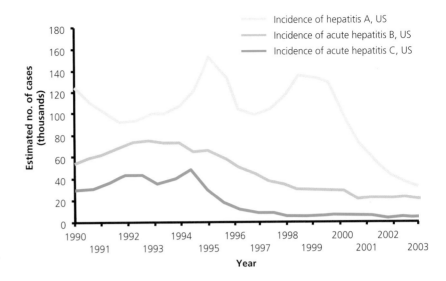

Figure 57.6 Disease burden of acute hepatitis A, B, and C as of 2003.

- Almost half of the world's population lives in an area with high HBV prevalence

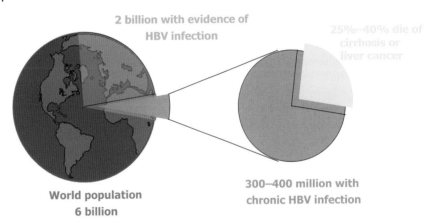

Figure 57.7 Hepatitis B: world burden of disease. HBV, hepatitis B virus.

▪ Eight HBV genotypes (based on complete HBV genome):

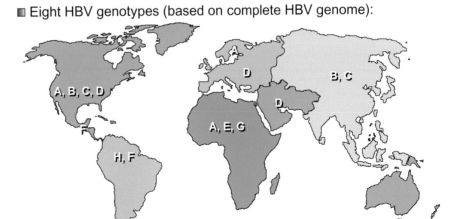

Figure 57.8 Hepatitis B virus: genotype distributions worldwide. HBV, hepatitis B virus.

58 Hepatitis C virus infection

Aijaz Ahmed, Emmet B. Keeffe

Chronic hepatitis C virus (HCV) infection is a major global public health problem, with an estimated 170 million individuals infected worldwide. Data from population-based studies demonstrates that HCV infection is the etiology of 40% or more of cases of chronic liver disease. Chronic hepatitis C is the most common chronic bloodborne infectious disease in the United States, even though the annual incidence rate has declined from 180 000 cases per year in the late 1980s to an estimated 26 000 cases in 2004. The overall national prevalence of antibody to HCV (anti-HCV) based on a US survey from 1999 to 2002 was 1.6%, which corresponds to an estimated 4.1 million individuals having been infected with HCV from various modes of transmission (Tables 58.1–58.3). In this updated survey, the age-specific prevalence rate moved from persons of 30–39 years of age to those of 40–49 years of age. Serum HCV RNA was detectable in 79.9% cases, which corresponds to an estimated 1.3% or 3.2 million actively infected individuals nationwide. Of these chronically infected individuals in the initial survey, 74% were infected with genotype 1, which is also the predominant genotype worldwide (Table 58.4).

New adult patients undergoing initial intake evaluation should be screened for a history of risk factors associated with HCV infection. During the history and physical examination, findings suggestive of chronic liver disease include encephalopathy, ascites, edema, spider angiomas, palmar erythema, a firm liver edge, and splenomegaly. The majority of patients with chronic hepatitis C have constitutional symptoms, such as fatigue and decreased energy level, which are nonspecific and thus not diagnostically helpful in suggesting the presence of chronic hepatitis C. A test for anti-HCV should be performed if an elevated alanine aminotransferase (ALT) level is found, if there is a positive history of risk factors for HCV infection, or if physical findings suggest the presence of chronic liver disease. A test for HCV RNA is warranted in patients who test positive for anti-HCV – particularly those with normal ALT levels or no HCV risk factors – to confirm HCV infection and rule out a false-positive test, or recovery from past HCV infection (Table 58.5 and Fig. 58.1). Serological testing for anti-HCV is the most practical screening test for HCV infection in hemodialysis patients, who often have normal ALT levels; however, serum HCV RNA is detectable in about 10% of HCV-seronegative patients, suggesting that patients in this high-risk population with negative anti-HCV testing should undergo a confirmatory HCV RNA test.

The primary goal of antiviral therapy in patients with chronic hepatitis C is long-term viral eradication as determined by an undetectable HCV RNA in serum and liver. Secondary objectives of treatment include normalization of ALT levels and reduced inflammation and fibrosis on liver biopsy, which logically should decrease progression to cirrhosis, hepatocellular carcinoma, and premature death. The National Institutes of Health consensus conference and other guidelines advocate a selective rather than routine role for liver biopsy. These guidelines recommended that a liver biopsy be performed when considering treatment for chronic hepatitis C to distinguish patients most likely to benefit from therapy, i.e., those with moderate histological disease, from those who may be less likely to benefit from therapy, i.e., those with mild disease and no or minimal fibrosis or those with advanced disease and cirrhosis. A decision to perform a liver biopsy may be influenced by many factors, such as patient preferences, cost-effectiveness, presence of contraindications, and suspicion of coexistent liver diseases (Table 58.6). Liver biopsy is the most reliable method of establishing the severity of liver disease due to chronic hepatitis C by determination of the stage of fibrosis and grade of inflammation. However, it provides no superiority to overall clinical and laboratory assessment in ruling out other unsuspected coexisting liver diseases. Based on cost-effectiveness considerations, the most suitable strategy in the management of chronic hepatitis C may be to initiate therapy in all patients without performing liver biopsy. Moreover, with recent

Atlas of Gastroenterology, 4th edition. Edited by Tadataka Yamada, David H. Alpers, Anthony N. Kalloo, Neil Kaplowitz, Chung Owyang, and Don W. Powell. © 2009 Blackwell Publishing, ISBN: 978-1-4051-6909-7

advances in antiviral therapy resulting from the addition of ribavirin to interferon-based therapy, patients with genotypes 2 and 3 have sustained virological response (SVR) rates of about 65% with regular interferon plus ribavirin and 80% or more with peginterferon plus ribavirin. Thus, the current role of liver biopsy is primarily to assess the stage of fibrosis in patients with genotype 1, whose likely SVR rate is approximately 45%; these patients may prefer to defer therapy if mild disease with no or minimal fibrosis is present.

The evolution of interferon-based therapy for chronic hepatitis C, particularly combination therapy with ribavirin and peginterferon, has resulted in incremental improvement in the SVR rates, i.e., 10%–15% with interferon monotherapy for 24 weeks, 15%–25% when interferon monotherapy was extended to 48 or 72 weeks, 40% with interferon plus ribavirin, and currently 55% with peginterferon plus ribavirin. Factors that predict a favorable response to antiviral therapy are shown in Table 58.7. The combination of peginterferon with ribavirin is the most efficacious antiviral therapy of chronic hepatitis C. Peginterferon alfa-2b at a weekly dose of 1.5 µg/kg plus ribavirin, 800 mg per day, showed a significantly higher response rate when compared with standard interferon plus ribavirin combination in a large pivotal trial. The SVR rate was 54% overall, 42% in patients with genotype 1, and 82% in patients with genotype 2 or 3 (Table 58.8). Secondary analysis of the data from the peginterferon alfa-2b plus ribavirin study suggested better efficacy with weight-based dosing of ribavirin. Results with peginterferon alfa-2a plus ribavirin were similar to those with peginterferon alfa-2b and ribavirin. The use of

peginterferon monotherapy is only appropriate if there are contraindications to ribavirin use or patients are not candidates for therapy (Table 58.9). Based on data from recent trials, peginterferon and ribavirin combination therapy is the standard of care in treating patients with chronic HCV infection (Fig. 58.2). Consensus recommendations regarding antiviral therapy of HCV infection in special populations are displayed in Table 58.10.

Patient should be informed that, although the risk of transmitting HCV infection by sexual contact is low (3%–5%), HCV is potentially transmissible. Patients should be careful about blood exposure of any type to partners and family contacts. Open wounds must be covered, and razors or toothbrushes should not be shared. Exposed persons should undergo postexposure baseline and follow-up testing (Table 58.11). Although sexual or intrafamilial HCV transmission is rare, testing sexual partners or other family members if there is a concern regarding infection usually provides reassurance. Patients with chronic hepatitis C should be counseled to avoid excessive consumption of alcohol, which can accelerate the progression of chronic hepatitis C when used in moderate or large amounts. It has been recommended that the less alcohol consumed the better, and that complete abstinence is ideal. In addition, acute hepatitis A or B may be more severe in patients with chronic hepatitis C, and thus it is recommended that HCV-infected patients without immunity to hepatitis A and B undergo vaccination (Table 58.12). Finally, a comprehensive strategy to prevent and control HCV infection, outlined in Table 58.13, is an important public health agenda over the next decade.

Table 58.1 Viral hepatitis in United States: CDC data from 1984 to 1994

	Hepatitis A	Hepatitis B	Hepatitis C
Acute hepatitis (×1000/year)	125–200	140–320	26–180
Fulminant hepatitis (deaths/year)	100	150	7
Chronic hepatitis (prevalence)	0	1–1.25 million (0.3%)	3–4 million (1.6%)
Chronic liver disease (deaths/year)	0	4–5 000	8–10 000

CDC, Centers for Disease Control.
From www.cdc.gov.

Table 58.2 Modes of transmission: risk factors for hepatitis C virus (HCV) infection

Illicit drug use
Injection drug use
Intranasal cocaine use

Sexual and vertical transmission
High-risk sexual activity (homosexual contact, multiple partners)
Children born to HCV-positive mothers

Health care-related transmission
Transfusion of blood or blood products before July, 1992
Recipient of solid organ transplant before July, 1992
Chronic hemodialysis
Health care and public safety workers with history of needle stick or
   mucosal exposure to HCV-positive blood
Receipt of injections in a third-world country

Miscellaneous
HIV infection
Body piercing or tattoos
Patients with elevated ALT levels independent of other risk factors

ALT, alanine aminotransferase; HIV, human immunodeficiency virus.

Table 58.3 Modes of transmission: percentage risk

Injection drug use	60%
Sexual	15%
Transfusion (before screening)	10%
Other (hemodialysis, health care worker, etc.)	5%
Unknown	10%

From Alter MJ, Kruszon-Moran D, Narnon OV, et al. The prevalence of hepatitis C infection in the United States 1988–1994. N Engl J Med 1999;341:556.

Table 58.4 Distribution of hepatitis C virus genotypes

Genotype	Geographical predominance
1a	USA and developed Western countries
1b	USA, Japan, and Europe
2	Developed countries
3	Developed countries
4	Middle East and North Africa
5	South Africa
6	Asia

Prevalence in USA: 74% genotype 1, 26% genotype 2 and 3.
Genotypes 1 and 4 are less responsive to antiviral therapy.

Table 58.5 Diagnostic tests for hepatitis C infection

Type of infection	ALT	EIA	RIBA	RT-PCR
Chronic hepatitis C	↑ or N	+	+	+
Recovered HCV infection	N	+	+	−
False positive anti-HCV	N	+	−	−

ALT, alanine aminotransferase; anti-HCV, antibody to HCV; EIA, enzyme immunoassay; HCV, hepatitis C virus; N, normal levels; RIBA, recombinant immunoblot assay; RT-PCR, reverse transcriptase polymerase chain reaction.
↑, elevated levels; −, negative; +, positive.

Table 58.6 Role of liver biopsy in HCV: selective vs routine

Arguments for routine liver biopsy
Determine fibrosis stage and need for therapy, i.e., treatment
   indicated for stages 2–4; treatment optional or not needed for
   stages 0–1 (particularly patients with genotype 1; may not apply
   for patients with genotypes 2 or 3)
Exclude coexisting unsuspected secondary liver diseases, such as
   autoimmune hepatitis or nonalcoholic fatty liver disease (not
   commonly found on biopsy)
Provide assistance in the management of side effects during antiviral
   therapy (use of adjunctive agents such as antidepressive drugs,
   epoetin alfa or G-CSF in patients with advanced stages of fibrosis)

Arguments for selective liver biopsy
Improved efficacy of antiviral therapy, particularly in patients with
   genotypes 2 and 3
Invasive procedure with risk of complications and death
Favorable cost-effectiveness analysis
Risk of sampling error
Clinical features indicating presence of cirrhosis
Patient preference

G-CSF, granulocyte colony-stimulating factor; HCV, hepatitis C virus.

Table 58.7 Favorable response determinants: peginterferon and ribavirin therapy

Host determinants
Female gender
White or Asian vs African or Hispanic
Age < 40 years
Absence of stage 3 or 4 fibrosis
HIV-negative status
Low hepatic iron levels
Absence of coexisting nonalcoholic fatty liver disease
Elevated ALT levels

Viral determinants
Genotype 2 and 3[a]
Low baseline serum HCV RNA level (<600 000–800 000 IU/mL)[a]
Short duration of infection
Small number of quasispecies
Mutation at interferon sensitivity determining site (NS5A)

Drug determinants
Ribavirin dose
Prolonged duration of treatment
Early response to therapy based on ALT and HCV RNA levels[a]

a Most important determinants.
ALT, alanine aminotransferase; HCV, hepatitis C virus; HIV, human immunodeficiency virus; RNA, ribonucleic acid.

Table 58.8 Peginterferon plus ribavirin therapy for chronic hepatitis C virus infection

Therapy	Overall	Genotype 1	Genotype 2,3
Peginterferon alfa-2a plus ribavirin	56%	46%	76%
Peginterferon alfa-2b plus ribavirin	54%	42%	82%
Peginterferon alfa-2b plus ribavirin (weight-based dosing)	61%	48%	88%

Table 58.9 Candidates for peginterferon monotherapy

Patients not eligible for ribavirin
    Severe anemia
    Coronary artery disease
    Renal failure (hemodialysis)
    Severe pulmonary disease
    Prior ribavirin toxicity
Patients receiving maintenance therapy

Table 58.10 Therapy for special HCV patient populations

Special HCV population	Therapy
Acute hepatitis C	Recommended
Children with HCV infection	Recommended
Histologically mild HCV infection	Recommended
Mixed cryoglobulinemia/glomerulonephritis	Recommended
Normal ALT levels	Individualized
Autoimmune hepatitis	Not recommended
HIV infection	Recommended
Compensated cirrhosis	Cautiously recommended
Decompensated cirrhosis	Clinical trial
Posttransplantation	Cautiously recommended

ALT, alanine aminotransferase; HCV, hepatitis C virus.

Table 58.11 Postexposure testing and follow-up for HCV infection

Source
Baseline testing for anti-HCV

Person exposed to HCV-positive source
Baseline anti-HCV and ALT

Follow-up testing for anti-HCV and ALT at 4–6 months; if earlier diagnosis of HCV infection is desired, testing for HCV RNA may be performed at 4–6 weeks. All EIA-based positive anti-HCV must be confirmed by PCR testing for HCV RNA. Prophylactic antiviral therapy not recommended

Anti-HCV, antibody to HCV; ALT, alanine aminotransferase; EIA, enzyme immunoassay; HCV, hepatitis C virus; PCR, polymerase chain reaction; RNA, ribonucleic acid.
From www.cdc.gov.

Table 58.12 Efficacy of hepatitis A and B vaccination in chronic hepatitis C

	Seroconversion rate	
	HAV vaccine	HBV vaccine
Patients		
Chronic hepatitis C		
Mild	Good	Good
Moderate	Good	Fair to good
Advanced (OLT candidates)	±[a]	Poor[b]
OLT recipients	±[a]	Poor[b]

a Data limited.
b Consider accelerated, high-dose regimen.
HAV, hepatitis A virus; HBV, hepatitis B virus; OLT, orthotopic liver transplantation.

Table 58.13 Comprehensive strategy to prevent and control hepatitis C virus infection

Primary prevention
Screening and testing of blood, plasma, organ, tissue, and semen donors
Virus inactivation of plasma-derived products
Risk-reduction counseling and services
Implementation and maintenance of infection-control practices

Secondary prevention
Identification, counseling, and testing of persons at risk
Medical management of infected persons

Professional and public education

Surveillance to monitor disease pattern and efficacy of prevention measures

From www.cdc.gov.

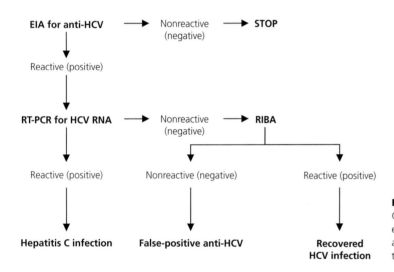

Figure 58.1 Diagnostic algorithm in patients with hepatitis C virus risk factors. Anti-HCV, antibody to hepatitis C virus; EIA, enzyme immunoassay; HCV RNA, hepatitis C virus ribonucleic acid; RIBA, recombinant immunoblot assay; RT-PCR, reverse transcriptase polymerase chain reaction.

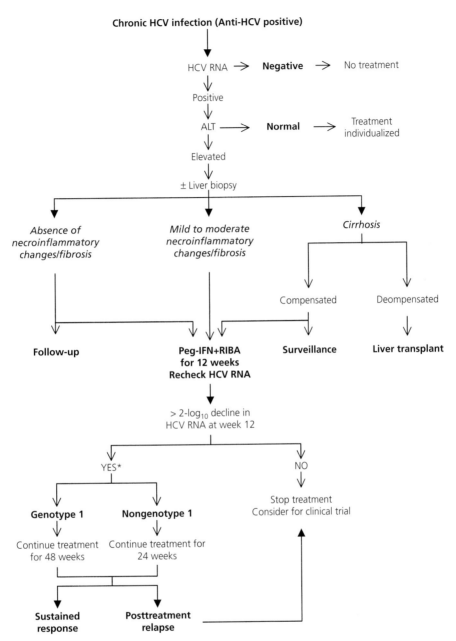

Figure 58.2 Treatment of chronic hepatitis C. *Patients with ≥ 2-log$_{10}$ decline in HCV RNA at week 12, but persistent viremia should undergo HCV RNA recheck at 24 weeks of therapy and treatment should be discontinued if there is still detectable virus. ALT, alanine aminotransferase; HCV RNA, hepatitis C virus ribonucleic acid; Peg-IFN+RIBA, peginterferon plus ribavirin combination.

59

Drug-induced liver disease

Frank V. Schiødt, William M. Lee

Drugs can cause hepatotoxicity in either a dose-dependent or a dose-independent (idiosyncratic) fashion. Both types of drug-induced liver injury are very frequent causes of acute liver failure with hepatic encephalopathy and coagulopathy (Fig. 59.1), although the proportion of cases of acute liver failure caused by drugs varies greatly worldwide (Table 59.1; Fig. 59.2).

Idiosyncratic drug reactions occur rarely (in 1:10 000–1:100 000 persons using the specific drug), and enzyme polymorphisms in one of the cytochrome P450 (*CYP*) or other genes undoubtedly play a role in many susceptible patients; however, the clinical role and value of pharmacogenetics are just beginning to emerge.

Acetaminophen (paracetamol) is probably the best example of a dose-dependent hepatotoxic drug. Acetaminophen is extremely safe when taken within the recommended doses (4 g/day), but doses of 8–10 g/day may cause severe liver necrosis. Figure 59.3 describes the metabolic pathways of acetaminophen. It is widely accepted that toxicity is ascribed to the highly reactive metabolite *N*-acetyl-*p*-benzoquinone imine (NAPQI). NAPQI can bind covalently to cellular proteins and cause blebbing and later lysis of the hepatocyte. Acetaminophen-induced acute liver failure is a hyperacute disease in which liver failure may develop only days after ingestion of the overdose. Biochemical characteristics include very high aminotransferase levels (5000–25 000 IU/L) and often also an elevated creatinine level because of a direct nephrotoxic effect of acetaminophen. Liver transplantation is not frequently performed for patients with acetaminophen-induced acute liver failure because the disease progresses too rapidly or medical or social contraindications preclude transplantation. In addition, the spontaneous (transplantation free) survival rate is better (approximately 70%) than for other causes of acute liver failure and liver transplantation is not needed for most patients. Cases of acetaminophen toxicity can be missed if the patient is encephalopathic on arrival or does not admit to use of acetaminophen. In these instances, a newly developed assay that can measure acetaminophen protein adducts is very effective in identifying the "smoking gun" (Fig. 59.4).

Idiosyncratic drug-induced liver injury differs from acetaminophen-induced acute liver failure in a number of ways, including a slower onset of symptoms and lower spontaneous (transplantation free) survival rates. Biochemical differences are also apparent in lower aminotransferase and creatinine levels and higher bilirubin levels. Unlike acetaminophen, which is a dose-related toxin, most idiosyncratic reactions do not appear to be dose related. As they occur very rarely (1:10 000–1:100 000 exposures), there must be some genetic predisposition to explain an altered metabolic pathway (Fig. 59.5), plus some other downstream events. One theory is that the initial alteration in cell proteins leads to the release of cytokines (the danger hypothesis, Fig. 59.6), which augment the initial pattern of injury. The mechanisms that result in damage to liver cells in cases of idiosyncratic toxicity are varied, as are the effects on the liver. Figure 59.7 describes some of the mechanisms that may be involved in this damage. As with acetaminophen, it is likely that drugs that cause significant liver injury lead to highly reactive intermediates that bind irreversibly to cell proteins, leading to formation of haptens that can then provoke an immune attack mediated by cytotoxic T cells and possibly B cells (autoantibody formation) as well.

Idiosyncratic drug-induced hepatotoxicity has been described for a very large number of drugs. Implicated agents include antibiotics (including isoniazid as the most commonly recognized), nonsteroidal agents, seizure medications, and a miscellaneous group. The proportion of drug-induced liver disease varies greatly among drug classes as evidence of class effect. The majority of reactions are directed against hepatocytes, but biliary injury and combined hepatocyte–biliary injury or damage to specific organelles can produce the different disease patterns observed (Fig. 59.7). Figure 59.8 displays some of the different

Atlas of Gastroenterology, 4th edition. Edited by Tadataka Yamada, David H. Alpers, Anthony N. Kalloo, Neil Kaplowitz, Chung Owyang, and Don W. Powell. © 2009 Blackwell Publishing, ISBN: 978-1-4051-6909-7

histological patterns of acute liver failure caused by drugs. One important issue is that of establishing causality. This is a process of guilt by association, establishing that the drug was given in an appropriate time interval in relation to the hepatic injury and that other causes were excluded (Table 59.2)

A number of drugs are approved after careful clinical trials only to be subsequently severely restricted or withdrawn by the US Food and Drug Administration (FDA) after identification of toxic reactions that had been unrecognized in the approval process (Table 59.3; Fig. 59.9). This is because, once approved, the exposure is much greater and the prescribing pattern much broader than that observed in the approval trial. A rare reaction (1:50 000) is unlikely to be identified during an approval trial involving 5000 patients.

One indicator of concern for FDA reviewers of phase III trials that is used for approval is if there is evidence of elevation of aminotransferase levels in a significant number of patients combined with any elevation of bilirubin. If jaundice attributable to the drug in question is observed in any patients during the trial, then with larger numbers of patient exposures there is likely to be hepatic failure in ~10% of those developing jaundice. This is sometimes referred to as Hy's Law in honor of Hyman Zimmerman, the father of the study of drug-induced liver injury (Fig. 59.10). A final word: drug toxicity from herbal medications is not uncommon and ranks near to drug toxicity from antibiotics in frequency. Studies are difficult to perform but it appears that herbal medication-related toxicity is increasing in this country (Fig. 59.11).

Table 59.1 The presumed etiology of acute liver failure in different parts of the world

	ACM (%)	HAV (%)	HBV (%)	Drug (%)	Shock (%)	Indeterminate (%)	Other (%)
Argentina 1996–2001 (n = 83)	0	8	22	14	0	25	31
Denmark 1973–1990 (n = 160)	19	2	31	17	3	15	13
France 1972–1990 (n = 502)	2	4	32	17	?	18	27
India 1987–1993 (n = 423)	0	2	31	5	0	0	62
Japan 1992–1999 (n = 38)	0	3	18	0	0	71	8
United Kingdom 1993–1994 (n = 342)	73	2	2	2	3	8	9
United States 1994–1996 (n = 295)	20	7	10	12	3	15	33
United States 1998–2006 (n = 1033)	46	3	7	12	4	15	13

All studies have cases of hepatitis A and hepatitis B, whereas acetaminophen-induced acute liver failure is a feature of studies in Western countries. Idiosyncratic drug reactions typically constitute 12%–17% of cases, with India, Japan, and the United Kingdom reporting fewer cases.
ACM, acetaminophen; drug, idiosyncratic drug reactions; HAV, hepatitis A virus; HBV, hepatitis B virus; shock, ischemic hepatitis.

Table 59.2 Components of the Roussel Uclaf Causality Assessment Method (RUCAM)

Points awarded for the following categories:
1. Time to onset
2. Course
3. Risk factors (age, alcohol)
4. Concomitant drugs
5. Search for nondrug causes
6. Previous information on hepatotoxicity of the drug
7. Response to readministration

Components of most causality assessment methods (CAMs) are similar. CAMs are efforts to codify the practice of "guilt by association." The most significant components are temporal relationship and exclusion of other causes. Most drugs cause injury at a delay from the initial dose (latency). The usual interval is 5–90 days, with drug reactions being very rare after 6 months of continuous ingestion. Response to rechallenge with a medication is seldom used as it is risky; however, it may be the most reliable evidence that a drug is implicated. It is undertaken only in extreme situations when the value and uniqueness of the drug are evident.

Table 59.3 Regulatory actions due to nonallergic hepatotoxicity[a]

Drug	Use	Regulatory action
Bromfenac	Analgesic	Withdrawn
Troglitazone	Diabetes	Withdrawn
Felbamate	Anticonvulsant	Restricted use
Pemoline	Central nervous system stimulant	Restricted use
Tolcapone	Parkinson disease	Restricted use
Trovafloxacin	Antibiotic	Restricted use
Acetaminophen	Analgesic	Warnings
Leflunomide	Immunomodulator	Warnings
Nefazodone	Antipsychotic	Warnings
Nevirapine	Antiviral (HIV)	Warnings
Pyrazinamide	Antituberculosis	Warnings
Rifampin	Antituberculosis	Warnings
Terbinafine	Antifungal	Warnings
Valproic acid	Anticonvulsant	Warnings
Zafirlukast	Asthma	Warnings

a Ximelagatran, anticoagulant, never approved; telithromycin, antibiotic, restricted use.
Data from Kaplowitz N. Idiosyncratic drug hepatotoxicity. Nat Rev Drug Disc 2005;4:489.

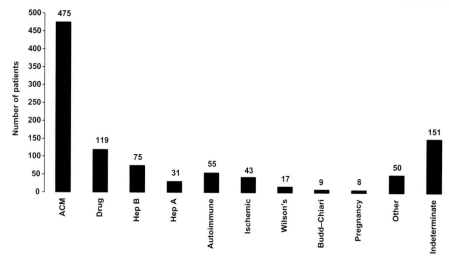

Figure 59.1 Prevalence of different etiologies in the registry of the US Acute Liver Failure Study Group from 1998 to 2006 (*n* =1033 patients). There has been a significant increase in the number of cases of acetaminophen poisoning since 1998. These very often involve narcotic–acetaminophen combinations. ACM, acetaminophen.

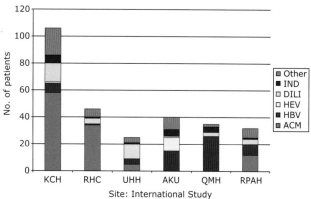

Figure 59.2 Prevalence of different etiologies of acute liver failure around the world as indicated by the number of patients seen at large referral centers over a one-year period. Acetaminophen and drug-induced liver injury predominate in developing countries while viral hepatitis is observed in Asia and the developing world. Etiologies: ACM, acetaminophen; DILI, drug-induced liver injury; HBV, hepatitis B virus; HEV, hepatitis E virus; IND, indeterminate. AKU, Aga Khan University, Karachi; KCH, Kings College Hospital, London; QMH, Queen Mary Hospital, Hong Kong; RHC, Rigshospitalet, Copenhagen; RPAH, Royal Prince Alfred Hospital, Melbourne; UHH, University Hospital, Hannover.

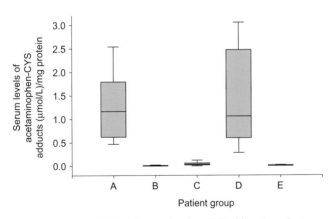

Figure 59.3 The metabolic pathways of acetaminophen. The major hepatic pathways include glucuronidation and sulfation **(left)**, which yield nontoxic water-soluble conjugates that are excreted by the kidney **(top right)**. A second pathway involves the cytochrome P450 (*CYP*) system, especially CYP2E1, by which acetaminophen is metabolized to the highly reactive metabolite *N*-acetyl-*p*-benzoquinone imine (*NAPQI*), which may bind covalently with hepatic proteins and cause cellular necrosis **(lower right)**. The toxic effect of NAPQI is eliminated by binding to the natural antidote glutathionine (*GSH*), yielding mercapturic acid, a nontoxic, water-soluble excretion product. *N*-acetylcysteine serves as an antidote by replenishing glutathione. Alcohol may enhance toxicity by induction of CYP2E1 or by depleting hepatic glutathione stores.

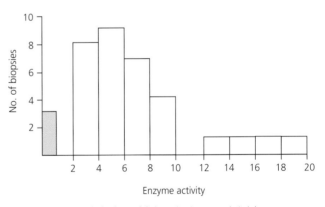

Figure 59.4 Serum levels of acetaminophen-CYS adducts in patient groups. A, patients with acute liver failure (ALF) secondary to known acetaminophen overdose. B, patients with ALF due to nonacetaminophen causes. C, patients with acetaminophen overdose but no ALF. D, patients with ALF of indeterminate etiology and detectable serum adducts. E, patients with ALF of indeterminate etiology and negative adducts. The boxes represent the 25th–75th interquartile range and the horizontal line represents the median. The extremes of the population are represented by the endmarks.

Figure 59.5 Genetic polymorphisms occur in cytochrome P450 (CYP450) enzymes. In this example, debrisoquine hydroxylase, CYP2D6, is present in several forms that differ greatly in their enzyme activity from nil to very high levels. These naturally occurring differences explain why individuals may metabolize drugs very differently.

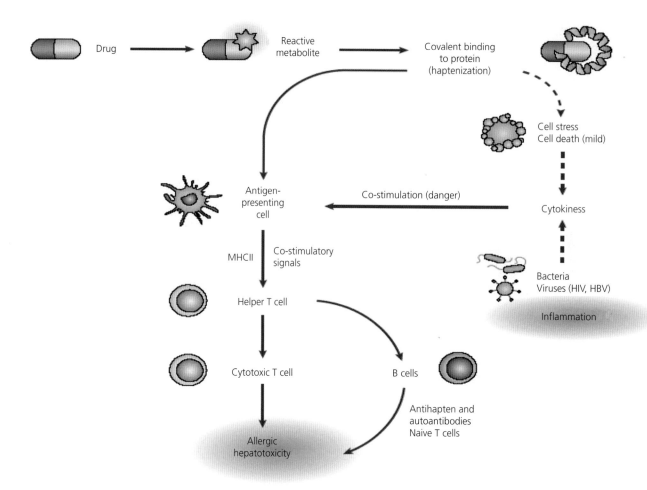

Figure 59.6 The danger hypothesis proposes that covalent binding to cell proteins (see **(c)** and **(d)** in Figure 59.7) initiates cytokine responses that then augment the injury to the cell in certain settings. HBV, hepatitis B virus; HIV, human immunodeficiency virus; MHCII, major histocompatibility complex II.

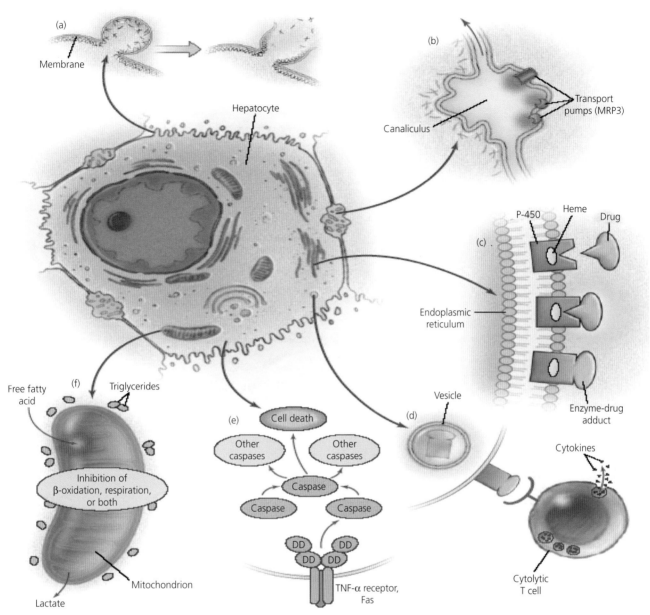

Figure 59.7 Proposed mechanisms of liver cell injury due to drugs.
(a) Disruption of the cytoskeletal filaments leading to blebbing and cell necrosis. **(b)** Damage to biliary canalicular transport mechanisms causes cholestasis. **(c)** Highly reactive intermediates that bind to cell proteins lead to hapten formation. **(d)** These neoantigens can be transported to the cell surface and evoke a cytotoxic immune response or autoantibody formation. **(e)** Apoptotic mechanisms can also take place.
(f) Mitochondrial disruption leads to accumulation of microvesicular fat in hepatocytes as well as lactic acid formation due to anaerobic metabolism.

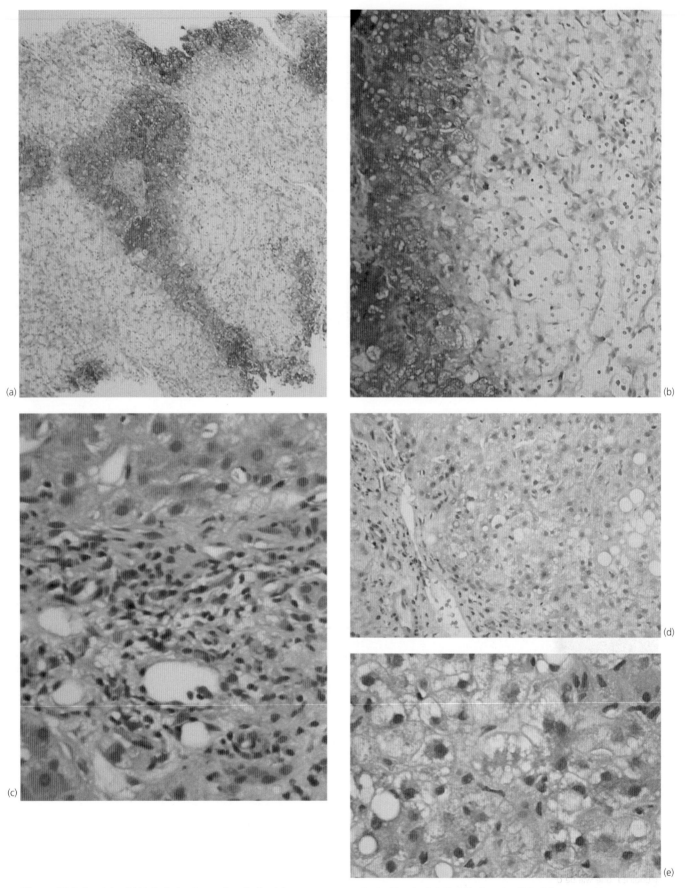

Figure 59.8 A variety of histological patterns of acute liver injury are caused by drugs. **(a)** Characteristic pattern of acetaminophen toxicity with acute necrosis–apoptosis of zones 2 and 3 (centrilobular region), with sparing of zone 1 (periportal region) (periodic acid–Schiff [PAS] stain; original magnification ×60). **(b)** Close-up view showing pattern of glycogen depletion and pyknotic nuclei in zones 2 and 3 (PAS stain; original magnification ×300). **(c)** Bile duct injury and eosinophilia in a patient with mixed cholestatic–hepatocellular injury caused by trimethoprim–sulfamethoxazole (H & E stain; original magnification ×240). **(d)** Diffuse cellular unrest with cell swelling and necrosis in a patient with fatal hepatitis caused by sulfasalazine (H & E stain; original magnification ×100). **(e)** Close-up view of cells with prominent ballooning degeneration in the same patient as shown in **(d)** (H & E stain; original magnification ×500).

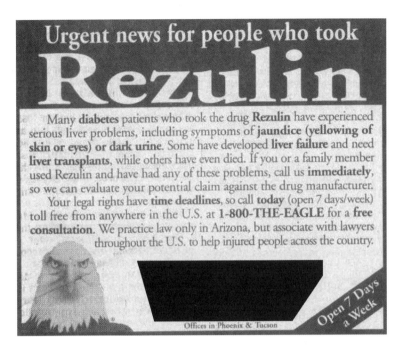

Figure 59.9 Rezulin was approved by the US Food and Drug Administration in 1999, only to be withdrawn more than 3 years later after more than 50 deaths or liver transplants. There are other ramifications to drug withdrawals as this nationally publicized advertisement indicates.

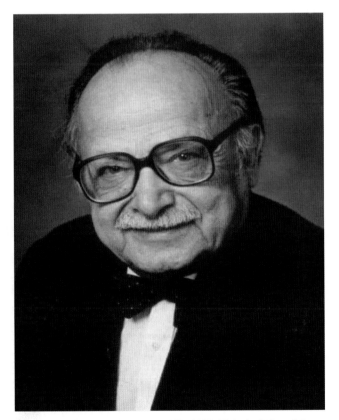

Figure 59.10 Hyman Zimmerman, MD, 1917–99, is the father of the field of drug-induced hepatotoxicity. Hy's Law suggests that if jaundice is observed in a clinical trial, the drug is likely to cause more severe toxicity when larger numbers of patients are exposed – once ten patients are jaundiced, one will be observed to have acute liver failure.

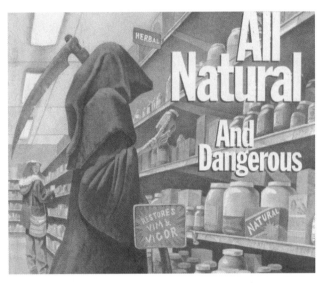

Figure 59.11 Health foods are not always healthy. After antibiotics, herbal medications are the second most common "drug class" implicated in hepatotoxicity. There is little quality control of nutraceuticals and herbs. In addition, patients often take excessive doses because of their implied promise of safety, and take a variety of herbs simultaneously. Assessing causality in this setting is particularly difficult.

60

Autoimmune hepatitis

E. Jenny Heathcote

When the disease entity autoimmune hepatitis (AIH) was first described, patients generally presented with decompensated cirrhosis. Now that liver enzymes are often checked at the time of a routine screen, it is apparent that AIH may be associated with a wide range of liver disease severity. Some individuals have no symptoms but the majority have various nonspecific symptoms with or without evidence of liver failure. Rarely, AIH presents as an acute fulminant hepatitis, although liver biopsy at the time often shows that cirrhosis is already present. Both asymptomatic and symptomatic patients may have underlying cirrhosis when first diagnosed.

This disease typically affects women more than men. All age groups and races may be affected. When symptoms are present they are nonspecific and consist of fatigue, anorexia, arthralgia, and secondary amenorrhea, with or without signs of liver failure. There is no specific hallmark(s) for AIH as there are for other autoimmune liver diseases. Laboratory test abnormalities include a variable degree of elevation in serum aminotransferase levels (5- to 10-fold elevation) and a minimally elevated alkaline phosphatase (ALP) level, with or without hyperbilirubinemia, hypoalbuminemia, and prolonged coagulation. The serological hallmarks of AIH are not definitive and include the nonorgan-specific antibodies antinuclear antibody (ANA) and smooth muscle antibody (SMA) in persons with type 1 AIH, and antiliver/kidney microsomal antibody type 1 (LKM-1) in those with type 2 AIH (Table 60.1). However, these first two autoantibodies may be detected in up to one-third of individuals with a wide range of chronic liver diseases, so they are not sufficient to make a diagnosis of AIH on their own. Hypergammaglobulinemia is a prerequisite, and levels need to be elevated more than 1.5 times normal; sometimes levels are very high (an immunoglobulin G [IgG] level elevated 1.5 times normal is

typical in cirrhosis of any etiology). In type 2 AIH, immunoglobulin levels are less elevated and the serum IgA level may even be low.

Any other hepatitis may mimic AIH, particularly drug-induced liver disease, chronic viral hepatitis B or C, and occasionally Wilson disease. Rarely, the laboratory findings in alcoholic hepatitis and nonalcoholic fatty liver disease may resemble AIH, but a liver biopsy clarifies this differential. Hence, in addition to a thorough history, tests for hepatitis B and C and serum ceruloplasmin should be performed as well as a liver biopsy.

It is necessary for a well-trained hepatopathologist to interpret the liver biopsy findings. Typically there is a lymphoplasmacytic infiltration of both the portal tracts and the liver parenchyma, with variable degrees of fibrosis (Fig. 60.1). It is a common mistake to misread bridging necrosis and collapse as fibrosis. Ischemic injury in zone 3 is another less common feature of AIH. Up to 50% of youngsters who present with typical AIH also have features of primary sclerosing cholangitis (PSC), and thus it is recommended that all children with AIH undergo examination of the biliary tract at diagnosis. The prevalence of this overlap in adults is uncertain but it may also occur.

When the diagnosis of AIH is uncertain, the AIH score may be helpful (Table 60.2). A score of 15 or more determines "definite" AIH. A score of 10–15 indicates "probable" AIH. It is best to calculate this score before institution of therapy. The score can be recalculated once the response to therapy is known.

Natural history

The majority of individuals recruited to the classical therapeutic trials initiated in the late 1960s had decompensated cirrhosis; it is improbable that they were asymptomatic. The natural history of asymptomatic AIH is poorly documented; some, but by no means all, patients subsequently develop symptomatic disease. The natural history of untreated symptomatic AIH (gleaned from the placebo groups in the early

Atlas of Gastroenterology, 4th edition. Edited by Tadataka Yamada, David H. Alpers, Anthony N. Kalloo, Neil Kaplowitz, Chung Owyang, and Don W. Powell. © 2009 Blackwell Publishing, ISBN: 978-1-4051-6909-7

therapeutic studies) indicates that survival without therapy is only 50% and 10% at 5 and 10 years respectively.

Generally, death is due to liver failure, often complicated by sepsis. With therapy, the 10-year survival rate of patients with AIH with or without cirrhosis is close to 100% at 5 years and 60%–80% at 20 years. Even when treatment is successful, cirrhosis may still develop in some and regress in others. The best outcomes are observed when treatment leads to complete normalization of serum aminotransferase levels.

Whereas fertility may be reduced in the untreated patient with AIH, women with well-controlled AIH may become pregnant and their ongoing therapy should be continued during the pregnancy. Therapy has no adverse effects on the fetus. Flareups may occur, most often but not always in the postpartum period. Portal hypertension and its complications are the greatest risk.

Treatment

Three well-conducted studies published in the early 1970s indicated that corticosteroid therapy markedly improved the survival of patients with AIH. Successful treatment was obtained with prednisone, alone or in combination with azathioprine (Imuran), but the latter was ineffective as monotherapy. A dose of 30 mg prednisone is generally sufficient to initiate therapy although the early trials used higher doses (60 mg/day), associated with marked side effects. Azathioprine, 1–2 mg/kg, may be started simultaneously or a little later. Once the serum aminotransferase values decrease to less than twofold elevated, the dose of prednisone should be reduced slowly. Alternatively, a fixed-dose reduction regimen may be employed. It is often possible to stop the administration of prednisone altogether and to maintain adequate disease suppression (normal alanine aminotransferase [ALT] values) with azathioprine 50–100 mg/day (Table 60.3). Few patients fail to respond to treatment, but relapse off treatment is frequent (83%). Those with cirrhosis at baseline and/or a marked lympho-plasmacytic infiltrate and very high IgG levels have the greatest risk of relapse. The optimal duration of immunosuppressive therapy required to induce and sustain remission is unknown, although it is generally advised that treatment be maintained for at least 1 year and up to 4 years after the ALT and immunoglobulin levels have returned to normal. Some clinicians advocate repeat liver biopsy before stopping therapy to ensure that there is no disease activity present. In those rare individuals who fail to respond to treatment, a higher dose of corticosteroid therapy may first be tried. Once doses greater than 40 mg/day are used, the side-effect profile is high and it is reasonable under these circumstances to attempt suppression of disease with other immunosuppressants, such as cyclosporin (ciclosporin), mycophenolate mofetil, methotrexate, or cyclophosphamide. In individuals who present with fulminant hepatitis, a liver transplant may be needed before the individual has a chance to respond to standard immunosuppressive therapy. Liver transplantation may also be required in individuals with burned-out, decompensated cirrhosis in whom immunosuppressive therapy is inappropriate. AIH may return in the transplanted liver, but this is not a reason to deny a transplant. It is not known whether those with asymptomatic AIH should receive immunosuppressive therapy, because their natural history is uncertain.

Immunosuppressive therapy frequently produces side effects. If there is time before the patient starts treatment with prednisone, baseline measurements of bone mineral density and blood glucose, and stool examination for ova and parasites in travelers, as well as measurement of systemic blood pressure and ophthalmological examination for glaucoma and cataracts, should be performed; subsequently monitoring of these same parameters during therapy is recommended. Patients should be warned to treat any infection and be advised appropriately about travel overseas. Because of the effect of the drug on the bone marrow, patients taking azathioprine should have their white blood count checked frequently. Pancreatitis and even hepatitis are rare complications of azathioprine, but gastrointestinal side effects are common and, when severe, may render the patient intolerant to this treatment. It is safe for women to conceive while taking prednisone or azathioprine. In individuals who are known to have cirrhosis and in all women who are pregnant, upper panendoscopy should be performed (during the second trimester in those who are pregnant) to check for the presence of esophageal varices. Prophylactic β-blocker therapy should be given to those with large varices.

Table 60.1 Comparison of the clinical and immunological features of types 1 and 2 autoimmune chronic active hepatitis

	Type 1 (antiactin)	Type 2 (anti-LKM)
Age at presentation (years)	10–25 and 45–70	Less than 15
Associated disorders (%)	10	17
Immunoglobulins	37 ± 11	23 ± 8
γ-Globulins		
IgG (g/L)	37 ± 16	25 ± 10.4
IgA (g/L)	3.7 ± 1.3	1.8 ± 0.9
IgM (g/L)	1.7 ± 1.1	2.4 ± 1.5
Autoantibodies		
Anti-SMA (%)	100	0
ANA (%)	33	2
AMA (%)	2	0
Progression to cirrhosis after 3 years (%)	43	82

AMA, antimitochondrial antibody; ANA, antinuclear antibody; Ig, immunoglobulin; LKM, antiliver/kidney microsome; SLA, soluble liver antigen.

Data from Johnson PJ, McFarlane IG, Eddleston AL. The natural course and heterogeneity of autoimmune-type chronic active hepatitis. Semin Liver Dis 1991;11:187.

Table 60.2 Summary of autoimmune hepatitis scoring, revised sheet

Parameters	Score
Gender: female	+2
Biochemistry	
(IU ALP:ULN ALP):(IU AST:ULN AST): <1.5, 1.5–3, >3	+2, 0, –2
Total globulin or IgG (fold elevation): >2, 1.5–2, 1–1.5, <1	+3, +2, +1, 0
Autoantibodies (ANA, SMA, LKM-1) titer: >1 : 80, 1 : 80, 1 : 40, <1 : 40 (IF)	+3, +2, +1, 0
Antimitochondrial antibody: AMA positive	–4
Viral hepatitis markers: IgM HAVAb, HBsAg, IgM HBcAb, anti-HCV, and HCV RNA, ?CMV/EBV Ab	Positive –3, negative +3
Hepatotoxic drug history (current)	Positive –4, negative +1
Average alcohol intake (current): < 25 g/day, > 60 g/day	+2, –2
Liver histology	
Interface hepatitis	+3
Mostly lymphoplasmacytic infiltrate	+1
Rosetting of liver cells	+1
None of the above	–5
Biliary changes	–3
Other changes	–3
Other autoimmune diseases in patients or first-degree relatives	+2
Optional additional parameters	
Seropositivity of other defined autoantibodies (pANCA, anti-LC1, anti-SLA, anti-ASGPR, anti-LP, antisulfatide)	+2
HLA DR3 or DR4	+2
Response to therapy	
Complete	+1
Relapse	+3

ALP, alkaline phosphatase; AMA, antimitochondrial antibody; ANA, antinuclear antibody; ASGPR, asialoglycoprotein receptor; AST, aspartate aminotransferase; CMV/EBV, cytomegalovirus or Epstein–Barr virus; HAVAb, hepatitis A virus antibody; HBcAb, hepatitis B virus core antibody; HBsAg, hepatitis B surface antigen; HCV, hepatitis C virus; HLA, human leukocyte antigen; IF, immunofluorescent; IgG, immunoglobulin G; IU, international unit; LC1, liver cytosol antibody type 1; LKM-1, antiliver/kidney microsomal antibody 1; LP, liver pancreas; pANCA, perinuclear antineutrophil cytoplasmic antibody; SLA, soluble liver antigen; ULN, upper limit of normal.

Data from Alvarez F, Berg PA, Blanchi FB, et al. International autoimmune hepatitis group report: review of criteria for diagnosis of autoimmune hepatitis. J Hepatol 1999;31:929.

Table 60.3 Suggested therapeutic regimen: autoimmune hepatitis

Initial therapy: prednisone 30–60 mg/day monotherapy or prednisone 30 mg/day and azathioprine 50–100 mg/day combined therapy

Dose reduction: slowly reduce prednisone (2.5–5 mg every 1–3 months) if ALT remains <1.5 ULN

Maintenance: minimum dose prednisone and/or azathioprine to maintain ALT <20 IU/L for women and < 30 IU/L for men

Stop therapy if ALT in normal range for 1–2 years and liver biopsy indicates inactivity

Treatment of relapse: reintroduce therapy as for initial treatment

Failure to respond: use either high-dose prednisone 40–60 mg/day and/or another immunosuppressant, or consider liver transplantation if appropriate

ALT, alanine aminotransferase; ULN, upper limit of normal; +/–, with/without.

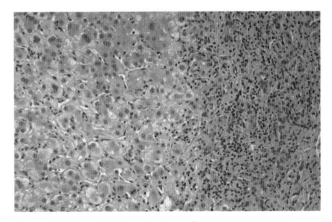

Figure 60.1 Typical histological picture of autoimmune hepatitis.

61

Primary biliary cirrhosis

Marlyn J. Mayo, Dwain L. Thiele

Primary biliary cirrhosis (PBC) is a chronic liver disease that is defined by its clinical presentation, histological features, and serological findings. The underlying abnormality in PBC is a slowly progressive, nonpurulent inflammatory destruction of the biliary epithelial cells lining the small to medium-sized interlobular ducts. Autoantibodies are a characteristic feature of the disease; over 90% of PBC patients have anti-mitochondrial antibodies (AMA) and about 50% have anti-nuclear antibodies (ANA). Loss of normal biliary drainage eventually leads to a clinical picture of chronic hepatic cholestasis and its potential complications.

Histology

Several authors have developed histological staging systems that group the histological abnormalities of PBC into four distinct stages (Fig. 61.1). Stage I is characterized by lymphocytes infiltrating the portal tracts (Fig. 61.2). Stage II is characterized by a greater degree of inflammation, extending beyond the limiting plate, and the presence of bile ductular proliferation (Fig. 61.3). Stage III is defined by the presence of bridging fibrosis (Fig. 61.4), and stage IV is represented by the presence of cirrhosis (Fig. 61.5). The most specific (although not pathognomonic) histological finding is the "florid duct lesion," in which the bile duct is surrounded by an intense lymphocytic or granulomatous infiltrate, and the basal integrity of the bile duct has been breached by individual lymphocytes (Fig. 61.6). Bile staining and cholate stasis with feathery degeneration of hepatocytes (Fig. 61.7) is evident in some patients, and Mallory hyaline may be found in the affected hepatocytes (Fig. 61.8). As the disease advances, ductopenia becomes evident. Results of staining for copper and copper-binding protein are often positive in studies of liver tissue affected by PBC (Fig. 61.9). The degree of copper retention correlates with

disease severity, and it may reach levels comparable to that seen in Wilson disease.

Clinical manifestations

The diagnosis of PBC is suspected when a patient presents with evidence of chronic cholestasis. In the early stages this may be an asymptomatic elevation of serum alkaline phosphatase and γ-glutamyltransferase levels. Over time, fatigue or clinical signs of chronic cholestasis such as pruritus or hypercholesterolemia may develop. Jaundice occurs late in the disease process and is a poor prognostic sign.

Xanthomas and hyperpigmentation are the primary skin findings expressed in patients with PBC. Xanthomas are most often seen around the eyes (xanthelasma) but may also develop over tendons and in palmar digital creases (Fig. 61.10). Hyperpigmentation (Fig. 61.11) results from increased melanin deposition and is most often found on the trunk and arms. Skin may also darken in areas that are repetitively scratched, which may result in a butterfly pattern of sparing in the middle of the back.

PBC is frequently accompanied by other extrahepatic conditions, many of which are also considered to be autoimmune in nature. The most common symptomatic comorbid condition is Sjögren syndrome, which occurs in 30%–58% of patients with PBC. Xerostomia and xerophthalmia of sicca syndrome are the usual manifestations. The CREST syndrome (calcinosis, Raynaud phenomenon, esophageal dysmotility, sclerodactyly, and telangiectasias) is present in about 5% of patients with PBC. The most common features seen are Raynaud phenomenon (Fig. 61.12) and telangiectasias (Fig. 61.13). Isolated Raynaud syndrome occurs in an additional 7%–14%.

Clinical course and therapy

PBC may exist for relatively long periods of time in an asymptomatic state. However, the majority of asymptomatic individuals eventually become symptomatic, and most individuals with established disease eventually progress to cirrhosis (Fig. 61.14). Clinical progression is foretold by worsening of specific biochemical parameters, particularly serum bilirubin levels.

Therapy with ursodeoxycholic acid (ursodiol) at a dose of 13–15 mg/kg/day has become the mainstay of therapy for PBC. Multiple large randomized double-blind controlled trials have demonstrated the beneficial effects of ursodeoxycholic acid therapy. Improvement in the results of serum liver tests usually occurs within the first 1–2 months of therapy, with a maximal response by about 6 months. Ursodiol is currently recommended as treatment for all stages of PBC; however, patients with early-stage disease appear to receive the most benefit. Patients with complicated cirrhosis or poor estimated survival should be considered for transplant referral.

Treatment of the symptoms and complications of chronic cholestasis comprises a significant portion of the management of patients with PBC (Fig. 61.15). Pruritus is a common and often a vexing symptom of patients with PBC. Bile acid sequestrants, such as cholestyramine and colestipol, are the first line of medical treatment for cholestatic pruritus. Other medications that have been demonstrated to relieve cholestatic itching in small controlled trials include rifampin (rifampicin), phenobarbital, opioid receptor blockers, and sertraline. Antihistamines, plasmapheresis, albumin dialysis, and phototherapy have also been anecdotally successful in ameliorating cholestatic pruritus. Finally, some patients have intractable itching, which has been an independent indication for liver transplantation.

Accelerated osteoporosis can be a devastating complication of chronic cholestasis, and careful monitoring and preventive treatment are warranted. The severity of bone disease correlates with the severity of the liver disease, and therefore patients with stage IV disease should be screened with bone densitometry at regular intervals. Calcium supplementation is well tolerated and widely used. The majority of postmenopausal patients with PBC can benefit from transdermal or low-dose oral estrogen replacement without experiencing a clinically significant increase in cholestasis. The ability of bisphosphonates to increase bone density has been demonstrated in patients with PBC, so these agents are indicated when bone density is already decreased.

Deficiencies in fat-soluble vitamins should be replaced. Because of potential toxicity from overdoses, levels of vitamin A and D should be monitored in patients receiving supplements.

Many patients with PBC have sicca syndrome and are troubled by xerophthalmia and xerostomia. Liberal use of moisturizers and regular evaluation by a dental professional are recommended.

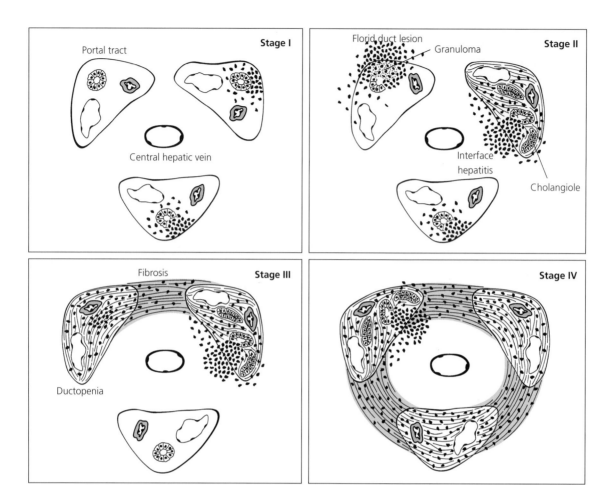

Figure 61.1 Diagrammatic illustration of the four stages of histological progression of primary biliary cirrhosis. Characteristic features of each stage are illustrated here, but the lesions are often patchy in nature. **Stage I**: mononuclear portal tract infiltrates, sometimes involving the bile duct. **Stage II**: intense mononuclear portal tract infiltrate with interface hepatitis, a florid duct lesion (granulomatous involvement of bile duct), and pseudoductular (cholangiolar) proliferation. **Stage III**: bridging fibrosis, mononuclear portal tract infiltrates with interface hepatitis, pseudoductular proliferation, and ductopenia. **Stage IV**: cirrhosis, mononuclear portal tract infiltrates with interface hepatitis, pseudoductular proliferation, and ductopenia.

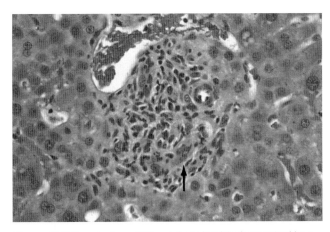

Figure 61.2 Stage I primary biliary cirrhosis (PBC) is characterized by a mononuclear cell portal tract infiltrate that does not extend beyond the limiting plate. The inflammatory infiltrate consists predominantly of T lymphocytes but it may also contain plasma cells and eosinophils. The arrow points to residual biliary epithelial cells of a native bile duct destroyed by the inflammatory process. Bile duct destruction suggests the diagnosis of PBC but may not be evident in biopsy specimens during stage I disease.

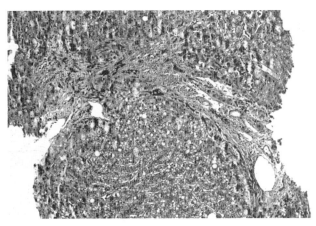

Figure 61.4 Stage III primary biliary cirrhosis is defined by the presence of bridging fibrosis. All of the features seen in stage II primary biliary cirrhosis (see Fig. 61.3) may be present, but ductopenia is more common in later stages of the disease. The diagnosis of ductopenia is often difficult to make because of a lack of sufficient diagnostic material. A minimum sample of four portal tracts (with all four portal tracts containing arterioles but no ducts) or ideally 20 portal tracts (with ≥10 portal tracts containing arterioles but no ducts) is needed to make a diagnosis of ductopenia.

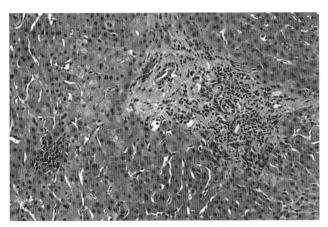

Figure 61.3 Stage II primary biliary cirrhosis (PBC) is characterized by a mononuclear cell infiltrate (predominantly of T lymphocytes, also plasma cells and eosinophils) of the portal tract that extends beyond the limiting plate. Bile ductules are usually found at the periphery of the portal tract (as opposed to the native bile ducts, which tend to be located adjacent to the portal arteriole) and they frequently have poorly defined basement membranes and lumens. Proliferation of bile ductules (pseudoducts or cholangioles) that arise from hepatic cell plates or putative stem cells under conditions of chronic cholestasis is a common feature of stage II disease. Nonsuppurative cholangitis, portal granulomas, and granulomatous cholangitis (see Fig. 61.6) are present in about 50% of stage II PBC biopsies. Septal fibrosis and ductopenia (not evident in this figure) may also be present. Foci of lobular hepatitis, as noted in the upper right corner of the photomicrograph, may also be seen in primary biliary cirrhosis.

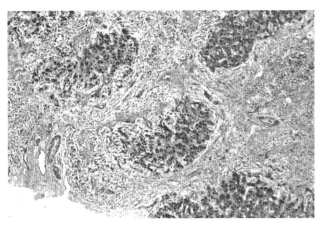

Figure 61.5 Stage IV primary biliary cirrhosis is defined by the presence of cirrhosis. Although any of the characteristic histological features of primary biliary cirrhosis may be present, they may also be absent if much of the liver has been replaced by fibrous tissue. Ductopenia is usually evident in stage IV primary biliary cirrhosis.

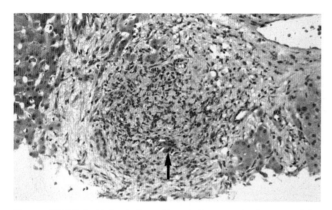

Figure 61.6 A florid duct lesion with granulomatous involvement of the bile duct is the most specific histological finding suggestive of the diagnosis of primary biliary cirrhosis. The granulomas in primary biliary cirrhosis are often poorly defined. Portal granulomas without bile duct involvement are also seen in primary biliary cirrhosis, but lobular granulomas are much less common.

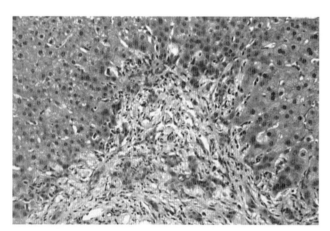

Figure 61.7 Biliary piecemeal necrosis in which there is death of periportal hepatocytes associated with an inflammatory infiltrate may also be evident in primary biliary cirrhosis. The injured hepatocytes appear swollen (feathery degeneration) as a result of cholate stasis.

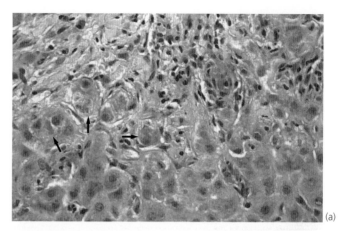
(a)

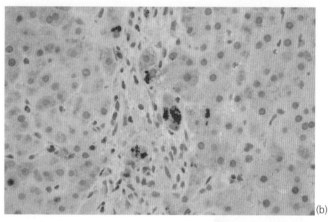
(b)

Figure 61.8 (a) Mallory bodies (arrows) may be seen in primary biliary cirrhosis. They are typically located in the periportal hepatocytes, as opposed to localization in the hepatic lobule in steatohepatitis. **(b)** Immunohistochemistry for ubiquitin (red pigment) highlights the presence of Mallory hyaline in liver tissue affected by primary biliary cirrhosis.

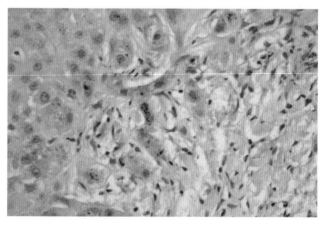

Figure 61.9 A rhodanine stain (red pigment) demonstrates copper granules in the liver tissue affected by primary biliary cirrhosis. Copper accumulates in the periportal hepatocytes as cholestasis progresses. It is often accompanied by Mallory hyaline (see Fig. 61.8) and is typically found in areas of cholate stasis (see Fig. 61.7).

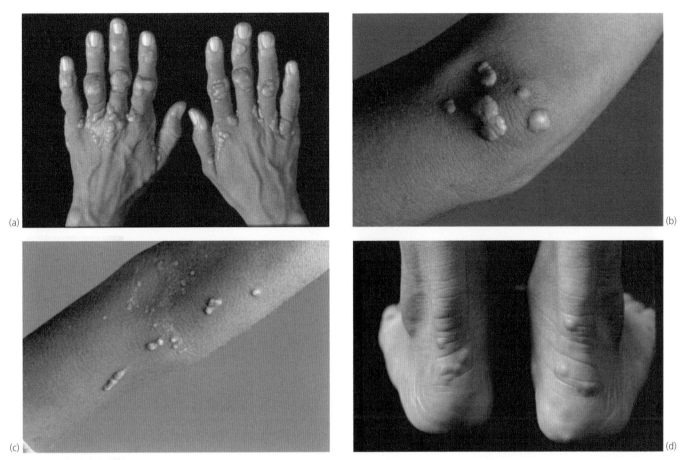

(a) (b)

(c) (d)

Figure 61.10 A patient with primary biliary cirrhosis with severe xanthomas. Xanthomas are most often seen around the eyes (xanthelasma) but they may also develop over tendons and in palmar digital creases. Shown here are xanthomas on the hands (**a**), antecubital fossae (**b**), elbow (**c**), and heels (**d**). Xanthomas occur more often in patients with primary biliary cirrhosis with prolonged cholestasis but they can also occur before the onset of cirrhosis.

Figure 61.11 Hyperpigmentation, which results from increased melanin deposition, occurs more often in patients with primary biliary cirrhosis with prolonged cholestasis but can also occur before the onset of cirrhosis. Pictured here is one patient with primary biliary cirrhosis with asymmetric hyperpigmentation of the hands. Hyperpigmentation is most often found on the trunk and arms. Skin may also darken in areas that are repetitively scratched, which may result in a butterfly pattern of sparing in the middle of the back.

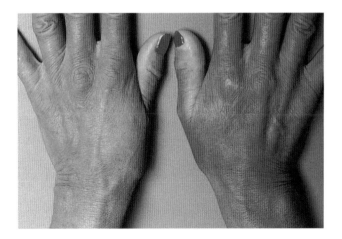

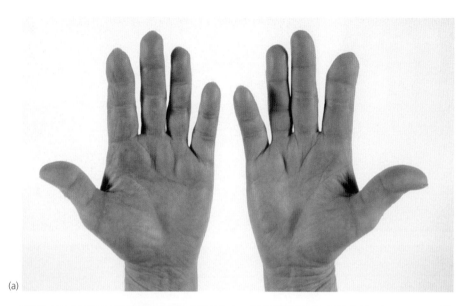

(a)

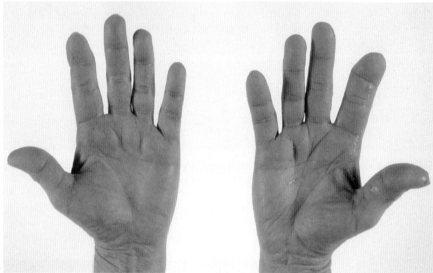

(b)

Figure 61.12 Raynaud phenomenon is present in about 15% of patients with primary biliary cirrhosis. It may be an isolated feature or part of the CREST (calcinosis, Raynaud phenomenon, esophageal dysmotility, sclerodactyly, telangectasias) syndrome. In (**a**), the patient's fingertips are cyanotic at room temperature. In (**b**), after she has soaked her hands in warm water, the bluish color disappears.

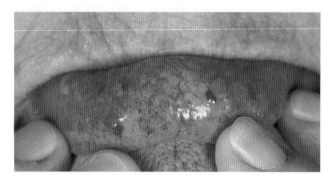

Figure 61.13 Telangiectasias are seen as part of the CREST (calcinosis, Raynaud phenomenon, esophageal dysmotility, sclerodactyly, telangiectasias) syndrome in 5%–7% of patients with primary biliary cirrhosis. Telangiectasias occur most commonly on the lips (shown here) and the fingertips.

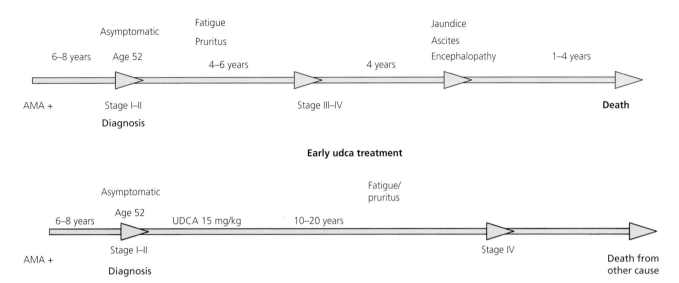

Typical* progression of a patient with primary biliary cirrhosis
natural history

Asymptomatic

Fatigue
Pruritus

Jaundice
Ascites
Encephalopathy

6–8 years   Age 52   4–6 years   4 years   1–4 years

AMA +   Stage I–II   Stage III–IV   **Death**
             Diagnosis

Early udca treatment

Asymptomatic

Fatigue/
pruritus

6–8 years   Age 52   UDCA 15 mg/kg   10–20 years

AMA +   Stage I–II   Stage IV   Death from
             Diagnosis   other cause

*Transition rates derived from Markov modeling and may differ substantially from individual cases.

Figure 61.14 The clinical course of primary biliary cirrhosis has improved over the past decade. Patients are more likely to be diagnosed at an earlier stage and to receive treatment with ursodeoxycholic acid (UDCA). AMA, antimitochondrial antibodies.

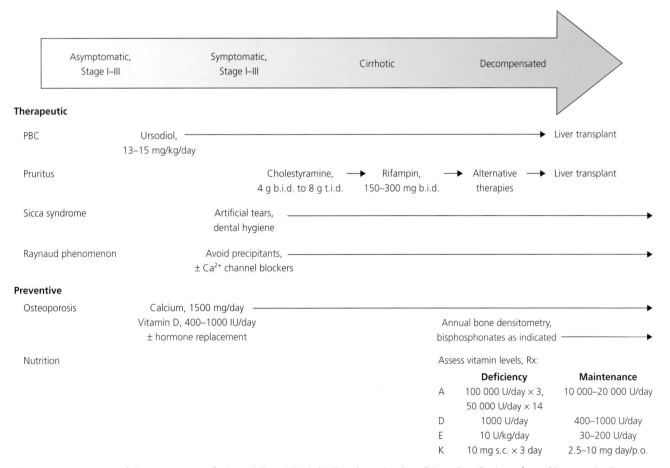

Asymptomatic,   Symptomatic,   Cirrhotic   Decompensated
Stage I–III   Stage I–III

Therapeutic

PBC   Ursodiol, —————————————————————————→ Liver transplant
                       13–15 mg/kg/day

Pruritus   Cholestyramine, ——→ Rifampin, ——→ Alternative ——→ Liver transplant
                                      4 g b.i.d. to 8 g t.i.d. 150–300 mg b.i.d. therapies

Sicca syndrome   Artificial tears, ——————————————————————————————→
                       dental hygiene

Raynaud phenomenon   Avoid precipitants, ————————————————————————————→
                       ± Ca^{2+} channel blockers

Preventive

Osteoporosis   Calcium, 1500 mg/day ————————————————————————————→
                       Vitamin D, 400–1000 IU/day
                       ± hormone replacement   Annual bone densitometry,
                                                        bisphosphonates as indicated ————————→

Nutrition   Assess vitamin levels, Rx:

	Deficiency	Maintenance
A	100 000 U/day × 3, 50 000 U/day × 14	10 000–20 000 U/day
D	1000 U/day	400–1000 U/day
E	10 U/kg/day	30–200 U/day
K	10 mg s.c. × 3 day	2.5–10 mg day/p.o.

Figure 61.15 Overview of the management of primary biliary cirrhosis (PBC) and associated conditions. Complications of portal hypertension (not shown) are managed in the same manner as in other forms of cirrhosis.

62

Hemochromatosis

Jacob Alexander, Kris V. Kowdley

Hemochromatosis is characterized by an inherited defect in the regulation of intestinal absorption of iron resulting in excessive accumulation of iron in different organs and tissues, predominantly liver, heart, endocrine glands, and joints.

Genetics

The C282Y mutation of the *HFE* gene has a population prevalence of 1:200–1:250 for homozygosity and 1:8–1:12 for heterozygosity in persons of northern European ancestry; homozygous C282Y mutations are responsible for 60%–90% of cases of phenotypic hemochromatosis in these populations. C282Y/H63D heterozygotes account for the majority of the rest of the cases, while mutations in other genes, many of them "private mutations" unique to a particular proband, are implicated in the remainder.

Pathophysiology

Several genes and proteins involved in iron homeostasis have been identified. Hepcidin, a 25-amino-acid peptide secreted from liver, is postulated to be the principal regulator of iron transport in enterocytes, macrophages, and placental cells. The roles of HFE and transferrin receptor 2 (TfR2) are not clearly elucidated, but they are hypothesized to influence hepatic expression of hepcidin in response to iron status.

Clinical manifestations

Clinical manifestations vary depending on the severity of iron overload. With the availability of *HFE* genotyping and

Atlas of Gastroenterology, 4th edition. Edited by Tadataka Yamada, David H. Alpers, Anthony N. Kalloo, Neil Kaplowitz, Chung Owyang, and Don W. Powell. © 2009 Blackwell Publishing, ISBN: 978-1-4051-6909-7

increased awareness, patients are increasingly diagnosed at earlier stages when they present with symptoms such as fatigue, malaise, or arthralgia; the classic triad of cirrhosis, diabetes, and skin pigmentation is now rare.

Diagnosis

Prompt evaluation of patients presenting with fatigue, malaise, arthralgia, hepatomegaly, or elevated serum aminotransferase levels is essential for the early diagnosis of hemochromatosis. Serum transferrin iron saturation (TS) is the preferred initial screening test and *HFE* gene testing is the preferred confirmatory test; liver biopsy is required only in selected cases.

Screening

Population surveillance for *HFE* gene mutations is not recommended as the overall risk of long-term complications of iron overload is perceived to be relatively low among those with pathogenic mutations and because of concerns of possible negative social, legal, and insurance consequences for identified individuals. However, phenotypic screening with TS is suggested to be suitable for identifying persons at risk of developing the complications of iron overload.

Treatment and prognosis

Phlebotomy, initially performed once or twice a week until the serum ferritin level is below 50 ng/mL and subsequently once every month to once every 4 months to maintain the serum ferritin level below 50 ng/mL, is the treatment of choice. Generally, phlebotomy is well tolerated and is effective in preventing long-term complications of iron overload and attaining normal life expectancy if initiated in the precirrhotic stage.

Table 62.1 Known coding region mutations in the *HAMP*, *HJV*, *TfR2*, and *FPN1* genes

HAMP	HJV	TfR2	FPN1
+14 alt Meti	Q6H	V22I	Y64N
Met50del	G66X	E60X	A77D
R56X	V74fsX113	R105X	G80S
R59G	C80R	M172K	N144H
C70R	S85P	Y250X	N144T
G71D	G99R	Q317X	N144D
C78T	G99V	R455Q	D157G
93delG	L101P	L490R	V162del
	Q116X	V561X	N174I
	C119F	AVAQ594-597del	Q182H
	R131fsX245	Q690P	Q248H
	R149fsX245		D270V
	A168D		G323V
	F170S		C326Y
	D172E		C326S
	W191C		R489S
	N196K		G490D
	S205R		Y64D
	I222N		G323T
	G250V		Q221Q
	N269fsX311		Q248H
	I281T		
	R288W		
	G319fsX341		
	G320V		
	C321X		
	R326X		
	S328fsX337		
	C361fsX366		
	R385X		
	G55G		
	insG69		
	S105L		
	S264S		
	I275I		
	E302K		
	A310G		
	R335Q		
	N372D		

Table 62.2 Key proteins involved in iron homeostasis

Protein	Function	Expression Site Crypt	Villus	Other cells	Effect of iron depletion
Dcytb	Reduction of iron from ferric to ferrous state on the apical plasma membrane of enterocytes	–	+	–	Increase
DMT1	Transport of ferrous iron across apical plasma membrane into the enterocyte	–	+	+ (many)	Increase
Ferritin	Storage protein for iron	+	+	+ (many)	Decrease
Ferroportin	Export of iron from enterocytes, macrophages, placental cells, and hepatocytes	–	+	+	Increase
Hephaestin	Oxidation of iron from ferrous to ferric state on the basolateral plasma membrane of enterocytes	–	+	+	No change
HFE	Facilitation of transferrin endocytosis; possible role in regulation of hepcidin expression	+	–	+	No change
Hepcidin	Inhibitory effect on iron export from enterocytes, macrophages, and placental cells	–	–	Liver	Decrease
TfR1	Transferrin endocytosis	+	+	+ (many)	Increase
TfR2	Transferrin endocytosis in hepatocytes; possible role in sensing iron status	?	?	Liver	No change
Transferrin	Transport protein for iron	–	–	Liver	Increase

Adapted from Morgan EH, Oates PS. Mechanisms and regulation of intestinal iron absorption. Blood Cells Mol Dis 2002;29:384.

Table 62.3 Classification of iron overload states

Hereditary hemochromatosis
HFE-related hemochromatosis (type 1 hemochromatosis)
   C282Y/C282Y
   C282Y/H63D
   Other HFE mutations
Non-HFE-related hemochromatosis
   Type 2 – juvenile hemochromatosis
      Subtype 2A – *HJV*-related hemochromatosis
      Subtype 2B – *HAMP*-related hemochromatosis
   Type 3 – *TfR2*-related hemochromatosis
   Type 4 – ferroportin-related iron overload

Other iron overload states
Iron-loading anemias
   Thalassemia major
   Sideroblastic anemia
   Chronic hemolytic anemia
   Aplastic anemia
   Pyruvate kinase deficiency
   Pyridoxine-responsive anemia
Parenteral iron overload
   Red blood cell transfusions
   Iron–dextran injections
   Long-term hemodialysis
Chronic liver disease
   Porphyria cutanea tarda
   Hepatitis C
   Hepatitis B
   Alcoholic liver disease
   Nonalcoholic steatohepatitis
   Following portocaval shunt
Dysmetabolic iron overload syndrome
Miscellaneous
   African iron overload
   Neonatal iron overload
   Aceruloplasminemia
   Congenital atransferrinemia

Adapted from Harrison SA, Bacon BR. Hereditary hemochromatosis: update for 2003. J Hepatol 2003;38(Suppl1):S14.

Table 62.4 Comparative overview of types of hemochromatosis

	HFE-related hemochromatosis	Juvenile hemochromatosis		*TfR2*-related hemochromatosis	Ferroportin-related iron overload
OMIM type	Type 1	Type 2, subtype 2A	Type 2, subtype 2B	Type 3	Type 4
Implicated gene and its chromosomal location	*HFE*, 6p21.3	*HJV*, 1q21	*HAMP*, 19q13.1	*TfR2*, 7q22	*FPN1*, 2q32
Gene product	HFE	Hemojuvelin	Hepcidin	Transferrin receptor 2	Ferroportin
Pattern of inheritance	Autosomal recessive	Autosomal recessive	Autosomal recessive	Autosomal recessive	Autosomal dominant
Biochemical tests of iron overload	Elevation of TS precedes elevation of ferritin	Elevation of TS precedes elevation of ferritin	Elevation of TS precedes elevation of ferritin	Elevation of TS precedes elevation of ferritin	Early elevation of ferritin
Distribution of iron accumulation	Parenchymal	Parenchymal	Parenchymal	Parenchymal	Reticuloendothelial
Potential for organ damage	Intermediate	High	High	Intermediate	Low
Age of onset of symptomatic organ disease	Fourth or fifth decade	Second or third decade	Second or third decade	Fourth or fifth decade	Fourth or fifth decade
Anemia	Absent	Absent	Absent	Absent	May be seen in menstruating women or after phlebotomy
Response to phlebotomy	Excellent: decrease in serum ferritin parallels TS; low risk of anemia	Excellent: decrease in serum ferritin parallels TS; low risk of anemia	Excellent: decrease in serum ferritin parallels TS; low risk of anemia	Excellent: decrease in serum ferritin parallels TS; low risk of anemia	Fair: rapid decrease in TS with persistently high serum ferritin; high risk of anemia

OMIM, online mendalian inheritance in man; TS, transferrin iron saturation.
Adapted from Pietrangelo A. Hereditary hemochromatosis – a new look at an old disease. N Engl J Med 2004;350:2383.

Table 62.5 Clinical features of hemochromatosis

Symptoms

Nonspecific, systemic symptoms

Weakness

Fatigue

Lethargy

Apathy

Specific, organ-related symptoms

Abdominal pain secondary to hepatomegaly

Arthralgia

Amenorrhea

Loss of libido, impotence

Congestive heart failure, arrhythmias

Signs

Asymptomatic

Hepatomegaly

Symptomatic

Liver: hepatomegaly; cutaneous stigmata of chronic liver disease; portal hypertension (splenomegaly, ascites, encephalopathy)

Joints: arthritis

Heart: dilated cardiomyopathy

Skin: increased pigmentation

Endocrine: testicular atrophy; hypogonadism; hypothyroidism

Adapted from Harrison SA, Bacon BR. Hereditary hemochromatosis: update for 2003. J Hepatol 2003;38(Suppl1):S14.

Table 62.6 Potential roles of liver biopsy in hemochromatosis

1. As confirmatory test for the diagnosis of hemochromatosis in either of the following situations:
   (a) Genotyping does not reveal C282Y homozygosity or C282Y/H63D compound heterozygosity
   (b) Genotyping is not available
2. To exclude coexistent or alternate causes of liver disease when noninvasive markers are equivocal
3. To exclude the presence of cirrhosis, for the purpose of prognostication

Table 62.7 Findings diagnostic of hemochromatosis in liver biopsy

1. Grade 4 stainable iron in hepatocytes, with periportal distribution, and sparing of Kupffer cells
2. Hepatic iron concentration (HIC) >80 µmol (4500 mg)/g dry weight
3. Hepatic iron index (HII = HIC in µmol/g ÷ age in years) >1.9

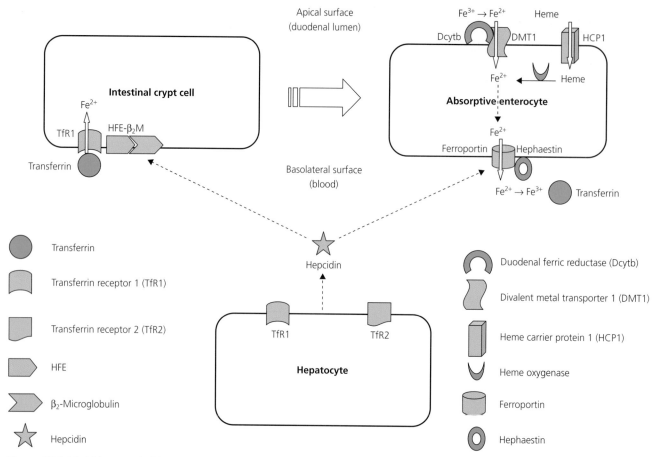

Figure 62.1 Model for control of iron absorption.

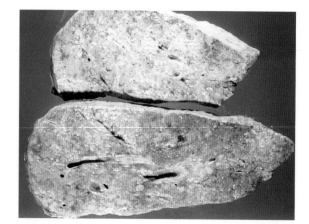

Figure 62.2 A cirrhotic liver from a patient with hemochromatosis. The **upper** specimen has been stained for iron, which appears blue, illustrating the diffuse iron distribution throughout the liver. Courtesy of L. W. Powell.

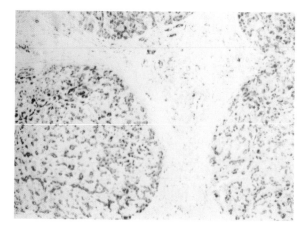

Figure 62.3 A liver biopsy specimen from an untreated C282Y homozygote with cirrhosis. The cirrhotic nodules are stained for iron (Prussian blue stain).

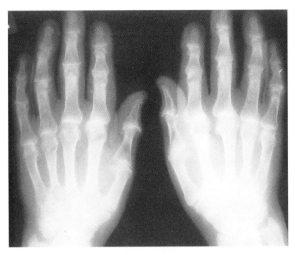

Figure 62.4 The arthropathy of the metacarpal phalangeal joints in hemochromatosis. In this case, a 55-year-old surgeon had to give up surgical practice because of severe disabling arthritis.

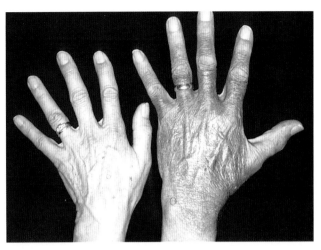

Figure 62.5 The skin pigmentation of hemochromatosis is illustrated in a patient with hemochromatosis **(right)** compared with his wife **(left)**.

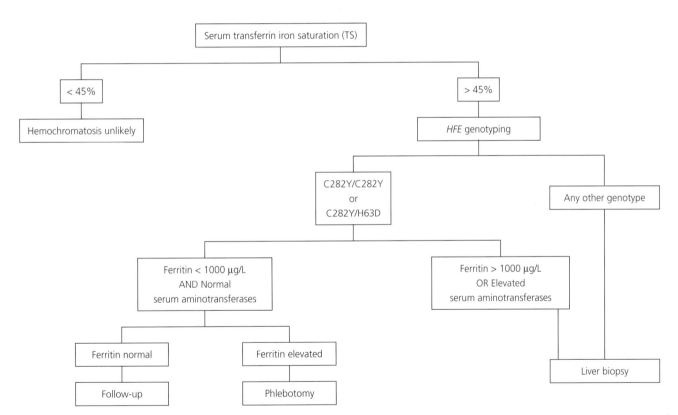

Figure 62.6 Algorithm for management of hemochromatosis.

63

Metabolic diseases of the liver

Ronald J. Sokol, Mark A. Lovell

Metabolic liver diseases comprise a diverse group of genetic disorders in which an enzyme or transport protein is deficient or dysfunctional. Most present during childhood with symptoms of neonatal cholestasis, chronic progressive hepatic fibrosis, or a metabolic syndrome (hypoglycemia, acidosis, encephalopathy, hyperammonemia). Identification of the precise etiology is possible through molecular, biochemical, or enzymatic testing and is important for the initiation of therapy to prevent irreversible injury to the liver, brain, kidneys, or other organs. Several of the most common and important metabolic liver diseases will be summarized and the histology of the liver illustrated.

Alpha-1-antitrypsin (A1AT) deficiency is an autosomal recessive disorder in which the ZZ or SZ phenotype of A1AT leads to liver involvement in 10%–20% of affected individuals and emphysema that is exacerbated by exposure to cigarette smoke. The incidence of A1AT deficiency varies with ethnic group, from 1 in 800 to 1 in 2000. Mutant A1AT, which accumulates in the endoplasmic reticulum of the hepatocyte, can be detected as periodic acid–Schiff (PAS)-positive, diastase-resistant globules, and is thought to be responsible for initiating injury to the hepatocyte (Fig. 63.1). There is no effective treatment for this liver disease; however, most patients do not have progressive disease. Liver transplantation is required for those patients with end-stage liver disease and is curative of all manifestations of A1AT deficiency as normal circulating levels are restored after transplantation.

Wilson disease is an autosomal recessive disorder of copper storage, primarily involving the liver, brain, eyes, and kidney, which has a prevalence of 1 in 30 000 individuals. It is caused by a mutation in the *ATP7B* gene, which codes for a P-type ATPase that is essential for copper transport out of the hepatocyte into bile and for incorporation of hepatic copper into ceruloplasmin, which is secreted into the sys-

temic circulation. In Wilson disease, copper first accumulates in the liver, leading to acute or chronic hepatitis, fulminant liver failure, or cirrhosis, and then in the brain, causing psychiatric symptoms and dystonic or pseudoparkinsonian symptoms. Liver lesions characteristically demonstrate steatohepatitis, glycogen-filled nuclei of periportal hepatocytes, varying degrees of portal tract inflammation, and periportal fibrosis advancing to cirrhosis (Fig. 63.2). Copper chelation and zinc therapies are effective; liver transplantation is required for acute fulminant cases and for those with advanced cirrhosis unresponsive to medical therapy.

Several physical findings suggest Wilson disease. The Kayser–Fleischer ring on the cornea is a hallmark of the disease (Fig. 63.3) and is a greenish-brown ring in the Descemet membrane at the periphery of the cornea on its posterior surface. It is best detected by slit-lamp examination by an experienced ophthalmologist, but can occasionally be seen by the naked eye, particularly in people with blue or green pigmentation of the iris. The ring, composed of granules rich in copper and sulfur, disappears during appropriate copper chelation therapy. Skin pigmentation may be increased, particularly on the anterior aspect of the lower leg, due to deposition of melanin (Fig. 63.4). Blue lunulae of the fingernails may also occur, presumably from deposition of copper (Fig. 63.5).

Glycogen storage diseases (GSD) are a heterogeneous group of defects in the degradation or synthesis of hepatic and muscle glycogen. Several GSD subtypes primarily affect the liver. In GSD type I, glucose-6-phosphatase is defective, leading to massive hepatomegaly, profound fasting hypoglycemia, lactic acidosis, hyperlipidemia, hyperuricemia, and growth failure. Liver biopsy (Fig. 63.6) shows swollen hepatocytes with clear cytoplasm (so-called "mosaic" appearance), macrovesicular and microvesicular steatosis, and a general lack of inflammation, cell death, or portal fibrosis. Treatment is aimed at maintaining normal blood sugar and includes frequent high-starch meals, oral doses of uncooked cornstarch throughout the day, and nocturnal nasogastric tube or gastrostomy tube drip feeding of a formula high in carbohydrate or awakening every 3–4 h at night to ingest

Atlas of Gastroenterology, 4th edition. Edited by Tadataka Yamada, David H. Alpers, Anthony N. Kalloo, Neil Kaplowitz, Chung Owyang, and Don W. Powell. © 2009 Blackwell Publishing, ISBN: 978-1-4051-6909-7

cornstarch. GSD type IX is a generally benign disease manifested by hepatomegaly without the metabolic symptoms of type I disease. Liver biopsy (Fig. 63.7) shows swollen hepatocytes with clear cytoplasm and varying degrees of periportal fibrosis. Occasional patients develop portal hypertension.

Reye syndrome, the prototypic mitochondrial hepatopathy, is called encephalopathy with fatty degeneration of the viscera. Its follows a viral infection (most often influenza or varicella) with the sudden onset of vomiting and lethargy in the absence of central nervous system infection, and elevated aminotransferase levels, prothrombin time, and ammonia levels but normal bilirubin levels, eventually progressing to coma. Most patients in the United States have been exposed to salicylates during the prodromal viral illness. Liver biopsy (Fig. 63.8) demonstrates diffuse, pan-lobular microvesicular steatosis characterized by swollen hepatocytes with central nuclei. Because the fat droplets may be so fine, the steatosis is frequently not appreciated

unless special fat stains are used (Fig. 63.8). There is no portal tract inflammation, although dead hepatocytes are occasionally observed. Special stains will demonstrate a marked decrease in mitochondrial enzyme activity (e.g., succinic acid dehydrogenase) with normal microsomal enzyme activity. Electron microscopy shows markedly swollen and pleomorphic mitochondria with hypodense matrices and loss of dense bodies. The hepatopathy is accompanied by cerebral edema, which becomes the primary clinical challenge in managing Reye syndrome as the liver injury eventually fully recovers. The diminished use of aspirin products in febrile children in the early 1980s after several government warnings about the association with Reye syndrome has been associated with a marked decline in the number of cases. Some of the cases, however, are probably now being correctly diagnosed as defects of mitochondrial fatty acid oxidation and related metabolic disorders that were possibly triggered in the past by viral infections and the effect of salicylates on mitochondrial oxidative phosphorylation.

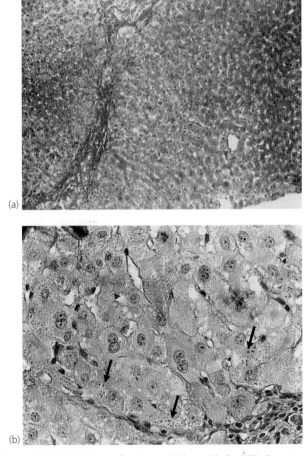

Figure 63.1 Liver biopsy of an 8-year-old boy with the PiZZ phenotype of alpha-1-antitrypsin deficiency. **(a)** Note the periportal bridging fibrosis with mild portal tract inflammation (trichrome stain; original magnification ×10) **(b)** Periodic acid–Schiff (PAS)–diastase staining reveals typical globules (arrows) of alpha-1-antitrypsin trapped within periportal hepatocytes (original magnification ×40).

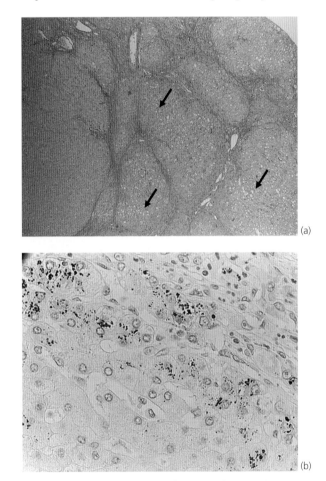

Figure 63.2 Liver removed at time of liver transplantation in a 12-year-old girl with acute fulminant presentation of Wilson disease. **(a)** Note the established cirrhosis with regenerative nodules and mild macrovesicular steatosis (arrows) (hematoxylin and eosin stain; original magnification ×4). **(b)** Rhodanine staining reveals increased copper-associated proteins (brownish pigment) present in hepatocytes (original magnification ×40).

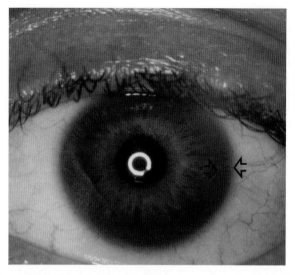

Figure 63.3 Kayser–Fleischer ring (between arrows) on the cornea of a 30-year-old man with Wilson disease.

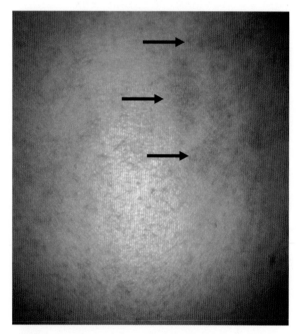

Figure 63.4 Increased brownish discoloration (arrows) of the skin over the tibia in a 10-year-old Cambodian boy with subfulminant Wilson disease.

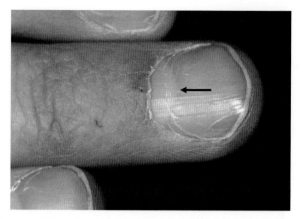

Figure 63.5 Blue lunulae of fingernails in a 10-year-old boy presenting with acute fulminant Wilson disease.

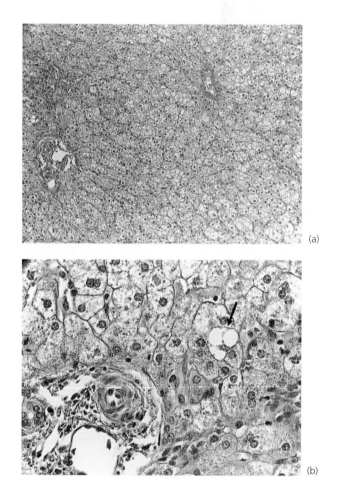

(a)

(b)

Figure 63.6 Liver biopsy from a 2-month-old Hispanic girl with glycogen storage disease type Ib. **(a)** Extensive hepatocyte ballooning with clear cytoplasm and lobular disarray are prominent; fibrosis and portal tract inflammation are absent (H & E stain; original magnification ×10). **(b)** Macrovesicular steatosis (arrow) is also present (H & E stain; original magnification ×40).

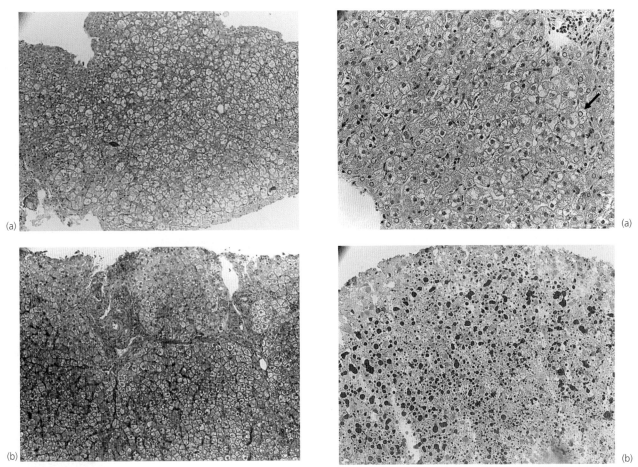

Figure 63.7 Liver biopsy from a 19-year-old man with glycogen storage disease type IX. **(a)** Note the swollen pale hepatocytes with clear cytoplasm exhibiting a "mosaic" appearance (hematoxylin and eosin (H & E) stain; original magnification ×10). **(b)** Mild periportal and early bridging fibrosis is present, although there is no indication of chronic inflammation or hepatocellular death (trichrome stain; original magnification ×10).

Figure 63.8 Liver biopsy from a 5-year-old boy with Reye syndrome. **(a)** Hepatocytes are swollen (arrow) with microvesicular steatosis that is difficult to discern on routine stains, absent portal tract inflammation, and no hepatocyte death. Bile ducts are normal (H & E stain; original magnification ×20). **(b)** Oil red O stain reveals extensive neutral lipid responsible for microvesicular steatosis (original magnification ×20).

64 Alcoholic liver diseases

Suthat Liangpunsakul, David W. Crabb

Epidemiology

In the United States, alcohol is the third leading cause of preventable mortality, behind cigarette smoking and obesity. Among all cirrhosis deaths in 2004, 47.5% were alcohol-related.

Alcohol misuse can be found in all age groups. The overall prevalence decreases with increasing age and always remains higher for men than for women. Alcohol intake is best quantified in terms of grams of ethanol per day. Each common unit of alcohol contains about 10–15 g of ethanol: 1 oz or shot of distilled spirits, a 12-oz bottle of beer, or a 4-oz glass of wine. There is no difference in risk of alcoholic liver disease (ALD) associated with use of any of these forms of beverage alcohol. There is general agreement that the risk of ALD increases with increasing alcohol consumption. The amount of ethanol that can be safely drunk is estimated to be up to 20 g (two drinks) per day for men and up to 10 g (one drink) per day for women. Women have a higher risk of developing cirrhosis than men, even at the lower daily alcohol intake and lower cumulative exposure to alcohol. In men, the risk of alcoholic cirrhosis increases with daily alcohol consumption of more than 60–80 g/day, whereas women have a lower threshold and are considered to be at risk with daily alcohol intake of more than 20 g/day. Additionally, there is a more rapid development of liver disease in women who abuse alcohol than in men. The peak incidence of ALD is in the age range of 40–55 years in men, but a decade earlier in women.

Metabolism of ethanol

In humans, more than 90% of ingested alcohol is eliminated by means of metabolic degradation in the liver, and 2%–

10% is eliminated in urine and breath. Ethanol is first metabolized into acetaldehyde through several enzymatic and nonenzymatic mechanisms, which include the alcohol dehydrogenase (ADH) pathway in the cytosol, the cytochrome P4502E1 (CYP2E1) pathway in the smooth endoplasmic reticulum, and the catalase pathway in peroxisomes (Fig. 64.1). Acetaldehyde is converted by aldehyde dehydrogenases (ALDH) to acetate, which is released from the liver and metabolized by the heart and muscle. The rate of ethanol metabolism by ADH and ALDH may be critical in determining its toxicity because the intermediates of this pathway are themselves potentially toxic.

Alcohol dehydrogenase

Alcohol dehydrogenase is responsible for the bulk of hepatic alcohol oxidation. Human ADHs are categorized into five classes on the basis of their structural and kinetic characteristics. Under physiological conditions, the main isoenzymes involved in human ethanol metabolism are ADHs from classes I, II, and IV. Class I ADH consists of three genes, *ADH1*, *ADH2*, and *ADH3* (renamed *ADH1A*, *ADH1B*, and *ADH1C* respectively). Among these genes, polymorphisms with physiological significance exist in the *ADH2* (*ADH1B*) and *ADH3* (*ADH1C*) loci. These polymorphic variants differ in their efficiency for ethanol oxidation. People of different racial backgrounds inherit different sets of ADH isoenzymes. African Americans who carry a copy of the *ADH2*3* (*ADH1B*3*) gene, encoding an enzyme with high maximum velocity, have a somewhat faster rate of alcohol metabolism.

Microsomal ethanol oxidizing system

Aside from the ADH pathway, ethanol can be metabolized by a microsomal ethanol oxidizing system (MEOS) involving mostly cytochrome P4502E1 (CYP2E1). It has a low ethanol catalytic efficiency compared with ADH and therefore is responsible for only a small part of total ethanol metabolism. CYP2E1 is inducible by chronic drinking, especially in the perivenular zone, and it may contribute to the increased rates of alcohol elimination in heavy drinkers. CYP2E1 is a major source of oxidative stress in the hepatocytes. Of

Atlas of Gastroenterology, 4th edition. Edited by Tadataka Yamada, David H. Alpers, Anthony N. Kalloo, Neil Kaplowitz, Chung Owyang, and Don W. Powell. © 2009 Blackwell Publishing, ISBN: 978-1-4051-6909-7

importance, this P450 enzyme also has the capacity to activate many xenobiotics to toxic metabolites, most notably acetaminophen (paracetamol).

Catalase

The enzyme catalase has also been shown to oxidize ethanol to acetaldehyde within the peroxisomes. Under normal physiological conditions it plays only a minor role in ethanol metabolism.

Aldehyde dehydrogenase

The second step of ethanol metabolism is mediated by ALDH. It converts acetaldehyde to acetate, which is released from the liver and metabolized by heart and muscle. However, only some of the ALDH isoforms are significantly involved in acetaldehyde metabolism, while others metabolize a variety of substrates. To date, a significant role in acetaldehyde oxidation has been identified for mitochondrial ALDH2. Similar to the class I ADH, the *ALDH2* gene is polymorphic and the variants demonstrate the vital role of ALDH2 in ethanol oxidation. The normal allele is termed *ALDH2*1*. The allele *ALDH2*2* has been thoroughly studied because it causes inactivation of the enzyme leading to acetaldehyde accumulation and thus flushing. *ALDH2*2* is found almost exclusively in populations of Asian origin.

Nonoxidative ethanol metabolism

In addition to the main oxidative pathways described above, ethanol is also metabolized, although to a minor extent, by a nonoxidative pathway to form fatty acid ethyl esters.

Pathogenesis

The pathogenesis of ALD is complex. The enzymes that metabolize alcohol, ADH and CYP2E1, generate potentially toxic substances (acetaldehyde and reactive oxygen species). The redox stress of alcohol oxidation contributes to the development of fatty liver, which may increase the sensitivity of the liver to endotoxin. Alcohol consumption is also associated with alterations in two transcription factors, peroxisome proliferator-activated receptor-α (PPAR-α) and sterol regulatory element binding protein 1 (SREBP-1), and the regulatory enzyme AMP-dependent protein kinase (AMPK), which leads to increased synthesis and decreased oxidation of fatty acids. Oxidative stress results in lipid peroxidation. Additional forms of toxicity include formation of protein adducts, dysfunction of the cytoskeleton, activation of Kupffer cells by endotoxin present in the portal blood, and ultimately activation of hepatic stellate cells with fibrosis and cirrhosis. These processes are summarized in Figure 64.1.

Clinical manifestations

Alcoholic liver disease represents a spectrum of clinical illness and pathological changes in individuals with chronic alcohol consumption. Patients may have minimal abnormalities from steatosis or may develop more severe signs and symptoms of liver disease associated with inflammation and fibrosis as seen in alcoholic hepatitis or cirrhosis. Clinical diagnosis of the three major stages of alcoholic liver injury is difficult in that these stages may occur in any combination in the same patient. A number of less common variants of ALD are listed in Table 64.1.

Alcoholic fatty liver is rarely diagnosed clinically because most patients are asymptomatic and do not seek medical attention. Another clinical variant of ALD is alcoholic sclerosing hyaline necrosis. It is characterized by a marked transient elevation of serum aminotransferases (especially aspartate aminotransferase [AST]) and hepatomegaly. The fibrosis forms around the central veins and extends out into the surrounding hepatocytes. It is associated with a poor prognosis, producing portal hypertension and ascites even in the absence of cirrhosis. Liver biopsies demonstrate an intact lobular architecture with centrilobular fibrosis and abundant Mallory bodies, an aggregation of perinuclear, eosinophilic, amorphous material (Fig. 64.2).

Alcoholic hepatitis is the most florid manifestation of ALD and is associated with a high mortality. Classically, alcoholic hepatitis presents with fever, jaundice, hepatomegaly, and signs of decompensated liver disease, such as ascites and hepatic encephalopathy. Fever is common and it is important to exclude other potential sources of infection. The common histological findings in alcoholic hepatitis are ballooning degeneration, focal hepatocyte necrosis, and neutrophilic infiltration. More than 30% of patients develop Mallory bodies (Fig. 64.3). These pathological findings may be indistinguishable from features seen in nonalcoholic steatohepatitis (NASH). Of importance, Mallory bodies are also seen in many other liver diseases (Table 64.2).

Alcoholic cirrhosis has similar clinical features to those of other types of cirrhosis. The pathological end-stage of ALD is characterized by fibrous bands connecting portal triads with central veins, and by regenerative nodules (Fig. 64.4).

It is important to recognize other medical problems related to the underlying alcoholism as well as ALD. Alcoholics are prone to fasting hypoglycemia, ketoacidosis, infections, alterations in mental status that are not due to acute alcohol intoxication (meningitis, hepatic encephalopathy, electrolyte abnormalities, withdrawal syndromes, inadvertent poisoning with methanol or ethylene glycol, and Wernicke–Korsakoff syndrome), and the toxicity of acetaminophen. Worsening liver disease in an alcoholic should prompt a search for other precipitating causes such as common bile duct stones, drug toxicity, acute viral hepatitis, and hepatoma.

Differential diagnosis

There are numerous pitfalls in the diagnosis of ALD, among them failing to consider ALD in patients not conforming to the alcoholic stereotype, and assuming that abnormal liver tests in an alcoholic patient are due to ALD. Alcoholic fatty liver needs to be differentiated from fatty liver that results from drug side effects, obesity, diabetes, and other conditions of insulin resistance, as well as numerous conditions that cause hepatomegaly. The clinical presentation of patients with alcoholic hepatitis may mimic that of NASH or that of cholangitis from choledocholithiasis. Alcoholic cirrhosis is usually micronodular but may sometimes be macronodular. The degree of fatty infiltration of the liver may decrease as cirrhosis develops.

Clinical course and prognosis of alcoholic liver disease

The course of alcoholic fatty liver is typically prompt resolution of hepatomegaly and liver test abnormalities when the patient stops drinking. However, it is important to note that 18% of patients with simple hepatic steatosis can progress to fibrosis or cirrhosis. Therefore, fatty liver is not a benign condition as previously thought. Alcoholic steatohepatitis, on the other hand, is associated with a high mortality. Several clinical scoring systems have been derived to predict the clinical outcome of patients with alcoholic hepatitis, such as the Child–Turcotte–Pugh score (CTP), the Maddrey discriminant function, the MELD (Model for End-stage Liver Disease) score, and most recently the Glasgow alcoholic hepatitis score. The development of infection, hepatic encephalopathy, or renal dysfunction is an ominous sign in patients with alcoholic hepatitis. Approximately 15%–20% of patients who chronically drink excessive amounts of alcohol will progress to cirrhosis in their lifetime, and the prognosis is poor in patients who continue to drink after the onset of liver disease.

Treatment

Fundamental to the treatment of ALD is control of alcoholism. Generally, treatment of alcohol disorders through the use of combinations of pharmacological and behavioral modalities may be more effective than single-modality approaches. Therefore, the current best therapy includes detoxification followed by behavioral or cognitive therapy to help the patient understand factors that precipitate relapse, ongoing involvement in Alcoholics Anonymous or other support programs, and, in some patients, the use of medications to reduce the risk or severity of relapse. Medications to facilitate abstinence, such as naltrexone and acamprosate, both singly and together, have been shown to be effective in some patients. The treatment of alcoholic fatty liver is abstinence from alcohol and lifestyle modification. Alcoholic hepatitis requires treatment if the patient is sufficiently ill. The Maddrey discriminant function (bilirubin + [4.6 × prolongation of the prothrombin time in seconds]), if greater than 32, predicts a more than 50% mortality at 30 days, and has been used as an indicator of the need for therapy. Infections are common in these patients and should be sought and treated. Corticosteroids reduce mortality by about 25%, but may also worsen infection in these patients. Pentoxifylline has been shown to improve short-term survival, largely through reduction in the frequency of hepatorenal syndrome. Most patients with alcoholic hepatitis suffer from protein-calorie malnutrition, which must be addressed. Several metaanalyses could not demonstrate any significant beneficial effects of propylthiouracil, S-adenosyl-L-methionine (SAMe), or vitamin E on any clinically important outcomes of patients with alcoholic hepatitis. Liver transplantation for patients with alcoholic hepatitis is not recommended according to the current guidelines. There are no medical treatments that have been demonstrated to have proven benefit in alcoholic cirrhosis. In an appropriate patient, liver transplantation is the best treatment in decompensated alcoholic cirrhosis. The outcome after liver transplantation for ALD is comparable to that of patients transplanted for other conditions. One important issue in patients who undergo liver transplantation for ALD is the higher rate of late deaths due to lung and oropharyngeal cancer. This is likely because alcohol and tobacco use commonly co-occur, with at least 90% of those with an alcohol problem also using tobacco. Currently, there are no recommendations for posttransplant surveillance for such malignancies.

Table 64.1 Less common pathological features of alcoholic liver disease

Alcoholic fatty liver with perivenular fibrosis
Alcoholic foamy degeneration (alcoholic microvesicular steatosis)
Sclerosing hyaline necrosis
Alcoholic cirrhosis with chronic hepatitis[a]
Cholestasis
Hepatic iron overload
Lipogranuloma
Massive hepatic necrosis (due to acetaminophen ingestion)
Focal fatty liver or focal fat sparing

a A significant proportion of these patients likely have concomitant hepatitis B or C infection.

Table 64.2 Differential diagnosis of liver diseases exhibiting Mallory hyaline

Alcoholic cirrhosis (especially with continued drinking)[a]

Steatohepatitis
  Alcoholic steatohepatitis[a]
  Nonalcoholic steatohepatitis[a]

Chronic hepatitis C

Parenteral nutrition-induced liver disease

Drug-induced liver disease (e.g., griseofulvin, nifedipine, nicardipine, didanosine, diethylstilbestrol, tamoxifen, tetracycline, valproic acid, vitamin A, diltiazem, glucocorticoids, methotrexate, or amiodarone)

Chronic cholestatic disorders
  Primary biliary cirrhosis[a]
  Primary sclerosing cholangitis
  Chronic biliary obstruction
  Extrahepatic biliary atresia

Copper overload conditions
  Wilson disease[a]
  Indian childhood cirrhosis[a]
  Congenital hepatic fibrosis
  Copper-associated liver disease of childhood

Hepatocellular neoplasms/masses

Hepatocellular carcinoma
  Hepatic adenoma
  Dysplastic hepatocellular nodule
  Focal nodular hyperplasia
  Adenomatous hyperplasia

a Indicates that Mallory bodies are found occasionally to commonly; in the other conditions they are rare.

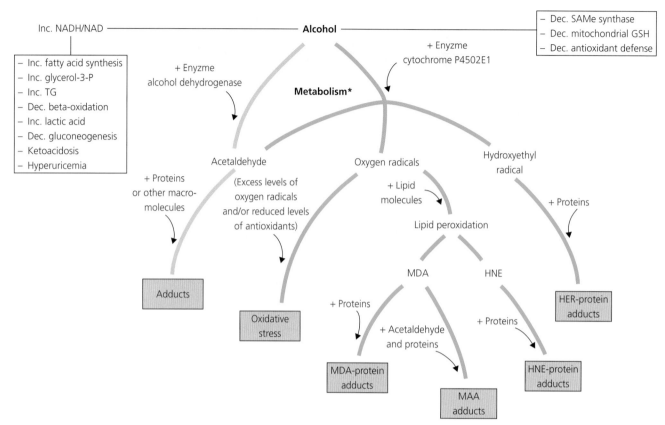

Figure 64.1 Pathway of alcohol metabolism and its effect on metabolism of hepatocytes. Ethanol is first metabolized into acetaldehyde by the major alcohol-metabolizing enzymes alcohol dehydrogenase (ADH) and cytochrome P4502E1 (CYP2E1). Acetaldehyde is then oxidized by aldehyde dehydrogenase (ALDH). The ADH and ALDH reactions generate reduced nicotinamide adenine dinucleotide (NADH). The increased NADH–NAD ratio modifies many metabolic pathways, which leads to increased fatty acid synthesis and decreased fatty acid oxidation. Acetaldehyde can react with other proteins in the cell to generate hybrid molecules known as adducts. CYP2E1 also generates acetaldehyde, as well as highly reactive oxygen-containing molecules called oxygen radicals, including the hydroxyethyl radical (HER) molecule. Elevated levels of oxygen radicals can generate oxidative stress, and oxygen radicals can also interact with lipids in the cell in a process known as lipid peroxidation. Other effects of alcohol include depletion of antioxidants such as SAMe (S-adenosyl-L-methionine) and glutathione. Ethanol may influence the activity of peroxisome proliferator-activated receptor-α (PPAR-α), sterol regulatory element binding protein 1 (SREBP-1), and AMP-dependent protein kinase (AMPK). These effects in turn activate lipogenic pathways, inhibit fatty acid oxidation pathways, and increase the concentration of malonyl-CoA. Malonyl-CoA inhibits the entry of free fatty acids (FFA) into the mitochondria and blocks fatty acid oxidation in mitochondria. Ethanol consumption increases the absorption of lipopolysaccharide (LPS, endotoxin) from the gut. LPS in turn stimulates endotoxin receptors on Kupffer cells (KC), which then activates numerous inflammation-related genes, notably tumor necrosis factor-α (TNF-α), interleukin-6, and transforming growth factor-β (TGF-β1). These cytokines have effects on hepatic stellate cells (HSC) leading to retinoid loss, collagen synthesis, and fibrosis, and may also affect hepatocyte lipid metabolism. Dec., decrease; GSH, glutathione; HNE, 4-hydroxynonenal; Inc., increase; MAA, malonaldehyde–acetaldehyde adduct; MDA, malondialdehyde; TG, triglyceride; SAMe, S-adenosylmethionine.

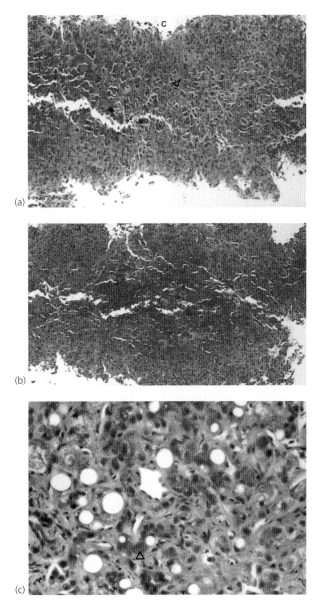

Figure 64.2 Alcoholic sclerosing hyaline necrosis is another variant of alcoholic liver disease. **(a)** The patient can present with the complications of portal hypertension in the absence of cirrhosis because of the extensive fibrosis (arrowhead) around the central vein (C) extending out into the surrounding hepatocytes. Liver biopsies usually demonstrate an intact lobular architecture **(b)** and abundant Mallory bodies **(c)** (arrowhead). Courtesy of Dr Oscar Cummings, Department of Pathology and Laboratory Medicine, Indiana University.

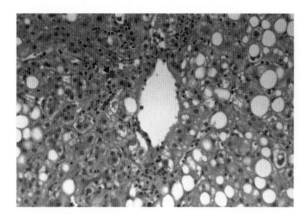

Figure 64.3 Alcoholic hepatitis is the most florid manifestation of alcoholic liver disease and is associated with a high mortality. This biopsy specimen shows evidence of macrovesicular fat, ballooning degeneration, focal hepatocyte necrosis, and neutrophilic infiltration. More than 30% of patients develop Mallory bodies, an aggregation of perinuclear, eosinophilic, amorphous material (arrowhead). Courtesy of Dr Oscar Cummings, Department of Pathology and Laboratory Medicine, Indiana University.

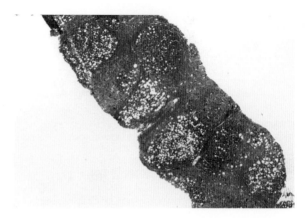

Figure 64.4 Alcoholic cirrhosis. This biopsy, at a lower magnification, shows persistent macrovesicular fat, as well as the formation of fibrous septae. Liver architecture is disrupted, hence this represents a cirrhotic nodule. There is little evidence of inflammation to suggest concurrent alcoholic hepatitis. This biopsy does not distinguish between alcoholic cirrhosis and cirrhosis secondary to a number of other liver diseases. Courtesy of Dr Oscar Cummings, Department of Pathology and Laboratory Medicine, Indiana University.

65

Nonalcoholic fatty liver disease

Arun J. Sanyal, Onpan Cheung

Nonalcoholic fatty liver disease (NAFLD) is the most common cause of chronic liver disease in North America, affecting up to 30% of the general population. Its spectrum of histological changes range from isolated macrovesicular steatosis (nonalcoholic fatty liver) to nonalcoholic steatohepatitis (NASH). NASH can progress to cirrhosis in 15%–20% of patients. The histological diagnosis of NASH is made by the presence of pericentral steatosis, cytological ballooning, and neutrophilic and lymphocytic intralobular infiltration with or without Mallory hyaline or pericellular fibrosis. NAFLD is now considered the hepatic manifestation of the metabolic syndrome and is strongly associated with insulin resistance and obesity.

Pathophysiology

The pathophysiology of NAFLD/NASH is multifactorial and not completely understood. However, insulin resistance has been shown to be one of the major mechanisms involved in disease occurrence and progression. The potential mechanisms that contribute to hepatocellular injury in NASH include oxidative stress, cytokines, mitochondrial injury, and free fatty acid toxicity. The hepatocellular unfolded protein response (UPR) secondary to endoplasmic reticulum stress (ER stress) has been implicated to play a major role in the pathogenesis and severity of NAFLD/NASH.

Diagnosis

The diagnosis of NAFLD and NASH is made by liver biopsy demonstrating either a fatty liver or steatohepatitis and a history of either no alcohol consumption or consumption of less than 20 g/day in women and less than 30 g/day in men. Most people are initially diagnosed with fatty liver because of abnormal results of liver tests performed for unrelated issues or when the liver is felt to be enlarged during a routine physical checkup. Initially, blood tests should be performed to exclude other liver diseases. An ultrasound image, a computed tomography (CT) scan, obtained or a magnetic resonance imaging (MRI) scan may also be obtained to look for hepatic steatosis. However, none of the existing imaging modalities distinguishes between a fatty liver and NASH. Therefore, the only definite way to accurately diagnose NAFLD and determine its severity with precision is to perform a liver biopsy.

Treatment

The prognosis of NAFLD and NASH depends on the risk factors associated with the metabolic syndrome. Weight loss with exercise and diet modifications along with good diabetic control may help reverse hepatic fatty infiltration. Bariatric surgery has shown promising results in improving both hepatic and metabolic abnormalities and is recommended for patients with a body mass index (BMI) of more than 40 kg/m^2 or for those with a BMI of more than 35 kg/m^2 and obesity-related comorbidities. Regimens of lipid-lowering agents and antioxidants contribute to some improvements in biochemical parameters although no obvious improvement in liver histology has been noted. Studies of various insulin-sensitizing agents including metformin and pioglitazone are in progress; their beneficial effects in NASH are yet to be determined.

Atlas of Gastroenterology, 4th edition. Edited by Tadataka Yamada, David H. Alpers, Anthony N. Kalloo, Neil Kaplowitz, Chung Owyang, and Don W. Powell. © 2009 Blackwell Publishing, ISBN: 978-1-4051-6909-7

Table 65.1 Drugs used for the treatment of nonalcoholic steatohepatitis

---

Insulin sensitizers
    Metformin
    Pioglitazone
    Rosiglitazone
Antioxidants
    Vitamin E
    Silymarin
    Vitamin C
Hepatoprotective agents
    Betaine
    S-adenosyl methionine
    Ursodeoxycholic acid
Hypolipidemic drugs
    Fibrates, e.g., gemfibrozil
    Statins
Anti-TNF regimens
    Pentoxifylline
    Adiponectin
Angiotensin receptor blockers
    Losartan

TNF, tumor necrosis factor.

Grade 1: 5%–33% Grade 2: 34%–66% Grade 3: > 67%

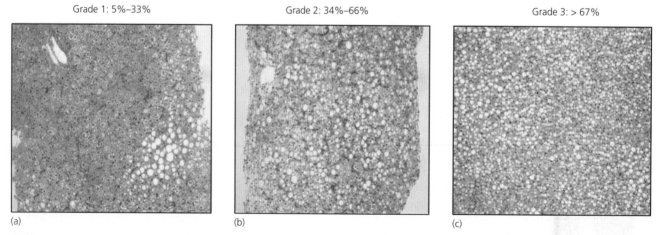

(a)   (b)   (c)

Figure 65.1 Macrovesicular hepatic steatosis with a single large vacuole within the hepatocyte cytoplasm resulting in peripheral displacement of the nucleus. The extent of steatosis is graded based on the percentage of total hepatocytes involved. **(a)** Grade 1 is defined as 5%–33% of parenchymal involvement by steatosis. **(b)** Grade 2 is 34%–66% involvement. **(c)** Grade 3 is > 67% involvement (hematoxylin and eosin stain; original magnification ×20). Courtesy of David E. Kleiner, MD. Histology definition and scoring system are based on the nonalcoholic steatohepatitis Clinical Research Network criteria.

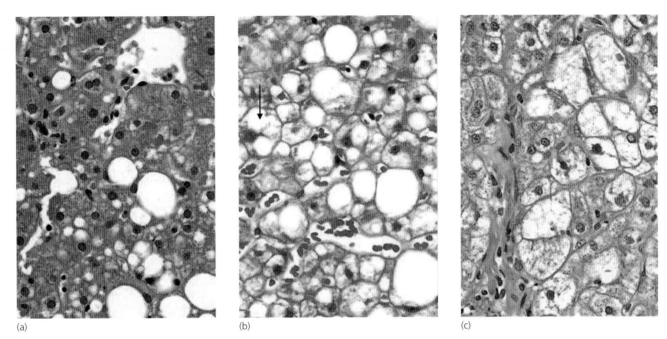

(a)

(b)

(c)

Figure 65.2 Cytological ballooning is a structural manifestation of microtubular disruption and severe cell injury and ballooned cells are often intermixed in areas of steatosis. The ballooned cells are swollen and enlarged (two times normal size) with a pale cytoplasm that appears finely granular or reticulated. **(a)** Mild steatosis without ballooning degeneration. **(b)** This field shows a ballooned cell (arrow) with the characteristics of a scalloped margin, filamentous-appearing intracytoplasmic material, and an accentuated nuclear membrane and prominent nucleoli. **(c)** More prominent ballooning injury (H & E stain; original magnification ×40). Courtesy of David E. Kleiner, MD. Histology definition and scoring system are based on the nonalcoholic steatohepatitis Clinical Research Network criteria.

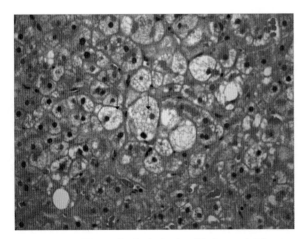

Figure 65.3 Membranes of paired mitochondria fuse and defuse to form megamitochondria (arrows). They appear as hepatocellular, cytoplasmic, discrete eosinophilic bodies, often 3–10 μm in diameter, and have a globoid or, less often, needle-like shape (H & E stain; original magnification ×40). Courtesy of David E. Kleiner, MD. Histology definition and scoring system are based on the nonalcoholic steatohepatitis Clinical Research Network criteria.

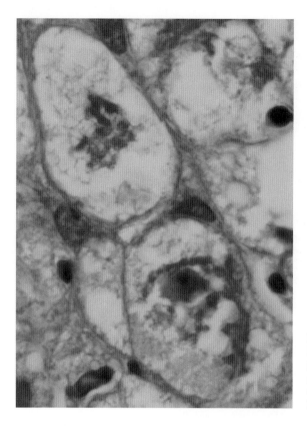

Figure 65.4 Mallory hyaline is seen at the center of the field within a ballooned hepatocyte. On routine H & E-stained sections it is recognized as intracytoplasmic, perinuclear eosinophilic material that ranges in shape from short coarsely clumped masses to elongated rope-like cords (H & E stain; original magnification ×40). Courtesy of David E. Kleiner, MD. Histology definition and scoring system are based on the nonalcoholic steatohepatitis Clinical Research Network criteria.

- (a): Lobular inflammation

  - 0 None

  - 1 <2 foci/20x field

  - 2 2–4 foci/20x field

  - 3 >4 foci/20x field

- (b): Portal inflammation

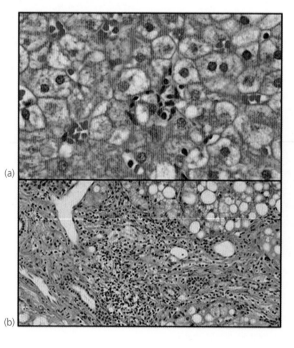

(a)

(b)

Figure 65.5 Inflammation. **(a)** A small cluster of inflammatory cells consisting mainly of lymphocytes is seen. The extent of lobular inflammation is scored as follows: score of 0 is defined as no inflammatory foci; score of 1 indicates fewer than two foci per 20× field; score of 2 indicates two to four foci per 20× field; and score of 3 indicates greater than four foci per 20× field. **(b)** Greater than minimal portal inflammation with predominantly lymphocytic infiltration is also seen, although neutrophils, eosinophils, and plasma cells may be present as the disease activity progresses (hematoxylin and eosin stain; original magnification ×40). Courtesy of David E. Kleiner, MD. Histology definition and scoring system are based on the nonalcoholic steatohepatitis Clinical Research Network criteria.

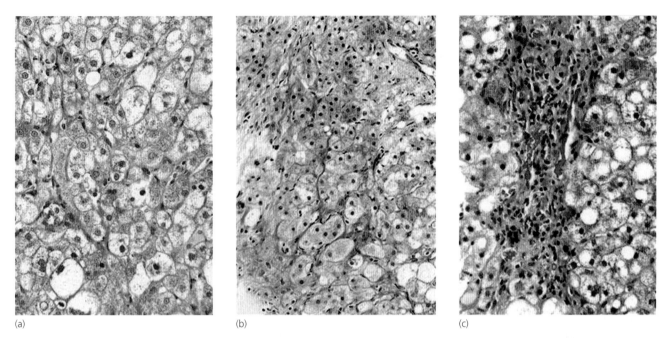

(a)   (b)   (c)

Figure 65.6 Pericellular fibrosis stage 1. **(a,b)** The Masson trichrome stain for collagen highlights perisinusoidal or periportal fibrosis. The collagenous tissue (shown in blue) surrounds individual hepatocytes, producing a chicken-wire appearance. **(c)** In another field the pericellular fibrosis is noted around several ballooned hepatocytes (Masson trichrome; original magnification ×40). Courtesy of David E. Kleiner, MD. Histology definition and scoring system are based on the nonalcoholic steatohepatitis Clinical Research Network criteria.

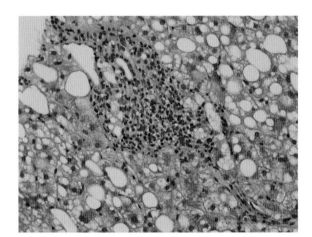

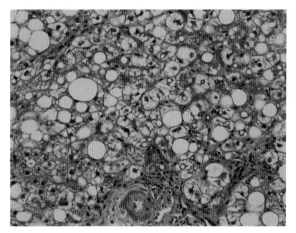

Figure 65.7 This photograph illustrates extensive inflammation with polymorphonuclear leukocytes and lymphocytes surrounding some hepatocytes with both macro- and microvesicular steatosis (H & E stain; original magnification ×40). Courtesy of David E. Kleiner, MD. Histology definition and scoring system are based on the nonalcoholic steatohepatitis Clinical Research Network criteria.

Figure 65.8 Portal fibrosis. Progressive injury in nonalcoholic steatohepatitis (NASH) results in portal fibrosis as shown here. This field illustrates fibrous expansion of portal fields with fibrosis extension along the terminal centriacinar portal vein (Masson trichrome; original magnification ×40). Courtesy of David E. Kleiner, MD. Histology definition and scoring system are based on the NASH Clinical Research Network criteria.

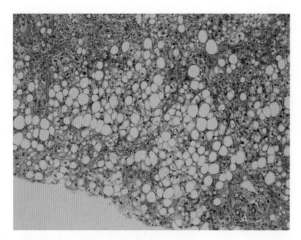

Figure 65.9 Bridging fibrosis. This field illustrates an early stage 3 bridging fibrosis. Note the condensed reticulin connecting two portal tracts (Masson trichrome; original magnification ×40). Courtesy of David E. Kleiner, MD. Histology definition and scoring system are based on the nonalcoholic steatohepatitis Clinical Research Network criteria.

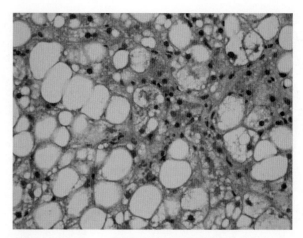

Figure 65.11 Patterns of nonalcoholic steatohepatitis (NASH) as evidenced by the presence of hepatic steatosis, lobular inflammation with lymphocytic infiltration, and hepatocellular ballooning (H & E stain; original magnification ×40). Courtesy of David E. Kleiner, MD. Histology definition and scoring system are based on the NASH Clinical Research Network criteria.

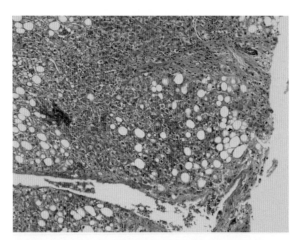

Figure 65.10 Cirrhosis in evolution. Extensive fibrosis with distortion of overall architecture and formation of a regenerative nodule surrounded by dense fibrous tissue. Note the absence of a central vein or portal tracts within the regenerative nodule (Masson trichrome; original magnification ×40). Courtesy of David E. Kleiner, MD. Histology definition and scoring system are based on the nonalcoholic steatohepatitis Clinical Research Network criteria.

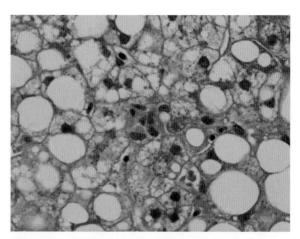

Figure 65.12 Pigment-laden macrophages are seen in the center of the field (H & E stain; original magnification ×40). Courtesy of David E. Kleiner, MD. Histology definition and scoring system are based on the nonalcoholic steatohepatitis Clinical Research Network criteria.

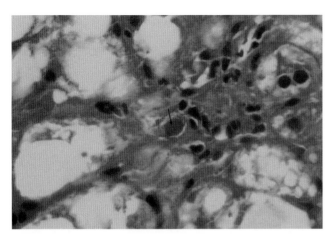

Figure 65.13 Acidophil body (arrow) is seen as well-demarcated, small eosinophilic cytoplasmic globules, either anuclear or possessing nuclear fragments, lying within the lobules, sinusoids, or in periportal areas. In addition to cytological ballooning, hepatocellular injury in nonalcoholic steatohepatitis (NASH) may also manifest as apoptotic (acidophil) bodies (H & E stain; original magnification ×40). Courtesy of David E. Kleiner, MD. Histology definition and scoring system are based on the NASH Clinical Research Network criteria.

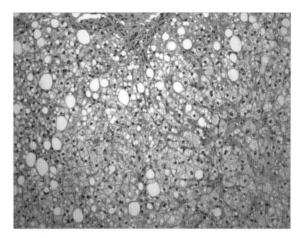

Figure 65.15 Histology highlighting the hepatic glycogenosis and macrovesicular steatosis. The hepatocytes are enlarged by accumulating glycogen, resulting in compression of sinusoids. In addition, mild macrovesicular steatosis is present (H & E stain; original magnification ×40). Courtesy of David E. Kleiner, MD. Histology definition and scoring system are based on the nonalcoholic steatohepatitis Clinical Research Network criteria.

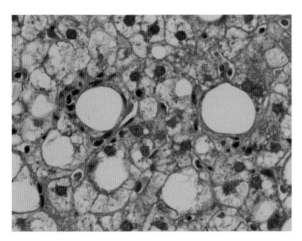

Figure 65.14 Formation of lipogranuloma around a fat cell. Lipogranulomas often occur in nonalcoholic steatohepatitis (NASH) although this finding is neither specific for nor diagnostic of steatohepatitis. They result from the rupture of a lipid-laden hepatocyte, which eventually leads to the development of a foreign body-type granulomatous reactive response. They are composed of steatotic hepatocytes surrounded by mononuclear cells, Kupffer cells, and occasionally eosinophils (H & E stain; original magnification ×40). Courtesy of David E. Kleiner, MD. Histology definition and scoring system are based on the NASH Clinical Research Network criteria.

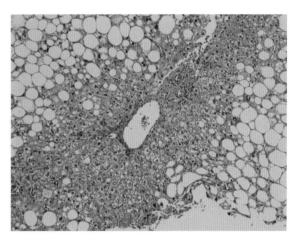

Figure 65.16 Numerous glycogenated hepatocyte nuclei are seen as enlarged, with a prominent nuclear membrane and clear nuclear inclusions. This is often seen in patients with diabetes mellitus and is a common finding in nonalcoholic steatohepatitis (NASH) (H & E stain; original magnification ×40). Courtesy of David E. Kleiner, MD. Histology definition and scoring system are based on the NASH Clinical Research Network criteria.

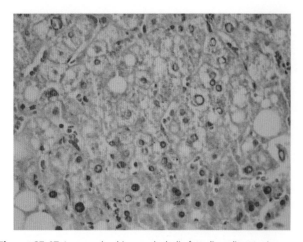

Figure 65.17 Iron overload in nonalcoholic fatty liver disease. A Prussian blue iron stain demonstrates the blue granules of hemosiderin in hepatocytes (Prussian blue; original magnification ×40). Courtesy of David E. Kleiner, MD.

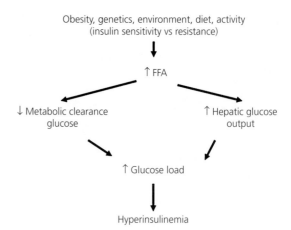

Figure 65.18 The metabolic consequences of insulin resistance. There is an impairment of insulin-mediated suppression of lipolysis in adipose tissue resulting in a net increase of lipolysis and release of free fatty acids (FFA) into the circulation. FFA impair insulin signaling in striated muscle and liver causing impaired glucose uptake and increased gluconeogenesis respectively. These increase the glucose load. The pancreas senses the glucose and FFA load and increases insulin production. Thus, hyperinsulinemia is a hallmark of the early stages of insulin resistance. Over time, as pancreatic function fails, the relative insulin levels drop and are unable to sustain normal blood sugar levels, leading to overt diabetes.

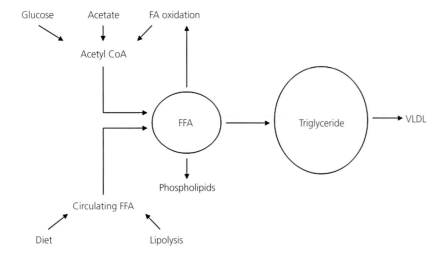

Figure 65.19 A pathophysiological view of hepatic steatosis. Fat accumulates because of either increased production or impaired output/oxidation. Triglycerides are formed from either de novo lipogenesis or reesterification of free fatty acids (FFA) taken up from the circulation. The availability of FFA for triglyceride synthesis is further affected by their utilization for phospholipid synthesis or oxidation to ketone bodies. Triglycerides are packaged into very-low-density lipoproteins (VLDL) by the addition of apolipoprotein B-100 in a step requiring the microsomal transfer protein.

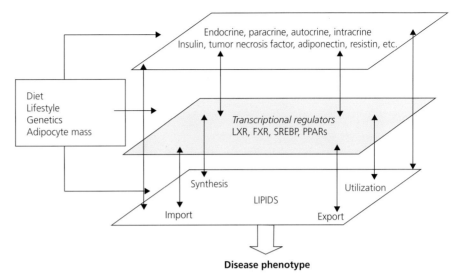

Figure 65.20 The ultimate phenotype of steatosis is subject to modulation by a variety of factors that interact to produce lipid accumulation in the liver. Triglyceride accumulation represents a breakdown in lipid homeostasis, which involves synthesis, import, oxidation, and export. These processes are normally closely regulated by a number of transcriptional factors, which are in turn regulated by cytokines, hormones, etc. Diet, lifestyle, genetic background, and adipocyte mass/distribution can affect all of these steps, thus creating a complex biological system. FXR, farnesoid X receptor; LXR, liver X receptor; PPAR, peroxisome proliferator-activated receptors; SREBP, sterol regulatory element binding protein.

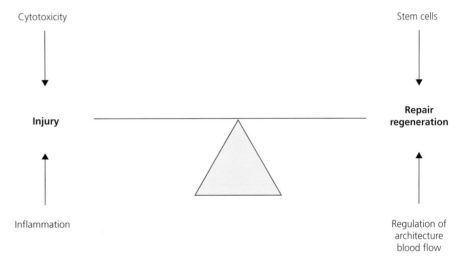

Figure 65.21 Progression of nonalcoholic steatohepatitis to cirrhosis is a function of cell injury and death vs repair and regeneration. Cell injury can result from metabolic disturbances secondary to insulin resistance or from the proinflammatory milieu within the liver. Cell repair and regeneration are still not well understood but presumably involve stem cells derived from the circulation as well as the liver and changes in regulation of hepatic architecture and microcirculation.

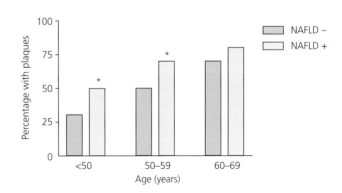

Figure 65.22 Subjects with nonalcoholic fatty liver disease (NAFLD) are more likely to have carotid plaques than matched control subjects who do not have NAFLD. This is particularly true for younger age groups. *The difference between the two groups had a P-value ≤0.05 and is statistically significant.

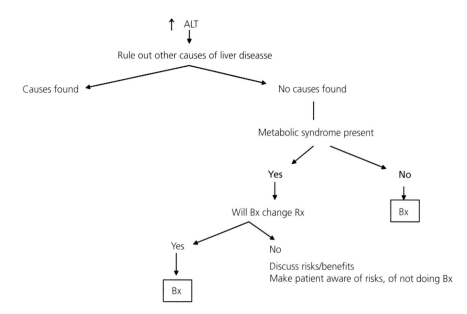

Figure 65.23 A diagnostic algorithm to determine the need for liver biopsy in asymptomatic subjects with persistently elevated liver enzymes. It should be noted that there are other indications for biopsy including the assessment of the stage of the disease. ALT, alanine aminotransferase; Bx, biopsy; Rx, treatment.

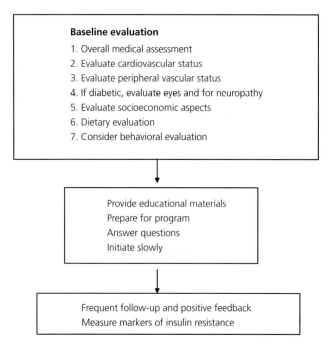

Figure 65.24 A suggested plan for initiation of weight management in subjects with nonalcoholic fatty liver disease.

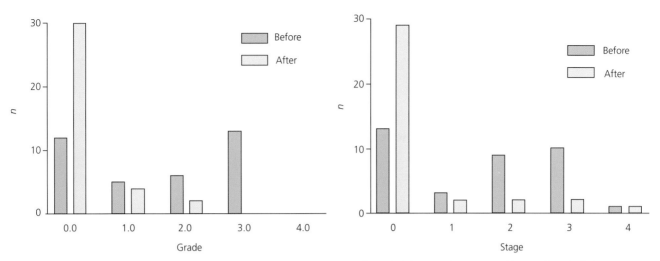

Figure 65.25 The effects of vertical banded gastroplasty on the grade and stage of nonalcoholic steatohepatitis in subjects with morbid obesity. After surgery there was a significant improvement in both the grade and the stage (fibrosis) of the disease.

Figure 65.26 The relative effects of vitamin E (400 IU/day) vs pioglitazone (30 mg/day) and vitamin E on the histological parameters of nonalcoholic steatohepatitis in one pilot study. Although both regimens improved steatosis, the combination was superior to vitamin E alone for improvement in cytological ballooning, Mallory bodies, and pericellular fibrosis. However, only the differences in steatosis reached significance. This is probably because of the small sample size and a type II error in a pilot study. The bar indicates a *P*-value of ≤0.05 and that the difference is statistically significant.

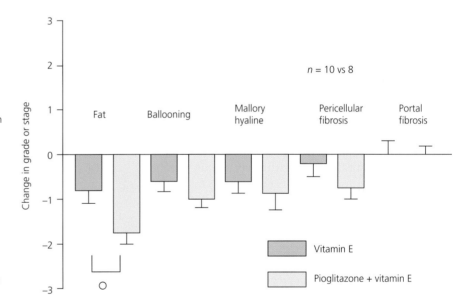

66

Central nervous system and pulmonary complications of end-stage liver disease

Javier Vaquero, Andres T. Blei, Roger F. Butterworth

End-stage liver disease and portal hypertension result in the exposure of vital organs to blood that has not been detoxified by the liver, as a result of both defective liver function and portosystemic shunting. Hepatic encephalopathy (HE), hepatopulmonary syndrome (HPS), and portopulmonary hypertension (POPH) are the result of the exposure of brain and lungs to bloodborne toxins and mediators. Together with variceal bleeding, ascites, and hepatorenal syndrome, they are major manifestations of advanced liver disease and cause significant deterioration of quality of life, with increased morbidity and mortality.

Hepatic encephalopathy

Hepatic encephalopathy refers to the presence of neuropsychiatric abnormalities in patients with liver dysfunction after other known brain diseases have been excluded (Table 66.1). The current multiaxial classification of HE distinguishes three major types depending on the type of hepatic dysfunction and the neurological manifestations (Table 66.2). Common neuropsychiatric symptoms of HE include shortened attention span, anxiety, depression, sleep abnormalities, and motor incoordination progressing through lethargy to stupor and coma. Whereas symptoms are frequently undulating and progress relatively slowly in type C HE, the course is rapid and coma may develop within hours in patients with acute liver failure (type A HE). Routine clinical grading of HE is performed using the West Haven criteria (Table 66.3). Neurological changes in patients with stupor or coma may be better assessed using the Glasgow Coma Scale (Table 66.4). In patients with minimal HE, the diagnosis and quantification of the impairment requires the use of psychometric and neurophysiological tests, such as number connection tests (Fig. 66.1) or auditory- and visual-evoked potentials. Electroencephalographic (EEG) changes charac-

teristic of HE include a bilateral synchronous decrease in wave frequency, increased amplitude, and loss of normal α-rhythm (Fig. 66.2).

The astrocyte is the cell in the central nervous system that demonstrates most alterations in HE. The principal neuropathological finding in type C HE is the "Alzheimer type II" astrocyte, but the presence of low-grade astrocytic edema has also been suggested (Fig. 66.3). There are no alterations pathognomonic of HE in neuroimaging studies, but T1-weighed magnetic resonance imaging reveals bilateral signal hyperintensities in the globus pallidus in over 80% of cases, probably related to manganese accumulation (Fig. 66.4). Studies using positron emission tomography (PET) and $^{13}NH_3$ have shown increases of the cerebral metabolic rate for ammonia and of the blood–brain barrier permeability to ammonia (Fig. 66.5), although the latter remains controversial.

Chronic liver failure results in altered interorgan trafficking of ammonia and hyperammonemia (Fig. 66.6), which is thought to cause the astrocytic alterations. Other cerebral alterations potentially involved in the development of HE are the deposition of manganese in basal ganglia, and diverse abnormalities of brain glucose utilization and cerebral blood flow. Defects in multiple neurotransmitter systems may also underlie many of the neuropsychiatric symptoms of HE (Table 66.5). Finally, the development of oxidative/nitrosative stress and a synergistic effect of inflammation have also been postulated to contribute to the development of HE.

Liver transplantation is the only treatment considered to be curative for HE in patients with end-stage liver disease, generally resulting in improvement of neuropsychiatric status and neuroimaging and neurospectroscopic abnormalities. Medical therapy for HE in end-stage liver disease may attenuate the symptoms, but recurrence is common. In patients with an acute episode or worsening of HE, treatment should begin with the identification and correction of potential precipitating factors (Table 66.6). The general management of HE consists of supportive care and measures directed to lower hyperammonemia (Fig. 66.7). Dietary protein intake should initially be withheld in patients with

Atlas of Gastroenterology, 4th edition. Edited by Tadataka Yamada, David H. Alpers, Anthony N. Kalloo, Neil Kaplowitz, Chung Owyang, and Don W. Powell. © 2009 Blackwell Publishing, ISBN: 978-1-4051-6909-7

severe HE, followed by a prompt and progressive reintroduction as the neurological status improves. Dietary protein should be preferably based on vegetable and dairy products, and long-term protein restriction should be avoided. Vitamin and mineral deficiencies, especially of zinc and thiamine, should be corrected. Nonabsorbable disaccharides (lactulose, lactitol) constitute the first choice to lower hyperammonemia. These agents lower colonic pH and increase fecal nitrogen excretion, and should be titrated to achieve two to three soft stools per day. Common adverse effects include flatulence, abdominal cramps, and diarrhea. As a second-line treatment, antibiotics can also lower hyperammonemia by inhibiting bacterial ammonia production. Neomycin has been commonly used, but the associated risk of nephrotoxicity and ototoxicity is prompting the use of alternatives such as rifaximin. Other agents capable of lowering ammonemia are acarbose, probiotics, L-carnitine, and agents that stimulate ammonia fixation such as L-ornithine–L-aspartate. Neuropharmacological agents such as L-DOPA, bromocriptine, antihistamines, and flumazenil have been tested in patients with HE, with variable and inconsistent effects. Flumazenil (1 mg intravenous bolus), an antagonist of benzodiazepine receptors, may be useful in some patients, particularly in those with suspected benzodiazepine drug ingestion.

Hepatopulmonary syndrome

Hepatopulmonary syndrome distinguishes a group of patients with liver disease and/or portal hypertension who present with alterations of arterial oxygenation because of the development of intrapulmonary vascular dilations (Table 66.7). HPS is relatively common in patients with advanced cirrhosis (prevalence of ~10%–20% in candidates for liver transplantation), but it may appear at any stage and in patients with noncirrhotic portal hypertension. Progressive deterioration of arterial oxygenation occurs in most cases. HPS is associated with increased mortality, particularly if PaO_2 is less than 60 mmHg.

Pulmonary vascular dilations constitute the anatomical basis of HPS. The mechanisms of hypoxemia in HPS include ventilation/perfusion mismatch (predominant mechanism in mild–moderate HPS), diffusion impairment with a perfusion–diffusion defect, and true vascular shunt (Fig. 66.8). Hypoxemia due to ventilation/perfusion mismatch or diffusion impairment characteristically has a good response to breathing 100% oxygen.

HPS develops as a consequence of altered regulation of pulmonary vascular tone, vascular remodelling, and angiogenesis. Increased synthesis of nitric oxide in the pulmonary vasculature, which has been related to specific derangements of the endothelin-1 system, may drive the pulmonary vasodilation in HPS. Induction of heme oxygenase-1 leading to production of carbon monoxide, another vasodilatory molecule, has also been implicated in the pathogenesis of HPS, as well as bacterial translocation and inflammatory mediators.

Patients with HPS may be asymptomatic or present with diverse degrees of dyspnea. Platypnea, spider angiomata, cyanosis, and finger clubbing may also be present. Arterial blood gas measurements show hypoxemia or a widened age-corrected alveolar–arterial oxygen pressure gradient, and orthodeoxia is relatively common. The degree of hypoxemia is used to stage disease severity (Table 66.7). In the diagnostic workup of HPS (Fig. 66.9), transthoracic contrast-enhanced echocardiography is the preferred method to detect the presence of intrapulmonary vascular dilations, but lung perfusion scanning using technetium 99m-labeled macroaggregated albumin ([99mTc]-MAA) particles can also be used (Fig. 66.10). The latter method is particularly useful if coexisting intrinsic pulmonary disease is present. Pulmonary angiography may be performed when discrete pulmonary arteriovenous communications are suspected (poor response of hypoxemia to breathing 100% oxygen).

Medical therapy of HPS basically consists of oxygen supplementation as there are currently no effective pharmacological agents. Pulmonary angiography with embolization of pulmonary arteriovenous communications may improve oxygenation in selected patients. Relieving portal hypertension by emplacement of transjugular portosystemic shunts is not an established therapy for HPS as evidence of the efficacy of this approach is conflicting.

Liver transplantation is currently the only effective therapy for HPS. The risk of mortality after liver transplantation, however, is increased in patients with HPS, particularly when hypoxemia is severe (PaO_2 <50 mmHg) and the [99mTc]-MAA shunt fraction is ≥20%.

Portopulmonary hypertension

Portopulmonary hypertension is characterized by a pathological obstructive process occurring in the pulmonary vasculature of patients who have portal hypertension, resulting in increased resistance to blood flow and pulmonary arterial hypertension (Table 66.7). The prevalence of POPH in candidates for liver transplantation is approximately 5%–6%. Diagnosis of POPH carries a dreadful prognosis, especially when a low cardiac index reflecting severe right cardiac function impairment is present.

The pathology of POPH is similar to that of idiopathic pulmonary arterial hypertension and is characterized by small pulmonary arteries exhibiting vasoconstriction, medial smooth muscle hypertrophy, endothelial and adventitial proliferation or fibrosis, and plexiform lesions (Fig. 66.11). These alterations are the consequence of the hyperdynamic circulation and portosystemic shunting of blood that occur in portal hypertension, but the precise mechanisms and vasoactive mediators involved are currently unknown.

Patients with POPH are frequently asymptomatic. Dyspnea is the most common symptom, but hypoxemia is rare and usually mild. Transthoracic Doppler echocardiography with estimation of right ventricular systolic pressure (RVSP) is the most common approach for screening for POPH (Fig. 66.9). A value of RVSP of 40–50 mmHg should prompt the performance of right heart catheterization with a complete hemodynamic workup, which is required to confirm the diagnosis (Table 66.7). An increase in mean pulmonary arterial pressure (MPAP) alone is not sufficient to make the diagnosis of POPH; it is essential to also demonstrate an increase in pulmonary vascular resistance. MPAP measurement has prognostic value and is used to stage the severity of POPH. If POPH is confirmed, an acute vasodilator test should be performed to help assess the potential response to treatment.

In addition to the avoidance of circumstances that worsen portal hypertension, pulmonary vasoconstriction or stress to the heart, the management of POPH includes oxygen therapy in hypoxemic patients. The evolution of POPH after liver transplantation is uncertain and, therefore, POPH is not considered an indication for this procedure. Furthermore, the presence of POPH significantly increases the mortality of patients undergoing liver transplantation, particularly when MPAP is greater than 35 mmHg. Specific vasodilator therapy with epoprostenol should be considered in patients with moderate-to-severe POPH (MPAP > 35 mmHg) who would otherwise be considered acceptable candidates for liver transplantation. Other pulmonary vasodilators, such as endothelin receptor antagonists or phosphodiesterase inhibitors, have also been tested and found to be effective in small series of patients.

Table 66.1 Differential diagnosis of hepatic encephalopathy

Metabolic encephalopathies
  Hypoglycemia
  Electrolyte imbalance
  Hypoxia
  Carbon dioxide narcosis
  Azotemia
  Ketoacidosis

Toxic encephalopathies
  Alcohol: acute intoxication; withdrawal syndrome; Wernicke–Korsakov syndrome
  Psychoactive drugs
  Salicylates
  Heavy metals

Intracranial lesions
  Subarachnoid, subdural, or intracerebral hemorrhage
  Cerebral infarction
  Cerebral tumor
  Cerebral abscess
  Meningitis
  Encephalitis
  Epilepsy or postseizure encephalopathy
  Neuropsychiatric disorders

Adapted from Riordan SM, Williams R. Treatment of hepatic encephalopathy. N Engl J Med 1997;337:473.

Table 66.2 Classification of hepatic encephalopathy

Type A	Encephalopathy associated with acute liver failure
Type B	Encephalopathy associated with portosystemic bypass and no intrinsic hepatocellular disease
Type C	Encephalopathy associated with cirrhosis and portal hypertension or portosystemic shunts:
	1. Episodic hepatic encephalopathy:
	(a) precipitated
	(b) spontaneous
	(c) recurrent
	2. Persistent hepatic encephalopathy:
	(a) mild
	(b) severe
	(c) treatment dependent
	3. Minimal hepatic encephalopathy

Table 66.3 West Haven criteria for clinical grading of hepatic encephalopathy

Stage 0	No abnormality detected
Stage I	Trivial lack of awareness, euphoria or anxiety
	Shortened attention span
	Impairment of addition or subtraction
Stage II	Lethargy
	Disorientation for time
	Obvious personality change
	Inappropriate behavior
Stage III	Somnolence to semistupor, but responsive to stimuli
	Confusion
	Gross disorientation
	Bizarre behavior
Stage IV	Coma
	Tests of mental state not possible

Table 66.4 Glasgow Coma Scale

	Points awarded
Eyes open:	
Spontaneous (eyes open does not imply awareness)	4
To speech (any speech, not necessarily a command)	3
To pain (should not use supraorbital pressure for pain stimulus)	2
Never	1
Best verbal response:	
Oriented (to time, person, place)	5
Confused speech (disoriented)	4
Inappropriate (swearing, yelling)	3
Incomprehensible sounds (moaning, groaning)	2
None	1
Best motor response:	
Obeys commands	6
Localizes pain (deliberate or purposeful movement)	5
Withdrawal (moves away from stimulus)	4
Abnormal flexion (decortication)	3
Extension (decerebration)	2
None (flaccidity)	1

Table 66.5 Alterations in neurotransmitter systems described in human and experimental hepatic encephalopathy

System	Abnormalities	Activity/tone of the system	Potential consequences
Glutamate	↓ Astrocytic glutamate uptake Alterations of glutamate binding sites in neurons and astrocytes	Diverse derangements	Impaired mental function; astrocytic edema; seizure activity
Serotonin	↑ Tryptophan in CSF ↑ 5-HIAA in brain ↑ Serotonin turnover in brain ↑ Activity and mRNA of MAO-A ↑ Density of postsynaptic serotonin receptors (5-HT$_2$)	Serotonin synaptic deficit	Serotonin synaptic deficit; behavioral abnormalities; sleep disorders
GABA	↑ GABAergic tone, without alterations of brain GABA concentration, GABA-related enzyme activities or densities, and affinities of GABA binding sites ↑ Benzodiazepine-like substances ↑ Densities of PTBRs ↑ Synthesis of neurosteroids	↑ GABAergic tone	Decreased consciousness
Histamine	↑ Hypothalamic concentration of histamine and its metabolites ↑ Histamine H$_1$ receptors	↑ Histaminergic tone	Circadian rhythm alterations; sleep disorders
Dopamine	↑ Concentration of homovalinic acid (dopamine metabolite) ↓ Density of postsynaptic dopamine (D$_2$) receptors	Dopamine deficit	Extrapyramidal manifestations
Opioids	↑ Sensitivity to morphine ↑ Circulating levels of endogenous opioids ↑ Brain levels of β-endorphin Region-selective ↑ of μ- and δ-opioid receptor sites	↑ Opioidergic tone	Decreased consciousness

CSF, cerebrospinal fluid; GABA, γ-aminobutyric acid; 5-HIAA, 5-hydroxyindoleacetic acid; MAO-A, monoamine oxidase-A; PTBR, peripheral-type benzodiazepine receptors.

Table 66.6 Precipitating factors for hepatic encephalopathy

Precipitating factor	Possible mechanism	Diagnosis	Therapeutic interventions
Constipation	Ammonia generation by enteric flora	Clinical history	Laxatives (lactulose, lactitol)
Large dietary protein intake	Nitrogen load, hyperammonemia	Clinical history	Correction of dietary habits; laxatives (lactulose, lactitol)
Infection	Protein catabolism, hyperammonemia	Clinical history and physical examination; chest radiograph; urinalysis; microbiological cultures (urine, blood)	Hygienic measures; antibiotics
Gastrointestinal bleeding	Nitrogen load, hepatic hypoperfusion, tissue hypoxia	Clinical history; hematemesis/melena; anemia, hypotension; endoscopy	Endoscopy with variceal ligation or sclerotherapy; acid suppression therapy if indicated
Hypokalemia	Ammonia generation	Blood chemistry	Avoid diuretics and laxatives; correct electrolyte abnormalities
Dehydration	Hepatic hypoperfusion	Physical examination; blood chemistry and renal function analysis	Avoid diuretics, laxatives, and large paracentesis; correct circulatory volume alterations
Azotemia	Increased ammonia production (urealysis)	Blood chemistry and renal function analysis	Correct etiological agents; correct circulatory volume
Acute hepatitis	Impairment of liver function	Clinical history and physical examination; elevation of aminotransferases in blood analysis	Avoid hepatotoxic drugs; general supportive care; consider liver transplantation
Benzodiazepines and psychoactive drugs	Increased CNS sensitivity	Clinical history; blood toxicology screen	Flumazenil or naloxone challenge
Surgery	Impairment of liver function	Clinical history	Avoid hepatotoxic insults; correct dehydration and electrolyte disturbances
Portosystemic shunts	Reduced hepatic metabolism, hyperammonemia	Clinical history (TIPS placement) and radiological examinations	Shunt occlusion or shunt diameter reduction

CNS, central nervous system; TIPS, transjugular intrahepatic portosystemic shunt.

Table 66.7 General characteristics and diagnostic criteria of hepatopulmonary syndrome and portopulmonary hypertension

	Hepatopulmonary syndrome	Portopulmonary hypertension
Anatomical substrate	Pulmonary vasodilation; intrapulmonary vascular dilation	Pulmonary vasoconstriction; obstruction to pulmonary blood flow
Clinical characteristics	Asymptomatic or dyspnea; platypnea, orthodeoxia; spider nevi, digital clubbing, cyanosis; significant hypoxemia	Asymptomatic or dyspnea; chest pain, syncope; signs of right heart failure; hypoxemia uncommon or only mild
Screening test	Arterial blood gases	Echocardiogram
Diagnostic criteria	Chronic liver disease and/or portal hypertension; alteration of arterial oxygenation (widened age-corrected alveolar–arterial O_2 gradient with or without hypoxemia); evidence of intrapulmonary vascular dilation	Portal hypertension with or without cirrhosis. MPAP >25 mmHg at rest; PCWP <15 mmHg; PVR >240 dynes/s/cm^5
Confirmatory diagnostic tools	Arterial blood gas (demonstration of altered arterial oxygenation); contrast-enhanced echocardiography or radionuclide lung perfusion scanning (demonstration of intrapulmonary vascular dilations)	Right heart catheterization with hemodynamic study
Disease staging	PaO$_2$ (mmHg): ≥80 Mild 60–79 Moderate 50–59 Severe <50 (or <300 on 100% O$_2$) Very severe	MPAP (mmHg): <25 Normal 25–34 Mild 35–44 Moderate ≥45 Severe
Liver transplantation	Usually curative	Frequently contraindicated; effect uncertain

MPAP, mean pulmonary arterial pressure; PCWP, pulmonary capillary wedge pressure; PVR, pulmonary vascular resistance; PaO$_2$, oxygen partial pressure in arterial blood.

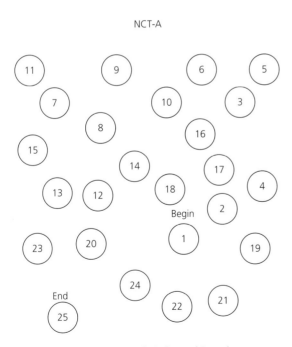

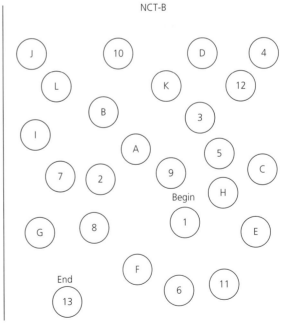

Figure 66.1 Number connection tests (NCTs) A and B used to assess minimal hepatic encephalopathy (MHE). The subject must connect the scattered circles in the correct order as quickly as possible. In NCT-A the sequence consists of numbers from 1 to 25, and in NCT-B the sequence consists of alternating numbers and letters (1-A, 2-B to 13-L). The time in seconds taken to complete each part, including the time needed to correct mistakes, is the score. A previous practice with a sample test is useful to reduce the training bias in follow-up testing. The sensitivity and specificity for detecting MHE is estimated to be 56% and 100%, respectively, for NCT-A (using an upper normal threshold of 30 s), and 68% and 99.2%, respectively, for NCT-B (using an upper normal threshold of 100 s).

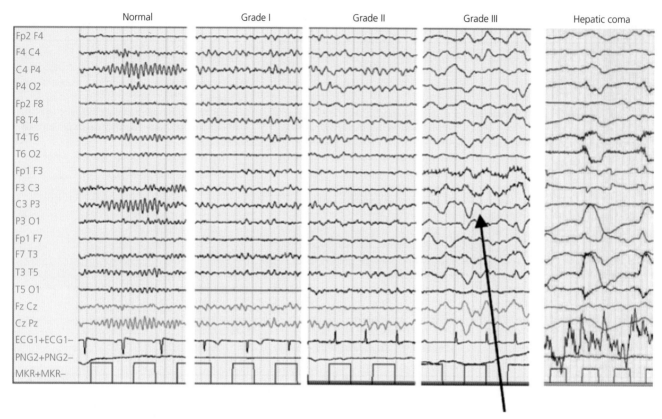

Figure 66.2 Normal electroencephalographic (EEG) tracing from a normal subject (left panel) and altered EEG tracings from patients with hepatic encephalopathy (**middle** and **right** panels). A progressive slowing of the EEG is characteristically observed, and sporadic triphasic waves (arrow) may appear superimposed on the basic slowed rhythm. The last panel shows marked suppression of EEG activity in a patient with severe hepatic coma; the high voltage waves are artifacts due to gasping.

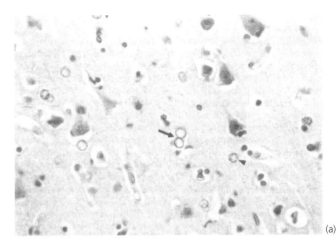

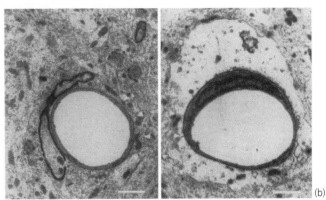

Figure 66.3 Altered morphology of astrocytes is the major neuropathological feature of hepatic encephalopathy. **(a)** Light micrograph of cerebral cortex from a patient with cirrhosis who died in hepatic coma showing Alzheimer type II astrocytosis, with large, pale (watery-looking) nuclei, margination of the chromatin, and prominent nucleoli. The nuclei can take on a variety of shapes from round (in cerebral cortex) to irregular or lobulated forms (in basal ganglia), and they frequently occur in pairs or triplets suggestive of hyperplasia (arrow). A normal astrocyte nucleus is shown for comparison (arrowhead). **(b)** Electron micrographic examination of the brain of a portacaval-shunted rat, an experimental model of chronic hepatic encephalopathy. Compared with the thin astrocytic processes surrounding a brain capillary in a sham-operated animal **(left)**, note the marked swelling of the astrocytic processes surrounding a comparable capillary in a portacaval-shunted rat **(right)**. Bars are 2 μm.

Figure 66.4 (a) Typical bilateral signal hyperintensities in the pallidum on T1-weighted magnetic resonance imaging of a 47-year-old cirrhotic patient with minimal hepatic encephalopthy. Signal hyperintensities resolved following liver transplantation. **(b)** Increased pallidal manganese concentrations in autopsied brain tissue from cirrhotic patients who died in hepatic coma.

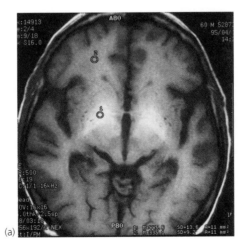

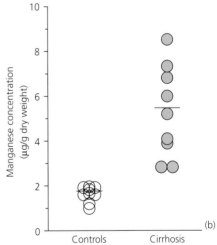

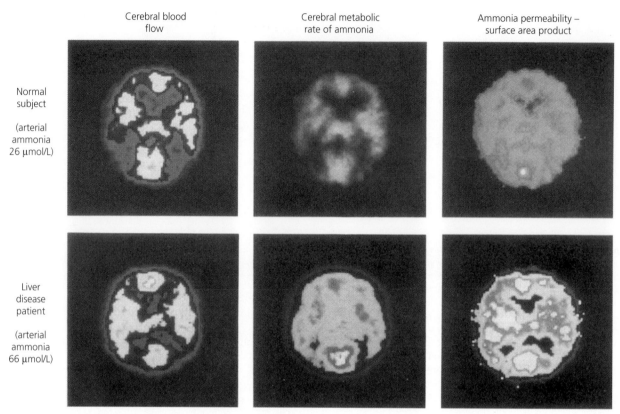

Cerebral blood flow

Cerebral metabolic rate of ammonia

Ammonia permeability – surface area product

Normal subject

(arterial ammonia 26 µmol/L)

Liver disease patient

(arterial ammonia 66 µmol/L)

Figure 66.5 Images of cerebral blood flow, cerebral metabolic rate for ammonia and apparent permeability–surface area product from a normal subject **(upper row)** and from a patient with chronic liver disease and moderate hyperammonemia **(lower row)** studied by positron emission tomography. The patient with liver disease demonstrates an increased cerebral metabolic rate for ammonia and an increased ammonia permeability–surface area product, suggesting increased ease of ammonia transfer into the brain in patients with hepatic encephalopathy.

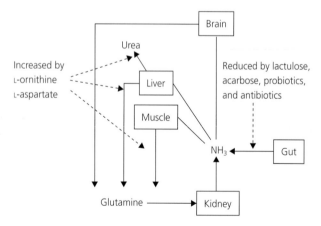

Figure 66.6 Interorgan trafficking of ammonia. Under normal physiological conditions, ammonia (NH$_3$) produced by the gut and kidney is removed primarily by the liver (as urea and glutamine) and to a lesser extent by muscle and brain (as glutamine). In liver failure, liver urea and glutamine production is severely impaired, and muscle (not brain) becomes the organ principally responsible for removal of circulating ammonia. Ammonia production in the gut is lowered by treatment with lactulose, acarbose, probiotics, and antibiotics. Hepatic ammonia removal as urea and glutamine together with muscle ammonia removal (as glutamine) are stimulated with L-ornithine–L-aspartate.

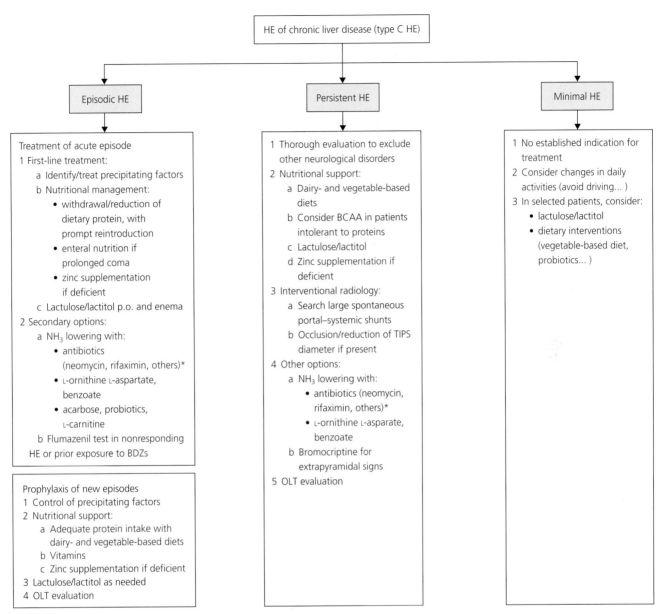

Figure 66.7 General management of hepatic encephalopathy (HE) of chronic liver disease (type C HE). No therapy has been conclusively shown to improve HE compared with placebo in randomized clinical trials. A majority of patients with HE, however, are effectively managed by following the present orientation scheme. The management of the recurrent type of episodic HE would be similar to that of persistent HE. BCAA, branched-chain amino acids; BDZ, benzodiazepine; OLT, orthotopic liver transplantation; TIPS, transjugular intrahepatic portosystemic shunt. *Neomycin for chronic use requires periodic monitoring to avoid nephrotoxicity and ototoxicity.

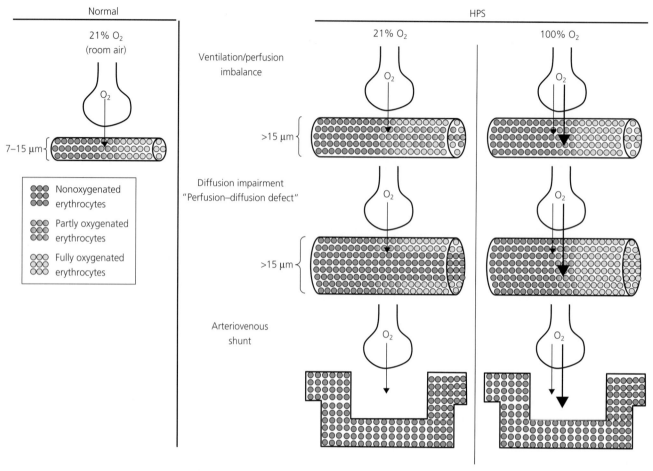

Figure 66.8 Schematic representation of the major mechanisms of hypoxemia in hepatopulmonary syndrome (HPS) and the response to breathing 100% oxygen.

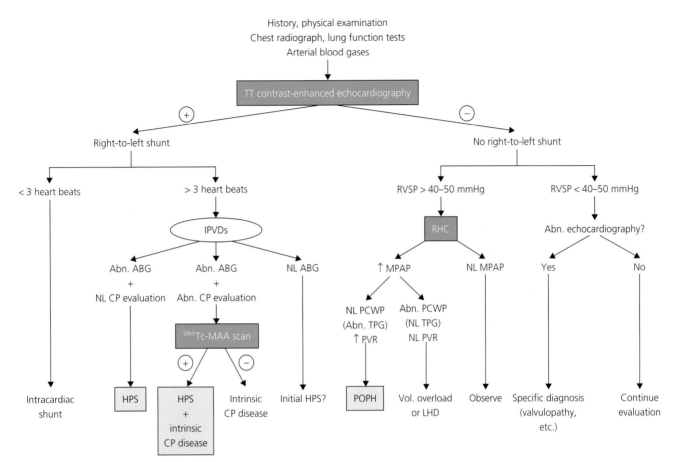

Figure 66.9 General diagnostic approach for hepatopulmonary syndrome (HPS) and portopulmonary hypertension (POPH). Patients with liver disease and/or portal hypertension presenting with respiratory symptoms or specific signs should be evaluated. All patients being evaluated for major surgical procedures (including liver transplantation) should undergo screening for HPS and POPH, even if asymptomatic. ABG, arterial blood gases; Abn., abnormal; CT, cardiopulmonary; IPVD, intrapulmonary vascular dilation; LHD, left heart dysfunction; MPAP, mean pulmonary arterial pressure; NL, normal; PCWP, pulmonary capillary wedge pressure; PVR, pulmonary vascular resistance; RHC, right heart catheterization; RVSP, right ventricular systolic pressure; TPG, transpulmonary gradient; TT, transthoracic; Vol., volume.

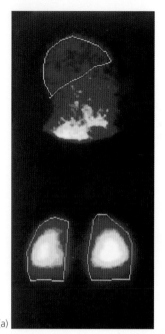
(a)

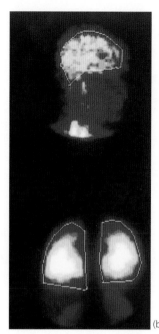
(b)

Figure 66.10 Radionuclide lung perfusion scanning. Technetium 99m-labeled macroaggregated albumin particles (^{99m}Tc-MAA) are injected via a peripheral vein. In normal subjects **(a)**, the albumin particles are trapped in the lungs and less than 6% of the total ^{99m}Tc-MAA activity can be detected in extrapulmonary organs such as the brain. The test is considered positive if ^{99m}Tc-MAA activity in extrapulmonary tissues is greater than 6% of the total. In the sample shown from a patient with hepatopulmonary syndrome **(b)**, the shunt fraction calculated from the ^{99m}Tc-MAA activity in the brain was 50%. Regions of interest are drawn around the posterior lungs and cerebrum. The radioactive intensity is coded as red (low), yellow (moderate), and white (high).

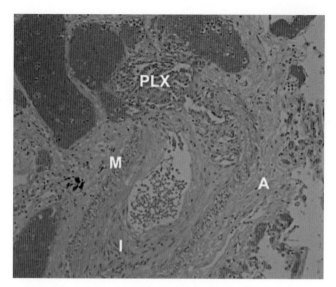

Figure 66.11 Plexiform lesion (PLX) adjacent to a small muscular pulmonary artery from a patient with portopulmonary hypertension. The plexiform lesion is characterized by development of in situ thrombosis and intralumenal endothelial proliferation with formation of narrow slit-like channels. A, adventitia; I, intima; M, media.

67

Liver transplantation

Francis Y.K. Yao, Nathan M. Bass

Liver transplantation is a highly successful treatment for patients with life-threatening, advanced liver disease and is performed in 137 centers across the United States. The success of this procedure is attributed to improved patient selection and pretransplant management, advances in surgical technique, improved organ preservation, new immunosuppressive agents and effective prophylaxis against and management of infectious complications and recurrent disease. The conventional liver transplant procedure matches the recipient to a donor of compatible ABO blood type and body size and involves orthotopic transplantation of the donor organ, i.e., in the normal anatomical location. The bile duct is most commonly anastomosed in a direct duct-to-duct fashion or by a Roux-en-Y choledocojejunostomy. The latter is used mainly in patients with pre-existing bile duct abnormalities (e.g., PSC and biliary atresia), in the anastomosis for a living donor segmental organ graft or when technical difficulty is encountered with a conventional anastomosis.

The 1-year patient survival for all deceased donor adult liver transplants in the United States is 87% (United Network for Organ Sharing [UNOS] data from 1996 to 2005) and many centers have achieved 1-year patient survival rates of about 90%, and 5-year survival rates of 70%–80% (Fig. 67.1). Liver transplantation improves the quality of life in patients with end-stage liver disease, and facilitates return to gainful employment in over 50%. The applicability of liver transplantation as a therapy is, however, limited by donor organ shortage. The total number of transplants performed yearly has increased steadily over the last 10 years, reaching 6441 procedures in 2005. This rise is mainly attributable to deceased donor liver transplantation (DDLT), the number of which increased by 30% since 2001 after rising more slowly over the previous decade (Fig. 67.2a). The size of the waiting list for a liver transplant has increased con-

tinuously, with a peak in 2001 at 14 897 patients (Fig. 67.3). The interruption of this rise in 2002 coincided with the implementation of the allocation system based on the Model for End-stage Liver Disease and Pediatric End-stage Liver Disease (MELD/PELD). A total of 12 822 candidates were actively listed in 2005 compared with 12 650 in 2003. Although the death rate among patients on the waiting list has declined steadily over the past decade (174.3 deaths per 1000 patient-years at risk in 1996 vs 125.5 deaths per 1000 patient-years at risk in 2005), since 1999 there have been approximately 2000 deaths per year among recipients on the waiting list. The continued disparity between cadaveric donor organ supply and recipient demand has undoubtedly contributed to these deaths.

The critical shortage of donor livers has led to strategies that make use of high risk, or "expanded criteria" donors including hepatitis B core antibody positive (HBcAb$^+$) donors, Centers for Disease Control and Prevention (CDC) high risk donors, donation after cardiac death (DCD) donors (for all recipients) and hepatitis C antibody positive donors (for hepatitis C antibody positive recipients). There has also been increased use of segmental grafts, which includes splitting of cadaveric livers between two recipients, and the use of living donors. The number of living donor liver transplants performed annually rose steadily from 1996 to 2001, when it peaked at 519 (Fig. 67.2b). The number of LDLT dropped sharply afterward and plateaued at about 300 procedures per year since 2003. The two reasons commonly cited for the drop since 2001 are the much-publicized deaths of two living liver donors and the introduction of the MELD allocation system around that time. In the case of pediatric liver recipients a left lateral segment is usually obtained from a blood type-compatible parent. In adults, the procedure usually involves removing the right lobe from the donor and transplanting it orthotopically into the recipient (Fig. 67.4). In both the donor and the recipient, there is rapid regeneration of the liver, with full size regained over 6–8 weeks. A right hepatic donor hepatectomy carries inherent risks for the healthy donor, the full extents of which are not yet fully known. There have been at least two known donor deaths

Atlas of Gastroenterology, 4th edition. Edited by Tadataka Yamada, David H. Alpers, Anthony N. Kalloo, Neil Kaplowitz, Chung Owyang, and Don W. Powell. © 2009 Blackwell Publishing, ISBN: 978-1-4051-6909-7

among close to 1000 adult-to-adult living donor liver transplants performed in the United States. The American Society of Transplant Surgeons has established practice guidelines for LDLT.

Liver transplantation should be considered for patients with complications of cirrhosis (end-stage liver disease), fulminant hepatic failure and certain metabolic disorders (Table 67.1). Patients with portal hypertensive bleeding or refractory ascites as the main complications of cirrhosis may undergo transjugular intrahepatic portosystemic shunt (TIPS) as a bridging procedure. Although there are no formal minimal listing criteria for listing patients as candidates for liver transplantation, a useful guideline is that patients with significant complications of end stage liver disease or who have a Child-Turcotte-Pugh [CTP] score of 7 or greater, or a MELD score of 10 or greater are considered reasonable candidates for placement on the liver transplant waiting list, and should be referred for evaluation. The MELD/PELD disease severity scoring systems, for adult and pediatric recipients, respectively, was implemented by UNOS in 2002 as the means for prioritizing organ allocation to candidates on the waiting list (Table 67.2). Since 2005, UNOS policy also requires that donor livers be allocated to local candidates with MELD <15 only if there are no regional candidates with MELD ≥ 15. Patients with fulminant liver failure who are at greatest risk for short-term mortality are classified in a separate category and listed at the highest priority (status 1).

The approach to the evaluation of patients for liver transplantation typically involves a multidisciplinary team including hepatologists, transplant surgeons, transplant nurse coordinators, social workers and individuals with expertise in substance abuse issues (Fig. 67.5). Major items that are addressed during evaluation include the presence of appropriate indications and absence of contraindications (Table 67.3) for transplantation, cardiopulmonary fitness to undergo major surgery, abstinence from substance abuse and appropriate rehabilitation, and adequacy of social support.

The relative frequencies of transplantation for major diagnoses are shown in Figure 67.6. While the numbers of patients transplanted yearly over the past decade for cholestatic liver diseases such as primary biliary cirrhosis and primary sclerosing cholangitis have remained relatively constant, the numbers transplanted for cirrhosis secondary to viral hepatitis and for hepatocellular carcinoma have increased, with 8.4% of liver transplants performed for the latter diagnosis in 2005 compared with 2.4% in 1996.

Although the outcomes for liver transplantation have been excellent for most indications, recurrent disease is a limiting factor in long term graft and patient survival and quality of life. The most significant problem in this respect is recurrent hepatitis C infection that is almost universal following transplantation and for which currently available options for prophylaxis and treatment are limited and poorly effective. Treatment with interferon plus ribavirin is commonly used, but is poorly tolerated and results for the control of recurrent hepatitis C disease have been suboptimal. Severe recurrent liver disease occurs in up to 25% of patients transplanted for end-stage hepatitis C, with 10%–20% progressing to cirrhosis within the first 5 years after liver transplantation. Long-term survival is also adversely impacted in these patients by the recurrent disease. Factors predictive of more severe recurrent disease and worse outcome after liver transplantation have not been clearly elucidated. Prevention and treatment of recurrent hepatitis B is currently achieved in most patients with a combination of currently available nucleoside analogues (i.e., lamivudine, entecavir and adefovir dipivoxil) and high dose intravenous or intramuscular hepatitis B immunoglobulin (HBIG). Recurrence of autoimmune diseases (autoimmune hepatitis, primary biliary cirrhosis and primary sclerosing cholangitis is usually mild, but infrequently causes graft loss. The results of transplantation for hepatocellular carcinoma have improved substantially with careful patient selection. Currently, patients can be listed for transplantation if they meet criteria for stage T2 disease (Fig. 67.7) with overall 5-year survival rates of 70%–75% and tumor recurrence rates of less than 15%.

A major focus of management following transplantation is the prevention and treatment of rejection, which is commonly based on a triple drug regimen of calcineurin inhibitors (cyclosporine or tacrolimus), a nucleoside analogue (azathioprine and or mycophenolate mofetil) and prednisone. Rapamycin (sirolimus), a nonnephrotoxic immunosuppressive has been used in place of the calcineurin inhibitors in selected patients with impaired renal function. Most patients can be maintained on lower doses of immunosuppression with time and in the absence of acute rejection. Lower levels of maintenance immunosuppression are used, in general, for patients transplanted for chronic hepatitis B or C, whereas higher levels are often used in patients with autoimmune hepatitis, primary biliary cirrhosis and possibly fulminant hepatic failure. Prednisone can be withdrawn with close monitoring in some patients at 6 months to 1 year after liver transplantation.

Acute cellular rejection occurs in 30%–60% of all liver transplant recipients within the first year after transplantation, and most commonly within the first 6 weeks after surgery. A single episode of mild acute rejection has not been shown to exert an overall detrimental impact on patient and graft survival but patients with an episode of severe rejection are at increased risk for death or re-transplantation. Initial treatment for acute cellular rejection is usually a high dose, and subsequently tapering corticosteroid regimen. Steroid-resistant rejection is treated with murine monoclonal antibody to the CD3 receptor on T lymphocytes (Muromonab-CD3, OK-T3) or thymoglobulin.

Chronic rejection is characterized by small bile duct loss (chronic ductopenic rejection) and is seen in about 10% of all liver transplant recipients. It usually occurs beyond 60 days after transplantation and is characterized by progressive loss of interlobular bile ducts and an obliterative arteriopathy. Chronic rejection may also result in diffuse bile duct stricturing in the allograft.

Graft dysfunction and loss following liver transplantation occurs mainly secondary to rejection, recurrent primary disease, vascular complications (mainly hepatic artery thrombosis), biliary complications (anastomotic and non-anastomotic strictures, bile leaks), and primary graft non-function. Liver re-transplantation, especially for severe acute or chronic rejection and recurrent primary disease, is associated with worse survival compared with primary liver transplantation. There are significant medical risks associated with the use of immunosuppressive drugs used in liver transplantation, and these are listed in Table 67.4. The most important short- and long-term complications of immunosuppression are infections (bacterial and opportunistic viral and fungal), malignancies (including post-transplant lymphoproliferative disease), as well as cardiovascular, renal and metabolic disease. Hypertension, obesity, altered lipid profiles and impaired glucose tolerance, are all aggravated by immunosuppressive drugs and contribute to an increased risk of ischemic heart disease and stroke in many patients after liver transplantation. Long-term follow-up data regarding the risks and incidence of cardiovascular events and mortality following liver transplantation are only beginning to emerge, and strategies to correct potentially reversible cardiovascular risk factors following liver transplantation will be an important challenge for the future.

Table 67.1 Indications for liver transplantation

Complications of end-stage liver disease
Failure of hepatic synthetic function
Ascites
Spontaneous bacterial peritonitis
Hepatorenal syndrome
Hepatic encephalopathy
Hepatopulmonary syndrome
Refractory portal hypertensive bleeding

Fulminant hepatic failure
Drug-induced liver failure
Viral hepatitis
Wilson disease
Idiopathic
Acute fatty liver of pregnancy
Primary liver graft nonfunction

Primary hepatic malignancy
Hepatocellular carcinoma
Hepatoblastoma
Epithelioid hemangioendothelioma

Impaired quality of life secondary to liver disease
Complications of cholestatic liver disease:
    Intractable pruritus
    Symptomatic osteopenia
    Xanthomatous neuropathy
    Recurrent bacterial cholangitis
Nutritional failure/failure to thrive

Extrahepatic complications of metabolic diseases
Familial amyloid polyneuropathy
Severe familial hypercholesterolemia
Primary oxaluria
Methylmalonic aciduria
Crigler–Najjar syndrome

Table 67.2 The MELD scoring system determining disease severity and priority for organ allocation

	3-month mortality according to the MELD score[b]				
MELD score[a]	≤9	10–19	20–29	30–39	≥40
Hospitalized cirrhotic patients	4% (6/148)	27% (28/103)	76% (16/21)	83% (5/6)	100% (4/4)
Outpatient cirrhotics	2% (5/213)	6% (14/248)	50% (15/30)	–	–

a The MELD calculator is available via the Internet: http://calc.med.edu/UNOS.htm.
b Data from Wiesner RH, McDiarmid SV, Kamath PS, et al. MELD and PELD: application of survival models to liver allocation. Liver Transpl 2001;7:567.
MELD risk score = $10 \times [0.957 \times \log e \text{ (creatinine mg/dL)} + 0.378 \times \log e \text{ (bilirubin mg/dL)} + 1.120 \times \log e \text{ (INR)}] + 6.43$. Current calculation of a MELD score uses a minimum value for the creatinine of 1.0 mg/dL, bilirubin of 1.0 mg/dL, and INR of 1.0. A maximum value of 4.0 mg/dL applies to creatinine. The scores are rounded to the nearest whole number with a score range of 6 (minimum) to 40 (maximum).

Table 67.3 Contraindications to liver transplantation

Absolute contraindications

Severe, irreversible comorbid medical illnesses that adversely impact short-term life expectancy

Severe pulmonary hypertension (mean PAP ≥50 mmHg; PVR >3 Wood Units)[*]

Extrahepatic malignancy (excluding some skin cancers)

Extensive hepatocellular carcinoma or with macrovascular or lymph node invasion[a]

Cholangiocarcinoma[a]

Uncontrolled systemic sepsis

Extensive portal vein and mesenteric vein thrombosis

Active alcohol or drug abuse

Noncompliance

Unacceptable risks for recidivism from drugs or alcohol

Lack of social support

Severe, uncontrolled psychiatric disease

AIDS (HIV[a])

Relative contraindications

Moderate pulmonary hypertension (mean PAP between 35 and 50 mmHg)[a]

Severe hepatopulmonary syndrome with PaO_2 of ≤50 mmHg

Severe obesity (body mass index ≥35)

Poor social support

Advanced age (≥70 years)

a Liver transplantation has been performed in some centers under an experimental treatment protocol.

PAP, pulmonary arterial pressure; PVR, pulmonary vascular resistance.

Table 67.4 Side effects of immunosuppressive drugs

Corticosteroids	Azathioprine	Mycophenolate mofetil	Rapamycin
Infection	Leukopenia	Leukopenia	Leukopenia
Poor wound healing	Thrombocytopenia	Thrombocytopenia	Thrombocytopenia
Osteonecrosis	Hepatotoxicity	Gastrointestinal	Hyperlipidemia
Cataracts	Gastrointestinal	Nausea/vomiting	Intersitial
Diabetes	Pancreatitis	Abdominal pain	Pneumonitis
Cushingoid habitus	Cough	Ulceration/gastritis	
Peptic ulcer	Arthralgia	Pancreatitis	
Hypertension	Retinopathy	Arthralgia	
Obesity	Hypersensitivity		
CNS symptoms			
Growth retardation			

	Cyclosporine	Tacrolimus
Nephrotoxicity	++	++
CNS toxicity	++	++
Headaches		
Tremor		
Paresthesia		
Confusion		
Nightmares		
Seizure		
Hypertension	++	+
Glucose intolerance	++	++
Hyperkalemia	+	++
Hypomagnesemia	++	++
Hyperuricemia	+	+
Gastrointestinal	++	++
Diarrhea		
Nausea/vomiting		
Abdominal pain		
Anorexia		
Hirsutism	++	–
Alopecia	–	+
Gingival hyperplasia	+	–
Hyperlipidemia	++	+

CNS, central nervous system.

Figure 67.1 Unadjusted patient and graft survival for all deceased (DDLT) and living donor (LDLT) recipients in the United States between 1996 and 2005. Patient survival following deceased donor liver transplantation was 93% at 3 months, 87% at 1 year, 79% at 3 years and 73% at 5 years. The corresponding patient survival was slightly better for recipients of LDLT (96%, 92%, 83% and 77%, respectively). A similar pattern is evident when analyzing graft survival.

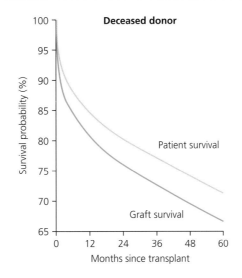

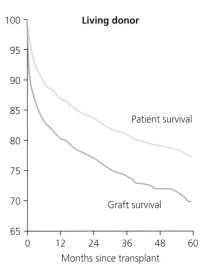

(a)

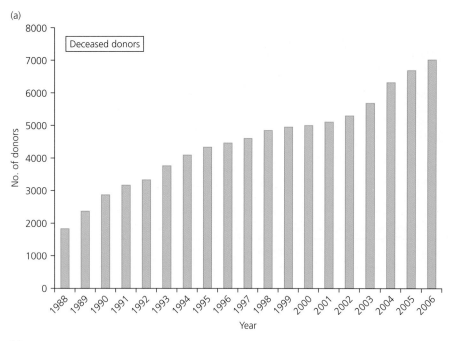

(b)

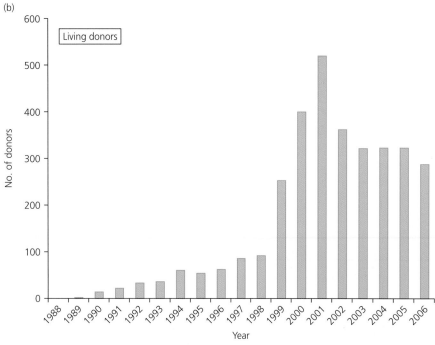

Figure 67.2 Donors recovered in the United States between 1988 and 2006. **(a)** Deceased donors; **(b)** living donors.

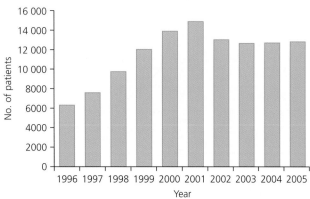

Figure 67.3 Number of patients on the active liver waiting list, 1996–2005.

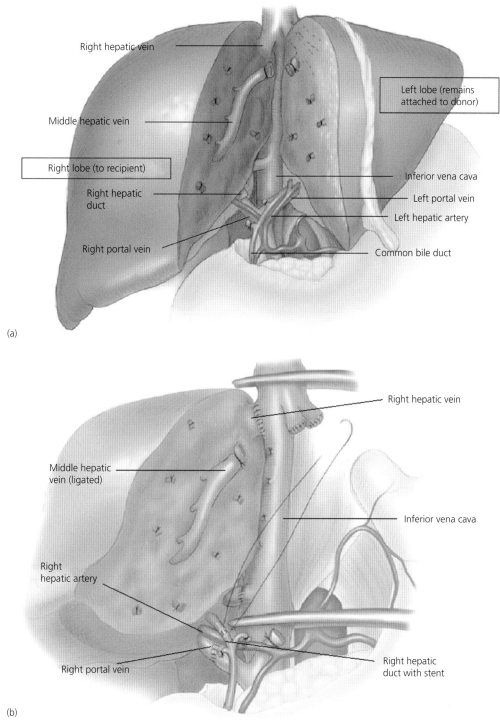

Right hepatic vein

Middle hepatic vein

Right lobe (to recipient)

Right hepatic duct

Right portal vein

Left lobe (remains attached to donor)

Inferior vena cava

Left portal vein

Left hepatic artery

Common bile duct

(a)

Right hepatic vein

Middle hepatic vein (ligated)

Inferior vena cava

Right hepatic artery

Right portal vein

Right hepatic duct with stent

(b)

Figure 67.4 Illustration of technique of living donor liver transplantation. **(a)** Right donor hepatic lobectomy; **(b)** right lobe implantation into recipient. Courtesy of John P. Roberts, Department of Surgery, University of California, San Francisco.

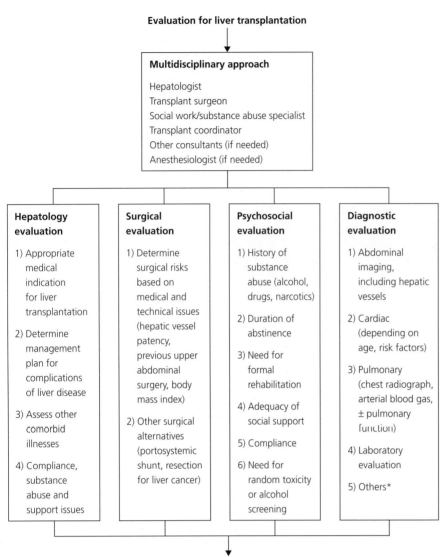

Figure 67.5 Principles in the evaluation of potential candidates for liver transplantation. *Renal function and biopsy, hematological or neurological consultation as indicated in selected cases.

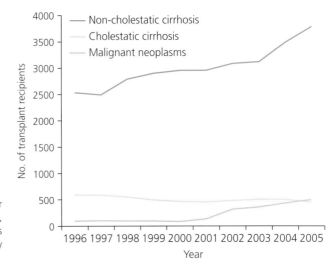

Figure 67.6 Liver transplantation in the United States according to major primary diagnoses. Noncholestatic cirrhosis includes viral hepatitis C and B, alcoholic and cryptogenic cirrhosis. Cholestatic liver disease/cirrhosis includes primary biliary cirrhosis and primary sclerosing cholangitis (but not biliary atresia). Malignant neoplasms consist mainly of hepatocellular carcinoma.

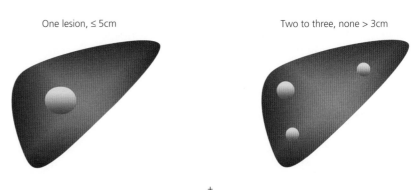

Figure 67.7 United Network for Organ Sharing (UNOS) ("Milan") criteria for transplantation of hepatocellular carcinoma.

G LIVER

68

Hepatocellular carcinoma

Lewis R. Roberts

Epidemiology of hepatocellular cancer

Hepatocellular cancer (HCC) is the fifth most common cancer and the third most common cause of death from cancer worldwide, with an estimated 626 000 new cases per year (Table 68.1). The incidence in the United States is 5.5 per 100 000 persons per year in males and 2.0 per 100 000 persons per year in females and has doubled over the past 25 years. There are strong etiological associations with cirrhosis caused by chronic hepatitis B virus (HBV) infection, chronic hepatitis C virus (HCV) infection, alcohol, hemochromatosis and other causes of chronic liver disease, and dietary aflatoxin exposure. Consequently, the worldwide geographic distribution of HCC cases parallels the distribution of chronic HBV infection, chronic HCV infection, and chronic dietary aflatoxin exposure. The regions with the highest incidence of HCC are in Asia and sub-Saharan Africa (Table 68.2, Fig. 68.1).

Pathogenesis of hepatocellular carcinoma

The pathogenesis of malignant primary liver tumors has been intensively explored. The hepatocellular injury and inflammation that characterize chronic HBV and HCV infection presumably result in cycles of liver cell death and regeneration, which lead to accelerated hepatocellular senescence, telomeric crisis, and chromosomal and genomic instability that contribute to carcinogenesis. Molecular pathways implicated in liver carcinogenesis include the p53/p21 pathway, the p16/cyclin D1/pRB pathway, multiple receptor tyrosine kinases that activate the MAPK and PI3K/AKT pathways, the NF-κB pathway, the Wnt/wingless signaling pathway, and the hedgehog signaling pathway. In addition, multiple growth factors (including TNF-α and TGF-β), oncogenes (particularly c-*myc*), and tumor suppressor genes (including

IGF2R, *SMAD2*, *SMAD4*, *DLC-1*, *SULF1*, and *KLF6*) have been implicated in hepatocarcinogenesis. The molecular mechanisms involved in hepatocarcinogenesis include promoter hypermethylation, deletions, and mutations. Mechanisms specific to HBV-induced HCC include HBV integration, which leads to the production of novel fusion transcripts, the interruption of genes, genomic instability with secondary insertion and deletion events, and transactivation of cellular genes by HBV proteins, particularly the X and pre-S gene products. HCV, which is an RNA virus, does not integrate into the host genome; however, the HCV core protein and nonstructural proteins NS4B and NS5A have been shown to have potentially tumorigenic effects. Chronic aflatoxin exposure predisposes to mutations in *TP53*, the gene coding for p53, in particular a G to T transversion at codon 249. In populations exposed to aflatoxin, approximately 50% of HCCs contain the G249T transversion.

Quantitative and qualitative alterations of β-catenin, a member of the Wnt/wingless signal transduction pathway, have been reported in HCC. Mutations in exon 3 of the β-catenin gene disrupt the serine/threonine phosphorylation sites normally phosphorylated by glycogen synthetase kinase-3β (GSK-3β). This interferes with the proteasomal degradation of β-catenin, leading to its accumulation in cells. Aberrantly accumulated β-catenin translocates to the nucleus and binds to members of the T-cell factor/lymphoid enhancer factor protein family; the resulting complexes then activate target genes such as c-*myc* and the gene coding for cyclin D1 that regulate cellular growth and apoptosis. Because β-catenin gene mutations are only observed in a portion of the liver tumors with β-catenin accumulation, it is reasonable to expect that defects in other molecules that disrupt the normal β-catenin pathway may also be responsible for tumorigenesis in liver cancers.

Diagnosis, growth patterns, and nature of the spread of hepatocellular carcinoma

The prognosis of untreated HCC depends on the extent of disease at the time of diagnosis. As current treatment of

Atlas of Gastroenterology, 4th edition. Edited by Tadataka Yamada, David H. Alpers, Anthony N. Kalloo, Neil Kaplowitz, Chung Owyang, and Don W. Powell. © 2009 Blackwell Publishing, ISBN: 978-1-4051-6909-7

early HCC is effective, high-risk patients should be under regular surveillance to allow for early diagnosis of the tumor. In the United States, many HCCs occur in patients without known risk factors, in whom the tumor is usually detected at a late stage because of a lack of symptoms or signs of early HCC. The high-risk population includes those with chronic HBV (with or without cirrhosis), chronic HCV with cirrhosis, hereditary hemochromatosis with cirrhosis, alcoholic cirrhosis, primary biliary cirrhosis, alpha-1-antitrypsin deficiency, and cryptogenic cirrhosis, which in many cases may be related to nonalcoholic steatohepatitis. Histopathological findings placing the patient with cirrhosis at high risk for HCC include dysplasia (Fig. 68.2), positive immunohistochemistry for proliferating cell nuclear antigen, and the presence of argyrophilic nucleolar organizer regions, macroregenerative nodules, and irregular regeneration. High-risk individuals have an incidence rate of HCC of 2%–8% per year. Histological variants of HCC include trabecular, pseudoglandular (Fig. 68.3), scirrhous, and fibrolamellar types (Fig. 68.4). Macroscopically, HCCs usually present as an expansile mass with a fibrous capsule (Fig. 68.5). Often, a high-grade focus arises within a low-grade early stage tumor, leading to a nodule-in-nodule appearance (Fig. 68.6). Spread of HCCs usually occurs by invasion into blood vessels, most often the portal vein (Fig. 68.7). Intrahepatic metastases are predominantly due to tumor spread via portal vein branches. Extrahepatic metastasis is most frequently to the lungs, regional lymph nodes, and bones.

Periodic liver ultrasonography is the recommended screening tool for HCC (Fig. 68.8). Ultrasonography has been shown to be cost-effective at incidence rates greater than or equal to 1.5% per year. Current guidelines are for liver ultrasonography in high-risk patients every 6 months. Positive ultrasounds are usually followed up with multiphasic spiral computed tomography (CT) or gadolinium contrast-enhanced magnetic resonance image (MRI) scanning (Figs 68.8 and 68.9). If possible, many experienced centers avoid the use of biopsy for the diagnosis of HCC because of a 0.5%–1% risk of needle track seeding. Radiographic and laboratory criteria for the diagnosis of HCC without biopsy include the presence of cirrhosis and characteristic findings on contrast-enhanced imaging of arterial phase enhancement and portal venous phase washout seen on two imaging modalities for a mass between 1 and 2 cm in size and on one imaging modality for a mass greater than or equal to 2 cm in size. The presence of a serum alpha-fetoprotein level greater than 400 ng/mL also has high specificity for the diag-

nosis of HCC. The serum alpha-fetoprotein level is currently not recommended for surveillance of patients at high risk for HCC, except where high-quality ultrasonography is not available. The alpha-fetoprotein level has an overall sensitivity of 39%–64%, a specificity of 76%–91%, and a positive predictive value of only 9%–32%. Because alpha-fetoprotein is seldom elevated in small HCCs (< 2 cm), its usefulness as a screening tool is limited. The serum alpha-fetoprotein level is most useful for identifying a high-risk group of patients who require close follow-up. Newer serum markers for HCC that are currently under investigation include des-gamma-carboxyprothrombin (DCP) and glypican 3.

Treatment options for hepatocellular carcinoma

The selection of an appropriate treatment strategy for patients with HCC depends on careful tumor staging and assessment of the underlying liver disease (Fig. 68.10). The best prognostic group are patients with performance status 0 with no constitutional symptoms, Child A cirrhosis, no vascular invasion, and no extrahepatic spread. All patients with localized HCC (involvement of one single lobe, no vascular invasion or extrahepatic disease) should be evaluated for the potentially curative therapy options of partial hepatectomy or orthotopic liver transplantation (OLT). Candidates for partial hepatectomy must have no liver disease or Child A cirrhosis, normal portal pressure, and normal serum bilirubin, typically with a Model for End-stage Liver Disease (MELD) score of 8 or less. For patients not meeting these criteria, OLT should be considered if there is a solitary lesion of less than 5 cm or fewer than three lesions of less than 3 cm. Local ablative therapies such as percutaneous ethanol injection (PEI), radiofrequency ablation (RFA), transarterial chemoembolization (TACE), and transarterial radioembolization (TARE) offer palliation for patients with contraindications to surgical approaches (Fig. 68.8). PEI and RFA are minimally invasive and can be used on an outpatient basis, usually for tumor nodules of less than 3 cm. When used for small tumors, the survival rates can be similar to those achieved by partial hepatectomy. RFA, PEI, TACE, or TARE may be used as an interim treatment for patients waiting for OLT. Sorafenib, a Raf kinase and vascular endothelial growth factor (VEGF) receptor kinase inhibitor, has recently been shown to prolong survival in advanced, unresectable HCC.

Table 68.1 Estimated worldwide annual mortality from major cancers 2002

Men			Women			Both genders		
Site	Number	Percentage	Site	Number	Percentage	Site	Number	Percentage
1. Lung	848 000	22.3	1. Breast	411 000	14.0	1. Lung	1 179 000	17.5
2. Stomach	446 000	11.7	2. Lung	331 000	11.3	2. Stomach	700 000	10.4
3. Liver	417 000	11.0	3. Cervix uteri	274 000	9.4	3. Liver	598 000	8.9
4. Colon/rectum	278 000	7.3	4. Stomach	254 000	8.7	4. Colon/rectum	529 000	7.9
5. Esophagus	261 000	6.9	5. Colon/rectum	251 000	8.6	5. Breast	411 000	6.1
6. Prostate	221 000	5.8	6. Liver	181 000	6.2	6. Esophagus	385 000	5.7
7. Leukemia	125 000	3.3	7. Ovary, etc.	125 000	4.3	7. Cervix uteri	274 000	4.1
8. Pancreas	120 000	3.2	8. Esophagus	124 000	4.2	8. Pancreas	227 000	3.4
9. Bladder	108 000	2.8	9. Pancreas	107 000	3.7	9. Leukemia	222 000	3.3
10. Non-Hodgkin lymphoma	99 000	2.6	10. Leukemia	97 000	3.3	10. Prostate	221 000	3.3
11. Oral cavity	81 000	2.1	11. Non-Hodgkin lymphoma	73 000	2.5	11. Non-Hodgkin lymphoma	172 000	2.6
12. Larynx	79 000	2.1	12. Brain/nervous system	62 000	2.1	12. Bladder	145 000	2.2

Table 68.2 World age-standardized incidence of hepatocellular carcinoma

	Male	Female	Male–female ratio
World	15.8	5.8	2.72
Eastern Africa	21.1	8.6	2.45
Middle Africa	27.8	13.4	2.07
Northern Africa	4.2	2.2	0.22
Southern Africa	7.0	2.5	2.80
Western Africa	15.3	5.6	2.73
Caribbean	8.2	4.5	1.82
Central America	4.9	4.9	1.00
South America	3.7	2.8	1.32
Northern America	5.3	2.0	2.65
Eastern Asia	36.9	13.4	2.75
Southeastern Asia	18.3	5.7	3.21
South Central Asia	2.6	1.4	1.86
Western Asia	4.6	2.0	2.30
Eastern Europe	5.3	2.4	2.21
Northern Europe	3.4	1.7	2.00
Southern Europe	11.6	4.0	2.90
Western Europe	6.2	1.7	3.65
Australia/New Zealand	3.9	1.3	3.00
Melanesia	16.9	8.2	2.06
Micronesia	8.5	3.2	2.66
Polynesia	12.3	4.0	3.08

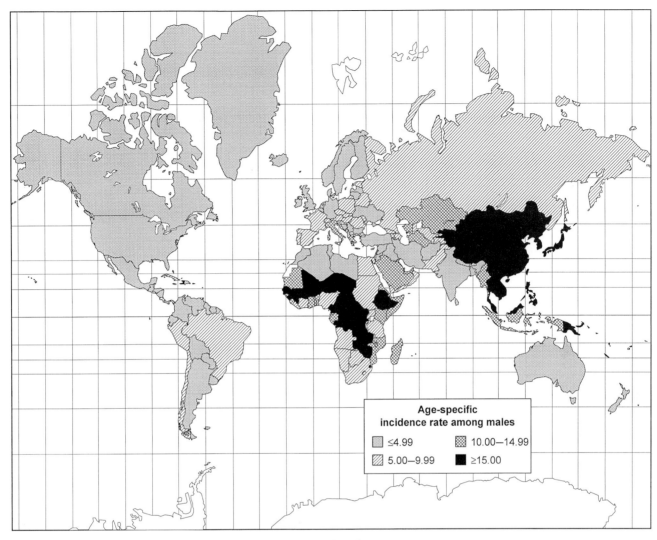

Figure 68.1 Worldwide age-specific incidence of hepatocellular carcinoma in males.

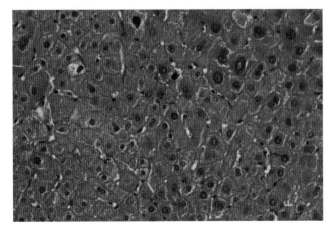

Figure 68.2 Liver cell dysplasia. This nodule from a patient with posthepatitis cirrhosis shows a moderate increase in cell density, an irregular trabecular pattern, and increased cellular atypia.

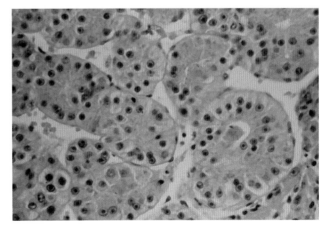

Figure 68.3 Hepatocellular carcinoma. The tumor has a mixed pseudoglandular and trabecular pattern with bile plugs. The sinusoid-like blood spaces show variable dilation.

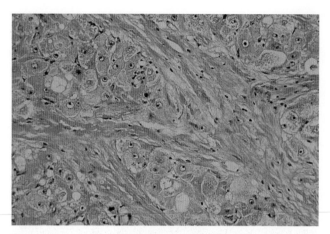

Figure 68.4 Fibrolamellar hepatocellular carcinoma is characterized by sheets of large polygonal tumor cells separated by hyalinized collagen bundles with a lamellar pattern. This variant of hepatocellular carcinoma usually affects adolescents or young adults who have no known risk factors for hepatocellular carcinoma.

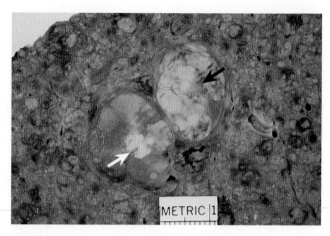

Figure 68.6 Nodule-in-nodule type of hepatocellular carcinoma. A lighter colored, higher grade focus of hepatocellular carcinoma (black arrow) has arisen within the upper right nodule and is compressing the original lower grade tumor towards the pseudocapsule. There is a small high-grade focus of hepatocellular carcinoma arising in the center of the lower left nodule (white arrow), surrounded by well-differentiated tumor.

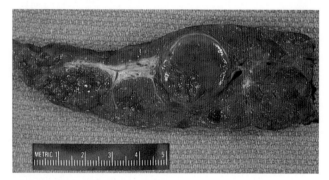

Figure 68.5 Nodular type of hepatocellular carcinoma. The tumor is expansile with a fibrous pseudocapsule. Prominent bile production gives the tumor its green color. The surrounding liver is cirrhotic, with multiple regenerative nodules.

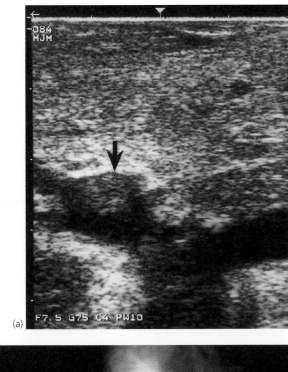

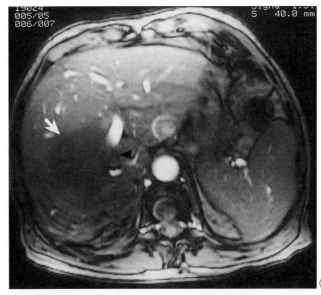

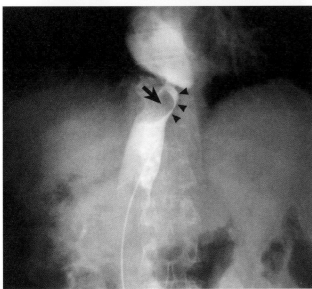

Figure 68.7 Vascular invasion is a hallmark of hepatocellular carcinoma. Over 70% of patients with advanced hepatocellular carcinoma develop tumor thrombi in the portal vein, which lead to intrahepatic dissemination of the tumor. **(a)** Ultrasound image showing extension of hepatocellular carcinoma into the portal vein (black arrow).

(b) Magnetic resonance image scan demonstrating a tumor mass (white arrow) and an abrupt cutoff of the right portal vein (arrowhead).
(c) Angiogram showing near occlusion of the inferior vena cava (arrowheads) by hepatocellular carcinoma within the lumen (black arrow).
(d) Histology of hepatocellular carcinoma invading a portal vein branch.

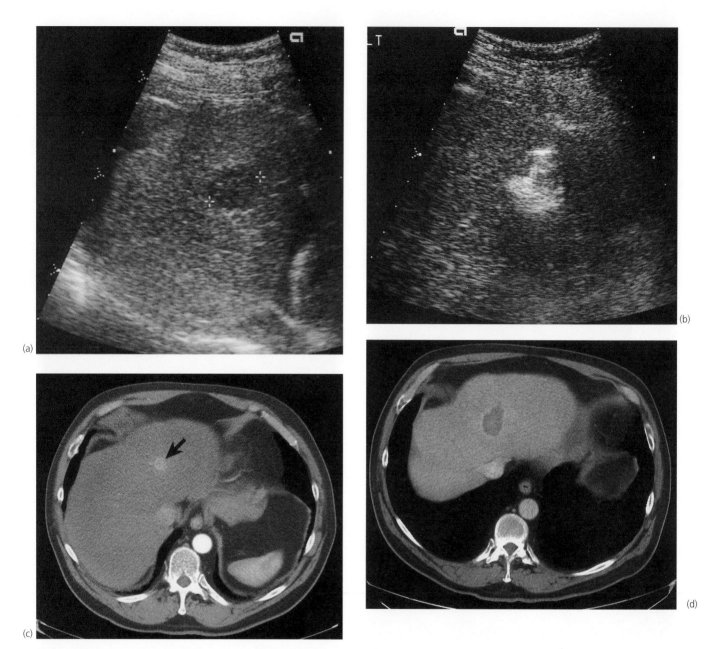

Figure 68.8 Imaging of hepatocellular carcinoma. **(a)** Ultrasound image of a 2.2-cm small hepatocellular carcinoma (marked by asterisks). **(b)** Ultrasound image immediately after percutaneous ethanol injection for treatment of the hepatocellular carcinoma in **(a)**. The tissue injury resulted in an enhanced echogenic signal. **(c)** Computed tomography scan of a 1.8-cm small enhancing hepatocellular carcinoma (arrow). **(d)** Computed tomography image after treatment of the hepatocellular carcinoma in **(c)** by radiofrequency ablation.

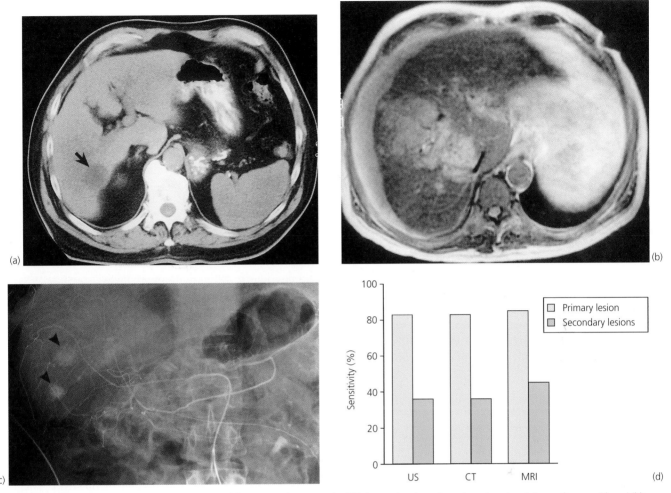

Figure 68.9 Imaging of hepatocellular carcinoma. **(a)** Computed tomography (CT) image showing a hypodense hepatocellular carcinoma with a visible capsular rim (arrow). **(b)** Magnetic resonance image (MRI) showing a large hepatocellular carcinoma located centrally within the liver. **(c)** Angiogram demonstrating two enhancing hepatocellular carcinoma lesions in the right lobe of the liver (arrowheads). **(d)** Ultrasound (US), CT, and MRI each have a sensitivity of over 80% for primary lesions and about 40% for secondary lesions.

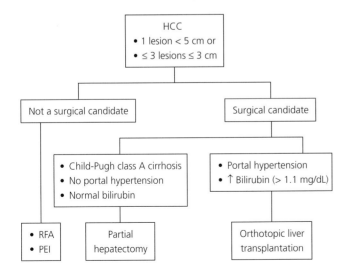

Figure 68.10 Current algorithm for the management of hepatocellular carcinoma (HCC). PEI, percutaneous ethanol injection; RFA, radiofrequency ablation.

69

Liver abscess

David S. Raiford

Amebic vs pyogenic abscess

Although there is considerable overlap in the clinical presentation and imaging characteristics of amebic and pyogenic abscesses, differences in epidemiology, associated conditions, treatment, and prognosis underscore the need for the physician to distinguish these entities. Effective management depends critically upon prompt and correct definition of the abscess type.

Epidemiology

Because intestinal amebiasis is a necessary prelude to hepatic amebic abscess, persons with amebic abscess typically have emigrated from or traveled to areas where intestinal amebiasis is prevalent. In contrast, the ethnicity and travel history of patients with pyogenic abscess does not differ from that of the general hospital population. Over the last few decades, biliary obstruction, both benign and malignant, has emerged as the most common etiology of pyogenic liver abscess, and accounts for 50%–60% of cases.

Symptoms

Fever and right upper quadrant pain are the principal symptoms of hepatic abscess, both amebic and pyogenic. Fever is evident in virtually all patients. Although spiking fever and chills favor pyogenic abscess, these may be seen with amebic abscess. Pain is reported by 75%–90% of patients, is usually constant, is of variable intensity, and may exhibit pleuritic features with radiation to the right shoulder if diaphragmatic involvement is present. The majority of patients will have symptoms for less than 2 weeks before seeking medical care.

Nonspecific symptoms such as weakness, anorexia, nausea, and weight loss are common. Approximately one-third of those with either type of liver abscess will report diarrhea and one-fourth will have a nonproductive cough.

Physical findings

On physical examination, sequential measurements of body temperature should be made to detect fever. Hepatic enlargement and tenderness are typical but not invariably present. Jaundice is rare in amebic abscess and, when present, should suggest biliary tract obstruction with pyogenic infection and underlying chronic liver disease. Percussion dullness, diminished breath sounds, or other chest findings at the right lung base are evident in 20%–30% of patients and suggest involvement of the superior portion of the right hepatic lobe. Occasionally, signs of weight loss, dehydration, and anemia will be evident.

Imaging modalities in diagnosis

The clinical constellation of fever, right upper quadrant discomfort, and hepatic enlargement with tenderness should prompt an imaging study early in the diagnostic assessment. Depending on the age of the patient and level of clinical suspicion for cholelithiasis or biliary obstruction, either ultrasonography (US) or computed tomography (CT) will be performed. These techniques facilitate discrimination of liver abscess from cholecystitis, bile duct obstruction, or pancreatitis. Both US and CT are sensitive for small lesions (< 3 cm in size) and offer precision in localizing lesions that may require percutaneous aspiration or drainage. Of note, lesions near the dome of the right hepatic lobe may be difficult to visualize by US. Typically on US, abscesses appears as hypoechoic lesions, sometimes with internal echoes (Fig. 69.1). CT scanning will identify abscesses as low-density lesions (Fig. 69.2), often with peripheral enhancement after intravenous contrast administration, and may provide better

Atlas of Gastroenterology, 4th edition. Edited by Tadataka Yamada, David H. Alpers, Anthony N. Kalloo, Neil Kaplowitz, Chung Owyang, and Don W. Powell. © 2009 Blackwell Publishing, ISBN: 978-1-4051-6909-7

definition of extrahepatic pathology associated with pyogenic abscess (e.g., appendiceal or diverticular abscess). Although both modalities are sensitive for detecting abscesses and biliary obstruction, neither can distinguish reliably between amebic and pyogenic abscesses. Although less widely used, magnetic resonance imaging (MRI) also has high sensitivity for the detection of hepatic abscess. Characteristically, liver abscesses are hypointense on T1-weighted and hyperintense on T2-weighted images, and wall enhancement soon after gadolinium infusion is typical. As CT and MRI techniques permit multiplanar imaging, these may be useful if US findings are ambiguous or when coronal or sagittal images will help guide management of a lesion. The majority of abscesses, both amebic and pyogenic, occur in the right hepatic lobe. The presence of multiple abscesses strongly suggests pyogenic infection, as does identification of concomitant biliary tract obstruction. Abscess-associated thrombosis within the portal vein (Fig. 69.3) or a hepatic vein is associated with anaerobic infections and may lead to residual portal hypertension or the Budd–Chiari syndrome after otherwise successful treatment of the abscess. Chest radiographs in patients with an abscess adjacent to the diaphragm may show elevation of the right diaphragm, subpulmonic effusion, and right lower lobe atelectasis or infiltrate. Note that hepatic tumors may present with necrosis and secondary infection, mimicking a primary abscess.

Needle aspiration

Key to diagnosis and treatment of liver abscess is identification of the organism(s) in the abscess. Needle aspiration of an abscess is the best and most direct method to distinguish amebic from pyogenic abscess. Material from an amebic abscess will be brown-red in color and typically is not particularly malodorous (Fig. 69.4). A pyogenic abscess will yield material that is creamy, tan-green in color, and often putrid, reflecting anaerobic infection. Gram stains of amebic abscess contents will show neutrophils but no bacteria, unless secondary infection is present. Smears of pyogenic abscess contents will usually identify at least one bacterial form. Meticulous handling of aspirated material to avoid exposure to air enhances recovery and identification of anaerobic species. Reliable and complete identification of infectious agents ensures proper selection of an antibiotic treatment regimen.

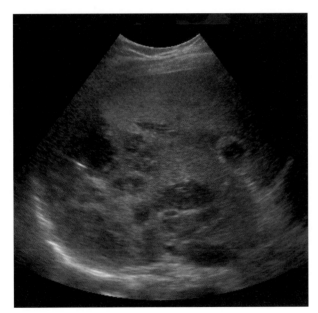

Figure 69.1 Sonogram of the right hepatic lobe showing multiple hypoechoic pyogenic abscesses. This image is from a 54-year-old man who developed multiple hepatic abscesses associated with sigmoid diverticulitis. Blood cultures obtained before antibiotic administration yielded *Bacteroides thetaiotaomicron*. Gram stain of abscess material obtained after antimicrobial therapy was initiated showed gram-positive cocci, gram-negative rods, and gram-positive rods. He was treated initially by percutaneous drainage and intravenous ceftriaxone and metronidazole. After clinical improvement he was discharged home and completed uneventfully a several-week course of oral ciprofloxacin and metronidazole.

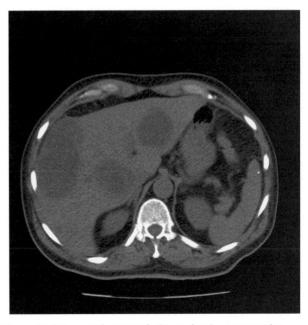

Figure 69.2 Computed tomography image showing numerous low-density lesions in both hepatic lobes in a 65-year-old man with colon carcinoma. *Streptococcus* (gamma-hemolytic) was cultured from fluid obtained by abscess aspiration. His liver lesions were treated by aspiration without drain placement and by administration of levofloxacin and metronidazole. He improved and subsequently tolerated resection of his colonic lesion.

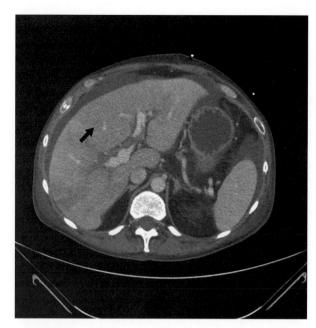

Figure 69.3 Computed tomography image showing filling defects within the intrahepatic portal vein, scattered hepatic hypodense lesions, and free fluid within the abdominal cavity (arrow). These findings are compatible with septic pylethrombophlebitis. This image is from a 44-year-old man who presented with sigmoid diverticulitis and pericolonic abscess. He was treated by segmental colectomy and his liver abscesses resolved without aspiration after prolonged antibiotic therapy. He was treated postoperatively with heparin and then warfarin (Coumadin). After 3 months of anticoagulation therapy, his portal vein thrombus resolved and there were no residual imaging abnormalities.

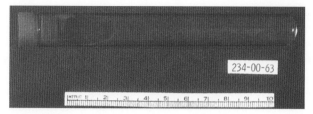

Figure 69.4 Material aspirated from a large right lobe amebic abscess in a 31-year-old man who had been ill for 2 weeks with fever and right upper quadrant pain. He recovered completely with chloroquine therapy.

70

Vascular diseases of the liver

Laurie D. DeLeve, Gary C. Kanel

This chapter reviews images of Budd–Chiari syndrome, sinusoidal obstruction syndrome (hepatic venoocclusive disease), nodular regenerative hyperplasia, and peliosis hepatis. These diseases are all thought to be primary circulatory problems that lead to secondary changes in the hepatic parenchyma.

In Budd–Chiari syndrome, the severity of the liver injury will depend on the extent of involvement of the hepatic veins, the time course over which the obstruction of the hepatic veins develops, and the duration of untreated disease. Slower development of the obstruction or occlusion allows the formation of collaterals to alleviate sinusoidal congestion as the obstruction progresses. These collaterals produce the characteristic spiderweb appearance shown in Figure 70.1. In acute Budd–Chiari syndrome there is perivenular and sometimes midzonal sinusoidal congestion, acute hemorrhage, and hepatocyte ischemia or dropout. Figure 70.2 demonstrates hemorrhage within the hepatic cords with red blood cells replacing the damaged hepatocytes. In chronic Budd–Chiari syndrome, chronic outflow obstruction may lead to bridging fibrosis between terminal hepatic venules with sparing of the portal tracts, and fibrosis that obliterates the terminal hepatic venules, as demonstrated in Figure 70.3.

Sinusoidal obstruction syndrome (SOS) is initiated by damage to sinusoidal endothelial cells. Figures 70.4 and 70.5 demonstrate the ultrastructural changes in the sinusoid that occur prior to "clinical" evidence of disease in the experimental model, notably formation of gaps in the sinusoidal endothelial cells and penetration of red blood cells through the gaps into the space of Disse. Figure 70.6 demonstrates the ultrastructural features of early SOS with denudation of the sinusoidal lining and loss of hepatocyte microvilli. The histological features of early SOS are shown in Figure 70.7 and include subendothelial and sinusoidal hemorrhage and perivenular necrosis. Occlusion of terminal hepatic venules is not present in all patients but is seen more commonly in

patients with more severe disease. Narrowing of terminal hepatic venules in early SOS is due to subendothelial accumulation of plasma and some formed elements or frank subendothelial hemorrhage. In late SOS there is fibrosis within perizonal sinusoids and adventitial or subendothelial fibrosis with narrowing or occlusion of the terminal hepatic veins (Fig. 70.8). Unlike more subtle changes in the sinusoid, venular occlusion is easily recognized on histology and this led to the previous name, hepatic venoocclusive disease. With the recognition that the disease is initiated in the sinusoid and that venular involvement is not present in a sizeable minority of patients, the disease was renamed sinusoidal obstruction syndrome.

It is thought that nodular regenerative hyperplasia is due to uneven perfusion of the liver. In areas of hypoperfusion hepatocytes atrophy or undergo apoptosis, with reactive hyperplasia in areas in which perfusion is maintained. Impaired perfusion may occur at the level of the portal vein or the sinusoids. Hypoperfusion resulting from obstruction of the portal vein may occur in collagen vascular diseases or immune complex diseases when inflammation of the hepatic artery leads to inflammatory destruction of adjacent portal veins. Nodular regenerative hyperplasia may accompany portal vein thrombosis caused by prothrombotic disorders such as agnogenic myeloid metaplasia, polycythemia vera, or antiphospholipid syndrome. Perfusion deficits at the level of the sinusoid are seen with toxicity to sinusoidal endothelial cells, such as by long-term azathioprine therapy in renal or liver transplantation patients or after conditioning therapy for hematopoietic stem cell transplantation. Figures 70.9 and 70.10 demonstrate small regenerative nodules, which are composed of cytologically benign hepatocytes. The nodules displace portal structures and are surrounded by areas with atrophic hepatocytes.

Patients with chronic wasting illnesses or who have been exposed to androgenic anabolic steroids or long-term azathioprine therapy may develop one or multiple peliotic lesions in the liver or spleen (Figs 70.11 and 70.12). The peliotic lesion consists of well-defined vascular cavities without a discrete endothelial lining (Fig. 70.13). In patients

Atlas of Gastroenterology, 4th edition. Edited by Tadataka Yamada, David H. Alpers, Anthony N. Kalloo, Neil Kaplowitz, Chung Owyang, and Don W. Powell. © 2009 Blackwell Publishing, ISBN: 978-1-4051-6909-7

with acquired immunodeficiency syndrome, peliosis may occur because of infection with *Bartonella* species (Fig. 70.14). Although it had been suggested that sinusoidal endothelial cells were the initial target in peliosis, this concept has been most clearly supported by studies of peliosis caused by *Bar-* *tonella* species. *Bartonella* bacilli can be detected by electron microscopy in sinusoidal endothelial cells. This leads to disruption of the sinusoidal endothelial cell barrier, with initial sinusoidal dilation and subsequent formation of peliotic cavities.

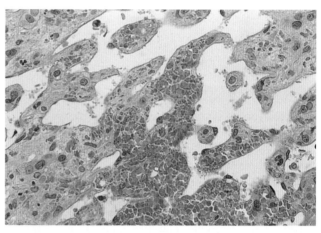

Figure 70.2 Budd–Chiari syndrome, acute. The sinusoids in the perivenular zone (zone 3 of Rappaport) show marked dilation and are virtually devoid of erythrocytes. The red blood cells are present within the hepatic cords, replacing the damaged hepatocytes.

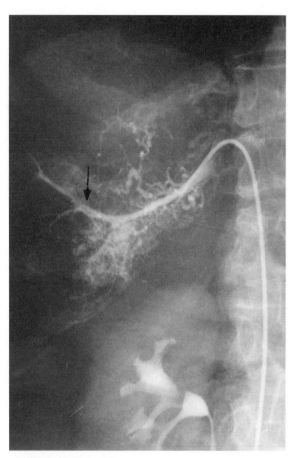

Figure 70.1 Budd–Chiari syndrome. The angiogram demonstrates the spiderweb pattern characteristic of Budd–Chiari syndrome. A residual, narrowed hepatic vein is indicated by the arrow. Courtesy of Dr Sue Ellen Hanks, University of Southern California.

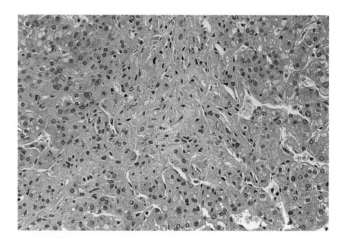

Figure 70.3 Budd–Chiari syndrome, chronic. The terminal hepatic venule has been replaced by intralumenal fibrosis, which has also extended into the perivenular zone.

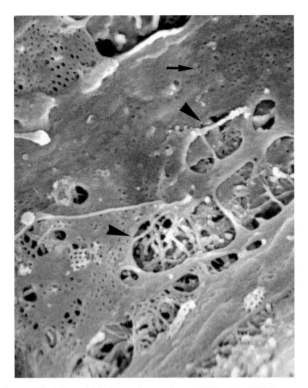

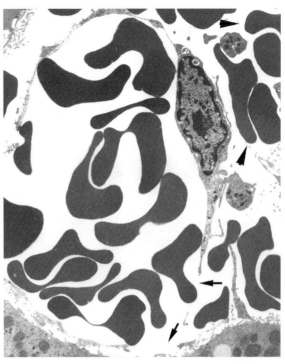

Figure 70.4 Sinusoidal obstruction syndrome (SOS), "pre-SOS." A scanning electron microscopy image was taken from the rat model of SOS 1 day after administration of monocrotaline. This demonstrates changes that occur before clinical or light microscopy images are observed in this model, i.e., pre-SOS: gaps in sinusoidal endothelial cells (arrowheads) that allow penetration of red blood cells into the space of Disse and loss of fenestrae organized as sieve plates (arrow) (original magnification ×10 300). Courtesy of Dr Robert McCuskey, University of Arizona.

Figure 70.5 Sinusoidal obstruction syndrome (SOS), "pre-SOS." A transmission electron microscopy image taken from the rat model of SOS demonstrates gaps in the sinusoidal endothelial cell (arrows) and red blood cells in the space of Disse (arrowheads) (original magnification ×10 300). Courtesy of Dr Robert McCuskey, University of Arizona.

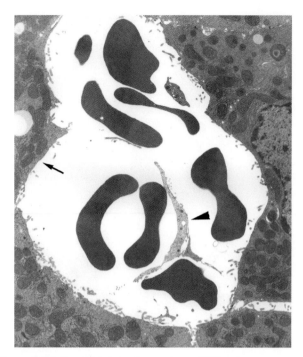

Figure 70.6 Sinusoidal obstruction syndrome (SOS), early. A transmission electron microscopy image taken from the rat model of SOS during early SOS demonstrates loss of sinusoidal lining and of microvilli on the hepatocyte (arrow) and a remnant of a sinusoidal endothelial cell in the lumen (arrowhead). Courtesy of Dr Robert McCuskey, University of Arizona.

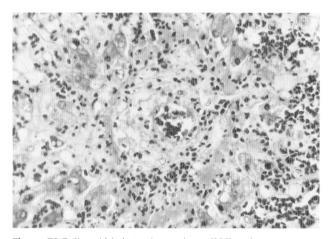

Figure 70.7 Sinusoidal obstruction syndrome (SOS), early. A photomicrograph demonstrates the changes of early SOS in a hematopoietic stem cell transplantation patient. Features demonstrated here are marked subendothelial and sinusoidal hemorrhage and perivenular necrosis. Courtesy of Dr Howard Shulman, Fred Hutchinson Cancer Research Center and the University of Washington.

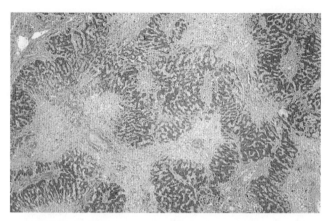

Figure 70.8 Sinusoidal obstruction syndrome, late. Marked sinusoidal and venular fibrosis is present in the perivenular zone in the liver of a patient 63 days after conditioning therapy for hematopoietic stem cell transplantation. Courtesy of Dr Howard Shulman, Fred Hutchinson Cancer Research Center and the University of Washington.

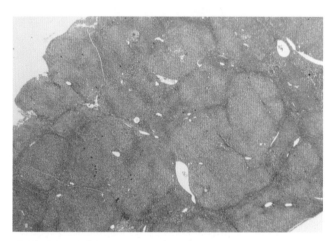

Figure 70.9 Nodular regenerative hyperplasia. A low-power photomicrograph shows small regenerative nodules ranging in size from 3 to 6 mm, displacing portal structures.

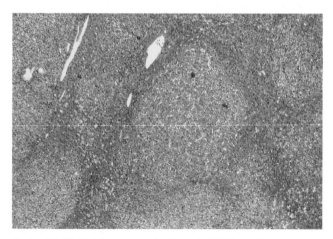

Figure 70.10 Nodular regenerative hyperplasia. This medium-power image shows the regenerative nodules to be composed of normal-appearing hepatocytes. No lobular inflammation is seen. A normal-sized portal tract is present towards the top of the field.

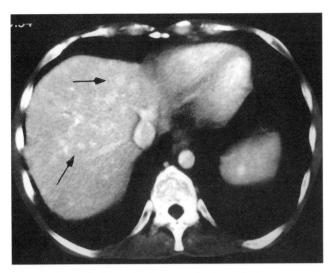

Figure 70.11 Peliosis hepatis. A computed tomography image demonstrates multiple peliotic lesions, two of which are indicated by arrows. Courtesy of Dr Randall Radin, University of Southern California.

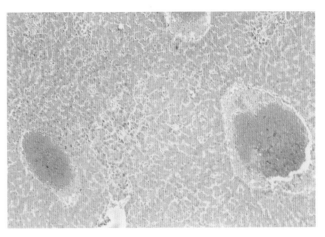

Figure 70.13 Peliosis hepatis. Scattered randomly within the hepatic parenchyma are well-defined vascular spaces filled with red blood cells. A closer inspection would show that the cysts have no discrete endothelial lining.

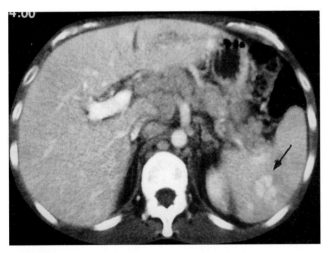

Figure 70.12 Peliosis hepatis. A computed tomography image demonstrates a large peliotic lesion in the spleen (arrow). Courtesy of Dr Randall Radin, University of Southern California.

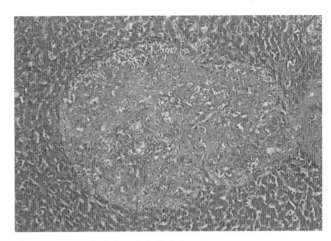

Figure 70.14 Peliosis hepatis. Peliosis hepatis may occur in immunocompromised patients caused by organisms from the rickettsial *Bartonella* (*Rochalimaea*) species, which can be identified as gram-negative bacilli in the lesion. The well-circumscribed lesion is composed of numerous vascular channels within a loose fibroconnective stroma.

71

Liver biopsy and histopathological diagnosis

Sugantha Govindarajan

Evaluation of liver biopsy requires that the pathologist recognize the architecture and identify the pathological changes, and correlate the changes with clinical and laboratory data. Although some histological diagnosis can be made without the help of the clinical or laboratory data, most meaningful information is obtained with a proper clinical–pathological correlation.

Special stains, such as Masson trichrome, demonstrate fibrosis or cirrhosis of the liver, an indication of a chronic process. Other routine stains include stains for iron, reticulin, and diastase-resistant periodic acid Schiff-positive material. Granulomas of the liver require special stains for the etiological agent such as acid-fast organisms and fungi. Shikata or orcein stain identifies hepatitis B surface antigen as well as copper-binding protein, metallothionein. Immunoperoxidase stains detect viral and nonviral protein in the biopsy material using specific antibodies directed against the proteins.

Routine hematoxylin and eosin stain sections are the most valuable tools in the diagnosis. Well-embedded (3-μm) sections with good hematoxylin and eosin stain will provide great cellular details of hepatocytes, such as inclusions in the cytoplasm or the nuclei, as well as features such as fat, cholestasis, or dysplasia.

Initial assessment of the architecture is followed by a closer review of the portal tract or the fibrous septa if cirrhosis is present. Elements to be examined are the bile ducts, epithelial abnormalities or their absence or proliferation, cellular types of the inflammatory infiltrates, and the infiltrates' involvement of the bile ducts, the parenchymal limiting plate, or the vessels (vasculitis). The portal tracts or the fibrous septa should also be examined under polarized light for foreign material in the macrophages, which is usually seen in patients with a history of intravenous drug addiction.

The parenchyma is examined for cord sinusoidal pattern; normal one-cell thickness is altered in hepatocellular carci-

noma to three to four or more cells that thicken the trabeculae. Parenchymal cytoplasmic inclusions such as Mallory bodies, mega-mitochondria, α_1-antitrypsin, or of groundglass cytoplasmic appearance are identified under higher magnifications in the review process. Areas of hepatocytolysis often appear as focal punched-out or spotty necrosis with an accumulation of Kupffer cells and lymphocytes, or as large areas of collapsed reticulin with loss of hepatocytes. Hepatocytolysis is often localized in the perivenular zones. Individual cell necrosis is seen as acidophil bodies or apoptotic cells.

Attention also should be paid to the sinusoidal lining cells, Ito cells, and the space of Disse. In alcoholic liver disease there is collagen deposition of the sinusoidal space, which stands out on Masson trichrome stain. Amyloid is also seen in this space, either as reticular or globular type, and is demonstrated by Congo red stain.

In addition to the histological diagnosis to confirm the clinical diagnosis, the liver biopsy has become a very important prognostic tool to assess the responses to treatment of chronic viral hepatitis B and C. The histological activity index (HAI) is measured using several standardized methods on pretreatment and 1- to 2-year follow-up biopsies. This quantitative measurement of necroinflammation and fibrosis either by Knodell or Ishak scoring (Table 71.1) has been applied to many long-term therapeutic protocols. Standardization of the scoring has been helpful in studies that compare different treatment modalities. Its application for individual cases also helps the clinician with patient follow up and monitoring of other serological viral markers.

Liver biopsies are also extremely valuable in post-liver transplant settings. Standard protocols of liver biopsies help confirm the clinical diagnoses from rejection to opportunistic infections. Post-liver transplantation management of patients is largely dependent on the liver biopsy interpretations in conjunction with the other laboratory studies.

With proper indications and carefully chosen technique, a needle biopsy of the liver is an invaluable tool. Most often, the biopsy provides the final diagnosis when the pathology interpretation is made using the combined expertise of the pathologist and the hepatologist.

Atlas of Gastroenterology, 4th edition. Edited by Tadataka Yamada, David H. Alpers, Anthony N. Kalloo, Neil Kaplowitz, Chung Owyang, and Don W. Powell. © 2009 Blackwell Publishing, ISBN: 978-1-4051-6909-7

Table 71.1 Histology Activity Index (HAI): Ishak score

Modified HAI grading necroinflammatory scores	Score
A. Periportal piecemeal necrosis	
Absent	0
Mild (focal, few portal areas)	1
Mild/moderate (focal, most portal areas)	2
Moderate (continuous around <50% of tracts or septa)	3
Severe (continuous around >50% of tracts or septa)	4
B. Confluent necrosis	
Absent	0
Focal confluent necrosis	1
Zone 3 necrosis in some areas	2
Zone 3 necrosis in most areas	3
Zone 3 necrosis + occasional portal–central (P–C) bridging	4
Zone 3 necrosis + multiple P–C bridging	5
Panacinar or multiacinar necrosis	6
C. Focal necrosis and focal inflammation	
Absent	0
One focus or less per 10× objective	1
Two to four foci per 10× objective	2
Five to ten foci per 10× objective	3
More than ten foci per 10× objective	4
D. Portal inflammation	
None	0
Mild, some, or all portal areas	1
Moderate, some, or all portal areas	2
Moderate/marked, all portal areas	3
Marked, all portal areas	4

Modified staging: fibrosis and cirrhosis	
Change	
No fibrosis	0
Fibrous expansion of some portal areas	1
Fibrous expansion of most portal areas	2
Fibrous expansion with occasional portal to portal (P–P) bridging	3
Fibrous expansion with marked bridging	4
Marked bridging with occasional nodules, incomplete cirrhosis	5
Cirrhosis, probable or definite	6

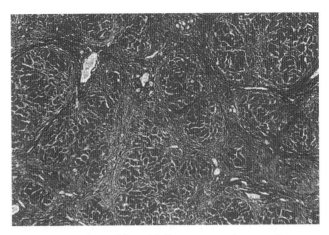

Figure 71.1 Cirrhosis of liver with fibrous septa and regenerative nodules. (Masson stain; original magnification ×40.)

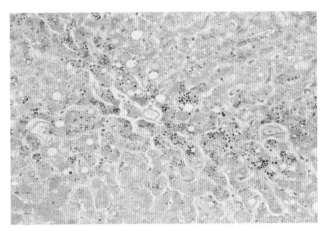

Figure 71.2 α_1-Antitrypsin globules in the periportal hepatocytes–diastase-resistant PAS-positive. (Di-PAS stain; original magnification ×200.)

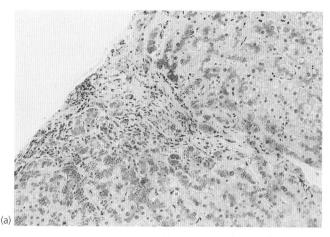

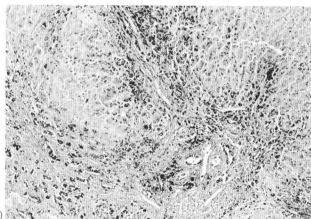

(a)

(b)

Figure 71.3 Perls' iron stain demonstrating bright blue granules in hepatocytes and duct epithelial cells in hemochromatosis. (Original magnification ×100.)

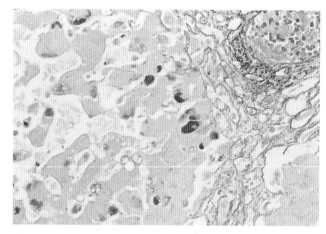

Figure 71.4 Shikata stain demonstrating the presence of HBsAg in the hepatocytes in chronic hepatitis B virus. (Original magnification ×200.)

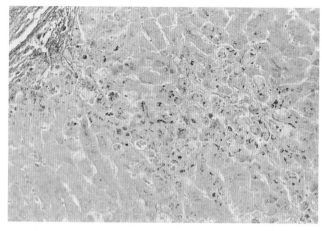

Figure 71.5 Shikata stain demonstrating dark black granules of copper binding protein in periseptal hepatocytes in Wilson disease. (Original magnification ×200.)

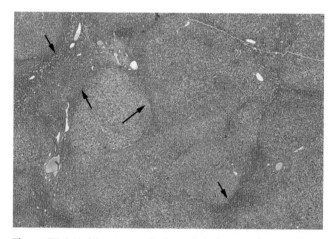

Figure 71.6 Nodular regenerative hyperplasia demonstrating regeneration of parenchyma compressing the surrounding parenchyma (arrows) without fibrous septa formation. (H & E stain; original magnification ×40.)

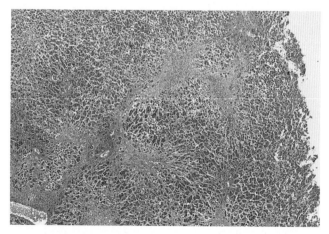

Figure 71.7 Submassive hepatic necrosis with collapsed perivenular reticulum network. (H & E stain; original magnification × 40.)

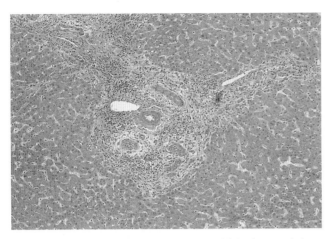

Figure 71.8 Portal area with prominent neutrophils in close proximity to the dilated interlobular bile duct in acute cholangitis. (H & E stain; original magnification ×100.)

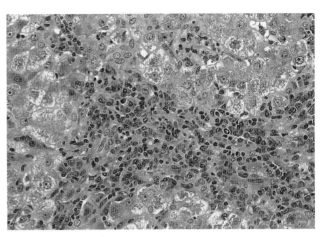

Figure 71.11 Prominent plasma cells among the infiltrates in the portal tract of autoimmune chronic hepatitis. (H & E stain; original magnification ×400.)

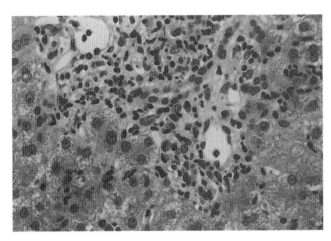

Figure 71.9 Portal area with prominent eosinophils among the inflammatory infiltrates in a case of Dilantin-induced hepatotoxicity. (H & E stain; original magnification ×200.)

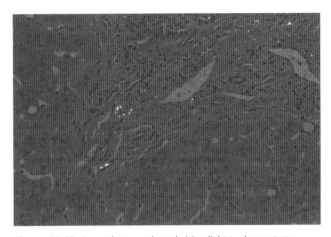

Figure 71.12 A portal area under polarizing light to demonstrate polarizable crystals in an intravenous drug user. (H & E stain; original magnification ×200.)

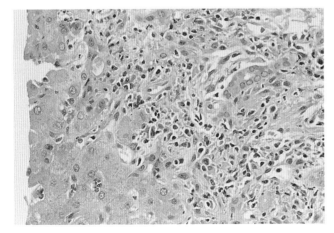

Figure 71.10 Portal area with increased number of eosinophils in a case of early rejection of orthotopic liver transplantation. (H & E stain; original magnification ×200.)

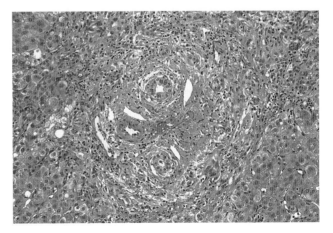

Figure 71.13 Lamellar periductal fibrosis in chronic bile duct obstruction. (H & E stain; original magnification ×100.)

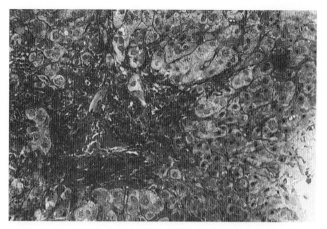

Figure 71.14 Arachnoid portal fibrosis with periportal extension of collagen in chronic alcoholic liver disease. (Masson trichrome stain; original magnification ×100.)

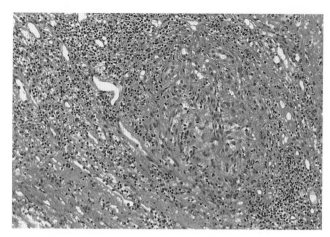

Figure 71.17 Primary biliary cirrhosis with granuloma. (Original magnification ×200.)

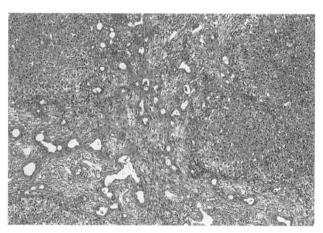

Figure 71.15 Portal area with marked cholangiolar proliferation in mechanical duct obstruction. (H & E stain; original magnification ×100.)

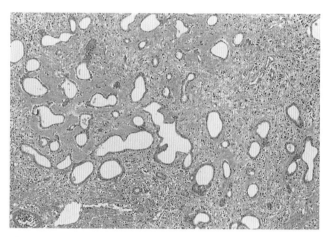

Figure 71.18 A few dilated duct structures with abnormal epithelium surrounded by loose collagen representing Meyenburg complex. (H & E stain; original magnification ×100.)

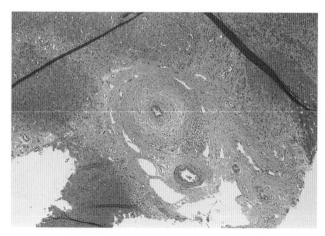

Figure 71.16 Primary sclerosing cholangitis with evidence of periductal fibrosis and chonic inflammatory infiltrate. (H & E stain; original magnification ×100.)

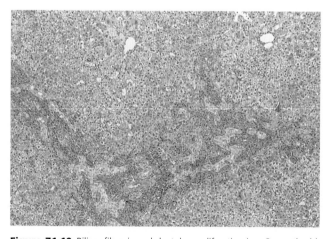

Figure 71.19 Biliary fibrosis and ductular proliferation in a 3-month-old infant with extrahepatic biliary atresia. (H & E stain; original magnification ×100.)

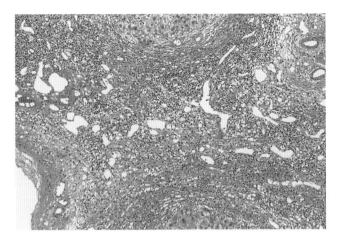

Figure 71.20 Increased number of thin-walled vascular structures representing portal venous radicles reflective of portal hypertension. (H & E stain; original magnification ×100.)

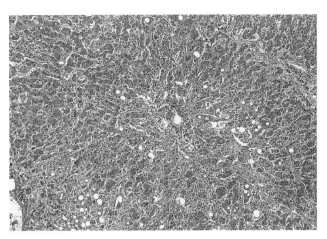

Figure 71.23 Marked perivenular fibrosis in alcoholic liver disease. (Masson trichrome stain; original magnification ×100.)

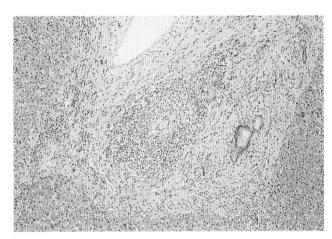

Figure 71.21 Severe necrotizing inflammatory reaction around hepatic arteriole in polyarteritis nodosa. (H & E stain; original magnification ×100.)

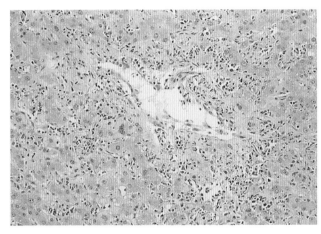

Figure 71.24 Endothelialitis showing inflammatory changes of a terminal hepatic venule in acute rejection of orthotopic liver transplantation. (H & E stain; original magnification ×200.)

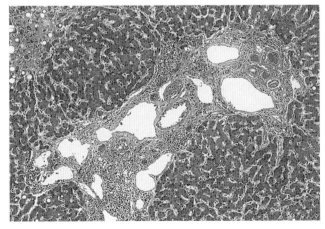

Figure 71.22 Increased number of abnormal vascular structures in a portal tract in Osler–Weber–Rendu syndrome. (H & E stain; original magnification ×100.)

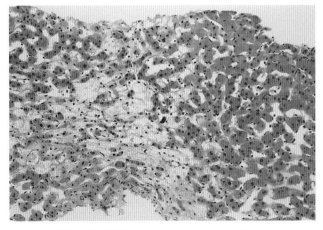

Figure 71.25 Budd–Chiari syndrome with perivenular hemorrhage, necrosis, and sinusoidal dilation. (H & E stain; original magnification ×200.)

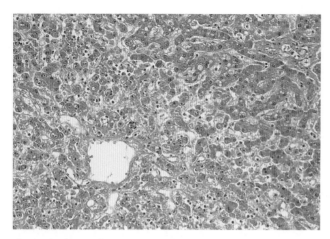

Figure 71.26 Confluent necrosis in the perivenular zone due to anoxia. (H & E stain; original magnification ×200.)

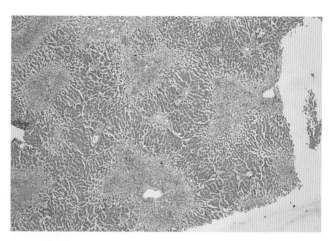

Figure 71.29 Acetaminophen toxicity resulting in perivenular coagulative necrosis without hepatocyte swelling. (H & E stain; original magnification ×100.)

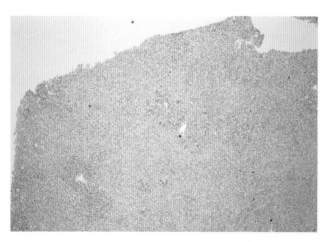

Figure 71.27 Massive hepatic necrosis involving the entire parenchyma with islands of portal tracts remaining. (H & E stain; original magnification ×40.)

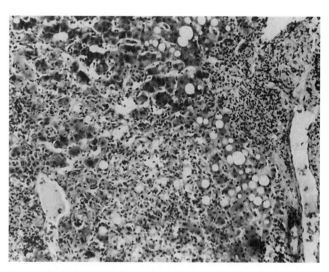

Figure 71.30 Halothane-induced perivenular and midzonal coagulative necrosis. (H & E stain; original magnification ×100.)

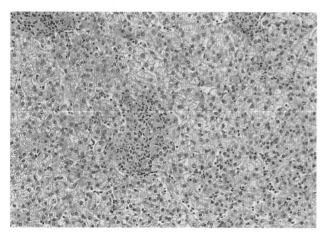

Figure 71.28 Punched-out granulomatous necrosis of the parenchyma in mononucleosis due to Epstein–Barr virus. (H & E stain; original magnification ×200.)

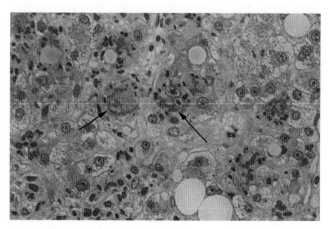

Figure 71.31 Perivenular hepatocytes containing Mallory hyaline (arrows) with neutrophilic reaction around them. (H & E stain; original magnification ×200.)

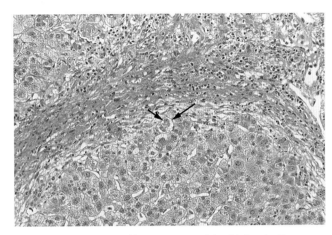

Figure 71.32 A periportal hepatocyte containing Mallory hyaline (arrows) in primary biliary cirrhosis. (H & E stain; original magnification ×200.)

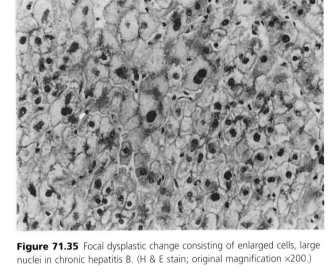

Figure 71.35 Focal dysplastic change consisting of enlarged cells, large nuclei in chronic hepatitis B. (H & E stain; original magnification ×200.)

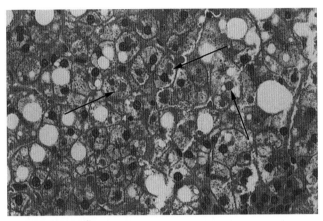

Figure 71.33 Hepatocytes containing spherical megamitochondria (arrows) in alcoholic liver disease. (H & E stain; original magnification ×200.)

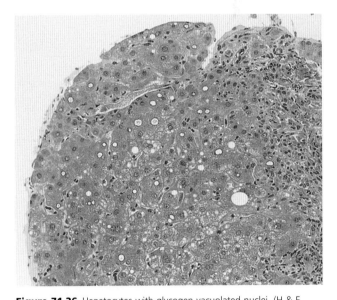

Figure 71.36 Hepatocytes with glycogen vacuolated nuclei. (H & E stain; original magnification ×200.)

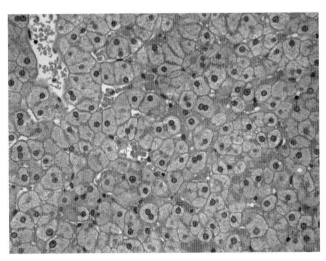

Figure 71.34 Focal regeneration with cobblestone arrangement of hepatocytes in chronic hepatitis. (H & E stain; original magnification ×200.)

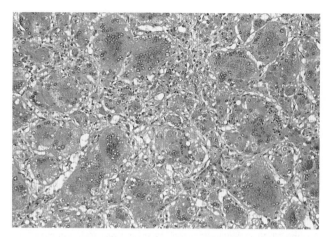

Figure 71.37 Syncytial hepatocytes in neonatal hepatitis. (H & E stain; original magnification ×200.)

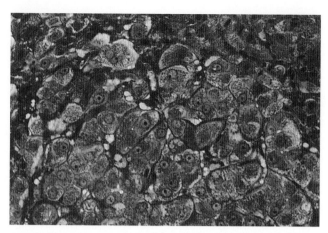

Figure 71.40 Collagen fibers along the sinusoids in the space of Disse in alcoholic liver disease. (Masson stain; original magnification × 200.)

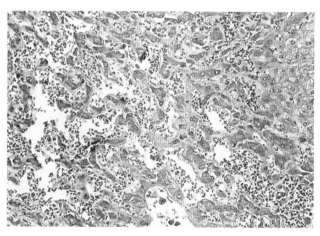

Figure 71.38 Chronic passive congestion causing perivenular sinusoidal dilation and atrophic hepatic cords. (Masson trichrome stain; original magnification ×400.)

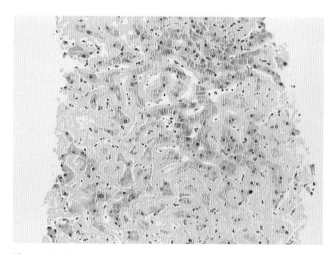

Figure 71.41 Reticular amyloid deposition in the space of Disse. (H & E stain; original magnification ×200.)

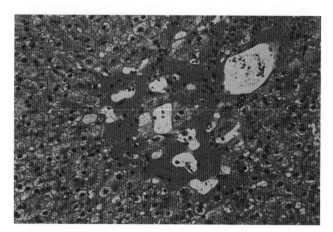

Figure 71.39 Perivenular hepatic parenchyma with dilated sinusoids and the presence of red blood cells within the hepatic cords in left-sided heart failure. (H & E stain; original magnification ×100.)

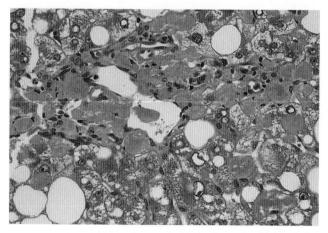

Figure 71.42 Globular amyloid deposition. (H & E stain; original magnification ×400.)

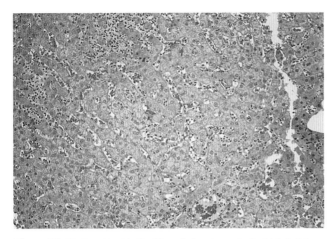

Figure 71.43 Hypertrophic Kupffer cells in salmonellosis. (H & E stain; original magnification ×200.)

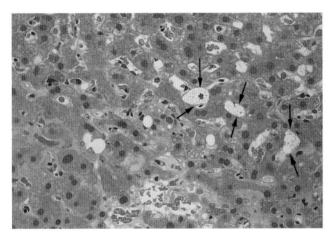

Figure 71.44 Ito cells with foamy fatty cytoplasm (arrows) along the sinusoidal surface in hypervitaminosis A. (H & E stain; original magnification ×400.)

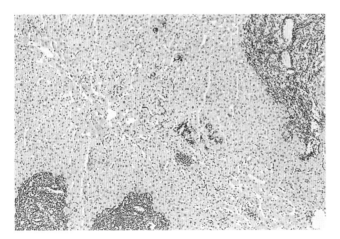

Figure 71.45 Leukemic cells in the sinusoidal blood space in a case of lymphocytic leukemia. (H & E stain; original magnification ×200.)

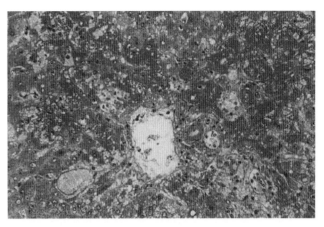

Figure 71.46 Periportal sinusoidal space filled with fibrin thrombi in toxemia of pregnancy. (H & E stain; original magnification ×100.)

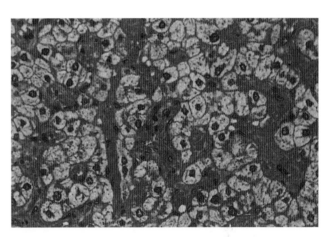

Figure 71.47 Clumps of sickled red blood cells packed in the sinusoidal spaces. (H & E stain; original magnification ×200.)

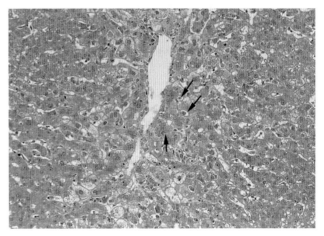

Figure 71.48 Cholestasis (arrows) in dilated canaliculi in zone 3 in chlorpromazine-induced liver disease. (H & E stain; original magnification ×200.)

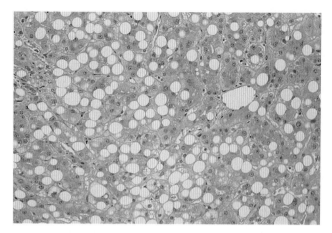

Figure 71.49 Macrovesicular fatty change of hepatocytes in alcoholic liver disease. (H & E stain; original magnification ×200.)

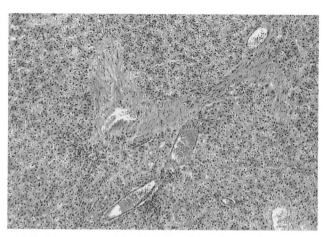

Figure 71.52 Liver cell adenoma with thick-walled vessels and lack of portal tracts. (H & E stain; original magnification ×100.)

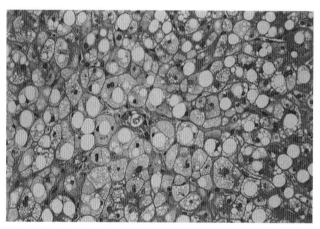

Figure 71.50 Diffusely enlarged hepatocytes with foamy fatty change in acute alcoholic liver disease. (H & E stain; original magnification ×100.)

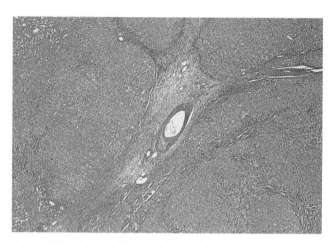

Figure 71.53 Focal nodular hyperplasia with central stellate scar. (H & E stain; original magnification ×40.)

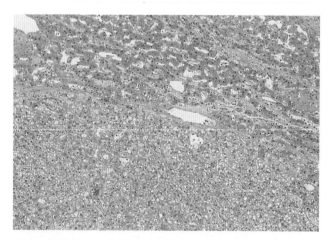

Figure 71.51 Liver cell adenoma with clear cells and the adjacent normal parenchyma. (H & E stain; original magnification ×100.)

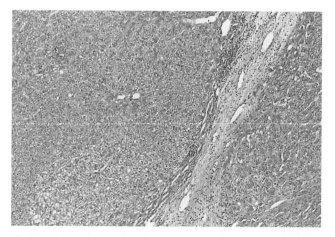

Figure 71.54 Focal nodular hyperplasia with the scar exhibiting lack of bile ducts and presence of vascular structures. Liver cells are uniform and regenerative in appearance. (H & E stain; original magnification ×100.)

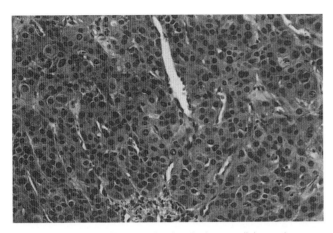

Figure 71.55 Well-differentiated trabecular hepatocellular carcinoma with endothelial lining. (H & E stain; original magnification ×100.)

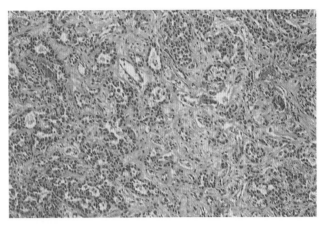

Figure 71.58 Neoplastic ductal structures with fibrous stroma in cholangiocarcinoma. (H & E stain; original magnification ×100.)

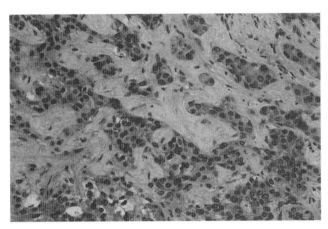

Figure 71.56 Sclerosing hepatic carcinoma with dense fibrous stroma. (H & E stain; original magnification ×100.)

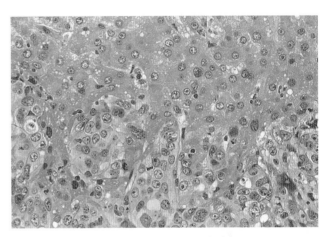

Figure 71.59 Metastatic, poorly differentiated adenocarcinoma infiltrating into the sinusoids. (H & E stain; original magnification ×200.)

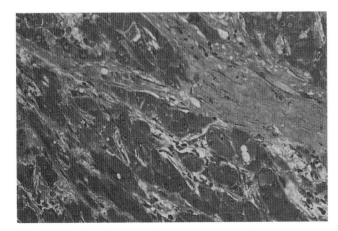

Figure 71.57 Eosinophilic neoplastic hepatocytes with lamellar fibrous stroma in fibrolamellar hepatocellular carcinoma. (H & E stain; original magnification ×100.)

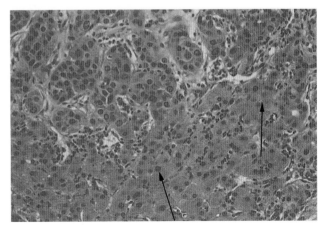

Figure 71.60 Junction of tumor and nontumor liver in hepatocellular carcinoma. The tumor cells grow into the hepatic cords (arrows). (H & E stain; original magnification ×100.)

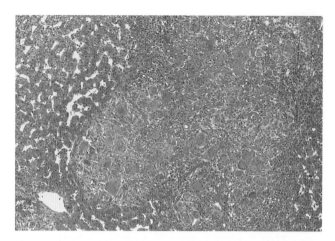

Figure 71.61 Partially segmented, exuberant epithelioid granuloma of sarcoidosis. (H & E stain; original magnification ×100.)

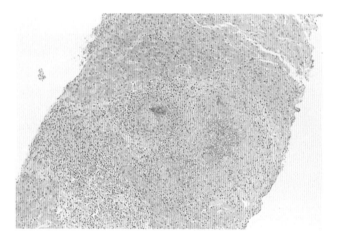

Figure 71.62 Epithelioid granuloma with Langhans giant cells in *Mycobacterium tuberculosis* infection of liver. (H & E stain; original magnification ×100.)

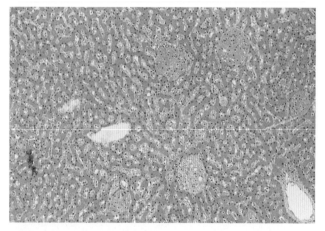

Figure 71.63 Well-circumscribed clusters of large foamy histiocytes in *Mycobacterium avium intracellulare* infection of the liver. These cells contain abundant acid-fast organisms on special stain (not shown). (H & E stain; original magnification ×100.)

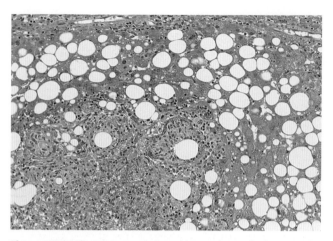

Figure 71.64 Granulomatous lesion with central vacuolization surrounded by a fibrin ring in Q fever. (H & E stain; original magnification ×200.)

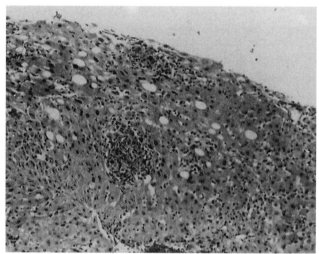

Figure 71.65 Small well-circumscribed granuloma in sulfonamide-induced hepatic necrosis. (H & E stain; original magnification ×100.)

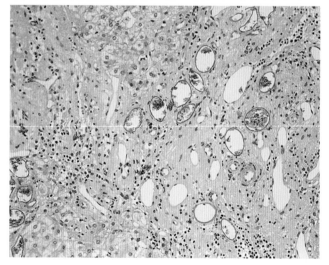

Figure 71.66 Remnants of ova of schistosomal organisms in a fibrous portal area. (H & E stain; original magnification ×200.)

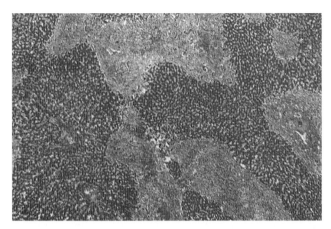

Figure 71.67 Jigsaw puzzle appearance of biliary cirrhosis. (Masson stain; original magnification ×40.)

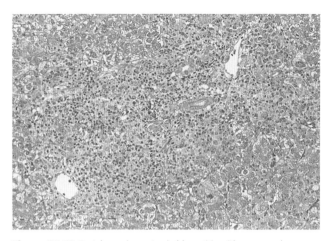

Figure 71.70 Portal area in acute viral hepatitis with mononuclear infiltration extending to the periportal regions. (H & E stain; original magnification ×200.)

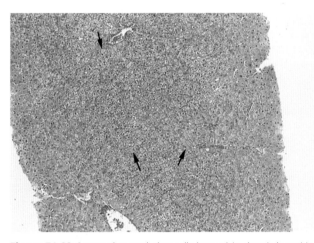

Figure 71.68 Scattered ground-glass cells (arrows) in chronic hepatitis, type B. (H & E stain; original magnification ×100.)

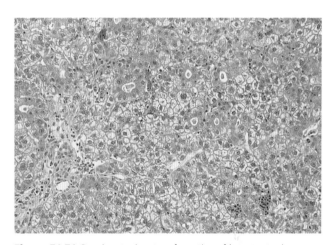

Figure 71.71 Prominent acinar transformation of hepatocytes in enterically transmitted acute hepatitis, type E. (H & E stain; original magnification ×200.)

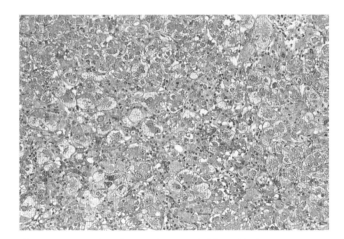

Figure 71.69 Perivenular zone in acute viral hepatitis demonstrating hydropic hepatocytes, hepatocytolysis, inflammatory exudate, and rare acidophilic bodies. (H & E stain; original magnification ×200.)

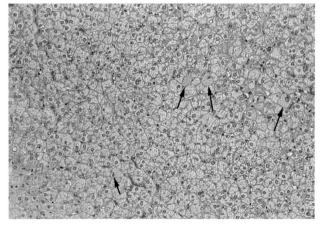

Figure 71.72 Uniform cobblestone appearance of parenchyma in chronic hepatitis, type B. A few ground-glass cells are seen (arrows). (H & E stain; original magnification ×200.)

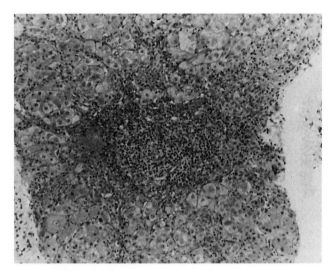

Figure 71.73 Portal areas with fibrosis and mononuclear inflammation extending to the parenchyma exhibiting piecemeal necrosis in chronic hepatitis. (H & E stain; original magnification ×100.)

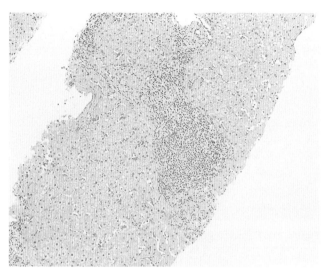

Figure 71.75 Chronic hepatitis C showing portal fibrosis and inflammation, macrovesicular fat, and inflammation in the adjacent parenchyma. (H & E stain; original magnification ×100.)

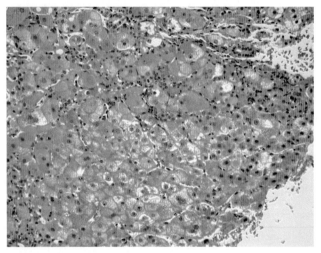

Figure 71.74 Inflammatory cells are seen cuffing around the hepatocytes in chronic hepatitis. (H & E stain; original magnification ×100.)

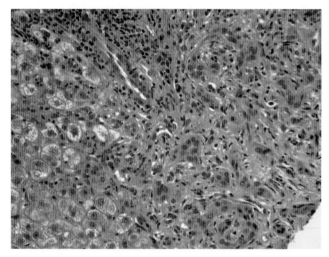

Figure 71.76 Atypical bile ducts in a portal tract of chronic hepatitis C. (H & E stain; original magnification ×200.)

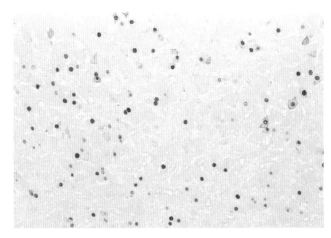

Figure 71.77 Immunoperoxidase stain demonstrating hepatitis D antigen in the nuclei of hepatocytes in chronic hepatitis D. (Original magnification ×100.)

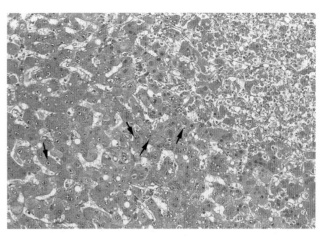

Figure 71.80 Intranuclear inclusions (arrows) of Cowdry type A of herpes simplex seen in hepatocytes. (H & E stain; original magnification ×200.)

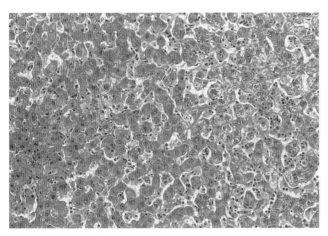

Figure 71.78 Striking sinusoidal lymphocytosis of atypical type in Epstein–Barr virus-induced mononucleosis. (H & E stain; original magnification ×200.)

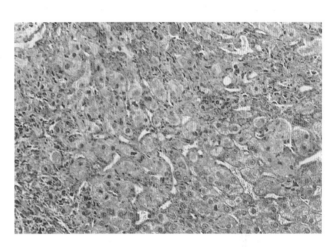

Figure 71.81 Diffuse interstitial fibrosis in chronic alcoholic liver disease. (Masson stain; original magnification ×100.)

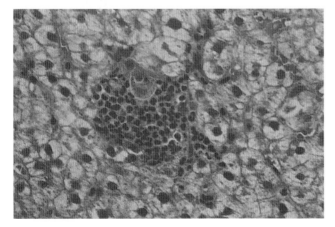

Figure 71.79 Intranuclear and cytoplasmic inclusions of cytomegalovirus (CMV) in a hepatocyte surrounded by polymorphonuclear leukocytes in an orthotopic liver transplant infected with CMV. (H & E stain; original magnification ×200.)

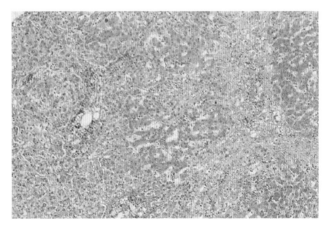

Figure 71.82 Marked perivenular fibrous scarring with mild portal fibrosis and lack of regenerative nodules in progressive perivenular fibrosis of alcoholic etiology. (Masson stain; original magnification ×100.)

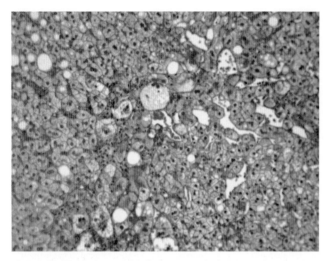

Figure 71.83 Perisinusoidal collagen in nonalcoholic steatohepatitis. (Masson trichrome stain; original magnification ×100.)

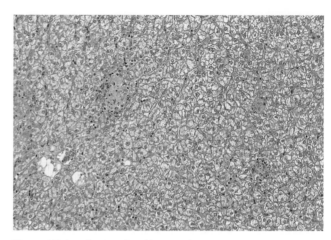

Figure 71.86 Dilantin-induced hepatic changes resembling mono-nucleosis. (H & E stain; original magnification ×100.)

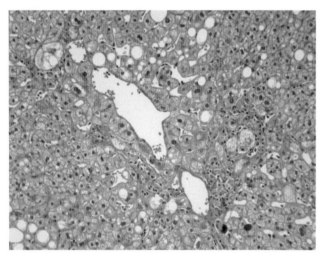

Figure 71.84 Hepatocytes with ballooning change and Mallory bodies in nonalcoholic steatohepatitis (H & E stain; original magnification ×100.)

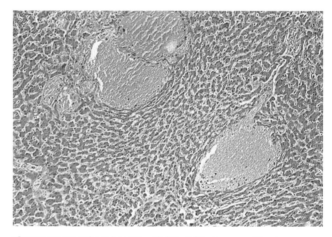

Figure 71.87 Peliosis hepatis with blood-filled spaces without endothelial lining. (H & E stain; original magnification ×100.)

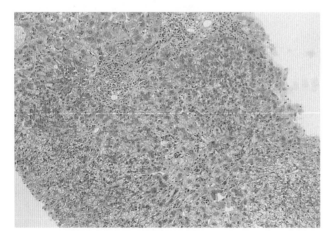

Figure 71.85 Hepatitis-like activity resembling acute viral hepatitis in Aldomet-induced hepatotoxicity. (H & E stain; original magnification ×200.)

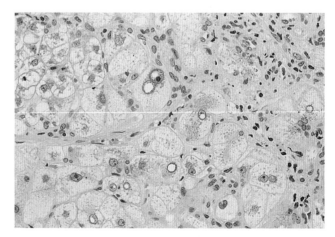

Figure 71.88 Sinusoidal fibrosis and nuclear dysplastic changes in methotrexate toxicity. (H & E stain; original magnification ×400.)

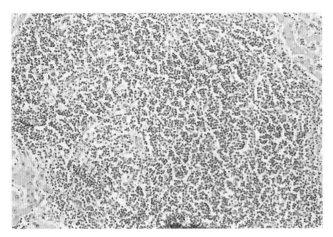

Figure 71.89 Portal infiltrate in non-Hodgkin lymphoma. (H & E stain; original magnification ×100.)

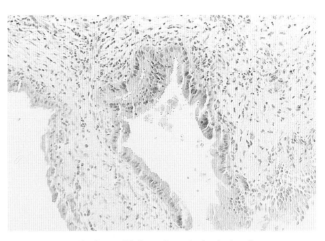

Figure 71.92 Bile duct epithelium along the luminal surface demonstrates the presence of cryptosporidiosis of 3- to 4-μm size. (H & E stain; original magnification ×400.)

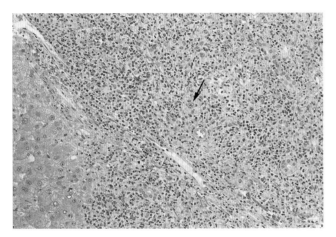

Figure 71.90 Portal infiltrate in Hodgkin lymphoma with an atypical Reed–Sternberg cell (arrow). (H & E stain; original magnification ×200.)

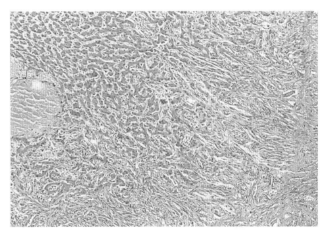

Figure 71.93 Kaposi sarcoma involving the liver. (H & E stain; original magnification ×100.)

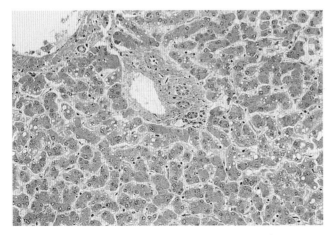

Figure 71.91 Portal area with lymphopenia in a patient with AIDS. (H & E stain; original magnification ×200.)

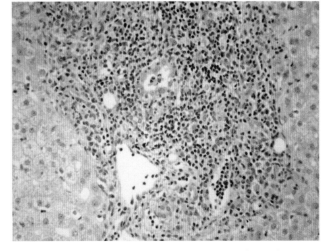

Figure 71.94 Portal inflammatory infiltrate, changes of interlobular bile ducts, and endothelialitis of portal vein radicles in acute rejection. (H & E stain; original magnification ×200.)

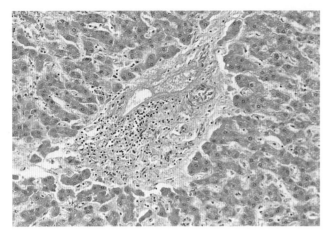

Figure 71.95 Portal inflammatory infiltrate with loss of bile ducts in chronic rejection. (H & E stain; original magnification ×200.)

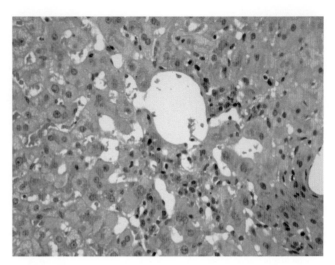

Figure 71.97 Perivenular zone with necroinflammatory changes in recurrent acute hepatitis B infection of allograft. (H & E stain; original magnification ×200.)

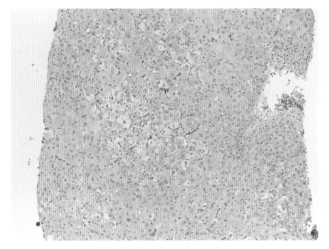

Figure 71.96 Marked ballooning of the hepatocytes in acinar zone 3 representing harvest injury. (H & E stain; original magnification ×100.)

72

Abdominal cavity: anatomy, structural anomalies, and hernias

Sareh Parangi, Richard A. Hodin

Embryology of the abdominal cavity

The abdominal cavity

An understanding of the embryology of the abdominal contents is imperative to understanding the pathophysiology of the various congenital and structural anomalies of the abdominal cavity. The abdominal cavity in the adult is defined by the diaphragm superiorly, the abdominal walls laterally, and the pelvis inferiorly. The peritoneal covering is the endodermal investment of the surface of the organs of the abdominal cavity. The pancreas, parts of the duodenum, right and left colon, and the rectum, which are all retroperitoneal, are covered only anteriorly by peritoneum.

Congenital anomalies

In the embryo, the abdominal cavity is too small to accommodate the intestines, and a physiological herniation occurs into the umbilical cord with return of the intestines to the abdominal cavity by the 10th week. An *omphalocele* results from failure in the growth of the celomic walls with a large herniation of the abdominal viscera into the base of the umbilical cord. The herniated viscera are covered by a sac composed of amnion. *Gastroschisis* is a similar anomaly, but the defect in the abdominal wall is located lateral to the umbilicus, and is caused by failure of closure of the abdominal wall. No sac is present to cover the herniated intestines and the size of the defect is often smaller.

Congenital diaphragmatic hernias

The diaphragm appears in the third week of development

as a septum transversum that separates the thorax from the abdomen. A diaphragmatic hernia is one of the more common malformations of the newborn and is most frequently caused by failure of the pleuroperitoneal membranes to completely separate the peritoneal and pleural cavities posteriorly.

Posterolateral hernia defects (hernia of Bochdalek) are usually large and on the left side; the intestinal loops, stomach, spleen, and part of the liver may enter the thoracic cavity (Fig. 72.1a). The presence of abdominal viscera in the chest results in compression of the heart and hypoplasia of the lung (Fig. 72.1b). Lung hypoplasia results in acute respiratory distress and is the main cause of death in these patients. Mortality depends on the age of the patient, associated malformations, and most importantly, the degree of lung hypoplasia.

Occasionally, a small part of the muscular fibers of the diaphragm fails to develop, and a hernia may remain undiscovered until later in life. Such a defect is seen in the anterior portion of the diaphragm and is known as a *parasternal hernia* (hernia of Morgagni). These hernias are usually small and can contain stomach, omentum, colon or small intestine with a peritoneal covering.

Hernias of the abdominal cavity in adults

Hernia is a protrusion of any viscus from its proper cavity (Sir Astley Cooper, 1804).

Hernias are composed of a herniated viscus, the hernia sac, and the opening of the hernia (the hernial ring).

A *reducible hernia* occurs when the hernial sac contents return to the abdominal cavity either spontaneously or with external manipulation. An *incarcerated hernia* occurs when the hernial contents cannot be dislodged from the sac. A hernia, reducible or incarcerated, becomes a *strangulated hernia* when the blood supply to the herniated viscus is compromised.

Atlas of Gastroenterology, 4th edition. Edited by Tadataka Yamada, David H. Alpers, Anthony N. Kalloo, Neil Kaplowitz, Chung Owyang, and Don W. Powell. © 2009 Blackwell Publishing, ISBN: 978-1-4051-6909-7

Diagnostic considerations

Most hernias are detected using history and physical examination. Radiographic studies are rarely needed, but may be useful in cases where the abdominal wall fat layer prevents accurate diagnosis. Ultrasound is rarely helpful, but in some cases can delineate the abdominal wall musculature and note the presence of air or peristalsing bowel. Computed tomography (CT) is good at detecting abdominal and pelvic defects; use of the Valsalva maneuver may sometimes be helpful during imaging. In some cases, attenuation of the abdominal fascia can be seen in the midline with no herniation; this is termed diastasis of the rectus muscle (Fig. 72.2).

Epigastric hernias

Epigastric hernias occur in the midline of the abdominal wall between the umbilicus and the xiphoid in 5% of the population.

Umbilical hernias

Umbilical hernias in adults often occur in obese multiparous women and patients with ascites. The diagnosis is usually self-evident with a protuberant mass at the umbilicus (Fig. 72.3).

Ventral hernias

Ventral hernias occur in the midline of the abdominal wall and can enlarge slowly. If the history and physical examination do not provide an accurate diagnosis, a computed tomography (CT) scan of the abdomen can be performed and will show a defect with herniated viscera (Fig. 72.4).

Groin hernias

Hernias of the groin are the most common of all hernias. An example of a giant inguinal hernia containing nearly all the small intestine is seen in Figure 72.5. The inferior epigastric artery serves as an important defining anatomic landmark. Indirect hernias originate lateral to this artery and protrude into the inguinal canal along the spermatic cord. Direct hernias are located medial to the inferior epigastric artery and come through a weakened inguinal floor composed of the transversalis aponeurosis and fascia. Figure 72.6 shows an example of an incarcerated inguinal hernia causing small bowel obstruction.

Pelvic hernias

The intestine can herniate through the pelvic floor (weakness, perhaps, from multiparity or previous trauma) in areas such as the obturator foramen, the greater or lesser sciatic foramina, or through the perineal muscle. The most common of these hernias is the *obturator hernia*. *Sciatic hernias* are extremely rare, and can present with a slowly enlarging mass in the gluteal fold area.

Lumbar hernias

The posterior abdominal wall has two naturally weak areas. Lumbar hernias should be surgically repaired when first noted as they tend to enlarge, and larger hernias are more difficult to repair.

Spigelian hernias

A spigelian hernia is rare, occurring through the linea semilunaris, lateral to the rectus abdominis, with protrusion through the external oblique fascia (Fig. 72.7). Spigelian hernias occur in the elderly, are often small and difficult to diagnose, and always present below the arcuate line of Douglas. Symptoms include local pain or discomfort worsened by increased intraabdominal pressure.

Diaphragmatic hernias

Acquired diaphragmatic hernias are the result of blunt or penetrating trauma. Most hernias occur on the left, and herniated viscera can include stomach, spleen, colon, or the left lobe of the liver (Fig. 72.8).

Internal hernias

An internal hernia is a protrusion of any intraperitoneal viscous into a compartment within the abdominal cavity. There is no hernia sac, and most often the herniated viscus is entering a known anatomical space or foramen; some hernias occur in surgically created or congenital defects.

Incisional hernias

Incisions of the abdominal wall result in future herniation 2%–5% of the time. Multiple factors are responsible for a postoperative incisional hernia, including defective suture material, undue tension on the sutured fascia, obesity, previous incisions, infections, seromas or hematomas, malnutrition, and smoking (Fig. 72.9). The diagnosis of an incisional hernia is usually evident by history as well as physical examination. The hernial ring is often palpable with the edges of the muscle retracted laterally. Incisional hernias often incarcerate but tend not to strangulate. Small hernias, such as laparoscopic port site hernias, can be difficult to diagnose on physical examination and will often strangulate because the opening is small (Fig. 72.10). Operative repair should be undertaken in most patients. For many years, the repair of incisional hernias was associated with a high recurrence rate. The introduction of synthetic prosthetic materials has provided the opportunity to perform a tension-free repair, thereby reducing the rate of recurrence. Note that recurrent herniation can occur even with mesh in place (Fig. 72.11).

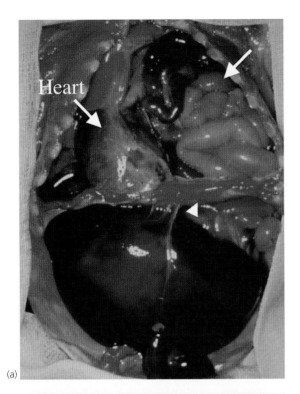

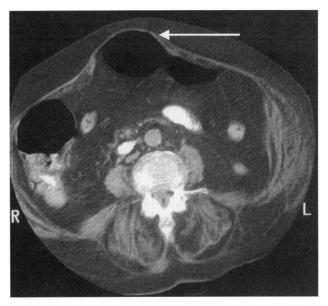

Figure 72.2 Diastasis recti (arrow). Computed tomography scan of the abdomen shows that the rectus muscle is attenuated in the midline, but there is no fascial defect; this is not a hernia. Courtesy of J. Kruskal, MD.

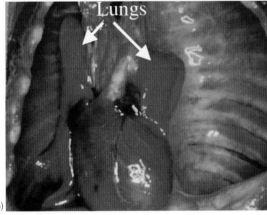

Figure 72.1 Congenital diaphragmatic hernia. **(a)** A posterolateral diaphragmatic hernia (hernia of Bochdalek) is seen in autopsy pictures of a newborn baby. Note the intestinal loops (arrow) present in the left chest cavity. The diaphragmatic defect is marked with the arrowhead. The presence of abdominal viscera in the chest results in compression of the heart and hypoplasia of the lungs. **(b)** The pulmonary hypoplasia associated with this condition. Courtesy of J. Wilson, MD.

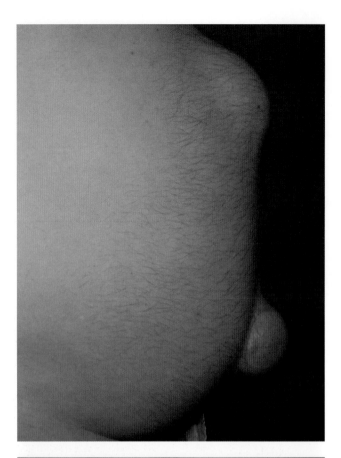

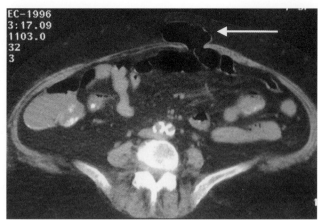

Figure 72.4 Ventral hernia seen on computed tomography scan of the abdomen. Note the gas-filled loop of intestine (arrow) going through the fascial defect and presenting in the subcutaneous tissue of the anterior abdominal wall. Courtesy of J. Kruskal, MD.

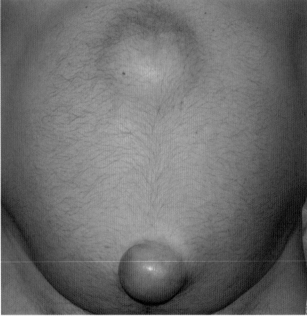

Figure 72.3 Subxiphoid hernia (superior) and umbilical hernia (inferior) in the same patient.

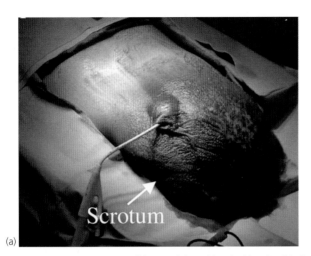

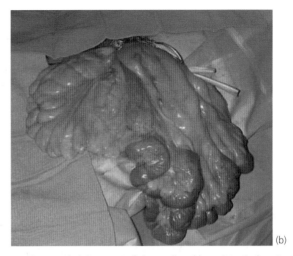

(a)

(b)

Figure 72.5 Giant inguinal hernia. **(a)** Large bilateral inguinal hernia. **(b)** The operation revealed that most of the small and large intestinal contents were present in the hernia sac in the scrotum. Repair was performed with polypropylene mesh.

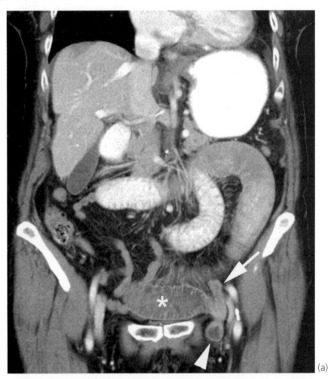

(a)

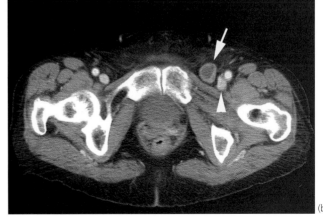

(b)

Figure 72.6 Incarcerated inguinal hernia with small bowel obstruction. Computed tomography of the abdomen in a patient with an incarcerated left inguinal hernia (reconstructed images in **(a)** and traditional transverse images in **(b)**). Reconstructed tomographic images are very helpful when available and in this patient show the incarceration, which is the point of intestinal obstruction (arrow), as well as the dilated small bowel (white star). Note the location of the hernia (arrowhead) medial to the femoral vessels in (b). Courtesy of I. Pedrosa, MD.

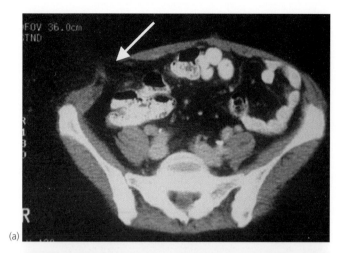

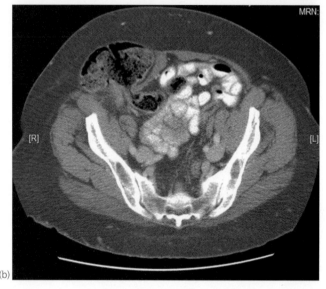

Figure 72.7 Spigelian hernia. Computed tomography scans of the abdomen demonstrating two examples **(a, b)** of spigelian hernias. These hernias are rare and occur through the linea semilunaris (arrow), lateral to the rectus abdominis, with protrusion through the external oblique fascia. (a) Courtesy of J. Kruskal, MD.

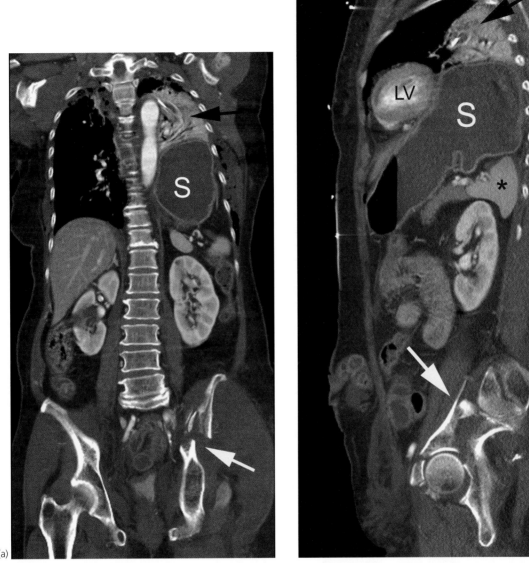

Figure 72.8 Traumatic diaphragmatic hernia. Reconstructed views of computed tomography of the abdomen reveal a traumatic rupture of the left hemidiaphragm with herniation of the stomach (S) into the left chest resulting in severe pulmonary compromise (black arrow). These patients often suffer from additional injuries such as fractures of the bony pelvis (white arrow). LV, left ventricle. Courtesy of I. Pedrosa, MD.

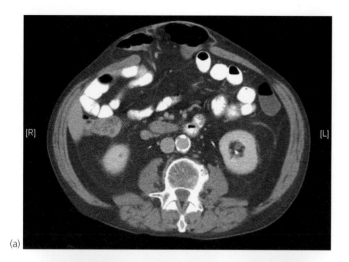

(a)

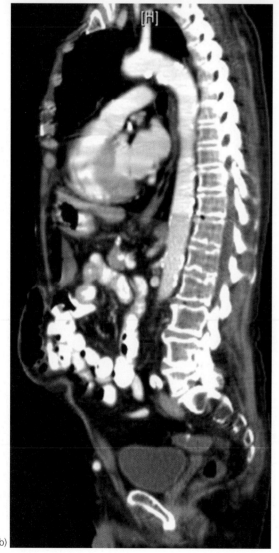

(b)

Figure 72.9 Large incisional hernia. Computed tomography scans show transverse **(a)** and longitudinal **(b)** images. Delay in repair can lead to intestinal ischemia. Courtesy of I. Pedrosa, MD.

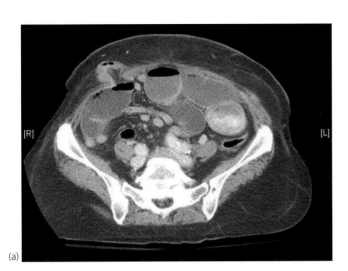

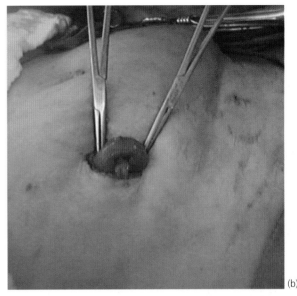

Figure 72.10 A laparoscopic port-site hernia of the anterior abdominal wall. **(a)** A small hernia in the right lower quadrant of the abdomen was seen on computed tomography performed for small bowel obstruction. Smaller port-site hernias such as this one may be difficult to distinguish on physical examination. **(b)** Intraoperative photograph of the incarcerated small bowel. Courtesy of V. Sanchez, MD.

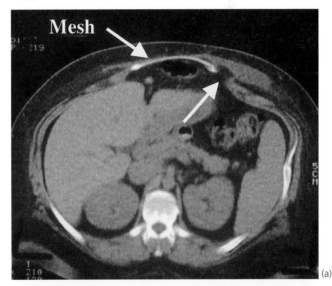

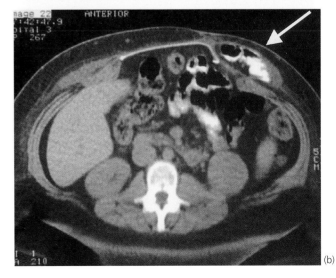

Figure 72.11 Recurrent ventral hernia after mesh repair. Computed tomography scan of the abdomen in a patient with a bulge 1 year after ventral hernia repair with polypropylene mesh. **(a)** A fascial defect (arrow) can be seen lateral to the mesh. **(b)** A loop of intestine filled with contrast is seen in the subcutaneous tissue of the abdomen lateral to the mesh (arrow). Courtesy of J. Kruskal, MD.

73

Intraabdominal abscesses and fistulae

Paul Knechtges, Ellen M. Zimmermann

Intraabdominal abscesses and fistulae are complications that arise from a variety of abdominal and pelvic processes. They should be approached as specific clinical entities, with close attention to the underlying etiology. In the past, most abscesses and fistulae required open surgical therapy. However, the modern therapeutic approach includes sophisticated diagnostic imaging, percutaneous or endoscopic aspiration and drainage, and medical therapy, leaving fewer cases requiring aggressive surgery. To appropriately utilize cross sectional and other imaging modalities, it is important to consider relevant anatomy including the peritoneal and retroperitoneal compartments consisting of a series of communicating compartmentalized potential spaces that determine the site and clinical symptoms associated with gastrointestinal abscesses and fistulae (Fig. 73.1).

Multiple imaging modalities are available to aid in evaluation of suspected or established intraabdominal abscesses and fistulae. Computed tomography (CT) has become the imaging method of choice to evaluate intraabdominal abscesses. Several findings on CT are highly suggestive of an intraabdominal abscess, including loculation, ring enhancement, and gas (Fig. 73.2). After an intraabdominal abscess is identified by CT, either CT or ultrasound can be used, if indicated, to guide imaging for needle aspiration or catheter drainage (Figs 73.3–73.5).

Others modalities, such as magnetic resonance imaging (MRI) and nuclear imaging, can play important roles in complex cases or in specific clinical situations. Exquisite detail of the retroperitoneal and pelvic structures can be provided by MRI and it is a superb imaging modality for perianal abscesses and fistulae (Fig. 73.6). While taking a secondary role to CT and MRI for evaluation of intraabdominal abscesses, nuclear medicine imaging is occasionally useful. [111]Indium-labeled leukocytes are the most appropriate for the localization of intraperitoneal abscesses, because it does not demonstrate physiological uptake in a normal bowel. While spatial resolution is limited, it can provide important physiological data about the infectious or inflammatory status of fluid collections and soft tissue stranding seen on CT (Fig. 73.7).

A hybrid approach combining cross-sectional imaging studies (e.g., CT and MRI) with more traditional studies (e.g., fistulography and contrast fluoroscopy) can provide complementary information. Such a hybrid/multimodality approach to fistula imaging is becoming more common as imaging technology advances (Figs 73.8–73.10).

Atlas of Gastroenterology, 4th edition. Edited by Tadataka Yamada, David H. Alpers, Anthony N. Kalloo, Neil Kaplowitz, Chung Owyang, and Don W. Powell. © 2009 Blackwell Publishing, ISBN: 978-1-4051-6909-7

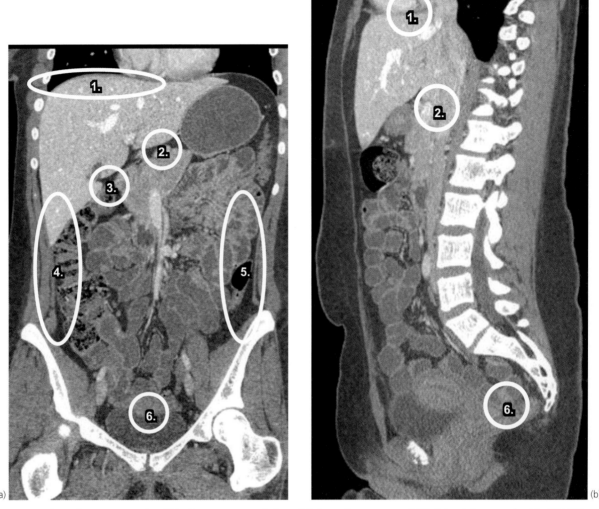

Figure 73.1 Peritoneal compartments in which abscesses commonly form. **(a)** Coronally reconstructed CT of the abdomen and pelvis. **(b)** Midline sagittally reconstructed CT of the abdomen and pelvis. (*Continued on next page.*)

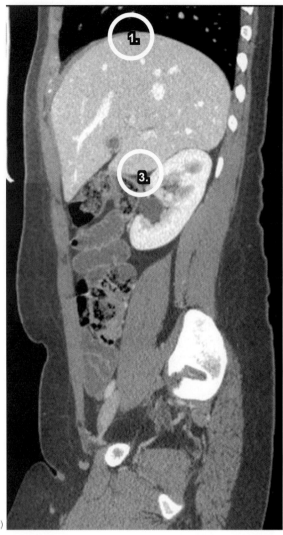

(c)

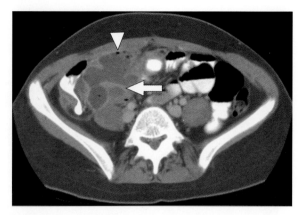

Figure 73.2 Right lower quadrant abscess in a patient with perforated appendicitis. This multiloculated, rim-enhancing fluid collection contains tiny gas bubbles (arrowhead) and enhancing septae (arrow).

Figure 73.1 *Continued* **(c)** Right paramidline sagittally reconstructed CT of the abdomen and pelvis. 1, subphrenic space; 2, lesser sac; 3, subhepatic space (Morison pouch); 4, right paracolic gutter; 5, left paracolic gutter; 6, rectouterine space in this female patient (rectovesical space in males).

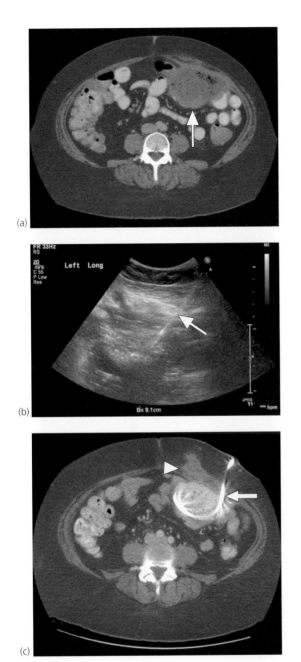

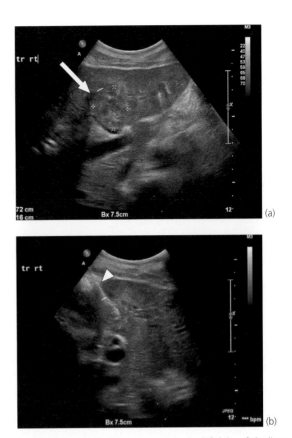

Figure 73.4 (a) Ultrasound of an abscess in the left lobe of the liver. Although bowel gas limits the ability of ultrasound to detect abscesses in between or among bowel loops, it can be very helpful for detecting abscesses in solid organs that have no intervening gas or bone between the ultrasound probe and the organ in question. The appearance of hepatic abscesses varies considerably on ultrasound depending on the amount of solid and fluid components. The differential diagnosis of such a finding includes abscess, hematoma, cyst, and cystic or necrotic neoplasm. **(b)** Interventions performed under real-time ultrasound guidance (arrowhead, needle), can be used for aspiration and catheter drainage.

Figure 73.3 (a) A patient with a prior history of diverticulitis presents with a rim-enhancing fluid collection containing mottled gas in the left lower quadrant, consistent with an abscess (arrow). **(b)** Under ultrasound guidance **(top right)** a needle (arrow) was introduced into the abscess and brown turbid fluid was aspirated. A drainage catheter was subsequently placed. **(c)** A follow-up CT scan reveals the drainage catheter in the abscess cavity. There is now oral contrast in the abscess cavity consistent with interval fistulization with adjacent bowel.

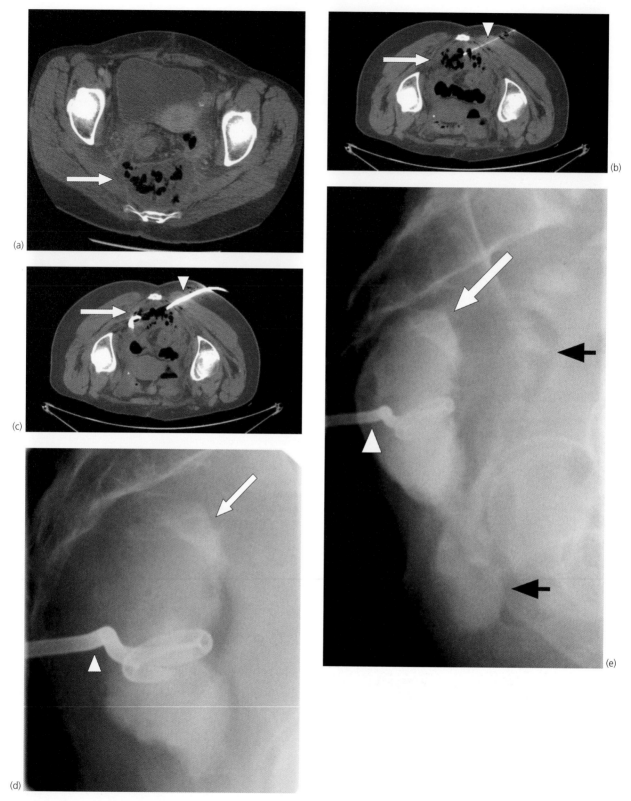

Figure 73.5 **(a)** CT of a patient status post low anterior resection and colorectal anastomosis with a presacral rim-enhancing abscess containing mottled gas and fluid (arrow). **(b)** The patient was placed in prone position and, under CT guidance, a needle (arrowhead) was introduced in to the abscess (arrow) and the collection was aspirated. **(c)** A drainage catheter (arrowhead) was subsequently inserted into the abscess cavity (arrow). **(d)** During a follow-up study, the patient was imaged under fluoroscopy performed in the lateral position. The drainage catheter (arrowhead) was injected and the abscess cavity (white arrow) filled with water-soluble contrast. **(e)** Upon further instillation of contrast, the contrast began to be seen in the rectum and sigmoid colon (black arrows). This finding confirmed that the abscess was secondary to an anastomotic leak.

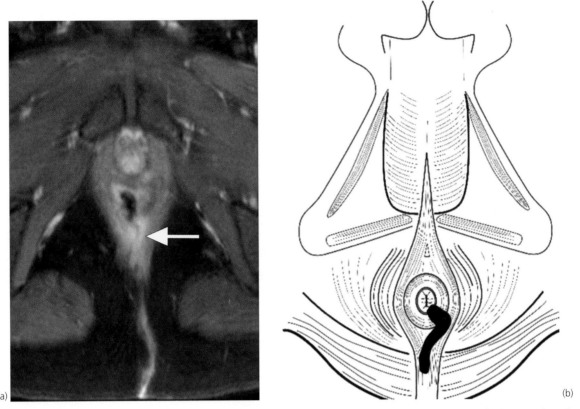

Figure 73.6 (a) Axial MR image (post-contrast spoiled gradient echo with fat saturation) demonstrates a trans-sphincteric fistula-in-ano (arrow) originating at the posterior anal mucosa and traversing the internal and external anal sphincters before emerging in the perianal skin. **(b)** An accompanying diagrammatic representation shows the fistula in black traversing the internal and external anal sphincters.

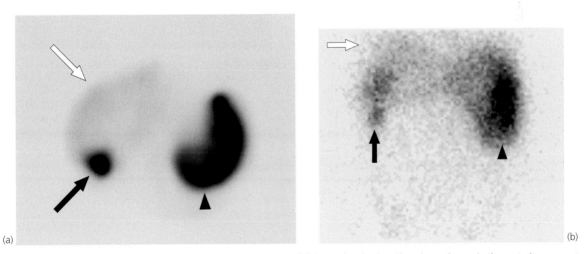

Figure 73.7 Indium-111 oxine-labeled leukocyte study. **(a)** Axial projection. **(b)** Coronal projection. There is an abscess in the posterior segment of the right lobe of the liver (black arrow) resulting in increased uptake of Indium-111 labeled leukocytes. Please note the intense normal physiological uptake of indium-111 labeled leukocytes in the spleen (arrowhead) and the lesser amount of physiological uptake in the normal liver parenchyma (white arrow).

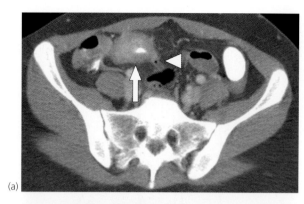

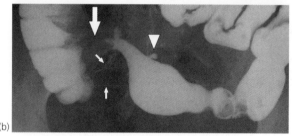

Figure 73.8 (a) Inflamed terminal ileum (arrow) demonstrating marked wall thickening in a patient with Crohn's disease. There is an enhancing gas-containing tract (arrowhead) between the terminal ileum and the sigmoid colon, which raised suspicion of an enterocolic fistula. **(b)** A small bowel followthrough was performed, which demonstrated that the tract seen on the CT was a blind-ending sinus tract (arrowhead). The small bowel followthrough was able to detect subtle ileocecal fistulae (small arrows) that were not visible on this conventional CT of the abdomen and pelvis. The terminal ileum is markedly narrowed secondary to Crohn's involvement (large arrow).

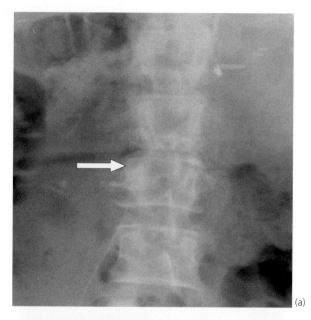

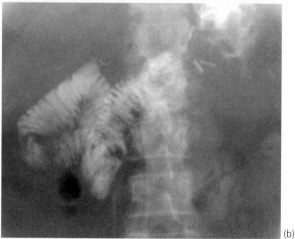

Figure 73.9 (a) Fistulography. Patient status post Whipple procedure developed an enterocutaneous fistula. The cutaneous orifice was cannulated with a small catheter (arrow). **(b)** Water-soluble contrast was then gently instilled under gravity drip. Contrast filled the afferent limb and refluxed into the patient's stomach confirming the presence of an enterocutaneous fistula communicating with the afferent limb.

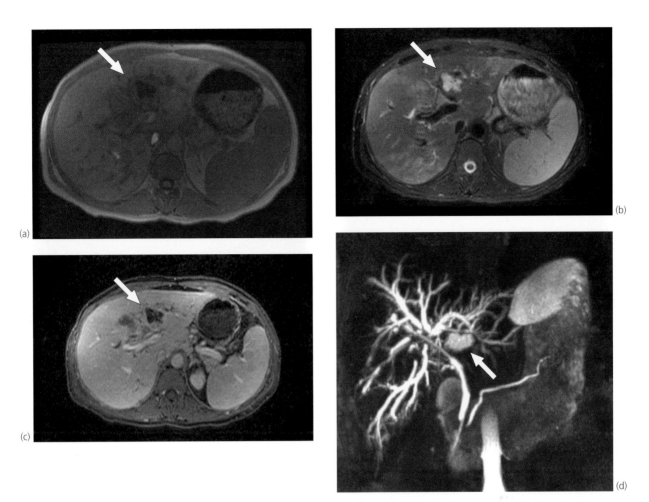

Figure 73.10 MRI of a patient with recurrent cholangitis and multifocal liver abscesses. **(a)** Axial T1-weighted in-phase dual gradient echo imaging demonstrates a low signal (dark) in the left lobe of the liver and an adjacent area of low signal in the medial segment of the right lobe of the liver consistent with another abscess. **(b)** Axial T2-weighted imaging with fat saturation demonstrates high signal (fluid) in the abscess cavity and an adjacent area of high signal in the medial segment of the right lobe of the liver, consistent with another abscess. The other geographic peripheral areas of increased signal intensity on T2-weighted imaging correspond to inflammation of the patient's intrahepatic biliary tree secondary to the patient's cholangitis. **(c)** Axial post-contrast spoiled gradient echo with fat saturation demonstrates rim enhancement of these lesions. **(d)** The abscess in the left lobe of the liver on the previous figure appears to communicate with the biliary tree on the magnetic resonance cholangiopancreatogram (MRCP). The arrow indicates the abscess on all images.

74

Diseases of the peritoneum, retroperitoneum, mesentery, and omentum

Shawn D. Larson, B. Mark Evers

The peritoneum is the mesothelial lining of the peritoneal cavity that covers the walls (parietal peritoneum) and the combined viscera (visceral peritoneum) of the peritoneal cavity. Diseases of the peritoneum include inflammation of the peritoneal lining (peritonitis), primary mesothelioma, and pseudomyxoma peritonei.

Peritonitis involves a local or generalized inflammatory condition of the parietal and visceral peritoneum. Management of peritonitis includes operative management to control the source of peritoneal contamination. If the source of infection is not completely eliminated with the initial operation, a planned reoperation with further debridement and irrigation is performed. In this situation, opening and closing of the abdominal cavity may be facilitated by means of placement of a large abdominal zipper (Fig. 74.1).

Granulomatous peritonitis, characterized by inflammation and granuloma formation, can be caused by diseases such as tuberculosis. Tuberculous peritonitis is usually associated with a primary focus elsewhere (most commonly the lung), with spread to the abdomen in approximately 1% of cases (Fig. 74.2). A computed tomography (CT) scan may identify thickened bowel and ascites (Fig. 74.3).

Other conditions that may affect the peritoneum include the rare malignant process, primary mesothelioma, which is linked to asbestos exposure. The diagnosis may be obtained by means of ultrasound and CT studies (Figs 74.4 and 74.5).

Pseudomyxoma peritonei is another rare condition that can involve the peritoneal cavity and omentum. Characteristic CT findings of pseudomyxoma peritonei include scalloping of the hepatic and intestinal margins caused by extrinsic compression by ascitic spaces containing gelatinous material (Fig. 74.6).

The retroperitoneum is the space behind the abdominal cavity that extends superiorly from the diaphragm and inferiorly to the levator muscles of the pelvis. Diseases of the retroperitoneum include retroperitoneal hemorrhage, inflammation, fibrosis, and neoplasia.

The most common cause of retroperitoneal bleeding is traumatic injury to the pelvis, vertebral column, or kidneys (Figs 74.7–74.9). Retroperitoneal infections may be caused by diseases of the surrounding abdominal organs, the urinary tract, or the vertebral column (Figs 74.10 and 74.11).

Retroperitoneal fibrosis is an uncommon disease characterized by progressive nonspecific inflammation and fibrosis of connective and adipose tissue in the retroperitoneal space. A useful imaging study for establishing the diagnosis is intravenous pyelography, in which the triad of findings is hydronephrosis, narrowing of the ureters, and medial displacement of the ureters (Fig. 74.12). CT scanning and magnetic resonance imaging (MRI) are useful in the diagnosis and follow-up management of this condition (Fig. 74.13).

Tumors of the retroperitoneal space arise from mesodermal, neuroectodermal, or embryonic remnants (Fig. 74.14). CT scanning is a useful imaging modality to identify the mass, determine the size and origin, and assess the relation to and possible invasion of surrounding structures. MRI has become an increasingly important diagnostic tool in the management of retroperitoneal neoplasms. It allows a better degree of definition between the mass and surrounding muscle groups and vascular structures than is obtained with CT scanning.

The mesentery or omentum may become involved in a variety of disease processes, most of which originate in adjacent visceral organs. These include inflammatory and vascular processes, mesenteric/omental cysts, and tumors (benign, malignant, and metastatic) (Table 74.1).

Mesenteric and omental cysts are uncommon lesions representing benign proliferation of ectopic lymphatics lacking

Atlas of Gastroenterology, 4th edition. Edited by Tadataka Yamada, David H. Alpers, Anthony N. Kalloo, Neil Kaplowitz, Chung Owyang, and Don W. Powell. © 2009 Blackwell Publishing, ISBN: 978-1-4051-6909-7

communication with the normal lymphatic system. Ultrasonography, CT, and MRI may demonstrate the multilocular or unilocular nature of the cysts, which may have homogeneous or nonhomogeneous contents. Of the three imaging modalities, ultrasonography probably yields the most infor-

mation for the least expense (Fig. 74.15). The definitive diagnosis and treatment of these lesions is with surgical resection. Most types of mesenteric cyst simply can be excised (Fig. 74.16).

Table 74.1 Classification of mesenteric and omental diseases

Mesenteric diseases	Omental diseases
Primary mesenteric inflammatory diseases	Mass lesions
Mesenteric panniculitis	Primary tumors and cysts
Retractile mesenteritis	Metastatic disease
Mesenteric cysts	Vascular lesions damaging blood supply
Embryonic and developmental cysts	Torsion
Traumatic or acquired cysts	Primary
Neoplastic cysts	Secondary: hernia, adhesion, tumor
Infective and degenerative cysts	Infarction
Mesenteric tumors	Primary
Benign tumors	Secondary: torsion, incarceration in
Lipoma	hernia
Hemangioma	
Leiomyoma	
Ganglioneuroma	
Malignant tumors	
Leiomyosarcoma	
Liposarcoma	
Rhabdomyosarcoma	
Metastatic disease	
Mesenteric fibromatosis	

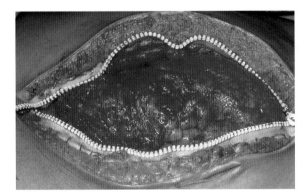

Figure 74.1 Patient with severe necrotizing pancreatitis with abscess requiring multiple reoperations for debridement, irrigation, and packing. An abdominal zipper was placed to facilitate abdominal opening and closing. It was removed at definitive fascial closure.

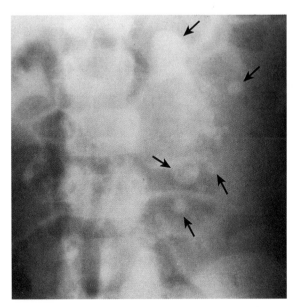

Figure 74.2 Abdominal radiograph of a patient with tuberculous peritonitis shows extensive calcification of the peritoneum, omentum, and lymph nodes (arrows). Courtesy of Dr Luis B. Morettin.

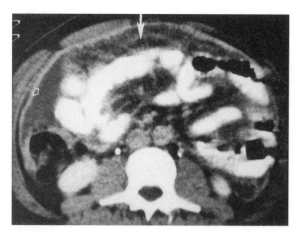

Figure 74.3 Computed tomographic scan demonstrates ascites (open arrow) and small bowel thickening (closed arrow) in a patient with tuberculous peritonitis. Courtesy of Dr Charles J. Fagan.

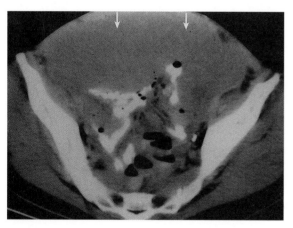

Figure 74.4 Computed tomographic scan of a patient with peritoneal mesothelioma demonstrates diffuse mesenteric and peritoneal involvement of a soft tissue mass (arrows) causing displacement of intraabdominal organs. Courtesy of Dr Eric van Sonnenberg.

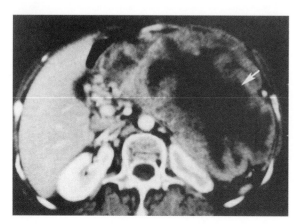

Figure 74.5 Computed tomographic scan demonstrates diffuse mesenteric and peritoneal involvement of a soft tissue mass (arrow) causing displacement of intraabdominal organs in a patient with peritoneal mesothelioma. Courtesy of Dr Charles J. Fagan.

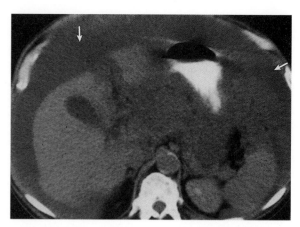

Figure 74.6 Computed tomographic scan of a patient with pseudomyxoma peritonei caused by adenocarcinoma of the appendix demonstrates a large amount of high-density gelatinous fluid (arrows) compressing the surrounding bowel. Courtesy of Dr Luis B. Morettin.

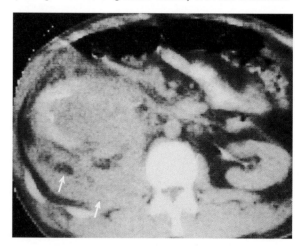

Figure 74.7 Computed tomographic scan demonstrates a large retroperitoneal hematoma (arrows) caused by hemorrhage from renal carcinoma. Courtesy of Dr Luis B. Morettin.

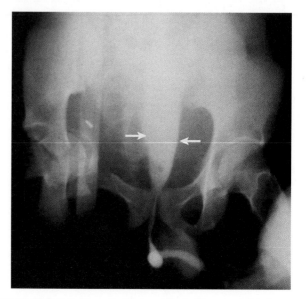

Figure 74.8 Cystogram of a trauma patient with severe pelvic fracture and large retroperitoneal hematoma compressing the bladder (arrows).

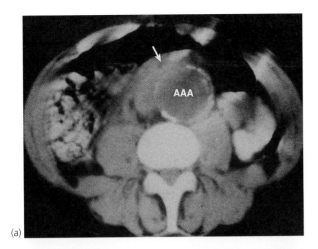

(a)

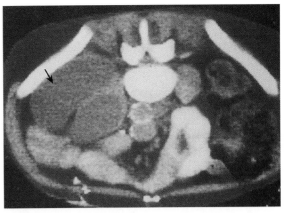

Figure 74.10 Computed tomographic scan shows a large retroperitoneal abscess (arrow) originating from an infection of a previously placed aortobifemoral graft. Courtesy of Dr Luis B. Morettin.

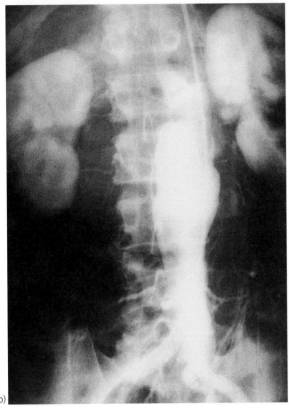

(b)

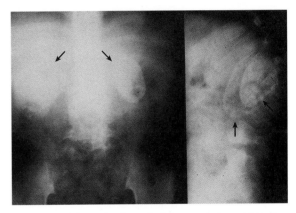

Figure 74.11 Abdominal radiographs (anteroposterior and lateral) demonstrate bilateral calcified psoas abscesses (arrows) caused by tuberculosis. Courtesy of Dr Luis B. Morettin.

Figure 74.9 (a) Computed tomographic scan demonstrates a large abdominal aortic aneurysm (AAA) with calcification in the wall of the aneurysm. A contained retroperitoneal hematoma is shown (arrow). **(b)** Arteriogram demonstrates the abdominal aortic aneurysm shown in (a). On arteriograms one often underestimates the size and extent of the aneurysms. Courtesy of Dr Luis Morettin.

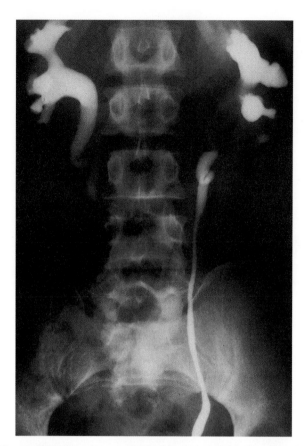

Figure 74.12 Intravenous pyelogram of a patient with retroperitoneal fibrosis demonstrates bilateral hydronephrosis, ureteral dilation, and narrowing without complete obstruction. Courtesy of Dr Luis B. Morettin.

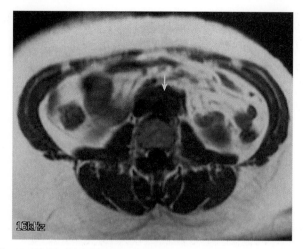

Figure 74.13 Axial T1-weighted magnetic resonance image of a patient with retroperitoneal fibrosis demonstrates a periaortic soft-tissue mass (arrow) that obliterates the fat plane. Courtesy of Dr Greg Chalchub.

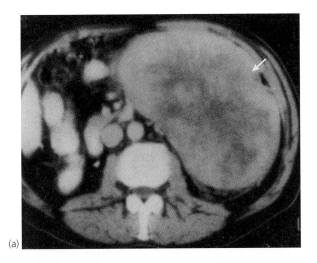

(a)

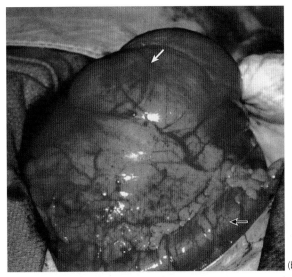

(b)

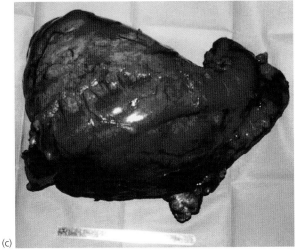

(c)

Figure 74.14 **(a)** Computed tomographic scan demonstrates a large left retroperitoneal mass (arrow). **(b)** Intraoperative view of the large retroperitoneal tumor shown in **(a)**. The tumor (white arrow) is contiguous with but does not invade the left kidney and descending colon (black arrow). **(c)** Retroperitoneal tumor after resection. The kidney and descending colon were resected en bloc with the tumor, which was a hemangiopericytoma.

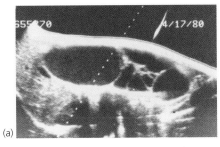

(a)

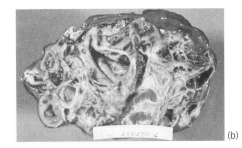

(b)

Figure 74.15 Sonographic appearance of a lymphangioma with gross specimen correlation. **(a)** As in this sagittal section of the right abdomen, the loculi of a lymphangioma can be anechoic and contain echogenic debris and fluid–fluid levels. **(b)** The corresponding gross specimen demonstrates the multilocular nature of a lymphangioma and the different kinds of fluid contained in the loculi, ranging from hemorrhagic to serous.

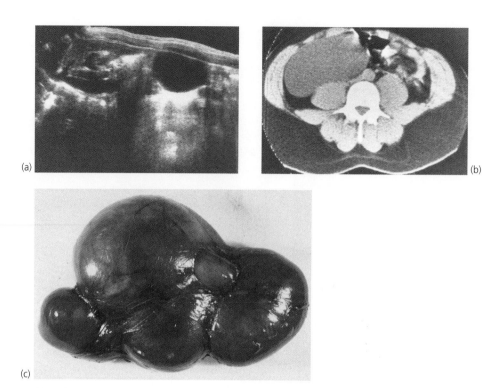

(a)

(b)

(c)

Figure 74.16 Sonographic and computed tomographic (CT) appearance of a mesothelial cyst with a pathological correlation. **(a)** A longitudinal abdominal sonogram (sagittal section, to the right of the midline) reveals an anechoic mass with acoustic enhancement. The anterior location suggests an omental location. **(b)** A CT scan of another patient demonstrates a fluid-filled mass in the right lower abdomen. There is no discernible wall. **(c)** Specimen corresponding to (b) shows elongated thin-walled cysts.

75

Complications of AIDS and other immunodeficiency states

Phillip D. Smith, Nirag C. Jhala, C. Mel Wilcox, Edward N. Janoff

The acquired immunodeficiency syndrome (AIDS) and other cellular and humoral immunodeficiency states are associated with an array of gastrointestinal complications. The complications associated with AIDS are caused predominantly by infection. Parasitic (mainly protozoal), viral, bacterial and fungal pathogens cause a spectrum of mucosal disease, depending on the location and severity of infection and the degree of immunosuppression induced by human immunodeficiency virus-1 (HIV-1), the causative agent of AIDS. These pathogens are considered opportunistic in immunosuppressed persons because they occur more frequently, cause more severe disease and are associated with more prolonged or recurrent infection. Opportunistic pathogens in patients with advanced HIV-1 disease more fre-

quently develop resistance to antimicrobial agents than do the same pathogens in immunocompetent persons. Gastrointestinal complications are also associated with allogeneic haematopoietic stem cell and solid organ transplantation. Graft-versus-host disease, which must be differentiated from infectious processes, is the most common gastrointestinal complication of haematopietic stem-cell transplantation. Opportunistic enteric infections, particularly cytomegalovirus, also commonly complicate solid organ transplantation. This chapter focuses on endoscopic and histological features of gastrointestinal infections associated with AIDS, hepatic complications of AIDS and intestinal involvement in graft-versus-host disease.

Atlas of Gastroenterology, 4th edition. Edited by Tadataka Yamada, David H. Alpers, Anthony N. Kalloo, Neil Kaplowitz, Chung Owyang, and Don W. Powell. © 2009 Blackwell Publishing, ISBN: 978-1-4051-6909-7

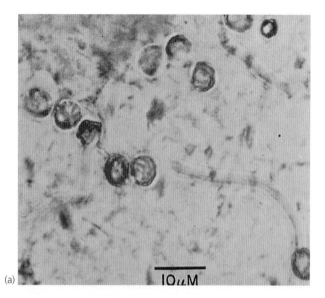

(a)

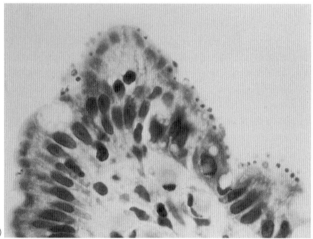

(b)

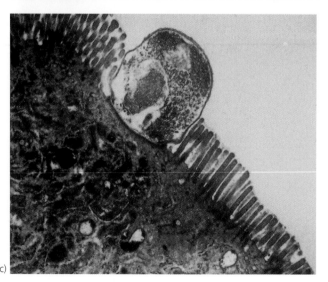

(c)

Figure 75.1 *Cryptosporidium parvum* is a parasitic protozoa that causes prolonged, often profuse, watery diarrhea among immunosuppressed persons with HIV-1 infection, particularly in the developing world. **(a)** Acid-fast stained stool specimen shows round *Cryptosporidium* oocysts 4-6 μm in diameter (modified Kinyoun stain; magnification × 630). **(b)** Light microscopic image shows *Cryptosporidium* protozoa lining the lumenal surface of the epithelium in an intestinal biopsy specimen from a patient with chronic diarrhea (hematoxylin and eosin; magnification × 400). **(c)** Electron micrograph of an intestinal biopsy section shows a *Cryptosporidium* trophozoite that has displaced the microvilli to attach to the apical surface of an epithelial cell (magnification × 12 500).

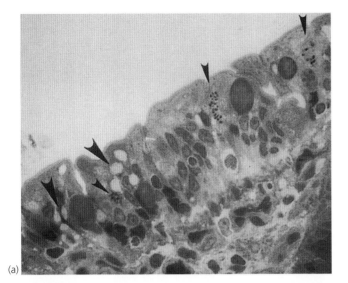

(a)

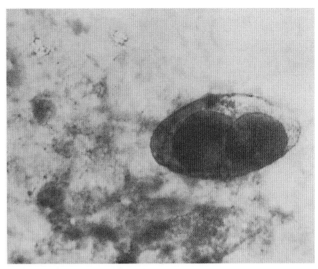

Figure 75.3 The coccidian protozoan *Isospora belli* causes a mild, self-limited diarrheal illness among immunocompetent persons but prolonged diarrhea among immunosuppressed persons. Infection with *I. belli* is diagnosed by identification of large (20–30 μm by 10–19 μm), oval, acid-fast oocysts that contain two sporoblasts in a fresh stool specimen (modified Kinyoun stain; magnification × 630).

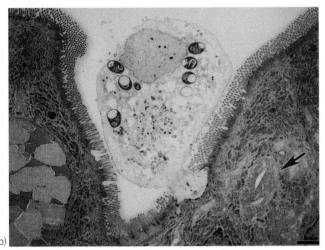

(b)

Figure 75.2 *Microsporida* protozoa in the small intestine of persons with HIV-1 infection is associated with a chronic diarrheal illness that clinically resembles cryptosporidiosis. **(a)** The intensity of infection is greatest in the jejunum, where densely stained elliptical spores are detected in the epithelial cell cytoplasm by light microscopic examination (semi-thin plastic section, methylene blue-azure II, basic fuchsin stain; original magnification × 630). **(b)** Electron micrograph shows a necrotic intestinal enterocyte in the final stage of being sloughed into the lumen; the enterocyte contains six microsporidian spores (magnification × 10 000). Courtesy of Dr Jan M. Orenstein.

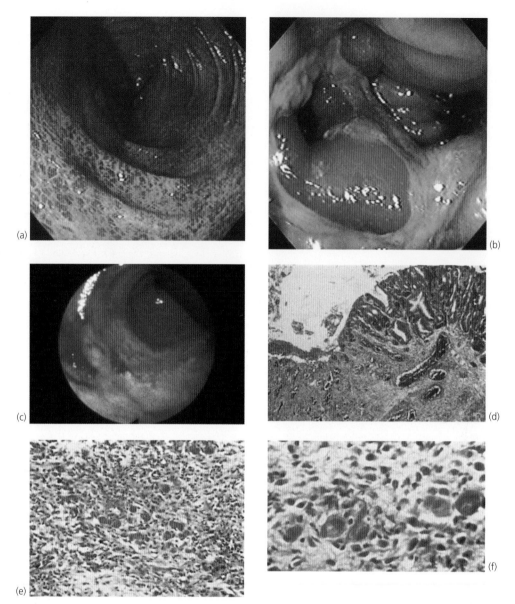

Figure 75.4 Colitis is the most common gastrointestinal manifestation of cytomegalovirus disease in AIDS. **(a)** Endoscopic view of diffuse colitis with prominent subepithelial hemorrhage in a patient with cytomegalovirus colitis. **(b)** Endoscopic visualization of a large well-circumscribed ulcer involving the ileocecal valve in a patient with cytomegalovirus colitis. **(c)** Endoscopic view of mucosal inflammation, ulceration and bleeding in a patient with cytomegalovirus colitis. **(d)** Light microscopic examination of a colon biopsy specimen from the patient in **(c)** shows ulceration and hemorrhage, **(e)** infiltration by large numbers of inflammatory cells, and **(f)** numerous cytomegalic inclusion cells, which are pathognomonic of the infection. (d, e, f hematoxylin and eosin; d, magnification × 30; e, magnification × 62; f, magnification × 125).

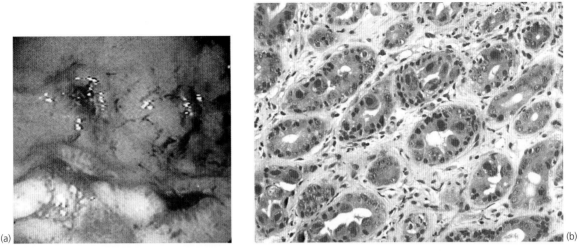

Figure 75.5 Cytomegalovirus infection may cause inflammation and ulceration in any organ of the gastrointestinal tract in immunosuppressed persons. **(a)** Endoscopic view of an antral ulcer in the gastric antrum in a woman with AIDS, who presented with nausea, vomiting, and weight loss. **(b)** Biopsy of the ulcer shows both nuclear and cytoplasmic inclusions, which are characteristic of cytomegalovirus infection, in cells of the glands, lamina propria, and vascular endothelium.

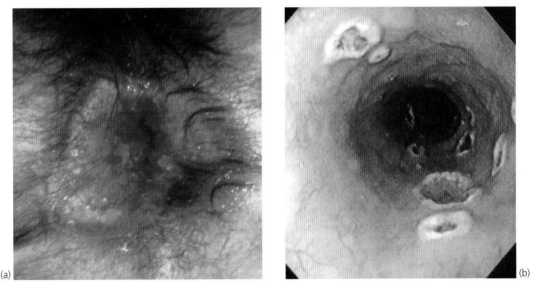

Figure 75.6 Herpes simplex virus is a latent infection among immunocompetent persons, but in persons infected with HIV-1, the virus can cause severe inflammation and ulceration of the anus, perianal region, and esophagus (esophagitis). **(a)** The perianal ulceration of this severely immunosuppressed patient with HIV-1 infection caused pain, tenesmus, and bleeding. Culture of a biopsy of the ulcer bed revealed herpes simplex virus. **(b)** Multiple small, well-circumscribed, shallow ulcers are typical for herpes simplex virus esophagitis.

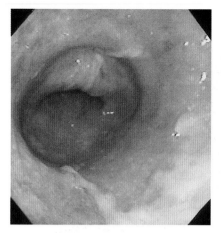

Figure 75.7 Bacterial infections with *Salmonella* spp., *Shigella flexneri,* and *Campylobacter jejuni* cause a similar clinical illness in persons infected with human immunodeficiency virus-1. This is characterized by recurrent or chronic diarrhea that is commonly associated with fever and abdominal cramps. Unlike infections with these pathogens in otherwise healthy persons, the infections in patients with HIV-1/AIDS are more often complicated by bacteremia. Endoscopic visualization of the colon of an HIV-1-infected patient shows superficial erosions, erythema, pus, and loss of the normal vascular pattern. A biopsy specimen of the area grew *C. jejuni.*

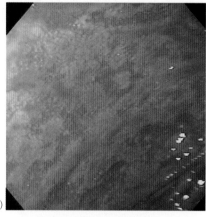

(a)

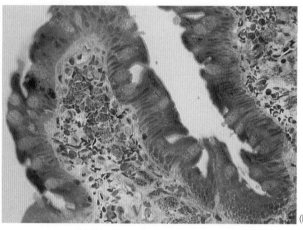

(b)

Figure 75.8 *Mycobacterium avium* complex is one of the most common bacterial pathogens identified in the gastrointestinal tracts of immunosuppressed patients with human immunodeficiency virus-1. Gastrointestinal involvement usually indicates disseminated infection and is associated with diarrhea, weight loss, fever, and a high bacterial burden in tissues. **(a)** Endoscopic image of the duodenum in a patient with AIDS and *M. avium* complex infection. The patient presented with diarrhea, abdominal pain, weight loss, and fever. The image shows multiple small yellow plaques, some of which have coalesced in the second portion of the duodenum. **(b)** Light micrograph of a biopsy section from the duodenum shows numerous lamina propria macrophages engorged with mycobacteria (methylene blue-azure II, basic fuchsin; magnification × 100).

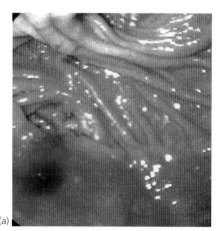

(a)

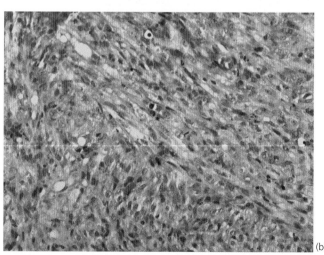

(b)

Figure 75.9 Kaposi sarcoma, a neoplasm associated with human herpes virus type 8 infection, may involve any region of the gastrointestinal tract. As a consequence of the widespread use of highly active antiretroviral therapy, Kaposi sarcoma has become uncommon in AIDS in the United States and Europe. **(a)** Endoscopic view of the stomach in a patient with AIDS shows a bleeding Kaposi sarcoma lesion; although the tumor is quite vascular, Kaposi sarcoma lesions bleed infrequently. **(b)** Biopsy of the stomach shows the characteristic proliferation of neoplastic spindle cells, some of which contain intracytoplasmic eosinophilic material (magnification × 40).

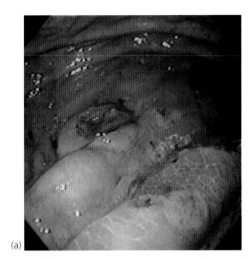

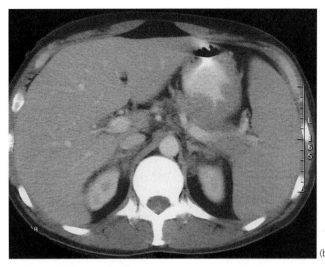

(a)

(b)

Figure 75.10 (a) Endoscopic view of the stomach from a patient with AIDS and non-Hodgkin gastric lymphoma shows thickened mucosal folds with superficial erosions and edema. **(b)** Abdominal CT scan with contrast from the same patient shows markedly thickened gastric mucosa; gastric distention was limited owing to mucosal infiltration by tumor. Although the overall survival of patients with AIDS and non-Hodgkin lymphoma has increased since the introduction of highly active antiretroviral therapy, the incidence of this B-cell tumor among these patients has not decreased significantly as has that of many opportunistic infections.

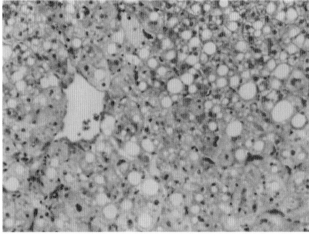

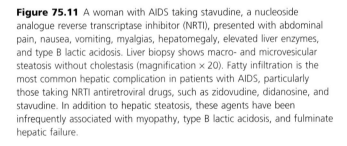

Figure 75.11 A woman with AIDS taking stavudine, a nucleoside analogue reverse transcriptase inhibitor (NRTI), presented with abdominal pain, nausea, vomiting, myalgias, hepatomegaly, elevated liver enzymes, and type B lactic acidosis. Liver biopsy shows macro- and microvesicular steatosis without cholestasis (magnification × 20). Fatty infiltration is the most common hepatic complication in patients with AIDS, particularly those taking NRTI antiretroviral drugs, such as zidovudine, didanosine, and stavudine. In addition to hepatic steatosis, these agents have been infrequently associated with myopathy, type B lactic acidosis, and fulminate hepatic failure.

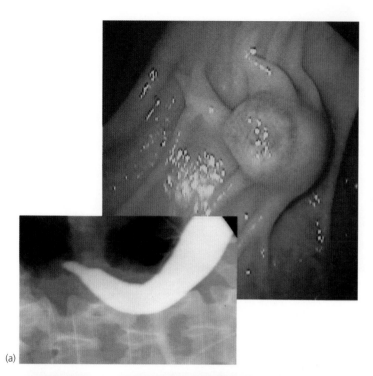

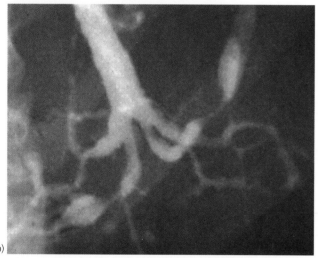

(a)

(b)

Figure 75.12 AIDS cholangiopathy is caused by inflammation of the biliary tract mucosa in patients infected with HIV-1 and is most commonly due to *Cryptosporidium*, cytomegalovirus, and microsporidia. **(a)** Endoscopic view of the ampulla of Vater in a patient with AIDS, abdominal pain and an elevated alkaline phosphatase shows an edematous, erythematous and partially exudative papilla. Insert shows endoscopic retrograde cholangiogram of the patient's stenotic distal common bile duct. Biopsy of the ampulla of Vater revealed *Cryptosporidium*. **(b)** Endoscopic retrograde cholangiogram in a patient with AIDS and cholangiopathy shows an irregular and distorted biliary tree with multiple areas of dilation and stricture.

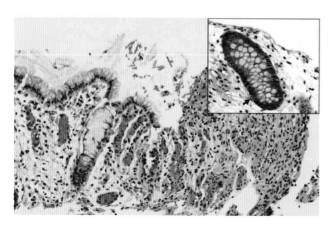

Figure 75.13 Acute graft-versus-host disease usually occurs within 3–4 weeks after stem cell transplantation and may involve the skin, liver, lung, and intestine. The clinical features of intestinal disease include watery diarrhea, anorexia, nausea, vomiting, abdominal pain, and bleeding. Intestinal biopsy from a patient with graft-versus-host disease shows flattening of crypts, crypt degeneration, edema, ulceration (magnification × 20) **(top right)** and typical epithelial cell apoptosis with (arrow) apoptotic bodies, necrotic epithelial cells and minimal inflammatory cell infiltration (magnification × 40).

76

Gastrointestinal manifestations of immunological disorders

Fergus Shanahan, Stephan R. Targan

Immunodeficiency

Immunodeficiency disorders are a heterogeneous group of conditions that may be classified broadly into primary and secondary syndromes. Selective immunoglobulin A (IgA) deficiency and common variable hypogammaglobulinemia (Figs 76.1 and 76.2) are the most common primary immunodeficiency syndromes among adults. Secondary immunodeficiencies are much more common than primary disorders. Causes include malnutrition, protein-losing enteropathy (Fig. 76.3), cancer, and iatrogenic immunosuppression. The most important secondary immunodeficiency disorder is acquired immunodeficiency syndrome (AIDS) caused by human immunodeficiency virus (HIV) (see Chapter 75).

The gastrointestinal tract is a primary target organ in both primary and secondary immunodeficiency disorders because of its large surface area and constant exposure to environmental pathogens. The principal gastrointestinal consequence of immunodeficiency is increased susceptibility to infection. This includes infection with unusual agents, atypical manifestations of infection with commonly encountered pathogens, and bacterial overgrowth with organisms normally present in the gastrointestinal tract. There is also an increased prevalence of autoimmune disorders or chronic inflammatory conditions such as atrophic gastritis and celiac disease. In some immunodeficiency states there is an increased incidence of malignant tumors, particularly lymphoma. Benign diffuse nodular lymphoid hyperplasia may occur among some patients, whereas lymphoid atrophy may be a feature among others. Patients with severe immunodeficiency may have graft-versus-host disease caused by transplacentally acquired maternal lymphocytes or unintentional transfusion of nonirradiated blood products. It is important

for the clinician to know, however, that patients with mild or selective forms of immunodeficiency, such as selective IgA deficiency, frequently are free of infections or other manifestations.

Nodular lymphoid hyperplasia

Diffuse nodular lymphoid hyperplasia occurs among approximately 20% of patients with common variable hypogammaglobulinemia. The lymphoid nodules are in the lamina propria and submucosa and produce a nodularity that is visible on barium radiographic studies (Fig. 76.4) and at endoscopy. They are most prevalent in the small bowel, in some cases extend into the colon, and rarely extend into the stomach. At microscopic examination, the nodules consist of large lymphoid follicles with germinal centers (Fig. 76.5). Plasma cells are usually absent. Lymphoid hyperplasia is believed to be caused by proliferation of B cells that are unable to undergo full differentiation to immunoglobulin secretion and therefore are unresponsive to feedback regulation of proliferation. Unlike the situation with common variable hypogammaglobulinemia, nodular lymphoid hyperplasia does not occur in X-linked hypogammaglobulinemia, probably because there is defective pre-B-cell to B-cell differentiation with hypoplasia of peripheral lymphoid tissue and a paucity of mature B cells. It is important to recognize that localized forms of nodular lymphoid hyperplasia, particularly in the large bowel, may occur among apparently healthy immunocompetent persons. Small nodules of lymphoid tissue on a background of normal folds of small bowel are normal and are a common finding among children and young adults.

Eosinophilic gastroenteritis

The term eosinophilic gastroenteritis is used to describe a group of poorly defined disorders characterized by diffuse

Atlas of Gastroenterology, 4th edition. Edited by Tadataka Yamada, David H. Alpers, Anthony N. Kalloo, Neil Kaplowitz, Chung Owyang, and Don W. Powell. © 2009 Blackwell Publishing, ISBN: 978-1-4051-6909-7

eosinophilic infiltration of a portion of the gastrointestinal tract in the absence of other disorders, such as intestinal parasitism, vasculitis, neoplasia, and other causes of eosinophilia and eosinophilic tissue infiltration (Figs 76.6 and 76.7). Thus, disorders known to be associated with eosinophilia and eosinophilic tissue infiltration must be excluded before the diagnosis of eosinophilic gastroenteritis is made. The cause of this disorder is unclear. Although an allergic basis has been considered, the evidence for this hypothesis is limited. Clinical manifestations depend on the site primarily affected and the layer of bowel wall predominantly involved. Mucosal involvement presents itself in a similar way to other forms of inflammatory bowel disease, submucosal infiltration tends to lead to intestinal obstruction, and serosal involvement may be associated with eosinophilic ascites.

Graft-versus-host disease

Gastrointestinal complications occur among virtually all patients at some stage during recovery from bone marrow transplantation. In addition to graft-versus-host disease, causes of gastrointestinal symptoms after bone marrow transplantation include the effects of chemotherapy and chemoradiation therapy given before bone marrow grafting and opportunistic infections that may be caused by the immunosuppressive protocol or the immunodeficiency associated with graft-versus-host disease. The gastrointestinal and liver damage associated with chemoradiation therapy usually resolves within 20–30 days after transplantation. Opportunistic infections may occur at any stage after bone marrow transplantation; bacterial and fungal infections tend to be more common during the first month, and viral infections more common thereafter.

The clinical severity and extent of gastrointestinal involvement with acute and chronic graft-versus-host disease are highly variable. Acute graft-versus-host disease usually occurs 20–60 days after transplantation and primarily affects the skin, liver, and gastrointestinal tract. Chronic graft-versus-host disease is a multisystem disorder with clinical features resembling those of sicca syndrome and systemic sclerosis. Gastrointestinal involvement occurs particularly in the oral mucosa (mucositis), esophagus, and small bowel. Chronic graft-versus-host disease usually occurs 80–400 days after transplantation.

The earliest morphological feature of acute intestinal graft-versus-host disease at light microscopic examination is apoptosis of individual cells in the intestinal crypts (Fig. 76.8). This characteristic finding is diagnostic if obtained from normal-appearing mucosa at least 20 days after transplantation (when the effects of chemoradiation therapy have resolved). Inflammatory cells or microorganisms are not present in adjacent mucosa. Later, the histopathology can progress to total denudation of the mucosa; the apoptotic lesion is no longer evident, and changes are not specific.

The radiographic appearance of graft-versus-host disease also varies with the severity and with the stage of the disease. During the acute phase there is mucosal and submucosal edema, particularly in the distal small bowel. The barium is often diluted because of excess lumenal fluid loss, and transit is rapid. In addition to thickening of the bowel wall there may be mucosal ulceration, sloughing, and pneumatosis cystoides intestinalis. The changes are not specific and may be mimicked by coexisting cytomegalovirus (CMV) infection. The radiological changes of intestinal graft-versus-host disease may resolve completely or occasionally may progress to a striking ribbon-like pattern of diffuse or segmental involvement of the jejunum and ileum. This finding appears to be unique to intestinal graft-versus-host disease (Fig. 76.9).

The endoscopic appearance of acute graft-versus-host disease may be normal, show patchy erythema, or show extensive mucosal sloughing, particularly in the ileum, cecum, and ascending colon, with relative sparing of the rectal and gastric mucosa. In contrast, esophageal involvement is particularly common in chronic graft-versus-host disease. Lesions include desquamation of the upper esophagus and upper esophageal webs; the distal esophagus usually is spared.

Cytomegalovirus infection

Gastrointestinal infection with CMV occurs in several clinical settings. It may be associated with primary or secondary immunodeficiency states, particularly when there is defective cell-mediated immunity. CMV infection is seen increasingly among patients with iatrogenic immunosuppression associated with cancer therapy, transplantation, or chronic inflammatory disorders such as lupus or inflammatory bowel disease. Infection with CMV occurs in as many as one-third of patients undergoing transplantation. After oroesophageal candidiasis it is probably the most common gastrointestinal infection among patients with AIDS. CMV infection has also been described among apparently immunocompetent persons with a variety of disorders including hypertrophic gastropathy, self-limited colitis, and ulcerative colitis, particularly when complicated by development of toxic megacolon. Although the manifestations of gastrointestinal CMV infection are highly variable, severity tends to correlate with the degree of immunosuppression. Inflammation with ulceration may be focal or diffuse (Fig. 76.10a), superficial or deep (Fig. 76.10b), and may lead to bleeding and perforation. Any part of the esophagus and small or large intestine may be involved. Multifocal involvement with CMV is usual among patients with AIDS, whereas CMV often is limited to the cecum (typhlitis) and ascending colon after transplantation.

Endothelial cells are the most frequent cell types infected (Fig. 76.10c,d). Smooth muscle cells and the myenteric plexus occasionally are involved. Infected macrophages also may be seen in the lamina propria, whereas epithelial cells are seldom involved. CMV-infected cells are large with a granular cytoplasm and nuclei that are filled with intranu-

clear (Cowdry type A) inclusions, often with a periinclusion halo. Unlike cells infected with herpes simplex virus, which tend to be superficial, characteristic CMV-infected cells usually are found in the deeper layers of resected or biopsy specimens (Fig. 76.10e). Identification of CMV infection may be facilitated by in situ hybridization or immuno-cytochemical analysis with virus-specific antibodies (see Fig. 76.10d,e).

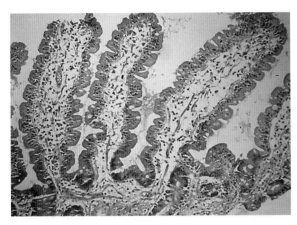

Figure 76.1 Small-bowel biopsy specimen from a patient with hypogammaglobulinemia shows a paucity of plasma cells in the lamina propria. Among patients with selective immunoglobulin A (IgA) deficiency, the absence or paucity of IgA-producing cells is compensated for by an increase in IgM-producing cells. Courtesy of Dr Klaus Lewin.

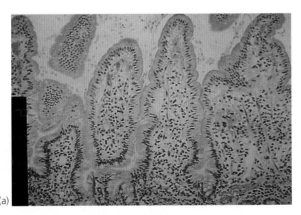

(a)

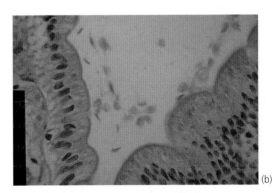

(b)

Figure 76.2 (a,b) Giardiasis (*Giardia lamblia*) is the most common gastrointestinal parasitic infection in primary immunodeficiency syndromes. It occurs most frequently among patients with common variable hypogammaglobulinemia. Giardiasis usually does not distort the villous structure but may do so among patients with immunodeficiencies. Although the diagnosis of giardiasis can be made from inspection of

histological sections of small bowel, finding the organism by means of this method is difficult and tedious when the infection is scanty. The diagnosis is made more conveniently by examination of the stools for cysts, or identification of the trophozoite form in intestinal fluid or smears of mucus adherent to the biopsy specimen.

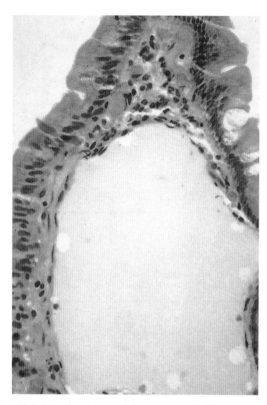

Figure 76.3 Secondary immunodeficiency – intestinal lymphangiectasia. Immunodeficiency caused by enteric protein loss may be a component of any severe inflammatory disorder of the gastrointestinal tract. The most severe cases of gastrointestinal protein loss occur with lymphangiectasia, which may be primary or secondary to lymphatic obstruction. Protein loss from the gastrointestinal tract is nonselective, and hypogammaglobulinemia is always accompanied by hypoalbuminemia. Among patients with lymphangiectasia there is also loss of lymphocytes, particularly T cells, and immunoglobulins.

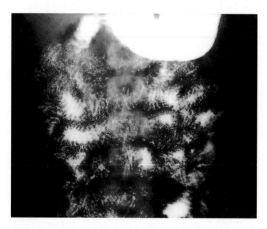

Figure 76.4 Upper gastrointestinal barium study of a patient with common variable hypogammaglobulinemia shows multiple diffuse filling defects caused by nodular lymphoid hyperplasia.

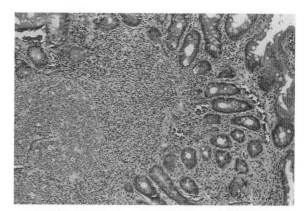

Figure 76.5 Histological features of diffuse nodular lymphoid hyperplasia in a patient with immunodeficiency. This jejunal biopsy specimen contains lymphoid tissue with germinal centers. Plasma cells were not identified. Radiographic evidence of nodular lymphoid hyperplasia was present. A cluster of *Giardia* organisms is present (top right).

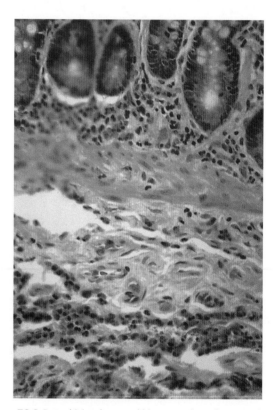

Figure 76.6 Peroral jejunal mucosal biopsy specimen from a patient with typical clinical findings of eosinophilic gastroenteritis. The biopsy specimen includes an involved area of submucosa that contains a characteristic band-like infiltrate of eosinophils.

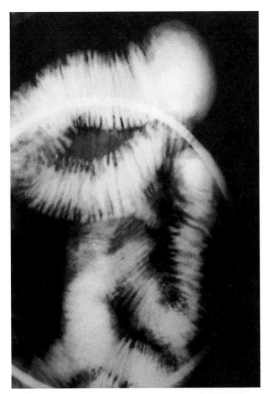

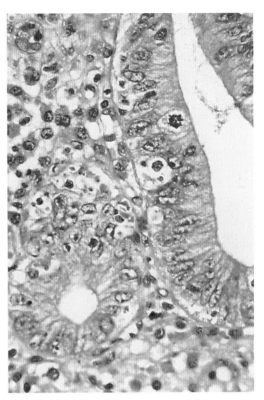

Figure 76.7 Upper gastrointestinal barium study of a patient with diffuse eosinophilic gastroenteritis. The thickening of jejunal folds with a "stack of coins" pattern is characteristic of submucosal infiltration but is not specific. It may occur with any cause of submucosal fluid (edema or blood) accumulation such as ischemia, hemorrhage, or inflammation. Depending on the depth of bowel wall involved, the folds may be irregular and nodular. There may be separation of bowel loops. The radiographic appearance of eosinophilic gastroenteritis may be difficult to differentiate from that of other infiltrative or inflammatory disorders, such as Crohn's disease.

Figure 76.8 Rectal biopsy specimen from a patient with acute graft-versus-host disease after bone marrow transplantation. The individual crypt cell apoptosis (karyolytic debris in vacuoles near crypt base) is characteristic if found after day 20, when damage from chemoradiation therapy has resolved. Courtesy of Dr Klaus Lewin.

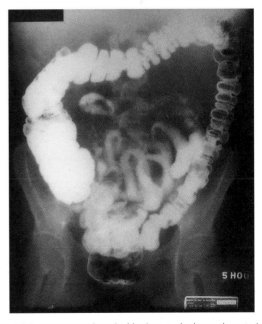

Figure 76.9 Upper gastrointestinal barium study shows characteristic ribbon-like pattern of small bowel that may occur among some patients with graft-versus-host disease if the early intestinal lesions do not resolve completely. This change is diagnostic and represents submucosal fibrosis and edema.

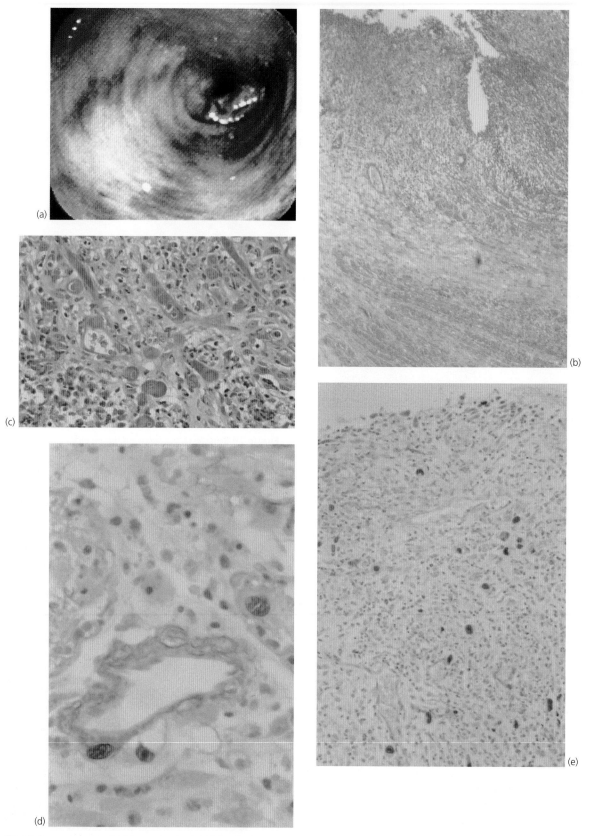

Figure 76.10 Cytomegalovirus (CMV)-associated colitis. **(a)** Endoscopic appearance of patchy erythematous mucosa with linear streaks. **(b)** Histopathological section of surgically resected colonic tissue shows penetrating ulceration with transmural inflammation in an immunodeficient patient with bloody diarrhea, abdominal pain, and peritoneal signs. **(c)** High-power light microscopic image of resected colonic tissue shown in **(b)** shows CMV-infected cells with characteristic nuclear inclusions within the lamina propria and submucosa. CMV has a propensity to infect endothelial cells, although smooth muscle cells, macrophages, and the myenteric plexus may be involved. **(d)** Immunocytochemical analysis with CMV-specific monoclonal antibody shows CMV within endothelial cells. **(e)** Full-thickness resected tissue stained immunocytochemically with viral-specific antibody shows that CMV-infected cells are usually found in the deeper layers of gastrointestinal specimens.

77

Parasitic diseases: protozoa

Ellen Li, Samuel L. Stanley Jr

The intestinal parasitic protozoa are being increasingly recognized as important causes of diarrheal illness worldwide. Infestation with *Entamoeba histolytica*, the causative agent of amebic dysentery and amebic liver abscess, is primarily a disease of developing countries. Infestation with *Giardia lamblia*, *Cryptosporidium parvum*, and *Cyclospora cayetanensis*, however, poses serious threats to public health in the United States and the rest of the world. Physicians (gastroenterologists in particular) must consider these pathogens in the differential diagnosis of acute and chronic diarrhea and should be familiar with the optimal diagnostic (Table 77.1) and therapeutic approaches to these diseases. Because conventional microscopic examination of the stool for ova and parasites is time consuming and expensive, special requests for microscopic examinations may need to be made to the laboratory. In some hospitals, only fecal immunoassay(s) directed against *Giardia* and *Cryptosporidium* species may be performed when stool ova and parasite testing is requested.

Amebiasis

Improved sanitation conditions have greatly reduced the number of cases of amebiasis in the United States. Disease in the United States is probably most commonly detected among immigrants and should be considered for all persons with dysentery and an appropriate travel or exposure history. *E. histolytica* trophozoites can be seen in wet mounts of stool, ulcer scrapings, or intestinal aspirates obtained during endoscopy and in fixed specimens stained with trichrome (Fig. 77.1). An important diagnostic problem is that *E. histolytica* is morphologically identical to the genetically distinct nonpathogenic *Entamoeba dispar* species. New antigen detection enzyme-linked immunosorbent assays (ELISA) that

specifically recognize *E. histolytica* and not *E. dispar* in stool may replace microscopic examination as the test of choice for the diagnosis of intestinal amebiasis.

E. histolytica trophozoites invade the colonic mucosa and cause discrete ulcers covered with yellowish-white exudate (Fig. 77.2a), multiple well-defined ulcers (Fig. 77.2c), diffuse erythema and ulceration (Fig. 77.2d), and, rarely, heaped-up inflammatory and granulation tissue that forms an ameboma (Fig. 77.2b). Pseudomembrane formation can be seen.

The most frequent extraintestinal manifestation of *E. histolytica* infestation is amebic liver abscess. Patients usually have the triad of fever, right upper quadrant pain and tenderness, and a space-occupying lesion in the liver. As illustrated in Fig. 77.3, an initial clue to the presence of amebic liver abscess may be an abnormal chest radiograph showing elevation of the right hemidiaphragm, right pleural effusion, and possibly a right basilar infiltrate. Amebic liver abscesses are often visible on computed tomographic (CT) scans as large, generally homogenous, low-attenuation lesions (Fig. 77.4). However, multiple abscesses can develop.

Blastocystis hominis

Blastocystis hominis is one of the protozoan organisms frequently detected in stools (Fig. 77.5). The pathogenicity of this organism continues to be controversial.

Giardiasis

G. lamblia has been the most common intestinal parasitic cause of diarrhea in the United States in recent years. Groups at high risk for giardiasis include children in day-care facilities and their adult contacts, travelers, and those who consume contaminated water. Abundant *Giardia* trophozoites may be seen in biopsy samples from the small intestine of these persons (Fig. 77.6). The diagnosis of *G. lamblia* infestation is based primarily on detection of trophozoites and

Atlas of Gastroenterology, 4th edition. Edited by Tadataka Yamada, David H. Alpers, Anthony N. Kalloo, Neil Kaplowitz, Chung Owyang, and Don W. Powell. © 2009 Blackwell Publishing, ISBN: 978-1-4051-6909-7

cysts in the stool by means of microscopic analysis of stained stool specimens (Fig. 77.7). Antigen detection tests are available that permit detection of *G. lamblia*, as well as *E. histolytica* and *C. parvum*; these tests may be valuable as initial screening tests for individuals with diarrhea. Immunofluorescence assays (MeriFluor, Meridian Bioscience, Cincinnati, OH) can be used to detect both *G. lamblia* cysts and *C. parvum* oocysts (Fig. 77.8).

Dientamoeba fragilis

Dientamoeba fragilis, a species of flagellated protozoa, is ameboid in shape and ranges in size from 5 to 15 μm; the flagella are not visible (Fig. 77.9). There is no known cyst form. Symptoms ascribed to this organism include mild diarrhea, abdominal pain, anorexia, and fatigue.

Balantidiasis

Balantidium coli is a ciliate parasite that can invade the colonic mucosa (Fig. 77.10) and cause colonic ulceration. Diagnosis is made by observation of the large motile trophozoites in saline mounts of stool.

Coccidia (*Cryptosporidium, Isospora, and Cyclospora*)

Since the onset of the acquired immunodeficiency syndrome (AIDS) epidemic, coccidial organisms from the genera *Cryptosporidium, Cyclospora,* and *Isospora* have emerged not only as important gastrointestinal protozoan pathogens among immunocompromised hosts but also as causative agents of diarrhea among immunocompetent hosts. *C. parvum* is a common cause of diarrhea among patients with AIDS in the United States and is one of the leading causative agents of waterborne disease outbreaks in the United States. *Cyclospora* and *Isospora* are seen less commonly in the United States but are prevalent in developing countries and should be suspected among travelers returning from endemic areas.

These organisms are intracellular pathogens with similar life cycles (Fig. 77.11), which may account for their similar clinical manifestations.

The diagnosis of these parasitic diseases generally is made by examination of the stool. The acid-fast stain may be the most useful stain for detecting these organisms (Figs 77.12 and 77.13). Some laboratories may not routinely search for these organisms, and the physician may need to submit special requests to the laboratory. The organisms differ in size and shape (see Figs 77.12 and 77.13; Table 77.1). *Cryptosporidium* and *Cyclospora* are particularly difficult to differentiate from each other, and measurements must be made to confirm the size difference. Smears and biopsies of small intestinal aspirates may be useful for the diagnosis of infestation with these organisms (Figs 77.14–77.16; see Table 77.1). Cryptosporidia can be easily detected on routine light microscopic examination as 4-μm basophilic dots on the apical surface of enterocytes and are typically located within crypt cells (see Fig. 77.14). The organism is intracellular but extracytoplasmic (see Fig. 77.15). A direct fluorescence assay allows screening by fluorescent microscopic examination, which can provide rapid and accurate results (see Fig. 77.8). *Isospora* organisms can be detected on light microscopic examination as 20-μm inclusions within the enterocyte and are typically located within villous enterocytes (see Fig. 77.16). With a heavy organism burden, *Cyclospora* organisms have been identified on light microscopic examination of duodenal biopsy specimens, but transmission electron microscopic examination may be a more sensitive approach.

Table 77.1 Morphological features of human gastrointestinal protozoan parasites

Type of parasite	Stool	Intestinal biopsy
Extracellular ameboid		
Entamoeba histolytica	Trophozoite 10–20 μm with pale, round nucleus with small central karyosome; cyst 9–25 μm with four nuclei Morphologically indistinguishable from *Entamoeba dispar*; immunoassays for detection of trophozoite antigen can differentiate *E. histolytica* from *E. dispar*; serological testing may be a useful adjunct	Trophozoites but not cysts seen invading colonic mucosa causing colonic ulcerations
Blastocystis hominis (pathogenicity is controversial)	Organisms 6–40 μm, round with large central body or vacuole	
Flagellates		
Giardia lamblia	Trophozoite pear shaped, 10–20 μm long, characteristic face-like image because of two nuclei, each with prominent karyosome Cyst oval, 7–10 μm long; direct fluorescence antibody test available in many laboratories for detection of cysts Fecal immunoassays are routinely used to detect *Giardia* in many US hospitals	Trophozoites seen most commonly on duodenal mucosal surface, but also on jejunal and ileal biopsy specimens Histological features usually normal, but villous atrophy seen in severe infections
Dientamoeba fragilis	Appears ameboid in shape, 10–15 μm, with flagella not visible, one or two nuclei No known cyst form	
Ciliate		
Balantidium coli (rare)	Trophozoite 50–200 μm in length, motile Cysts are rarely seen in stool and are 50–75 μm in diameter	Trophozoites can invade into colonic mucosa causing ulceration
Intracellular coccidia		
Cryptosporidium parvum	Modified acid-fast stain: oocysts stain uniformly, are round, 4–6 μm, contain four sporozoites that may or may not be visible Direct fluorescence assay may be helpful in detecting cysts Fecal immunoassays are used for detection of *Cryptosporidium* in many hospitals	Intracellular forms seen as 4-μm extracytoplasmic dots on the apical surface of enterocytes; distribution may be patchy
Isospora belli	May be observed on wet preparation May need to submit special request to laboratory Modified acid-fast stain: oocysts stain uniformly, appear oval, 20–30 μm, with two sporocysts, each containing four sporozoites	Intracellular forms seen as 20-μm intracytoplasmic inclusions within the enterocyte on light microscopic examination; distribution may be patchy
Cyclospora cayetanensis	May be observed on wet preparation May need to submit special request to laboratory Modified acid-fast stain: oocysts stain variably, resemble *Cryptosporidium* oocysts but are larger (8–10 μm), contain two sporocysts, each with two sporozoites Oocysts autofluoresce under ultraviolet light (365 nm)	Intracellular forms difficult to see on light microscopic examination but have been seen on electron microscopic examination as intracytoplasmic inclusions

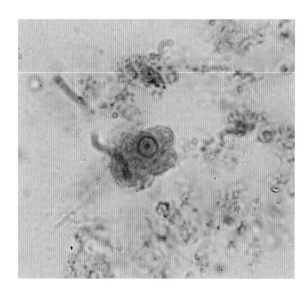

Figure 77.1 *Entamoeba histolytica* trophozoite in stool. This trophozoite is approximately 20 μm in diameter and has the characteristic round nucleus with a small, centrally placed karyosome. Courtesy of Patrick Murray, PhD.

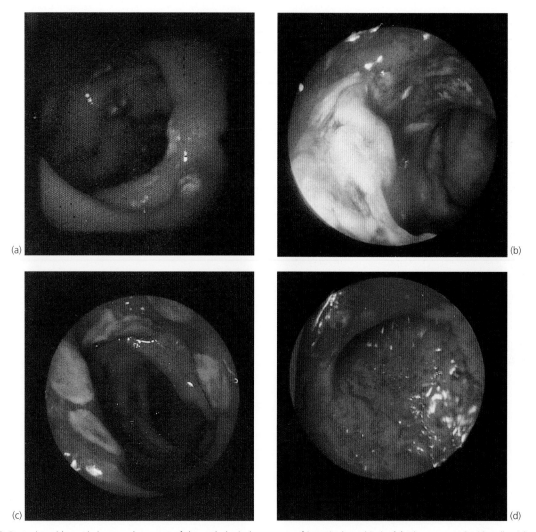

(a)

(b)

(c)

(d)

Figure 77.2 Rectosigmoidoscopic images show part of the pathological spectrum of intestinal amebiasis. **(a)** Ulcers covered with yellowish-white secretion. **(b)** Heaped-up granulation tissue forming an ameboma. **(c)** Multiple well-defined ulcers. **(d)** Diffuse erythema and ulceration.

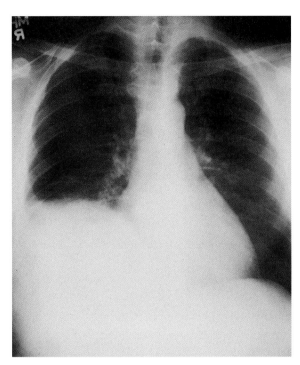

Figure 77.3 Chest radiograph of a patient with amebic liver abscess that has ruptured into the right pleural space. Elevated right hemidiaphragm, pleural effusion, and basilar infiltrate are depicted. This patient was initially thought to have bacterial pneumonia and empyema.

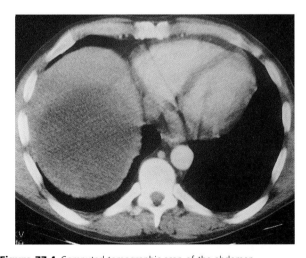

Figure 77.4 Computed tomographic scan of the abdomen demonstrates a large amebic liver abscess in the right lobe of the liver.

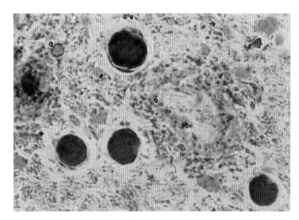

Figure 77.5 Trichrome stain of *Blastocystis hominis.*

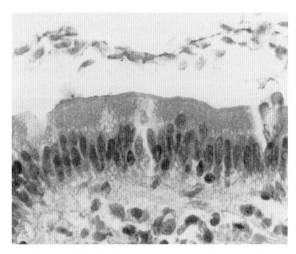

Figure 77.6 Multiple *Giardia lamblia* trophozoites that were lying on the surface of the duodenal mucosa.

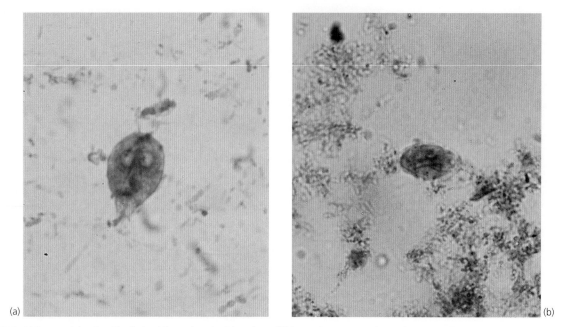

(a)

(b)

Figure 77.7 Trichrome stain of a *Giardia lamblia* trophozoite **(a)** and cyst **(b)** in stool. Courtesy of Patrick Murray, PhD.

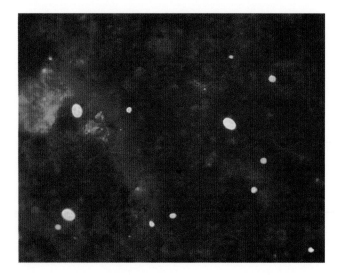

Figure 77.8 *Giardia lamblia* cysts (larger, ellipsoid, with some internal detail present) and *Cryptosporidium parvum* oocysts (smaller, spherical) in a stool sample are revealed by direct fluorescence assay. Courtesy of Meridian Diagnostics.

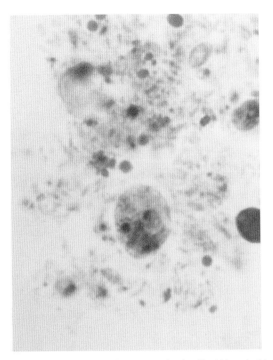

Figure 77.9 Trichrome stain of *Dientamoeba fragilis*. Although this organism is a flagellate, its appearance mimics that of amebas.

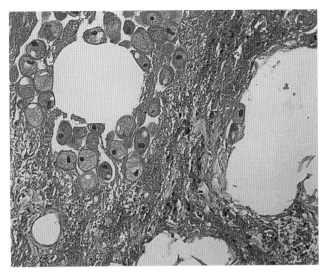

Figure 77.10 Balantidiasis. Numerous large trophozoites in the wall of the intestine in a patient with acquired immunodeficiency syndrome.

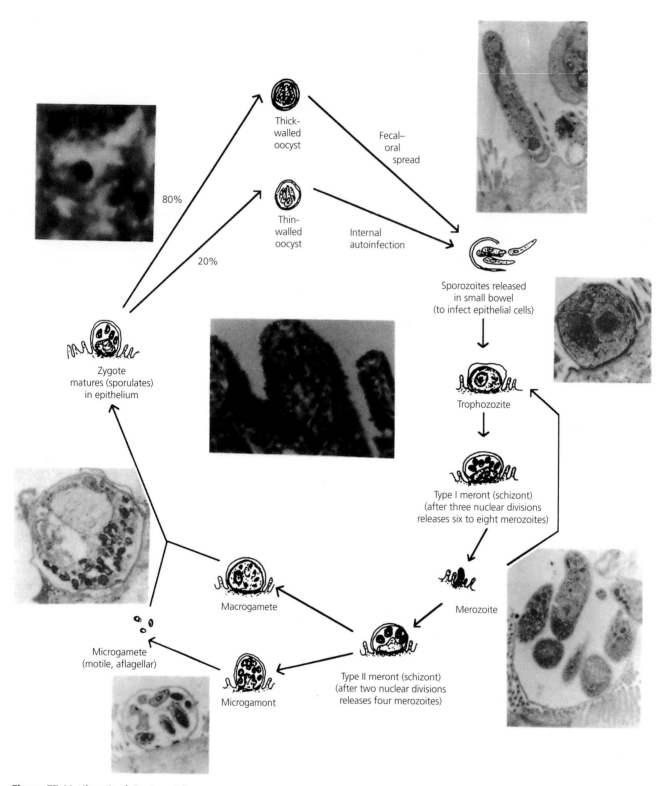

Figure 77.11 Life cycle of *Cryptosporidium*.

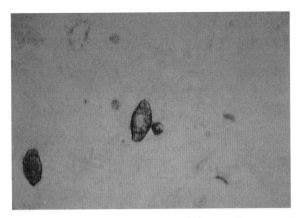

Figure 77.12 Acid-fast stain of an *Isospora belli* oocyst (large oocyst) and a *Cryptosporidium* oocyst (small oocyst) in a patient from Haiti. Courtesy of Dr Madeline Boncy and Dr Rosemary Soave.

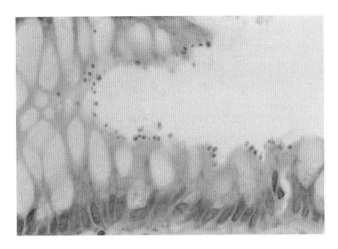

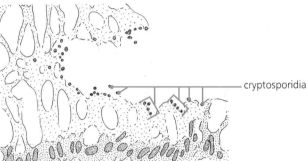

cryptosporidia

Figure 77.14 Cryptosporidia are seen as 4-μm dots on the apical surface of enterocytes.

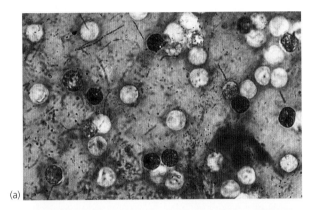

(a)

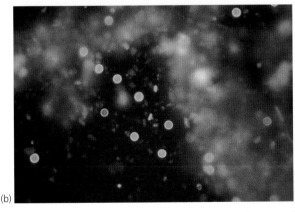

(b)

Figure 77.13 *Cyclospora cayetanensis.* **(a)** Modified acid-fast stain of *Cyclospora* oocysts shows multiple well-stained, poorly stained, and unstained oocysts within the same field. **(b)** Autofluorescence of *Cyclospora* oocysts. Courtesy of Earl G. Long.

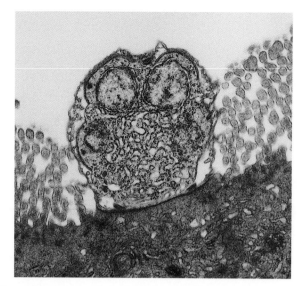

Figure 77.15 Transmission electron micrograph of a schizont stage of *Cryptosporidium parvum* attached to the intestinal epithelium. The organism is surrounded by the enterocyte plasma membrane but is separated from the cytoplasm by the membrane of a parasitophorous vacuole. Courtesy of Dr Paul Swanson.

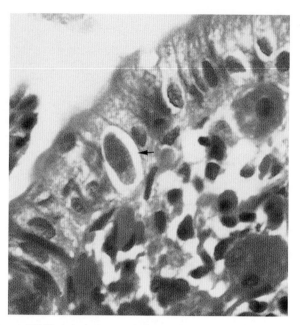

Figure 77.16 A single *Isospora belli* organism (arrow) appears as a 20-μm inclusion within an enterocyte.

78

Parasitic diseases: helminths

Alejandro Busalleu, Martin Montes, A. Clinton White Jr

Helminth parasites are multicellular eukaryotic organisms that are common inhabitants of the human gastrointestinal tract. Throughout human history, infestation with intestinal helminths has been a normal part of the human condition. Helminths are categorized into three major groups: nematodes, trematodes, and cestodes. Nematodes are round worms with a tubular gut, including both a mouth and anus. There are two groups of flatworms: trematodes and cestodes. Trematodes, or flukes, are flat leaf-shaped organisms with a blind gut. All trematodes require an obligate freshwater snail host. The cestodes, or tapeworms, typically have two distinct forms. The adult forms a tapeworm in the gut of the defini-

tive host with an attachment organ, the scolex, and segments, termed proglottids. While not having a separate gut, the external surface shares many features with the mammalian digestive tract. The proglottids are hermaphroditic, containing both ovaries and testes. The larval forms develop as cystic lesions in the tissues of the intermediate host. Some species have a second intermediate host. As members of the animal kingdom, helminths are multicellular organisms with their own organs and are large enough to be visible to the human eye at some point in their life cycle. Thus, it is not uncommon to encounter these organisms during endoscopic procedures performed on high-risk populations.

Atlas of Gastroenterology, 4th edition. Edited by Tadataka Yamada, David H. Alpers, Anthony N. Kalloo, Neil Kaplowitz, Chung Owyang, and Don W. Powell. © 2009 Blackwell Publishing, ISBN: 978-1-4051-6909-7

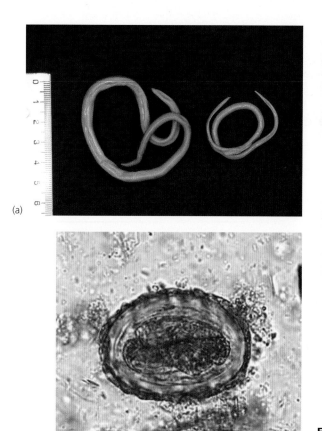

(a)

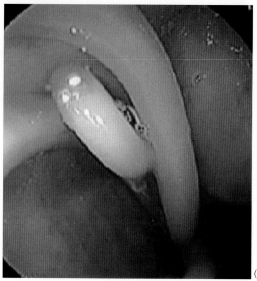

(b)

(c)

Figure 78.1 *Ascaris lumbracoides*. The mature adult worms are large with males and females up to 31 cm in length, similar in size to an earthworm. **(a)** Adult worms that have been passed by a patient. **(b)** An *Ascaris* adult identified during endoscopic gastroduodenoscopy. **(c)** *Ascaris* ova are often bile-stained and typically have an external mammillated layer of thickened shell.

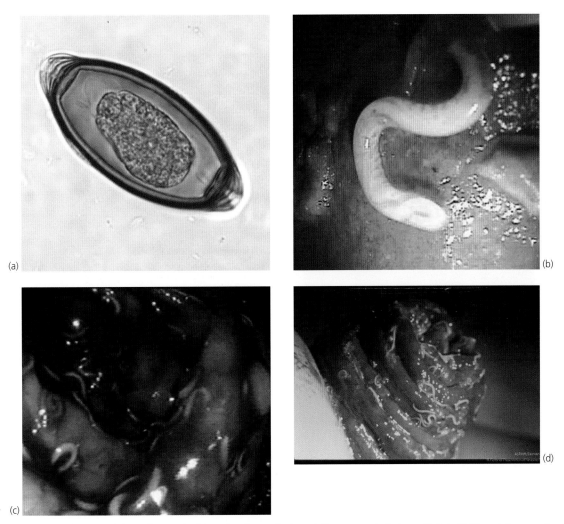

Figure 78.2 *Trichuris trichiura* ova **(a)** are characterized by polar plugs at both ends (from www.dpd.cdc.gov/DpDx). **(b)** The adult worms live in the colon and can be noted incidentally at colonoscopy. Courtesy of Richard Goodgame. The thin anterior end is often buried in the mucosa and the wider posterior end is frequently noted forming a curved shape in the colon. **(c)** Massive infection can be associated with diarrhea and colonic bleeding or **(d)** rectal prolapse. Courtesy of Zaiman H/ASTMH, "A pictoral presentation of parasites."

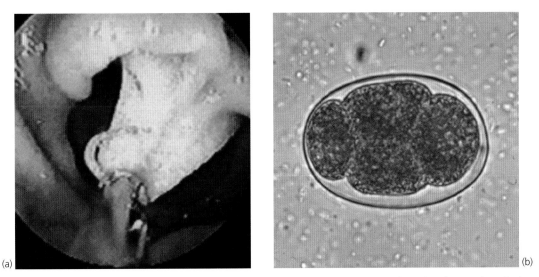

Figure 78.3 Human hookworms, *Necator americanus* and *Ancylostoma duodenalis*, are common intestinal parasites that attach to the intestinal villi and feed on blood. Low burden infections are typically asymptomatic, but heavy infection may cause iron deficiency. **(a)** The adult worms can be visualized at EGD. Courtesy of Richard Goodgame. **(b)** Ova typically display segmented larvae within a thin clear shell.

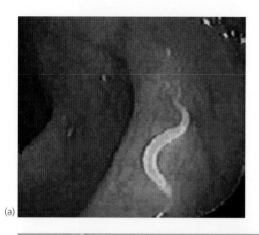

(a)

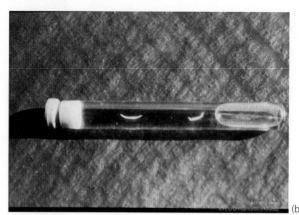

(b)

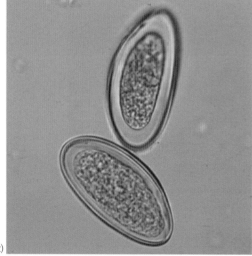

(c)

Figure 78.4 (a) The adult pinworms, *Enterobius vermicularis,* live attached to the colon. Courtesy of Richard Goodgame. **(b)** At night, the adult worms emerge and lay ova on the perianal skin, From Zaiman H/ASTMH, "A pictoral presentation of parasites." **(c)** The ova, which are found on the perianal skin, are flattened on one side.

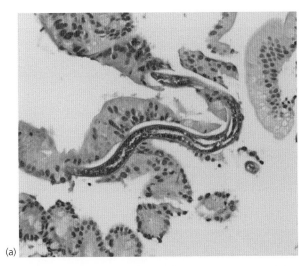

(a)

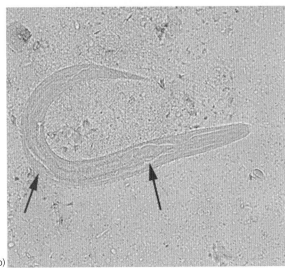

(b)

Figure 78.5 (a) *Strongyloides stercoralis* differs from the other intestinal helminth in that the adult females live within the duodenal mucosa, where they shed their ova. **(b)** The ova hatch in the intestinal wall and the rhabditiform larvae, rather than ova, are shed in the stool.

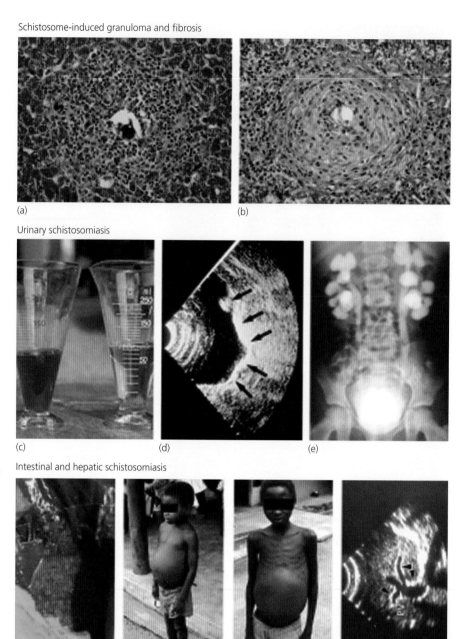

Schistosome-induced granuloma and fibrosis

(a)   (b)

Urinary schistosomiasis

(c)   (d)   (e)

Intestinal and hepatic schistosomiasis

(f)   (g)   (h)   (i)

Figure 78.6 The blood flukes of the genus *Schistosoma* cause intestinal, liver, and urinary disease. **(a)** Acute and **(b)** chronic fibrosis develops surrounding the ova (in this case in mouse liver). **(c)** Urinary involvement with *S. haematobium* can lead to hematuria, **(d)** bladder polyps, and **(e)** hydronephrosis. **(f)** Involvement of the gastrointestinal tract by *S. mansoni*, *S. japonicum*, *S. mekongi*, and *S. intercalatum* can lead to bloody diarrhea and portal fibrosis. **(g)** Portal fibrosis presents with hepatosplenomegaly, ascites, varices, and **(h)** growth retardation and **(i)** characteristic clay pipe fibrosis on ultrasound. Reproduced from Gryseels B, Polman K, Clerinx J, Kestens L. Human schistosomiasis. Lancet 2006;368(9541):1106. (*Continued on next page.*)

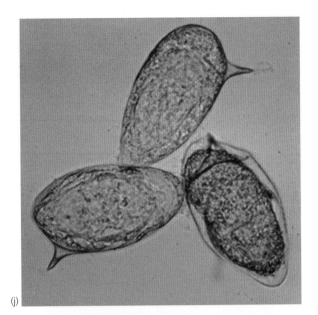

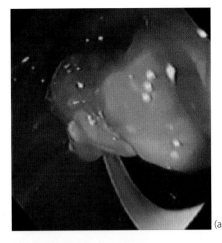

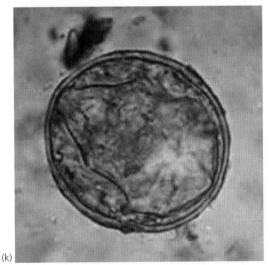

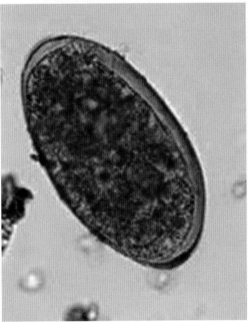

Figure 78.7 *Fasciola hepatica* adult worms live in the biliary tract. Adult worms are flat leaf-shaped organisms and are typically stained by bile. **(a)** An adult worm being removed from the biliary tract. **(b)** The ova are oval with a barely visible operculum at one end.

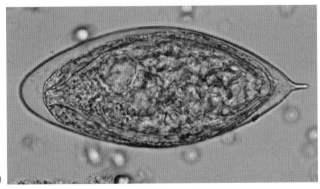

Figure 78.6 *Continued* **(j)** Ova of *S. mansoni* have a characteristic lateral spin. **(k)** Ova of *S. japonicum* are more rounded and have only a vestigial spine. **(l)** The spine on *S. haematobium* is found at one end of the ovum (a terminal spine).

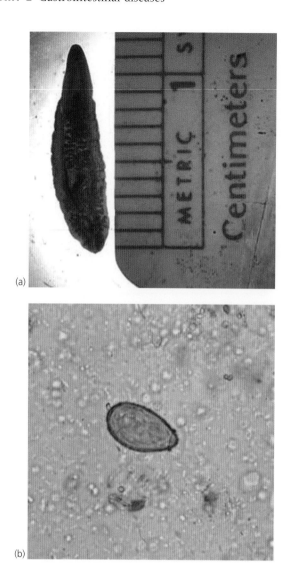

(a)

(b)

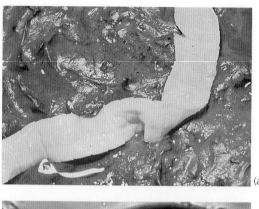

(a)

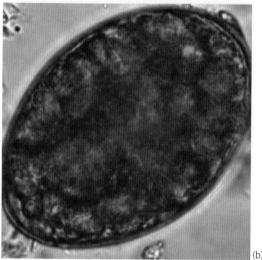

(b)

Figure 78.9 *Diphyllobothrium latum.* Adult tapeworms appear as ribbons of segments termed proglottids. **(a)** The proglottids are broad and off-white in color. **(b)** The ova are non-descript, but have a barely visible operculum on one end and a knob on the opposite end.

Figure 78.8 The adult worms of liver flukes, *Clonorchis sienensis* and *Opisthorchus* species live in the biliary tract. **(a)** The adult worm of *Clonorchis sienensis* are flat leaf-like. **(b)** The ova are oval and operculated on one end.

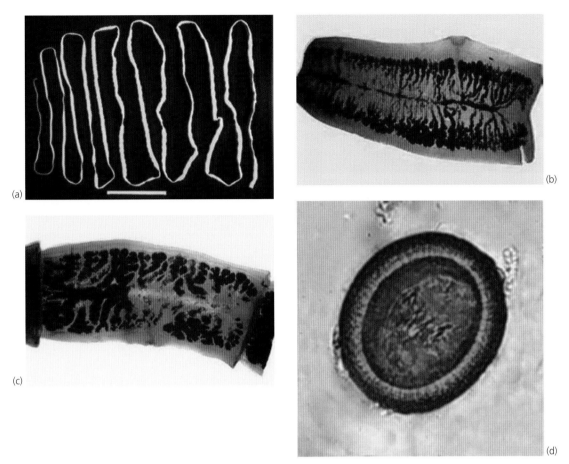

Figure 78.10 *Taenia saginata* and *Taenia solium* are the major human tapeworms acquired from beef and pork. **(a)** The adult worms form ribbon-like chains of proglottids that can reach lengths of up to 30 feet. The proglottids have a similar appearance, but can be distinguished based on the number of major uterine branches. **(b)** *T. saginata* has 12–30 main lateral branches compared with **(c)** *T. solium*, with 8–13 branches. **(d)** The ova for these two species are identical.

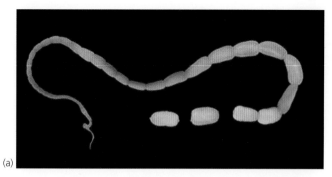

(a)

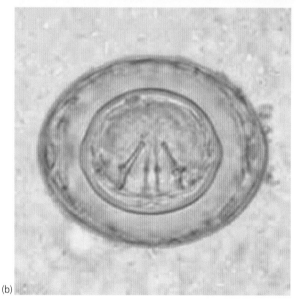

(b)

Figure 78.11 Other tapeworms. The dog and cat tapeworms of the genus *Dipyllidium* occasionally infect humans. **(a)** The proglottids resemble grains of rice, but are motile. *Hymenolepis nana* is a common human infection, but is usually asymptomatic. **(b)** The ova are surrounded by a striated outer membrane separated by a clear space from the internal membrane containing the larvae, which have six hooks.

Type of cyst

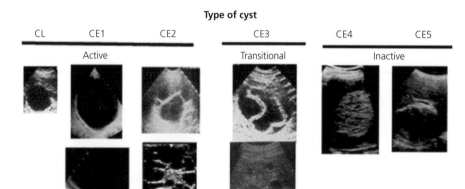

CL	CE1	CE2	CE3	CE4	CE5
Active			Transitional	Inactive	

Figure 78.12 *Echinococcus granulosus* and related organisms cause cystic hydatid disease. Ultrasound staging can separate organisms into groups. Reproduced from WHO Informal Working Group on Echinococcosis. International classification of ultrasound images in cystic echinococcosis for application in clinical and field epidemiological settings.

79

Gastrointestinal manifestations of systemic diseases

Joel S. Levine

Many systemic disorders have gastrointestinal manifestations caused by inflammatory infiltration. Granulomas are specialized, focal inflammations that form around poorly degradable foreign substances. The inciting factor may be either antigenic or a bland foreign body. Granulomas sequester toxic and antigenic materials released from the inciting nidus. They also wall off and destroy the nidus and eliminate the debris.

Granulomas are complex, dynamic lesions composed of a variety of inflammatory cells. As illustrated in Figures 79.4–79.12, granulomas that form in response to various inciting factors may have distinctive morphological features. The following six case reports are unusual and are good examples of how systemic illness can manifest problems in the gastrointestinal tract (Figs 79.13–79.18).

Case 1

A 23-year-old Hispanic woman with achy upper abdominal discomfort was referred because of hepatomegaly and abnormal liver tests. She did not drink alcohol and her mother had died of complications of cirrhosis. The patient was obese (100 kg), her liver span was 21 cm at the midclavicular line, and she had no stigmata of chronic liver disease. The alanine aminotransferase (ALT) level was 110 IU (normal < 40 IU) and the aspartate aminotransferase (AST) level was 140 IU (normal < 35 IU). The prothrombin time and bilirubin and alkaline phosphatase levels were normal. Viral hepatitis studies, urine copper excretion, and the serum iron level were normal. The patient had mild diabetes. A liver biopsy was performed. A low-power view of the liver (Fig. 79.13a) showed marked steatosis. At higher power (Fig. 79.13b) the prominent macrovesicular fat with fibrosis and focal inflammatory change was evident. The patient had nonalcoholic steatonecrosis.

Atlas of Gastroenterology, 4th edition. Edited by Tadataka Yamada, David H. Alpers, Anthony N. Kalloo, Neil Kaplowitz, Chung Owyang, and Don W. Powell. © 2009 Blackwell Publishing, ISBN: 978-1-4051-6909-7

Case 2

A 60-year-old woman with long-standing rheumatoid arthritis was found to have a rock-hard, 20-cm liver at physical examination. Liver biochemical findings were normal. A computed tomographic scan of the liver showed focal filling defects that suggested cancer. A liver biopsy was performed. A low-power view (Fig. 79.14a) showed multiple homogeneous eosinophilic densities in the liver surrounding the blood vessels. A high-power view (Fig. 79.14b) showed expansion of the portal area. The eosinophilic material is amyloid protein. Nodular deposition of amyloid is unusual.

Case 3

A 22-year-old man had fever and abdominal pain. His liver was large and painful. A white blood cell count demonstrated 45 000 cells/mL with immature myelocytes. Bone marrow examination was diagnostic of acute myelogenous leukemia. Combination chemotherapy was begun, but the patient died of overwhelming sepsis within 2 days. At autopsy the liver (Fig. 79.15) demonstrated leukemic cells throughout the sinusoids.

Case 4

A 50-year-old man arrived in the emergency department with a 3-day history of "easy bruising," fever, and new onset of hematemesis. Physical examination revealed multiple areas of characteristic palpable purpura without necrosis (Fig. 79.16a,b). The platelet count and bleeding time were normal. Upper gastrointestinal endoscopy revealed multiple similar lesions (Fig. 79.16c) in the stomach. Skin biopsy revealed leukocytoclastic vasculitis compatible with Henoch–Schönlein purpura. A cause was not identified. Lesions resolved with time and steroid therapy. There were no recurrences.

Case 5

A 29-year-old man arrived at the emergency department and reported passing dark red blood through the rectum. He said that this had been happening episodically over the past 4 years. He explained that multiple needlesticks on his arms were related to a recent hospital admission. He had undergone multiple tests in a variety of different hospitals in the area and in four surrounding states without receiving a diagnosis. He passed a large amount of dark clotted blood in the emergency room, was found to have a hematocrit of 24%, and was admitted to the intensive care unit.

While the patient was being admitted the attending gastroenterologist obtained the names of several hospitals that the patient had visited and called the medical records departments. During 2 h on the phone the physician found 19 admissions for rectal bleeding that led to transfusion of 42 units of blood, 20 colonoscopic examinations, 7 angiographic studies, 19 upper gastrointestinal endoscopic examinations, 15 tagged red blood cell scans, 10 Meckel scans, and an exploratory laparotomy. The colonoscopic examinations always demonstrated blood in the colon, but no cause was ever identified.

After conducting the phone research the attending gastroenterologist sent the patient to the radiology suite. In the presence of the hospital attorney, the patient's room was searched, and the objects shown in Figure 79.17 were found among the patient's possessions. Included were multiple syringes and needles containing clotted blood, lancets, and a plastic bag containing clotted blood. When confronted with the findings, the patient refused further treatment and left the hospital against medical advice. The blood in the plastic bag was later found to be from nonhuman sources. It was hypothesized that this patient had a case of factitious hematochezia caused by rectal insertion of both self-derived and animal blood compatible with the diagnosis of Munchausen syndrome.

Case 6

A 42-year-old woman was referred for endoscopy by her general internist because of chronic recurrent food impactions. She described episodic solid food dysphagia felt in the upper chest for 10 years. At times she needed to induce vomiting to get the food out. By chewing her food well and taking her time eating, she had reduced the number of these episodes to 1–2 per year. She denied any heartburn, indigestion, gastrointestinal bleeding, or weight loss. She had mild chronic fatigue that was attributed to her active lifestyle of work and caring for her three children. She had no other health problems. Her physical examination was normal. An upper endoscopy was performed. Multiple esophageal webs (Fig. 79.18) were identified, and were the only findings. The webs were dilated. The dysphagia resolved. A blood count revealed a microcytic anemia and iron studies confirmed her iron deficiency. With oral iron therapy her anemia resolved and she has had no further dysphagia. This was a case of Plummer–Vinson syndrome.

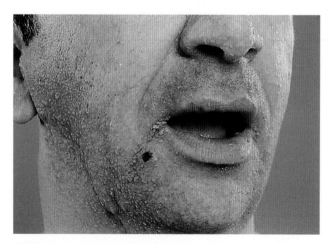

Figure 79.1 Verrucous and papillomatous papules on the face of a patient with Cowden syndrome. Courtesy of Dr Garry A. Neil and Dr Joel V. Weinstock.

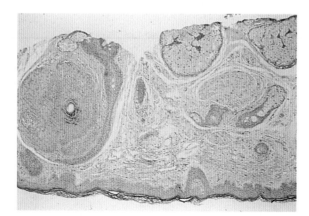

Figure 79.2 Skin biopsy specimen from a patient with Cowden syndrome demonstrates cutaneous trichilemmoma. Courtesy of Dr Garry A. Neil and Dr Joel V. Weinstock.

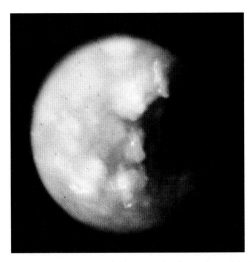

Figure 79.3 Endoscopic view of the stomach of a patient with Cowden syndrome reveals multiple hamartomatous polyps. Courtesy of Dr Garry A. Neil and Dr Joel V. Weinstock.

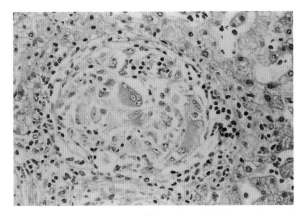

Figure 79.4 Sarcoidosis. One well-formed epithelioid granuloma with a thin lymphocytic halo is present in an otherwise normal-appearing liver (H & E stain; original magnification ×100). Courtesy of Dr Garry A. Neil and Dr Joel V. Weinstock.

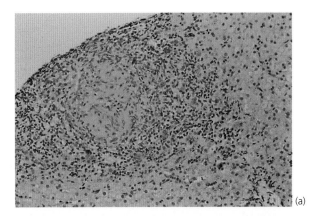

(a)

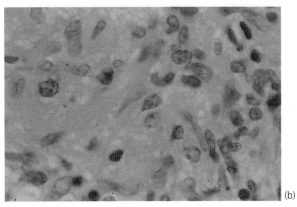

(b)

Figure 79.5 (a) Liver granuloma of tuberculosis; **(b)** acid-fast stain of granuloma in (a) demonstrates *Mycobacterium tuberculosis* (H & E stain. (a) Original magnification ×50, (b) original magnification ×330). Courtesy of Dr Garry A. Neil and Dr Joel V. Weinstock.

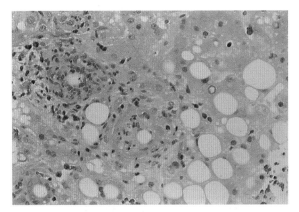

Figure 79.6 Characteristic hepatic ring granuloma of Q fever; the fibrin ring encircles a central vacuole (H & E stain; original magnification ×100). Courtesy of Dr Garry A. Neil and Dr Joel V. Weinstock.

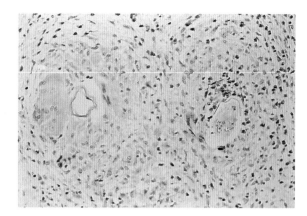

Figure 79.7 Eosinophilic hepatic granulomas induced by ova of *Schistosoma mansoni* (H & E stain; original magnification ×100). Courtesy of Dr Garry A. Neil and Dr Joel V. Weinstock.

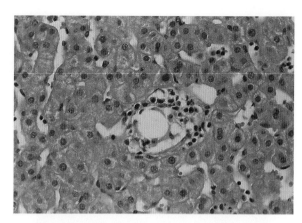

Figure 79.8 Lipogranuloma located in hepatic parenchyma near a central vein. The granuloma contains distinctive fat vacuoles (H & E stain; original magnification ×100). Courtesy of Dr Garry A. Neil and Dr Joel V. Weinstock.

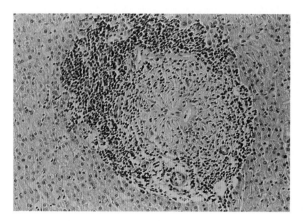

Figure 79.9 Portal granuloma from a patient with primary biliary cirrhosis. The relationship of the granuloma to a damaged bile duct is depicted (H & E stain; original magnification ×100). Courtesy of Dr Garry A. Neil and Dr Joel V. Weinstock.

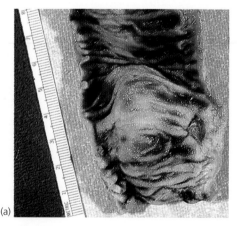

(a)

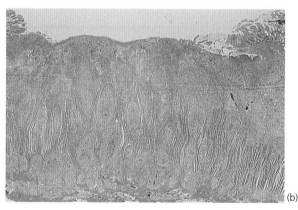

(b)

Figure 79.10 Enteric tuberculosis. **(a)** Photograph of specimen from colonic resection reveals a tuberculous ulcer; **(b)** tuberculous ulcer underlying focal granulomas (H & E stain; original magnification ×10). Courtesy of Dr Garry A. Neil and Dr Joel V. Weinstock.

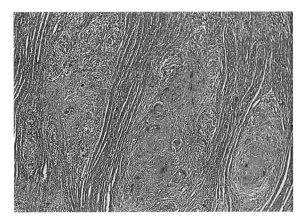

Figure 79.11 Enteric tuberculosis. Lesion depicted in Figure 79.10b reveals granulomas with central necrosis and large giant cells (H & E stain; original magnification ×40). Courtesy of Dr Garry A. Neil and Dr Joel V. Weinstock.

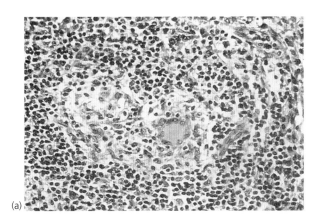

(a)

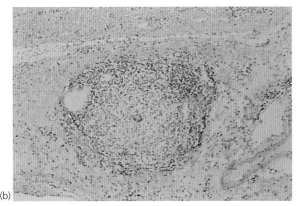

(b)

Figure 79.12 Crohn's disease. **(a)** Loosely aggregated ileal granuloma. **(b)** Mature ileal granuloma. Courtesy of Dr Garry A. Neil and Dr Joel V. Weinstock.

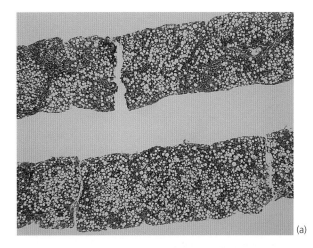

(a)

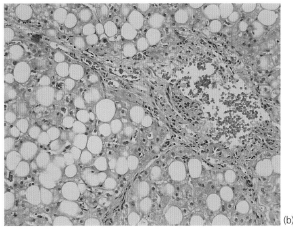

(b)

Figure 79.13 Nonalcoholic steatonecrosis in a patient with diabetes. **(a)** Low-power view of liver biopsy specimen shows marked fatty infiltration. **(b)** High-power view of biopsy specimen depicted in (a); mild fibrosis and inflammatory changes are visible.

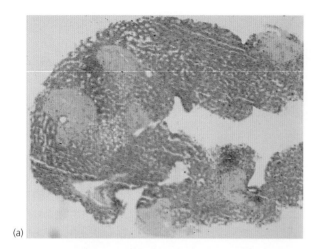

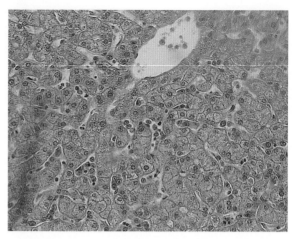

Figure 79.15 Liver biopsy specimen from patient with acute myelogenous leukemia. Formed blood elements are present within the sinusoids.

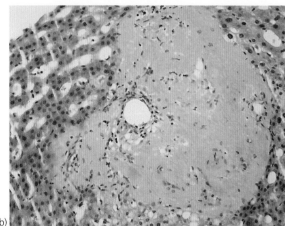

Figure 79.14 Liver biopsy specimen of a patient with rheumatoid arthritis. **(a)** Low-power view of liver biopsy specimen shows nodular eosinophilic infiltration. **(b)** High-power view of biopsy specimen depicted in (a); the pale eosinophilic extracellular deposits surrounding blood vessels are consistent with the presence of amyloid.

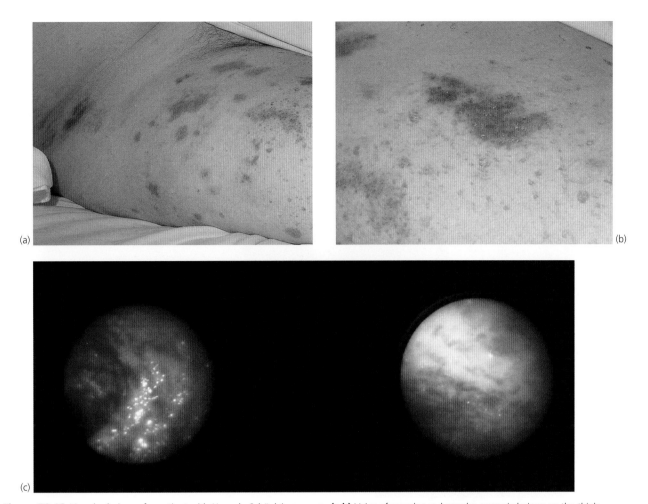

Figure 79.16 Vascular lesions of a patient with Henoch–Schönlein purpura. **(a,b)** Veins of macular and papular purpuric lesions on the thigh. **(c)** Endoscopic view of gastric mucosa demonstrates purpura.

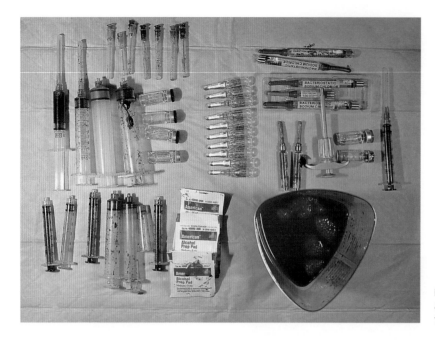

Figure 79.17 View of needles and syringes used by a patient with Munchausen syndrome to produce the factitious presentation of colonic bleeding.

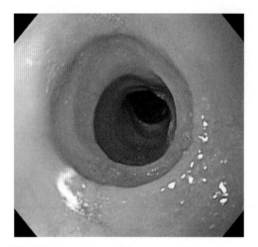

Figure 79.18 Endoscopic view of the upper esophagus demonstrating multiple webs in a patient with Plummer–Vinson syndrome.

Matilde Iorizzo, Joseph L. Jorizzo

80

Skin lesions associated with gastrointestinal and liver diseases

Skin lesions may be a presenting sign of conditions involving the gastrointestinal tract or liver, as in the case of pyoderma gangrenosum, dermatitis herpetiformis, or the skin changes of cryoglobulinemia. Primary skin diseases occasionally may involve the gastrointestinal tract directly, as in the case of blistering diseases. In some situations, examination of the skin, hair, and nails during evaluation of gastrointestinal symptoms may help provide an important clue to internal diseases. On the other hand, it is important to maintain an objective, morphological approach to diagnosis of skin lesions for such patients.

The keys to diagnosis of some of the conditions shown here are to:

- take the time to listen to the patient's possible incidental concerns
- perform a thorough examination of the skin, hair, and nails
- recognize disease associations or common skin and gastro-intestinal pathological conditions, and
- perhaps most important, have the cutaneous diagnosis confirmed by a dermatologist.

Figures 80.1–80.76 illustrate examples of occasional and rare cutaneous involvement of disease processes.

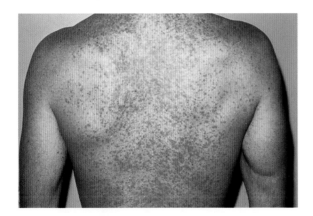

Figure 80.1 Generalized morbilliform erythema caused by penicillin allergy.

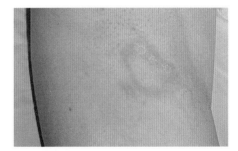

Figure 80.2 Erythema annulare centrifugum without identified precipitant.

Atlas of Gastroenterology, 4th edition. Edited by Tadataka Yamada, David H. Alpers, Anthony N. Kalloo, Neil Kaplowitz, Chung Owyang, and Don W. Powell. © 2009 Blackwell Publishing, ISBN: 978-1-4051-6909-7

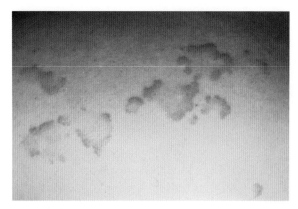

Figure 80.3 Urticaria. Note the variation in configuration. Each lesion resolved within 24 h.

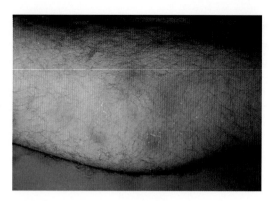

Figure 80.6 Panniculitis presenting as tender erythematous nodules on a patient with pancreatitis.

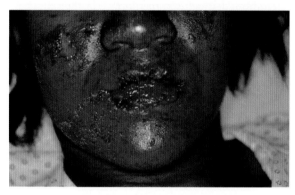

Figure 80.4 Erythema multiforme. Typical target lesions.

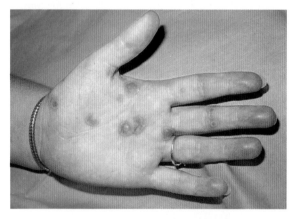

Figure 80.7 Stevens–Johnson syndrome. Note crusted lip involvement.

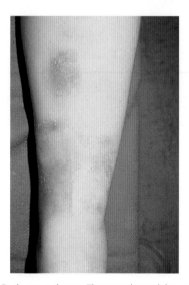

Figure 80.5 Erythema nodosum. These tender nodules occurred in association with ulcerative colitis.

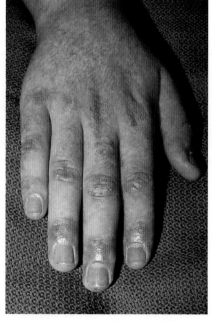

Figure 80.8 Dermatomyositis. Note the erythematous shiny papules involving the knuckles (Gottron sign).

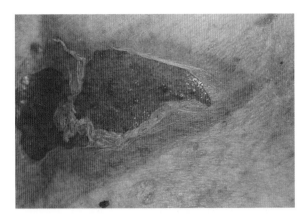

Figure 80.9 Toxic epidermal necrolysis caused by allopurinol reaction.

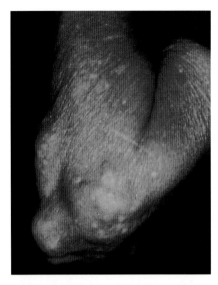

Figure 80.12 Rheumatoid nodules of the elbow.

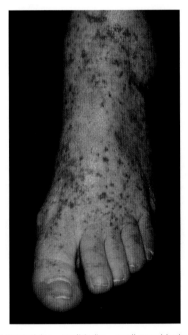

Figure 80.10 Necrotizing venulitis (i.e., small-vessel leukocytoclastic vasculitis), which was idiopathic in this patient and confined to the skin.

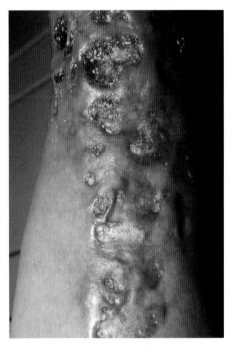

Figure 80.13 Superficial ulcerating necrobiosis in a patient with severe rheumatoid arthritis.

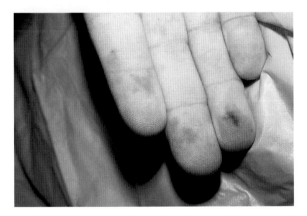

Figure 80.11 Polyarteritis nodosum. Note the necrotizing changes in multiple digits.

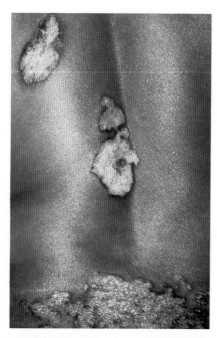

Figure 80.14 Chronic cutaneous lupus erythematosus. Note the typical discoid lesions that are well marginated and show central scarring.

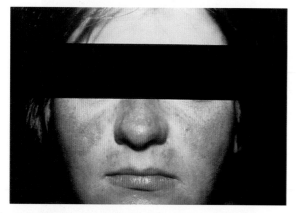

Figure 80.15 Systemic lupus erythematosus. Note the malar poikiloderma (i.e., hyperpigmentation and hypopigmentation, telangiectasia, and epidermal atrophy).

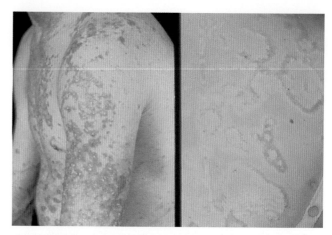

Figure 80.16 Subacute cutaneous lupus erythematosus. Note both the annular and the papulosquamous forms of the disease. Courtesy of Dr Richard Sonthelmer.

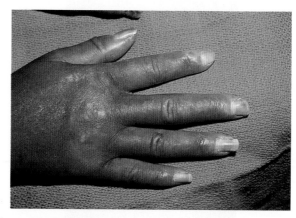

Figure 80.17 Scleroderma, CREST (calcinosis, Raynaud phenomenon, esophageal dysfunction, sclerodactyly, telangiectasia) type. Note "salt and pepper" dyspigmentation over sclerotic areas.

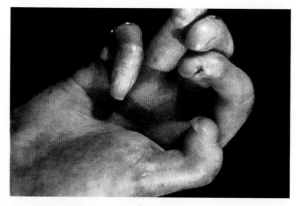

Figure 80.18 Scleroderma. This patient with progressive systemic scleroderma had a truncal pattern of onset and associated severe deformity of the hands.

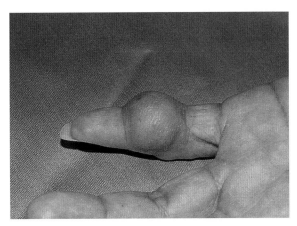

Figure 80.19 Blue rubber bleb nevus syndrome. Note the large vascular malformation.

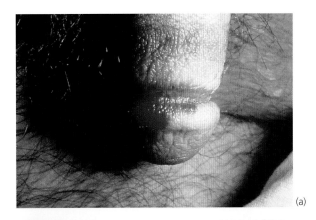

(a)

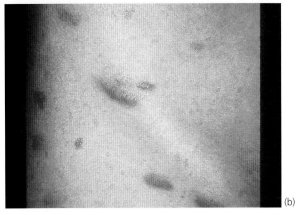

(b)

Figure 80.22 (a,b) Kaposi sarcoma in patients with acquired immunodeficiency syndrome.

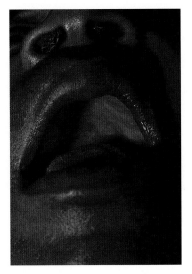

Figure 80.20 Typical telangiectasia of Osler–Weber–Rendu disease.

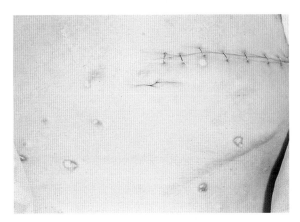

Figure 80.23 Degos disease. Note the typical cutaneous lesions with "porcelain" centers and the scars from management of gastrointestinal bleeding.

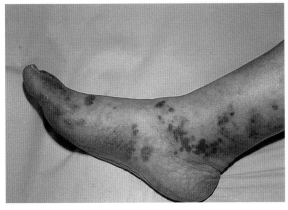

Figure 80.21 Kaposi sarcoma, classic type. Note the vascular tumors in a typical dependent site.

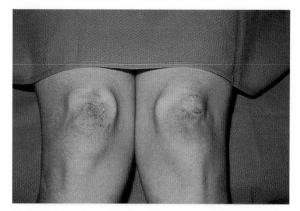

Figure 80.24 Ehlers–Danlos syndrome. Note the "fish mouth" scars and "pseudotumors" on the knees. This patient died of aortic rupture during her pregnancy.

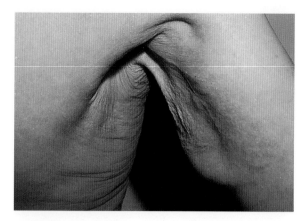

Figure 80.27 Pseudoxanthoma elasticum. Note the "chicken skin" appearance of the axillary skin.

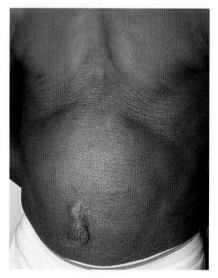

Figure 80.25 Cutis laxa. Note the skin "too large for the body" of this young boy.

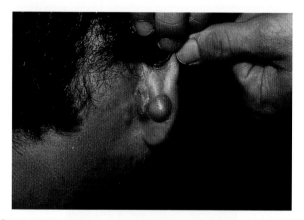

Figure 80.28 Gardner syndrome. Note the typical epidermal inclusion cyst. This patient had multiple other cystic nodules, particularly on the scalp.

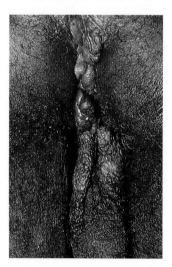

Figure 80.26 Amyloidosis. Note the perirectal amyloid nodules of this patient with multiple myeloma.

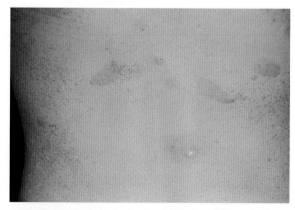

Figure 80.29 Neurofibromatosis. Note the café-au-lait macules and neurofibroma on this patient's back.

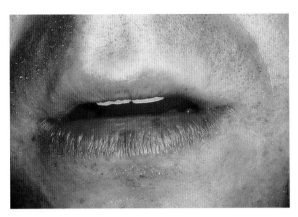

Figure 80.30 Peutz–Jeghers syndrome. Note pigmented macules on the lips that cross the vermilion border. Courtesy of Dr Jeffrey P. Callen.

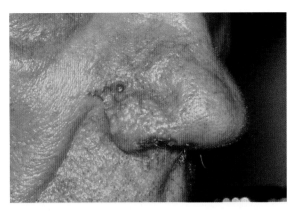

Figure 80.33 Muir–Torre syndrome. Note sebaceous adenomas of the nose. Courtesy of Dr Jeffrey P. Callen.

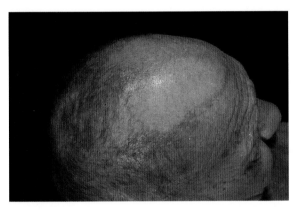

Figure 80.31 Cronkhite–Canada syndrome. Note the alopecia and hyperpigmentation.

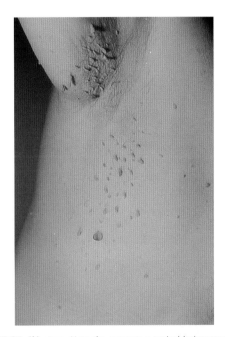

Figure 80.34 Skin tags. Note the numerous typical lesions near the axilla.

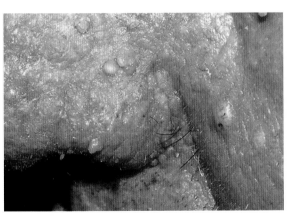

Figure 80.32 Cowden disease (multiple hamartoma syndrome). Note multiple tricholemmomas on the nose. Courtesy of Dr Jeffrey P. Callen.

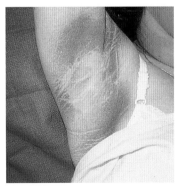

Figure 80.35 Acanthosis nigricans in a nonobese adult patient.

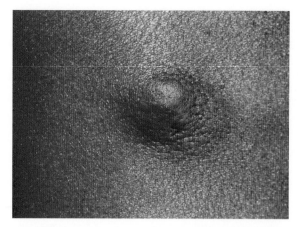

Figure 80.36 Metastatic nodule with primary adenocarcinoma of the colon.

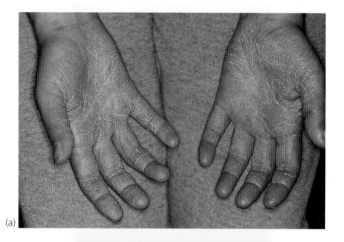

(a)

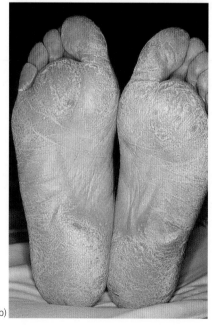

(b)

Figure 80.37 (a,b) Acquired palmar–plantar keratoderma of a patient found to have carcinoma of the esophagus.

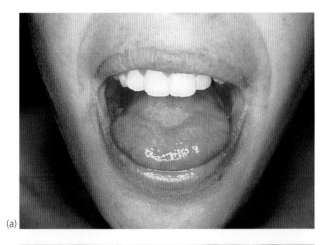

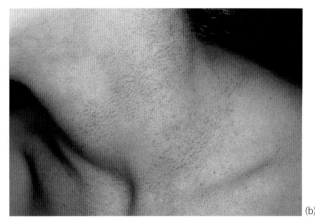

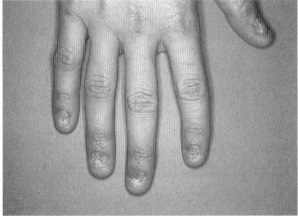

Figure 80.38 (a–c) Dyskeratosis congenita. White keratotic lesions of the tongue, reticulated neck pigmentation, and dystrophic nails of a boy.

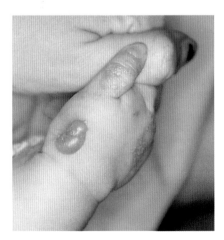

Figure 80.39 Epidermolysis bullosa, dystrophic type. Note scarring on the thumb and dorsal hand of this infant.

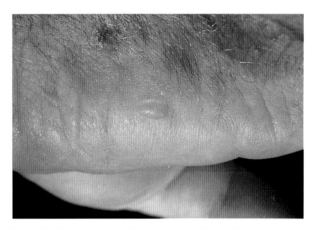

Figure 80.40 Epidermolysis bullosa acquisita. The bullous lesion is not inflamed.

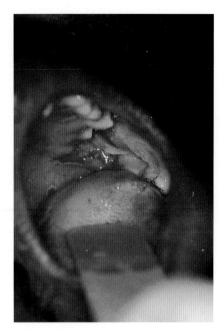

Figure 80.41 Pemphigus vulgaris. Oral erosions may be the initial manifestation.

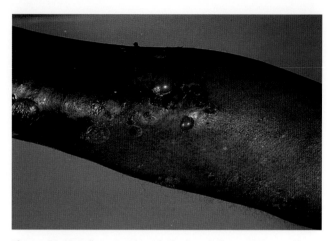

Figure 80.43 Bullous pemphigoid. The large bullae are tense and leave circular healing sites.

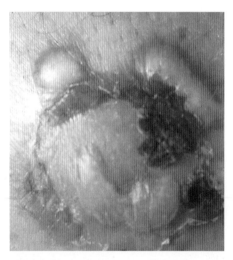

Figure 80.42 Pemphigus vulgaris. Note multiple bullous lesions and crusted erosions.

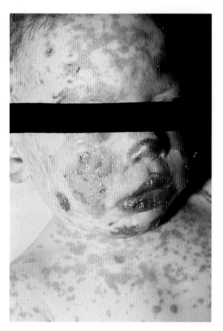

Figure 80.44 Erythema multiforme (Stevens–Johnson syndrome). Lip crusting is typical.

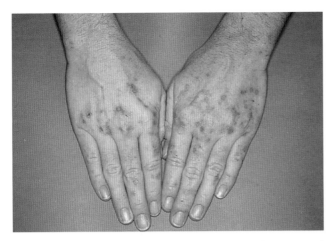

Figure 80.45 Variegate porphyria. Scarring and erosions in sun-exposed sites may be more prominent than intact blistering. The clinical features are the same as those of porphyria cutanea tarda.

Figure 80.46 Angiokeratoma. The patient has Fabry disease.

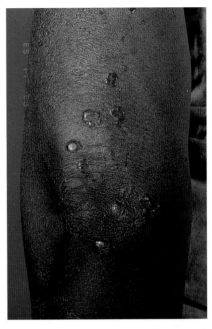

Figure 80.48 Eruptive xanthoma. New onset of multiple shiny papules over extensor surfaces of diabetic patient with a triglyceride level greater than 50 mmol/L.

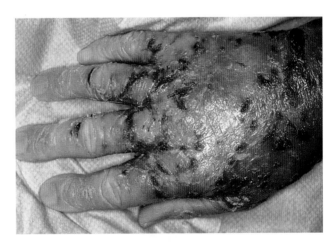

Figure 80.49 Pellagra. Erosions and crusting on sun-exposed site of a patient with chronic ethanol intake and poor nutrition.

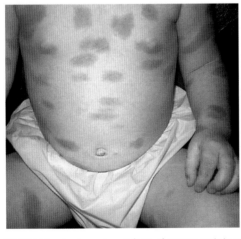

Figure 80.47 Urticaria pigmentosum form of mastocytosis in an infant.

Figure 80.50 Scurvy of a patient with poor nutrition. Note perifollicular hemorrhage.

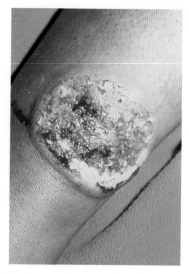

Figure 80.53 Pyoderma gangrenosum of a patient with Crohn's disease.

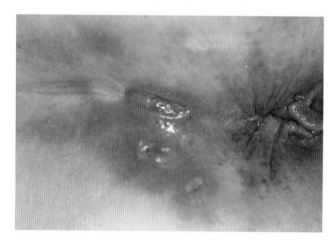

Figure 80.51 Herpes simplex. Persistent perianal erosions that were culture positive. Patient is immunosuppressed.

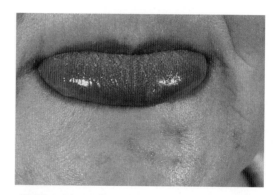

Figure 80.54 Aphthous ulcer involving the tongue of a patient with Behçet disease.

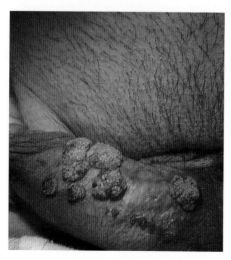

Figure 80.52 Condyloma acuminatum. Typical verrucous papules and nodules in the genital area.

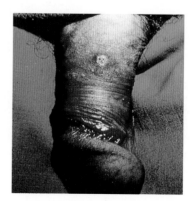

Figure 80.55 Behçet disease. Note early genital aphtha showing features of pustular vasculitis.

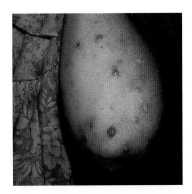

Figure 80.56 Bowel-associated dermatosis–arthritis syndrome. Pustular vasculitis lesions on a patient with a blind loop after a Billroth II operation.

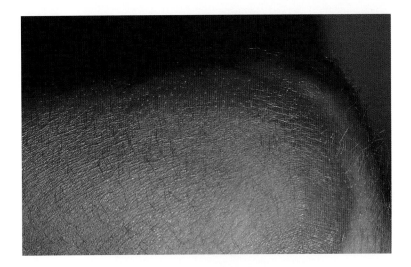

Figure 80.57 Typical lesions over the joints in a patient with erythema elevatum diutinum.

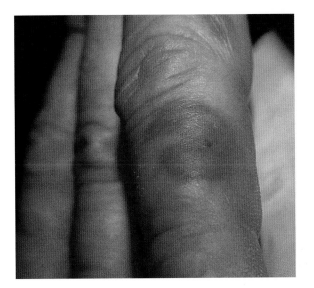

Figure 80.58 Tender erythematous papules and plaques on the upper extremities of a patient with Sweet syndrome.

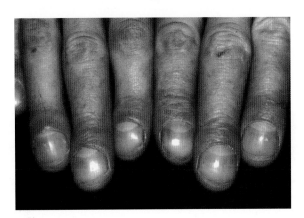

Figure 80.59 Finger clubbing.

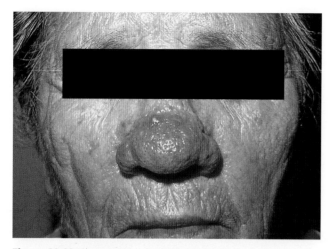

Figure 80.60 Characteristic telangiectasia, acneiform papules, and rhinophyma of a patient with rosacea.

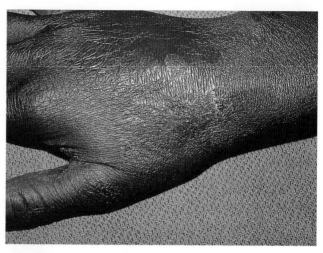

Figure 80.61 Scaling and thickened leathery skin of a patient with pellagra.

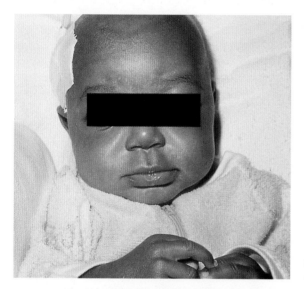

Figure 80.62 Patches of dry, scaly, eczematous skin in a young patient with acrodermatitis enteropathica.

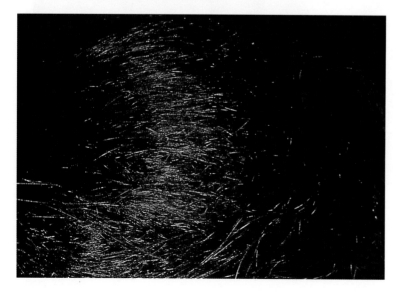

Figure 80.63 Flag sign in kwashiorkor.

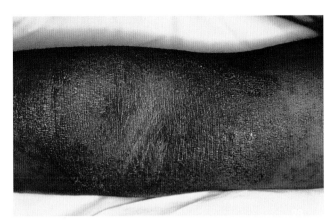

Figure 80.64 Pruritus of liver disease. Chronic scratching produces hyperpigmentation and lichenification.

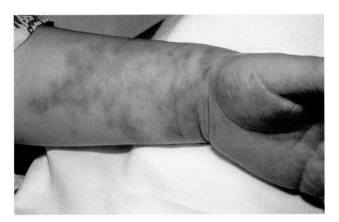

Figure 80.65 Polyarteritis nodosa. Livedo reticularis and tender subcutaneous nodules are characteristic.

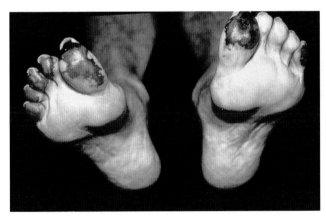

Figure 80.66 Cryoglobulinemia produces acral vasculitic infarcts. Hepatitis C is a leading cause.

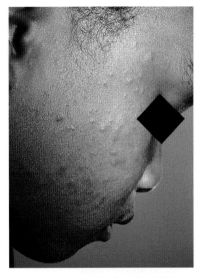

Figure 80.67 Papular acrodermatitis of childhood (Gianotti–Crosti syndrome) produces asymptomatic papules on the face and extremities of children. It was first noted in association with hepatitis B infection.

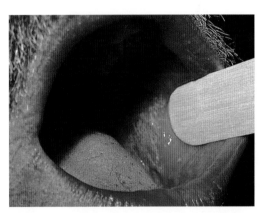

Figure 80.68 Lichen planus produces lacy mucosal plaques and pruritic papules on the skin. Patients should be evaluated for hepatitis C infection.

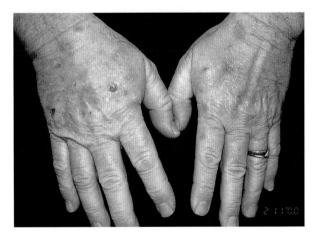

Figure 80.69 Porphyria cutanea tarda, with bullae, erosions, and scarring on the hands, can occur with many forms of liver disease.

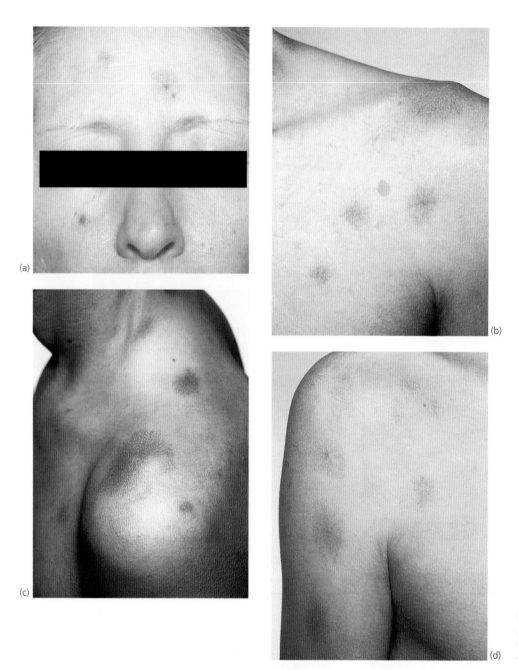

(a)

(b)

(c)

(d)

Figure 80.70 Cutaneous spider angiomas of cirrhosis on the face **(a)** and upper torso **(b–d)**. Courtesy of Dr Telfer Reynolds.

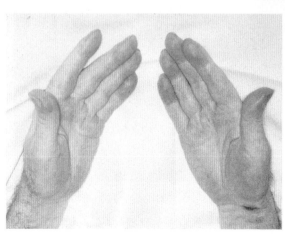

Figure 80.71 Palmar erythema of severe liver disease. Courtesy of Dr Telfer Reynolds.

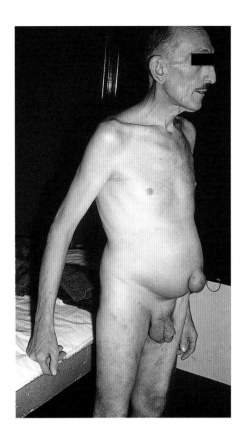

Figure 80.72 Severe muscle atrophy and malnutrition of chronic liver disease. The patient also has moderate ascites and a small umbilical hernia. Courtesy of Dr Telfer Reynolds.

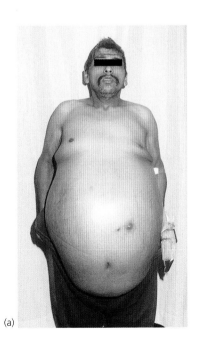

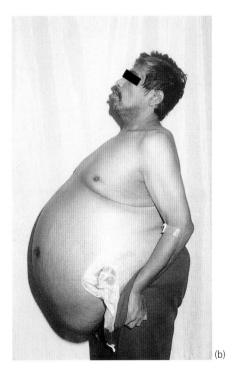

Figure 80.73 (a) Anterior and **(b)** side view of a cirrhotic patient with massive ascites. Courtesy of Dr Telfer Reynolds.

(a)

(b)

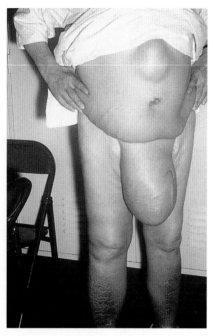

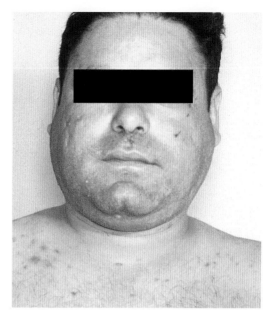

Figure 80.76 Parotid hypertrophy may be a clue to chronic alcoholism. Courtesy of Dr Telfer Reynolds.

Figure 80.74 This patient demonstrates three not-uncommon findings of cirrhosis with ascites: abdominal distention, umbilical hernia, and scrotal edema. Courtesy of Dr Telfer Reynolds.

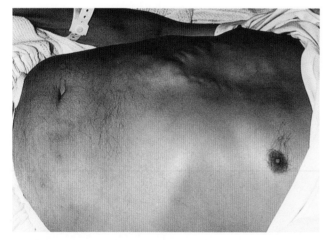

Figure 80.75 The caput medusae of cirrhosis with portal hypertension. Courtesy of Dr Telfer Reynolds.

81 Oral manifestations of gastrointestinal diseases

John C. Rabine, Timothy T. Nostrant

In patients with gastrointestinal symptoms, the oropharynx can provide diagnostic clues in disease processes ranging from rare hereditary syndromes, such as familial polyposis, to more frequently encountered entities, such as inflammatory bowel disease and gastroesophageal reflux. Oral manifestations of gastrointestinal disease may be secondary to vitamin deficiencies caused by accompanying malabsorption or poor dietary intake, caused by recurrent exposure of the oropharynx to gastric contents, or as a result of susceptibility to oropharyngeal infections in immunodeficiency states. In other cases, oropharyngeal features may be a primary manifestation of the gastrointestinal disorder such as the mucocutaneous lesions in Peutz–Jeghers syndrome or hereditary hemorrhagic telangiectasias.

Although often merely a cosmetic nuisance, oral lesions may impair mastication and swallowing, be a source of bleeding, or predispose to infectious processes and premature tooth decay. Figures 81.1–81.18 are illustrations of oral lesions seen in association with disease processes affecting the gut.

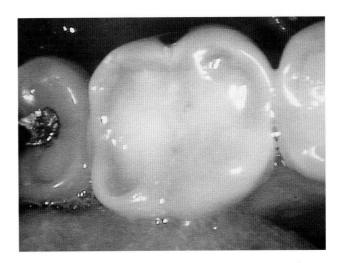

Figure 81.1 Dental erosion. Circumscribed yellowish regions correspond to exposed dentin in areas of enamel loss from repeated exposure to gastric contents secondary to chronic gastroesophageal reflux.

Atlas of Gastroenterology, 4th edition. Edited by Tadataka Yamada, David H. Alpers, Anthony N. Kalloo, Neil Kaplowitz, Chung Owyang, and Don W. Powell. © 2009 Blackwell Publishing, ISBN: 978-1-4051-6909-7

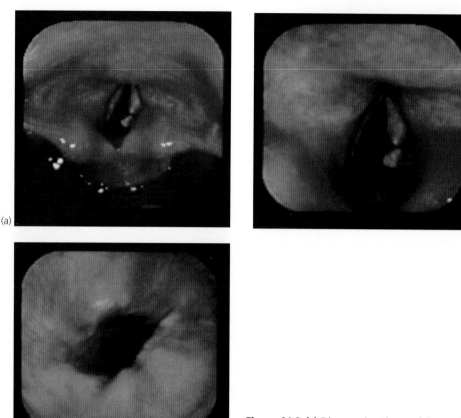

(a)

(b)

(c)

Figure 81.2 (a) Edema and erythema of the vocal cords and posterior glottis (reflux laryngitis), **(b)** vocal cord ulcer, and **(c)** vocal cord granuloma seen during upper endoscopy in a man with reflux symptoms.

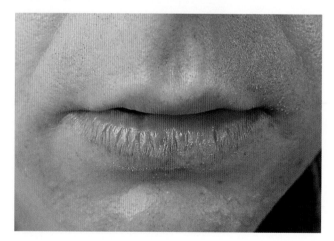

Figure 81.3 Melanin spots in a young male with Peutz–Jeghers syndrome.

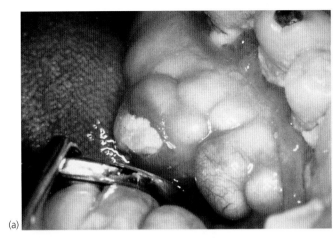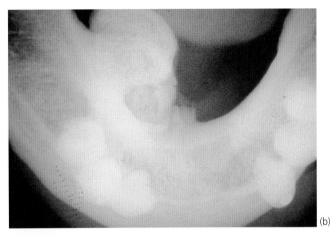

(a) (b)

Figure 81.4 (a) Mandibular osteoma in a patient with Gardner syndrome. **(b)** Radiograph of the mandible in this patient.

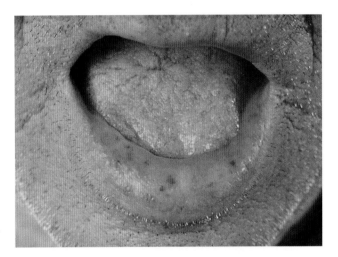

Figure 81.5 Multiple telangiectasias of the lower lip in a man with Osler–Weber–Rendu syndrome.

Figure 81.6 (a) Hemangioma of the oral cavity in a patient with blue rubber bleb nevus syndrome. The blue rubbery appearance is characteristic of the hamartomatous growths, which may be seen at any mucocutaneous site in this unusual disorder **(a, b)**.

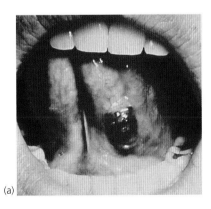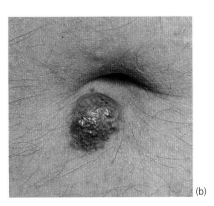

(a) (b)

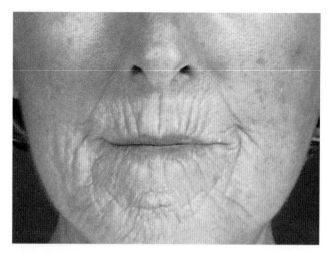

Figure 81.7 Degenerative changes and fibrosis of the perioral skin limit mobility of the mouth in progressive systemic sclerosis. Oral hygiene may be compromised in this setting.

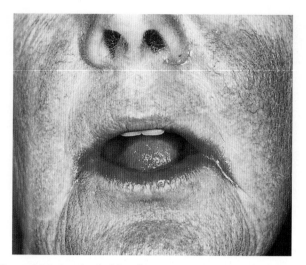

Figure 81.9 Angular cheilitis. Inflammation at the angles of the mouth is commonly associated with deficiencies of B vitamins such as riboflavin (B-2), niacin (B-3), and pyridoxine (B-6). Secondary infection with *Candida* or staphylococci may occur.

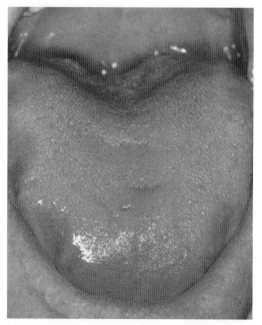

Figure 81.8 Macroglossia due to infiltration of the tongue in a patient with primary amyloidosis. Evidence of repeated tongue-biting is illustrated in this photograph.

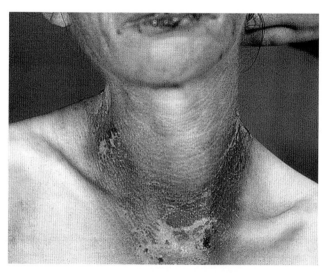

Figure 81.10 Pellagra develops from niacin and tryptophan deficiencies (because the latter can be synthesized into niacin) and is typically seen in alcoholism and severe malabsorption states. Dermatitis (usually in sun-exposed areas), diarrhea, dementia, and death are the classical sequelae of pellagra. The tongue and oral cavity may be painful and swollen.

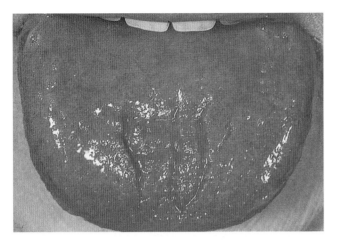

Figure 81.11 A raw, fissured tongue, especially in the setting of peripheral neuropathy, should raise the suspicion of vitamin B-12 deficiency. In later stages, the tongue may appear more atrophic with a bald, glistening surface.

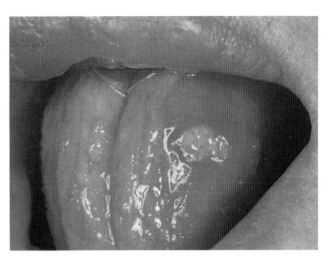

Figure 81.12 Aphthous ulcer. Aphthae appear as minute, shallow white ulcers distributed along mucous membranes. Although observed in normal individuals, multiple or persistent lesions mandate exclusion of an underlying disease process, such as inflammatory bowel disease or Behçet disease.

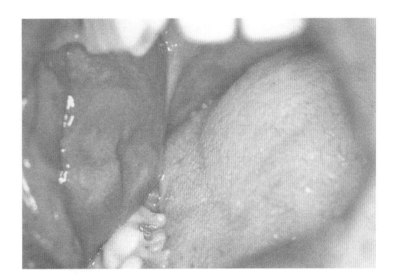

Figure 81.13 Orofacial granulomatosis diagnosed by biopsy from a patient with painful swelling of the mouth. This buccal abnormality is uncommonly seen in patients with Crohn's disease.

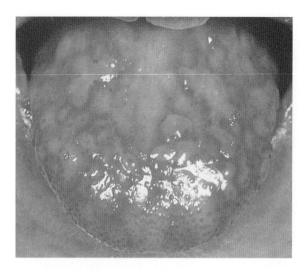

Figure 81.14 Ulcerated tongue in a patient with graft-versus-host disease following bone marrow transplantation. This phenomenon, whereby mature donor lymphocytes attack the recipient's tissues, consists of a tetrad of painful oral mucositis, enteritis, dermatitis, and hepatic dysfunction.

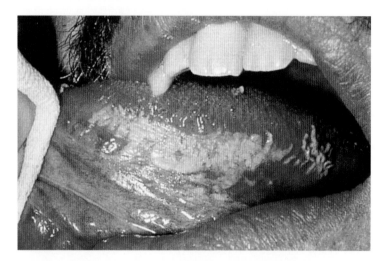

Figure 81.15 Oral hairy leukoplakia in a patient with acquired immunodeficiency syndrome. Painless whitish, verrucous excrescences along the lateral aspects of the tongue, that harbor the Epstein–Barr virus, are characteristic of this entity.

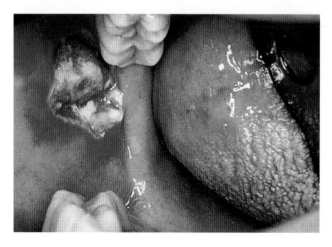

Figure 81.16 Necrotizing stomatitis. This is the most severe form of periodontal disease in the acquired immunodeficiency syndrome population, with extension of inflammation and necrosis from the gingiva and underlying bone to adjacent soft tissue and nonalveolar bone.

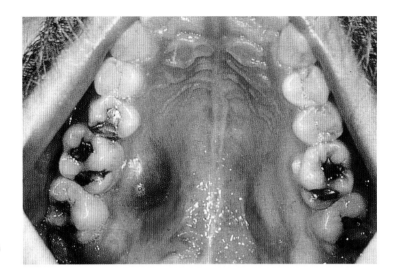

Figure 81.17 Kaposi sarcoma of the palate in an acquired immunodeficiency syndrome patient. These vascular tumors initially present as oval, poorly demarcated, rust-colored or violaceous plaques that rapidly progress to bulky lesions, which may affect mastication and swallowing.

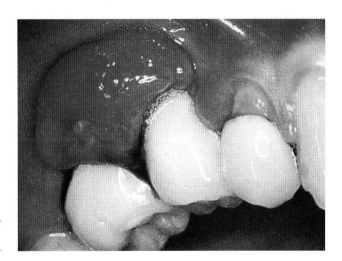

Figure 81.18 Oral lymphoma in an acquired immunodeficiency syndrome patient. These aggressive tumors typically present as firm, painless masses which progress to elevated, ulcerated regions marked by rapid proliferation.

82

Gastrointestinal vascular malformations or neoplasms: arterial, venous, arteriovenous, and capillary

Mitchell S. Cappell

Intrinsic vascular gastrointestinal lesions are divided according to pathophysiology into structural, neoplastic, and inflammatory; they are subdivided according to most affected vessel into arterial, arteriovenous, venous, and capillary. The structural vascular lesions are clinically important because of their propensity to bleed, whereas the neoplastic lesions are clinically important because of their tendency to bleed and metastasize. Inflammatory vascular lesions tend to cause mesenteric ischemia.

Structural vascular lesions

Dieulafoy lesion

Dieulafoy lesions cause about 1.5% of upper gastrointestinal bleeding and about 0.3% of lower gastrointestinal bleeding. Microscopic examination of the lesion reveals a thrombus attached to a large superficial artery at the base of a small mucosal erosion (Fig. 82.1). At endoscopy the lesion appears as a pigmented protuberance representing the vessel stump, with minimal surrounding erosion and no ulceration (Fig. 82.2). The Dieulafoy lesion most commonly occurs in the proximal stomach.

Angiodysplasia

Angiodysplasia account for about 3%–6% of lower gastrointestinal bleeding and about 2%–5% of upper gastrointestinal bleeding. Angiodysplasia most commonly cause chronic occult gastrointestinal bleeding, particularly in the elderly. They are usually diagnosed by endoscopy. At endoscopy angiodysplasia appear as dense, macular, and reticular networks of angiodysplastic vessels (vascular tufts), each of which is typically arranged in a fern tree, starburst, or stellate pattern (Figs 82.3 and 82.4). Angiodysplasia are intensely red because of the high oxygen content in erythrocytes

within vessels supplied by arteries without intervening capillaries. The vascular tuft is well demonstrated by microscopic analysis of a cleared preparation of gastrointestinal mucosa after silicone injection (Fig. 82.5). Sometimes, a prominent feeding artery or draining vein is observed (Fig. 82.6). Sometimes, a pale (anemic) mucosal halo is observed around angiodysplasia, attributed to shunting of blood (vascular steal) from surrounding mucosa by the low-resistance arteriovenous shunt (Fig. 82.7). Histologically, angiodysplasia consist of dilated, distorted, tortuous, and thin-walled vessels lined by endothelium with little or no fibrosis. Congenital arteriovenous malformations in young adults, unlike angiodysplasia in the elderly, typically have thick-walled arteries (Fig. 82.8). Angiodysplasia are often multiple. When multiple, they tend to be clustered (Fig. 82.9).

The angiographic hallmarks of angiodysplasia are a vascular tuft or tangle resulting from the local mass of irregular vessels, best visualized in the arterial phase; an early and intensely filling vein resulting from a direct arteriovenous connection without intervening capillaries; and persistent opacification beyond the normal venous phase (slowly emptying vein), possibly resulting from venous tortuosity (Fig. 82.10). Angiodysplasia occasionally bleed acutely (Fig. 82.11a). Sometimes, bleeding angiodysplasia are first injected with alcohol or epinephrine (adrenaline) to slow the bleeding, as was carried out in the illustrated case (see Fig. 82.11a). At esophagogastroduodenoscopy or colonoscopy, isolated actively bleeding angiodysplasia are treated by endoscopic argon plasma coagulation (APC), thermocoagulation, electrocoagulation, or photocoagulation (Fig. 82.11b).

Gastrointestinal telangiectasia

The endoscopic appearance of gastrointestinal telangiectasia in patients with hereditary hemorrhagic telangiectasia (HHT) may be identical to that of angiodysplasia, except that the lesions of HHT tend to be greater in number, occur in all bowel wall layers, and occur in all bowel segments (Fig. 82.12). Patients with these telangiectasia are also

Atlas of Gastroenterology, 4th edition. Edited by Tadataka Yamada, David H. Alpers, Anthony N. Kalloo, Neil Kaplowitz, Chung Owyang, and Don W. Powell. © 2009 Blackwell Publishing, ISBN: 978-1-4051-6909-7

distinguished from patients with angiodysplasia by the presence of a positive family history, epistaxis, and orocutaneous telangiectasia, which frequently occur on the lips, tongue, and oral mucosa (Fig. 82.13).

Patients with calcinosis, Raynaud phenomenon, esophageal dysmotility, sclerodactyly, and telangiectasia of the mucous membranes (CREST) syndrome sometimes have gastrointestinal telangiectasia, which tend to be punctate (1–5 mm wide), circular, and numerous (Fig. 82.14).

Gastric antral vascular ectasia

Endoscopy in gastric antral vascular ectasia reveals multiple, parallel, prominent, longitudinal folds that traverse the antrum and converge to the pyloric sphincter, and that contain intensely erythematous linear streaks at their apices (Fig. 82.15). The alternative name of watermelon stomach derives from the resemblance of these erythematous linear streaks to the stripes on a watermelon rind. Histological analysis of endoscopic biopsy samples taken from the apices of the longitudinal folds reveals hypertrophied mucosa, dilated and tortuous mucosal capillaries, often occluded by bland fibrin thrombi, and dilated and tortuous submucosal veins (Fig. 82.16).

Gastrointestinal varices

Although patients with portal hypertension most commonly develop esophageal varices, they sometimes develop gastric varices, and rarely develop varices in the small or large intestine that can cause severe gastrointestinal hemorrhage. At endoscopy, gastrointestinal varices, like esophageal varices, appear as purple, serpiginous, superficial vessels that are covered by normal-appearing mucosa and which project into the lumen (Figs 82.17 and 82.18). Occasionally, endoscopy reveals active bleeding or other stigmata of recent hemorrhage at these varices (Fig. 82.17). Intestinal varices can also be diagnosed by selective mesenteric angiography as dilated, tortuous portosystemic collaterals connecting mesenteric veins to retroperitoneal veins during the venous phase (Fig. 82.19).

Internal hemorrhoids

Hemorrhoids are the most common cause of bright red blood per rectum. At colonoscopy internal hemorrhoids characteristically appear as prominent, linear, purplish lesions radiating several centimeters proximally from the anorectum and protruding into the rectal lumen (Fig. 82.20).

Neoplastic vascular lesions

Hemangiomas

About one-half of intestinal hemangiomas are associated with cutaneous hemangiomas; the condition is called the blue rubber bleb nevus syndrome. Patients with the blue rubber bleb nevus syndrome classically present with multiple, violet-blue, slightly raised, and elastic cutaneous hemangiomas ranging in size from 0.5 to 5 cm in diameter (Fig. 82.21), together with multiple gastrointestinal hemangiomas (Fig. 82.22). The syndromic name is derived from the tactile and visual similarity of the hemangiomas to a rubber nipple. The cutaneous lesions have a wrinkled surface (see Fig. 82.21) and can be emptied of blood by manual pressure, leaving a wrinkled blue or white sac that slowly refills with blood after the pressure is released.

Abdominal radiographs or computed tomography demonstrates phleboliths from thrombosis and calcification in about one-half of intestinal hemangiomas. Typically, the phleboliths are arrayed as a cluster that outlines part of the bowel wall, and they maintain a constant distance between each other when the entire cluster shifts position within the abdomen when the patient is turned. At endoscopy, intestinal hemangiomas appear as bluish, compressible submucosal polyps that resemble the cutaneous lesions (Fig. 82.23).

Rarely patients present with intestinal hemangiomas as part of disseminated hemangiomatosis involving three or more organ systems. Patients typically present at birth with numerous cutaneous hemangiomas (Fig. 82.24).

Intestinal hemangiomas without cutaneous lesions present similarly to intestinal hemangiomas that are part of blue rubber bleb nevus syndrome, as described above.

Phlebectasia

Intestinal phlebectasia are venous varicosities consisting of a markedly dilated and tortuous vein with a normal vascular wall and scant connective tissue stroma. They are sometimes classified as multiple, small hemangioma. Phlebectasia may also occur in the oral cavity, mostly at the base of the tongue, where they are called caviar spots (varices) or sublingual phlebectasia (Fig. 82.25). Intestinal phlebectasia are dark bluish-black and range from several millimeters to 10 mm in size (Fig. 82.26). They are characteristically multiple, submucosal, soft, and compressible. They blanch with pressure. Although usually asymptomatic, they occasionally produce chronic occult or acute gross intestinal bleeding.

Nonhemangiomatous vascular neoplasms

Kaposi sarcoma

At endoscopy, gastrointestinal lesions of Kaposi sarcoma generally appear as purple or red nodules, sometimes with central ulceration, and occasionally appear as sessile masses or as hemorrhagic maculae (Fig. 82.27).

Table 82.1 Endoscopic appearance of gastrointestinal vascular malformations or neoplasms

Lesion	Endoscopic appearance
Arterial lesions	
Dieulafoy lesion	Pigmented, small (2–5 mm wide) protuberance (representing an unusually large submucosal end artery) with minimal surrounding erosion and no ulceration. Most commonly on lesser curve of proximal stomach
Vascular Ehlers–Danlos	Colonic diverticular bleeding, intramural gastrointestinal hematomas, and other forms of arterial gastrointestinal bleeding due to arterial wall and perivascular connective tissue weakness
Pseudoxanthoma elasticum	Bleeding from yellowish xanthomatoid papules (pseudoxanthomas) and petechiae in gastric fundus due to elastin degeneration in small gastric arteries
Arteriovenous communication or capillary lesions	
Angiodysplasia	Mucosal or submucosal, 2–8 mm wide, intensely red, dense, macular, reticular, network of vessels (vascular tuft); abrupt and irregular (stellate) border
Hereditary hemorrhagic telangiectasia	Endoscopic appearance identical to nonsyndromic angiodysplasia except that the lesions are numerous, are distributed in all layers of the bowel wall, and occur in all bowel segments. Patients typically also have orocutaneous telangiectasia and epistaxis
Gastric antral vascular ectasia (watermelon stomach)	Multiple parallel, prominent, intensely erythematous, longitudinal folds that traverse the antrum to converge on the pylorus. Histology: hypertrophied mucosa; dilated tortuous mucosal capillaries often occluded by bland fibrin thrombi; dilated tortuous submucosal veins; minimal inflammation
Venous lesions	
Cavernous hemangiomas	Moderately well-circumscribed, violet-blue, sessile, compressible polypoid lesions, most commonly in distal colon or rectum. Histology: large, dilated, thin-walled vessels
Blue rubber bleb nevus syndrome	Endoscopic appearance like that of cavernous hemangiomas. Often have numerous and diffuse gastrointestinal lesions. Associated with numerous similar cutaneous lesions
Klippel–Trenaunay syndrome	Extensive, infiltrative cavernous hemangioma of distal colon. Patients also have atretic deep veins and bony hypertrophy of one lower limb
Phlebectasias	Numerous, dark-bluish, soft, compressible, dilated submucosal veins of colon or jejunoileum. Histology: markedly dilated, tortuous veins with normal vascular walls
Neoplastic lesions	
Angiosarcoma (hemangiosarcoma)	Hemorrhagic ulcerated mass. Histology: numerous interconnecting vascular channels (vasoformative structures) irregular in size and shape, and atypical cells with mitosis. Immunoreactive for endothelial cell markers
Hemangiopericytoma	Solitary, circumscribed, submucosal polyp, covered by normal or ulcerated mucosa. Histology: tightly packed, spindle-shaped, neoplastic pericytes surrounding interconnecting vascular channels
Hemangioendothelioma	Intestinal mass. Histology: borderline malignancy with more cellularity and mitoses than hemangiomas, but less than that for angiosarcomas
Kaposi sarcoma	Purple or red submucosal nodules, sometimes with central ulceration or hemorrhagic nodules. Usually associated with human immunodeficiency virus infection

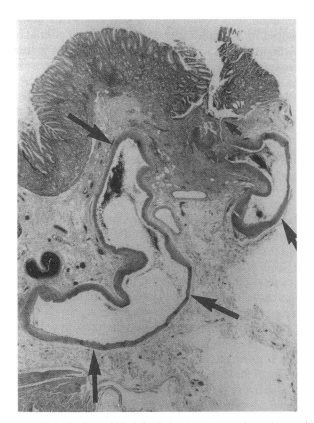

Figure 82.1 Histology of Dieulafoy lesion. Low-power photomicrograph shows the sinuous path of an enlarged caliber, but otherwise normal, artery (Dieulafoy lesion) in the submucosa (large arrows) of the gastric fundus. A recent thrombus is attached to the artery at the base of a deep mucosal erosion (small arrow). No enlarged vein accompanies the enlarged artery, as would occur in an arteriovenous malformation.

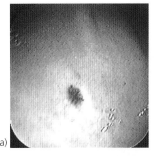 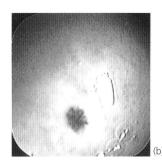

(a)　　　　　　　　　　　　　　　　　　　　(b)

Figure 82.3 Vascular tuft of angiodysplasia. Endoscopic videophotograph of the gastric antrum demonstrates the intense erythema and the complex internal reticular structure (in a starburst or stellate pattern) characteristic of an angiodysplasia in a far-away **(a)** and close-up **(b)** view. Note the irregular lesion margin (also in a stellate pattern).

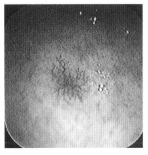 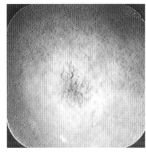

Figure 82.4 Arachnoid network of angiodysplasia. Endoscopic videophotograph showing an intensely red and complex reticular (arachnoid) network characteristic of an angiodysplasia in the antrum of a middle-aged woman presenting with epigastric pain.

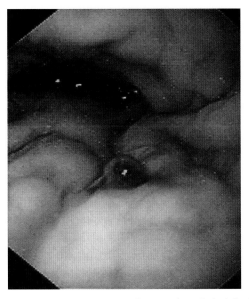

Figure 82.2 Endoscopic appearance of an esophageal Dieulafoy lesion. The lesion appears as a small, pigmented protuberance that represents the vessel stump, with no surrounding ulceration or erosion.

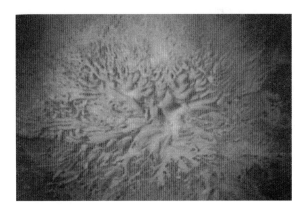

Figure 82.5 "Coral head" appearance of advanced angiodysplasia. Stereophotomicrograph shows the typical coral head appearance of a vascular tuft in an advanced right colonic mucosal angiodysplasia after arterial injection with silicone.

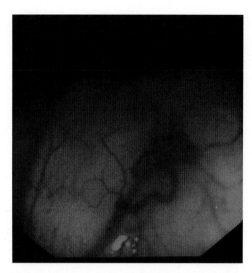

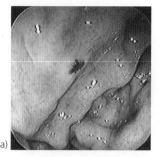
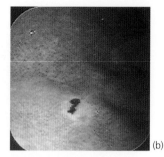

Figure 82.6 Supplying vessel of angiodysplasia. Endoscopic photograph showing a large vessel supplying an angiodysplasia in the ascending colon, and the well-defined internal structure (vascular tuft) of the angiodysplasia.

Figure 82.7 Anemic halo of angiodysplasia. Endoscopic videophotograph **(a)** showing an intensely red and complex finely reticular network characteristic of an angiodysplasia in the gastric antrum of an elderly man presenting with iron-deficiency anemia. The mucosa immediately around the angiodysplasia is pale **(b)**. This anemic halo is attributed to shunting of blood from the surrounding tissue by the low-resistance arteriovenous shunt. Note that the anemic halo is also apparent, although less conspicuous, in Figure 82.3, particularly in part (b) of the figure.

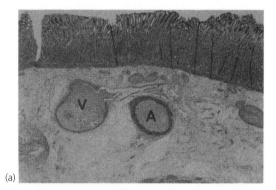
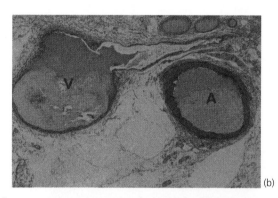

Figure 82.8 Histology of arteriovenous malformation. **(a)** Low- and **(b)** medium-power photomicrographs of a gastric fundal arteriovenous malformation. Note the dilated submucosal artery (A) and vein (V), the close proximity of the vein and artery, and the digitiform projection from the vein toward the artery. The arteries have a thick muscular wall and a continuous, prominent internal elastic membrane (stained black in the tunica media) (van Gieson–Verhoeff stain; original magnification ×20 and ×40 respectively).

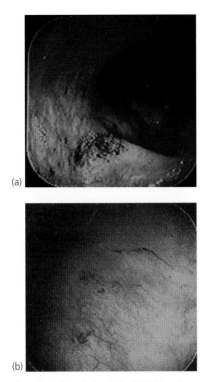

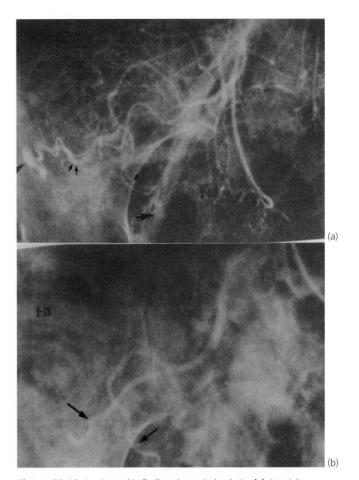

Figure 82.9 Clustering of angiodysplasia. **(a)** Videophotograph demonstrates that the multiple angiodysplasia were all clustered in the descending colon on colonoscopy in an elderly woman with iron-deficiency anemia. **(b)** Close-up views demonstrate the characteristic endoscopic appearance of angiodysplasia: an intensely red color, an intricate reticulonodular structure, and communication with prominent feeding arteries.

Figure 82.10 Angiographic findings in angiodysplasia. **(a)** Arterial phase, 6 s after contrast injection into the superior mesenteric artery, in a patient with vascular ectasia shows a vascular tuft (large arrow) and two early-filling veins (small arrows) that have filled with contrast before other veins. **(b)** Late phase, 14 s after contrast injection, from the same angiogram reveals two densely opacified, dilated, and tortuous late-draining cecal veins (arrows) that still retain contrast after other veins have cleared.

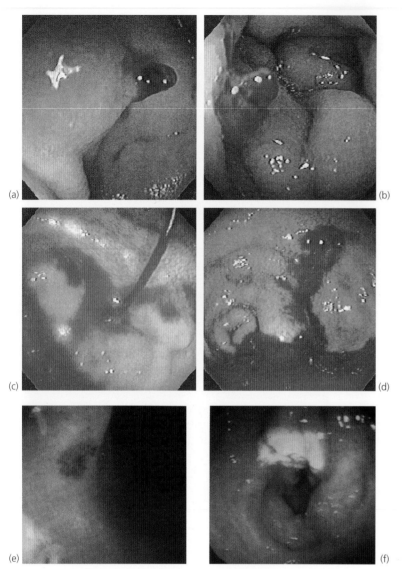

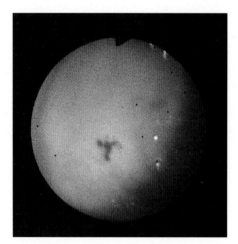

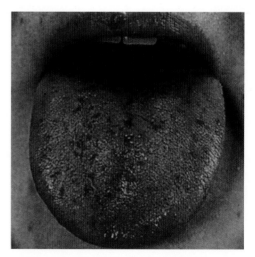

Figure 82.11 (a–d) Sclerotherapy for active bleeding from angiodysplasia. At colonoscopy, blood is oozing from a nonulcerated pigmented protuberance that appears to be a visible vessel in the cecum: **(a)**, profile view; **(b)**, close-up profile view. Lesion irrigation prior to electrocautery washes away an overlying clot and reveals blood spurting from a small elevated mound that resembles a Dieulafoy lesion: **(c)** en face view. The bleeding slows after sclerotherapy: **(d)**, en face view. Note in this videophotograph the appendiceal orifice at the 8 o'clock position, about 2 cm away from the lesion at the 1 o'clock position. Pathological examination of the resected specimen after subsequent segmental colonic resection reveals an angiodysplasia and not a Dieulafoy lesion. **(e)** and **(f)** Endoscopic electrocoagulation of angiodysplasia. Endoscopic videophotographs show an angiodysplasia in the duodenal bulb (e). A white coagulum is present after Gold Probe (Microvasive, Boston Scientific Corporation, Watertown, MA) electrocoagulation (f). (a–d) Courtesy of Dr Roger Mendes, Director of Gastroenterology Fellowship Training Program, and Dr Vanada Vedula, Long Island College Hospital and Woodhull Hospital, Brooklyn, New York.

Figure 82.12 Endoscopic appearance of gastric antral telangiectasia in hereditary hemorrhagic telangiectasia. Videophotograph shows the characteristic findings: intense erythema, well-demarcated maculae, fine internal reticular (fern-like) structure, and irregular stellate (fern-like) margin. The endoscopic appearance is virtually identical to that of nonsyndromic angiodysplasia. Courtesy of Dr Burton Shatz.

Figure 82.13 Mucocutaneous lesions in hereditary hemorrhagic telangiectasia. Photograph shows the typical appearance of telangiectasias on the lips and tongue in a patient with hereditary hemorrhagic telangiectasia as intensely red maculae with an abrupt but irregular (stellate) border.

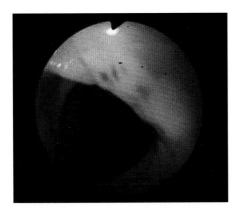

Figure 82.14 Endoscopic appearance of gastric antral telangiectasia in calcinosis, Raynaud phenomenon, esophageal dysmotility, sclerodactyly, and telangiectasia (CREST) syndrome. Videophotograph shows the characteristic endoscopic findings: intense erythema, well-demarcated maculae, fine internal reticular (fern-like) structure, and irregular stellate (fern-like) margin. The endoscopic appearance closely resembles that of nonsyndromic angiodysplasia.

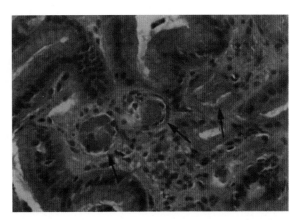

Figure 82.16 Histology of gastric antral vascular ectasia. Findings include multiple dilated capillaries, many of which contain bland fibrin thrombi (arrows), and normal capillary endothelium (H & E stain; original magnification ×200).

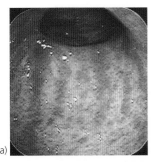 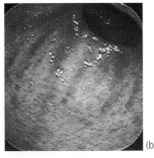

(a) (b)

Figure 82.15 Endoscopic appearance of gastric antral vascular ectasia (GAVE). Videophotograph shows the characteristic endoscopic finding in GAVE of linear, intensely erythematous lesions at the apices of longitudinal antral folds radiating to the pylorus. The alternative lesion name of watermelon stomach derives from the resemblance of these erythematous linear streaks to the stripes on a watermelon rind.

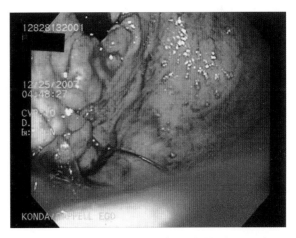

Figure 82.17 Endoscopic appearance of actively bleeding gastric varices. Esophagogastroduodenoscopy in a cirrhotic patient with exsanguinating upper gastrointestinal hemorrhage reveals the characteristic endoscopic findings of superficial, purplish, serpiginous lesions in the very proximal stomach from fundal varices. Active bleeding is evidenced by the spurting of blood from a varix and the adjacent pooling of bright red blood. In this retroflexed view, the endoscopic shaft is seen adjacent to the fundal varices exiting from the gastroesophageal junction **(top, left)**. Courtesy of Dr Mitchell S. Cappell, Chief, Division of Gastroenterology, and Dr Amulya Konda, Gastroenterology Fellow, William Beaumont Hospital, Royal Oak, MI.

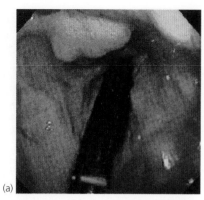
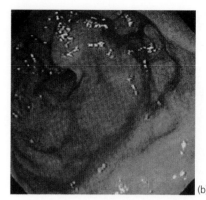

(a)　　　(b)

Figure 82.18 Endoscopic appearance of rectal varices. **(a)** Rectal varices at colonoscopy appear as superficial serpiginous bluish lesions covered by normal mucosa that project from the mucosa into the lumen, as shown on direct colonoscopic view. **(b)** Same varices shown on colonoscopic rectal retroflexion in an elderly woman with cirrhosis from chronic hepatitis C infection. Courtesy of Dr Roger Mendes, Director of Gastroenterology Fellowship Training Program, and Dr Vanada Vedula, Long Island College Hospital and Woodhull Hospital, Brooklyn, New York.

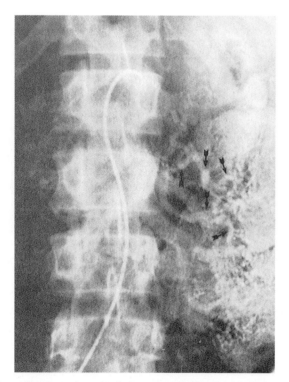

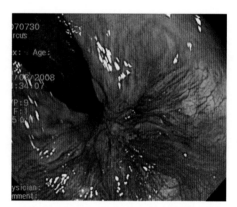

Figure 82.20 Endoscopic appearance of internal hemorrhoids. Rectal retroflexion during colonoscopy reveals the characteristic findings of internal hemorrhoids of prominent linear purplish lesions radiating from the anorectal junction and protruding into the rectal lumen. The patient had presented with postdefecatory bright red blood per rectum. Note the presence of the distal colonoscopic shaft in this retroflexed view.

Figure 82.19 Angiographic findings in intestinal varices. Contrast injection via a catheter in the superior mesenteric artery shows in the venous phase dilated tortuous portosystemic collaterals (arrows) communicating between the superior mesenteric vein and a massive network of retroperitoneal veins in a patient with jejunal varices proven at laparotomy.

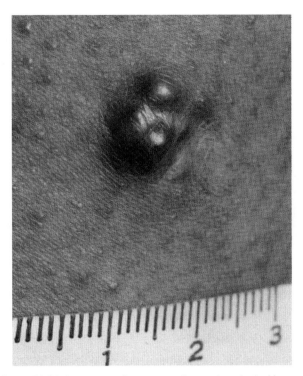

Figure 82.21 Appearance of a cutaneous hemangioma in the blue rubber bleb nevus syndrome. Close-up view of a dark blue, nodular, and rubbery skin lesion on the left thigh in a patient with the blue rubber bleb nevus syndrome.

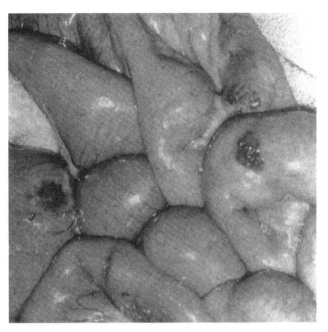

Figure 82.22 Intraoperative appearance of intestinal hemangiomas. At laparotomy, multiple hemangiomas appear as bluish, round, smooth, and well-demarcated sessile polypoid lesions on the serosal surface of the small intestine.

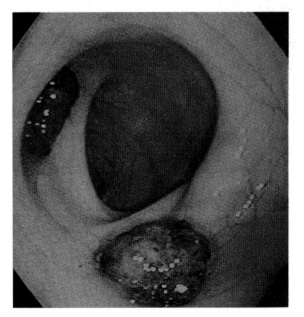

Figure 82.23 Endoscopic appearance of a colonic hemangioma in the blue rubber bleb nevus syndrome. Lesion appears as a bluish, round, smooth, and well-demarcated sessile polypoid lesion.

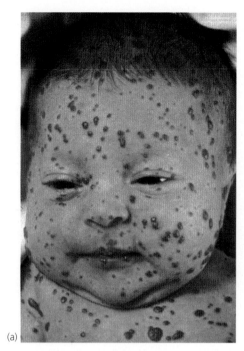

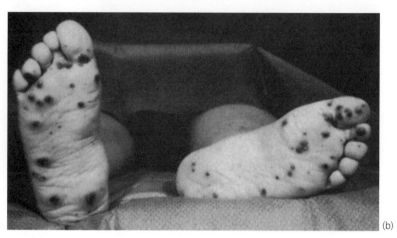

(a)

(b)

Figure 82.24 (a) Disseminated cutaneous hemangiomas. Numerous bluish, nodular, and rubbery cutaneous lesions occur on the face of a child with disseminated hemangiomatosis. Patients characteristically have multiple intestinal hemangiomas. **(b)** Photograph of numerous bluish-black, nodular, and rubbery skin lesions on the plantar surface of both feet in a child with diffuse hemangiomatosis.

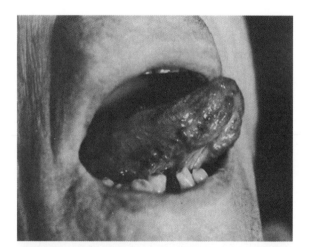

Figure 82.25 Sublingual phlebectasia (caviar spots). Curling and extension of the tongue demonstrates multiple purplish or bluish-gray nodular to oblong venous varicosities on the undersurface of the tongue.

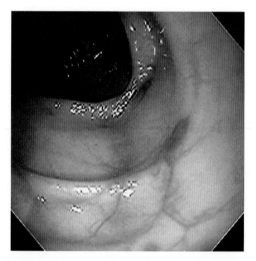

Figure 82.26 Endoscopic appearance of phlebectasia. Phlebectasia appear at endoscopy as bluish oblong venous varicosities. In this case a cluster of these lesions was localized to the transverse colon.

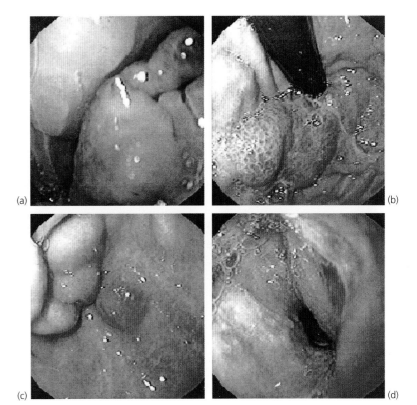

Figure 82.27 (a–d) Spectrum of the endoscopic appearance of upper gastrointestinal Kaposi sarcoma. Esophagogastroduodenoscopy reveals a reddish-purple oral mass near several teeth **(a)**, a multinodular cardial mass with superficial punctate erythema noted on gastric retroflexion **(b)**, a small reddish nodular mass at the pylorus **(c)**, and a violaceous circumferential mass with an overlying whitish exudate producing irregular constriction of the descending duodenum **(d)**. Courtesy of Dr Roger Mendes, Director of Gastroenterology Fellowship Training Program, and Dr Vanada Vedula, Long Island College Hospital and Woodhull Hospital, Brooklyn, New York.

83

Intestinal ischemia

Julián Panés, Josep M. Piqué

Intestinal ischemia represents a broad spectrum of diseases with various clinical, radiological, and pathological manifestations, which range from localized transient ischemia to extensive necrosis of the gastrointestinal tract. Diagnosis before the occurrence of intestinal infarction is the most important factor in improving survival for patients with intestinal ischemia.

Anatomy of the intestinal circulation

The celiac artery arises from the abdominal aorta and branches into the left gastric, the common hepatic, and the splenic arteries (Fig. 83.1). The left gastric artery supplies the stomach, and the common hepatic artery divides into the hepatic artery, the right gastric artery, and the gastroduodenal artery. The superior mesenteric artery (SMA) arises from the aorta and courses inferiorly and toward the right to terminate at the level of the cecum as the ileocolic artery (Fig. 83.1). The inferior mesenteric artery (IMA) is the smallest of the mesenteric vessels and branches into the left colic artery, several arteries that supply the sigmoid and descending colon, and the superior rectal artery. The venous system generally parallels the arterial distribution.

Mechanisms of ischemic injury

The mechanisms that are believed to participate in ischemic and reperfusion injury include the infiltration of postischemic tissues by inflammatory cells, an increased production of reactive oxygen species (ROS), alterations in vascular permeability, and inhibition of local cytoprotective mechanisms (Fig. 83.2).

Atlas of Gastroenterology, 4th edition. Edited by Tadataka Yamada, David H. Alpers, Anthony N. Kalloo, Neil Kaplowitz, Chung Owyang, and Don W. Powell. © 2009 Blackwell Publishing, ISBN: 978-1-4051-6909-7

Clinical syndromes

Acute insufficiency of the blood supply to the intestine can result from emboli, arterial and venous thrombi, or vasoconstriction secondary to low-flow states. Embolization to the SMA accounts for 50% of all cases of acute mesenteric ischemia (AMI) (Fig. 83.3). The most common precipitant of thrombus dislodgment and embolization is a cardiac arrhythmia. Thrombosis accounts for about 15% of cases of acute intestinal ischemia. Thrombosis of the SMA or celiac artery is generally associated with a preexisting stenosis, usually at the origin of the arteries (Fig. 83.4). Mesenteric ischemia without anatomic arterial or venous obstruction is due to mesenteric vasospasm that can occur during periods of relatively low mesenteric flow (Fig. 83.5). Thrombosis of the superior mesenteric vein (SMV) is more common than symptomatic inferior mesenteric vein (IMV) thrombosis because of the larger caliber and flow of the SMV. Chronic mesenteric ischemia is the result of repeated transient episodes of insufficient intestinal blood flow. Ischemic colitis is the most common form of ischemic injury to the gut and occurs more frequently in elderly people.

Diagnosis

Radiology
Subtle signs of AMI on plain abdominal radiographs include adynamic ileus and distended, air-filled loops of bowel (Fig. 83.6). More specific radiographic findings occur in 25% of cases, usually with advanced disease. These findings include mural thumbprinting resulting from edema or hemorrhage (Fig. 83.7). In advanced stages of ischemia, pneumatosis of the bowel wall can be detected (Fig. 83.8). Specifically, portal vein gas on abdominal radiography portends an extremely poor prognosis (Figs 83.9 and 83.10). After an ischemic episode, contrast radiology may be helpful in identifying residual stenotic lesions (Fig. 83.11).

Duplex ultrasonography can document proximal stenoses in the SMA (Fig. 83.12) or celiac axis or complete occlusion of these vessels (Fig. 83.13).

Single-detector helical computed tomography (CT) is of limited use in the diagnosis of AMI, except in patients suspected of having SMV thrombosis (Fig. 83.14). Nonspecific findings in a contrast-enhanced CT scan examination may include the presence of bowel wall thickening and diffuse mesenteric haziness due to edema (Fig. 83.15). The presence of portal venous gas and pneumatosis intestinalis are seen only after infarction has developed (Figs 83.16 and 83.17). In patients with chronic mesenteric ischemia, CT scan may demonstrate the presence of calcified atheromatous lesions (Fig. 83.18) and collateral circulation (Fig. 83.19).

Multidetector-row CT provides increased spatial resolution, high-quality three-dimensional reconstructions (Figs 83.20 and 83.21), and shorter examination times. It has thus confirmed a fundamental role for CT in the diagnosis of AMI, achieving a sensitivity of 80%–96% and a specificity of 94%–98%. CT enables the site of the vascular obstruction to be visualized, appearing as a site of defective opacification of the lumen of the vessel (Fig. 83.22). It is most easily recognized when the occlusion is at the level of the main trunks. Thrombosis of the main vessels can easily be seen on axial imaging, often with associated collateral vessels, depending on its chronicity (Fig. 83.23).

Selective catheter angiography has long been the gold standard for diagnosis of AMI. In cases of SMA embolization, most emboli are impacted 3–10 cm from the origin of the SMA, distal to the origin of the middle colic artery (Fig. 83.3). The classic meniscus sign can often be visualized at the point of occlusion, which is different from the planar defect produced by a thrombus (Fig. 83.4). Symptomatic thrombosis of the SMA is generally associated with a high-grade stenosis or occlusion of the celiac axis (Fig. 83.24). The stenosis usually slowly progresses and permits reconstitution of vascular flow because of development of collaterals (Fig. 83.25). Aortography is essential in these patients to evaluate potential inflow and outflow sites for bypass grafts as well as to clarify the extent and location of other atherosclerotic lesions in the iliac and inferior mesenteric arteries (Fig. 83.26). In patients suffering nonocclusive mesenteric ischemia (NOMI), angiography usually reveals multiple areas of narrowing and irregularity in major branches. The small and medium arterial branches may be decreased or absent producing a "pruned" arterial tree, and there is also impaired intramural vascular filling (Fig. 83.5).

Endoscopy

Colonoscopy or flexible sigmoidoscopy is the method of choice for the diagnosis of ischemic colitis, as it allows direct visualization of the mucosa and tissue sampling. The mucosa of the affected segment usually appears edematous, hemorrhagic, friable (Fig. 83.27), and ulcerated (Figs 83.28 and 83.29). When bowel necrosis is present, colonoscopy reveals cyanotic, gray, or black mucosa.

Histopathology of intestinal ischemia

When infarction occurs, the bowel becomes edematous and plum colored (Fig. 83.30). Microscopic examination of specimens with early mucosal lesions usually shows a patchy distribution with almost normal mucosa surrounding diseased areas in which crypts show necrosis, and with the formation of a surface membrane composed of mucus, fibrin, blood cells, and necrotic tissue (Fig. 83.31). There is vascular congestion with edema and occasional hemorrhages in the submucosal layer (Fig. 83.32). It is common to see fibrin thrombi within the blood vessels. With increasing severity of ischemia the deeper layers of the bowel wall become affected (Fig. 83.33). Infarction is manifested by hemorrhage into the bowel wall, particularly the submucosa, with intravascular thrombosis and mucosal ulceration (Fig. 83.34).

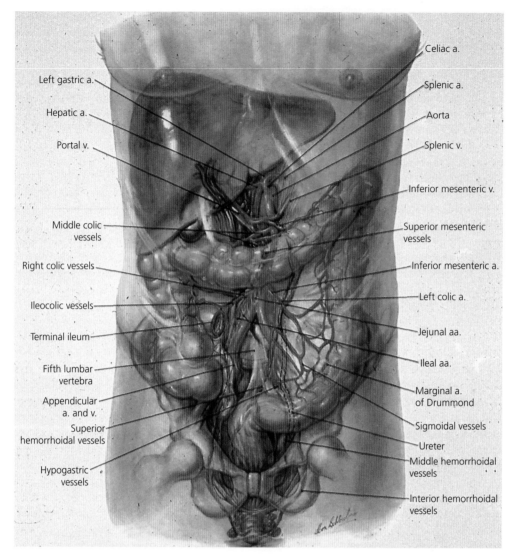

Celiac a.

Left gastric a.

Splenic a.

Hepatic a.

Aorta

Portal v.

Splenic v.

Inferior mesenteric v.

Middle colic
vessels

Superior mesenteric
vessels

Right colic vessels

Inferior mesenteric a.

Left colic a.

Ileocolic vessels

Jejunal aa.

Terminal ileum

Ileal aa.

Fifth lumbar
vertebra

Marginal a.
of Drummond

Appendicular
a. and v.

Sigmoidal vessels

Superior
hemorrhoidal vessels

Ureter

Middle hemorrhoidal
vessels

Hypogastric
vessels

Interior hemorrhoidal
vessels

Figure 83.1 Anatomy of the intestinal circulation. The celiac artery arises from the abdominal aorta and branches into the left gastric, common hepatic, and splenic arteries. The superior mesenteric artery (SMA) exits the aorta 1 cm below the celiac artery. It supplies the entire small intestine except for the superior part of the duodenum, and supplies the right and transverse colon and part of the pancreas. Branches include the inferior pancreaticoduodenal artery, numerous jejunal and ileal branches, the ileocolic artery, and the middle colic artery. The inferior mesenteric artery (IMA) arises from the aorta 3 cm proximal to the aortic bifurcation. The artery branches into the left colic, several sigmoid (inferior left colic) arteries, and the superior rectal (hemorrhoidal) artery. The arcades of the SMA and IMA interconnect at the base and border of the mesentery. The connection at the base of the mesentery provides a potential collateral channel between SMA and IMA called the arc of Riolan. The connection along the mesenteric border provides another potential collateral channel called the marginal artery of Drummond. a., artery; v., vein.

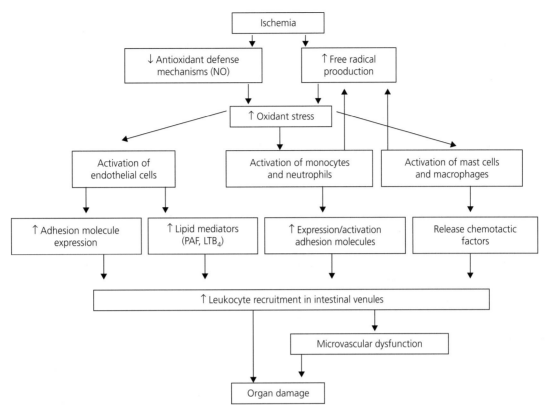

Figure 83.2 Mechanisms involved in ischemia-induced intestinal damage. Ischemia results in an increased production of oxidants, with a corresponding reduction in the synthesis of nitric oxide (NO) by endothelial NO synthase (eNOS). The enhanced generation of oxidants results in the activation of endothelial cells and leukocytes. Firm adhesion of leukocytes, which is mediated by β-2 integrins (CD11/CD18), is induced by engagement of activated leukotriene B$_4$ (LTB$_4$) and platelet-activating factor (PAF) with their receptors on rolling leukocytes. Sustained rolling and adhesion of leukocytes on endothelial cells are ensured by an oxidant-dependent synthesis of endothelial cell adhesion molecules, such as P-selectin and intercellular adhesion molecule-1 (ICAM-1). The inflammatory responses to ischemia are further amplified by oxidants derived from reduced nicotinamide adenine dinucleotide phosphate (NADPH) oxidase in leukocytes, and by mediators released from mast cells and macrophages that normally reside in close proximity to postcapillary venules.

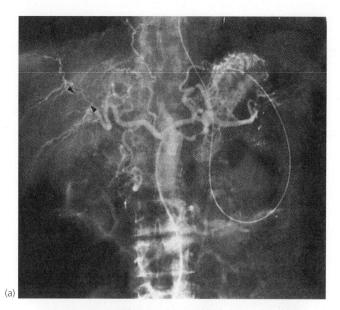

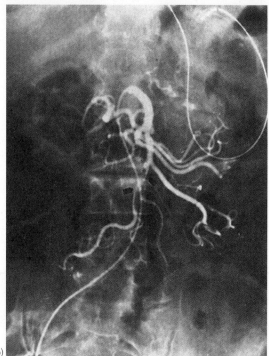

Figure 83.3 Visceral embolic disease. Arteriographic demonstration of splanchnic embolic disease. These two views of the same patient demonstrate emboli in two different splanchnic vessels. **(a)** Hepatic artery embolus (arrowheads). **(b)** Superior mesenteric artery embolus (arrow).

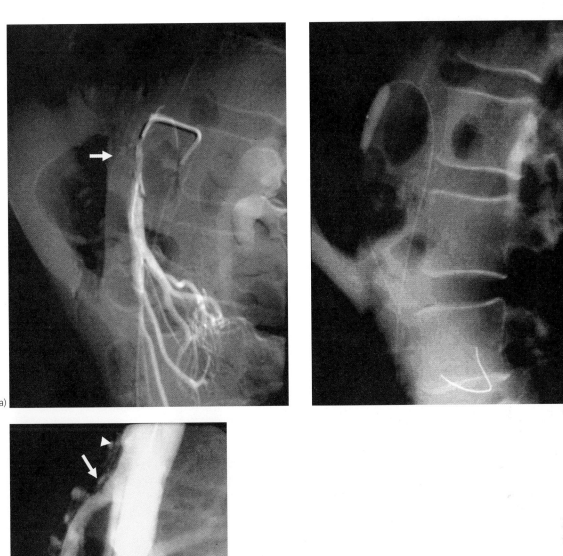

(a)

(b)

(c)

Figure 83.4 Abdominal angiogram of a 70-year-old patient with severe periumbilical pain of sudden onset. **(a)** Selective angiogram of the superior mesenteric artery (SMA) demonstrating an 80% occlusion of the lumen (arrow) with poor filling of distal branches. An abdominal angiogram showed total obstruction of the celiac trunk. **(b)** Translumenal angioplasty. Balloon inflated at the level of the SMA stenosis. No residual waste in the balloon is present. **(c)** Abdominal angiogram after translumenal angioplasty shows a good perfusion of the SMA (arrow) and persistence of proximal occlusion of the celiac trunk (arrowhead).

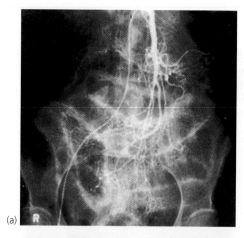

(a)

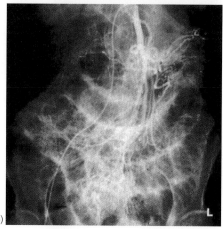

(b)

Figure 83.5 Nonocclusive intestinal ischemia, arteriographic findings. **(a)** Initial mesenteric arteriogram of a patient with nonocclusive intestinal ischemia shows vasospasm and irregularities of the celiac and superior mesenteric arteries. The normal arterial blush of the intestinal wall is lost. **(b)** After infusion of papaverine, substantial vasodilation is visible at both the macrovascular and microvascular levels. This radiograph is compatible with a normal superior mesenteric arteriogram but is diagnostic for nonocclusive mesenteric ischemia when compared with (a).

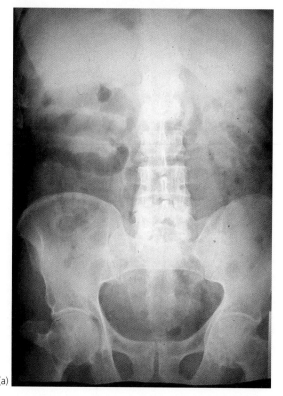

(a)

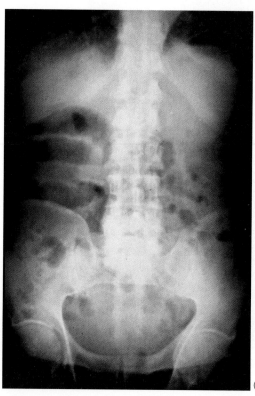

(b)

Figure 83.6 A 58-year-old patient with abdominal pain. **(a)** Plain abdominal radiograph showing three horizontal distended air-filled loops with mural thickening on the right upper quadrant. **(b)** A second abdominal radiograph of the same patient taken after a 3-h interval shows persistence of the same distended loops. This finding is suggestive, although not pathognomonic, of intestinal ischemia. The patient underwent urgent surgery because peritoneal signs were present. Necrosis of 70 cm of the ileum associated with a thrombosis of the superior mesenteric artery was diagnosed.

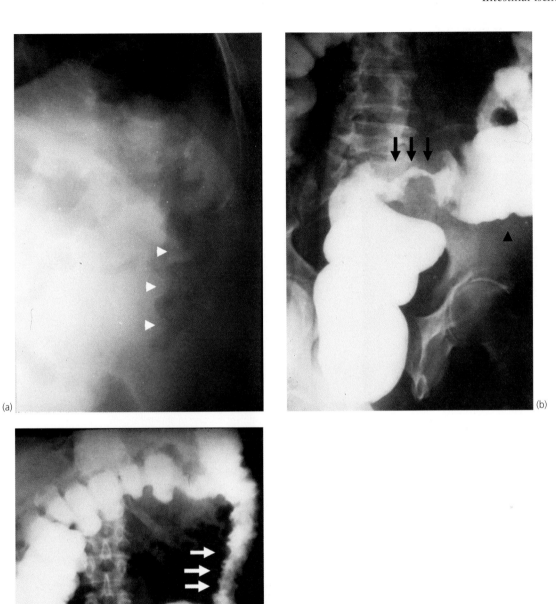

(a)

(b)

(c)

Figure 83.7 Patient with a sigmoid stricturing neoplasm with distention of the proximal colon and secondary ischemic lesions. **(a)** Thumbprinting, a characteristic radiological feature of ischemic colitis, is observed in the descending colon (arrowheads). Projections of the intestinal wall toward the intestinal lumen result from edema or hemorrhage. **(b)** Barium enema examination discloses the stricturing sigmoid neoplasm (arrows) and proximal distention (arrowhead). **(c)** Thumbprinting lesions on the wall of the ascending colon are confirmed by the barium study (arrows).

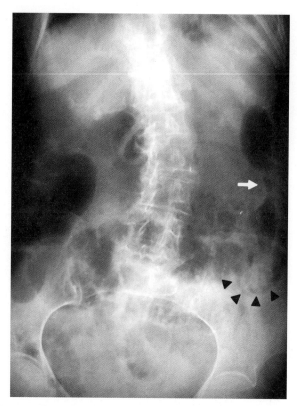

Figure 83.8 A 75-year-old woman with ischemic colitis. Intramural air (pneumatosis) is present in the lower part of the descending colon (arrowheads). There is tapering of the lumen in the midportion of the descending colon (arrow).

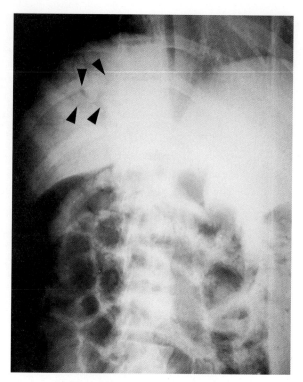

Figure 83.9 A 53-year-old man with atrial fibrillation who came to the emergency department because of abdominal pain. Plain abdominal radiograph shows a generalized dilation of the small and large intestine and presence of gas in the portal branches (arrowheads). Arteriography demonstrated an embolus lodged in the superior mesenteric artery. At surgery, lesions of transmural bowel necrosis affecting the distal ileum and right colon were observed.

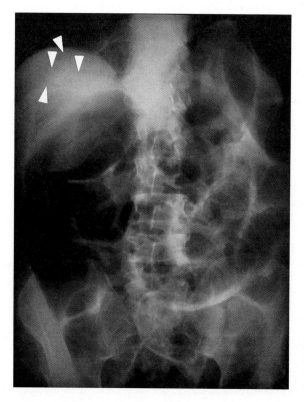

Figure 83.10 A 72-year-old man with superior mesenteric artery ischemia caused by thrombosis. The plain abdominal radiograph demonstrated a marked dilation of the colon and small intestine, along with presence of gas in intrahepatic branches of the portal vein (arrowheads).

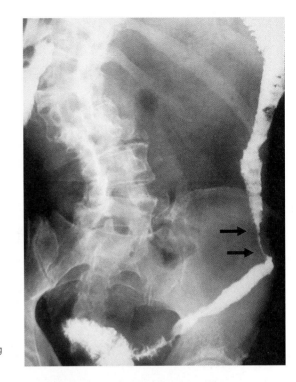

Figure 83.11 Barium enema of a 76-year-old woman who had suffered ischemic colitis, resolved with conservative measures. The patient had episodes of left-sided abdominal pain that were relieved by defecation. Barium enema was performed 2 months after the ischemic episode and revealed a stricturing lesion in the descending colon that corresponds with the location of the ischemic region (arrows).

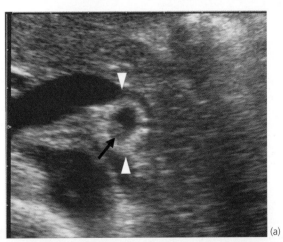

(a)

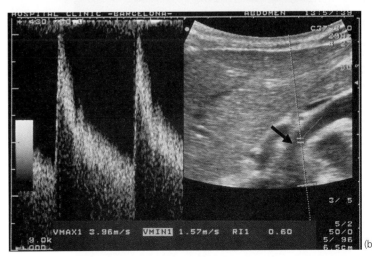

(b)

Figure 83.12 Ultrasound examination in a patient with celiac artery occlusion and superior mesenteric artery (SMA) stenosis. **(a)** Gray-scale ultrasound showing a partial thrombus at the origin of the SMA (arrowheads) occluding 50% of the arterial lumen (arrow shows thrombus). **(b)** Pulsed Doppler study of the SMA origin in the same patient. **Left half** reveals a very high peak systolic velocity (3.84 m/s) resulting from the SMA stenosis (**right half,** arrow).

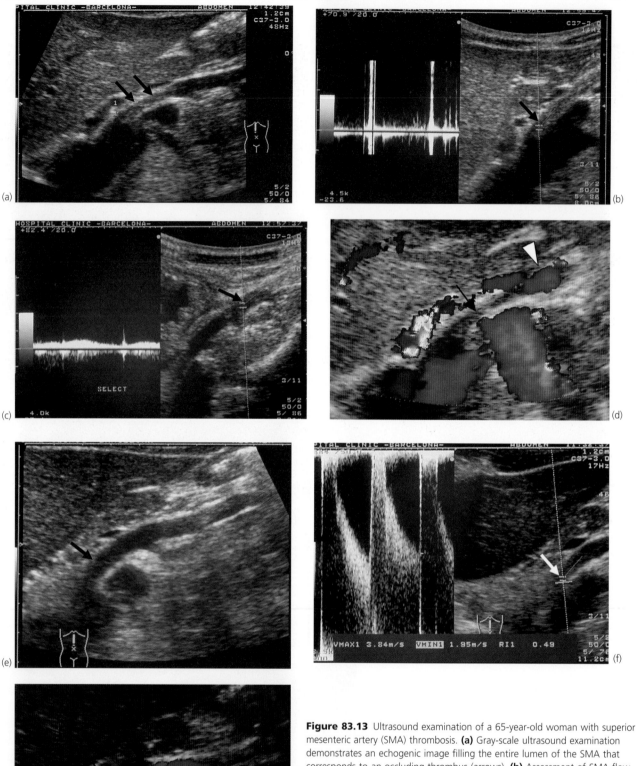

Figure 83.13 Ultrasound examination of a 65-year-old woman with superior mesenteric artery (SMA) thrombosis. **(a)** Gray-scale ultrasound examination demonstrates an echogenic image filling the entire lumen of the SMA that corresponds to an occluding thrombus (arrows). **(b)** Assessment of SMA flow by pulsed Doppler reveals absence of flow **(left half)** in the thrombosed area (arrow). **(c)** A low flow is detected in more distal branches (arrow); arteriography examinations demonstrated distal filling from the celiac axis through the pancreaticoduodenal branches. **(d)** Color Doppler ultrasound confirms the absence of flow signal in the thrombosed area (arrow), along with presence of flow in the more distal segment (arrowhead). **(e)** Ultrasound examination of the same patient following percutaneous angioplasty. The echogenic signal in the lumen of the SMA has disappeared (arrow). **(f)** Doppler ultrasound demonstrates pulsatile flow **(left half)** in the region previously thrombosed (arrow). **(g)** Color Doppler also confirms patency of the SMA (arrows), with normal caliber of the vessel.

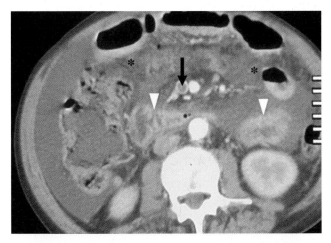

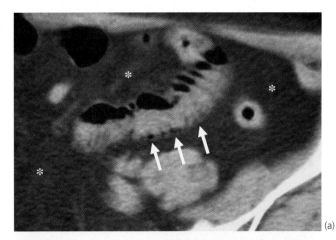

(a)

Figure 83.14 Contrast-enhanced computed tomography (CT) scan of the abdomen in a patient with acute pancreatitis and mesenteric venous thrombosis. CT scan shows mural thickening of small bowel loops (arrowheads) and a hypoattenuating thrombus of the superior mesenteric vein (arrow). Ascites is also present (asterisks).

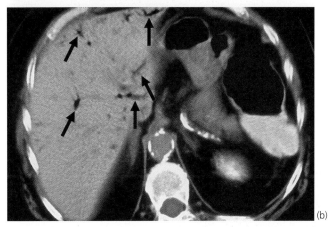

(b)

Figure 83.16 Contrast-enhanced computed tomography (CT) scan in a 72-year-old man with intestinal infarction caused by a superior mesenteric artery embolus. **(a)** Intestinal pneumatosis (arrows) and extensive infiltration of the mesentery (asterisks) are present. **(b)** CT scan obtained at an upper level shows presence of gas in numerous portal branches (arrows).

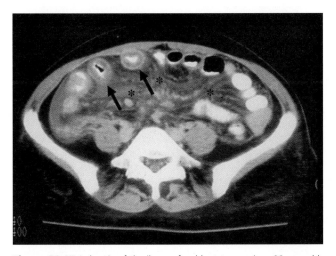

Figure 83.15 Ischemia of the ileum after blunt trauma in a 66-year-old woman. Contrast-enhanced computed tomography scan shows bowel wall thickening (arrows) in the ileum with diffuse mesenteric haziness caused by edema (asterisks).

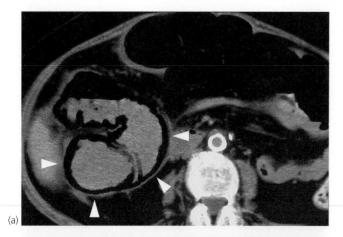

(a)

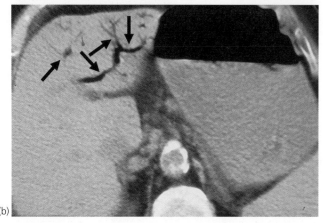

(b)

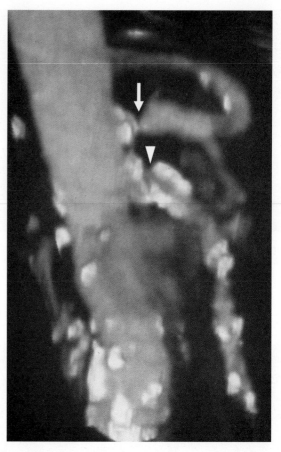

Figure 83.17 Severe ischemic colitis in a patient with septic shock.
(a) Transverse computed tomography scan shows extensive pneumatosis
in the colonic wall (arrowheads). **(b)** Transverse section obtained at an
upper level shows the presence of portal venous gas (arrows).

Figure 83.18 Lateral computed tomography angiogram of a 81-year-
old patient with chronic intestinal ischemia. Calcified atheromatous
plaques are widely distributed in the wall of the aorta, celiac axis, and
superior mesenteric artery. A 95% reduction of the lumen of the origin
of the celiac axis is observed (arrow), along with a 60% decrease in the
lumen of the proximal superior mesenteric artery (arrowhead).

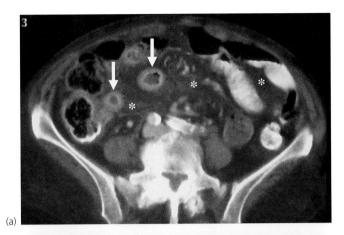

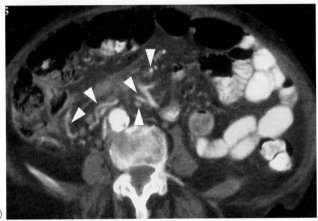

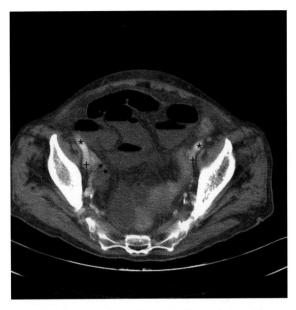

Figure 83.20 Contrast-enhanced computed tomography, axial projection. Contrast is present in the iliac arteries (*) and veins (+), whereas the walls of the dilated intestinal loops remain unenhanced and with air–fluid levels.

Figure 83.19 Contrast-enhanced computed tomography scan in a 72-year-old woman with chronic intestinal ischemia. **(a)** Mural thickening of the ileal intestinal loops (arrows) and regional mesenteric haziness caused by edema (asterisks) are present. **(b)** Abundant collateral circulation through aberrant vessels (arrowheads) is observed in this image obtained at an upper level. Angiogram (not shown) demonstrated complete occlusion of the celiac axis and an 80% occlusion of the superior mesenteric artery.

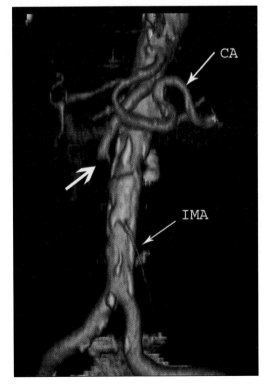

Figure 83.21 Volume-rendered three-dimensional computed tomography image of abdominal aorta in frontal projection showing occlusion of the superior mesenteric artery (thick arrow) with patency of the celiac axis (CA) and inferior mesenteric artery (IMA).

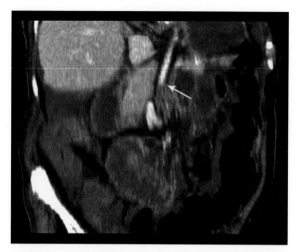

Figure 83.22 Contrast-enhanced computed tomography (multiplanar reconstruction). Oblique projection showing embolic occlusion of the superior mesenteric artery (SMA) (arrow).

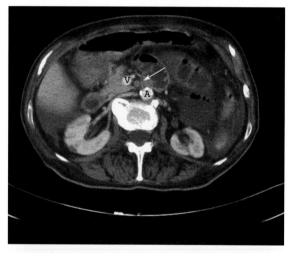

Figure 83.23 Axial contrast-enhanced computed tomography. Thrombosed (unenhanced) mesenteric artery (arrow) in the presence of a well-perfused aorta (A) and mesenteric vein (V).

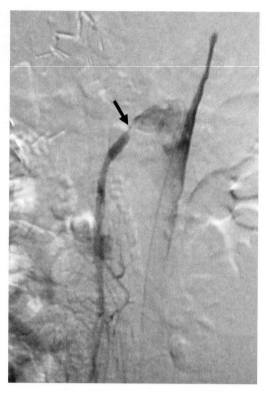

Figure 83.24 Arteriography of the superior mesenteric artery in a 59-year-old man with chronic abdominal pain. Selective injection demonstrates a 90% proximal stenosis (arrow) with poor filling of the distal branches.

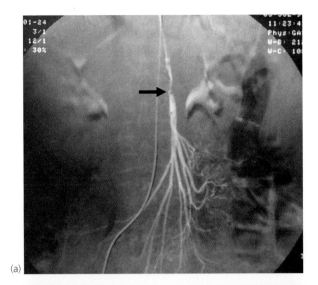

(a)

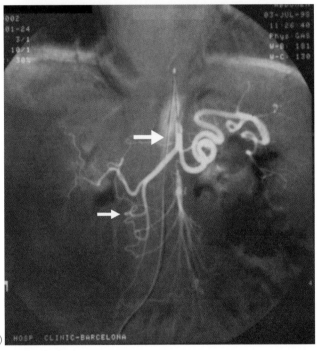

(b)

Figure 83.25 (a) Selective digital subtraction angiography (DSA) of the superior mesenteric artery (SMA) showing a long and high-grade stenosis of the proximal artery (arrow). **(b)** DSA injection of the celiac axis (thick arrow) in the same patient demonstrating collateral filling of the distal SMA through pancreaticoduodenal collaterals (thin arrow).

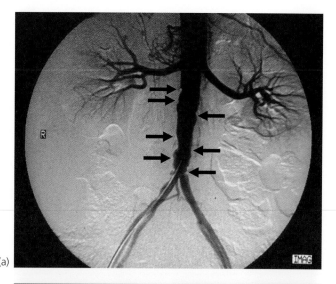

(a)

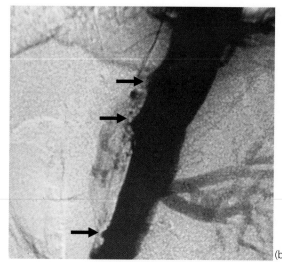

(b)

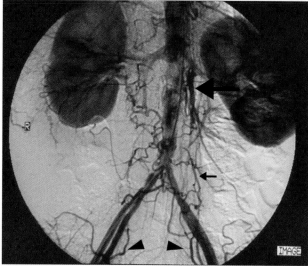

(c)

Figure 83.26 A 66-year-old man with long-standing postprandial abdominal pain and significant weight loss. **(a)** Aortography shows diffuse atheromatous lesions in the abdominal aorta (arrows). **(b)** The three mesenteric vessels (celiac axis, superior mesenteric artery, and inferior mesenteric artery) have a proximal thrombotic occlusion (arrows).
(c) Profuse collateral circulation fills the superior mesenteric artery (thick arrow) and inferior mesenteric artery (thin arrow) through the hypogastric vessels (arrowheads).

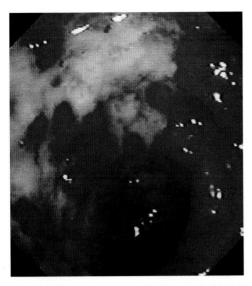

Figure 83.27 An 83-year-old woman who presented with abdominal pain and bloody diarrhea. Colonoscopy revealed the presence of large ulcerations in the splenic flexure. Biopsies were compatible with the diagnosis of ischemic colitis. This region is commonly affected in colonic ischemia because of its relatively low perfusion (watershed area). Colonoscopy is the method of choice for the diagnosis of ischemic colitis, because it allows direct visualization of the mucosa and tissue sampling.

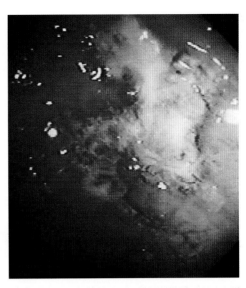

Figure 83.29 Endoscopic findings in a 62-year-old woman with ischemic colitis associated with a low-flow state (sepsis). The mucosa of the affected segment appears edematous, hemorrhagic, friable, and ulcerated.

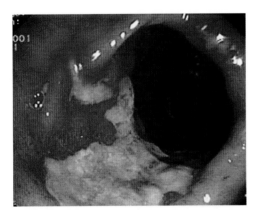

Figure 83.28 Large ulceration in the sigmoid region caused by ischemia. The sigmoid colon is another area that is particularly susceptible to ischemic lesions because of its relatively low perfusion. Although this lesion can be reached by sigmoidoscopy, complete colonoscopy should be performed in patients suspected of having ischemic colitis because 50% of the ischemic lesions are proximal to the sigmoid colon.

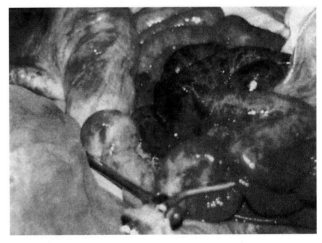

Figure 83.30 Gross findings at laparotomy in a patient with nonocclusive mesenteric ischemia. Although the bowel wall is mottled, it remains viable. The patient had undergone angiography and vasodilator infusion, but irreversible bowel necrosis had already occurred, necessitating laparotomy and resection.

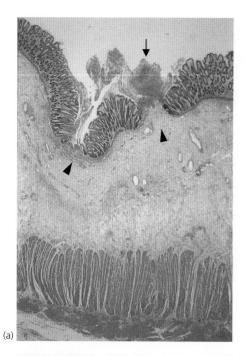

(a)

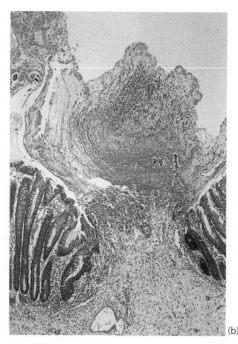

(b)

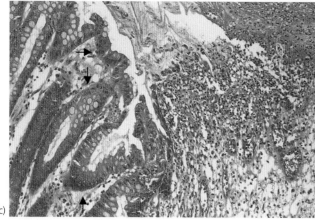

(c)

Figure 83.31 Early stages of intestinal ischemic damage. **(a)** There are two well-delimited erosions of the mucosa (arrowheads), with formation of a pseudomembrane (arrow). The remaining mucosa is normal. The submucosa has a marked edema and discrete infiltration by inflammatory cells. **(b)** Close-up view of the pseudomembrane composed of fibrin and leukocytes. **(c)** Detail of inflammatory cell infiltration at the erosion site. At this magnification, reactive changes in the mucosal epithelium can be observed (arrows).

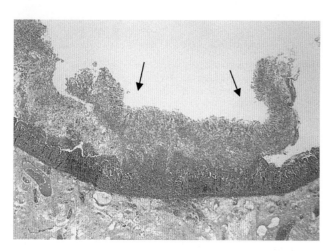

Figure 83.32 More extensive ischemic damage with formation of a surface exudate (arrows). There is vascular congestion and the presence of an inflammatory infiltrate in the lamina propria, and edema of the submucosa.

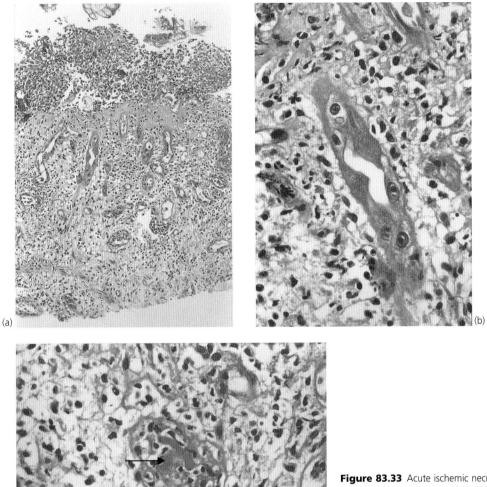

(a)

(b)

(c)

Figure 83.33 Acute ischemic necrosis. This illustrates a more advanced stage of ischemic damage. **(a)** Villi have completely disappeared and are replaced by a membrane composed of fibrinous exudate, necrotic epithelial cells, and inflammatory cells. **(b)** The crypts are severely affected and only the most basal parts have survived; at higher magnification reactive changes can be observed in the remaining portions of the crypts. **(c)** A fibrin thrombus in one of the submucosal small vessels (arrow).

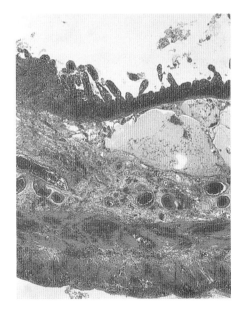

Figure 83.34 Transmural hemorrhagic necrosis in a patient with superior mesenteric vein thrombosis. The mucosa, submucosa, and muscularis have congestive dilated vessels, and extravasated red cells infiltrating the tissue. There is marked edema of the submucosa and muscularis propria layers.

84

Radiation injury in the gastrointestinal tract

Steven M. Cohn, Stephen J. Bickston

The gastroenterologist will continue to encounter and treat patients with gastrointestinal or hepatic complications resulting from the therapeutic use of ionizing radiation. The histopathological analysis of tissue specimens can often aid in establishing the diagnosis and excluding other etiologies for a patient's symptoms. The histological appearance of lesions observed in tissue specimens is often characteristic of acute or delayed radiation injury. However, no individual histological feature is pathognomonic for radiation-induced damage. Therefore, histological findings may mimic other pathological conditions and must be interpreted carefully within the appropriate clinical context for a given patient. Patients may present with acute symptoms days or weeks after radiation therapy is initiated or with delayed clinical syndromes that may occur years after therapy. The early effects primarily involve the mucosa, which is lined by rapidly proliferating epithelial cells that are sensitive to the acute effects of radiation injury. Clinical symptoms include odynophagia, diarrhea, nausea, vomiting, or gastrointestinal bleeding; the symptoms depend on the location of the radiation field, the dose of irradiation, and the fractionation schedule. The delayed effects of therapeutic irradiation are more likely to present with chronic diarrhea, fibrosis, ulcer formation, or bleeding, and are thought to be secondary to damage to the vasculature of the organs involved. The figures that follow illustrate selected histopathological features of acute and chronic radiation injury in the gastrointestinal tract and liver.

The histopathological features of acute radiation injury are dominated by evidence of acute injury to the mucosa. Apoptosis of lamina propria lymphocytes and epithelial cells and the cessation of epithelial cell replication occur within hours of a radiation dose. Mature, differentiated epithelial cells continue to be lost in the absence of replacement by replication of the progenitor cells within these epithelia, resulting in the subsequent loss of mucosal function. Acute diarrhea may result under these circumstances. Mucosal and submucosal edema may also be observed within the radiation field as a result of endothelial dysfunction.

Specimens from patients with acute hepatic injury secondary to therapeutic irradiation for solid neoplasms are rarely obtained. However, venoocclusive disease is not uncommon in bone marrow transplant patients following cytoreductive therapy with combined chemotherapy and irradiation (see below). Onset of venoocclusive disease in this setting usually occurs before 5 weeks posttransplant. Changes in hepatic histology include vascular congestion that is most prominent in centrilobular areas, subendothelial edema, endothelial destruction, sinusoidal dilation, and centrizonal hepatocyte necrosis with attenuation of the hepatocellular cords.

Evidence of vascular injury and regeneration is a hallmark of chronic radiation injury and is often observed in pathological specimens. Myointimal proliferation in medium-sized muscular arteries may lead to chronic ischemic injury and ulceration caused by the marked decrease in the luminal diameter of these vessels. The presence of lipophages or foamy macrophages in the intima of small arterioles is also a characteristic finding of delayed radiation injury, although these lesions may also result from other etiologies. Telangiectatic vessels in the lamina propria or submucosa are another frequent finding and account for the diffuse bleeding sometimes observed in radiation enteritis. Sclerosis or medial fibrosis indicative of healing vasculitic lesions may also be observed.

Changes in the mucosa and submucosa are also frequently observed in chronic radiation injury and are thought to be secondary to the chronic vascular changes described above. Cellular atypia may be observed in the epithelium lining any region of the alimentary tract that was within the radiation field. Mucosal atrophy resulting in impaired mucosal function is also sometimes observed. Fibrosis may be confined to the submucosa or extend through the muscularis propria and accounts for luminal strictures seen in chronic radiation injury. These strictures may occur within any irradiated region of the alimentary tract. The appearance of these fibrotic lesions in the small intestine may resemble that of Crohn's disease both on gross inspection and on radiological examination, although fistulae and creeping fat are rarely observed.

Atlas of Gastroenterology, 4th edition. Edited by Tadataka Yamada, David H. Alpers, Anthony N. Kalloo, Neil Kaplowitz, Chung Owyang, and Don W. Powell. © 2009 Blackwell Publishing, ISBN: 978-1-4051-6909-7

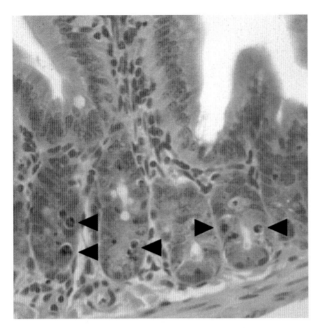

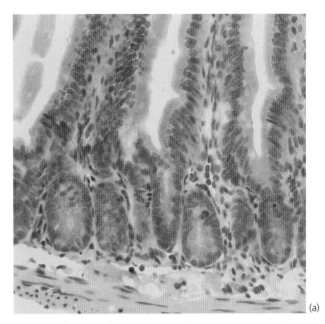

(a)

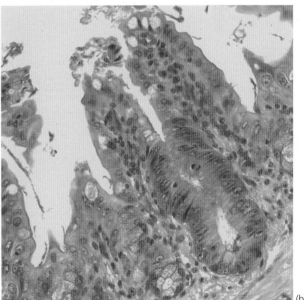

(b)

Figure 84.1 Acute radiation injury 6 h after 8 Gy γ-irradiation. Apoptotic cells (programmed cell death; arrowheads) appear within the small intestinal crypt epithelium by 3–6 h after irradiation (FVB/N inbred mouse strain; H & E stain; original magnification × 200). The remaining crypt epithelial cells undergo cell cycle arrest and migrate onto the villi, depleting the crypt of cells over the next 24 h. This experimental sample is from the laboratory mouse because tissue is rarely obtained during this time frame after irradiation in humans.

Figure 84.2 Acute radiation injury 3 days after 14 Gy γ-irradiation. **(a)** The architecture of normal epithelium in the adult mouse small intestine. **(b)** The histological features found in the small intestine 3 days after irradiation. Note the marked shortening of the intestinal villi, which results from cessation of crypt epithelial replication and lack of replacement of villous epithelial cells after irradiation. The loss of differentiated epithelial cells associated with villous blunting can result in impaired mucosal absorptive function. Expanded regenerative crypts first appear at this time and are composed of rapidly proliferating basophilic cells that are somewhat larger than those found in normal uninjured crypts (H & E stain; original magnification × 400). As in Figure 84.1, this experimental sample was obtained from the laboratory mouse to illustrate the regenerative process after irradiation because tissue is rarely obtained during this time frame after irradiation in humans.

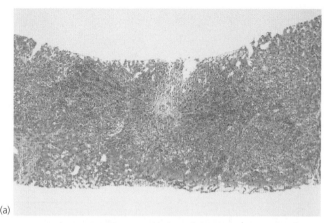

(a)

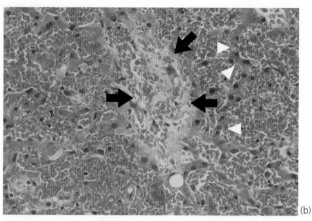

(b)

Figure 84.3 Hepatic venoocclusive disease occurring in a 24-year-old woman after cytoreductive therapy for bone marrow transplantation with combined chemotherapy and irradiation. **(a)** A low-power view of a core biopsy that shows sinusoidal congestion with increased numbers of red blood cells in the centrolobar region (H & E stain; original magnification

× 40). Courtesy of Dr Christopher Moskaluk. **(b)** A higher-power view of the same biopsy that demonstrates fibrinous deposits in a central vein (arrows), atrophy of the hepatic cords (arrowheads), and congestion of the sinusoids, which are packed with red blood cells (H & E stain; original magnification × 200). Courtesy of Dr Christopher Moskaluk.

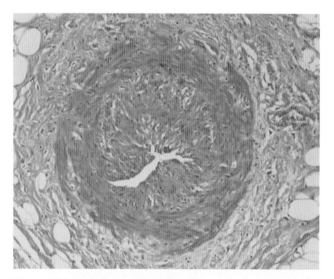

Figure 84.4 Myointimal proliferation nearly occludes the lumen of a moderate-sized mesenteric artery. This process usually occurs over several years after radiation injury and may lead to chronic ischemic injury caused by the marked decrease in the lumenal diameter of these vessels. Ulceration of the overlying mucosa can occur in areas of localized ischemia (H & E stain; original magnification × 100). Courtesy of Dr Christopher Moskaluk.

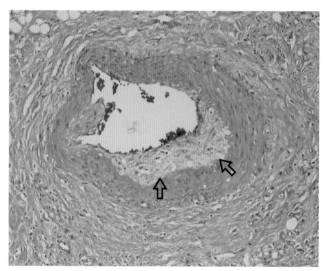

Figure 84.5 Intimal lipophage accumulation in intestinal arteriole following irradiation. These foam cells (arrows) may be seen in the intima of small arteries and arterioles of the intestine several years after irradiation, and may contribute to lumenal narrowing of these vessels and subsequent ischemic injury to the mucosa (H & E stain; original magnification × 100). Courtesy of Dr Christopher Moskaluk.

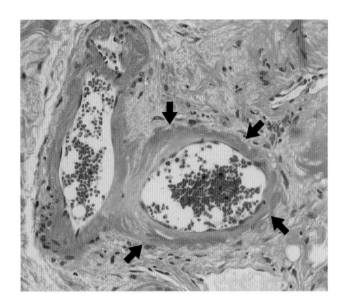

Figure 84.6 Radiation-induced sclerosis of small- to medium-sized blood vessels in the mesenteric vasculature. Sclerosis or medial fibrosis is a histological feature associated with healing vasculitic lesions. Note the hyalinization of the vessel walls (arrows) with prominent vascular ectasia (H & E stain; original magnification × 200). Courtesy of Dr Christopher Moskaluk.

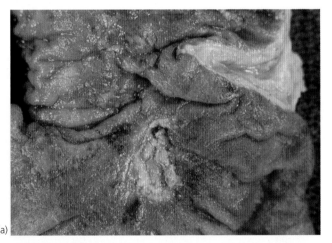

(a)

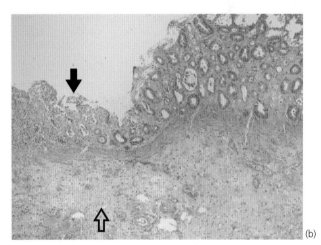

(b)

Figure 84.7 Radiation-induced ulceration in the colon. **(a)** The gross appearance of a well-demarcated ulcer present in the rectum years after external radiation for an adjacent neoplasm. **(b)** The histological appearance with chronic ulceration, mucosal necrosis similar to that seen in ischemic injury (closed arrow), and dense submucosal fibrosis (open arrow). The fibrosis may be confined to the submucosa or extend through the muscularis propria, and accounts for the thickening or strictures noted on gross examination. These strictures may occur within any irradiated region of the alimentary tract. The lesion is notable because of the absence of a prominent inflammatory infiltrate (H & E stain; original magnification × 20). Courtesy of Dr Christopher Moskaluk.

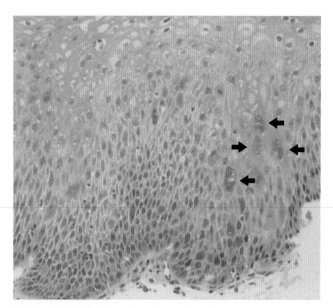

Figure 84.8 Epithelial atypia in the esophagus secondary to chronic radiation injury. Note the presence of enlarged atypical nuclei with irregular nuclear contours (arrows). Hyperchromasia of these atypical cells is rare in contrast to the cellular atypia that is characteristic of neoplastic processes and is an important histological feature distinguishing these two processes (H & E stain; original magnification × 800). Courtesy of Dr Christopher Moskaluk.

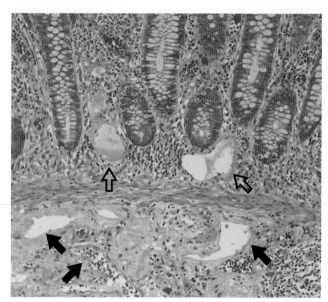

Figure 84.10 Telangiectasias are frequently observed in delayed radiation injury. Dilated venules and lymphatic channels may be seen in the lamina propria (open arrows) or in the submucosa (solid arrows) underlying relatively normal appearing colonic epithelium. These lesions likely account for the diffuse bleeding sometimes observed in chronic radiation enteritis (H & E stain; original magnification × 40). Courtesy of Dr Christopher Moskaluk.

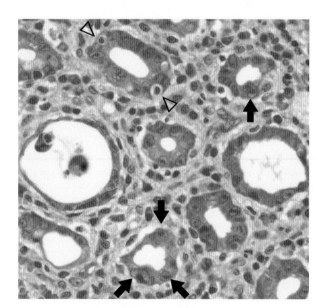

Figure 84.9 Epithelial alterations in the colon secondary to chronic radiation injury. Note the cells with enlarged irregular nuclei with prominent nucleoli (arrows). As in the esophagus in Figure 84.8, the epithelial cellular atypia characteristic of chronic radiation injury is not associated with the nuclear hyperchromasia that is commonly observed in atypia associated with neoplastic processes. Apoptotic cells are noted in some glands (arrowheads). Atrophic glands with flattened and sloughing epithelial cells are also prominent (H & E stain; original magnification × 400). Courtesy of Dr Christopher Moskaluk.

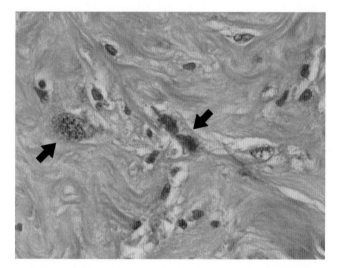

Figure 84.11 Atypical fibroblasts in radiation injury. Bizarre appearing fibroblasts with large pyknotic nuclei (arrows) are frequently seen in delayed phase of radiation injury in the alimentary tract. Although these atypical fibroblasts are frequently observed, their presence is not specific for radiation injury (H & E stain; original magnification × 400). Courtesy of Dr Christopher Moskaluk.

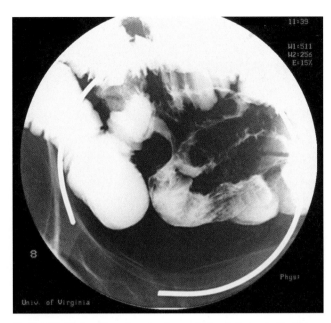

Figure 84.12 Small bowel spot radiograph of radiation enteritis. String-like stricturing and separation of bowel loops seen may give an appearance of Crohn's disease. Courtesy of Dr H. Shaffer.

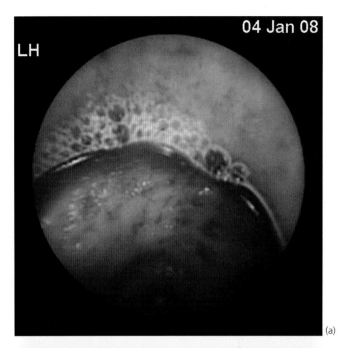
(a)

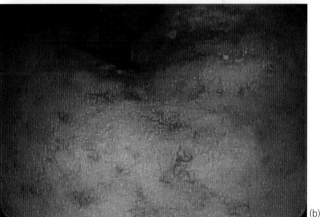
(b)

Figure 84.13 Endoscopic appearance of mucosal radiation damage. **(a)** Endoscopic image of radiation proctitis. Note the mucosal telangiectasias. **(b)** Capsule endoscopic image of the small intestine showing telangiectasia. Courtesy of Dr G.S. Raju, Galveston, TX.

85

Upper gastrointestinal endoscopy

Field F. Willingham, William R. Brugge

The father of modern endoscopy is Rudolf Schindler. He pioneered the use of gastroscopy through the use and development of a semi-rigid gastroscope. The first endoscope, of a kind, was developed in 1806 by Philip Bozzini with his introduction of a "Lichtleiter" (light conductor) "for the examinations of the canals and cavities of the human body." However, the Vienna Medical Society disapproved of such curiosity. Apparently an endoscope was first introduced into a human in 1853. The use of electric light was a major step in the improvement of endoscopy. The first such lights were external. Later, smaller bulbs became available, making internal light possible. Jacobeus has been given credit for early endoscopic explorations of the abdomen and the thorax with laparoscopy (1912) and thoracoscopy (1910). For diagnostic endoscopy, Basil Hirschowitz invented a superior glass fiber for flexible endoscopes. The technology resulted in not only the first useful medical endoscope, but the invention revolutionized other endoscopic uses and led to practical fiberoptics.

Technical considerations

Upper gastrointestinal endoscopy is a highly technical procedure that requires a close cooperative arrangement between physicians and nurses. A well-organized facility will optimize patient safety and the ability to provide the appropriate techniques. With only a few exceptions, upper GI endoscopy will be performed in a hospital or a medical care facility that can provide a reliable set of highly trained personnel and specialized equipment. In addition to a wide array of endoscopes and processors, the procedure unit should be equipped with an organized set of accessories used during endoscopy.

In addition to procedure rooms, it is critical to have a travel cart that will enable endoscopists to provide endoscopic procedures at sites remote from an endoscopy unit.

Atlas of Gastroenterology, 4th edition. Edited by Tadataka Yamada, David H. Alpers, Anthony N. Kalloo, Neil Kaplowitz, Chung Owyang, and Don W. Powell. © 2009 Blackwell Publishing, ISBN: 978-1-4051-6909-7

Well-maintained, controlled access storage is essential for the endoscopic accessories. There must be a well-designed area for endoscope disinfection and preparation of accessories for sterilization. It is also critical to have preparation and recovery areas for the evaluation and monitoring of patients.

Electrocautery devices are critical to the performance of many endoscopic procedures. In many units, the devices are not installed in each procedure room. Since these devices are frequently used, it is critical that they be readily available during procedures and properly maintained by qualified personnel.

Videoendoscopes

Videoendoscopy, introduced in the mid-1980s, has dramatically improved and expanded the field of endoscopy. Videoendoscopy is now used almost universally. The endoscopic image is generated electronically using a charge-coupled device (CCD) located in the tip of the endoscope. Endoscope processors manage the images and display them on video monitors. Prior to video endoscopy, fiberoptics generated the images on small hand-held eye pieces.

The first videoendoscopes used black and white CCDs that required a color wheel. Green, red, or blue light was sequentially sent down the illumination bundle of the endoscope and activated the CCD at the tip. A color image was reconstructed using the three sets of images generated by the colored lights. The videoprocessor displayed a full-color image of the gastrointestinal tract lining, although with apparent image flickering during rapid movement. Most current videoendoscopes use a color CCD that obtains the image in color on the tip of the endoscope. These devices provide 30 000–850 000 pixels of resolution. By incorporating high-pixel density charged-coupled devices, high-resolution endoscopes provide images that display vivid mucosal detail. High-resolution endoscopes are capable of discriminating objects 10–70 microns in diameter, compared to the naked eye, which is capable of discriminating objects 125–165 microns in diameter. The videoendoscope has controls for air, water, and suction; knobs for up-and-down and right-and-left bending of the tip. The instrument channel is shared for the passage of accessories and suction. There are also buttons on the videoendoscope control handle to activate digital video recording, image capture and recording video images.

Video endoscopy has greatly expanded the viewing capabilities of procedures. Multiple monitors in the procedure room provide bright vivid images that enable many procedure personnel to participate in procedures. The live video images can also be distributed remotely to sites within an institution or to remote sites for teaching, research, and demonstration. The teaching, instruction, and training of endoscopy has improved dramatically with the use of video endoscopy. Documentation of procedures is provided by the saving, retrieval, and reviewing of stored digital images. Stored images can be recalled from a central image storage system and sent to any location in the endoscopy service. The storage drives can be used for image processing and management as well as a reliable storage of endoscopic images and information on PACS (picture archiving and communication system). The hardware and software are now available for the capture, editing, and storage of video clips. This type of material will further improve teaching and patient care.

Introducing the endoscope

Most small-diameter videoendoscopes can be easily passed under direct vision through the upper esophageal sphincter.

The tip of the instrument is advanced in the midline into the direction of the closed cricopharyngeal sphincter. The patient is asked to swallow, and under direct vision the tip of the instrument is passed from the epiglottis and larynx into the proximal esophagus. In the past, endoscopes were passed blindly aided by the swallowing action. The direct vision technique allows an inspection of the pharynx, epiglottis, and vocal cords prior to insertion. Furthermore, direct imaging may decrease the risk of the inadvertent passage of the endoscope into a proximal esophageal diverticulum. Small-diameter videoendoscopes can also be passed transnasally and may provide the opportunity to perform unsedated endoscopy.

Endoscopes are designed with the endoscopic controls (e.g., air, water, and suction valves; tip direction wheels) to be controlled with the left hand. The right hand is used to advance the instrument and use the tip control knob. Torque of the endoscope is accomplished by rotating the instrument control handle with the right hand, which results in rotation of the entire shaft and tip of the endoscope. A central instrument channel is used for a wide variety of devices and accessories. The instrument channel is variable in diameter and there may be two instrument channels in some instruments.

Upper gastrointestinal endoscopy is the basis for many of the diagnostic and therapeutic procedures offered by endoscopists and gastroenterologists. Identification of normal mucosa and normal endoscopic anatomy is critical for determining what is abnormal. This chapter demonstrates normal and pathological endoscopic findings in the esophagus, stomach, and duodenum.

Figure 85.1 Normal distal esophagus. The impression of the vertebral column can be seen in the inferior aspect.

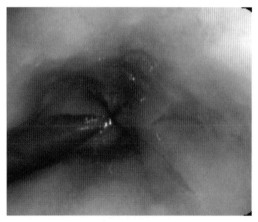

Figure 85.2 Normal distal esophagus and lower esophageal sphincter.

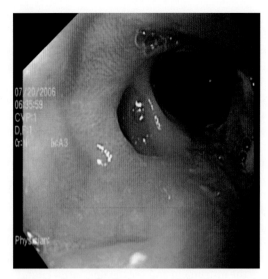

Figure 85.3 Esophageal diverticulum. A small diverticulum can be seen on the left in the distal esophagus.

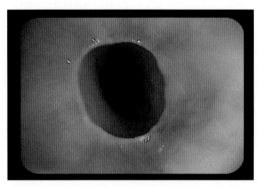

Figure 85.4 A Schatzki ring can be appreciated here in the distal esophagus. The junction between the squamous mucosa of the esophagus and the columnar mucosa of the stomach occurs in the vicinity of the ring.

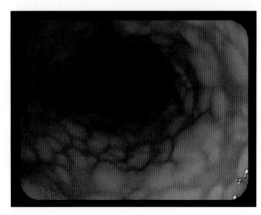

Figure 85.5 Diffuse glycogenic acanthosis. These white nodules represent esophageal glycogenic acanthosis which is usually sparse and of little clinical significance. This patient has Cowden syndrome, with a marked diffuse presentation.

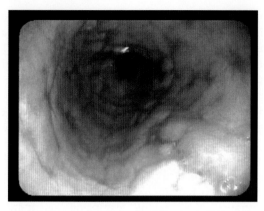

Figure 85.6 Reflux esophagitis. Savary–Miller Grade III (circumferential lesion, erosive or exudative) reflux type esophagitis can be seen in this image. Multiple erosions in the lower third of the esophagus can be seen in this image.

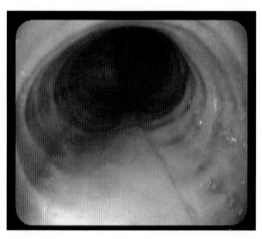

Figure 85.7 Feline esophagus refers to the endoscopic finding of a fine stacked concentric ring appearance in the esophagus. Feline esophagus is suggestive of eosinophilic esophagitis, which was proven by biopsy in this 36-year-old man.

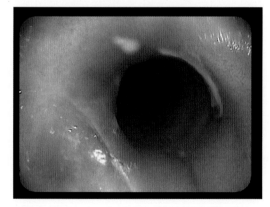

Figure 85.8 Endoscopic view of a benign appearing intrinsic esophageal stenosis in a patient with a history of photodynamic therapy for Barrett esophagus.

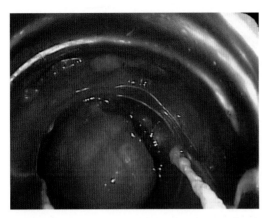

Figure 85.9 Endoscopic mucosal resection. A nodule was found in a region of Barrett esophagus with known high-grade dysplasia. The nodule is being removed here with an endoscopic mucosal resection. Pathological examination revealed intramucosal adenocarcinoma.

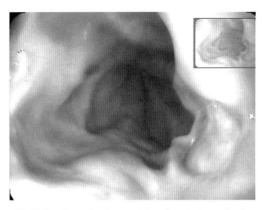

Figure 85.12 Esophageal varices post banding. Endoscopic appearance of esophageal varices healing after banding. One persistent varix column can be seen inferiorly. Scarred obliterated varices can be seen distally. At the lower right, a healing site of prior banding can be seen. With serial banding, all the varices will be obliterated.

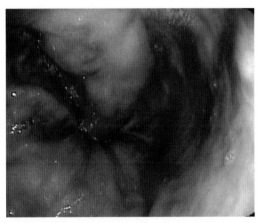

Figure 85.10 Esophageal varices. Endoscopic image of large esophageal varices in a patient who presented with hematemesis. The patient had a history of liver injury secondary to the use of Chinese herbal supplements.

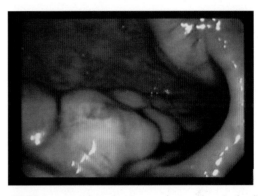

Figure 85.13 Large esophageal varices can be seen here in the distal esophagus. At approximately 7 o'clock, a fibrin cap overlies the varix and may have been the source of the bleeding.

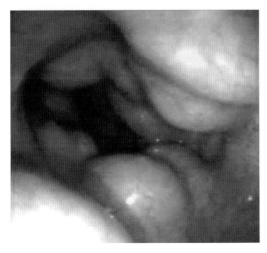

Figure 85.11 In a patient presenting with dysphagia, multiple submucosal masses were discovered on endoscopy. These masses were esophageal leiomyomata.

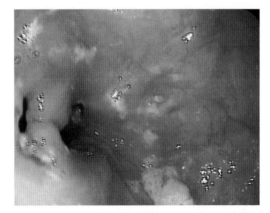

Figure 85.14 In this image, an esophageal perforation with fistula can be seen. This patient had squamous cell carcinoma of the lung invasive to the esophagus.

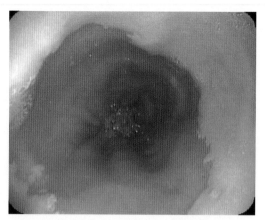

Figure 85.15 This image demonstrates the characteristic salmon pink mucosa of Barrett esophagus extending proximally from the gastroesophageal junction. The normal esophageal squamous mucosa is pearly white and can be seen here in the proximal portion of the esophagus.

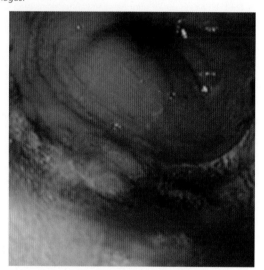

Figure 85.16 Chromoendoscopy involves staining the gastrointestinal mucosa for better endoscopic visualization, usually for the detection of malignant or pre-malignant lesions. In this image, Lugol solution has been used to stain the distal esophaus. Negative staining of nodular mucosa can be seen. Biopsy confirmed Barrett esophagus with mild dysplasia. Courtesy of Dr Moises Guelrud.

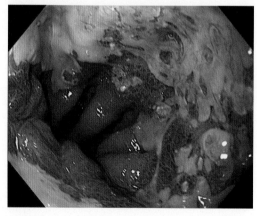

Figure 85.17 Narrow band imaging (NBI) is a high resolution endoscopic technique that may enhance the visualization of the fine vasculature and mucosal morphology. In this patient with Barrett esophagus, high-grade dysplasia, and squamous overgrowth, NBI demonstrates dysmorphic glands and vasculature. Courtesy of Drs Herbert C. Wolfsen and Michael B. Wallace.

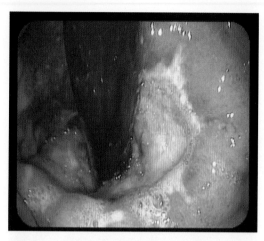

Figure 85.18 Esophageal adenocarcinoma. Endoscopic appearance of an ulcerated gastroesophageal junction mass, which revealed poorly differentiated esophageal adenocarcinoma on biopsy. In this image, the mass can be seen extending from the gastroesophageal junction in a retroflexed view.

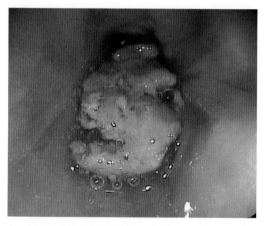

Figure 85.19 Food impaction. Food bolus in the distal esophagus proximal to an esophageal stricture in a patient with Barrett esophagus.

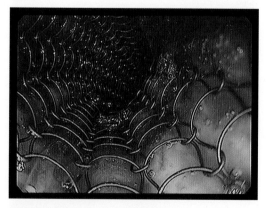

Figure 85.20 Esophageal stent. Metal stent placement for palliation of obstructing gastroesophageal junction adenocarcinoma. The wire mesh of the stent can be seen in this image overlying and compressing a fungating and ulcerated mass.

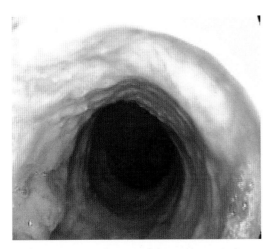

Figure 85.21 Squamous cell cancer of the esophagus. In the midesophagus, an irregular nodular plaque was observed in a patient with a history of alcohol and tobacco use. Biopsies revealed moderately differentiated squamous cell cancer of the esophagus.

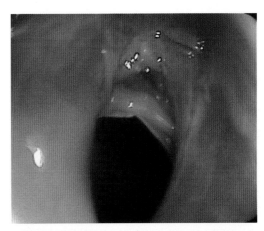

Figure 85.24 Esophageal web. A thin membrane can be seen in the superior aspect of the image. This patient had a cervical esophageal web, which was dilated with passage of the endoscope.

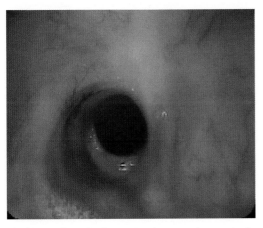

Figure 85.22 Esophageal stricture. A stricture can be seen in the upper esophagus. This patient had a history of esophageal squamous cell cancer, which had been treated with chemotherapy and radiation six years prior to this endoscopy.

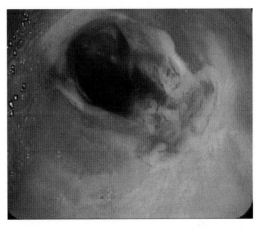

Figure 85.25 Radiation esophagitis. Distal esophageal circumferential ulceration and esophagitis in a patient who had received full-dose radiation therapy for regionally advanced adenocarcinoma.

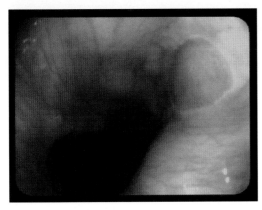

Figure 85.23 Esophageal inlet patch. This lesion in the right superior aspect of the image has the typical appearance of an inlet patch. An inlet patch is an area of heterotopic gastric mucosa, characteristically found in the cervical esophagus.

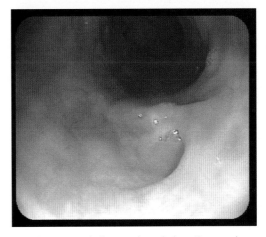

Figure 85.26 Cytomegalovirus esophageal ulcer. Upper endoscopy in a patient with AIDS and dysphagia revealed a distal esophageal ulceration. An immunohistochemical stain for cytomegalovirus was positive.

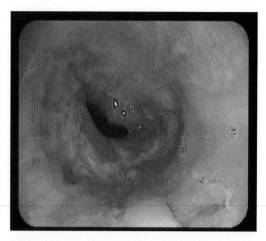

Figure 85.27 Herpetic esophageal ulcer. The earliest manifestation of herpes simplex esophagitis may be vesicular, though this is rarely seen. The herpetic lesions may coalesce. On endoscopy, a well-circumscribed, volcano appearance has been described. In this case, HSV-1 was cultured from esophageal biopsies.

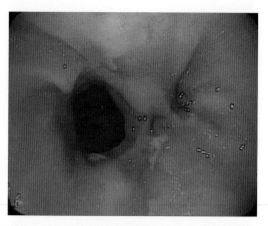

Figure 85.30 This patient had an esophagojejunal anastomosis after gastrectomy for gastric cancer. He presented with dysphagia, and a stricture at the anastomosis can be seen here.

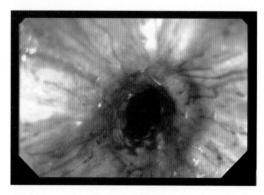

Figure 85.28 Caustic esophagitis. Severe caustic injury to the entire esophagus in a patient with a history of a suicide attempt by alkaline ingestion.

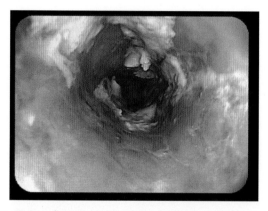

Figure 85.31 Inflammation with thick, white adherent plaques in a patient with AIDS and candidal esophagitis. Fluconazole-sensitive *Candida albicans* was cultured from the esophageal brushing.

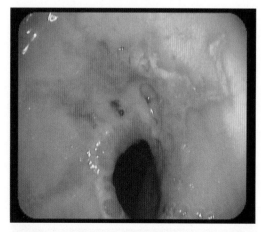

Figure 85.29 Esophagogastric anastomosis. Endoscopic appearance of the esophagogastric anastomosis in a patient who had previously had an Ivor–Lewis esophagectomy for high-grade dysplasia with intramucosal carcinoma arising in an area of Barrett esophagus.

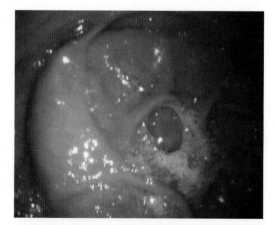

Figure 85.32 Normal gastric body. The appearance of the normal stomach with a prominent splenic impression. A prominent splenic impression may be noted in patients with a low body mass index.

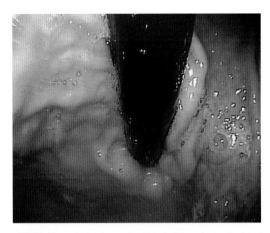

Figure 85.33 Normal gastric cardia. This is the endoscopic view in retroflexion of the normal gastric cardia. The proximal portion of the scope is seen exiting from the gastroesophageal junction.

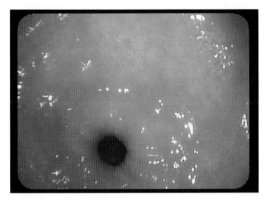

Figure 85.34 Normal gastric antrum. The muscular pylorus is in the lower mid portion of the image.

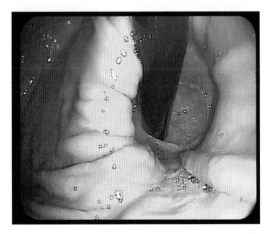

Figure 85.35 Large hiatal hernia. This patient was 86 years old and, on retroflexed view, a large hiatal hernia can be appreciated.

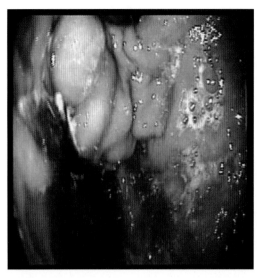

Figure 85.36 Gastric varices. Large gastric varices on retroflexed view of the gastric cardia. This patient had cirrhosis and presented with massive upper gastrointestinal bleeding.

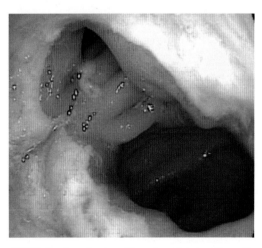

Figure 85.37 Anastomotic ulcer. Circumferential ulceration with overlying fibrinous material at the anastomosis in a patient status post Roux-en-Y gastric bypass surgery. This patient ultimately underwent a redo gastrojejunostomy with ulcer excision.

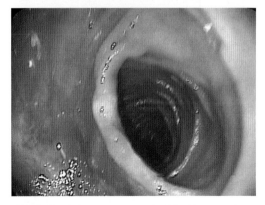

Figure 85.38 Gastric bypass anastomosis. A healthy appearing gastrojejunal anastomosis can be seen here in a woman who underwent a Roux-en-Y gastric bypass for obesity with multiple comorbid conditions.

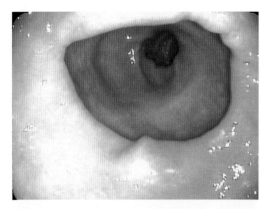

Figure 85.39 This image demonstrates a Bilroth type I anastomosis, where following antrectomy, the duodenum is anastomosed to the proximal stomach. Antrectomy was common in the years prior to antisecretory therapy for peptic ulcer disease.

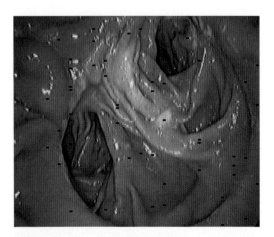

Figure 85.40 This image demonstrates a Bilroth type II anastomosis. In a Bilroth II procedure, a gastrojejunostomy is created. Both the afferent limb (which drains upstream pancreatobiliary secretions) and efferent limb (which allows food and secretions to flow downstream) are visible here.

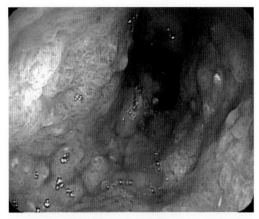

Figure 85.41 This patient with hypoalbuminemia presented with markedly enlarged gastric folds. Biopsies revealed edematous gastric mucosa with foveolar hyperplasia and no evidence of malignancy, confirming Ménétrier disease; however, years later he developed gastric leiomyosarcoma.

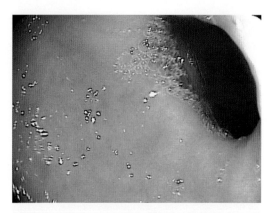

Figure 85.42 This patient had diffuse atrophic gastritis. The image of the antrum reveals thin mucosa with visible submucosal vessels. Biopsy confirmed chronic antral gastritis with marked intestinal metaplasia consistent with atrophic gastritis.

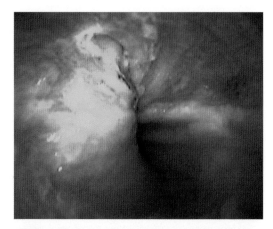

Figure 85.43 Mallory–Weiss tear in a 27-year-old man who presented with emesis followed by hematemesis. Mallory–Weiss tears are longitudinal intramural mucosal lacerations occurring in the distal esophagus and proximal stomach. They are usually associated with forceful retching.

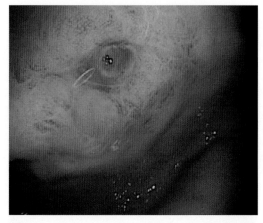

Figure 85.44 A Dieulafoy lesion is an uncommon cause of upper gastrointestinal bleeding, resulting from an aberrant dilated submucosal artery eroding through the mucosa in the absence of a primary ulcer. A large Dieulafoy lesion can be seen here in the gastric body.

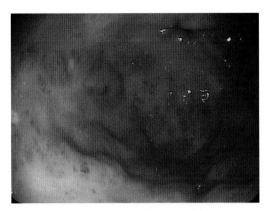

Figure 85.45 Gastric antral vascular ectasia presenting with typical erythematous lesions in the antrum of the stomach. These lesions may require repeated treatments with argon plasma coagulation or electrocautery to prevent recurrent gastrointestinal bleeding.

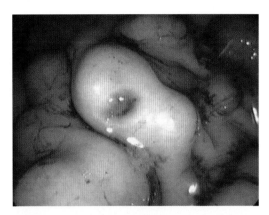

Figure 85.48 In this patient, markedly enlarged gastric folds in the cardia represent gastric varices. Endoscopic ultrasound can confirm the presence of varices if the diagnosis is in question.

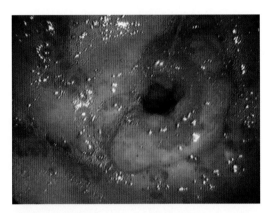

Figure 85.46 Watermelon stomach, another term for gastric antral vascular ectasia (GAVE), refers to the watermelon-like appearance of the antrum in the presence of the striped lines of GAVE. In this patient, multiple bleeding angioectasias can be seen in the gastric antrum. These were treated with argon plasma coagulation with successful hemostasis.

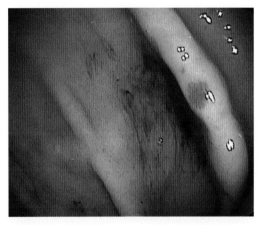

Figure 85.49 Endoscopic appearance of a gastric angioectasia on a rugal fold in the stomach. This patient presented with bleeding, and hematin (altered blood) can be seen adjacent to the angioectasia.

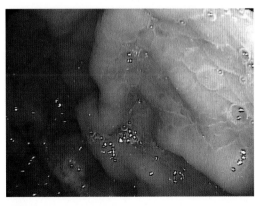

Figure 85.47 Endoscopic appearance of portal hypertensive gastropathy in a 55-year-old man with cirrhosis. Note the characteristic snakeskin appearance of the gastric mucosa.

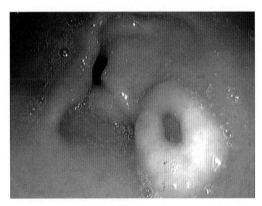

Figure 85.50 Pancreatic rest. Ectopic pancreatic tissue in the gastric antrum with characteristic apical dimpling. A rudimentary ductal system may empty into this depression.

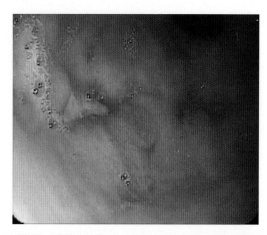

Figure 85.51 Gastric peptic ulcer. Antral gastric ulcer in a patient with a history of heavy nonsteroidal antiinflammatory drug (NSAID) exposure. The patient discontinued her NSAID use and, on repeat upper endoscopy, the ulcer had resolved.

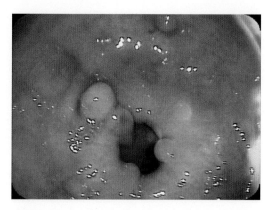

Figure 85.54 Gastric polyps. In the antrum, polyps can be seen in a patient with Cowden syndrome. Cowden syndrome is characterized by multisystem involvement, with gastrointestinal lesions including gastric and small bowel hamartomatous polyposis with esophageal glycogenic acanthosis.

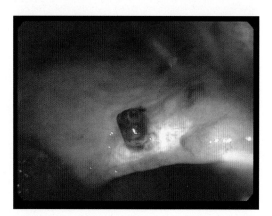

Figure 85.52 Gastric ulcer with adherent clot. This gastric ulcer was located on the incisura. The adherent clot is an endoscopic finding associated with an increased risk of rebleeding.

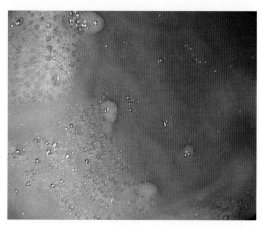

Figure 85.55 These small sessile polyps distributed in the body and fundus in a patient with a history of proton pump inhibitor therapy are characteristic of fundic gland polyps.

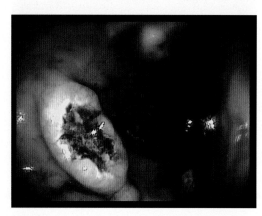

Figure 85.53 Malignant gastric ulcer. This large cratered gastric ulcer had heaped margins and a chronic appearance. Biopsies from this ulcer revealed a signet ring cell adenocarcinoma with ulceration and candidal overgrowth.

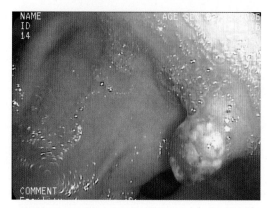

Figure 85.56 An inflamed hyperplastic polyp is seen here in the antrum of the stomach. Hyperplastic polyps are the most common type of gastric polyp and, while they have a low malignant potential, should be removed at the time of endoscopy.

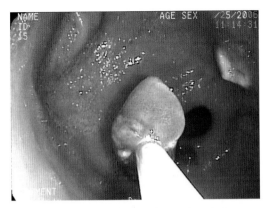

Figure 85.57 Endoscopic appearance of polyp tissue being removed after snare polypectomy in the gastric antrum.

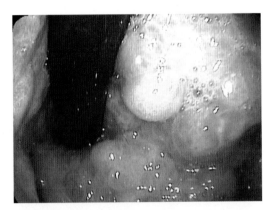

Figure 85.58 Gastric carcinoid tumor. A large fungating and submucosal noncircumferential mass was found in the cardia in this patient with multiple endocrine neoplasia type 1. Biopsies confirmed a low-grade carcinoid tumor.

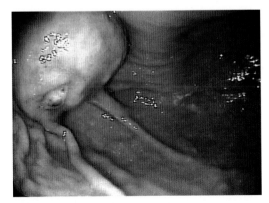

Figure 85.59 Endoscopic appearance of a 3.4-cm gastrointestinal stromal tumor (GIST) in the stomach. These submucosal tumors may have an overlying ulceration as seen here.

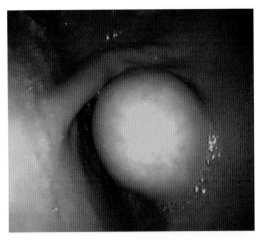

Figure 85.60 Gastric antral lipoma. A submucosal mass is seen here in the antrum. After resection, the pathological examination revealed a lipoma.

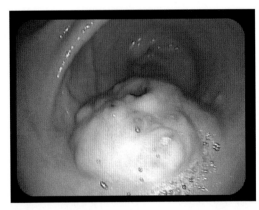

Figure 85.61 Glomus tumor. Endoscopic image of a glomus tumor in the antrum of the stomach. Glomus tumors are benign lesions originating from the modified smooth muscle cells of the glomus body and are rarely seen in the stomach. These submucosal lesions may present with overlying mucosal ulceration as seen here.

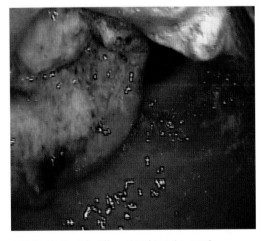

Figure 85.62 Moderately differentiated invasive gastric adenocarcinoma. An ulcerated mass in the antrum of the stomach seen here in an 84-year-old Korean woman with iron deficiency anemia. Stomach cancer is the most prevalent malignant neoplasm in Korea.

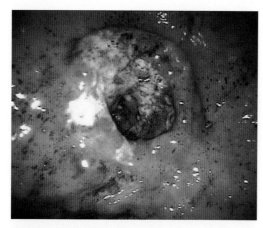

Figure 85.63 Gastric adenocarcinoma. Irregular fungating ulcerated pyloric channel mass. The mass was an invasive poorly differentiated adenocarcinoma on biopsy.

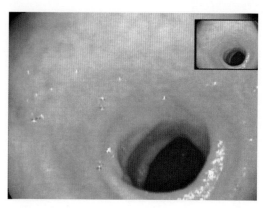

Figure 85.66 Normal duodenal bulb. The first portion of the duodenum, just after the pylorus, is referred to as the duodenal bulb.

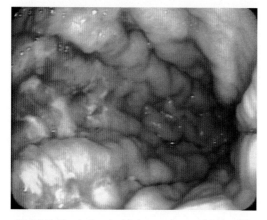

Figure 85.64 Linitis plastica. In this image, the rugal folds of the stomach are thickened diffusely. This patient was found to have poorly differentiated metastatic adenocarcinoma of the breast.

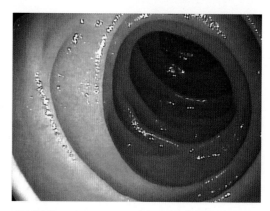

Figure 85.67 Normal appearance of the second portion of the duodenum.

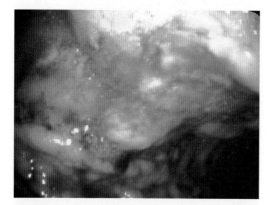

Figure 85.65 Gastric mucosa associated lymphoid tissue (MALT) lymphoma. Friable ulcerated mucosa on the lesser curvature of the stomach. Biopsies revealed a dense lymphoid infiltrate with focal ulceration consistent with low-grade marginal zone MALT B-cell lymphoma.

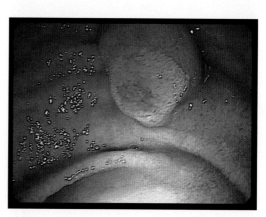

Figure 85.68 Using a side viewing endoscope, the papilla can usually be easily seen. The ampulla was normal in this patient.

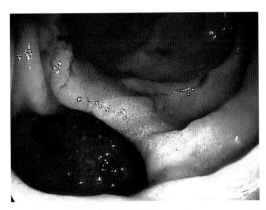

Figure 85.69 A large duodenal diverticular cavity can be seen in the lower left aspect of the image.

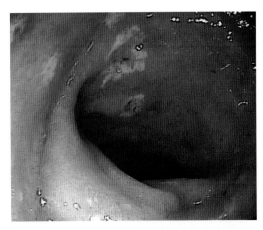

Figure 85.72 Duodenal erosions. White patches in the distal duodenal bulb can be seen. Erosions are differentiated from ulcers by the depth of penetration. In contrast to ulcers, erosions remain superficial to muscularis mucosa.

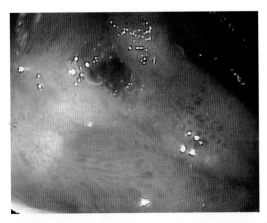

Figure 85.70 A duodenal ulcer with a pulsatile visible vessel was found in the duodenal bulb in a patient who presented with melena. The presence of a visible vessel is an endoscopic feature that is associated with an increased risk of recurrent bleeding.

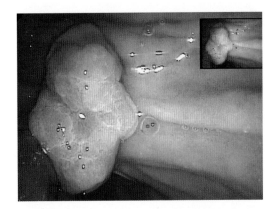

Figure 85.73 Endoscopic view of a large periampullary mass with clear yellow bile draining from the central portion of the lesion. After resection, this mass was found to be a tubular adenoma.

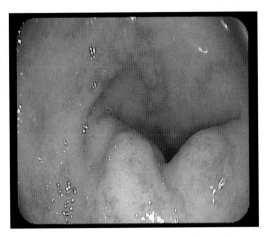

Figure 85.71 Prominent duodenitis characterized by erythema and mild edema in the bulb of the duodenum. This patient had a history of heavy nonsteroidal antiinflammatory drug use.

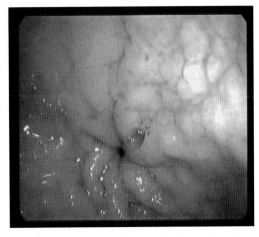

Figure 85.74 Duodenal mucosa in the bulb with a scalloped mosaic appearance in a patient with celiac disease. This patient had a high titer of antiendomysial and tissue transglutaminase antibodies. Small bowel biopsies confirmed villous blunting, crypt hyperplasia, and markedly increased intraepithelial lymphocytes.

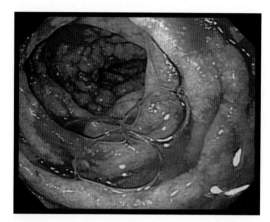

Figure 85.75 Endoscopic appearance of diffuse intestinal lymphangiectasia. The white papules arising from the duodenal mucosa represent lymph in dilated lacteals in the mucosa.

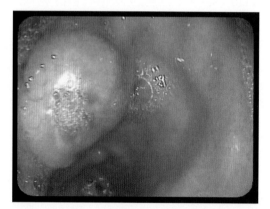

Figure 85.76 Duodenal metastatic tumor. A mass was found in the duodenal bulb in a patient with hepatocellular carcinoma. Biopsies confirmed metastatic hepatocellular carcinoma.

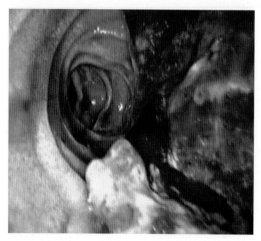

Figure 85.77 Malignant melanoma metastatic to the duodenum. A large fungating pigmented mass with minimal bleeding can be seen here involving the second portion of the duodenum. The ampulla was not involved.

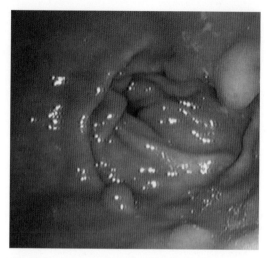

Figure 85.78 Benign appearing polypoid lesions can be seen here in the bulb of the duodenum. These are consistent with Brunner gland hyperplasia.

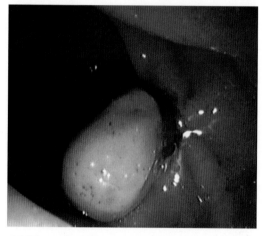

Figure 85.79 Duodenal lipoma. A submucosal mass can be seen in the second portion of the duodenum. Pathological examination confirmed the clinical impression of a lipoma.

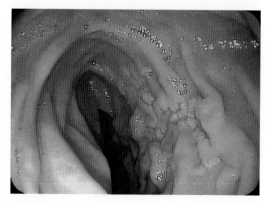

Figure 85.80 Duodenal adenoma. A mass can be appreciated in the second portion of the duodenum. Biopsies confirmed that the mass was a tubulovillous adenoma.

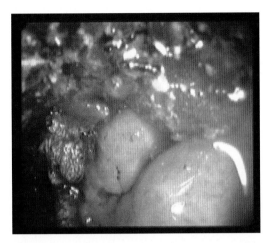

Figure 85.81 Duodenal lymphoma. A firm mass can be seen here in the fourth portion of the duodenum. This patient had a history of kidney transplant, and biopsies confirmed a diffuse large B-cell lymphoma.

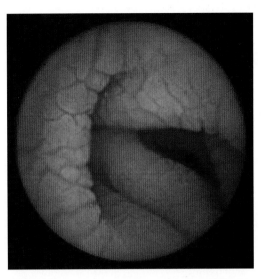

Figure 85.83 Video capsule endoscopy – celiac disease. Capsule endoscopy in a patient with celiac disease reveals scalloping of the small intestinal mucosa. Courtesy of Dr Myles D. Keroack.

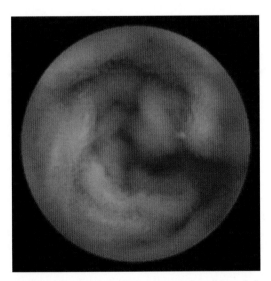

Figure 85.82 Video capsule endoscopy – normal small bowel. Capsule endoscopy involves ingestion of a capsule-sized device that obtains images of the gastrointestinal tract and transmits data to a recorder worn by patients during the study. This image reveals the typical appearance of the normal small bowel folds and villi. Courtesy of Dr Myles D. Keroack.

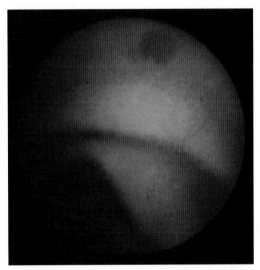

Figure 85.84 Video capsule endoscopy – angioectasia. Capsule endoscopy may be indicated in some patients with obscure gastrointestinal bleeding. This image reveals an angioectasia in the small intestine. Courtesy of Dr Myles D. Keroack.

86

Colonoscopy and flexible sigmoidoscopy

Jerome D. Waye, Christopher B. Williams

Colonoscopy provides visual inspection of the mucosal surface of the large intestine, where most of the colon pathology occurs. The most readily recognized abnormalities are elevated lesions and changes in the topographic anatomy. Inflammation of the colon is commonly encountered during colonoscopy. The cause of inflammatory changes ranges from infection to idiopathic inflammatory bowel disease. The process may be acute or chronic and may be localized or diffuse. No matter what the cause, the colon does not respond differently to each inflammatory insult. The result is that most inflammatory reactions can be categorized into two main types of surface changes caused by either ulcerative colitis or Crohn's disease.

If mild inflammatory disease affects the mucosa, edema causes the superficial layer to become opaque, hiding the normal branching vascular pattern of the submucosa from view. As vascular congestion proceeds, the surface lining may become hyperemic, erythematous, or may bleed whenever the endoscope contacts the mucosa. This pattern of response is most often seen with ulcerative colitis, which may progress to both small and large ulcerations. In contrast to the diffuse type of mucosal response in ulcerative colitis, the inflammatory component of Crohn's disease typically originates in the submucosa, and as the inflammation burrows onto the mucosal surface, individual aphthous ulcerations form, which are the hallmark of granulomatous colitis. This type of discrete ulceration with intervening normal mucosa is never seen with ulcerative colitis but may be present with amebiasis, tuberculosis, and other inflammatory processes in the large bowel.

With prolonged inflammation, ulcerations can become deeper and may interlink; with healing, the intervening islands of inflamed but not ulcerated mucosa exhibit a different growth pattern than the thin, reepithelialized mucosa that regenerates over ulcerated segments. This difference in growth pattern may cause elevated protusions to appear. These are postinflammatory polyps that have no malignant potential and are frequently called "pseudopolyps." A cap of white slough suggests that a polyp is inflammatory, although some juvenile (hamartomatous) polyps may have similar features. Inflammatory polyps that are small, shiny, and worm-like may be diagnosed as inflammatory on visual grounds alone, although biopsies may be necessary when there is any question about the nature of polyps observed at colonoscopy.

The terminal ileum can be intubated in most patients, and entry into the small bowel may be especially important in the differential diagnosis of inflammation of the large bowel. For the most part, patients with ulcerative colitis have completely normal-appearing small bowel. Among patients with Crohn's disease of the ileum, however, the small bowel has an appearance similar to that of the large bowel, ulcers being the most prominent feature. Inflammatory polyps may occur with either ulcerative colitis or Crohn's disease but are rarely seen in the terminal ileum.

In contrast to the ulcerations of inflammatory bowel disease, pseudomembranous colitis caused by *Clostridium difficile* infection may cause patchy clumps of creamy plaques on the mucosal surface. When the history is consistent with previous exposure to antibiotics, the endoscopic appearance is virtually diagnostic and mandates bacteriological or toxin studies in addition to routine histological examination.

Diverticulosis is common among patients older than 50 years. Diverticular orifices may range from small in size to a size that admits the tip of an endoscope. Muscular hypertrophy may be pronounced in some instances, causing the lumen to become narrow with spasm and marked tortuosity. Intubation may be difficult and tedious. Severe muscular hypercontractility often may result in a superficial subepithelial hematoma, which can become a small nidus of intra- or submucosal blood that can lead to further blood accumulation as a result of muscular hypercontractility. This may result in a cycle of further bleeding, hematoma, and with peristaltic activity, even appearance of a polypoid mass. When a diverticular red fold is seen, the surface mucosa is red or magenta. As red blood corpuscles break down in the tissue, hemosiderin is formed. A biopsy allows differentiation from adenoma. A request for the pathologist to stain

Atlas of Gastroenterology, 4th edition. Edited by Tadataka Yamada, David H. Alpers, Anthony N. Kalloo, Neil Kaplowitz, Chung Owyang, and Don W. Powell. © 2009 Blackwell Publishing, ISBN: 978-1-4051-6909-7

for hemosiderin in the tissue often assists in the differential diagnosis.

Ischemic colitis presents a wide array of mucosal appearances depending on the elapsed time from the ischemic episode to endoscopic examination. The ischemic segment may be quite friable and purplish-black in its initial phase, in which the mucosa has lost its blood supply. In less severe cases, erythema alone may be encountered in the area of the descending colon or splenic flexure. Subsequent sloughing of the edematous mucosa may be associated with local or widespread ulceration. The involved segments tend to heal rapidly, leaving superficial ulcerations that may appear similar to the lesions of Crohn's disease. Biopsies often provide the correct histopathological diagnosis when ischemia of the bowel is suspected.

Vascular abnormalities of the mucosa tend to be present at opposite ends of the large bowel, with radiation changes in the rectum and vascular ectasia in the right colon. Telangiectasia caused by radiation is more frequently encountered in the rectum, because the diagnosis of prostate cancer is being made earlier, and patients are undergoing radiation therapy for tumor ablation. Radiation changes are confined to the area of radiation therapy. They consist of multiple, small, interlacing blood vessels. Biopsies are not necessary for confirmation of this diagnosis. For patients whose radiation is delivered by means of radioactive seed implantation, an extremely localized segment of telangiectasia may occur over the area of the prostate. External beam radiation may be associated with diffuse damage to the rectal mucosa. Radiation telangiectasia most often occurs after a latent period following radiation therapy treatment. Persistent surface bleeding may ensue, which can be quite resistant to therapeutic endeavors. Angiodysplasia or focal vascular ectasia, probably of degenerative origin, may develop in the proximal colon of elderly patients. These may be a cause of bleeding or anemia and may be single or multiple. They vary from small, flat blebs to large, elevated collections of blood vessels with a span of 15 mm. A draining vein often is visible at endoscopic examination and represents the hallmark angiographic descriptor of this vascular malformation.

Polypoid protuberances above the normally flat surface mucosa are a common finding at colonoscopy. Such elevations may be on or underneath the surface mucosa. If the protusion is mucosal in origin it is called a "polyp" and if covered by normal mucosa it is termed a "submucosal tumor." A biopsy specimen usually has to be submitted to a pathologist for correct designation of structure and significance. The most common submucosal tumor of the colon is a lipoma, which usually has a broad base and is covered by normal mucosa, often with a recognizable surface vascular pattern with a slightly yellowish hue caused by the underlying fatty tissue. The surface indents easily with a biopsy forceps (pillow sign), and fat may be extruded from the surface during the course of obtaining multiple, progres-

sively deeper biopsy specimens. Small, discrete submucosal nodules in the rectum may be carcinoid tumors. These firm tumors often are adherent to the superficial mucosa, so a biopsy of the surface often leads to the proper diagnosis. Diffuse submucosal nodules are uncommon but may be present in lymphoma or in pneumatosis coli. Deep biopsies may cause air cysts to collapse, as may aspiration with a needle.

Hyperplastic polyps are elevated above the flat surface lining, but they arise from the mucosa and are most commonly pale and translucent. Large hyperplastic polyps may occur in the right colon. In this location, the polyps frequently look like an ear with a small, narrow footprint. Hyperplastic polyps have no stroma. In the rectum, they may disappear with air insufflation, which causes mucosal stretching, but they can be revisualized as air is aspirated from the rectum.

Adenomas may occur singly or in any distribution throughout the colon. When more than 100 adenomas are present, the diagnosis of familial adenomatous polyposis (FAP) can be made, even if there is no family history of polyposis. Other than sheer number of polyps, there is nothing about the configuration of polyps that would set aside patients with FAP from those with sporadic adenomas. There is no need to remove any of these polyps except to confirm that they are adenomatous. Among patients without FAP, removal of small and pedunculated polyps can be accomplished with the snare and cautery technique, but larger sessile polyps may be more easily and safely removed after submucosal injection of fluid at the base of the polyp. This technique is especially useful in the right colon, where the wall is thin. Placing a fluid load into the submucosa provides an additional safety factor for polypectomy by increasing the distance between snare application (and thermal tissue injury) and the serosal surface of the bowel. A sufficient volume of fluid should be given to elevate the polyp away from the wall, after which the polyp is removed with electrocautery current.

Dye spray may be used to add definition to the extent of a polyp or to enhance the surface topology. This technique, called chromoendoscopy, generally involves applying dye (indigo carmine 0.1% or methylene blue 1%) onto the surface of a polypoid lesion. Because hyperplastic polyps and adenomas have different surface configurations, dye spraying may enhance the visual ability to differentiate various types of polyps. It may also aid delineation of the edges of polyps to ensure total endoscopic ablation. A magnifying colonoscope helps in assessment of surface structure.

The location of lesions in the colon may be permanently marked with a tattoo accomplished by injecting carbon particles into the submucosa, either with a sterilized India ink solution or by injecting a pure carbon suspension. This will ensure the location for a subsequent surgical operation or for the endoscopist to reidentify the site at subsequent endoscopic examinations. Submucosal injection of carbon particles results in a stain that lasts for the life of the patient.

Bleeding during polypectomy may be controlled with various techniques, including injection with dilute epinephrine. A loop ligature can be placed on a bleeding pedicle or can be used to ensure hemostasis for patients with a bleeding diathesis. Hemostasis also may be achieved with application of clips to the surface through the channel of the colonoscope. Endoscopic clips are relatively easy to apply and have been found to be efficacious in the control of postpolypectomy bleeding.

Malignant tumors of the colon grow in a haphazard manner. Ulceration is a frequent finding, as is sloughing of a portion of the surface. The endoscopic appearance may vary from an apparent indentation on the top of a polyp to an obvious, fungating tumor. The cancer may be bulky or may ulcerate and become relatively flat in configuration. After colonic resection, most anastomoses are identifiable as a ridge with surrounding increased vascularity. Sometimes staples or sutures may be identified at the margin of the anastomosis.

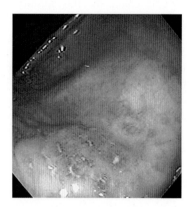

Figure 86.1 Crohn's disease. Multiple aphthous ulcerations in an area of otherwise unremarkable mucosa.

Figure 86.4 Crohn's disease of the terminal ileum with aphthous ulcers.

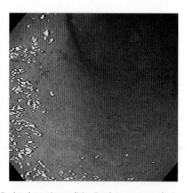

Figure 86.2 Early ulcerative colitis. Erythema, granularity, loss of the normal vascular pattern, and slight friability.

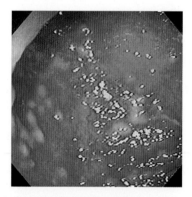

Figure 86.5 Antibiotic colitis pseudomembranes.

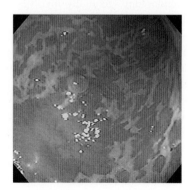

Figure 86.3 Severe ulcerative colitis. Linear ulcerations, erythema, and multiple interlacing ulcers.

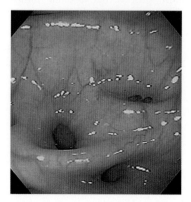

Figure 86.6 Diverticulosis. Multiple diverticular orifices. Highlights indicate that the lumen is at the 12 o'clock position.

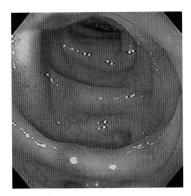

Figure 86.7 Reddened folds related to intramucosal bleeding from muscular activity in diverticular disease. Redness on several folds is associated with muscular hypertrophy.

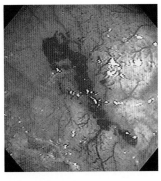

Figure 86.10 Vascular malformation.

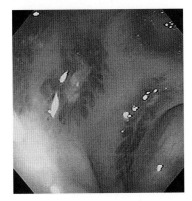

Figure 86.8 Ischemic bowel disease. Marked edema and erythema.

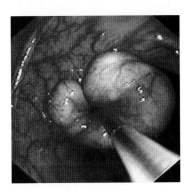

Figure 86.11 Lipoma. Fatty tumors can be indented with a biopsy forceps, resulting in a cushion or pillow sign.

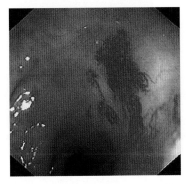

Figure 86.9 Radiation "colitis." Radiation therapy effect in the rectum caused by an implant for cervical carcinoma.

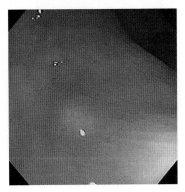

Figure 86.12 Submucosal rectal polyp: a carcinoid tumor.

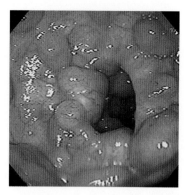

Figure 86.13 Pneumatosis cystoides intestinalis: multiple gas cysts.

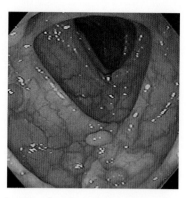

Figure 86.15 Familial polyposis. Multiple polyps of varying sizes throughout the colon.

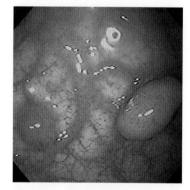

Figure 86.14 Hyperplastic polyps in the rectum.

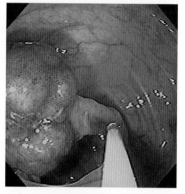

Figure 86.16 Pedunculated polyp on a slender pedicle (with snare).

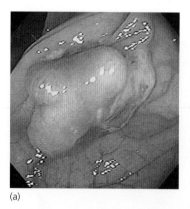

(a)

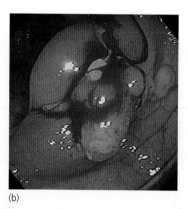

(b)

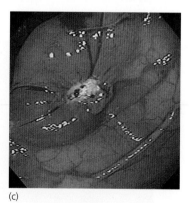

(c)

Figure 86.17 Submucosal injection polypectomy. **(a)** Sessile polyp. **(b)** After large-volume saline submucosal injection. **(c)** Polypectomy site. A small amount of residual tissue is present at the edge of the polypectomy site, which was removed with another snare application.

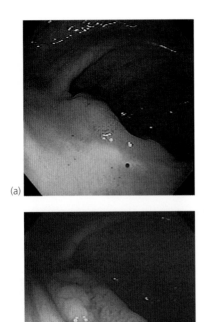

(a)

(b)

Figure 86.18 Dye spray. **(a)** Polyp in the right colon. **(b)** The extent of the same polyp is easier to see after using methylene blue dye spray.

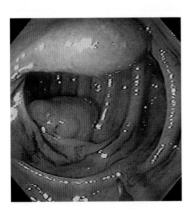

Figure 86.19 India ink stain. Blebs from India ink immediately after injection of mucosa near colon cancer.

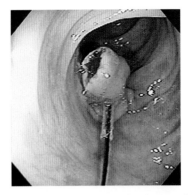

Figure 86.20 Endoscopic loop on pedicle that began to bleed after snare polypectomy.

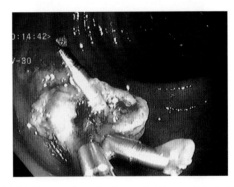

Figure 86.21 Three endoscopic clips applied to a pedicle that bled immediately after transection.

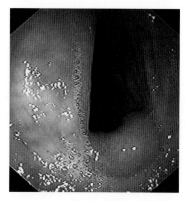

Figure 86.22 Cancer. Small bean-shaped carcinoma in the transverse colon.

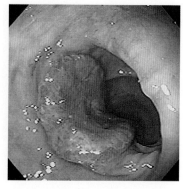

Figure 86.24 Cancer. Flat, saucer-shaped carcinoma.

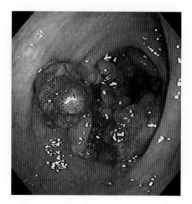

Figure 86.23 Cancer. Fungating carcinoma.

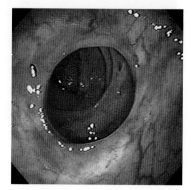

Figure 86.25 Colonic anastomosis. Normal stapled anastomosis.

A ENDOSCOPIC

87

Endoscopic retrograde cholangiopancreatography, endoscopic sphincterotomy and stone removal, and endoscopic biliary and pancreatic drainage

Tony E. Yusuf, David L. Carr-Locke

Endoscopic retrograde cholangiopancreatography (ERCP) is an advanced and interventional endoscopic procedure that involves evaluation and management of various disorders of the pancreatobiliary system. Over the past three decades, ERCP has evolved from a diagnostic to a therapeutic endoscopic modality. These techniques include endoscopic papillectomy, sphincter of Oddi manometry, biliary sphinc-terotomy, pancreatic sphincterotomy, stone removal, tissue sampling, stenting, and drainage of peripancreatic fluid collections. Image capturing and video recording during the procedure are essential for documentation and record keeping. It is equally important for teaching purposes. In the following images, sample illustrations of selected findings and maneuvers used during ERCP are shown.

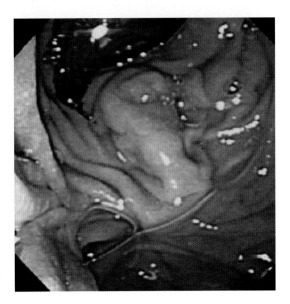

Figure 87.1 A prominent major duodenal papilla seen endoscopically through a duodenoscope in a patient with HNPCC. This was a biopsy-proven ampullary adenoma. Endoscopic ultrasound demonstrated the lesion to be superficial. Endoscopic ampullectomy was planned.

Atlas of Gastroenterology, 4th edition. Edited by Tadataka Yamada, David H. Alpers, Anthony N. Kalloo, Neil Kaplowitz, Chung Owyang, and Don W. Powell. © 2009 Blackwell Publishing, ISBN: 978-1-4051-6909-7

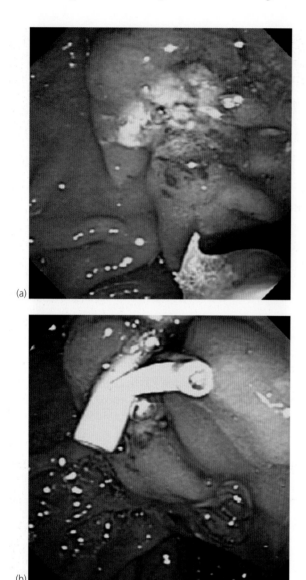

(a)

(b)

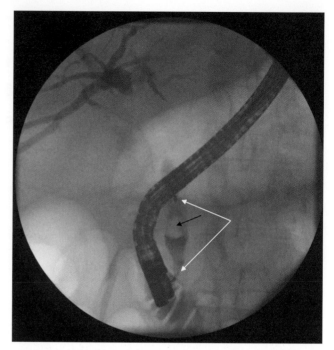

Figure 87.3 A filling defect in the distal common bile duct consistent with a stone (black arrow). After a generous biliary sphincterotomy, the stone could not be removed with an extraction balloon. The stone was then entrapped in a wire basket mechanical lithotripter (white arrows) and crushed followed by extraction.

Figure 87.2 Same patient as in Figure 87.1. The major duodenal papilla was resected endoscopically with a snare using electrosurgical current and here you can see the postresection appearance **(a)**. A 10F biliary plastic stent was placed to facilitate drainage and a 7F plastic stent was placed in the pancreatic duct to minimize the risk of postprocedural pancreatitis **(b)**. The stents are usually removed endoscopically at 1 month post procedure and the site is inspected for residual adenoma.

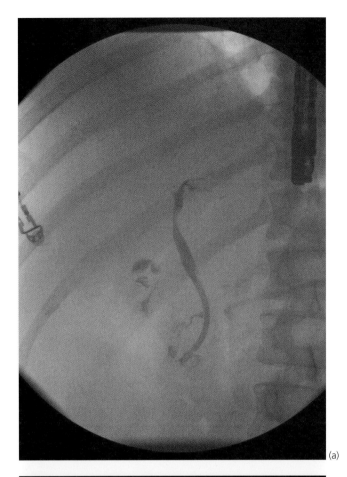

(a)

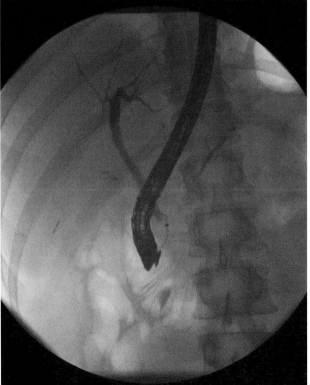

(b)

Figure 87.4 A young female patient underwent laparoscopic cholecystectomy for gallstone disease. Postoperatively, the patient complained of abdominal pain and increased bile drainage seen through a Jackson-Pratt (JP) drain. Bile leak was suspected. Endoscopic retrograde cholangiogram revealed extravasation of contrast at the level of cystic duct stump and plastic biliary stent placed **(a)**. Six weeks later, repeat cholangiogram revealed healing of bile leak **(b)**.

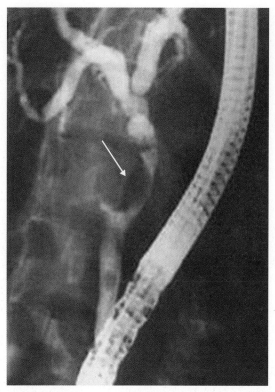

Figure 87.5 Large stone (white arrow) in the neck of the gallbladder seen compressing the common bile duct and resulting in proximal biliary dilatation. This is type I Mirizzi syndrome.

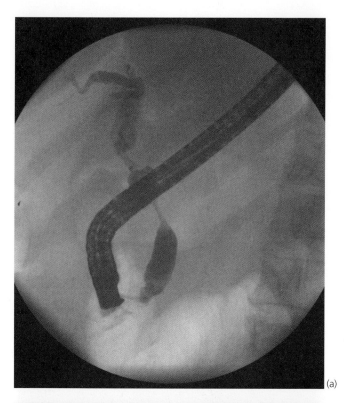

(a)

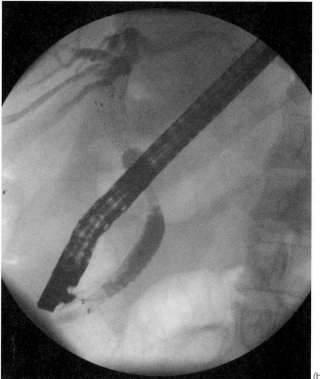

(b)

Figure 87.6 An elderly patient presenting with right upper quadrant pain, jaundice, and weight loss. Later diagnosed with unresectable gallbladder cancer. ERCP performed and demonstrated common bile duct and common hepatic duct strictures **(a)**. Self-expandable uncovered metal stent was successfully deployed across both strictures **(b)**.

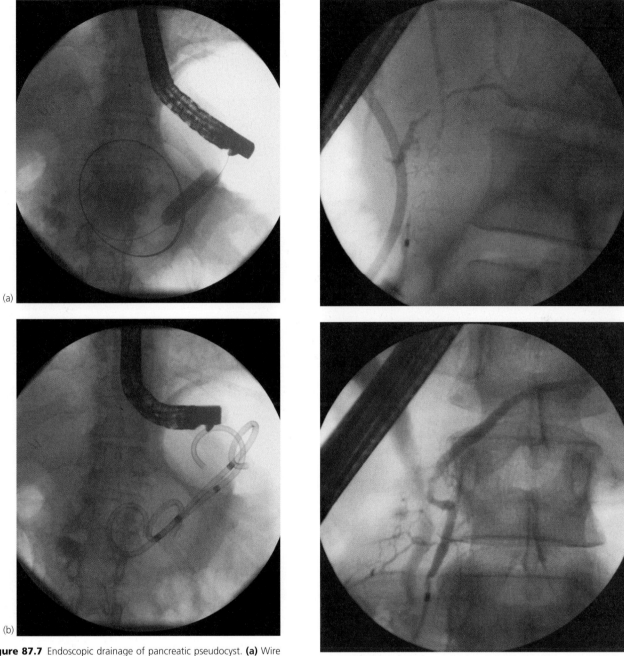

Figure 87.7 Endoscopic drainage of pancreatic pseudocyst. **(a)** Wire looping into the cyst cavity and balloon dilation of cystgastrostomy tract as seen fluoroscopically. **(b)** Placement of two double pigtail stents between the cyst cavity and gastric lumen.

Figure 87.8 A 36-year-old female patient presented with recurrent pancreatitis and obstructive jaundice. On ERCP, there was multifocal stricturing of the pancreatic duct and no ductal dilation as seen in autoimmune pancreatitis **(a)**. A common bile duct stricture was also seen. There was significant improvement of the pancreatogram **(b)** and clinically after a course of oral steroid therapy.

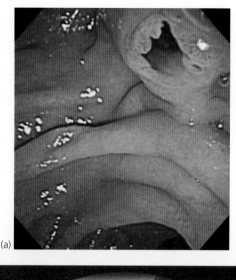

(a)

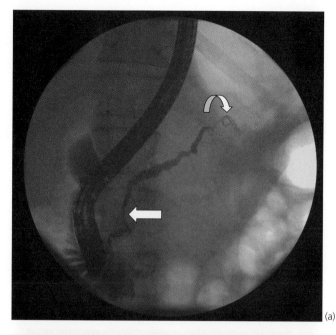

(a)

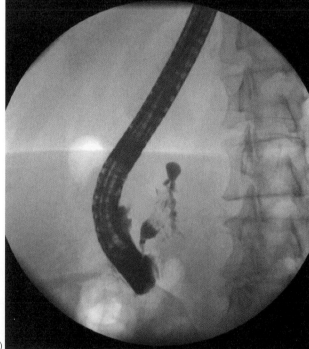

(b)

Figure 87.9 "Gaping" or "fish mouth" endoscopic appearance of the major duodenal papilla and pancreatic ductal dilation with filling defects, consistent with main-duct intraductal papillary mucinous neoplasm (IPMN).

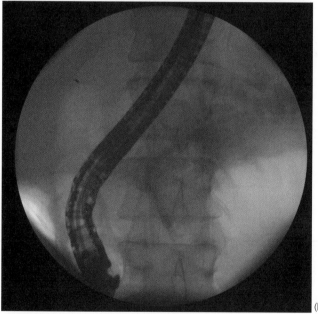

(b)

Figure 87.10 Patient with chronic pancreatitis with **(a)** stricture in the head of the pancreas (straight arrow) and leak in the tail (curved arrow) and **(b)** status-post (s/p) stent placement.

A ENDOSCOPIC

88

Gastrointestinal dilation and stent placement

James D. Lord, Drew B. Schembre, Richard A. Kozarek

Although dilation of gastrointestinal strictures has been limited historically to the esophagus and anorectum, the development of polyethylene balloons has expanded the endoscopist's therapeutic horizons. Passed over a guidewire or directly through an endoscope, such balloons allow access to stenotic lesions of the stomach, small intestine, colon, and pancreaticobiliary tract. Paralleling our ability to dilate previously inaccessible stenoses has been the development of newer dilating systems for use in the esophagus. For bougienage, polyvinyl dilators have virtually supplanted the Eder–Puestow metal olives (Pauldrach Medical, Garben, Germany), and lesions previously considered "undilatable" have been recategorized. More recent modifications, such as over-the-scope bougies, or balloons with a controllable expansion radius, may further improve the safety and efficacy of dilation.

Consequently, these expanded capabilities have led endoscopists into widespread dilation therapy for a variety of stenoses, despite the absence of data or contradictory studies regarding the risks and benefits of dilation compared with more conventional therapy such as surgery. Similarly, as pharmacological and radiation therapies evolve, it is unclear whether dilation provides a desirable alternative or adjuvant to these treatments. For example, stenoses with deep ulcerations caused by Crohn's disease, which would have historically necessitated surgery, are increasingly being dilated by endoscopists. Whether these dilations may be made more successful, or even obviated, by new immunomodulatory treatments for inflammatory bowel disease (IBD) remains unknown.

As with dilation, technological advances have driven the increased use of, and indications for, endolumenal stents in the alimentary canal. Expandable stent therapy has virtually supplanted conventional prosthesis placement in the esophagus, given the relative ease of placement and improved safety profile during insertion. Nevertheless, critical evaluation of this technology suggests that the need for intervention actually may increase after placement of expandable esophageal stents. This reintervention is a direct consequence of stent design: uncovered stents elicit granulation tissue and allow tumor ingrowth, and completely covered prostheses have a penchant for migration. All prostheses have the capability of causing erosion with fistulization, gastrointestinal bleeding, or occlusion by food bolus.

Even though expandable stent technology has at least the potential to open obstructed lumenal orifices for patients at high risk and patients with widespread metastases, and to open nonesophageal locations, the exact role of the technology remains ill-defined. Part of this uncertainty reflects the paucity of controlled studies regarding placement of these stents into locations other than the esophagus or biliary tract. Another part of the uncertainty includes the ongoing evolution of the various stents themselves and their respective delivery systems. Finally, additional uncertainty revolves around the cost of this technology – from US$1000 to US$2000 per device depending on stent design and length. It is hoped that, in the future, the various stent types can be better placed into perspective with each other and with other potential therapies.

Atlas of Gastroenterology, 4th edition. Edited by Tadataka Yamada, David H. Alpers, Anthony N. Kalloo, Neil Kaplowitz, Chung Owyang, and Don W. Powell. © 2009 Blackwell Publishing, ISBN: 978-1-4051-6909-7

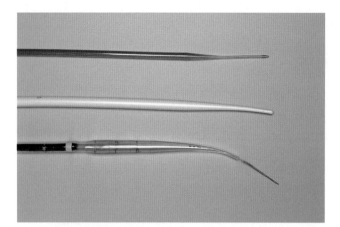

Figure 88.1 Dilating systems: Savary–Gilliard **(top)**, American **(middle)**, and Optical **(bottom)** dilators. All these are wire-guided, with the Optical dilator also admitting an endoscope for direct visualization.

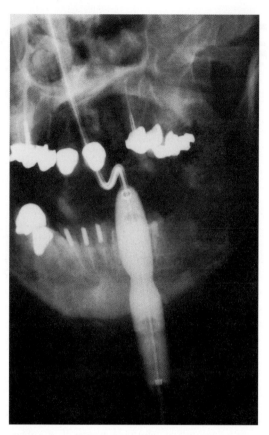

Figure 88.3 Balloon dilation of a radiation stricture at the cervical inlet. Location of stenosis precludes use of through-the-scope technology. The waist is present near the midportion of the balloon.

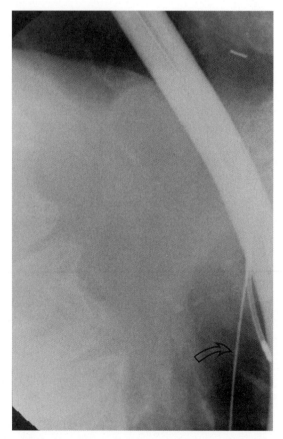

Figure 88.2 Barium-impregnated Savary-type dilator (American Dilator; Bard, Mentor, OH) passed over a guidewire (arrow shows distal portion of free guidewire in stomach) and through an obstructing distal esophageal cancer. Wire-guided polyvinyl dilators are the preferred treatment modality for acutely angulated, complex stenoses of the esophagus.

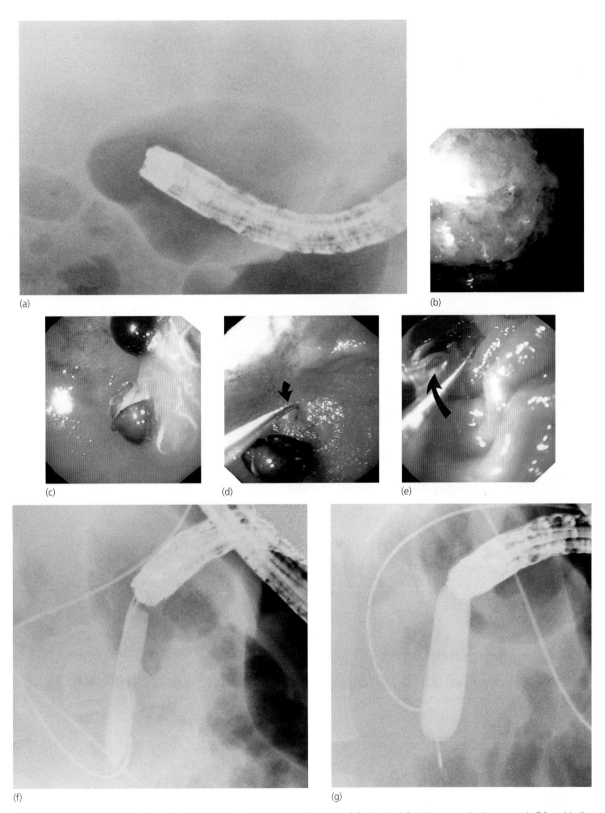

(a)

(b)

(c)

(d)

(e)

(f)

(g)

Figure 88.4 Dilated duodenal bulb of a patient with high-grade stricture of the apex **(a)**. Retained food is present in the stomach **(b)** and bulb **(c)**. A guidewire (small arrow) is inserted through the stricture **(d)** to allow proper positioning of the balloon (Microvasive, Natick, MA) (large arrow) **(e)**. Radiograph shows balloon dilation **(f,g)**. (*Continued on next page.*)

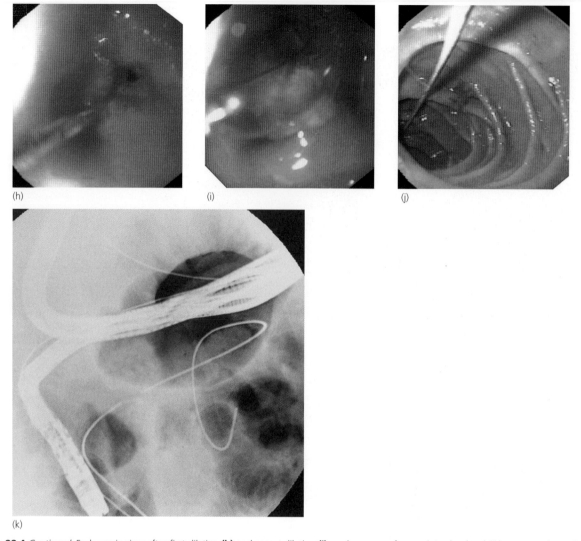

(h)   (i)   (j)

(k)

Figure 88.4 *Continued* Endoscopic view after first dilation **(h)** and repeat dilation **(i)**, and passage of scope into duodenal C loop on endoscopic image **(j)** and radiograph **(k)**.

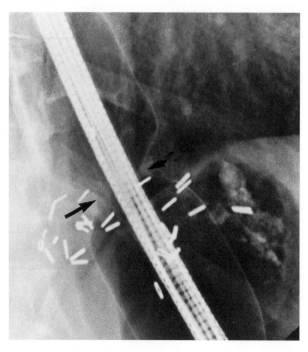

Figure 88.5 Witzel pneumatic dilator (Endo-Flex, Voerde, Germany) placed across the esophagogastric junction for patient with intractable dysphagia after laparoscopic antireflux operation. The dilator is a balloon hybrid with a central channel in the balloon accepting a pediatric endoscope to ensure proper positioning. The balloon waist is also shown (arrows).

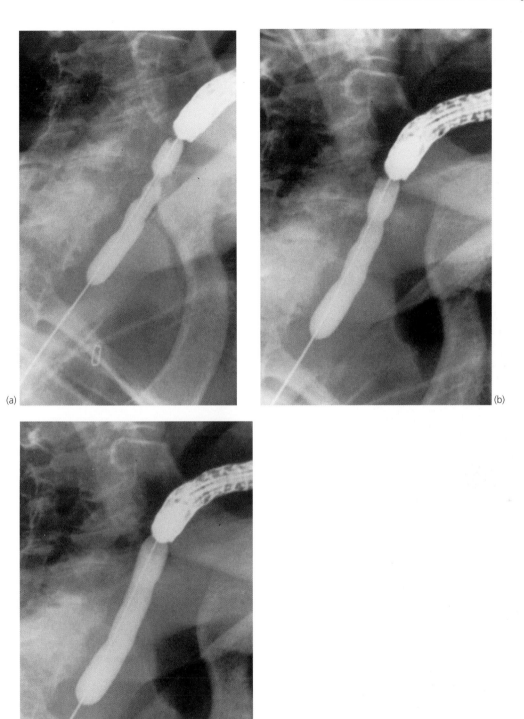

(a)

(b)

(c)

Figure 88.6 (a–c) Fluoroscopic views of 8-, 9-, and 10-mm controlled radial expansion (CRE) balloons (Microvasive, Natick, MA) used to treat tight irradiation stricture of the esophageal inlet.

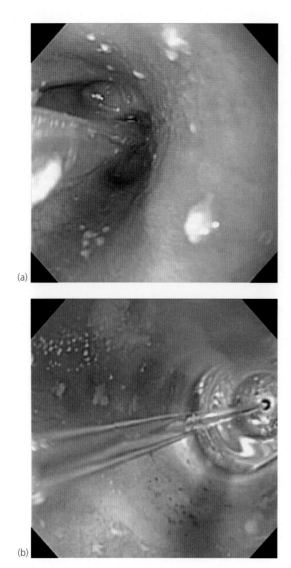

(a)

(b)

Figure 88.7 Endoscopic views of balloon dilation. An esophageal stenosis was cannulated with a deflated balloon **(a)** and then visualized directly through the balloon during inflation **(b)** by placing the inflated balloon against the endoscope tip.

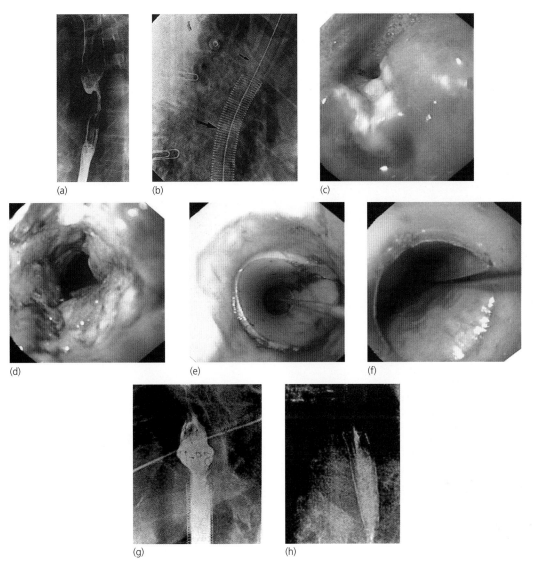

(a)　　　(b)　　　(c)

(d)　　　(e)　　　(f)

(g)　　　(h)

Figure 88.8 Conventional esophageal prosthesis placement. A stricture caused by midesophageal squamous cell carcinoma **(a)** was managed with a conventional prosthesis (Wilson-Cook, Winston-Salem, NC) (large arrow) pushed into position with a Drummond introducer (small arrows) **(b)**. Endoscopic photographs show original neoplasm **(c)**, appearance after dilation **(d)**, and proximal **(e)** and distal **(f)** stent margin. Proper proximal **(g)** and distal **(h)** stent position and function at barium swallow.

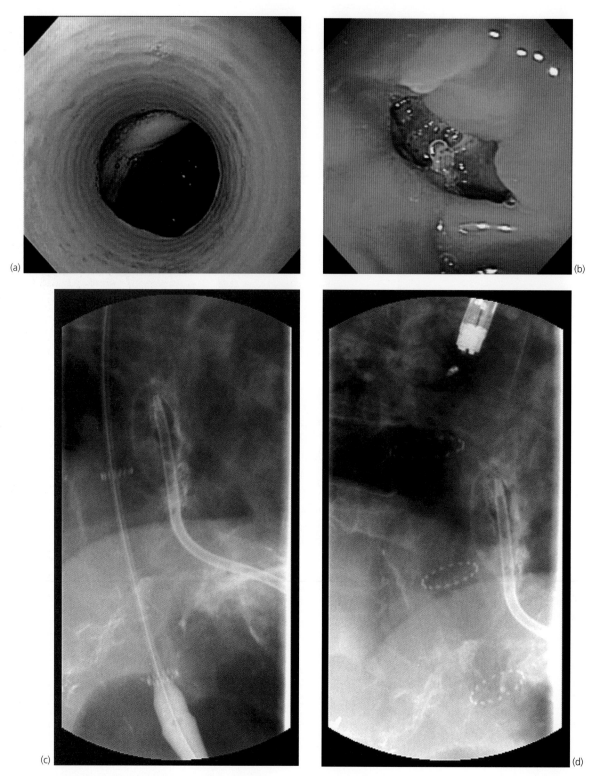

Figure 88.9 Treatment of a benign esophageal leak with a covered expandable stent. Endoscopic views of a previously placed conventional Celestin esophageal prosthesis **(a)** covering a persistent esophageal leak from previous Boerhaave syndrome. The prosthesis was removed revealing an esophageal defect **(b)**. Residual contrast from a previous study allows fluoroscopic visualization of the defect (containing drain tip) while a temporary Polyflex stent (Willy Rusch GmbH, Kernen, Germany) is positioned across it within a large catheter **(c)** and then deployed as the catheter is withdrawn **(d)**.

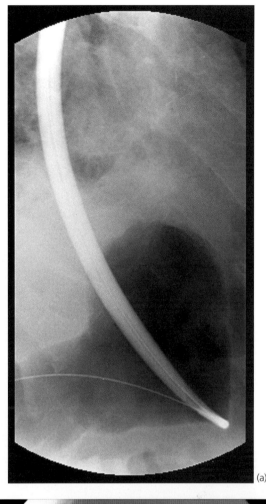

(a)

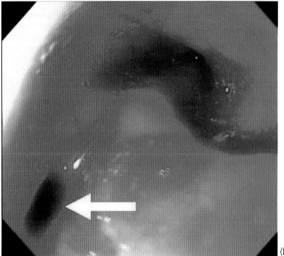

(b)

Figure 88.10 Esophageal dilation with perforation treated by subsequent expandable prosthesis placement. Patient with a malignant distal esophageal stricture underwent dilation with a wire-guided Savary dilator **(a)**, resulting in mucosal abrasion and a small perforation (arrow) **(b)**. (*Continued on next page.*)

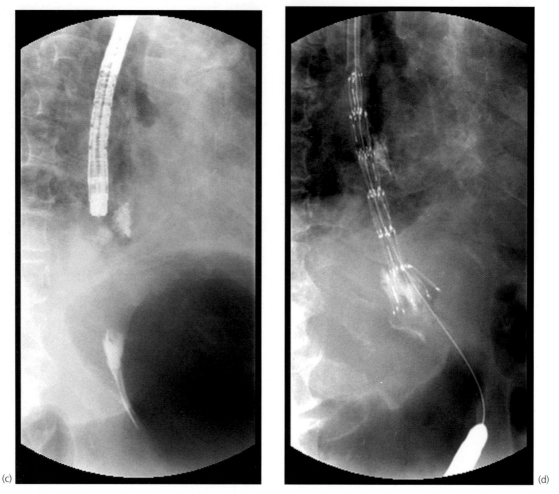

(c)

(d)

Figure 88.10 *Continued* Stricture margins were endoscopically marked with contrast **(c)** to facilitate placement of a covered Z stent (Wilson-Cook, Winston-Salem, NC), seen gradually expanding after deployment **(d)**. (*Continued on next page.*)

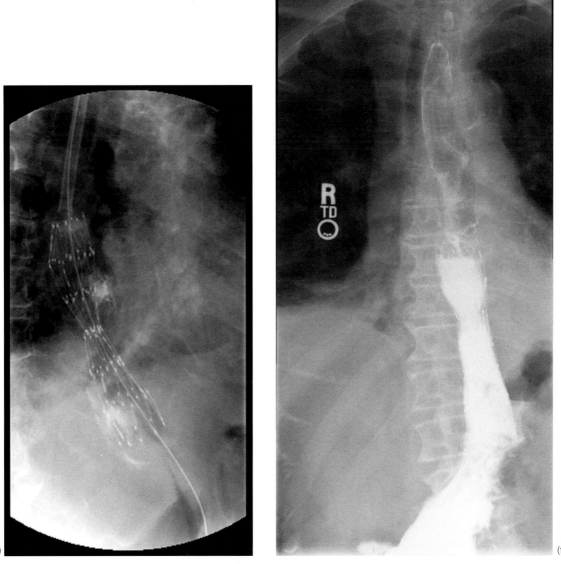

(e)   (f)

Figure 88.10 *Continued* Placement of a covered Z stent (Wilson-Cook, Winston-Salem, NC), seen gradually expanding after deployment **(e)**. Subsequent barium esophagram revealed good flow with no contrast extravasation **(f)**.

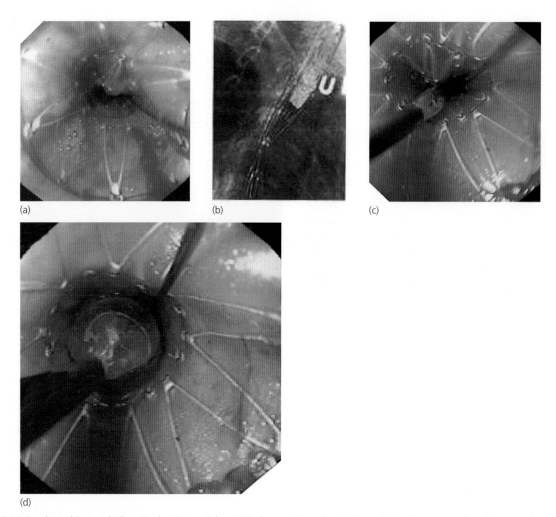

(a)

(b)

(c)

(d)

Figure 88.11 Esophageal Z stent (Wilson-Cook, Winston-Salem, NC) placement in patient with mediastinal metastases from breast carcinoma. Persistent extrinsic compression after stent delivery **(a,b)** requires balloon dilation **(c–d)** to achieve full expansion.

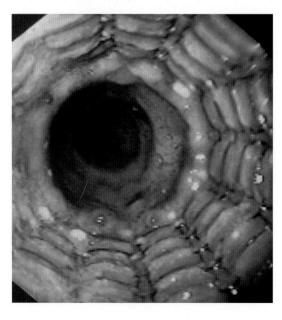

Figure 88.12 Endoscopic image of an Ultraflex (Microvasive, Natick, MA) esophageal stent 1 month after insertion. Granulation tissue is present at the distal end and a Schatzki ring is visible in the distance.

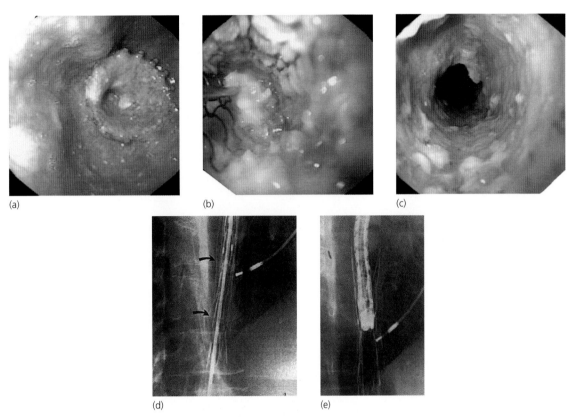

(a)   (b)   (c)

(d)   (e)

Figure 88.13 Problems encountered with expandable esophageal prostheses. Endoscopic photographs of a patient with esophageal cancer treated with an Ultraflex stent (Microvasive, Natick, MA) depict foodstuff **(a)**, tumor ingrowth **(b)**, and reactive inflammatory changes **(c)**. Tumor ingrowth was managed by means of insertion of a Gianturco-Rösch (European) Z stent (Wilson Cook, Winston-Salem, NC) **(d)**. An Ultraflex stent through which the Z stent has been inserted is shown (arrows). The pacemaker wire is visible. Deployment was followed by endoscopic visualization **(e)**.

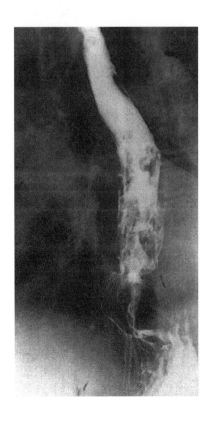

Figure 88.14 Tumor overgrowth through both ends of a completely covered Z stent (Wilson-Cook, Winston-Salem, NC) in a patient with Barrett esophagus and distal adenocarcinoma of the esophagus.

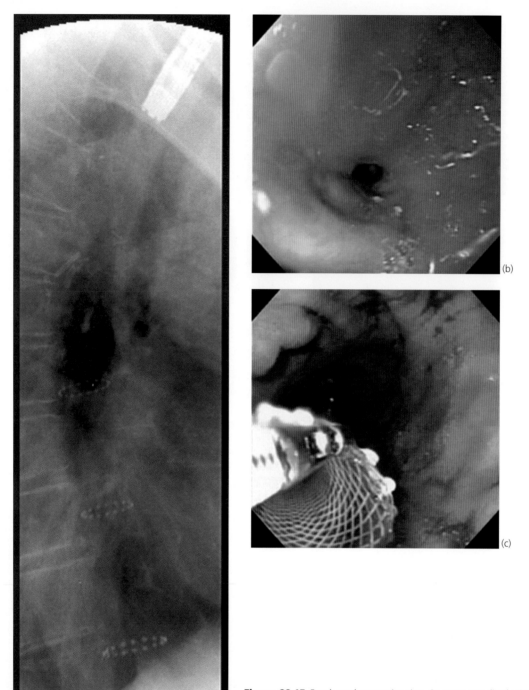

Figure 88.15 Esophageal stent migration. Spontaneous distal migration of a Polyflex stent (Willy Rusch GmbH, Kernen, Germany) into the gastric pull-up **(a)** of an esophagectomy recipient with an anastomotic stricture **(b)**. The stent was retrieved endoscopically with forceps **(c)**. (*Continued on next page.*)

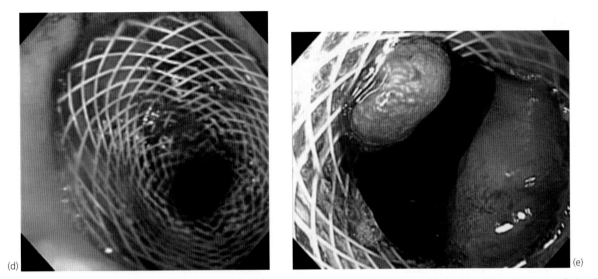

(d)

(e)

Figure 88.15 *Continued* The stent was replaced with another Polyflex stent **(d)**. Three months later, repeat endoscopy demonstrates granulation tissue growing over the distal end of the prosthesis **(e)**, reducing the risk of another stent migration, but increasing the risk of obstruction.

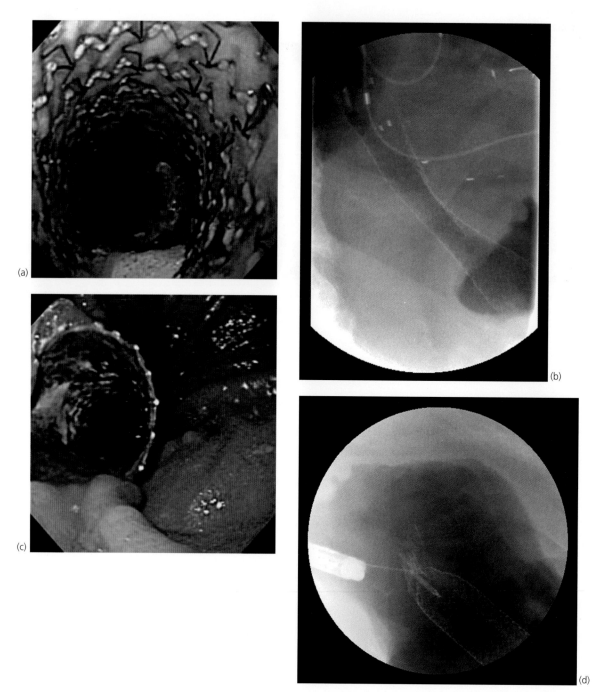

Figure 88.16 Placement of a stent with an antireflux valve. An Alimaxx-E stent (Alveolus, Charlotte, NC) **(a)** migrated distally across the esophagogastric junction **(b)** and resulted in reflux esophagitis. By passing the endoscope around the migrated stent **(c)**, it was snared around its distal free end and pulled into the stomach, where it could then be inverted **(d)** and removed. (*Continued on next page.*)

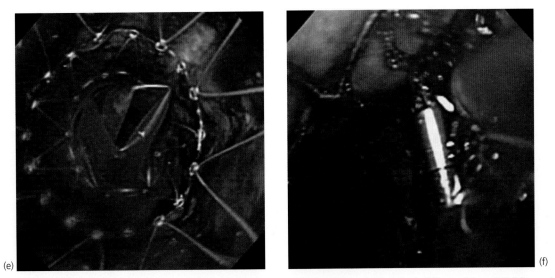

(e)

(f)

Figure 88.16 *Continued* **(e, f)** To reduce reflux, a Z stent with a Windsock/Dua antireflux valve (Wilson-Cook, Winston-Salem, NC) **(e)** was deployed, and a clip was endoscopically placed through its mesh into the mucosa **(f)** in an effort to prevent another stent migration.

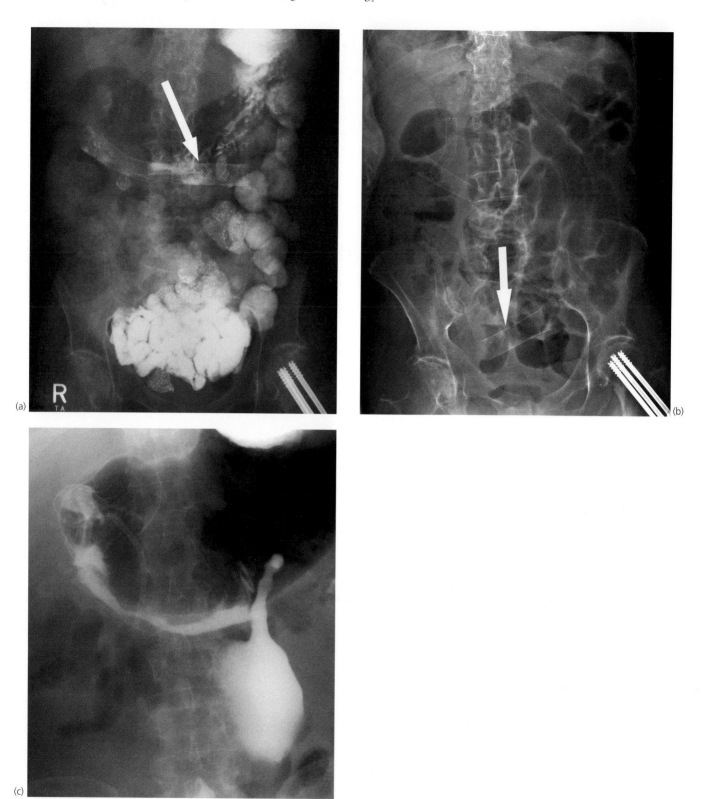

Figure 88.17 Problems encountered with extraesophageal prostheses. Radiographs show two tandem duodenally placed stents **(a)**, the distal one of which (arrows) later migrated distally **(b)**, resulting in intermittent small bowel obstruction, with dilated small bowel visible proximal to the migrated stent. In another patient, duodenal stent placement was complicated by bowel perforation, with extravasation of contrast into the peritoneum seen on fluoroscopy **(c)**.

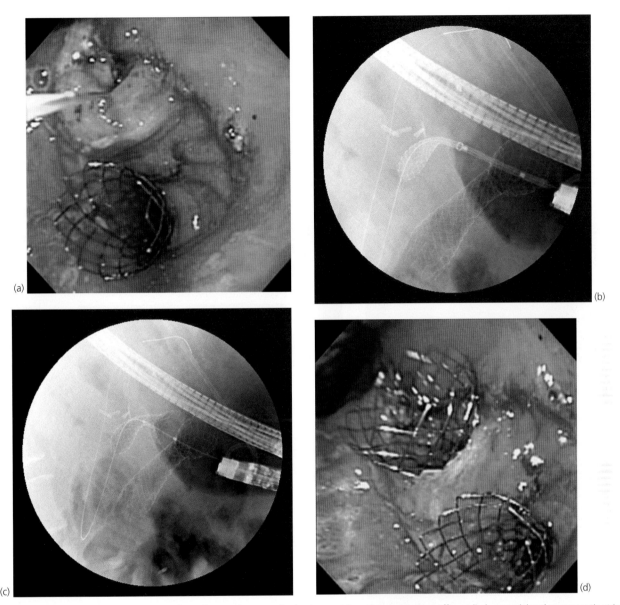

Figure 88.18 Transendoscopic extraesophageal stent placement for benign gastric outlet obstruction. Afferent limb gastrojejunal anastomotic stricture (cannulated with a wire) as seen on endoscopy just above the efferent limb anastomosis, in which a Wallflex (Microvasive, Natick, MA) stent was placed previously **(a)**. A second Wallflex stent was deployed through the endoscope across the afferent limb anastomosis **(b,c)**. Postplacement endoscopic view of both deployed Wallflex stents **(d)**.

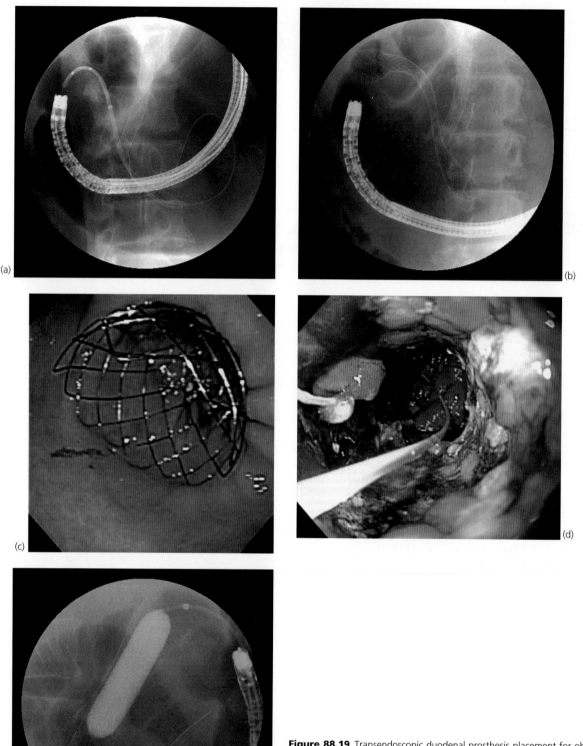

Figure 88.19 Transendoscopic duodenal prosthesis placement for obstructing pancreatic cancer. A Wallflex (Microvasive, Natick, MA) stent positioned through the endoscope over a wire across the stricture expands distally as its deployment catheter is withdrawn **(a)**. Note the permanent biliary stent placed previously, as biliary stents cannot usually be placed subsequent to duodenal stent placement. Deployed stent on fluoroscopy **(b)**, with proximal flange at the pylorus **(c)** to reduce stent migration. Three months later, considerable tumor ingrowth through the duodenal stent **(d)** necessitates balloon dilation **(e)**.

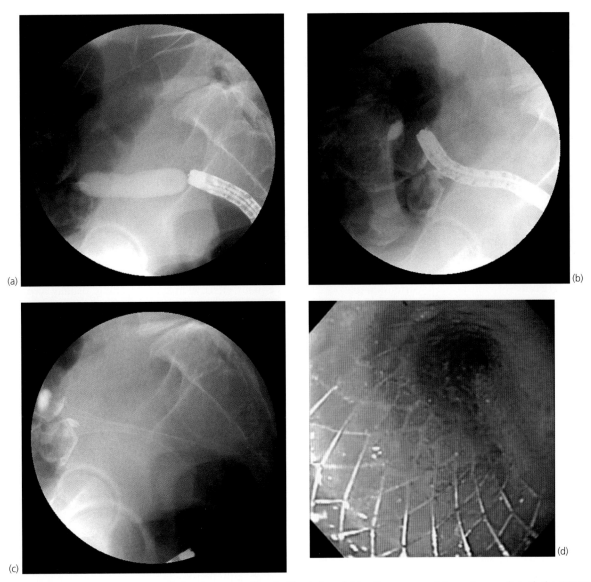

Figure 88.20 Colonic stent placement. A colonic stricture was dilated with a balloon **(a)** to allow passage of the endoscope through the stricture to mark its proximal end with contrast **(b)**. A colonic Wallstent (Microvasive, Natick, MA) was then deployed **(c)** and visualized endoscopically with passage of liquid stool **(d)**.

89

Management of upper gastrointestinal hemorrhage related to portal hypertension

Paul J. Thuluvath

The portal venous system is unique (Fig. 89.1). In addition to cirrhosis there are many other causes of portal hypertension, including portal vein thrombosis. Budd–Chiari syndrome is a rare cause of acute portal hypertension (Fig. 89.2). Three-dimensional computed tomography (CT) (Fig. 89.3) and magnetic resonance imaging (MRI) (Fig. 89.4) are reliable ways to assess the portal venous anatomy and large collaterals.

The pathophysiology of portal hypertension is illustrated in Figure 89.5. As portal hypertension advances, collaterals develop in the esophagus and stomach as shown in Figure 89.6. Esophageal varices are commonly seen in the distal esophagus but can also be seen in the middle and proximal esophagus. There are many grading systems of esophageal varices; a simple grading system is shown in Figure 89.7 (F0 = none, F1 = small, F2+ = medium, and F3 = large). Larger varices are more likely to bleed than smaller ones. Furthermore, the presence of "red signs" suggests a high risk of imminent bleeding (Fig. 89.8).

When varices are seen in the stomach they may occur as a continuation of esophageal varices in the cardia or fundus. Rarely, they are seen in the absence of esophageal varices. When fundal varices are seen without esophageal varices, splenic vein thrombosis should be considered in the differential diagnosis. The classification of gastric varices as proposed by Sarin et al. (Hepatology 1992;16:1343) is shown in Figure 89.9. The gastric varices may be small or large, and rarely may exhibit red signs (Fig. 89.10). Rarely, collaterals can be seen elsewhere, including gastric antrum, small bowel, stoma, and rectum (Fig. 89.11). The risk of bleeding is small from ectopic varices, but stomal varices (may be seen in patients with primary sclerosing cholangitis who have had a colectomy) may be an exception.

Bleeding from esophageal or gastric varices (Fig. 89.12) is associated with a very high mortality, and mortality is dependent on the severity of liver disease. Acute esophageal variceal bleeding can be controlled with medical therapy or endoscopic treatment. Endoscopic esophageal variceal banding is preferable (Figs 89.13–89.14), but sclerotherapy is equally effective in acute bleeding. Usually a combination of medical and endoscopic therapy is preferred to manage acute esophageal variceal bleeding.

Bleeding from gastric varices is more difficult to control because of the location, size of the varices, and poor visibility. Endoscopic band ligation or sclerotherapy with sodium morrhuate or similar substances is discouraged because of poor results and major complications. Bleeding should be initially (and preferably) controlled with medical therapy and balloon tamponade. The definitive treatment options include transjugular intrahepatic portosystemic shunt (TIPS) (Fig. 89.15), surgical shunt (Fig. 89.16), or injection of cyanoacrylate ("glue") (Fig. 89.17). It is important to exclude splenic vein thrombosis in isolated fundal varices, for which splenectomy would be the treatment of choice.

Patients with portal hypertension may also bleed from other sites including ectopic varices or portal hypertensive gastropathy. TIPS is a good option for bleeding ectopic varices, although rectal varices can be managed with local therapy. Bleeding from portal hypertensive gastropathy is usually mild and not a medical emergency, unlike esophageal or gastric variceal bleeding. When patients bleed from portal hypertensive gastropathy, the gastropathy is often severe (Fig. 89.18). Bleeding is usually self-limiting and the treatment of choice is nonselective β-blockers. TIPS may be effective in refractory bleeding from gastropathy. Mucosal changes similar to portal hypertensive gastropathy may be seen in other parts of the gastrointestinal tract including the colon (Fig. 89.19). To enable the best therapy to be given it is important to distinguish severe portal hypertensive gastropathy from gastric antral vascular ectasia (GAVE) (Fig. 89.20). Furthermore, both conditions may coexist (Fig. 89.21).

Atlas of Gastroenterology, 4th edition. Edited by Tadataka Yamada, David H. Alpers, Anthony N. Kalloo, Neil Kaplowitz, Chung Owyang, and Don W. Powell. © 2009 Blackwell Publishing, ISBN: 978-1-4051-6909-7

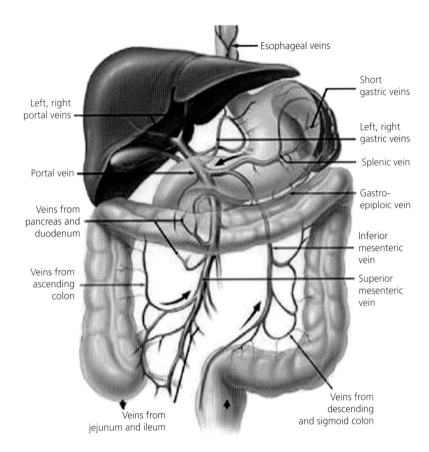

Figure 89.1 labels:
- Esophageal veins
- Short gastric veins
- Left, right gastric veins
- Splenic vein
- Gastro-epiploic vein
- Inferior mesenteric vein
- Superior mesenteric vein
- Veins from descending and sigmoid colon
- Veins from jejunum and ileum
- Veins from ascending colon
- Veins from pancreas and duodenum
- Portal vein
- Left, right portal veins

Figure 89.1 Anatomy of the portal venous system.

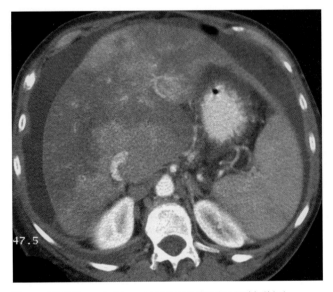

Figure 89.2 Computed tomography scan showing Budd–Chiari syndrome.

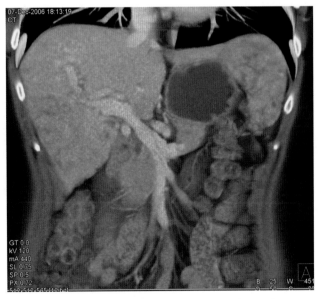

Figure 89.3 A three-dimensional computed tomography scan is a sensitive and reliable way to assess portal venous anatomy.

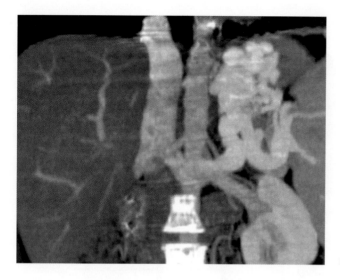

Figure 89.4 Magnetic resonance image showing large fundal varices.

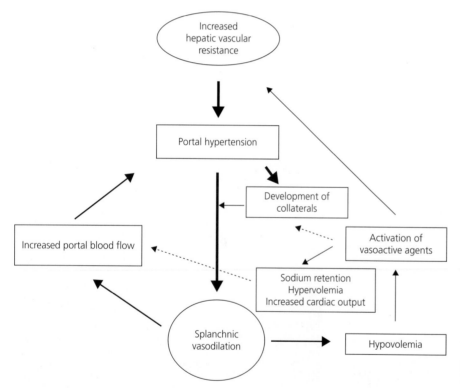

Figure 89.5 Pathophysiology of portal hypertension.

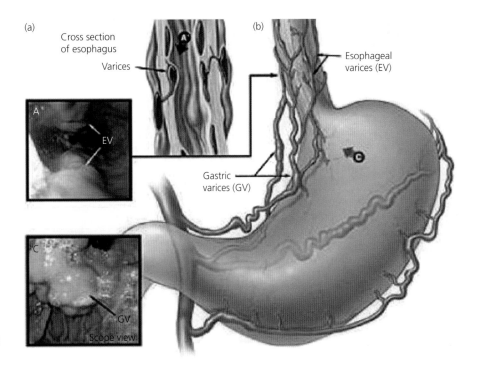

Figure 89.6 Collateral circulation in portal hypertension.

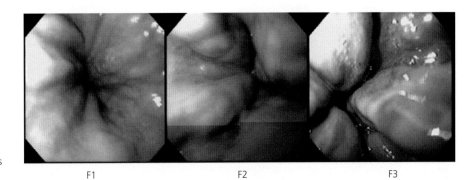

F1   F2   F3

Figure 89.7 Grading of esophageal varices based on the size.

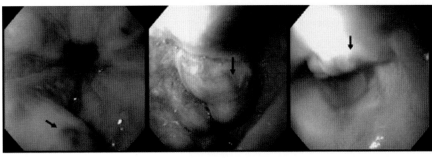

Red spots   Wale signs   Hematocystic spots

Figure 89.8 "Red signs" of esophageal varices.

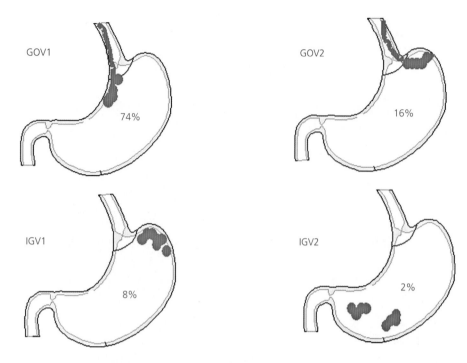

Figure 89.9 Sarin's classification of gastric varices.

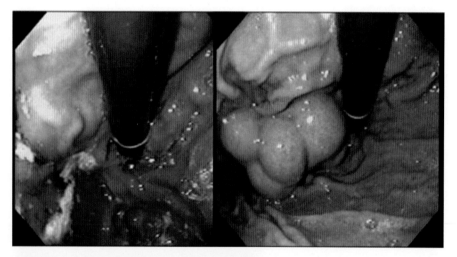

Figure 89.10 Small **(left)** and large **(right)** gastric varices.

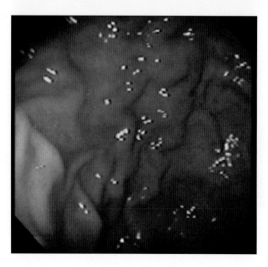

Figure 89.11 Rectal varices.

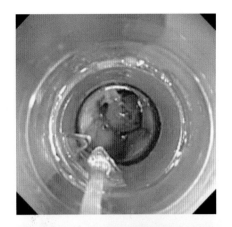

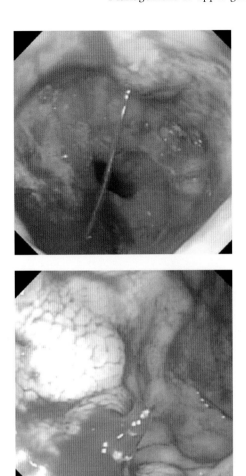

Figure 89.12 Bleeding esophageal and gastric varices.

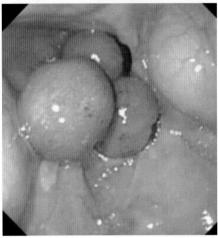

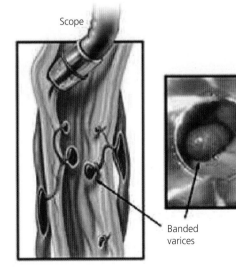

Figure 89.14 Multiple bands applied to esophageal varices.

Rubber band
ligation
system®

Scope

Banded
varices

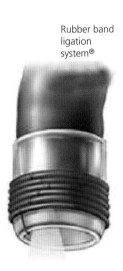

Figure 89.13 A cartoon showing
esophageal variceal banding.

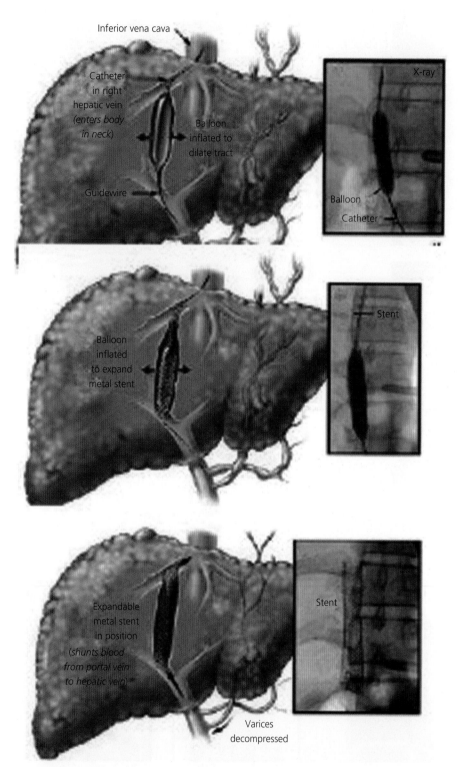

Figure 89.15 A cartoon showing the technique of transjugular intrahepatic portosystemic shunt (TIPS).

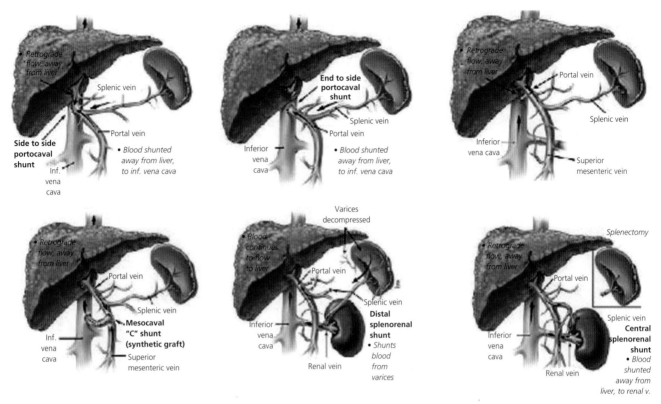

Figure 89.16 Various types of shunt surgery for the management of portal hypertension.

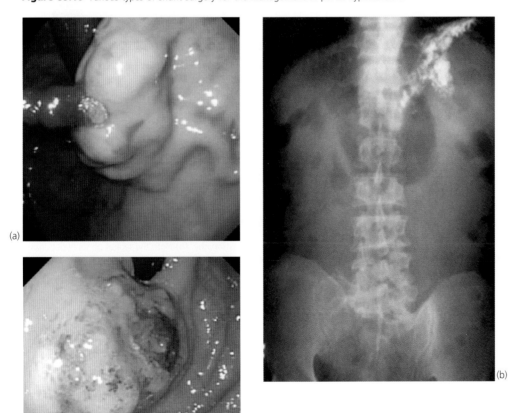

Figure 89.17 Injection of cyanoacrylate into gastric varice under fluoroscopic control. **(a)** Gastric varix with clotted blood oozing immediately after the glue injection. **(b)** Radiograph confirms that the glue mixed with lipiodol remains within the gastric varix. **(c)** Cast extruding from the varix several days after the glue injection.

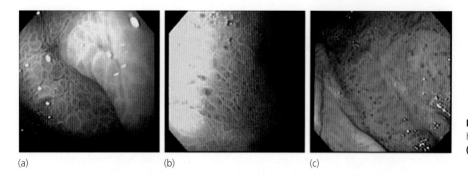

(a)   (b)   (c)

Figure 89.18 Grading of portal hypertensive gastropathy. **(a)** Mild; **(b)** moderate; **(c)** severe.

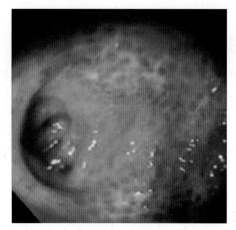

Figure 89.19 Portal hypertensive colopathy (cecum).

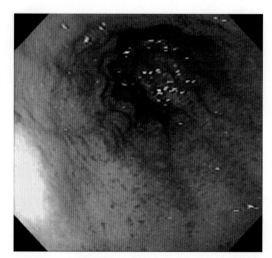

Figure 89.20 Gastric antral vascular ectasia.

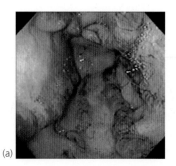
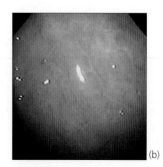

(a)   (b)

Figure 89.21 (a) Gastric antral vascular ectasia-like appearance in portal hypertensive gastropathy. **(b)** Note the typical portal hypertensive gastropathy in the background.

90

Endoscopic diagnosis and treatment of nonvariceal upper gastrointestinal hemorrhage

David J. Bjorkman

Upper gastrointestinal (UGI) bleeding from peptic ulcer disease and other nonvariceal causes is a frequent cause of hospitalization (250 000–300 000 hospital admissions per year in the United States). Advances in endoscopic diagnosis and therapy have not substantially affected the overall mortality rate of this disorder, which remains in the range of 5%–15% depending on age and comorbid medical conditions.

Initial treatment should focus on vigorous volume resuscitation. A combination of clinical characteristics and endoscopic findings can predict the risk for rebleeding and mortality. This allows the level of care to be tailored to the risk for the individual patient. In the setting of bleeding peptic ulcers the best predictor of persistent or recurrent bleeding, the need for surgical intervention, and mortality is the endoscopic appearance of the ulcer. Lesions with active bleeding or a visible vessel have a high likelihood of rebleeding (40%–55%) and a mortality rate that exceeds 10%. On the other hand, lesions with a clean base have a very low risk of rebleeding (< 5%) and a mortality rate that approaches 0%. Early endoscopic evaluation can, therefore, determine the optimal treatment approach for each patient.

Endoscopic therapy is indicated for all lesions that are considered to have a high risk of rebleeding (active bleeding or visible vessel). Ulcers with adherent clots that obscure the underlying lesions may benefit from careful endoscopic therapy.

Endoscopic therapies can be thermal (electrocoagulation, direct heat application, or laser therapy), involve injection with various agents, or employ mechanical compression of the bleeding site (hemostatic clips or bands). All of these methods have a high rate (90%) of success in stopping active bleeding, and significantly reduce the risk of rebleeding. Endoscopic therapy also reduces morbidity, mortality, transfusion requirements, and the costs of care. The technique of choice for a specific patient depends on the clinical situation, the location of the lesion, and the skill of the endoscopist.

This chapter demonstrates some of the endoscopic findings predictive of the outcome of a bleeding lesion, some of the devices used to treat the lesions, and the results of therapy.

Atlas of Gastroenterology, 4th edition. Edited by Tadataka Yamada, David H. Alpers, Anthony N. Kalloo, Neil Kaplowitz, Chung Owyang, and Don W. Powell. © 2009 Blackwell Publishing, ISBN: 978-1-4051-6909-7

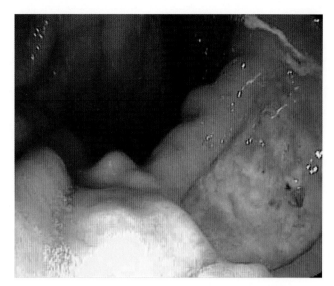

Figure 90.1 Deep gastric ulcer with flat pigmented spots in the base. This lesion, despite its depth, has a low (< 10%) risk of rebleeding and a mortality rate of less than 5%. Endoscopic therapy is not indicated for this lesion.

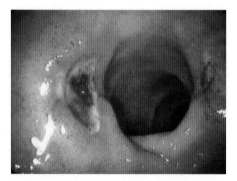

Figure 90.2 A duodenal ulcer with a central smooth-surfaced protuberance indicating a visible vessel. Despite the absence of active bleeding, the risk of rebleeding in this lesion is greater than 40% and the mortality rate is greater than 10%. Both of these figures can be considerably reduced by appropriate endoscopic therapy.

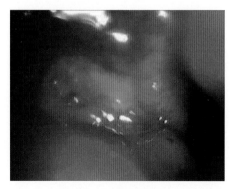

Figure 90.3 A large, deep duodenal ulcer with a visible vessel with bleeding is seen in the center of the base of the ulcer. The position of this lesion is ideal for direct application of thermal therapy to coagulate the vessel.

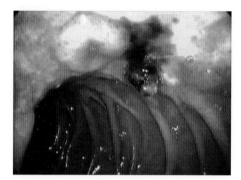

Figure 90.4 This large ulcer at the apex of the duodenal bulb shows a visible vessel extending into the lumen. The risk of rebleeding from this lesion is very high without endoscopic therapy.

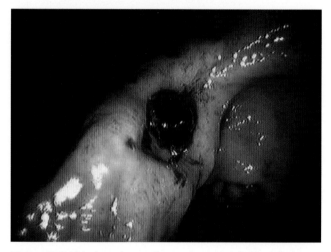

Figure 90.5 This deep ulcer on the gastric angularis has an adherent clot (remains after vigorous washing) that obscures the ulcer base. The risk of rebleeding in this setting depends on the underlying lesion. Removal of the clot may precipitate active bleeding. Optimal treatment of this lesion remains controversial. If the clot is removed to evaluate the underlying lesion, injection therapy with epinephrine (adrenaline) should be performed before clot manipulation to limit or prevent active bleeding.

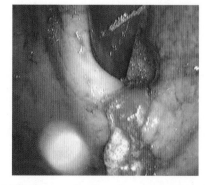

Figure 90.6 This clot extending from the gastroesophageal junction into the cardia of the stomach overlies and obscures a Mallory–Weiss tear. There is oozing at the superior aspect of the clot from the Mallory–Weiss tear. The endoscope is retroflexed with the proximal part of the scope seen entering the stomach from the esophagus. Although Mallory–Weiss tears usually stop bleeding spontaneously, endoscopic therapy is indicated for actively bleeding lesions such as this.

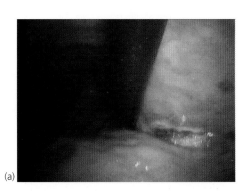

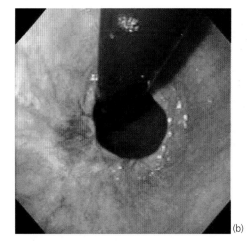

Figure 90.7 (a,b) Two Mallory–Weiss tears at the gastroesophageal junction are demonstrated in these images.

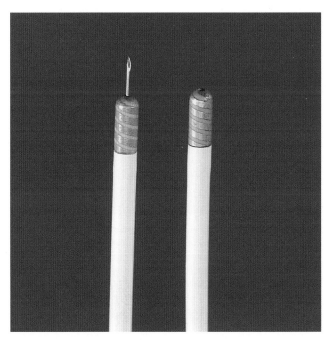

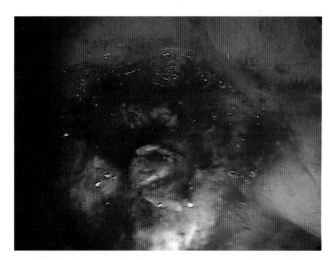

Figure 90.9 Active bleeding from a duodenal ulcer. Initial injection with saline or dilute epinephrine can control the bleeding. Subsequent thermal therapy can be applied to the specific bleeding site. Injection alone is not as effective as injection followed by thermal therapy.

Figure 90.8 Multipolar electrocoagulation catheter with electrodes that circle the end of the catheter and a central channel for vigorous water irrigation. This catheter also has a retractable central injection needle to allow combined electrocoagulation and injection therapy. The probe is inserted through the working channel of the endoscope and applied directly to the bleeding lesion while electrical energy is repeatedly passed between the electrodes through the tissue. The resistance of the tissue results in heat that cauterizes the lesion and seals the walls of the bleeding vessel together in what is called coaptive coagulation. Control of energy delivery and water irrigation is achieved by foot pedals attached to the electrical generator and the probe.

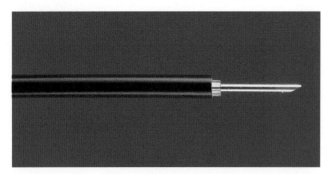

Figure 90.10 Endoscopic injection needle. This needle is attached to a syringe containing the desired solution for injection. The needle is retracted into the catheter and then passed through the working channel of the endoscope. The needle is then advanced out of the catheter and repeated injections are made around the bleeding lesion. When saline or dilute epinephrine is used, large volumes of injected fluid (10 mL or more) can be used to tamponade the bleeding lesion. Smaller volumes (0.1- to 0.2-mL aliquots) should be injected when absolute alcohol is used. Injection of saline or epinephrine is very helpful in slowing active bleeding in preparation for more definitive thermal or injection therapy. Data suggest that saline injection alone is not as effective as contact thermal methods in preventing rebleeding.

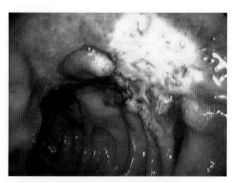

Figure 90.12 Appearance of a duodenal ulcer after successful thermal therapy. The bleeding site and the surrounding area have been successfully heated, leaving the white coagulated tissue behind with no evidence of a persistent visible vessel or bleeding. The surrounding edema is the result of thermal therapy and may also help reduce blood flow to the area.

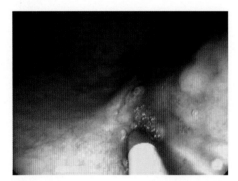

Figure 90.11 Direct application of a multipolar probe to a visible vessel in the base of a gastric ulcer. The central injection needle can be used to inject saline or dilute epinephrine around the vessel. The definitive thermal therapy can then be applied with firm pressure of the probe using long bursts of low energy.

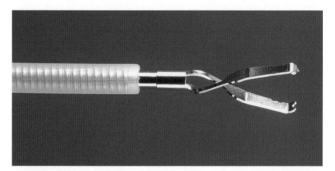

Figure 90.13 A hemostatic clip attached to the delivery catheter. The clip is similar to that used in surgery and is applied to a bleeding vessel to close it. After several days, the clip sloughs into the lumen and is passed. The clip can be rotated to provide a better position for application. The clip is then closed via the handle on the delivery catheter and released from the delivery device. Because the bleeding vessel is not always visible or accessible, multiple clips are often required to achieve the appropriate hemostatic effect.

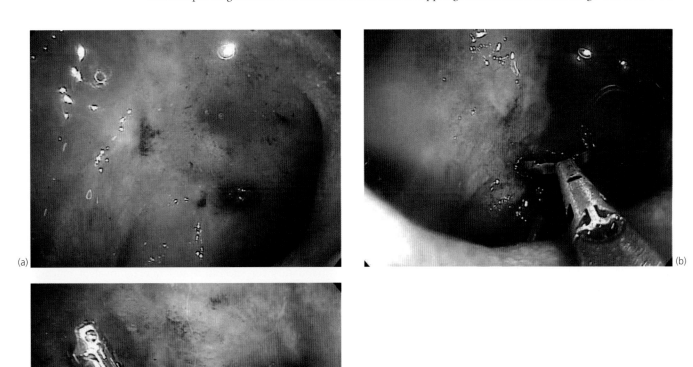

(a)

(b)

(c)

Figure 90.14 (a) Deep duodenal ulcer with a visible vessel in the base. This lesion has a high risk of rebleeding without treatment. **(b)** Application of a hemostatic clip to the ulcer seen in (a). The position of the ulcer facilitates the placement of the clip. Clips may be difficult to place in ulcers that are behind folds or when the ulcer base is extremely fibrotic. Manipulation of the visible vessel may precipitate active bleeding, as seen here. **(c)** Appearance of the same ulcer after successful placement of multiple hemostatic clips. The bleeding has been controlled.

91

Endoscopic therapy for polyps and tumors

Sergey V. Kantsevoy

Endoscopic resection of gastrointestinal polyps and tumors is an important addition to traditional surgical therapy. Endoscopic lesion removal has multiple advantages over open and laparoscopic surgery:

• Endoscopic lesion resection preserves the affected organ and is less traumatic and less risky than surgery.

• Endoscopic resection is usually done as out-patient procedure under sedation obviating the need for general anesthesia and hospital admission with significant cost saving.

• Endoscopic procedures provide faster patient recovery and early return to work and normal physical activity compared with traditional open and laparoscopic surgery.

Knowledge of proper technique and appropriate devices is mandatory for successful and safe removal of mucosal lesions. The following chapter will illustrate procedures and accessories most commonly used during endoscopic removal of large and small bowel lesions. Various complications encountered during endoscopic polypectomy are also demonstrated in this chapter.

Atlas of Gastroenterology, 4th edition. Edited by Tadataka Yamada, David H. Alpers, Anthony N. Kalloo, Neil Kaplowitz, Chung Owyang, and Don W. Powell. © 2009 Blackwell Publishing, ISBN: 978-1-4051-6909-7

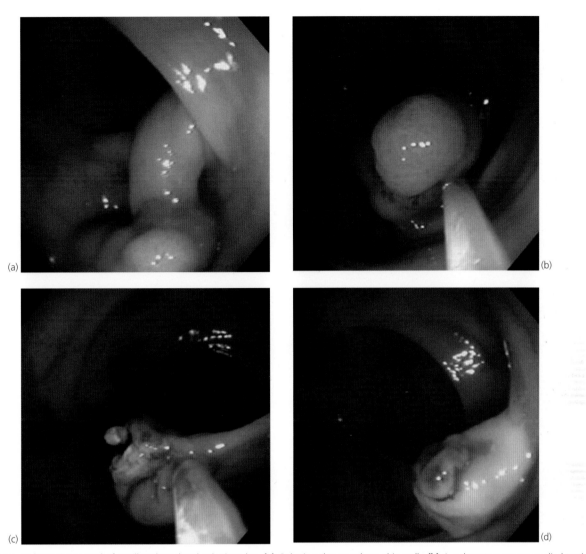

Figure 91.1 Endoscopic removal of small pedunculated colonic polyp. **(a)** Colonic polyp on a long, thin stalk. **(b)** A polypectomy snare applied to the stalk below the head of the polyp. **(c)** The polyp pulled away from the colonic wall to prevent electrical damage to the bowel wall when electrocautery was applied. **(d)** The stalk is transected by the snare without any bleeding from the remaining portion of the stalk. It is very important to leave at least a small portion of the stalk, which can be used for ligation or cautery if post-polypectomy bleeding occurs (as illustrated later in Figure 91.11).

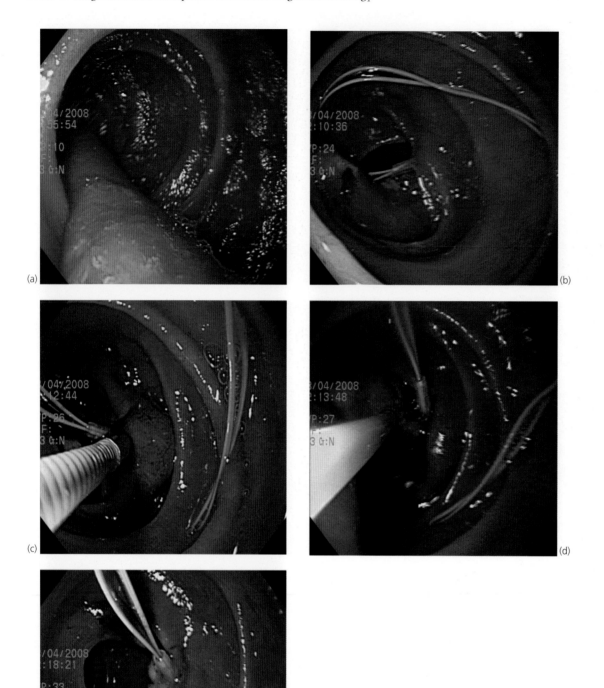

Figure 91.2 Use of detachable snare to prevent post-polypectomy bleeding following removal of a pedunculated polyp with a large (thick) stalk. **(a)** Pedunculated polyp with a large stalk (>1 cm in diameter) located in the second portion of the duodenum. **(b)** Detachable loop (PolyLoop® HX-400U-30, Olympus Optical Inc, Tokyo, Japan) is applied to the base of the stalk at the point of its attachment to the duodenal wall. **(c)** The future polypectomy site is tattooed using a submucosal injection of Spot® (GI Supply, Camp Mill, PA). **(d)** An endoscopic snare is applied to the stalk of the polyp above the previously deployed detachable loop. **(e)** The polyp is excised and removed. The detachable loop is clearly seen at the site of its application. There is no bleeding from the remnant of the stalk.

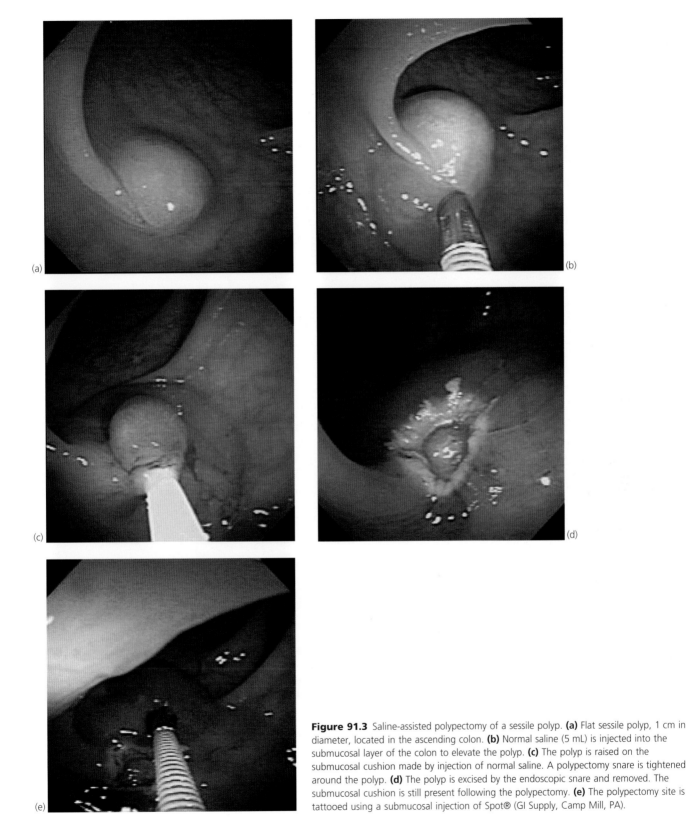

(a)

(b)

(c)

(d)

(e)

Figure 91.3 Saline-assisted polypectomy of a sessile polyp. **(a)** Flat sessile polyp, 1 cm in diameter, located in the ascending colon. **(b)** Normal saline (5 mL) is injected into the submucosal layer of the colon to elevate the polyp. **(c)** The polyp is raised on the submucosal cushion made by injection of normal saline. A polypectomy snare is tightened around the polyp. **(d)** The polyp is excised by the endoscopic snare and removed. The submucosal cushion is still present following the polypectomy. **(e)** The polypectomy site is tattooed using a submucosal injection of Spot® (GI Supply, Camp Mill, PA).

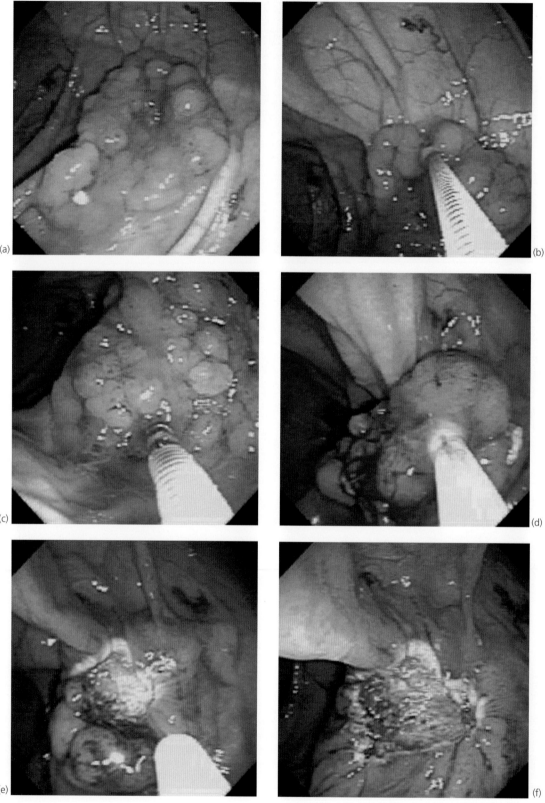

Figure 91.4 Piecemeal removal of a large, flat, sessile colonic polyp with saline-assisted injection technique. **(a)** A large sessile polyp is located in the proximal ascending colon. **(b)** Submucosal injection of normal saline performed in the most proximal portion of the polyp. **(c)** Submucosal injection into the most distal portion of the polyp completes creation of the submucosal cushion under the polyp. **(d)** The polypectomy snare is applied around the proximal portion of the polyp. **(e)** The proximal half of the polyp is removed. **(f)** The polypectomy is completed without technical problems or complications. (*Continued on next page.*)

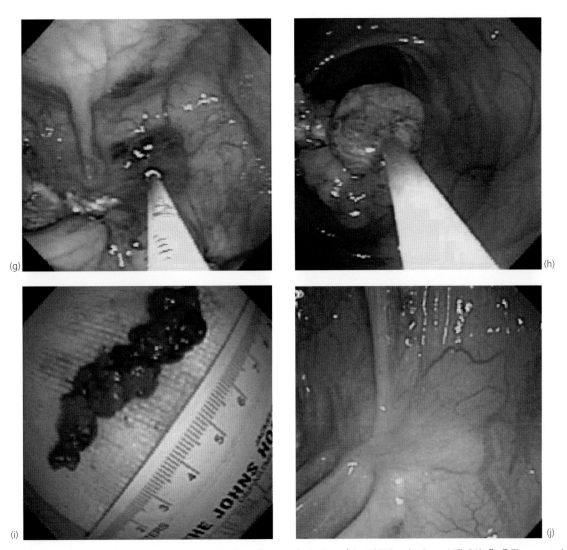

Figure 91.4 *Continued* **(g)** The polypectomy site is tattooed using submucosal injection of Spot (GI Supply, Camp Mill, PA). **(h, i)** The resected polyp is removed for pathological examination with a Roth Net® (US Endoscopy, Mentor, OH) retrieval net. **(j)** A repeat colonoscopy 3 months following initial removal demonstrates complete healing of the polypectomy site without any residual polypoid tissue.

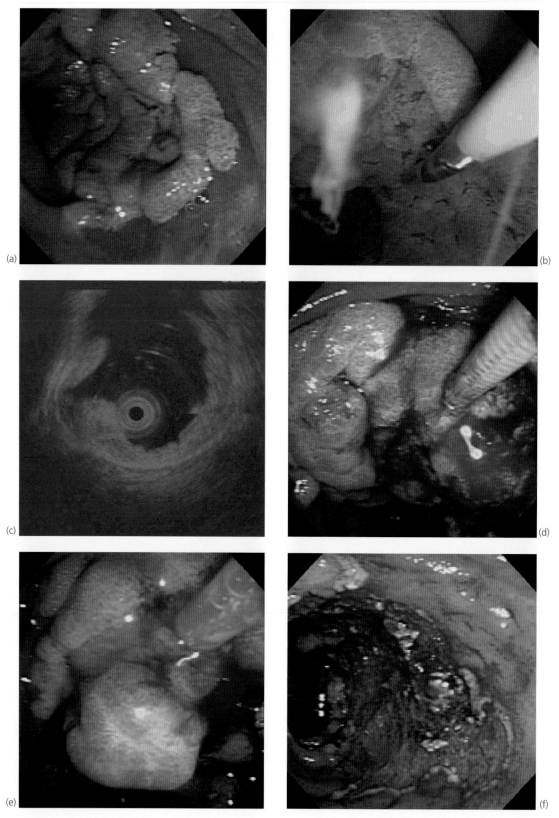

Figure 91.5 Endoscopic ultrasound for detection of the depth of the bowel wall involvement prior to endoscopic resection of a sessile polypoid lesion. **(a)** A large flat sessile polypoid lesion is seen in the second portion of the duodenum. **(b)** The duodenum is filled with water (to create acoustic interface for endoscopic ultrasound) and 20 MHz endoscopic ultrasound probe (Olympus Optical Ltd, Tokyo, Japan) is advanced toward the lesion. **(c)** Endoscopic ultrasound demonstrates polypoid thickening of the mucosal layer with intact submucosal layer of the duodenum. **(d)** Normal saline is injected into the submucosal layer to facilitate polypectomy. **(e)** The polypectomy snare is applied to the polyp. The polyp is excised by the piecemeal technique. **(f)** Final endoscopic view demonstrating the polypectomy site after complete resection of the polyp.

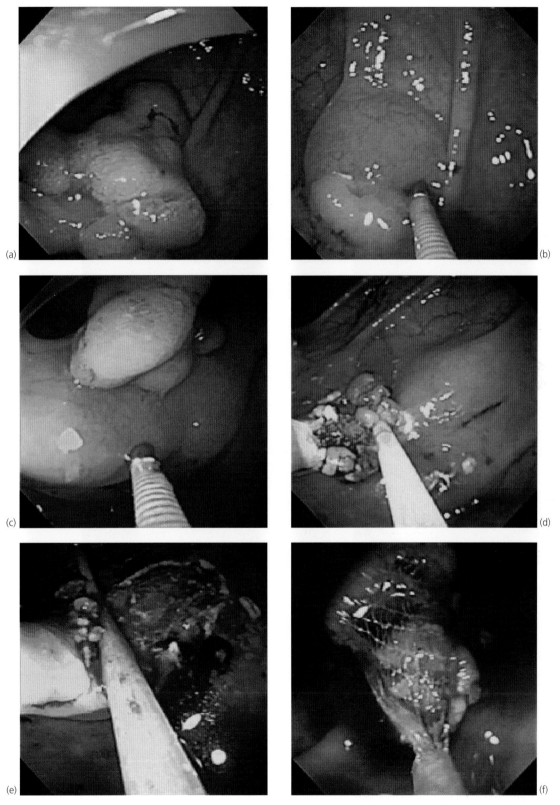

Figure 91.6 Removal of sessile colonic polyp located on an angulated fold in the area of fixed colonic turns can be technically difficult and cause perforation of the colonic wall. Submucosal injection prior to polypectomy facilitates removal of the lesion and decreases the risk of perforation. **(a)** Large fungating polyp with a broad base located in the hepatic flexure on top of the colonic fold. **(b)** Submucosal injection of normal saline solution started with the most proximal portion of the polyp. **(c)** Submucosal injection is completed when the polyp is elevated above the colonic fold. **(d)** The polyp is excised using the piecemeal technique with a polypectomy snare. **(e)** Polypectomy is completed without perforation or bleeding from the polypectomy site. **(f)** All resected parts of the polyp are collected with a Roth Net® (US Endoscopy, Mentor, OH) retrieval net.

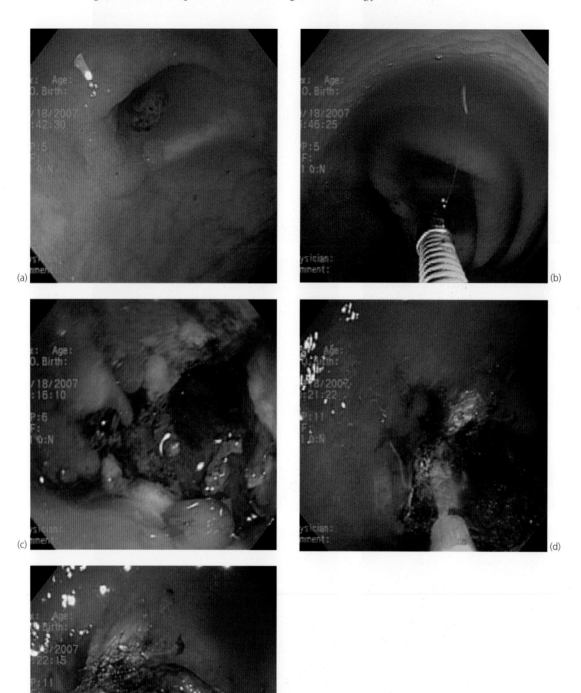

Figure 91.7 Argon plasma coagulation is frequently used to eliminate residual polypoid tissue at the margins and the base of the polypectomy site in order to prevent recurrence of the polyp after polypectomy. **(a)** Endoscopic view of the sessile polyp located inside the appendicular orifice. **(b)** The polyp is elevated with submucosal injection of normal saline solution. **(c)** The polyp is excised with an endoscopic polypectomy snare. **(d)** The base and margins of the polypectomy site are treated with the argon plasma coagulator to remove residual polypoid tissue at the margins and the base of the polypectomy site. **(e)** Final view of the polypectomy site with no visible residual polypoid tissue.

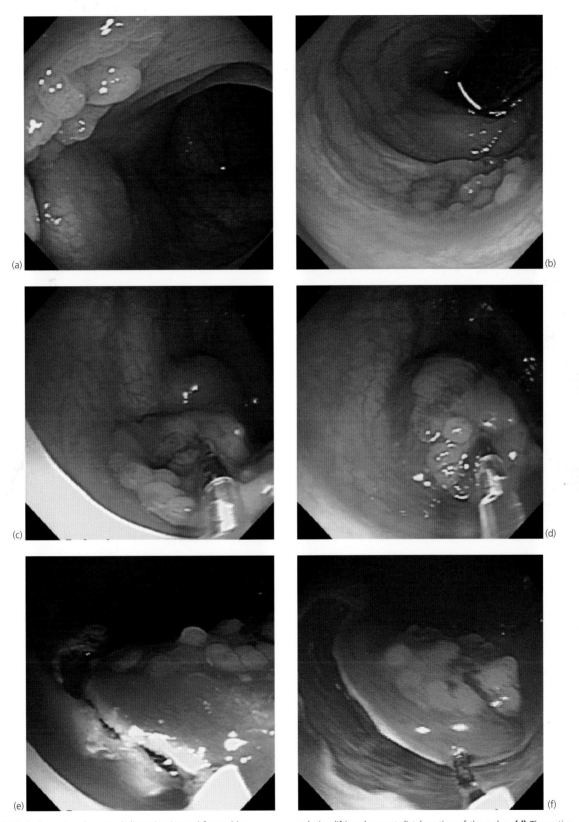

Figure 91.8 Endoscopic submucosal dissection is used for en bloc removal of sessile lesions of gastrointestinal tract. **(a)** Large, flat, sessile polyp located in descending colon. Please notice suboptimal visualization of the polyp on forward view due to its location behind the colonic fold. **(b)** Retroflex position of the colonoscope significantly improves visualization of the polyp. **(c)** Submucosal injection of normal saline solution lifting the most distal portion of the polyp. **(d)** The entire polyp is lifted with the submucosal injection of normal saline. **(e)** A circumferential incision is made around the polyp using the tip of a polypectomy snare. **(f)** The polyp is dissected from underlining muscularis layer using the tip of the polypectomy snare. (*Continued on next page.*)

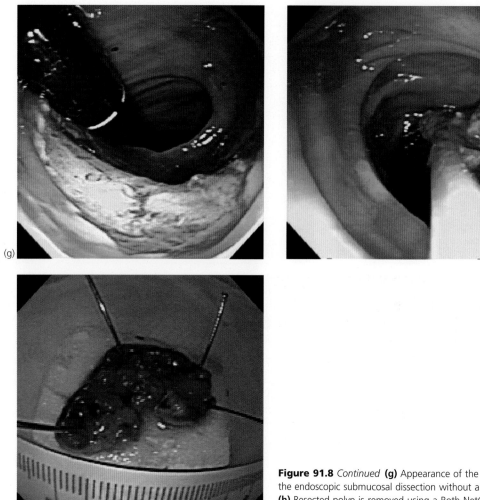

(g)

(h)

(i)

Figure 91.8 *Continued* **(g)** Appearance of the polypectomy site after completion of the endoscopic submucosal dissection without any evidence of bleeding or perforation. **(h)** Resected polyp is removed using a Roth Net® (US Endoscopy, Mentor, OH) retrieval net. **(i)** Pathological specimen demonstrating en bloc removal of the large (3 cm in diameter) polyp within the healthy tissues.

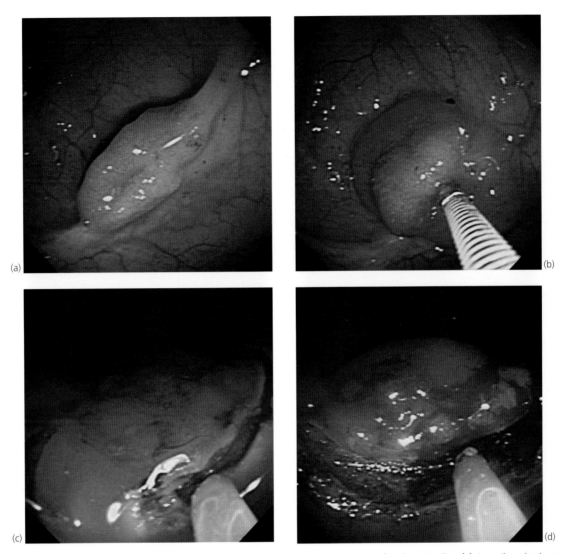

Figure 91.9 Small perforations after endoscopic submucosal dissection repaired with application of endoscopic clips. **(a)** A sessile polyp located on a colonic fold in the descending colon. **(b)** The polyp is raised with a submucosal injection of normal saline solution. **(c)** A circumferential incision around the polyp performed with the tip of an endoscopic polypectomy snare. **(d)** Endoscopic submucosal dissection is performed with the tip of an endoscopic polypectomy snare. (*Continued on next page*.)

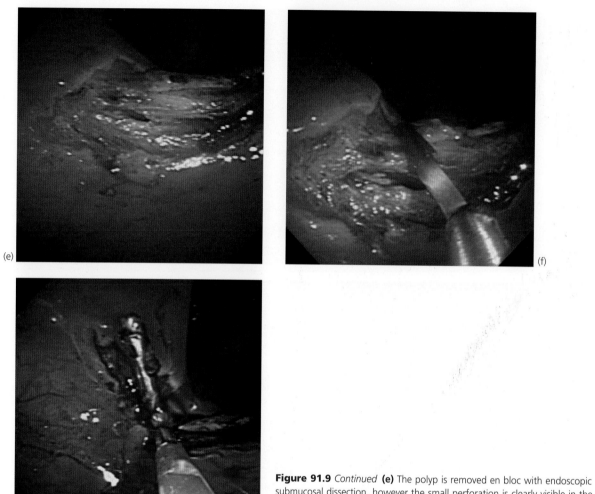

(e)

(f)

(g)

Figure 91.9 *Continued* **(e)** The polyp is removed en bloc with endoscopic submucosal dissection, however the small perforation is clearly visible in the muscularis layer of the colon. **(f)** Endoscopic clip (Resolution® Boston Scientific Microvasive, Natick, MA) is ready for application to close the perforation. **(g)** Application of two endoscopic clips to completely close the colonic perforation.

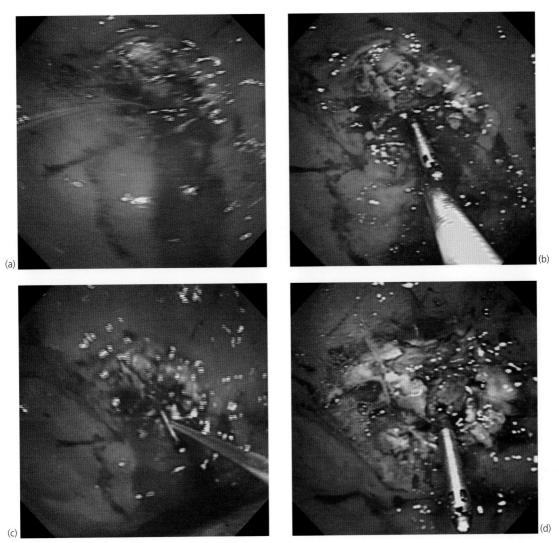

Figure 91.10 Bleeding following endoscopic polyp removal. Endoscopic hemostasis is usually successful in controlling the bleeding. **(a)** Active arterial bleeding from a polypectomy site. **(b)** Endoscopic clip (Resolution® Boston Scientific Microvasive, Natick, MA) is applied to the bleeding vessel. **(c)** The blood from the polypectomy site is washed away. **(d)** Final view of the polypectomy site demonstrating successful hemostasis without any active bleeding.

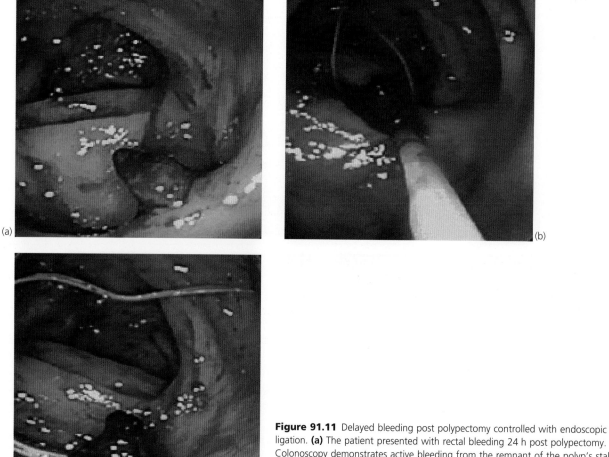

Figure 91.11 Delayed bleeding post polypectomy controlled with endoscopic ligation. **(a)** The patient presented with rectal bleeding 24 h post polypectomy. Colonoscopy demonstrates active bleeding from the remnant of the polyp's stalk post previous polypectomy. **(b)** Endoscopic detachable loop (PolyLoop® HX-400U-30, Olympus Optical Inc., Tokyo, Japan) is positioned around the remnant of the polyp's stalk. **(c)** Full deployment of the detachable loop with successful endoscopic hemostasis.

92

Laparoscopy and laparotomy

Wenliang Chen, David W. Rattner

Laparoscopy and laparotomy are surgical techniques that provide direct access to the abdominopelvic cavity for diagnosis and therapy. The word laparoscopy was compounded from two Greek roots, *lapara* (meaning the soft parts of the body between rib cage and hips) and *skopein* (*scope* in English, meaning to see or examine). Similarly, laparotomy was compounded from Greek roots *lapara* and *tome* (meaning to cut). Since most gastrointestinal (GI) organs reside in the abdominopelvic cavity, laparotomy has traditionally been the gold standard in diagnosing and treating GI conditions. However, in recent years, the dominance of laparotomy has been challenged by laparoscopy. Nowadays, laparoscopy has replaced laparotomy as the standard approach for gallbladder surgery, antireflux surgery, and weight-loss surgery. In colon surgery and hernia surgery, laparoscopic approaches are rapidly gaining popularity.

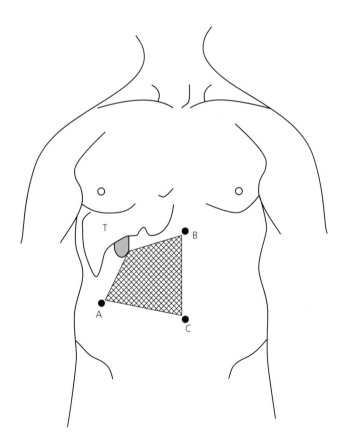

Figure 92.1 Optimal trocar placement in laparoscopic surgery. T, target organ, in this case the gallbladder; C, camera port; A and B, ports for laparoscopic instruments.

Atlas of Gastroenterology, 4th edition. Edited by Tadataka Yamada, David H. Alpers, Anthony N. Kalloo, Neil Kaplowitz, Chung Owyang, and Don W. Powell. © 2009 Blackwell Publishing, ISBN: 978-1-4051-6909-7

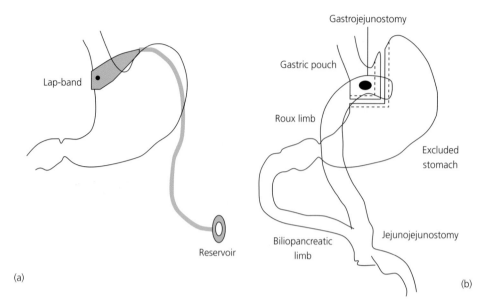

(a)

(b)

Figure 92.2 Weight-loss surgery. A, laparoscopic adjustable gastric band. B, Roux-en-Y gastric bypass.

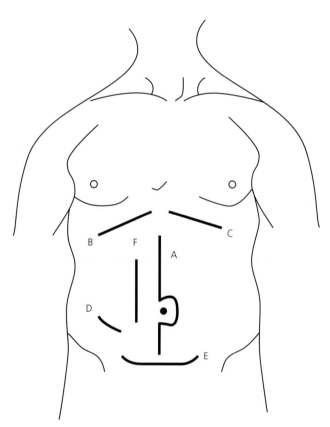

Figure 92.3 Laparotomy incisions. A, midline; B, right subcostal; C, left subcostal; D, McBurney; E, Pfannenstiel; F, right paramedian.

93

Plain and contrast radiology

Marc S. Levine, Stephen E. Rubesin, Hans Herlinger, Igor Laufer

Plain radiographs of the abdomen are useful for evaluating abdominal pain or distention, obstructive symptoms, or clinical signs of an acute abdomen. The combination of supine and upright or decubitus horizontal beam radiographs allows the diagnosis of ileus as opposed to obstruction of the small bowel or colon, free intraperitoneal air (pneumoperitoneum) (Fig. 93.1), ischemic or necrotic bowel with air in the bowel wall (pneumatosis) (Fig. 93.2), air in the bile ducts (pneumobilia), and portal venous gas (Fig. 93.3). Nevertheless, computed tomographic (CT) scanning has been recognized as a more sensitive modality for evaluating acute abdominal symptoms (see Chapter 96).

Double-contrast radiography is a valuable technique for diagnosing a wide spectrum of pathological processes in the gastrointestinal tract. Because this technique can delineate normal mucosal surface patterns in the pharynx, upper gastrointestinal tract, small bowel, and colon, it is particularly helpful in detecting a variety of inflammatory or neoplastic diseases involving the mucosa. In some cases, barium studies may demonstrate abnormalities that are missed or misinterpreted at endoscopic examination. The double-contrast study is also a less expensive and less invasive procedure than endoscopy. We therefore believe that double-contrast radiography and endoscopy should be considered as complementary procedures for evaluating suspected gastrointestinal disease.

Double-contrast radiography can delineate in detail the normal anatomic features of the pharynx (Fig. 93.4). As a result, inflammatory (Fig. 93.5) or neoplastic (Figs 93.6 and 93.7) lesions that disrupt or obliterate the normal anatomic landmarks can be demonstrated readily. In the upper gastrointestinal tract, double-contrast techniques allow detection of esophagitis caused by plaques or ulcers (Fig. 93.8), esophageal cancer (Fig. 93.9), benign gastric ulcer (Fig. 93.10), early gastric cancer (Fig. 93.11), duodenal ulcer (Fig. 93.12), erosive gastritis or duodenitis, and other inflammatory or neoplastic lesions. The small bowel enema (enteroclysis) has proved to be a much more sensitive technique than conventional small bowel follow-through examination for determining the site and cause of small bowel obstruction (Fig. 93.13) and a variety of other abnormalities in the small bowel (Figs 93.14–93.16). Double-contrast barium enema examination is a valuable technique for detecting colonic polyps or carcinoma (Fig. 93.17) and for diagnosing inflammatory bowel disease (granulomatous and ulcerative colitis) or its complications (Fig. 93.18). Double-contrast studies may also be performed to evaluate the colon after a surgical procedure (Fig. 93.19). Although rare, complications of these studies may be encountered (Fig. 93.20).

Atlas of Gastroenterology, 4th edition. Edited by Tadataka Yamada, David H. Alpers, Anthony N. Kalloo, Neil Kaplowitz, Chung Owyang, and Don W. Powell. © 2009 Blackwell Publishing, ISBN: 978-1-4051-6909-7

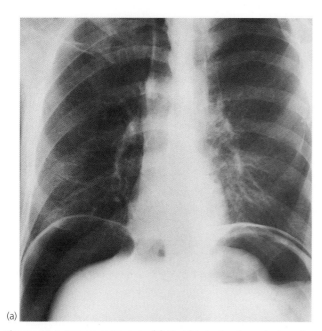

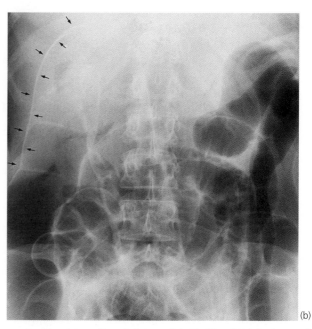

(a)

(b)

Figure 93.1 Pneumoperitoneum. **(a)** Upright chest radiograph shows large amounts of free intraperitoneal air beneath both sides of the diaphragm of this patient with a perforated duodenal ulcer. **(b)** Supine plain radiograph of the abdomen of another patient shows an indirect sign of pneumoperitoneum, air on both sides of the bowel wall (Rigler sign; arrows) after perforation at colonoscopy.

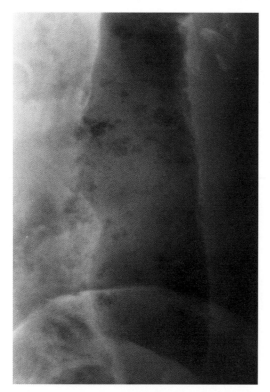

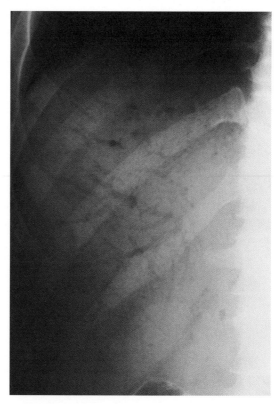

Figure 93.2 Pneumatosis caused by infarction of the left colon after a surgical procedure. Close-up view of supine plain radiograph of the abdomen shows tiny, mottled, and linear collections of gas in the wall of the descending colon.

Figure 93.3 Close-up view of the right upper quadrant on supine plain radiograph of the abdomen shows linear, branching collections of gas in the portal venous system caused by intestinal infarction. Gas shadows extend to the periphery of the liver. This appearance is characteristic of portal venous gas.

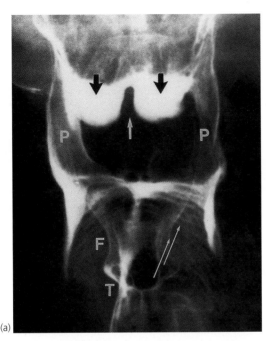

(a)

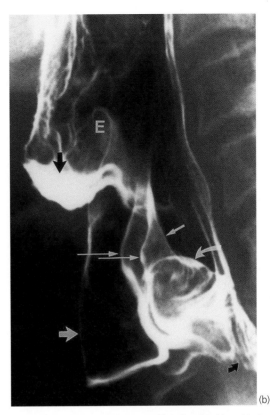

(b)

Figure 93.4 Normal pharyngeal anatomy. **(a)** Frontal view of pharynx shows cup-shaped valleculae (black arrows) separated by the median glossoepiglottic fold (short white arrow). More inferiorly, pyriform sinuses (P) form the anterior portion of lateral food channels. The arcuate line (long white arrows) is caused by normal laryngeal impression on the collapsed hypopharynx. In this case, both true (T) and false (F) vocal cords are outlined with aspirated barium in the larynx. **(b)** Lateral view during phonation shows the epiglottic tip (E), valleculae (short black arrow), aryepiglottic folds (medium-length white arrow), and anterior walls of pyriform sinuses (long white arrows). Redundant mucosal folds overlie the muscular process of the arytenoid (curved white arrow) and cricoid (curved black arrow) cartilages. Aspirated barium outlines the laryngeal vestibule (short white arrow) and ventricle.

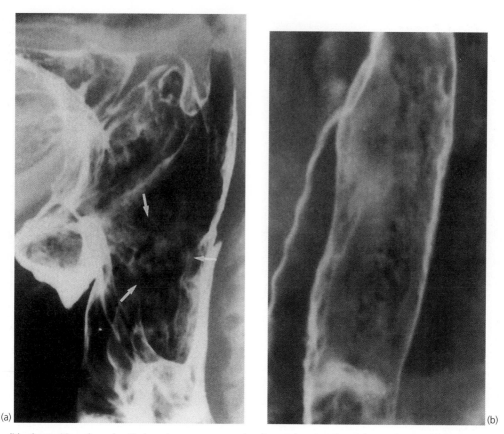

(a)

(b)

Figure 93.5 *Candida* pharyngitis and esophagitis in an immunosuppressed patient undergoing chemotherapy for metastatic breast cancer. **(a)** Lateral view of the pharynx shows small, sharply circumscribed plaques (arrows) in the hypopharynx. **(b)** Double-contrast esophagogram also shows multiple plaque-like lesions in the esophagus caused by concomitant *Candida* esophagitis.

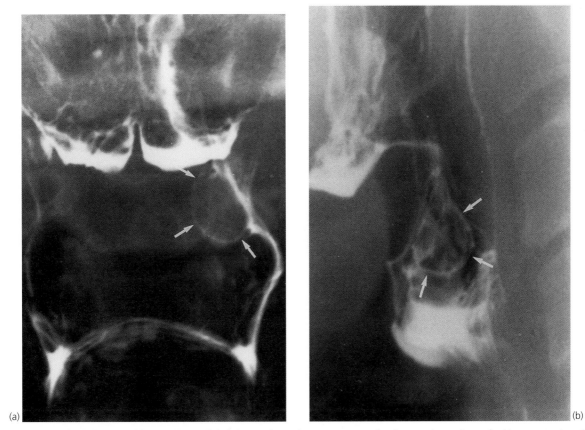

(a)

(b)

Figure 93.6 Aryepiglottic fold cyst. **(a)** Frontal view of the pharynx shows the cyst as a smooth submucosal mass (arrows) with an approximately 90° angle between the border of the mass and the adjacent pharyngeal wall. **(b)** Lateral view shows the lesion as a round, sharply circumscribed mass (arrows).

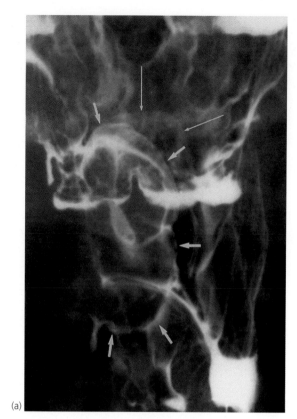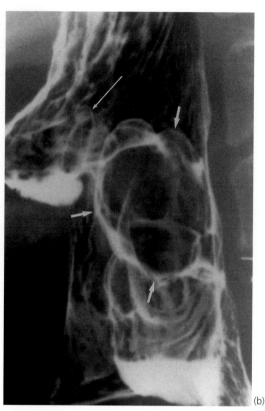

(a)

(b)

Figure 93.7 Squamous cell carcinoma of the hypopharynx. **(a)** Frontal view of the pharynx shows a large polypoid mass (short arrows) obliterating the right lateral wall of the hypopharynx. The tumor extends across the midline. Valleculae and the tip of the epiglottis (long arrows) are preserved. **(b)** Lateral view demonstrates a lobulated mass (short arrows) in the hypopharynx. The epiglottic tip (long arrow) is preserved.

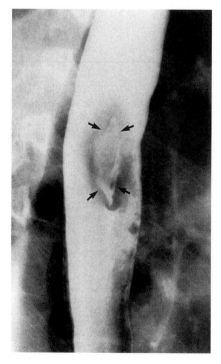

Figure 93.8 Single-contrast esophagram shows a giant, diamond-shaped ulcer (arrows) with a surrounding radiolucent rim of edema in the midesophagus. The patient has human immunodeficiency virus (HIV) infection and odynophagia. Endoscopic biopsy specimens, brushings, and cultures revealed no evidence of cytomegalovirus infection, so the ulcer probably was caused directly by HIV infection (idiopathic or HIV-related ulcer).

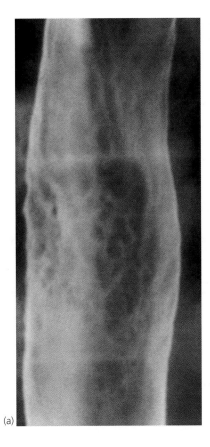

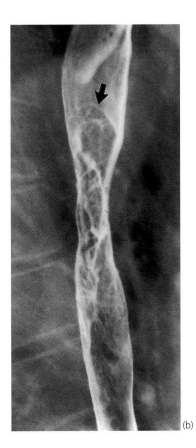

Figure 93.9 Esophageal carcinoma. **(a)** Superficial spreading carcinoma with focal nodularity of the midesophagus caused by tiny, coalescent nodules and plaques. **(b)** Advanced infiltrating esophageal carcinoma with irregular narrowing of the lumen. The tumor has an abrupt shelf-like proximal border (arrow).

(a)

(b)

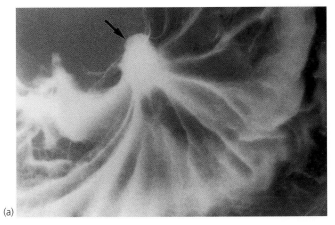

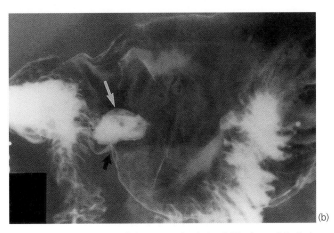

(a)

(b)

Figure 93.10 Benign gastric ulcers. **(a)** Lesser curvature ulcer (arrow). Smooth folds radiate to the edge of the crater. This lesion fulfils the radiological criteria for a benign gastric ulcer. **(b)** Greater curvature ulcer (white arrow) caused by aspirin ingestion. Deformity of the greater curvature (black arrow) is depicted adjacent to the ulcer.

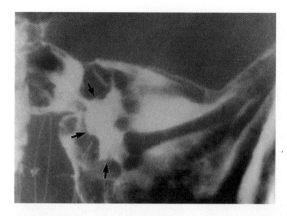

Figure 93.11 Early gastric cancer manifested by an irregular ulcer (arrows) on the posterior wall of the antrum with scalloped borders and nodular, clubbed folds surrounding the ulcer.

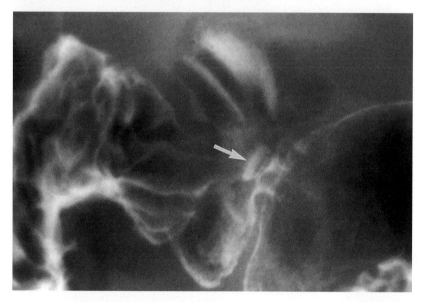

Figure 93.12 Linear duodenal ulcer (arrow) at the base of the bulb. Thickened folds are present above the ulcer.

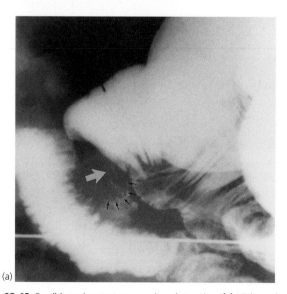

(a)

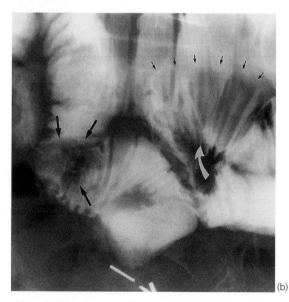

(b)

Figure 93.13 Small bowel metastases causing obstruction. **(a)** High-grade small bowel obstruction caused by annular metastasis from gastric carcinoma. Tight, constricted segment (white arrow) and distal mass effect (black arrows) are visible. **(b)** Partially obstructing metastases from sigmoid carcinoma. One metastasis causes spiculation and fixation of the small bowel wall (white arrow) with normal distensibility of the opposite wall (small black arrows). Another metastasis appears en face as a filling defect (large black arrows) causing distortion of folds.

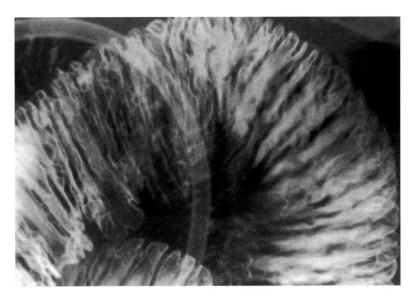

Figure 93.14 Intestinal lymphangiectasia manifested by thickened, mildly irregular folds and tiny nodules representing engorged villi.

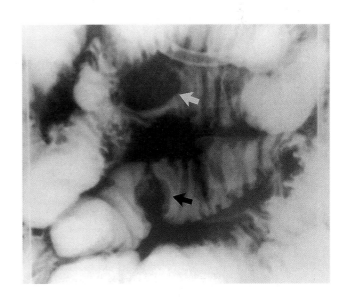

Figure 93.15 Carcinoid tumors in the ileum. The smaller, more distal lesion appears as a smooth submucosal mass (black arrow). However, a larger lesion (white arrow) is associated with outward extension into the mesentery.

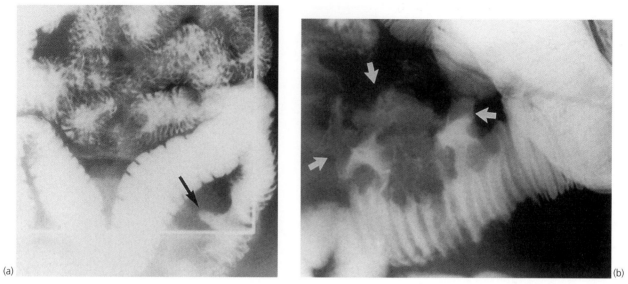

Figure 93.16 Non-Hodgkin lymphoma of the small bowel. **(a)** Radiograph from small-bowel follow-through study shows focal obliteration of folds of the small bowel with associated ulcer (arrow) on the mesenteric border of the bowel. Because of a history of systemic lupus erythematosus, these findings were attributed to lupus-related vasculitis. **(b)** Spot radiograph from small bowel enema examination performed during later hospital admission shows exoenteric excavation (arrows) from previously ulcerated area. This finding is characteristic of non-Hodgkin lymphoma involving the small bowel.

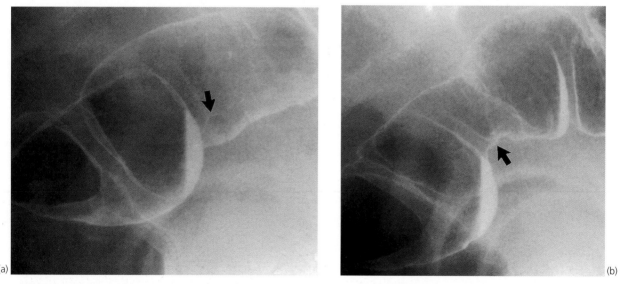

Figure 93.17 Development of colonic carcinoma. **(a)** Initial radiograph shows a small polypoid lesion (arrow) on the anterior wall of the distal sigmoid colon. **(b)** Repeat radiograph from double-contrast barium enema examination several years later shows how the polyp has developed into an infiltrating carcinoma (arrow).

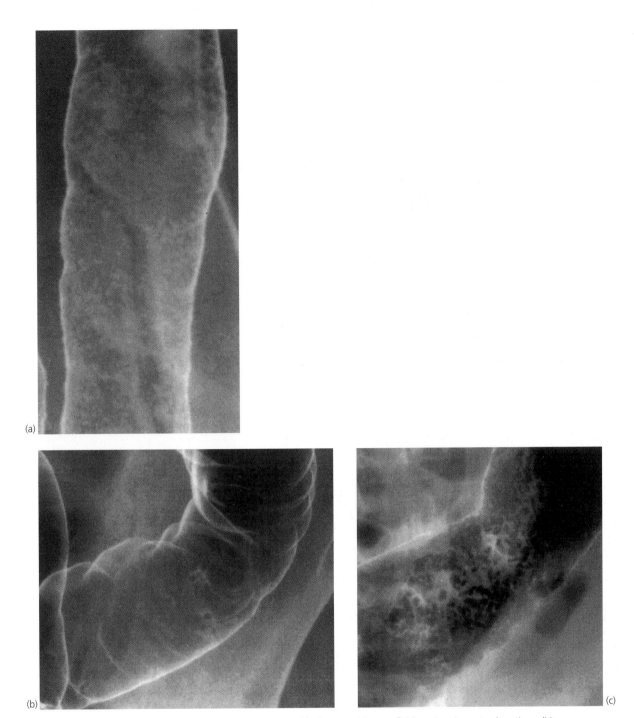

(a)

(b)

(c)

Figure 93.18 Ulcerative colitis. **(a)** Stippling of colonic mucosa caused by innumerable superficial erosions in acute ulcerative colitis.
(b) Postinflammatory (filiform) polyposis in a patient with quiescent colitis. **(c)** Epithelial dysplasia (precancerous) in a patient with chronic ulcerative colitis. Faceted, angular filling defects are characteristic of dysplasia. **(c)** Courtesy of Dr F.M. Kelvin.

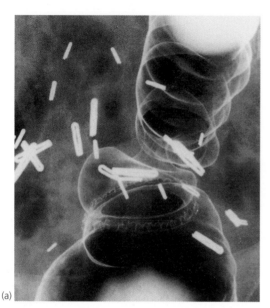

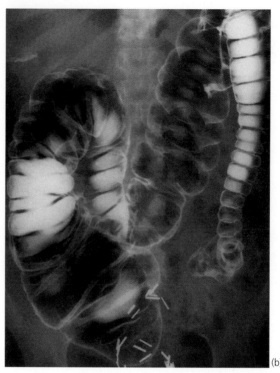

(a)

(b)

Figure 93.19 Postoperative colons of two patients. **(a)** Normal double-contrast appearance of colorectal anastomosis. The site of anastomosis is indicated by the staple line. **(b)** Radiograph from double-contrast colostomy enema examination shows a normal postoperative colon. This examination is important for detecting recurrent or metachronous carcinoma.

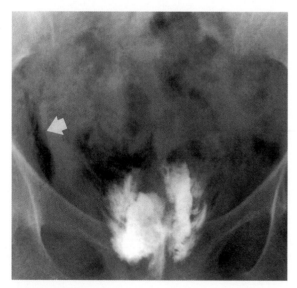

Figure 93.20 Complication of barium enema caused by laceration of the rectum by inflated rectal balloon. Radiograph shows extravasation of barium into perirectal tissue. Retroperitoneal air (arrow) is visible along the right lateral wall of the pelvis.

94

Diagnostic sonography

Philip W. Ralls, R. Brooke Jeffrey Jr, Robert A. Kane, Michelle L. Robbin

Diagnostic sonography is experiencing the most vigorous and revolutionary period of technological advancement in its history. Current systems make use of sophisticated technology to produce high-resolution pictures that incorporate anatomic and pathological features and color-coded blood flow into a single moving real-time image.

Doppler sonography

Doppler sonography is a virtually routine component of many modern sonographic examinations. It adds dynamic, real-time flow information to the morphological images provided by gray-scale imaging. Color Doppler sonography (CDS) passively and automatically superimposes color-coded flow information on all or a selected portion of gray-scale images. It also facilitates comparison of flow in different anatomic locations and minimizes the chance of missing flow in an unexpected area. Spectral Doppler sonography is used to acquire detailed flow information from a small area when quantitative information about flow velocity or fluctuation in flow is important.

Role of sonography in gastroenterology

Sonography is an important, often primary imaging modality for the biliary tract, liver, and pancreas. High-resolution transabdominal visualization of the gastrointestinal tract is vital in appendicitis and increasingly useful for the remaining gastrointestinal tract from esophagus to anus. Its abilities ensure an increasing role in evaluating gastrointestinal problems.

Strengths and weaknesses of sonography compared with other modalities

When sonography can depict the area of clinical interest, it is nearly an ideal modality. The ability of diagnostic sonography to display flow and soft tissue in real time is unique among imaging techniques. Unlike other modalities, ultrasound has no known adverse effects; it is completely safe. Its spatial resolution is superior to that of computed tomographic (CT) scanning and magnetic resonance imaging (MRI). Because diagnostic sonography is safe and tolerated well by patients, it can be performed serially when necessary to follow the progress of treatment. When needed, ultrasound examinations can be performed quickly and at the bedside.

Unfortunately, there are many circumstances in which optimal or even adequate images cannot be obtained. The single most important problem is the inability of sonography to show what is beyond gas–soft tissue or bone–soft tissue interfaces. This makes comprehensive survey scanning essentially impossible. Better survey modalities are CT scanning, in particular, and MRI. The other main limitation of sonography is its relatively poor contrast resolution, which provides a limited ability to display differences between normal and abnormal tissue. Also, CT scanning and MRI have inherently better contrast resolution, which is further improved with the use of oral and intravenous contrast agents. Contrast agents for non-cardiac ultrasound imaging, despite overwhelming evidence of their usefulness, have not been approved yet by the FDA for use in the United States. Many abnormalities displayed automatically on whole-body CT scans or magnetic resonance images are either impossible or very difficult to visualize with sonography.

Sonography often is superior to CT scanning and MRI in examinations of patients who are uncooperative, unable to hold their breath, or unable to remain relatively still. It is often superior in examinations of patients with little body fat. This makes sonography very useful in pediatric imaging, for example. Patient factors that impede optimal sonography include extreme obesity and factors that limit cutaneous acoustic access, such as burns, incisions, dressings that

Atlas of Gastroenterology, 4th edition. Edited by Tadataka Yamada, David H. Alpers, Anthony N. Kalloo, Neil Kaplowitz, Chung Owyang, and Don W. Powell. © 2009 Blackwell Publishing, ISBN: 978-1-4051-6909-7.

cannot be removed, and cutaneous gastrointestinal enterostomies.

The liver

Liver sonography has many uses as a primary and secondary imaging examination. Primary indications include suspected or known cirrhosis (Fig. 94.1), suspected abscess (Fig. 94.2), suspected tumor (Figs 94.3–94.5), suspected vascular abnormalities (Figs 94.6 and 94.7), trauma, and transplantation. Sonography can be used to characterize abnormalities found at other imaging examinations, such as CT scanning or MRI. Its safety and relatively modest cost make it an ideal means of assessment of the therapeutic response of known lesions or sequential follow-up evaluation of liver lesions of questionable importance.

Sonography is often a simple and effective way to guide percutaneous aspiration, drainage, biopsy, or tumor ablation. Unsuspected liver lesions often are incidental findings during sonography performed for nonhepatic indications. Sonography can guide further evaluation or management of these lesions. The main strengths of hepatic sonography are the ability to help characterize common benign lesions (cysts, hemangiomas) and guide percutaneous procedures, safety, excellent patient tolerance, and low cost. Weaknesses include inability to image the entire liver in some patients and inferiority to CT scanning in detecting extrahepatic disease.

Sonography, like CT scanning, can be used effectively to guide percutaneous procedures. Nuclear medicine studies and MRI lack this ability. When performed by an expert, sonographically guided liver biopsy often is quicker and easier than biopsy with CT guidance. Sonography can directly depict the needle tip as it is placed in the lesion, facilitating biopsy of small lesions and lesions in uncooperative patients. Ultrasound-guided biopsy is more efficient and cost effective, even when lesions are initially detected with another modality. Despite the advantages of sonography, CT biopsy is more popular with radiologists because it almost always shows the needle location. Sonographic needle visualization may be difficult or impossible when the liver is echogenic or when acoustic access is imperfect. Newer sonographic techniques that enhance needle-tip visualization and improved biopsy guides promise to make sonographically guided biopsy easier.

Sonography may be used to evaluate resectability of primary or metastatic liver tumors (see Fig. 94.3). The ability of sonography to provide images in any oblique plane often makes it superior to CT scanning and MRI in localizing lesions to an anatomic hepatic segment. Sonography can be used to guide biopsy of newly detected lesions that might preclude curative hepatic resection. Intraoperative sonogra-

phy is the most sensitive means of detecting focal liver lesions. At many centers where hepatic resections are performed, intraoperative sonography is routine before resection. When a questionable lesion is found at intraoperative ultrasound scanning, sonographically guided biopsy can be performed.

Although less sensitive than CT scanning or MRI, hepatic sonography can be used to seek focal lesions. When a liver abscess (see Fig. 94.2) is suspected clinically, sonography is the preferred screening modality. Hepatic sonography can be used to screen for metastases, if extrahepatic staging is not needed. When an optimal sonographic examination cannot be performed on an individual patient, CT scanning or MRI should be performed. CT scanning is preferred when extrahepatic staging is needed.

The gallbladder and biliary tract

Sonography is the imaging method of choice for the initial evaluation of all clinically suspected diseases of the gallbladder. It is particularly valuable to patients with acute right upper quadrant pain and possible acute cholecystitis. Sonography is highly reliable in the detection of tiny gallstones (Fig. 94.8) and is useful for evaluating focal or diffuse abnormalities of the gallbladder wall (Figs 94.9 and 94.10). Biliary sonography has several distinct advantages compared with scintigraphy and CT scanning. It is less expensive than both modalities and can be performed rapidly without patient preparation or use of contrast agents. Unlike biliary scintigraphy, sonography is not organ specific and may provide important diagnostic information regarding the liver, pancreas, and peritoneal cavity. Sonography can be performed readily on patients with abnormal liver tests, which often preclude scintigraphy. Finally, sonography may be used to guide percutaneous cholecystostomy in the care of critically ill patients at the bedside. When the gallbladder is normal, sonography can be used for a rapid survey of the remainder of the abdomen to search for an alternative cause of right upper quadrant pain.

One of the most important technical improvements in the last decade has been the increasing sensitivity of color Doppler imaging and the development of power Doppler sonography. Although some initial studies have suggested that mural hyperemia may accompany some cases of more advanced forms of acute cholecystitis, it remains to be seen whether color Doppler imaging will have a role in differentiating normal from abnormal gallbladder perfusion (see Fig. 94.9). The development of ultrasound contrast agents affords an opportunity to evaluate gallbladder perfusion much more easily. The most problematic area in gallbladder imaging is that of acalculous cholecystitis. It is unclear whether future developments will enhance diagnostic efficacy.

The ability of sonography to depict dilated bile ducts and the level of biliary obstruction makes it the technique of choice for examining patients with jaundice. Sonography can depict the cause of obstruction (Fig. 94.11), albeit with limited accuracy. Infectious cholangitis and conditions such as cholangiopathy caused by human immunodeficiency virus infection are instances for sonography. Sonography can be used to detect and assess, with the help of color Doppler imaging, the resectability of cholangiocarcinoma and other tumors of the bile ducts.

Sonography routinely displays the normal intra- and extrahepatic ducts. The internal diameter of the normal extrahepatic bile duct is 5 mm or less, although elderly patients and patients with gallstones may have ducts 6–9 mm in internal diameter. Ten or more millimeters is abnormal dilation. The distal common duct is usually seen within the pancreatic head and has a somewhat smaller caliber. The intrahepatic bile ducts may be ventral to the left and right portal veins. The normal internal diameter of the main left and right intrahepatic bile ducts is about 1 mm.

The pancreas

Sonography is indicated in the care of all patients with acute pancreatitis, not to evaluate the pancreas itself but to detect gallstones and biliary dilation. Complications of pancreatitis are best sought with CT scanning, but sonography may be used to detect and follow complications of acute pancreatitis (Fig. 94.12). Sonography can be used to guide biopsy, drainage, or aspiration of selected pancreatic lesions. Sonography is the primary imaging method to screen patients with jaundice or abdominal pain. Sonography may be used to detect acute or chronic pancreatitis or reveal pancreatic masses. Sonography may be more effective than CT scanning in determining whether a lesion is pancreatic or contiguous with the pancreas. Sonography occasionally is useful to characterize abnormalities found at CT scanning, to determine, for example, whether a lesion is cystic or solid.

Although CT scanning remains the most sensitive means of evaluating pancreatic disease, modern ultrasound technology and new scanning techniques (oral contrast administration, compression scanning) are reestablishing sonography as a useful and clinically relevant pancreatic imaging technique. Although sonography cannot be used to diagnose pancreatic necrosis, it can be used to follow known pancreatitis-associated fluid collections and guide interventional techniques to treat patients with pancreatitis. Color Doppler sonography shows great promise as a tool to assess the resectability of pancreatic tumors (Fig. 94.13), potentially lessening the role of both CT and endoscopic ultrasound scanning.

The gastrointestinal tract

The most common indication for gastrointestinal sonography is evaluation of right lower quadrant pain and possible appendicitis (Fig. 94.14). Sonography may be useful in the diagnosis of diverticulitis (Figs 94.15 and 94.16), obstruction of the small bowel (Fig. 94.17), and bulky mesenteric (Fig. 94.18) or gastrointestinal neoplasms. Not infrequently, a gastrointestinal tract abnormality is discovered incidentally during a screening examination of the upper abdomen or pelvis. High-resolution intralumenal probes routinely depict five discrete layers of bowel wall. With conventional abdominal transducers, however, it is not possible to resolve all five layers. The echogenic submucosal layer, however, is clearly visible and serves as a constant anatomic feature that is an extremely useful landmark to identify an intraabdominal structure as a bowel loop.

Pathological processes that cause ulceration and necrosis of the bowel lead to focal or global loss of visualization of the echogenic submucosa. Primary neoplasms involving the bowel wall may result in focal thickening of the bowel wall, referred to as the target sign or pseudokidney sign (Fig. 94.19). Tumor infiltrating the bowel wall appears as a hypoechoic mass (mimicking the cortex of the kidney). The echogenic mucosal surface lumen is preserved and mimics the fat-containing hilum of the kidney. Gas trapped within ulcerating lesions involving the bowel wall may result in high-amplitude echoes with acoustic reverberation artifacts within the submucosal layers of the bowel wall.

Color Doppler sonography may be a useful adjunct to gray-scale imaging in the evaluation of focal thickening of the bowel wall. Increased arterial flow within the involved segment suggests inflammation or infection; diminished flow or absence of flow suggests intramural hemorrhage (Fig. 94.20), ischemia, or infarction (Fig. 94.21). The vascularity of gastrointestinal tumors is variable, but adenocarcinoma typically is hypovascular.

The peritoneal cavity

The most common indication for evaluation of the peritoneal cavity with sonography is to search for intraperitoneal fluid collections such as ascites, abscesses, or hemorrhage. Sonography is useful not only to identify intraperitoneal fluid collections but also to guide percutaneous needle aspiration for definitive diagnosis. Solid peritoneal masses representing either primary or metastatic tumors may be detected on occasion. For patients with a clinical likelihood of peritoneal metastases, however, CT scanning is the preferred imaging modality.

Intraoperative ultrasound

Intraoperative ultrasonography (IOUS) provides indispensable information that influences clinical management and choice of surgical procedure. Several technical advances have made IOUS even more effective. These advances include miniaturization of transducers, use of spectral and color Doppler ultrasound, and the development of laparoscopic ultrasonography.

Optimal IOUS requires considerable technical expertise and, more important, experience in interpreting subtle real-time sonographic abnormalities. If surgeons perform intraoperative scanning, it is imperative that they be appropriately trained and sufficiently experienced to use IOUS effectively. In gastroenterology, IOUS is most often used in examining patients who are candidates for surgical resection of primary or metastatic malignant tumors of the liver. IOUS is essential for optimal detection of all liver lesions. It is far superior to all preoperative imaging modalities, including MRI and CT

portography. It is even better than surgical inspection and palpation (Fig. 94.22).

In intraoperative pancreatic imaging, IOUS is important to search for small occult tumors (Fig. 94.23), assess tumor extension, and detect metastatic disease in draining lymph nodes and the liver. Laparoscopic ultrasonography is important in gallbladder surgery; it has replaced intraoperative cholangiography at some centers. Laparoscopic ultrasonography also has been used to stage malignant bowel tumors, particularly gastric tumors.

Also, IOUS facilitates accurate and safe biopsy of deep-seated, nonpalpable lesions and small lesions adjacent to critical vascular structures; is an effective guide to drainage of cysts, pseudocysts, and other fluid collections encountered intraoperatively; and is useful for tumor ablation with cryosurgery, alcohol injection, or hyperthermic ablation with radio frequency, laser, or microwave energy sources. Increased awareness of the abilities of IOUS has resulted in the development of new applications.

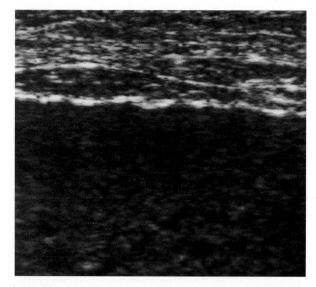

Figure 94.1 Cirrhosis with nodular liver surface. Image obtained with a high-resolution linear array transducer shows liver nodules several millimeters in size. The normal liver surface is smooth. This nodularity usually indicates cirrhosis. Micronodular cirrhosis may have a smooth-appearing surface on ultrasound scans. On occasion, subcapsular tumor nodules cause surface nodularity.

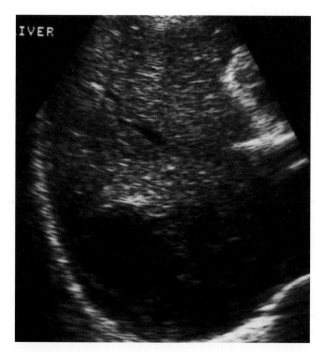

Figure 94.2 Pyogenic liver abscess. Transverse sonogram of the right lobe of the liver shows a mixed echogenicity, predominantly hypoechoic liver abscess at the hepatic dome. The lesion is not well defined medially, which is a sonographic feature of pyogenic liver abscess.

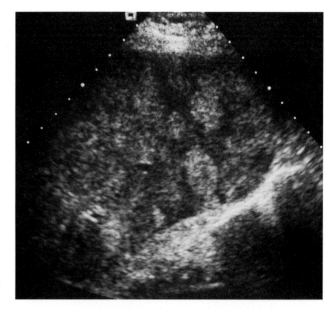

Figure 94.3 Echogenic liver metastases. Hepatic metastases can have any sonographic pattern. In this patient, the metastases are primarily hyperechoic compared with the normal liver parenchyma. Some hypoechoic lesions are present.

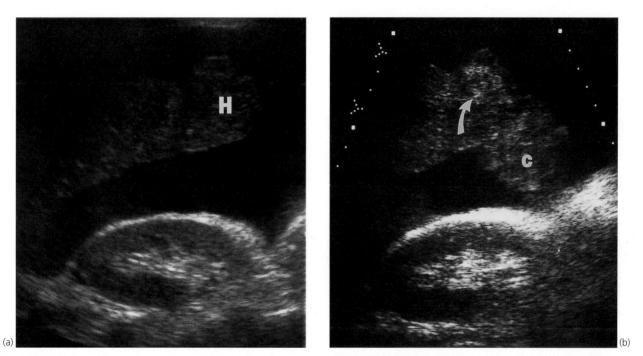

(a)

(b)

Figure 94.4 Hepatocellular carcinoma with acute intraperitoneal hemorrhage. **(a)** Longitudinal sonogram shows an exophytic hepatocellular carcinoma (H) extending out of the tip of the right lobe of the liver. **(b)** Sonogram performed 1 week later shows increased echogenicity within the lesion (curved arrow) and an acute clot (c). This represents acute hemorrhage of a hepatocellular cancer, a fairly common occurrence.

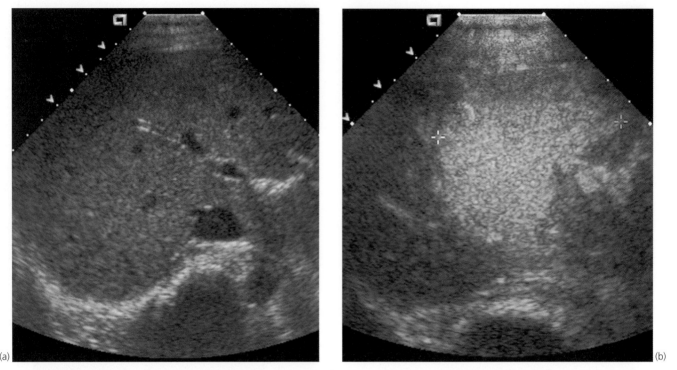

(a)

(b)

Figure 94.5 Focal nodular hyperplasia: transverse ultrasound image through the right lobe. **(a)** Precontrast gray-scale image does not demonstrate a definite mass. **(b)** Postcontrast gray-scale interval delay image shows the now easily visualized hypervascular mass (cursors).

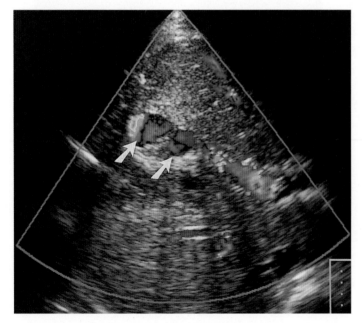

Figure 94.6 Hepatic pseudoaneurysm after gunshot wound. This patient had fever and pain 3 weeks after being released from the hospital after treatment of a liver injury associated with a gunshot wound. Color Doppler sonogram demonstrates two hepatic artery pseudoaneurysms (arrows). Color Doppler sonography is useful in the diagnosis of vascular abnormalities such as this. The patient later underwent therapeutic angiographic embolization.

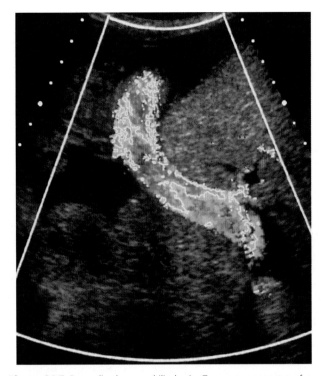

Figure 94.7 Recanalized paraumbilical vein. Transverse sonogram of a patient with cirrhosis, ascites, and portal hypertension shows an enlarged paraumbilical vein that serves as a hepatofugal collateral vessel. Paraumbilical veins are the easiest portosystemic collaterals to image because of their superficial location as they arise from the left portal vein to communicate with superficial abdominal collateral vessels. The most common type of collateral vessel, the left gastric-coronary vein, is extremely difficult to identify at sonography.

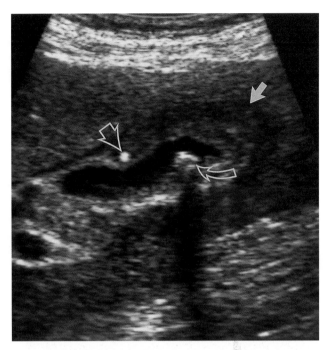

Figure 94.8 Gallstone in a patient with adenomyomatosis. An intralumenal gallstone (curved open arrow) is visible, and an intramural gallstone (straight open arrow) is present within a diffusely thickened gallbladder wall (arrow). Surgical findings confirmed gallstone disease and adenomyomatosis.

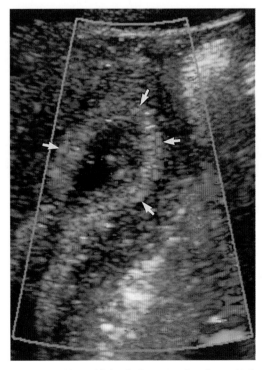

Figure 94.9 Hepatitis A with fundic flow. Not all patients with fundic color Doppler flow have acute cholecystitis. This image shows a patient with hepatitis A who has thickening of the gallbladder wall related to inflammation caused by the hepatitis. Mural color flow (small arrows) is displayed on the color Doppler image.

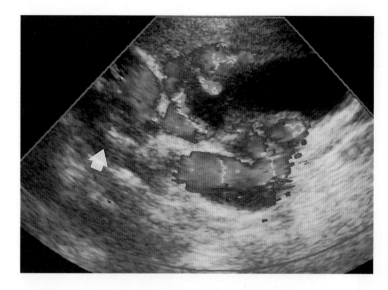

Figure 94.10 Prominent color-coded gallbladder wall varices in a patient with main portal thrombosis. The occluded portal vein is visible adjacent to the gallbladder (arrow). Hepatopetal collateral vessels after portal vein thrombosis may involve the gallbladder wall and produce gallbladder varices, as in this patient.

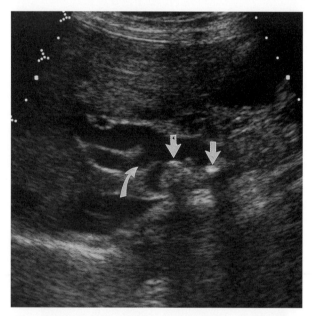

Figure 94.11 Common bile duct stone. Long-axis view of the intra- and extrahepatic bile ducts reveals two echogenic common duct stones (arrows). The cystic duct (curved arrow) enters the common duct dorsally.

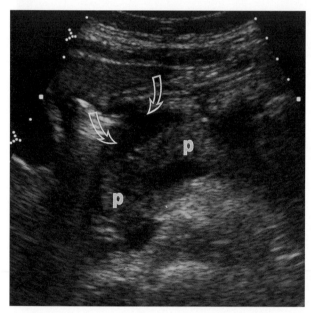

Figure 94.12 Acute pancreatitis with peripancreatic abnormality. Transverse sonogram reveals hypoechoic inflammation (curved open arrows) ventral to the pancreas (p). The pancreas itself appears normal. Peripancreatic abnormality may be the only sonographic evidence of acute pancreatitis.

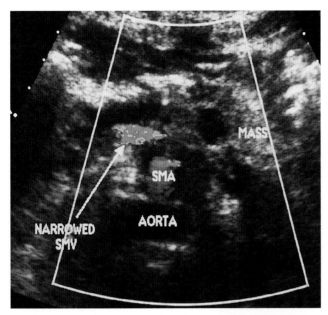

Figure 94.13 Pancreatic carcinoma encases the celiac artery. The hypoechoic pancreatic mass (MASS) encases the superior mesenteric artery (SMA) and narrows the superior mesenteric vein (long-tailed arrow). This renders the tumor unresectable. Sonography, especially with color Doppler imaging, is an effective tool in assessing resectability of periampullary neoplasms.

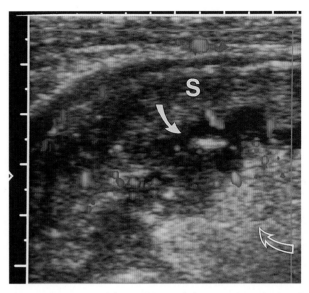

Figure 94.15 Sigmoid diverticulitis. Graded compression color Doppler scan of left lower quadrant reveals thickened sigmoid colon (S). Image shows echogenic sigmoid mesocolon (open curved arrow) and intramural abscess (closed curved arrow).

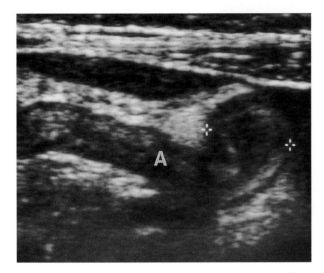

Figure 94.14 Acute appendicitis. Distended appendix (A) has a dilated tip (cursors).

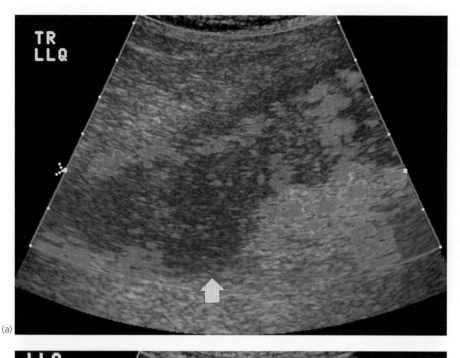

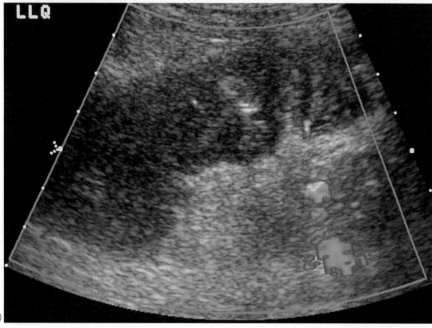

Figure 94.16 Diverticulitis with focal ischemia. **(a)** A transverse power Doppler sonogram obtained of the left lower quadrant reveals focal areas of hyperemia with a necrotic area where there is no flow (arrow). **(b)** Conventional-velocity color Doppler image is much less useful in showing flow and is essentially nondiagnostic for this patient.

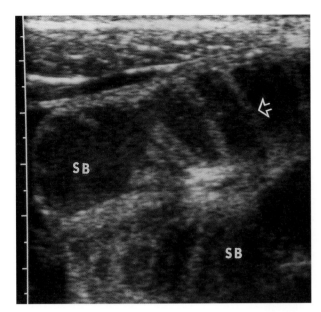

Figure 94.17 Closed-loop obstruction of the small bowel. Dilated U-shaped loop of small bowel (SB) represents closed-loop obstruction. The small bowel can be distinguished from other gastrointestinal viscera by identification of the valvulae conniventes (open arrow).

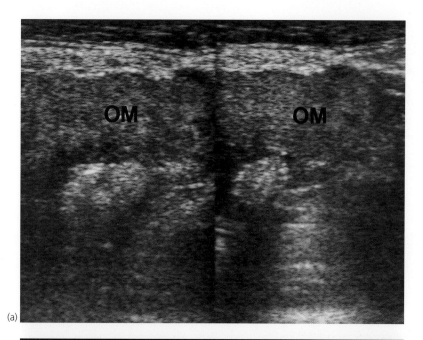

(a)

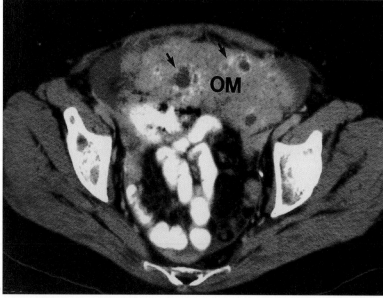

(b)

Figure 94.18 Omental metastases. **(a)** Sonogram demonstrates an echogenic omental "cake" (OM) from metastatic ovarian carcinoma. **(b)** Computed tomographic scan of the same patient as in **(a)**. Areas of calcification (arrows) within the omental cake (OM) are not apparent on sonogram.

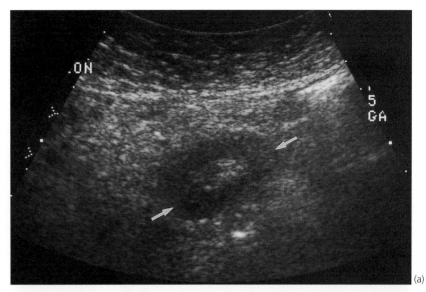

(a)

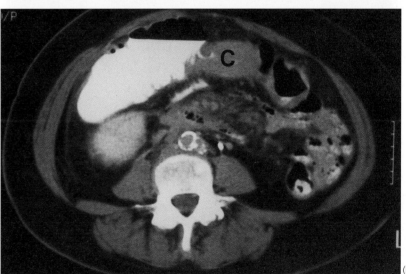

(b)

Figure 94.19 Pseudokidney sign of gastrointestinal tumor. **(a)** Sagittal sonogram of the midabdomen demonstrates a mass (arrows) that resembles a kidney. **(b)** Computed tomographic scan demonstrates circumferential carcinoma (C) obstructing hepatic flexure.

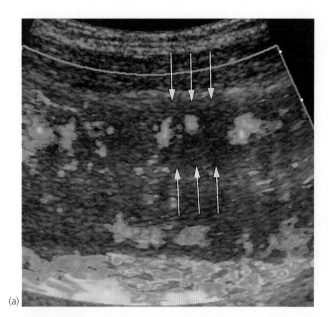

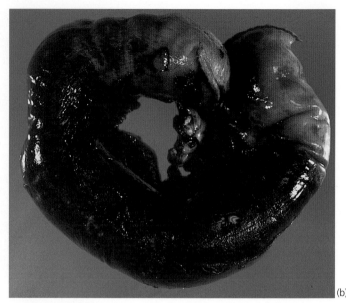

Figure 94.20 Intramural hemorrhage caused by warfarin therapy. **(a)** A longitudinal left lower quadrant image of the small intestine reveals diffuse thickening of the bowel wall (a portion of which is outlined between the arrows) but intact blood flow as manifest with power Doppler imaging. **(b)** Surgical specimen shows intramural hemorrhage in the same location.

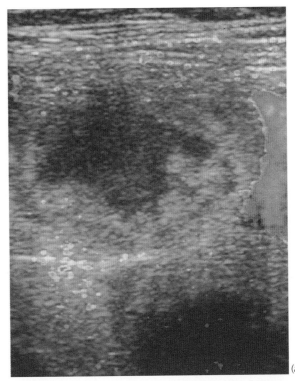

(a)

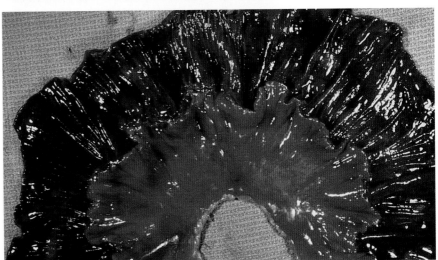

(b)

Figure 94.21 Infarction of the small bowel. **(a)** Power Doppler sonogram of the left upper quadrant shows little or no flow in the edematous loop of small intestine. **(b)** The pathological specimen confirms the sonographic diagnosis.

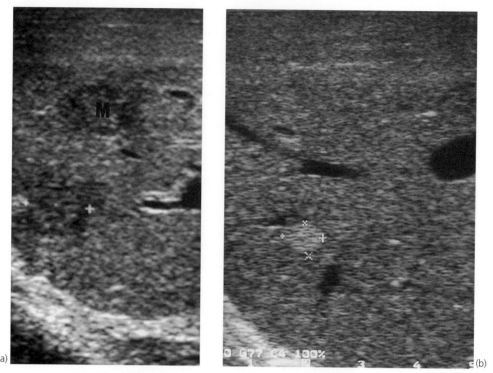

Figure 94.22 Intraoperative ultrasound scans show metastasis and hemangioma. **(a)** Sonogram shows hepatic metastasis (M). **(b)** Homogeneous hyperechoic hemangioma (outlined by cursors) in the same patient. A total of three hemangiomas were visualized in addition to the metastases.

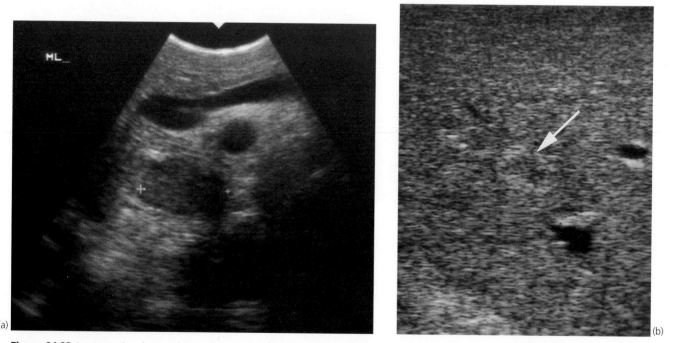

Figure 94.23 Intraoperative ultrasound scans show nonpalpable pancreatic insulinoma. **(a)** Intraoperative ultrasound scan of the pancreas demonstrates hypoechoic insulinoma (outlined by cursors) in the low head and uncinate process of the pancreas. **(b)** Intraoperative ultrasound scan of the liver shows a less than 1-cm liver nodule (arrow) in the same patient, which suggests metastasis. Intraoperative ultrasound-guided biopsy is required to confirm metastasis because other lesions, such as fibrosed hemangioma or focal nodular hyperplasia, can have a similar appearance.

95

Endoscopic ultrasonography

Marcia I. Canto, Sanjay B. Jagannath

Endoscopic ultrasonography (EUS) is an established diagnostic and therapeutic modality in gastroenterology. Although most gastroenterologists are not trained in the practice of EUS, it is important that they understand the principles of the technique and the indications for EUS in order to offer optimal patient care.

This chapter provides case vignettes with selected images that illustrate common diagnostic and therapeutic indications for EUS. A brief overview of the role of EUS in such indications is included. As a complete representation of images encountered in endosonography could not be provided here, the authors recommend that anyone interested in learning EUS should review textbooks dedicated to the practice of EUS and seek out an established EUS training program.

Types of echoendoscopes

There are two major types of echoendoscopes: radial imaging and linear imaging. Radial echoendoscopes provide cross-sectional anatomical imaging. Newer generations of the radial echoendoscope include electronic array, which allows for the addition of Doppler to the radial echoendoscope (Fig. 95.1a). Linear echoendoscopes transmit ultrasound waves in the same axis as the long shaft of the transducer, which allows for real-time therapeutic intervention, most commonly fine-needle aspiration (Fig. 95.1b). Figures 95.2–95.6 depict selected images of normal histology or anatomy as visualized by EUS. Case examples showing the use of EUS follow.

Case 1: A 57-year-old man with a history of reflux presents with 2 months of progressive dysphagia for solids more than liquids. He reports a 15 lb weight loss. A computed

Atlas of Gastroenterology, 4th edition. Edited by Tadataka Yamada, David H. Alpers, Anthony N. Kalloo, Neil Kaplowitz, Chung Owyang, and Don W. Powell. © 2009 Blackwell Publishing, ISBN: 978-1-4051-6909-7

tomography (CT) scan of the thorax reveals thickening of the distal esophagus. Upper endoscopy reveals a narrowed esophageal stricture (Fig. 95.7a). The EUS (Fig. 95.7b) shows an asymmetric hypoechoic image of the stricture region that reflects the mass at 40 cm from the incisors. The mass extends beyond the esophageal muscularis propria and invades the adjacent left pleura. A malignant periesophageal lymph node is identified that was not seen on the CT scan (Fig. 95.7c). EUS stage is T4N1Mx.

Case 2: A 43-year-old man with history of cystic fibrosis presents with hemoccult positive stools and mild anemia. Upper endoscopy reveals a polypoid mass in the distal esophagus (Fig. 95.8a). Biopsy confirms adenocarcinoma. EUS shows an asymmetric, hypoechoic mass with submucosal invasion (Fig. 95.8b). Endoscopic mucosal resection was performed as ablative therapy (Fig. 95.8c).

Case 3: A 65-year-old woman with weight loss undergoes CT of the abdomen. The CT scan shows a left adrenal mass. Upper endoscopy reveals a large gastric ulcer in the fundus (Fig. 95.9a). Radial EUS demonstrates a mass in the left adrenal (Fig. 95.9b) and a mass in the left upper lobe of the lung. The results of a fine needle aspiration confirmed the diagnosis of stage IV non-small cell lung cancer (Fig. 95.9c).

Case 4: A 47-year-old man with a history of gastroesophageal reflux undergoes upper endoscopy. A submucosal mass of about 3 cm is identified (Fig. 95.10a). Radial EUS demonstrates a well-circumscribed, hypoechoic mass originating from the muscularis layer of the stomach (Fig. 95.10b). Fine-needle aspiration demonstrates spindle-shaped cells that stain positive for C-kit protein. A gastrointestinal stromal cell tumor (GIST) was diagnosed.

Case 5: A 57-year-old woman undergoes upper endoscopy for epigastric pain. An ulcerated mucosa was identified from a biopsy, confirming adenocarcinoma (Fig. 95.11a). EUS revealed mucosal and submucosal infiltration (Fig. 95.11b). Curative subtotal gastrectomy was performed.

Case 6: A 68-year-old man presents with epigastric pain and weight loss. A CT scan shows pancreatic head enlargement without a discrete mass. EUS shows a hypoechoic mass (Fig. 95.12a), which is confirmed to be adenocarcinoma by EUS-guided fine-needle aspiration (Fig. 95.12b).

Case 7: A 49-year-old woman suffers from episodes of hypoglycemia. Prior imaging studies failed to identify a clinically suspected insulinoma. EUS reveals a 5-mm well-circumscribed hypoechoic lesion in the pancreatic tail (Fig. 95.13). Distal pancreatectomy was performed and symptoms were resolved.

Case 8: A 48-year-old man presents with steatorrhea and persistent abdominal pain. EUS demonstrates hyperechoic foci and strands, pseudolobulations and lobularity of the pancreatic gland (Fig. 95.14). Other features (not shown) included calcifications and an echogenic pancreatic duct.

These EUS features are most consistent with chronic pancreatitis.

Case 9: An asymptomatic 65-year-old man has a 2.5-cm pancreatic cyst. EUS reveals a multiseptated, well-circumscribed, anechoic lesion with posterior acoustic enhancement. Echogenic debris is noted within the cyst (Fig. 95.15). The results of a fine-needle aspiration confirm a mucinous tumor.

Case 10: A 29-year-old man with a history of rectal pain and bleeding. Colonoscopy reveals multiple polyps and an anorectal stricture that is nearly causing obstruction (Fig. 95.16a). EUS reveals an irregular hypoechoic mass with infiltration into adjacent soft tissue (EUS stage T4NxMx) (Fig. 95.16b).

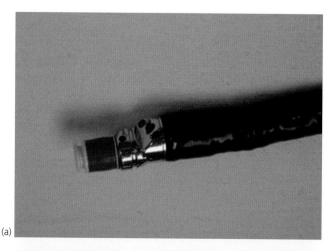

(a)

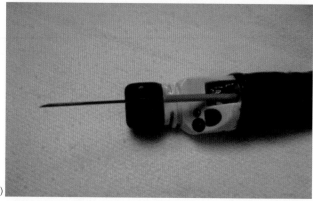

(b)

Figure 95.1 (a) Electronic radial echoendoscope (Olympus). **(b)** Linear echoendoscope with a protruding needle used for a fine-needle aspiration (Olympus).

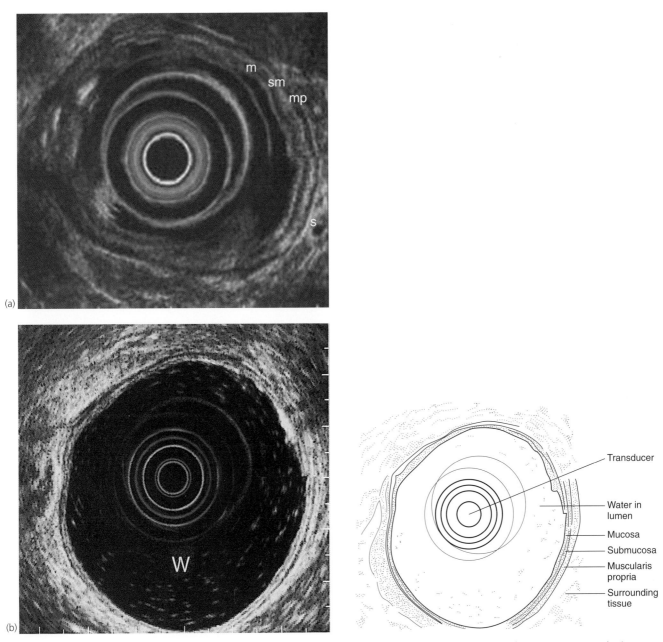

Figure 95.2 (a) Endoscopic ultrasonography showing the five layers of the stomach wall. The image showing normal anatomy was created using a 5.0 MHz radial scanning endoscope. m, mucosa, sm, submucosa, mp, muscularis propria, s, serosa. **(b)** A healthy stomach imaged with a 7.5 MHz radial scanning endoscope. Water (W) in the gastric lumen facilitates imaging of the wall layers that correspond to mucosa, submucosa, muscularis propria, and surrounding tissue.

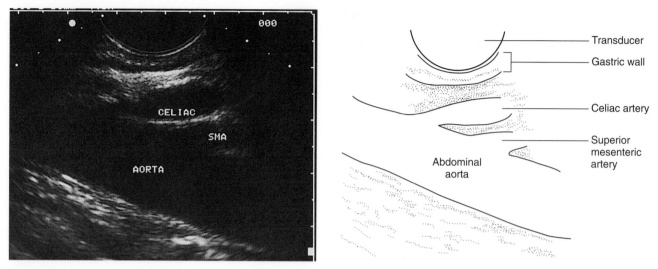

Figure 95.3 The abdominal aorta and the origins of the celiac and superior mesenteric arteries (SMA) imaged through the gastric wall with an electronic curvilinear-array ultrasound endoscope. This instrument also has Doppler capability for demonstration of blood flow in these vessels.

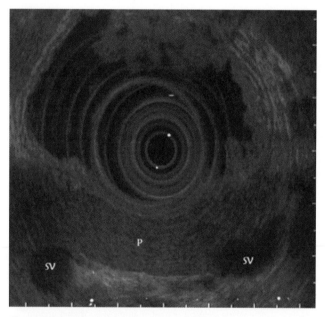

Figure 95.4 Radial endoscopic ultrasonography image showing characteristic normal "salt-and-pepper pattern" of the pancreas. P, body of the pancreas; SV, splenic vein.

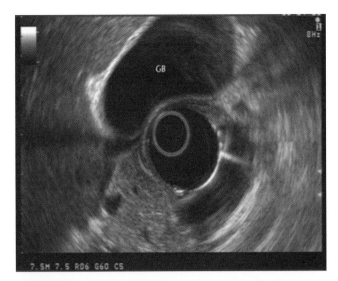

Figure 95.5 Radial endoscopic ultrasonography image showing image of a healthy gallbladder (GB).

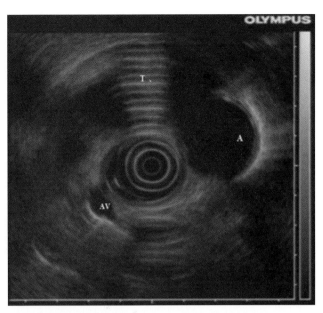

Figure 95.6 Radial endoscopic ultrasonography image showing normal mediastinal anatomy. A, aorta; T, trachea; AV, azygos vein.

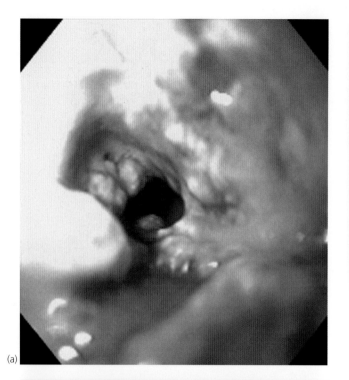
(a)

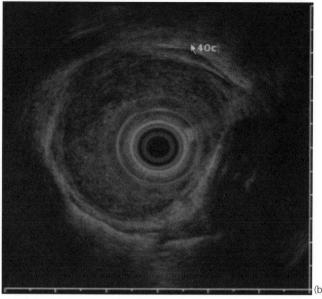
(b)

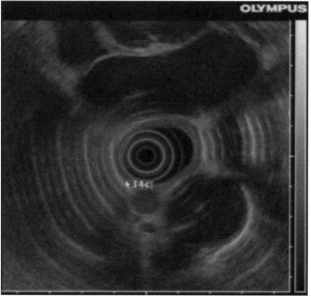
(c)

Figure 95.7 (a) Malignant stricture of the distal esophagus.
(b) Endoscopic ultrasonography image of esophageal carcinoma (T4) with pleural invasion. **(c)** EUS reveals a hypoechoic, sharply defined periesophageal lymph node suspicious for malignancy. EUS-guided fine-needle aspiration confirms malignant status of the lymph node.

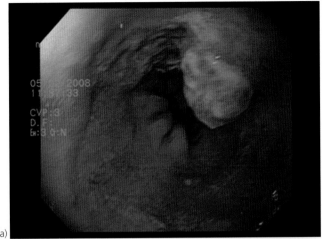

(a)

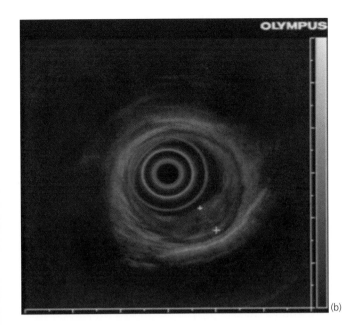

(b)

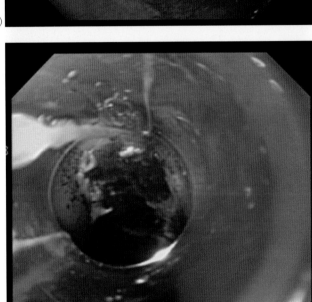

(c)

Figure 95.8 **(a)** Upper endoscopy image showing a polypoid lesion in the distal esophagus. The results of the biopsies confirmed adenocarcinoma. **(b)** Endoscopic ultrasonography image showing esophageal cancer. **(c)** Patient was treated with endoscopic mucosal resection.

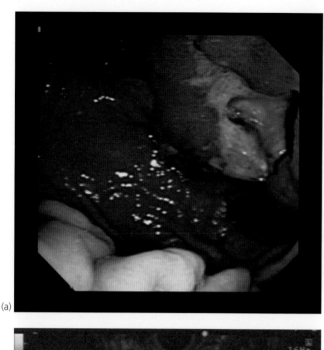

(a)

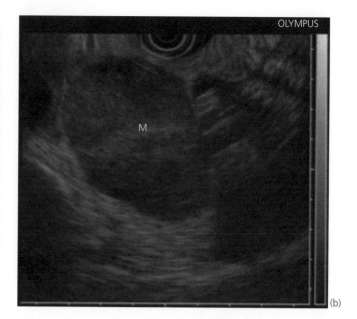

(b)

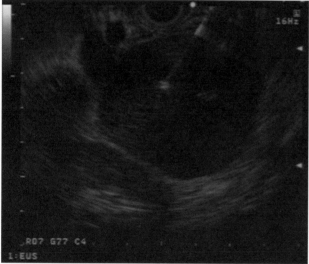

(c)

Figure 95.9 (a) Upper endoscopy image showing ulcerated gastric mass in fundus. **(b)** Radial endoscopic ultrasonography demonstrates a hypoechoic mass (M) of the left adrenal gland. **(c)** Fine-needle aspiration of the mass in (b).

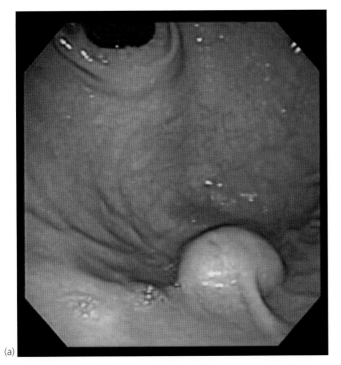

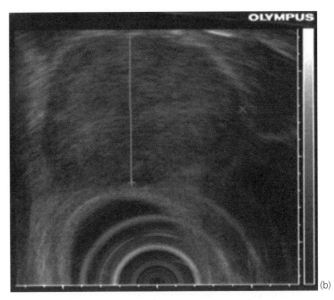

Figure 95.10 (a) An upper gastrointestinal endoscopy image of the stomach showing a submucosal mass. **(b)** Endoscopic ultrasonography demonstrates a hypoechoic mass originating from the gastric muscularis propria.

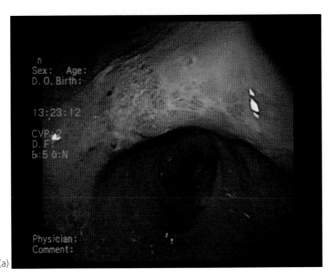

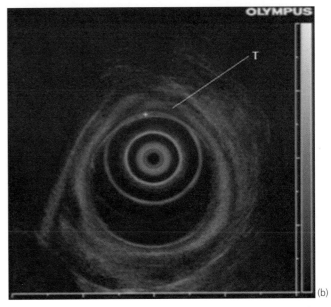

Figure 95.11 (a) Endoscopy revealing an ulcerated mucosa along the gastric incisura. **(b)** Endoscopic ultrasonography shows mucosal and submucosal thickening, which suggests T1N0 gastric malignancy. T, tumor.

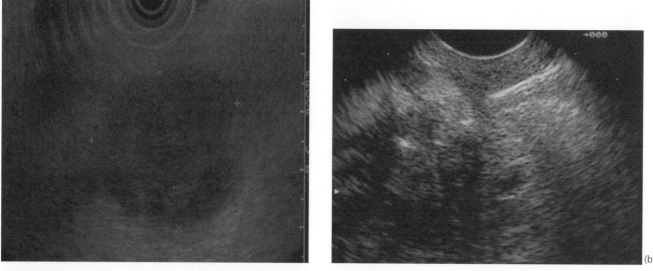

(a)   (b)

Figure 95.12 (a) Hypoechoic pancreatic mass. **(b)** Fine-needle aspiration needle entering pancreatic mass. The biopsy results confirmed adenocarcinoma.

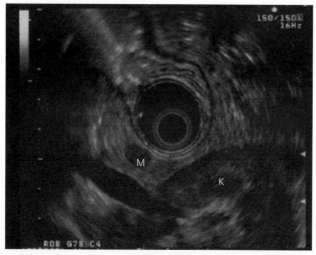

Figure 95.13 Endoscopic ultrasonography reveals 5-mm well-circumscribed hypoechoic lesion (M) in the pancreatic tail. K, left kidney.

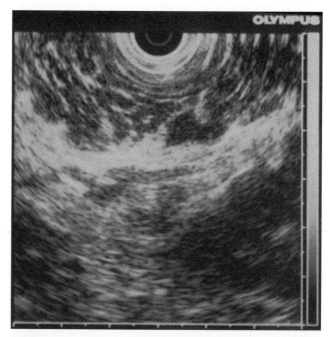

Figure 95.14 Endoscopic ultrasonography image of chronic pancreatitis.

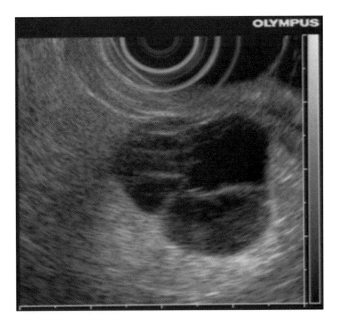

Figure 95.15 Endoscopic ultrasonography image showing a multiseptated, well-circumscribed, anechoic lesion with posterior acoustic enhancement. Echogenic debris is evident within the cyst.

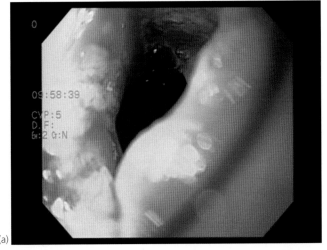

(a)

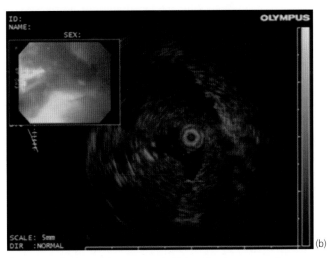

(b)

Figure 95.16 **(a)** Endoscopic image of an anorectal stricture. **(b)** Endoscopic ultrasonography image of an anorectal stricture (inset: corresponding endoscopic image).

B IMAGING

Applications of computed tomography to the gastrointestinal tract

Karen M. Horton, Pamela T. Johnson, Elliot K. Fishman, Alec J. Megibow

Introduction

Since its introduction in the late 1970s, computed tomography (CT) has made unparalleled technical advancements in both scanner hardware and software. Today's multidetector row CT (MDCT) scanners allow submillimeter collimation (0.6 mm) and fast scanning speeds (0.33 s per rotation). The resultant temporal and spatial resolution have greatly improved our ability to image the body. For example, 64-slice MDCT scanners can image the entire abdomen and pelvis in less than 10 s, using submillimeter slices. This narrow temporal window has directly impacted protocol design, enabling data acquisition during the phase of maximum lesion conspicuity. Consequently, specific acquisition phases have been delineated for pancreatic tumor and hepatocellular carcinoma detection using multislice technology. Following data acquisition, easy-to-use three-dimensional (3D) post-processing software is now widely available, which enables the radiologist to view the scan data in any imaging plane. Beyond improved image quality and diagnostic efficacy for existing applications, these advancements have facilitated the development of new CT applications, such as virtual colonoscopy and coronary CT angiography. In this chapter, a discussion of CT techniques for hollow visceral imaging is followed by a collection of cases demonstrating the utility of CT to image pathology of the hollow viscera, solid organs and peritoneal cavity.

The hollow viscera of the gastrointestinal tract

Techniques
Oral contrast

Identifying abnormalities of the luminal gastrointestinal tract, whether it be neoplastic or inflammatory, relies on the ability to adequately visualize the bowel wall. Optimal distension of the bowel is necessary for evaluation of the wall. There are a variety of CT contrast agents that can be administered orally or rectally. These are categorized as positive agents, neutral agents, or negative agents.

Positive agents appear "white" on CT and usually consist of diluted (1.5%–2%) iodinated water-soluble contrast or diluted (2%) barium suspensions. These are the agents traditionally used for routine CT scans of the abdomen.

Neutral contrast agents appear "gray" on CT and usually have a density similar to water. Currently used neutral agents include water, methylcellulose agents, and commercially available products such as Volumen (E-Z-Em; Lake Success, New York), which has a density value slightly greater than water.

Future studies are needed to determine which oral agent is best for specific CT applications. Neutral agents may be beneficial for detailed imaging of the stomach and small bowel because they allow excellent visualization of the enhancing wall that may otherwise be obscured by positive agents. In addition, if 3D imaging is performed, it is beneficial to use either neutral or negative contrast agents, as they will still allow 3D visualization of the vasculature without extensive post-processing to segment the bowel loops from the volume. When positive oral agents are used, these "white" loops need to be removed, as they will obscure the adjacent contrast enhanced vessels, particularly with maximum intensity projection.

Negative agents appear "black" on CT and usually consist of either gas granules administered orally to distend the stomach or insufflation of the colon with air or carbon dioxide for virtual colonoscopy. Other negative agents such as oil-based products (peanut oil) are not used routinely. In clinical practice, the choice of oral contrast depends on the clinical indication and will be reviewed under each subsection of this chapter.

Intravenous contrast

Intravenous (i.v.) contrast-enhanced images expand the diagnostic range of CT and have become essential for most clinical indications. Intravenous contrast enhancement

Atlas of Gastroenterology, 4th edition. Edited by Tadataka Yamada, David H. Alpers, Anthony N. Kalloo, Neil Kaplowitz, Chung Owyang, and Don W. Powell. © 2009 Blackwell Publishing, ISBN: 978-1-4051-6909-7

improves conspicuity of pathological processes in evaluation of the alimentary canal by increasing the level of confidence in diagnosing a thickened bowel loop as being truly diseased, as well as allowing assessment of bowel wall enhancement and the detection of small bowel masses. This refines the differential diagnosis by highlighting attenuation differences within the thickened loop, or by accentuating the "vascularity" of a bowel-related mass, thereby facilitating the determination of histological type and neoplastic potential. Variations in blood supply of pathological processes demand a tailored approach to intravenous contrast administration for evaluation of the alimentary tract.

Nonionic iodinated contrast agents are typically utilized for CT today. The protocol for administration will vary depending on the clinical indication. For example, in patients with suspected mesenteric ischemia, it is important to acquire images in both the arterial and venous phases, to ensure adequate visualization of both the mesenteric arteries and veins in addition to assessment of bowel wall enhancement. The radiologist will tailor the i.v. contrast injection rate and scan delay based on the clinical question. Therefore, it is essential that appropriate clinical information is provided by the ordering physician in order for scans to be performed correctly.

Scanning protocol

In general, CT imaging of the abdomen and the alimentary tract in particular, requires high-resolution volumetric datasets. Data acquisition parameters are dictated by the clinical question. For example, if 3D imaging is performed, it is helpful for the CT scan to be performed using the thinnest possible detectors. Today's state-of-the-art 64-slice scanners have detectors as narrow as 0.6 mm, which can be used to create 0.75-mm overlapping sections reconstructed every 0.5 mm to produce a volume data set that is ideal for 3D imaging. The data may also be reconstructed with 3 to 5-mm sections for axial review of the abdomen and pelvis. With respect to voltage and tube current, 120 kV and 270 effective milliamperes are usually adequate for 3D studies. For studies not requiring 3D imaging, thicker collimator settings can be used, such as 1.2 mm, and the tube current can be reduced appropriately.

Three-dimensional imaging

A comprehensive CT examination in patients with suspected gastrointestinal tract pathology may be aided by review of the dataset with 3D software. The interpretation is tailored to fit the specific clinical question, and different rendering algorithms may be needed to optimally display specific findings. Current 3D imaging software varies by vendor, but typically includes a combination of multiplanar reconstruction (MPR), volume rendering and maximum intensity projection (MIP). Multiplanar reconstructions are the most simple to use and allow scrolling through the dataset in any plane. However, volume rendering is the most robust 3D imaging tool for full analysis of the gastrointestinal tract and abdominal vasculature. Volume rendering allows the brightness, opacity, window width, and window level to be adjusted in real time in order to accentuate certain tissue types or selective viewing of the vasculature. Manipulating trapezoidal transfer functions interactively modifies the image contrast and the related pixel attenuations in the final image. This function allows color and opacity assignments to each voxel and can be adjusted to alter the display. Although initial volume rendering software was somewhat labor intensive, today's software packages are easy to use and can be adjusted in real-time. Also, the process can be simplified by creating presets, which can be applied quickly and then only minor adjustments are needed. The projection technique MIP displays the brightest voxel along a ray. This can be valuable using thin slabs of data to accentuate small vessels. The radiologist often utilizes a combination of these 3D tools to optimally display the relevant anatomy and pathology. In the last several years, specialized 3D software has been developed for specific CT applications, including virtual colonoscopy.

The images shown in this chapter relate to: the gastrointestinal tract (pp. 1006–1010); the liver (p. 1011); the pancreas (pp. 1012 and 1013); the biliary tract (p. 1014); the peritoneum (p. 1014) and; hernias (p. 1014).

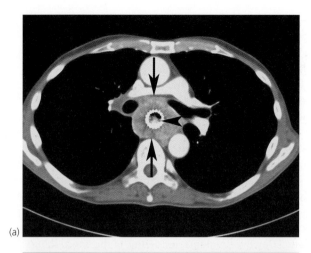

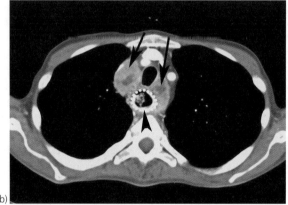

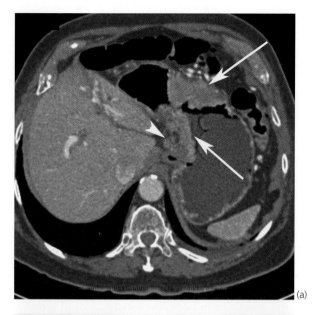

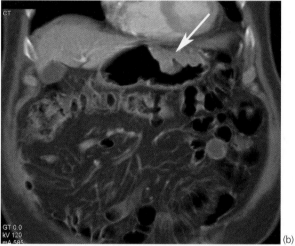

Figure 96.1 **(a)** Axial intravenous contrast-enhanced multidetector computed tomography (MDCT) image reveals a large circumferential esophageal mass (arrows). The mass splays the carina. An esophageal stent is in place (arrowhead). **(b)** Axial intravenous contrast-enhanced MDCT image demonstrates bulky mediastinal adenopathy (arrows). The esophageal stent is again noted (arrowhead).

Figure 96.2 **(a)** Axial intravenous contrast-enhanced multidetector computed tomography (MDCT) image in a patient with gastric adenocarcinoma shows an infiltrating mass in the gastric body (arrows). There is extension into the gastrohepatic ligament (arrowhead). **(b)** Coronal volume-rendered image nicely demonstrates the bulky gastric mass (arrow).

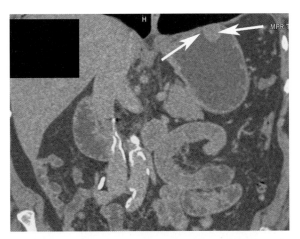

Figure 96.3 Intravenous contrast-enhanced coronal multiplanar reconstruction using water as oral contrast demonstrates a 1.3-cm intramural gastric mass (arrows) compatible with a gastrointestinal stromal tumor. This was an incidental finding.

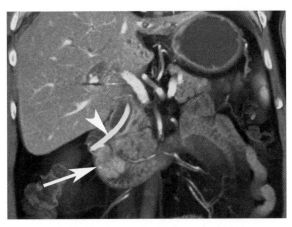

Figure 96.4 Intravenous contrast-enhanced coronal volume-rendered image using water as oral contrast demonstrates a 2-cm lobulated mass (arrow) in the second portion of the duodenum. A common bile duct stent is in place (arrowhead). The patient underwent Whipple surgery and pathology revealed adenocarcinoma arising in a tubular adenoma.

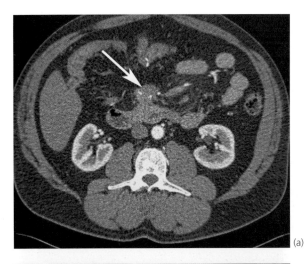

(a)

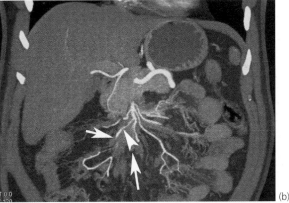

(b)

Figure 96.5 (a) Axial intravenous contrast-enhanced multidetector computed tomography (MDCT) image shows a 1.5-cm infiltrating mass (arrow) in the root of the mesentery, compatible with carcinoid. **(b)** Coronal maximum intensity projection nicely demonstrates encasement of the superior mesenteric artery branches (arrowhead) by the infiltrating tumor (arrows).

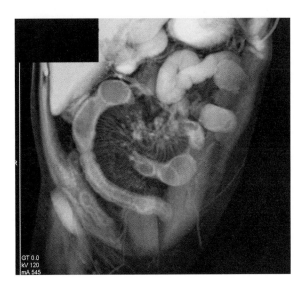

Figure 96.6 Coronal volume-rendered image from an intravenous and oral contrast-enhanced computed tomography (CT) in a patient with Crohn's disease demonstrates small bowel wall thickening, mucosal hyperemia, and engorgement of the vasa recta. This is an example of the comb sign, indicating active disease.

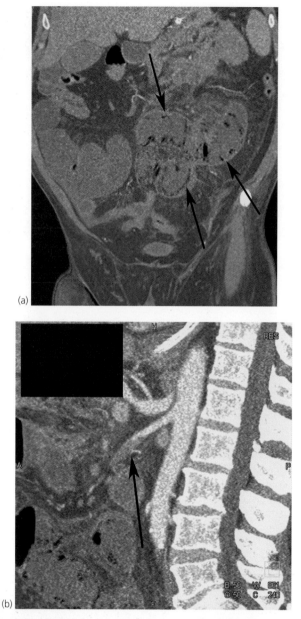

Figure 96.7 (a) Coronal multiplanar reconstruction (MPR) from intravenous contrast-enhanced computed tomography (CT) demonstrates dilated small bowel with pneumatosis (arrows). **(b)** Sagittal MPR demonstrates thrombosis in the superior mesenteric artery (arrow).

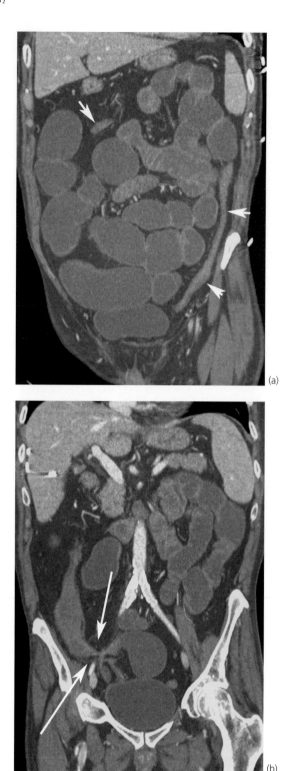

Figure 96.8 (a) Intravenous contrast-enhanced coronal multiplanar reconstruction (MPR) using water as oral contrast demonstrates moderate small bowel dilatation. The colon is decompressed (arrows). **(b)** Intravenous contrast-enhanced coronal MPR using water as oral contrast demonstrates multiple fistulae (arrows) in the distal small bowel and colon. This was the source of the small bowel obstruction in this patient with Crohn's disease.

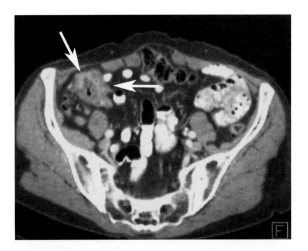

Figure 96.9 Axial intravenous and oral contrast-enhanced multidetector computed tomography (MDCT) image demonstrates a subtle mass (arrows) in the right colon. Colonoscopy and biopsy revealed adenocarcinoma.

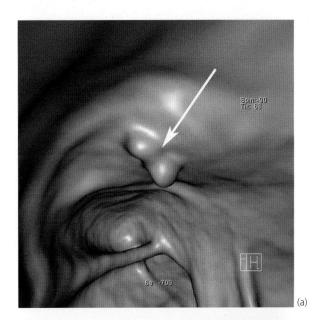

(a)

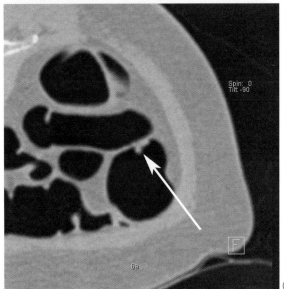

(b)

Figure 96.10 (a) Endolumenal fly-through view from virtual colonoscopy shows 8-mm polyp (arrow). **(b)** Axial prone image from virtual colonoscopy demonstrates an 8-mm polyp (arrow) in the right colon.

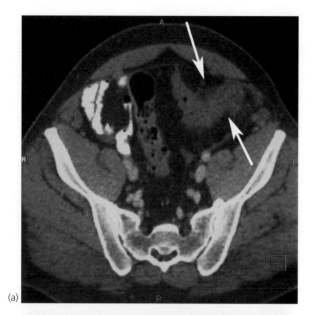

(a)

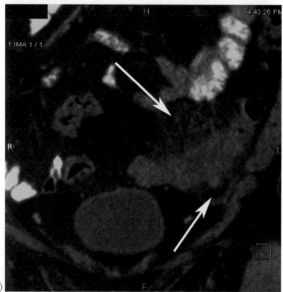

(b)

Figure 96.11 (a) Axial oral and intravenous contrast-enhanced multidetector computed tomography (MDCT) image reveals thickening of the sigmoid colon with pericolonic stranding (arrows) compatible with diverticulitis. **(b)** Coronal multiplanar reconstruction shows extensive inflammation and minimal fluid in the pericolonic fat (arrows) typical of diverticulitis.

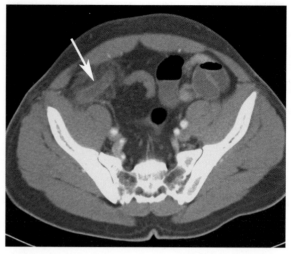

Figure 96.12 Axial intravenous contrast-enhanced multidetector computed tomography (MDCT) in a patient with right lower quadrant pain demonstrates an enlarged fluid-filled appendix (arrow) with moderate periappendiceal inflammation, compatible with acute appendicitis.

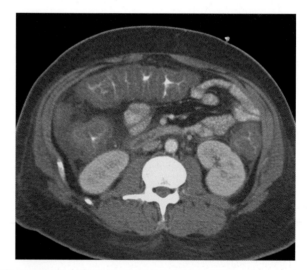

Figure 96.13 Axial intravenous and oral contrast-enhanced multidetector computed tomography (MDCT) demonstrates marked diffuse colonic thickening compatible with pseudomembranous colitis.

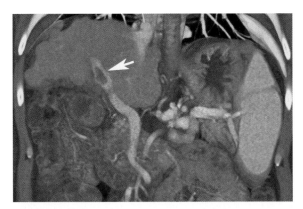

Figure 96.14 Coronal volume-rendered image from intravenous contrast-enhanced computed tomography (CT) demonstrates a small shrunken nodular liver compatible with cirrhosis. Splenomegaly reflects portal hypertension. Thrombus is present in the intrahepatic portal vein (arrow).

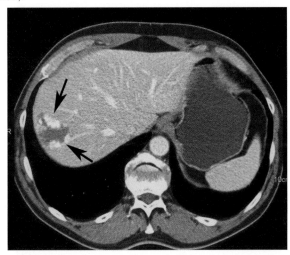

Figure 96.15 Intravenous contrast-enhanced axial multidetector computed tomography (MDCT) demonstrates a 2.5-cm mass (arrows) in the right lobe of the liver with peripheral nodular enhancement characteristic of a hemangioma.

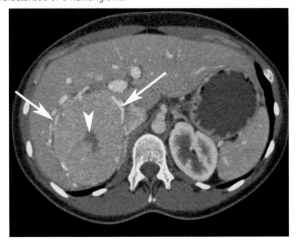

Figure 96.16 Axial intravenous contrast-enhanced multidetector computed tomography (MDCT) during portal venous phase of enhancement demonstrates a large mass in the right lobe of the liver (arrows), with a central scar (arrowhead). This is a typical CT appearance of focal nodular hyperplasia.

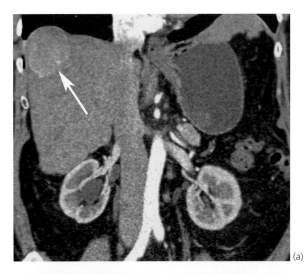

(a)

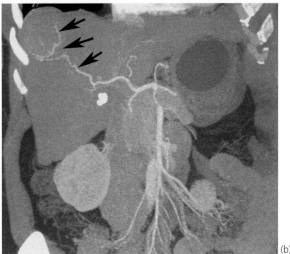

(b)

Figure 96.17 **(a)** Coronal intravenous contrast-enhanced multiplanar reconstruction from an arterial phase acquisition demonstrates a 4-cm enhancing hepatoma (arrow) in the dome of the liver. The liver is shrunken, compatible with cirrhosis. **(b)** Coronal maximum intensity projection demonstrates the arterial vessel (arrows) feeding the hepatoma.

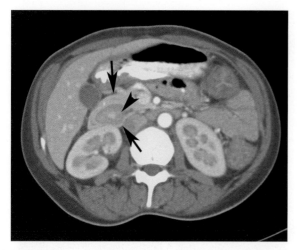

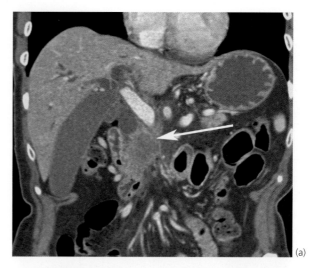

(a)

Figure 96.18 Oral and intravenous contrast-enhanced axial computed tomography (CT) demonstrates pancreatic tissue (arrows) surrounding the second portion of the duodenum (arrowhead), compatible with annular pancreas.

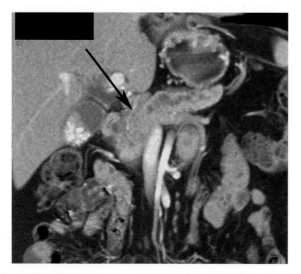

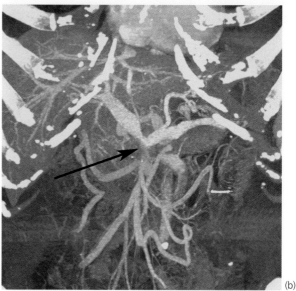

(b)

Figure 96.19 Intravenous contrast-enhanced coronal multiplanar reconstruction image demonstrates 1.5-cm pancreatic mass (arrow) with distal pancreatic ductal obstruction. At surgery this was an adenocarcinoma.

Figure 96.20 (a) Intravenous contrast-enhanced coronal multiplanar reconstruction image demonstrates a 4-cm mass (arrow) in the head of the pancreas causing common bile duct obstruction. The gallbladder is also distended. Biopsy revealed pancreatic adenocarcinoma. **(b)** Coronal maximum intensity projection demonstrates encasement of the superior mesenteric vein (arrow) with resulting collaterals. The patient was deemed unresectable.

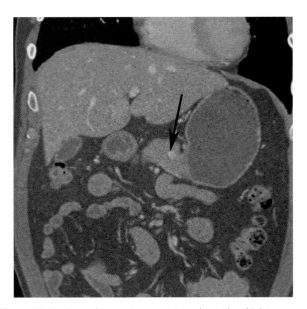

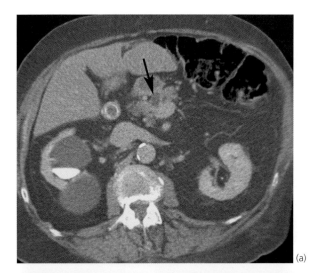

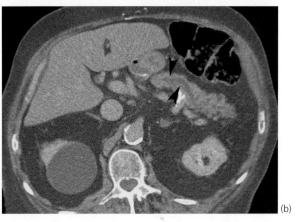

Figure 96.21 Coronal intravenous contrast-enhanced multiplanar reconstruction demonstrates a 5-mm enhancing lesion (arrow) in the body of the pancreas. This was an insulinoma.

Figure 96.22 **(a)** Axial intravenous contrast-enhanced multidetector computed tomography (MDCT) demonstrates a 1-cm cystic lesion (arrow) in the pancreatic neck. **(b)** Axial image also demonstrates pancreatic ductal dilatation (arrowheads). These findings are very suspicious for intraductal pancreatic mucinous neoplasm.

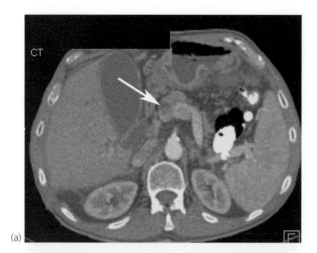

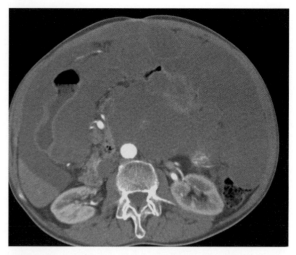

Figure 96.24 Intravenous contrast-enhanced axial computed tomography (CT) in a patient with pseudomyxoma peritonei demonstrates extensive low-density implants filling the peritoneal cavity.

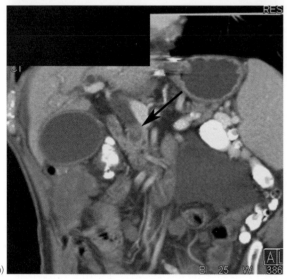

Figure 96.23 (a) Axial intravenous contrast-enhanced multidetector computed tomography (MDCT) in a patient with obstructive jaundice shows a subtle filling defect in the common duct (arrow). **(b)** Coronal multiplanar reconstruction better demonstrates the stone (arrow) in the distal common bile duct.

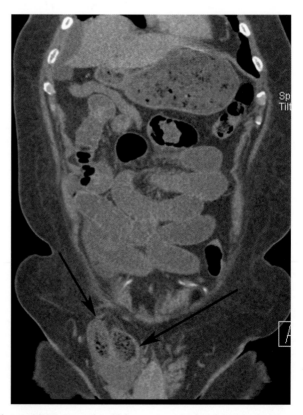

Figure 96.25 Coronal multiplanar reconstruction shows moderate dilatation of small bowel loops due to an obstructing right inguinal hernia (arrows).

97

Magnetic resonance imaging

Diane Bergin

Magnetic resonance imaging (MRI) allows a comprehensive evaluation of the intraabdominal solid organs including the liver, pancreas, and spleen and is the most sensitive noninvasive imaging modality for evaluating the biliary system.

Since the development of MRI, its applications for imaging the gastrointestinal tract have expanded rapidly. MRI of the abdomen was initially hampered because of artifacts associated with respiratory and bowel motion. The development of fast imaging techniques has overcome these effects of motion, enabling examination of structures and organs that were previously not reliably imaged.

MRI utilizes several parameters to characterize tissues including T1, T2, lipid content, and magnetic susceptibility. The generation of MR images involves the spatial localization of radiofrequency signals elicited from water- or fat-containing tissue in the body. The variation in grayscale on the image from white to black represents the strength of these signals and is called the signal intensity. Tissues and structures that are bright on the MR image are described as being of high signal intensity, and tissues and structures that are black on the image are of low signal intensity. When the specific technical parameters are changed on the MR magnet system, images can be generated that evaluate different tissue properties. Two tissue properties, T1 and T2, are examined on T1- and T2-weighted sequences respectively. The presence of lipid within tissue is identified using chemical shift images. Other properties, such as vascularity, biliary secretion, or macrophage activity, are imaged using a wide array of different contrast agents. Blood flow in vessels is selectively visualized with gradient-echo sequences called magnetic resonance angiography.

One of the most frequent applications of MRI of the abdomen is characterization of a liver lesion. The most common benign liver lesions are hepatic cysts (Fig. 97.1) and hepatic hemangiomas (Fig. 97.2), which have very high signal on T2-weighted sequences. Hemangiomas enhance from the periphery with a discontinuous nodular pattern. Hepatic cysts do not enhance. Arterial enhancing lesions that are commonly seen in women are focal nodular hyperplasia (Fig. 97.2). Hepatic lesions that are of moderately high signal intensity on T2-weighted images are malignant lesions, including hepatocellular carcinoma (Fig. 97.3) and hepatic metastases (Figs 97.4 and 97.5).

MRI can be used to diagnose diffuse liver disease such as cirrhosis, fatty infiltration, and hemochromatosis. Fatty infiltration is diagnosed using chemical shift imaging (Fig. 97.6). Iron deposition is characterized by marked low signal on T2 and gradient-echo sequences (Fig. 97.7). Cirrhosis is accurately diagnosed on MRI by visualization of the regenerating nodules, which are separated from each other by the fibrovascular septae. Larger regenerating nodules can be differentiated from small hepatocellular carcinomas on the basis of their arterial phase enhancement during dynamic scanning (Fig. 97.8).

MR cholangiography (MRC) and MR cholangiopancreatography (MRCP) are used for evaluating the biliary tract and pancreatic duct. They selectively image fluid in the abdomen, including bile and secretions in the biliary tract and pancreatic duct. Using these sequences and displaying them in a format similar to conventional endoscopic retrograde cholangiopancreatography or cholangiography, one can identify obstruction of the biliary duct and pancreatic duct. Filling defects such as calculi appear as low-signal abnormalities within the duct (Fig. 97.9). Characterization of obstructing lesions is aided by dynamic gadolinium-enhanced images. Cholangiocarcinoma typically demonstrates delayed enhancement (Fig. 97.10).

Atlas of Gastroenterology, 4th edition. Edited by Tadataka Yamada, David H. Alpers, Anthony N. Kalloo, Neil Kaplowitz, Chung Owyang, and Don W. Powell. © 2009 Blackwell Publishing, ISBN: 978-1-4051-6909-7

The normal pancreatic parenchyma is high signal on T1-weighted images (Fig. 97.11). Chronic pancreatitis is characterized by loss of this high T1 signal as well as irregular dilation of the pancreatic duct (Fig. 97.12). Pancreatic adenocarcinoma typically is hypoenhancing relative to the normal pancreas and depending on its location may cause secondary ductal dilation (Fig. 97.13).

The potential of MRI for evaluating the bowel has been explored. Bowel motion can be reduced by the intravenous injection of antiperistaltic agents such as glucagon. These techniques can differentiate bowel from pathological processes. Intrinsic intestinal wall abnormalities such as inflammatory bowel disease can be characterized (Fig. 97.14).

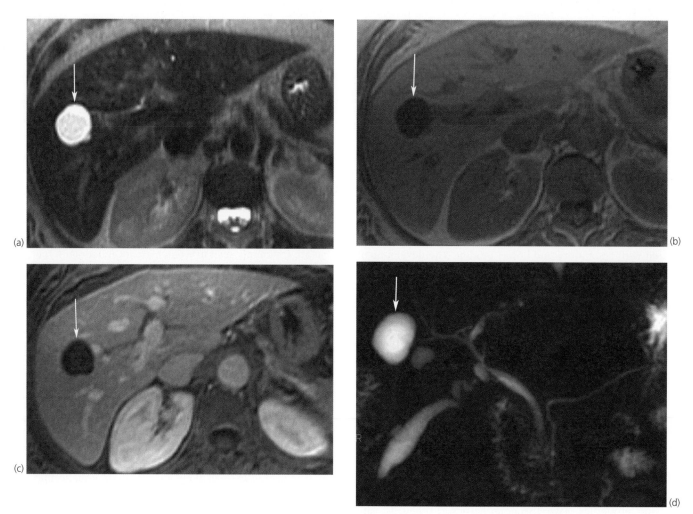

(a)

(b)

(c)

(d)

Figure 97.1 Simple hepatic cyst. Axial T2-weighted **(a)**, axial T1-weighted **(b)**, postcontrast three-dimensional gradient-echo **(c)**, and magnetic resonance cholangiopancreatography (MRCP) **(d)** images demonstrate a high T2 signal lesion (arrow) and low T1 signal nonenhancing lesion (arrow) consistent with simple hepatic cyst.

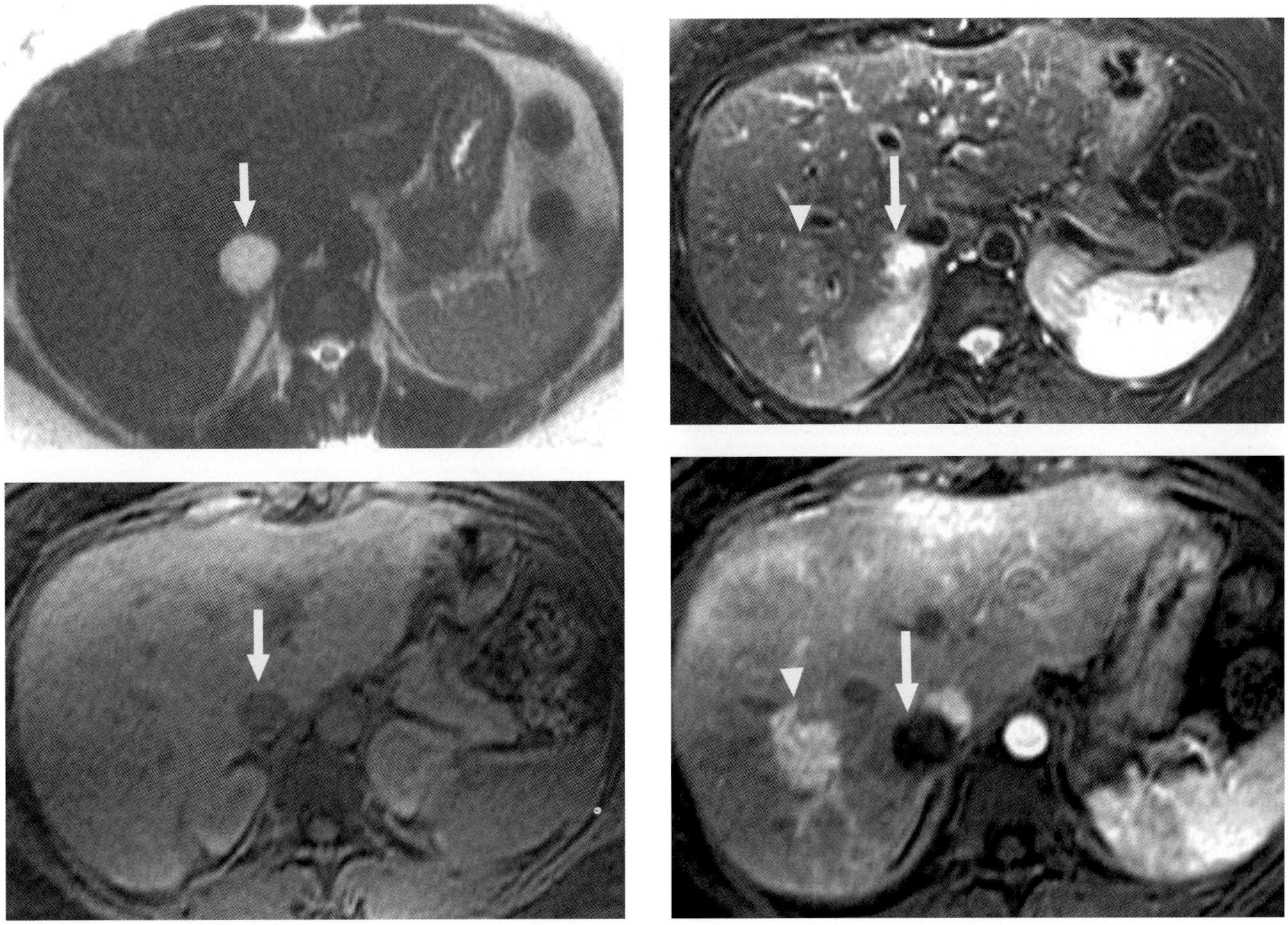

Figure 97.2 Hepatic hemangioma (arrow) and focal nodular hyperplasia (arrowhead). **(a)** Long time to echo (TE) (180 ms) and **(b)** intermediate TE (80 ms) axial T2-weighted images of the liver demonstrate a high T2 signal lesion (arrow) adjacent to the inferior vena cava (IVC). Of note, a second lesion (arrowhead) is also seen on the intermediate T2-weighted image **(b)** but not on the long T2-weighted image **(a)**. **(c)** Three-dimensional gradient echo image before contrast; **(d)** during arterial phase. Following contrast administration, the paracaval lesion (arrow) demonstrates discontinuous peripheral enhancement with progressive delayed enhancement consistent with a hemangioma. The second lesion (arrowhead) enhances avidly in the arterial phase and becomes isointense to hepatic parenchyma on subsequent imaging consistent with focal nodular hyperplasia.

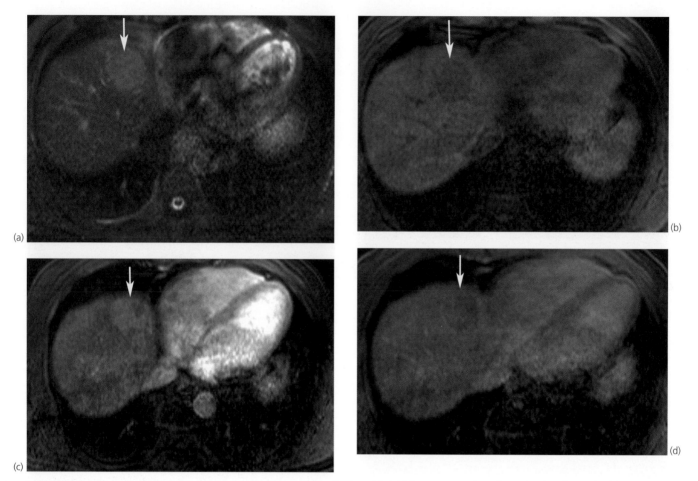

Figure 97.3 Hepatocellular carcinoma. Intermediate time to echo (TE) axial T2-weighted **(a)**, precontrast three-dimensional gradient-echo **(b)**, arterial phase **(c)**, and delayed postcontrast three-dimensional gradient-echo **(d)** images demonstrate a high T2 signal lesion with arterial hyperenhancement and washout on delayed images following contrast administration (arrows).

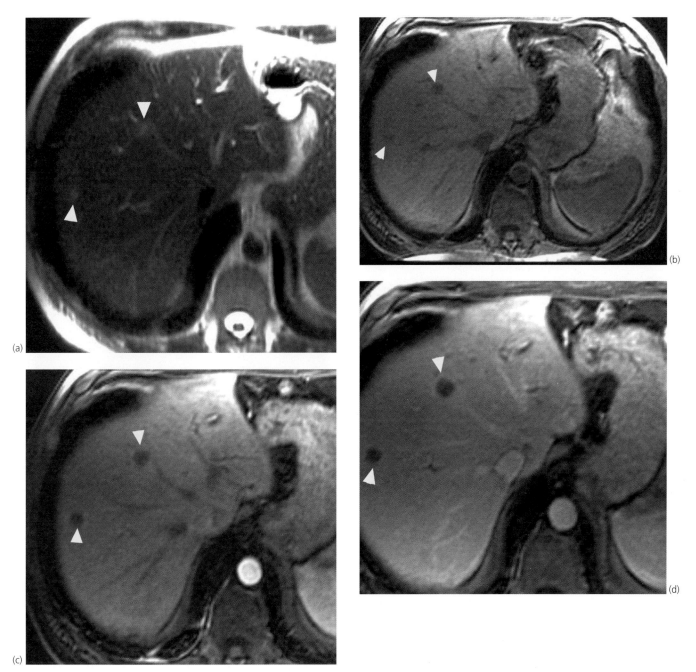

Figure 97.4 Hypovascular hepatic metastases. Axial T2-weighted **(a)**, precontrast three-dimensional gradient-echo **(b)**, arterial phase **(c)**, and postcontrast three-dimensional gradient-echo enhanced **(d)** images demonstrate hypoenhancing metastatic lesions (arrowheads) with rim enhancement in a patient with metastatic pancreatic carcinoma.

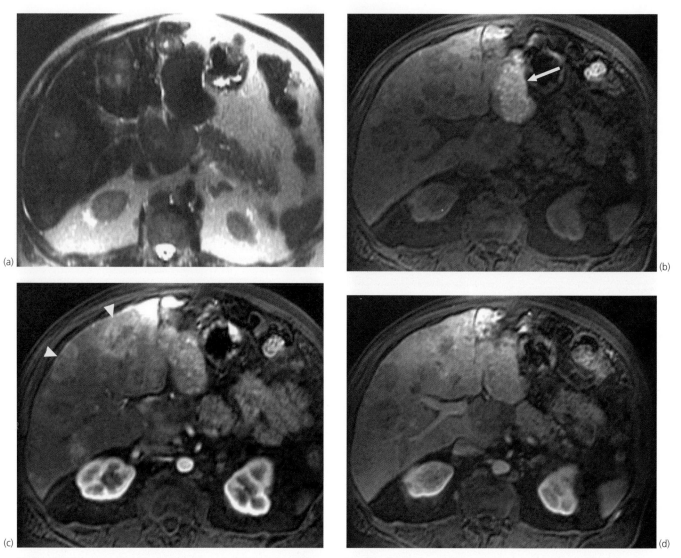

(a)

(b)

(c)

(d)

Figure 97.5 Hypervascular hepatic metastases. Axial T2-weighted **(a)**, precontrast **(b)**, arterial phase **(c)**, portal venous phase postcontrast three-dimensional gradient-echo **(d)** images demonstrate multiple arterial enhancing lesions (arrowheads) in this patient with melanoma metastases. Note the increased signal on precontrast T1-weighted images in the lesion in the lateral segment of the left lobe of the liver (arrow) secondary to melanin or hemorrhage.

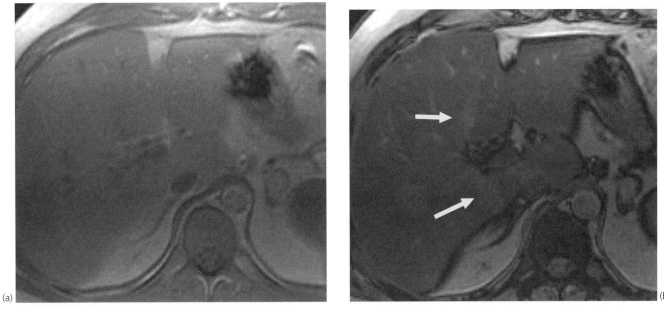

Figure 97.6 Hepatic steatosis. **(a)** Axial in-phase gradient-echo image with time to echo (TE) of 4.6 ms and **(b)** opposed-phase gradient-echo image with TE of 2.2 ms of the liver demonstrate a drop in signal of the liver parenchyma on opposed-phase images consistent with hepatic steatosis. There is a relative lack of a drop in signal near the gallbladder fossa (arrows) consistent with focal fatty sparing.

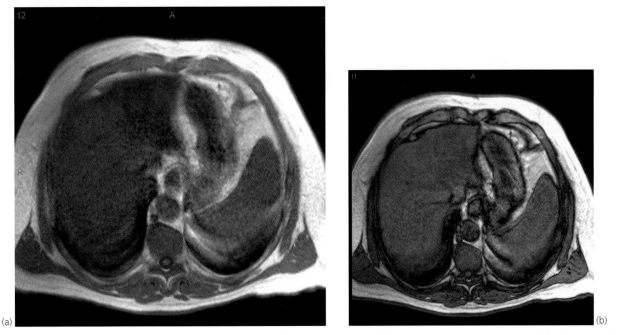

Figure 97.7 Secondary hepatic hemosiderosis. Axial in-phase **(a)** and opposed-phase **(b)** gradient-echo images with time to echo (TE) of 4.6 ms and 2.2 ms, respectively, demonstrate a relatively decreased signal on the in-phase images of the hepatic and splenic parenchyma consistent with secondary hemosiderosis.

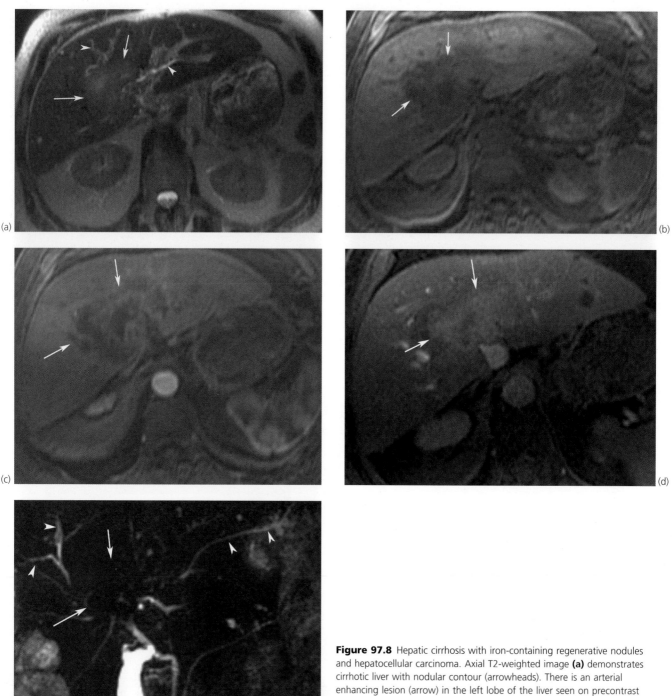

Figure 97.8 Hepatic cirrhosis with iron-containing regenerative nodules and hepatocellular carcinoma. Axial T2-weighted image **(a)** demonstrates cirrhotic liver with nodular contour (arrowheads). There is an arterial enhancing lesion (arrow) in the left lobe of the liver seen on precontrast **(b)** and arterial phase **(c)** three-dimensional gradient-echo images that demonstrates "washout" on portal venous phase imaging **(d)**. Two-dimensional gradient-echo in-phase image **(e)** demonstrates scattered subcentimeter low T1 signal lesions throughout the liver parenchyma consistent with iron-containing regenerative nodules.

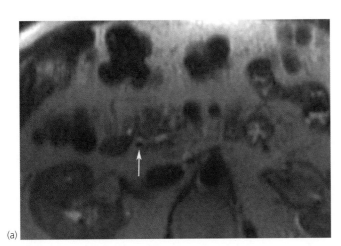

(a)

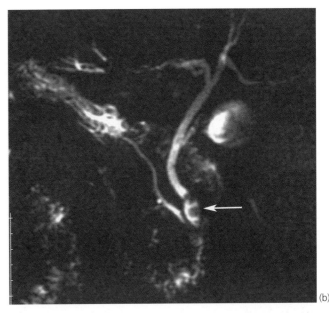

(b)

Figure 97.9 Choledocholithiasis. Axial T2-weighted **(a)** and magnetic resonance cholangiopancreatography (MRCP) **(b)** images show a low signal void (arrow) consistent with common bile duct calculi.

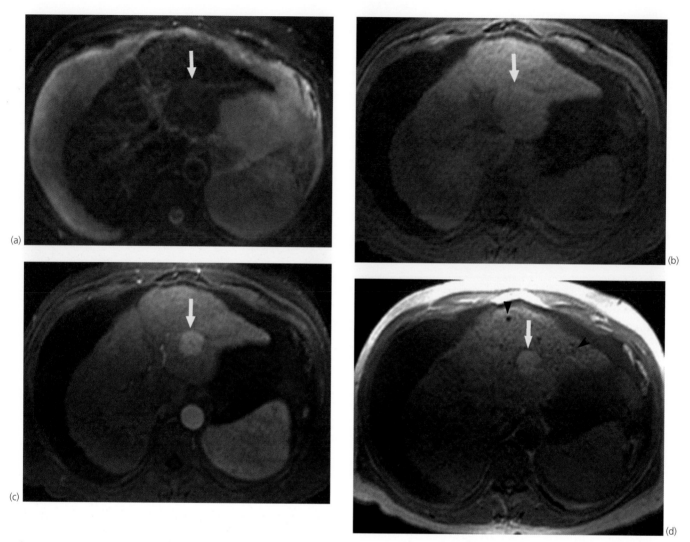

Figure 97.10 Cholangiocarcinoma. Axial T2-weighted **(a)**, precontrast **(b)**, arterial phase **(c)**, and delayed **(d)** three-dimensional gradient-echo images show a large central mass (arrow) that demonstrates delayed enhancement following contrast administration. There is mild peripheral intrahepatic biliary dilation (arrowheads) secondary to obstruction.

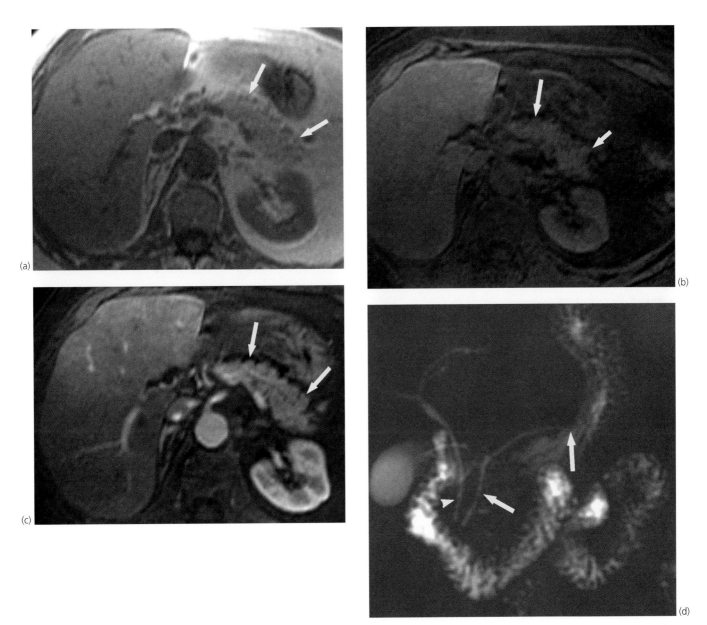

Figure 97.11 Normal pancreas. Axial two-dimensional gradient-echo **(a)** and precontrast three-dimensional gradient-echo fat-suppressed T1-weighted **(b)** images demonstrate a normal magnetic resonance imaging signal of the pancreatic parenchyma of the body and tail of pancreas, which is isointense or higher in signal than liver parenchyma. Axial three-dimensional gadient-echo arterial phase images **(c)** demonstrate normal peak enhancement of the pancreatic parenchyma in the arterial phase. Magnetic resonance cholangiopancreatography (MRCP) **(d)** demonstrates normal relative anatomy of the common bile duct (arrowhead) and the pancreatic duct (arrows).

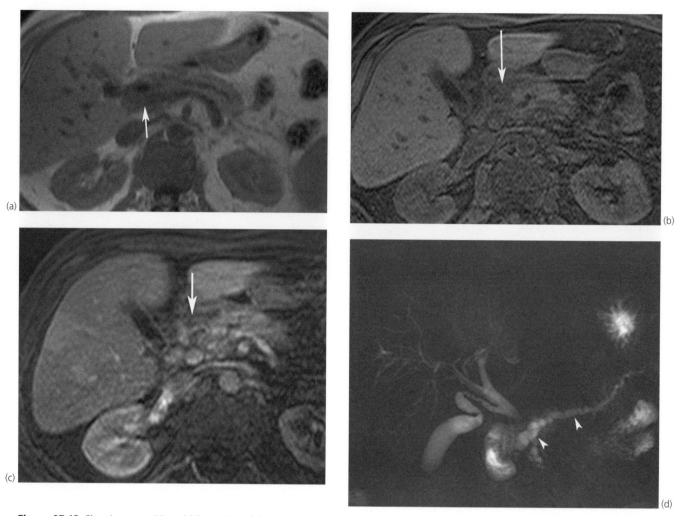

Figure 97.12 Chronic pancreatitis. Axial T1-weighted **(a)** and precontrast three-dimensional gradient-echo **(b)** images demonstrate a relatively low signal (arrow) in the region of the head of the pancreas with relative hypoenhancement following contrast administration on postcontrast images **(c)**. Magnetic resonance cholangiopancreatography (MRCP) **(d)** demonstrates associated diffuse dilation of the pancreatic duct (arrowheads).

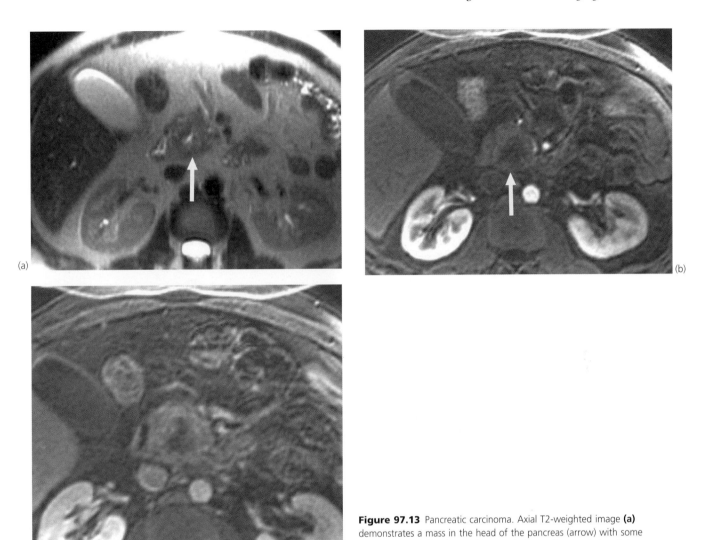

(a)

(b)

(c)

Figure 97.13 Pancreatic carcinoma. Axial T2-weighted image **(a)** demonstrates a mass in the head of the pancreas (arrow) with some central necrosis that hypoenhances relative to the remainder of the pancreas on postcontrast arterial three-dimensional gradient-echo **(b)** and portal venous (**c**) images.

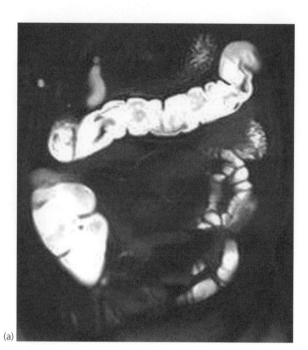
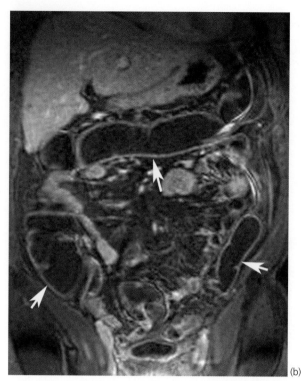

Figure 97.14 Magnetic resonance colonography. Coronal T2-weighted **(a)** and coronal three-dimensional gradient-echo (T1) **(b)** images demonstrate a fluid-distended normal colon (arrows). Courtesy of Thomas Lauenstein MD, Atlanta, GA.

98

Applications of radionuclide imaging in gastroenterology

Harvey A. Ziessman

The advantage of nuclear medicine imaging is that interpretation is based on physiology and function, information that is often quite different from that of anatomical imaging methods, e.g., ultrasonography, CT and MRI.

Acute cholecystitis

Cholescintigraphy has a high accuracy for the diagnosis of acute cholecystitis because it detects the specific underlying pathophysiology, i.e., obstruction of the cystic duct, manifested as non-filling of the gallbladder. Sensitivity for the diagnosis is greater than 95% and specificity 90%. Ultrasonography can be helpful for evaluation of hepatobiliary disease. However, the findings are insensitive and nonspecific for the diagnosis of acute cholecystitis. Direct comparison studies have shown the superiority of cholescintigraphy.

Although non-visualization of the gallbladder at 60 min after injection of the dimethyl iminodiacetic acid (HIDA) radiopharmaceutical, e.g., ^{99m}Tc mebrofenin (choletec), is abnormal; delayed gallbladder filling at 3 to 4 h rules out acute cholecystitis. An alternative to delayed imaging is to administer morphine sulfate, 0.04 mg/kg intravenously at 60 min if the gallbladder is not seen. The diagnosis can be confirmed or excluded 30 min later. Nonvisualization is consistent with acute cholecystitis. Visualization of the gallbladder rules out the disease (Fig. 98.1). Morphine contracts the sphincter of Oddi, increases intrabiliary pressure, and produces preferential bile flow towards and through the cystic duct, if patent.

A useful scintigraphic finding in acute cholecystitis is the "rim sign." Although it is insensitive occurring in only 25%–35% of patients with acute cholecystitis, it is very specific for the diagnosis and warns of late stage disease with an increased likelihood of complications, e.g., gangrene and perforation. This imaging sign is manifested as increased uptake of radiotracer in the liver adjacent to the gallbladder fossa (Fig. 98.2). The reason for the increased uptake is severe inflammation that has spread from the severely inflamed gallbladder to the adjacent liver, resulting in increased blood flow and extraction in that region.

Chronic cholecystitis

Chronic calculous cholecystitis is often easily diagnosed in a patient with recurrent biliary colic-like pain and evidence of cholelithiasis on anatomical imaging. These patients are usually directed to surgery. Occasionally, the pain is atypical and it is not certain whether the stones are actually incident and the pain caused by another factor. Cholecystokinin (CCK) cholescintigraphy can be helpful. A diseased gallbladder does not contract normally. Good gallbladder contraction in response to CCK or a fatty meal would suggest that the patient has asymptomatic cholelithiasis and another cause for pain should be sought. Poor gallbladder contraction would be consistent with symptomatic chronic cholecystitis.

Chronic acalculous gallbladder disease occurs in approximately 5%–10% of patients who have had cholecystectomy for symptoms of chronic cholecystitis. Recent laparoscopic literature suggests that the incidence may be higher. Chronic acalculous gallbladder disease is clinically and histopathologically indistinguishable from chronic calculous cholecystitis, except for the absence of gallstones. Symptoms resolve with cholecystectomy. The problem is in making the diagnosis noninvasively and preoperatively. CKK (sincalide) cholescintigraphy has proven accurate for making a diagnosis; the rationale is the same. Diseased gallbladders do not contract well and have a low gallbladder ejection fraction (GBEF) on CCK stimulated cholescintigraphy. More than 90% of patients with symptoms suggestive of chronic cholecystitis and a low GBEF are cured with cholecystectomy.

Atlas of Gastroenterology, 4th edition. Edited by Tadataka Yamada, David H. Alpers, Anthony N. Kalloo, Neil Kaplowitz, Chung Owyang, and Don W. Powell. © 2009 Blackwell Publishing, ISBN: 978-1-4051-6909-7

Normal values have not been established for 1- to 3-min infusions of sincalide; however, for longer infusions of 30–60 min, the lower limit of normal GBEFs is in the range of 30%–40%, depending on the specific method used (Fig. 98.3). Many studies have shown that the accuracy of CCK cholescintigraphy to diagnose chronic acalculous gallbladder disease is greater than 90%.

Biliary obstruction

In patients clinically suspected of having biliary obstruction, anatomical imaging (e.g., ultrasonography) is often confirmatory, by demonstrating dilated biliary ducts. However, early after the acute onset of obstruction caused by cholelithiasis, bile ducts may not be dilated. Dilation may take 24–72 h to become apparent. Early after onset of obstruction, HIDA imaging can confirm the diagnosis by showing the characteristic pathophysiology, i.e., increased intraductal pressure causing reduced bile flow. In high-grade biliary obstruction, cholescintigraphy demonstrates good hepatic extraction, but no biliary clearance; therefore, the images are of a persistent hepatogram (Fig. 98.4). This is a very specific pattern and diagnostic of high-grade obstruction.

Partial low-grade or intermittent biliary obstruction has a different imaging pattern. Bile ducts often do not become dilated because of the lower intraductal pressure and the intermittent nature of the process. The cholescintigraphic pattern shows good hepatic function, prompt secretion into biliary ducts, but retention of radiotracer in biliary ducts and delayed transit into the small intestines. Thus cholescintigraphy can also provide valuable diagnostic information in patients with the post-cholecystectomy syndrome. Common biliary causes for recurrent pain after cholecystectomy are residual or recurrent biliary duct stones, biliary stricture and sphincter of Oddi dysfunction. All have a scintigraphic picture of partial biliary obstruction. The combination of image analysis and quantification can be diagnostic of partial biliary obstruction (Fig. 98.5). If stones, tumor, and stricture have been eliminated by ERCP or MRCP, sphincter of Oddi dysfunction is likely. Manometry is then diagnostic and sphincterotomy indicated.

Esophageal motility

Esophageal transit scintigraphy is noninvasive, relatively simple to perform, and can provide clinically useful physiological information. During the ingestion of liquids or semisolids mixed with radiotracer it provides sequential images depicting esophageal transit. Qualitative image analysis with cinematic display is often sufficient to diagnose abnormal esophageal motility; however, a strength of the radionuclide method is quantification. Calculation of an esophageal transit time or the residual esophageal activity is performed. Semisolid food swallows have been reported to be more sensitive for abnormal motility than clear liquid swallows, although there is less data and they are less commonly used (Fig. 98.6). Although scintigraphy can serve as a sensitive screening test, it is done most commonly to evaluate response to therapy.

Gastric motility

The radionuclide gastric emptying study has been the standard noninvasive test for the evaluation of gastric motility for decades. Various radiolabeled meals have been used. Some form of egg meal, often a sandwich, is common. Solids empty differently than liquids. Clear liquids empty rapidly and in an exponential pattern, with a half-time of less than 20 min (Fig. 98.7). Solids empty slower. There is a delay before emptying begins (lag phase) which is the length of time required for the antrum to grind up food into particles small enough to pass through the pylorus. After the lag phase, solid emptying generally empties in a linear pattern, at least through 2 h (Fig. 98.8). Normal values used must be based on the specific meal and methodology.

Recent collaboration between the American Motility Society and the Society of Nuclear Medicine has resulted in a consensus publication (Abell, et al. Am J Gastroenterol 2008;103:753) recommending a standardized protocol based on a multinational normal database of 123 subjects. It was designed as a simplified screening test with only four imaging times, at 0, 1, 2, and 4 h. The meal is a ^{99m}Tc-labeled egg substitute sandwich with jam and water. The study length is based on published evidence that a 4-h study detects more abnormal emptying than a 2-h study.

Gastroesophageal reflux

The radionuclide gastroesophageal reflux study is a noninvasive sensitive method to detect reflux. This method was developed and successfully used for pediatric patients but it is also applicable to adults. The study's high sensitivity for reflux detection is owing to the rapid framing rate used during acquisition (10 s frames for 1 h) (Fig. 98.9). For children, formula or milk is mixed with ^{99m}Tc sulfur colloid (SC) and ingested. For adults, orange juice is commonly used. In addition to visual assessment, quantitative or semiquantitative methods can be helpful. A simple method is to count the number of reflux events, to note whether the events are long (greater than 10 s) or short, high (greater than half the distance to the mouth) or low, and then sum the results. For neonates, there are no normal values; however, this is unquestionably abnormal.

Somatostatin receptor imaging (OctreoScan)

Somatostatin receptor imaging plays an important role in imaging neuroendocrine tumors, e.g., gastroenteropancreatic and carcinoid tumors.

Gastroenteropancreatic tumors are highly differentiated, slow growing, and often quite small. Most have high concentrations of somatostatin receptors. Symptoms are often secondary to the hormonal activity expressed, e.g., hypoglycemia, gastric ulcers, severe diarrhea, and flushing. Frequently the tumors have metastasized by the time of diagnosis, to liver, lymph nodes, bone, lungs, and skin. *Gastrointestinal carcinoid tumors* are derived from the foregut, midgut, or hindgut. The midgut carcinoids with liver metastases cause the carcinoid syndrome with symptoms and signs of flushing, diarrhea, wheezing, and valvular right heart disease.

Normal distribution after intravenous injection of the radiopharmaceutical, Indium-111 pentreotide (OctreoScan), shows prominent uptake in the kidneys and spleen. The liver has lesser uptake and gallbladder clearance is variably seen. Whole body planar imaging and single photon emission computed tomography (SPECT) imaging of the region of interest is performed 24 h after injection. Hybrid SPECT/CT systems are increasingly used. Abnormal focal uptake is consistent with tumor.

Sensitivity for detection of carcinoid tumors and gastrinomas is high, approximately 80%–90%, lower for VIPomas and glucagonomas (75%), and poorest for insulinomas (50%). Conventional imaging, e.g., ultrasonography, MRI, and CT, have considerably lower tumor detection rates. Somatostatin receptor imaging is used at the time of initial diagnosis and also to evaluate response to therapy. It can be used to select patients likely to respond favorably to octreotide therapy. Scintigraphy is most useful for detection of metastases and can direct inoperable patients to other forms of therapy (Figs 98.10 and 98.11). OctreoScan imaging positively impacts patient management in 25%–45% of patients.

18-F FDG PET imaging of gastrointestinal malignancies

[18]F-labeled fluorodeoxyglucose (18-F FDG) PET (positron emission tomography) and hybrid PET-CT are experiencing rapid growth and today play an important role in the diagnosis, staging, restaging, and monitoring of response to therapy of many gastrointestinal malignancies. F-18 FDG is a radiolabeled glucose analog. It is transported into the cell and phosphorylated by the same mechanism as glucose but is unable to be metabolized further and is therefore trapped intracellularly. Unlike glucose, it is normally physiologically cleared through the kidneys and bladder. Most malignant tumor cells exhibit increased glucose metabolism compared to normal tissue cells and thus have increased uptake of F-18 FDG. Whole body cross-sectional imaging is routinely performed. Most PET scanners sold today are PET-CT cameras. The PET and CT images are obtained sequentially with the patient lying on a table that moves between the two adjacent scanners, and then the images are registered and fused (overlaid) for functional and anatomical correlation (Fig. 98.12).

In many cancers FDG PET is having an increasingly important role in diagnosis, staging, restaging, and evaluating response to therapy. In many gastrointestinal malignancies, including colorectal cancer, esophageal cancer, and pancreatic cancer, FDG uptake is quite high. Although not routinely used for primary diagnosis in colorectal cancer, it can be helpful in patients at high risk for metastases (Fig 98.12). When other imaging modalities are negative and the serum carcinoembryonic antigen (CEA) level is elevated, F-18 PET has been found very useful for detecting tumor recurrence. It also has an important role in evaluating patients with a single known liver metastasis that is potentially curable. Preoperative detection of distant metastases is poor by conventional methods. FDG PET can help to select patients for surgical resection. It has been shown to frequently change patient management and has a clinical impact in 30%–40% of patients. Finally, FDG PET can determine the effectiveness of chemotherapy and radiation therapy. Also, FDG PET is commonly requested for patients with a new diagnosis of esophageal and pancreatic cancer to screen for metastases. It also plays a useful role in evaluating response to therapy.

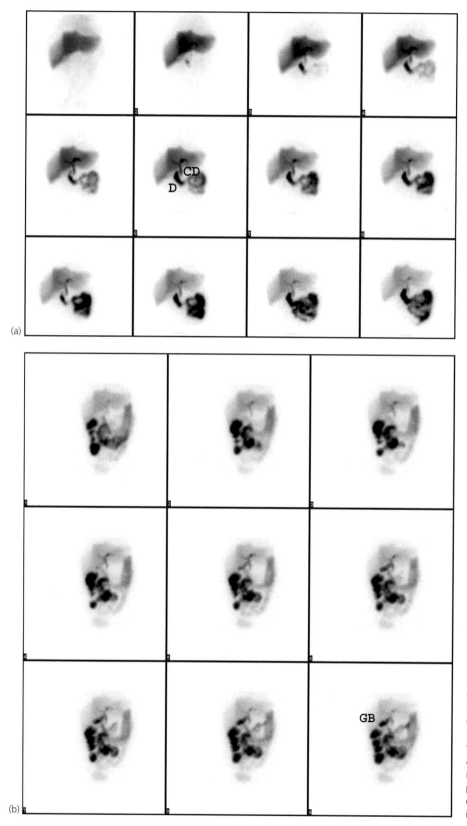

(a)

(b)

Figure 98.1 Delayed gallbladder visualization with intravenous morphine in a 45-year-old female referred for suspected acute cholecystitis. **(a)** Sequential images over 60 min. The right lobe has an abnormal appearance due to a loculated pleural effusion. There is normal hepatic uptake and biliary clearance of the radiotracer into the common duct (CD) and duodenum (D) and more distal small bowel. However, there is no filling of the gallbladder. **(b)** Thirty minutes of additional imaging after administration of morphine sulfate. The gallbladder (GB) progressively fills. This rules out acute cholecystitis. Transit of radiotracer can be seen in the ascending colon.

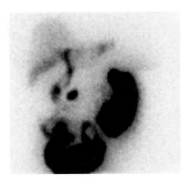

Figure 98.2 Rim sign in acute cholecystitis. This 40-year-old female was referred for suspected acute cholecystitis. The technetium 99m-labeled hepatic iminodiacetic acid ($[^{99m}Tc]$HIDA) study showed nonfilling of the gallbladder at 1 h (not shown). Further delayed images were obtained at 3 h. The image shows a "rim" sign with increased uptake in the liver adjacent to the gallbladder fossa along the inferior aspect of the right lobe. There is no gallbladder filling and normal transit to the small bowel. The rim sign is additional evidence that this is acute cholecystitis and suggests that there is severe inflammation and an increased likelihood of complications such as gangrene and perforation.

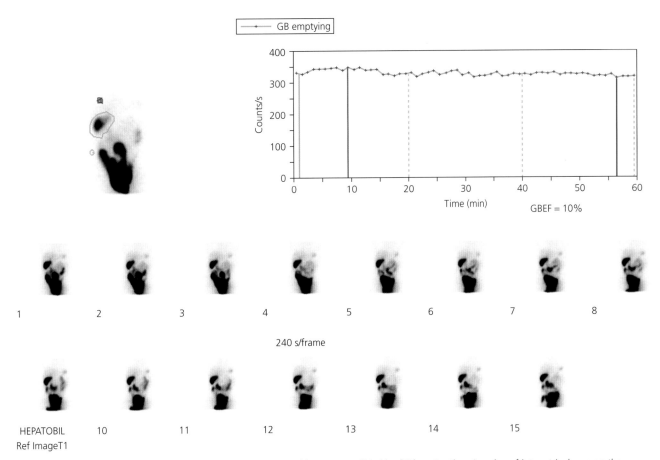

Figure 98.3 Chronic acalculous gallbladder disease in a 52-year-old patient with recurrent biliary-colic-like pain. Ultrasonography showed no stones. The gallbladder filled during the first 60 min of the study (not shown). Shown are sequential 2-min images made during the 60-min infusion of sincalide (cholecystokinin, CCK). Images show poor gallbladder (GB) contraction. A region of interest is drawn on the computer and a time–activity curve generated. The calculated gallbladder ejection fraction (GBEF) was 10% (normal ± 40%). The patient became asymptomatic postcholecystectomy and histopathology showed a chronically inflamed gallbladder.

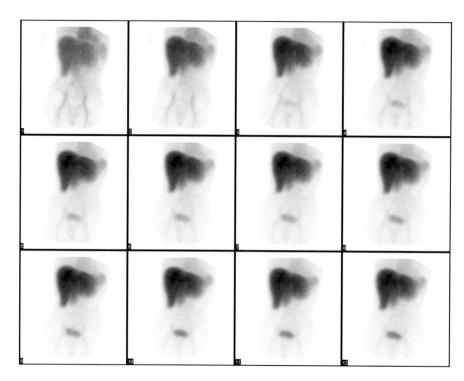

Figure 98.4 High-grade biliary obstruction. Technetium 99m-labeled hepatic iminodiacetic acid ([99mTc]HIDA) study for patient with recent onset of upper abdominal pain. Ultrasonography showed normal-sized biliary ducts and no biliary stones or mass. Sequential images over 1 h show prompt radiotracer extraction, but no biliary excretion into biliary ducts, consistent with high-grade biliary obstruction.

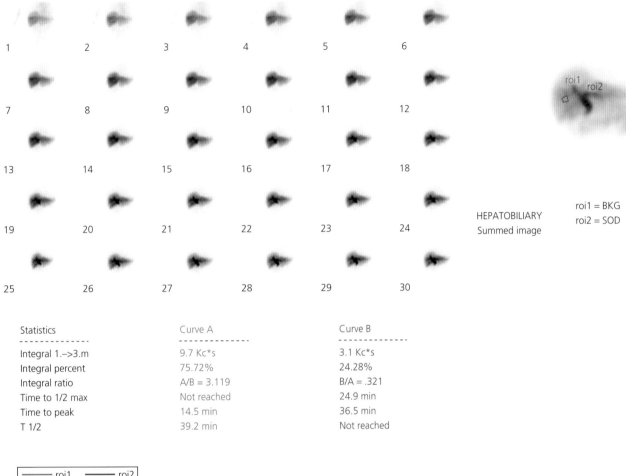

	roi1	roi2

HEPATOBILIARY
Summed image

roi1 = BKG
roi2 = SOD

Statistics	Curve A	Curve B
Integral 1.–>3.m	9.7 Kc*s	3.1 Kc*s
Integral percent	75.72%	24.28%
Integral ratio	A/B = 3.119	B/A = .321
Time to 1/2 max	Not reached	24.9 min
Time to peak	14.5 min	36.5 min
T 1/2	39.2 min	Not reached

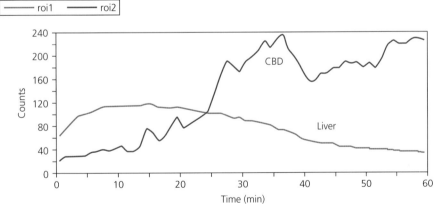

Figure 98.5 Sphincter of Oddi obstruction in a 38-year-old female with chronic recurrent biliary colic starting 5 months postcholecystectomy. Sequential technetium 99m-labeled hepatic iminodiacetic acid ([99mTc]HIDA) images over 1 h show persistent prominent activity in biliary ducts (best seen on image to right of time–activity curve) and little bile transit to the intestines (best seen on large image to right of sequential images). The common bile duct (CBD) time–activity curve shows a progressive rise. This is consistent with a partial biliary obstruction. No stones or biliary stricture were found on further evaluation and sphincterotomy was performed with subsequent symptom resolution.

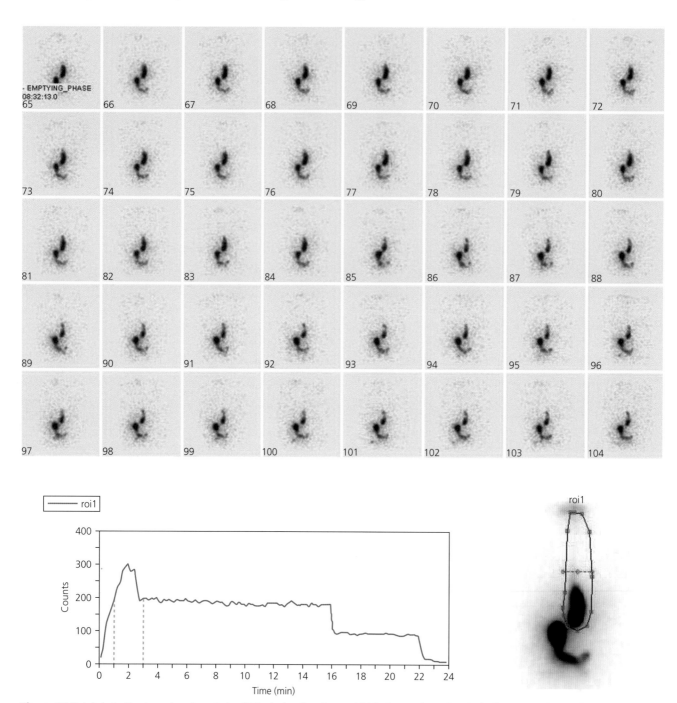

Figure 98.6 Achalasia. Esophageal swallow study of 24-min duration. Sequential 15-s images (posterior view) of ingestion of a cornflake and milk meal demonstrates delayed clearance from the esophagus. A region of interest (ROI) drawn around the esophagus generates a time–activity curve confirming the slow clearance and permits quantification. The drop in counts at 16 and 24 min is due to the ingestion of additional clear liquids.

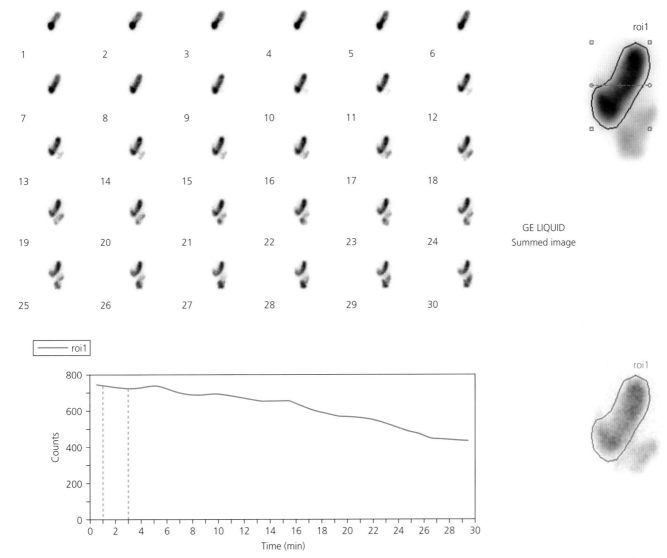

GE LIQUID
Summed image

Figure 98.7 Delayed liquid gastric emptying. The patient could not tolerate solid food. Water (500 mL) mixed with technetium 99m-labeled sulfur colloid was ingested and images acquired every minute for 30 min. A region of interest was drawn around the stomach. A time–activity curve shows delayed emptying. The extrapolated emptying half-time is approximately 45 min (normal 6–18 min).

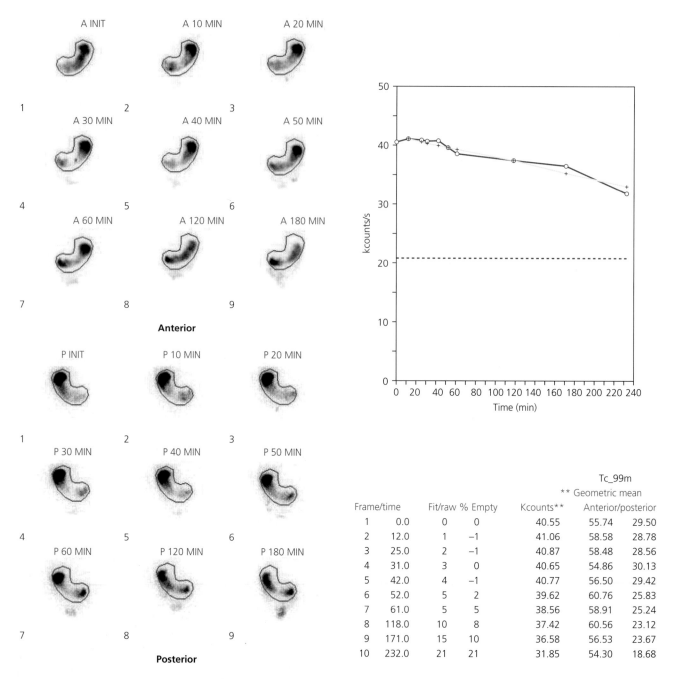

| | | Tc_99m | | |
| | | | ** Geometric mean | |
Frame/time		Fit/raw % Empty	Kcounts**	Anterior/posterior
1	0.0	0	0	40.55	55.74	29.50
2	12.0	1	−1	41.06	58.58	28.78
3	25.0	2	−1	40.87	58.48	28.56
4	31.0	3	0	40.65	54.86	30.13
5	42.0	4	−1	40.77	56.50	29.42
6	52.0	5	2	39.62	60.76	25.83
7	61.0	5	5	38.56	58.91	25.24
8	118.0	10	8	37.42	60.56	23.12
9	171.0	15	10	36.58	56.53	23.67
10	232.0	21	21	31.85	54.30	18.68

Figure 98.8 Delayed solid gastric emptying. Anterior and posterior images were acquired every 10 min during the first hour, then once per hour for 4 h. The purpose of early frequent imaging was to get an estimate of the lag phase, which is delayed. The horizontal dashed line represents 50% emptying. Overall emptying in this patient is markedly delayed with only 21% emptying at 4 h (normal > 90%). Without the images at 10, 20, 30, 40, and 50 min and the 3-h image, this would be similar to the Tougas et al. protocol.

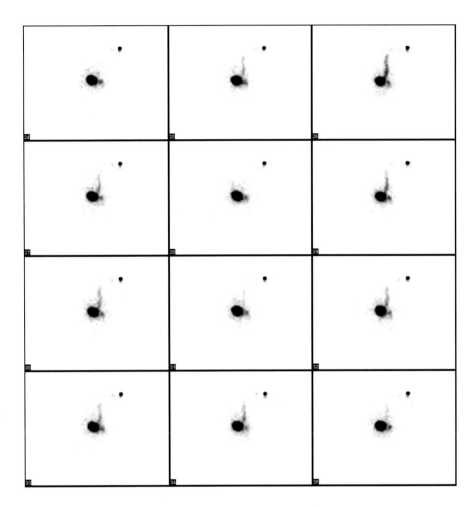

Figure 98.9 Gastroesophageal reflux. A neonate with failure to thrive ingested the usual formula meal with technetium 99m-labeled sulfur colloid. Ten-second sequential frames show frequent episodes of reflux of varying duration, but mostly high level. The hot dot in the right upper corner is a radioactive marker to show the level of the mouth.

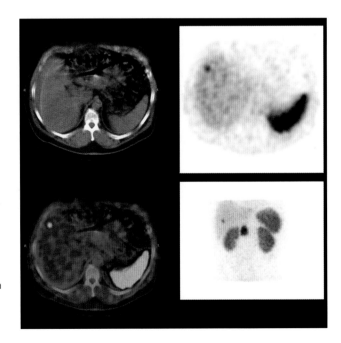

Figure 98.10 OctreoScan single photon emission computed tomography (SPECT) for a pancreatic islet cell tumor. This patient was imaged with indium 111-labeled OctreoScan on a SPECT–CT system, combining both imaging modalities. CT slice **(upper left)**, SPECT image **(upper right)**, fused SPECT–CT image **(lower left)**. The maximal intensity projection images (MIPS) image, a 3D reconstructed abdominal image **(lower right)**, shows normal high uptake in spleen and kidneys and focal hot uptake in a midline mass, which is the patient's islet cell tumor. Also a small focus of uptake due to a metastasis is seen in the anterior inferior portion of the liver on the MIPS view and the SPECT and fused images.

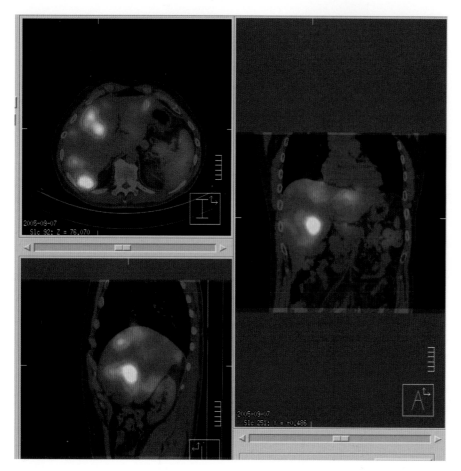

Figure 98.11 OctreoScan single photon emission computed tomography (SPECT)–computed tomography (CT) of carcinoid tumor. Fused SPECT and CT images with transverse **(upper left)**, sagittal **(lower left)**, and coronal **(right)** slices. Intense uptake is seen in multiple large carcinoid tumors metastatic to the liver.

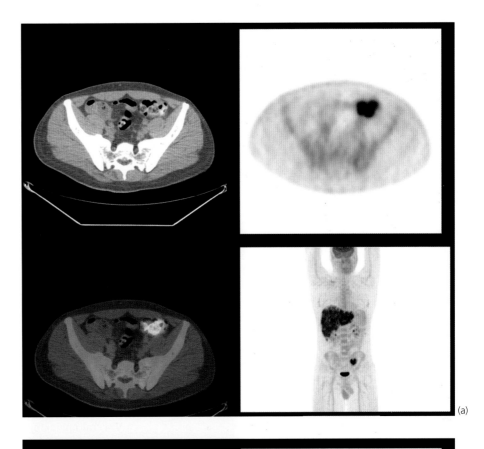

(a)

(b)

Figure 98.12 Fluorine 18-labeled fluorodeoxyglucose (^{18}F FDG) positron emission tomography (PET) of metastatic colon cancer: newly diagnosed adenocarcinoma of sigmoid colon. **(a)** Whole-body maximal image projection images view **(lower right)** shows the primary cancer in the left lower quadrant and extensive metastases to the liver. There is normal bladder clearance. Transverse cross-sectional FDG PET slice **(upper right)** shows intense FDG uptake in the primary malignancy that corresponds to the CT lesion **(upper left)** and fused CT and FDG images **(lower left)**. **(b)** Multiple regions of uptake in the liver consistent with metastases.

99 Angiography

Kyung J. Cho

Angiography is performed to establish a specific diagnosis of neoplasm and vascular lesions, to evaluate hepatoportal hemodynamics, and to obtain specific information about vascular anatomy and variation before radiological and surgical intervention. In this chapter the technique and use of angiography in the diagnosis and management of gastrointestinal, pancreatic, hepatic and splenic lesions are illustrated.

Percutaneous angiography

Gastrointestinal angiography is performed by means of percutaneous retrograde femoral arterial catheterization (Seldinger technique). The common femoral artery usually is punctured with a 21-gauge (0.032 inch) single-wall puncture needle. The Seldinger technique using the micropuncture set is shown in Figure 99.1. Most visceral angiography is performed with 4F or 5F catheters with preshaped configurations. Three commonly used preshaped catheter configurations for visceral angiography are the shepherd's hook, cobra, and sidewinder (Fig. 99.2).

Intraarterial digital subtraction angiography is currently used for visceral angiography. Conventional angiography using the cut-film technique is no longer used. Both iodinated contrast medium (nonionic or isosmolar contrast agents) and carbon dioxide (CO_2) are used. The preferred contrast agent for detection of gastrointestinal (GI) bleeding, wedged hepatic venography, and splenoportography is CO_2. The gas causes no known allergic reactions and nephrotoxicity.

The techniques used in visceral angiography are aortography, selective and superselective visceral angiography,

indirect portography (arterial portography), direct portography (transhepatic, transjugular or transumbilical approach), hepatic venography, and wedged hepatic venography. The coaxial catheterization method using a 3F microcatheter is used for superselective catheterization for embolization of GI bleeding, tumors, and vascular lesions.

Gastrointestinal angiography

Visceral angiography often begins with lateral aortography to visualize the origins of the celiac and superior mesenteric arteries in patients suspected of having mesenteric ischemia (Fig. 99.3). Visceral angiography includes the injection into the celiac and superior mesenteric arteries to demonstrate vascular anatomy (Figs 99.4–99.7). Visceral angiography is used for the diagnosis of arterial occlusive disease (Fig. 99.8), collateral circulation (Fig. 99.9), aneurysms (Fig. 99.10), arteriovenous fistulae (Fig. 99.11), and portal vein aneurysm (Fig. 99.12).

Angiography continues to play an important role in the diagnosis of upper and lower gastrointestinal bleeding (Figs 99.13–99.16). Angiography is especially important for the diagnosis of chronic gastrointestinal bleeding from tumors (Fig. 99.17), vascular malformations (Fig. 99.18), and colonic vascular ectasia (Fig. 99.19). Visualization of the portal venous system is important in the evaluation of cirrhosis, portal hypertension, and pancreatic, biliary, and hepatic tumors. The portal vein can be evaluated by means of indirect portography (arterial portography) (Figs 99.20 and 99.21) or direct portography (Figs 99.22 and 99.23). Angiography is used to differentiate occlusive from nonocclusive mesenteric ischemia. It is also useful in the diagnosis of carcinoid tumor (Fig. 99.24) and pancreatic (Fig. 99.25) and hepatic (Fig. 99.26) metastases. Diagnostic angiography is performed prior to balloon angioplasty of superior mesenteric artery stenosis and transcatheter embolization for control of upper and lower GI bleeding, and occlusion of splanchnic artery aneurysms.

Atlas of Gastroenterology, 4th edition. Edited by Tadataka Yamada, David H. Alpers, Anthony N. Kalloo, Neil Kaplowitz, Chung Owyang, and Don W. Powell. © 2009 Blackwell Publishing, ISBN: 978-1-4051-6909-7

Pancreatic angiography

Ultrasound and computed tomographic scanning are the initial diagnostic procedures for inflammatory and neoplastic pancreatic lesions. Endoscopic retrograde cholangiopancreatography with cytological examination is commonly performed for patients with suspected pancreatic cancer. Once pancreatic lesions have been demonstrated with the imaging methods, angiography is performed to obtain a specific diagnosis and to assess the vascular anatomy and resectability of the tumor before surgical intervention (Fig. 99.27).

Endoscopic ultrasound scanning is commonly used for localization of pancreatic islet cell tumors. When it reveals a pancreatic mass in a patient with hyperinsulinism, surgical therapy is provided without additional localization procedures. For occult insulinomas, selective arterial calcium stimulation is used to regionalize the source of hyperinsulinism with assay of insulin from the hepatic vein at 30 s and 60 s, following stimulation of the potential supplying arteries. Angiography is positive for insulinoma in about 60% of cases, and the tumor appears as a localized hypervascular mass within the pancreas (Fig. 99.28). Angiography is often negative for gastrinomas because they are usually hypovascular. Selective secretin injection is performed for localization of occult gastrinomas. Angiography is usually positive for other neuroendocrine tumors, including vasoactive intestinal polypeptide-secreting tumor (Vipoma), pancreatic polypeptide-producing tumor (PPoma), somatostatinoma, and glucagonoma (Fig. 99.29). Angiography is important in the diagnosis and management of gastrointestinal bleeding, complicating pancreatitis and pseudocysts (Fig. 99.30). Such bleeding may originate from an aneurysm or varices associated with portal or splenic venous thrombosis.

Hepatic angiography

Ultrasound and computed tomography (CT), magnetic resonance imaging (MRI), and radionuclide studies are used for the diagnosis of hepatic mass lesions. The most frequently used modality for the diagnosis of hepatic neoplasm is CT scanning, with and without contrast enhancement. Angiography is sensitive in detecting vascular tumors in the liver, including hepatoma, cavernous hemangioma (Fig. 99.31), focal nodular hyperplasia (Fig. 99.32), and bleeding associated with hepatic adenoma (Fig. 99.33).

Hepatic angiography plays an important role in the preoperative evaluation of resectability of tumors. Involvement of both lobes, regional lymph node metastases, and portal vein invasion indicate unresectability of the tumor (Fig. 99.34). The portal venous phase of high-dose superior mesenteric angiography is used to evaluate the portal venous system. Angiography is used for localization of lesions and treatment of patients with clinically significant hemobilia (Fig. 99.35) or bleeding after laparoscopic cholecystectomy (Fig. 99.36). Selective arterial embolization is effective in controlling bleeding from intrahepatic sources and eliminates the need for major surgical intervention.

Panhepatic angiography is an important preoperative procedure for portosystemic shunt operations and for endovascular interventions. It includes both arterial and venous examinations with manometry. Angiography is essential in the diagnosis of Budd–Chiari syndrome (Fig. 99.37). Hepatic venography with injection of contrast medium into the occluded hepatic vein or patent accessory vein usually demonstrates typical spider web collaterals. Angiographic methods used for the management of Budd–Chiari syndrome include percutaneous translumenal angioplasty, placement of metallic stents, and transjugular intrahepatic portacaval shunt (TIPS). Wedged hepatic venography and manometry is an important part of angiographic evaluation in patients with cirrhosis and portal hypertension. Wedged hepatic venography is performed to diagnose portal vein occlusion (Fig. 99.38), facilitate transjugular liver biopsy (Fig. 99.39), and to visualize the portal vein target for a TIPS procedure. In the absence of presinusoidal obstruction, wedged hepatic venous pressure reflects sinusoidal pressure.

Splenic angiography

The splenic artery is a branch of the celiac artery and rarely originates from the superior mesenteric artery. The splenic artery gives rise to the dorsal pancreatic, pancreatica magna artery, caudal pancreatic and left gastroepiploic arteries before branching into the segmental arteries of the spleen. Occasionally, it gives rise to accessory left gastric and superior polar splenic artery before entering the hilus of the spleen. The short gastric arteries arise from the splenic arterial branches in the upper pole of the spleen. All the branches of the splenic artery provide collateral pathways in occlusion of the celiac, superior mesenteric and splenic artery. The splenic artery is visualized with the injection of contrast medium into the celiac axis. Selective catheterization of the splenic artery can be performed by advancing a 4F or 5F catheter into the splenic artery over a guide wire. The coaxial catheterization method using a 3F microcatheter is useful for superselective catheterization of the splenic artery and its branches for transcatheter embolization. Splenic angiography is performed for the diagnosis of pancreatic tumor, aneurysm (Fig. 99.40 and Fig. 99.41), and splenic vein occlusion. The indications for splenic artery embolization include:
- Control of traumatic splenic hemorrhage (Fig. 99.42);
- Hypersplenism, using partial splenic artery embolization;

- Gastric variceal bleeding from isolated splenic vein occlusion;
- Prior to laparoscopic splenectomy in massive splenomegaly (Fig. 99.43); and
- Splenic artery aneurysm.

Percutaneous splenoportography is a useful method for evaluating the splenic and portal veins in patients with cirrhosis and portal hypertension, and splenic vein occlusion. Noninvasive imaging modalities and indirect splenoportography with the injection of large volume of contrast medium into the splenic artery have largely replaced splenoportography. CO_2 splenoportography with a skinny needle (22- to 25-gauge needle) is a safe, useful technique in visualizing the splenic and portal veins, and portosystemic collaterals.

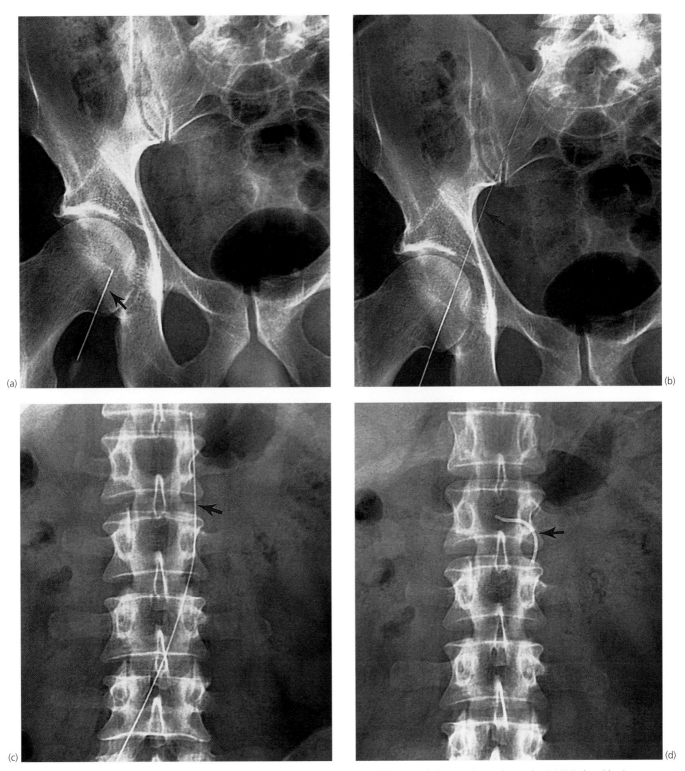

(a)

(b)

(c)

(d)

Figure 99.1 Seldinger technique for percutaneous angiography with micropuncture technique. **(a)** The common femoral artery is accessed with a 21-gauge needle (arrow). **(b)** The 0.018-inch (0.46-mm) guidewire (arrow) is introduced through the iliac artery into the aorta. **(c)** The 0.035-inch guidewire (arrow) is introduced into the aorta through a 4F coaxial dilator, which was advanced over the 0.018-inch guidewire. **(d)** The 5F shepherd's hook catheter (arrow) has been placed in the abdominal aorta for catheterization of the branches of the aorta. A pigtail catheter should be used for abdominal aortography with contrast medium whereas an end-hole catheter is used for CO_2 aortography.

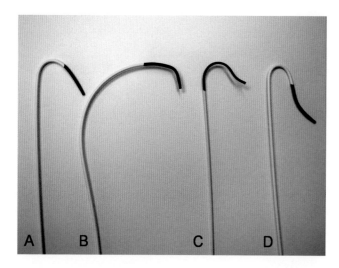

Figure 99.2 Shapes of distal bends for visceral angiography. **(a)** Simple curve. **(b)** Cobra. **(c)** Shepherd's hook. **(d)** Sidewinder.

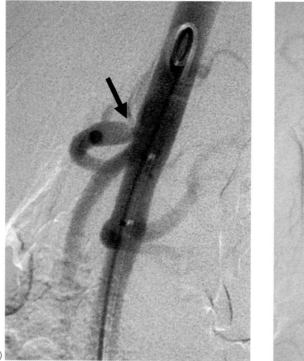

(a)

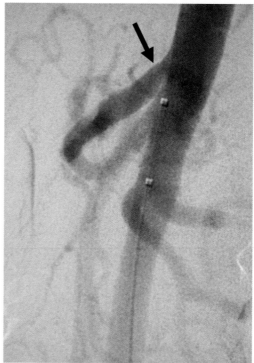

(b)

Figure 99.3 Median arcuate ligament compression of the celiac artery in a 28-year-old woman with postprandial abdominal pain. **(a)** Full expiration. The origin of the celiac axis has a 60% stenosis (arrow) caused by median arcuate ligament compression. **(b)** Full inspiration. The origin of the celiac axis shows no stenosis (arrow).

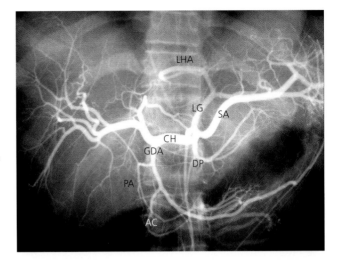

Figure 99.4 Celiac axis anatomy. The celiac axis gives off the splenic (SA), left gastric (LG), and common hepatic (CH) arteries. There is an aberrant left hepatic artery (LHA) originating from the left gastric artery. The common hepatic artery divides into the gastroduodenal artery (GDA) and proper hepatic arteries. The gastroduodenal artery gives rise to the posterior arcade (PA) and anterior arcade (AC) arteries, which join to form the inferior pancreaticoduodenal artery. The dorsal pancreatic (DP) artery originates from the celiac artery.

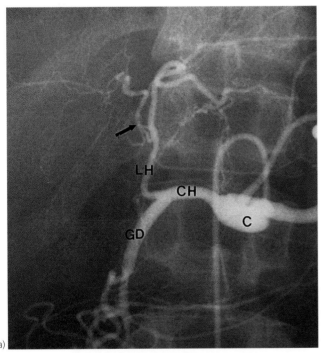

(a)

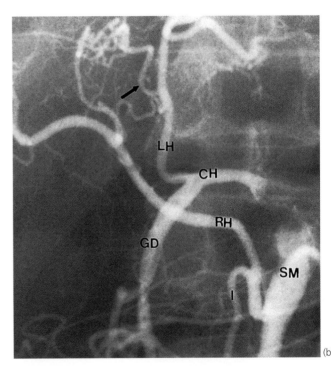

(b)

Figure 99.5 Aberrant right hepatic artery originating from the superior mesenteric artery. **(a)** The common hepatic artery (CH) divides into the gastroduodenal (GD) and left hepatic (LH) arteries. The middle hepatic artery (arrow) originates from the left hepatic artery (LH). **(b)** Arterial phase of superior mesenteric arteriogram of same patient. The replaced right hepatic (RH) originates from the superior mesenteric artery (SM), and the inferior pancreaticoduodenal (I) artery originates from the aberrant right hepatic artery. The gastroduodenal (GD) and left hepatic (LH) arteries are filled from the superior mesenteric artery because of celiac stenosis.

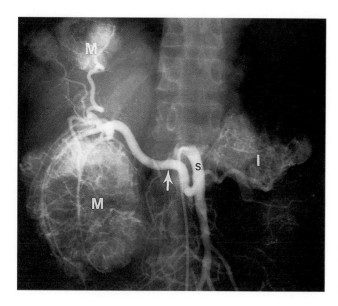

Figure 99.6 Hepatic artery variation. Superior mesenteric arteriogram of a patient with hepatic metastases (M) from nonfunctioning islet cell carcinoma of the pancreas (I). The right hepatic artery (arrow) is replaced from the superior mesenteric artery (S) and supplies hypervascular metastases (M) in the liver. The splenic, left gastric, and common hepatic arteries originate from the celiac axis (not shown).

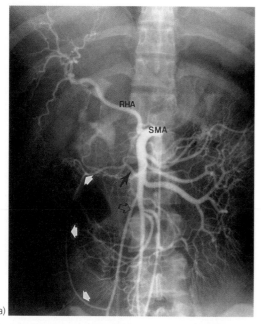

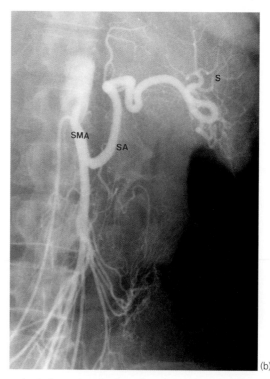

Figure 99.7 Celiac trunk variations. **(a)** Arterial phase of a superior mesenteric angiogram. The right hepatic artery (RHA) has a replaced origin from the superior mesenteric artery (SMA). The middle colic (black arrow) and right colic (black open arrow) arteries form the paracolic arcade (white arrows) along the ascending colon. The common hepatic and splenic arteries arise from the celiac trunk (not shown). **(b)** Arterial phase of a superior mesenteric angiogram. The splenic artery (SA) has a replaced origin from the superior mesenteric artery (SMA). In this patient, the celiac trunk gives off a left gastric artery and a common hepatic artery (not shown). S, spleen.

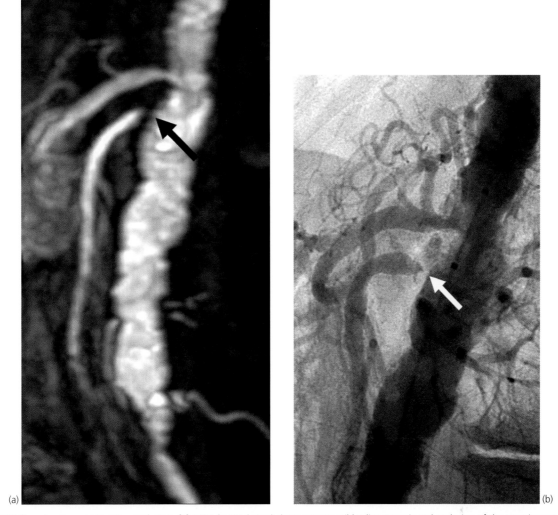

(a)

(b)

Figure 99.8 Superior mesenteric artery occlusion. **(a)** MRA (sagittal view) demonstrates mild celiac stenosis and occlusion of the superior mesenteric artery (arrow). **(b)** Lateral aortogram. The superior mesenteric artery is occluded (arrow).

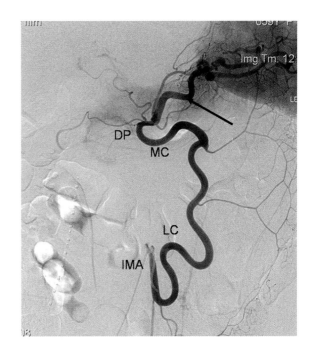

Figure 99.9 Collateral circulation from interior mesenteric artery in celiac artery occlusion. The left colic branch (LC) of the inferior mesenteric artery (IMA) is markedly dilated. Blood flows through this artery to the middle colic (MC), to the dorsal pancreatic (DP) and to the splenic artery (arrow).

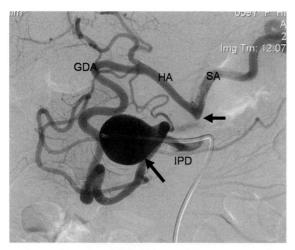

Figure 99.10 Pancreatic artery aneurysm. Arteriogram with the injection of contrast medium into the inferior pancreaticoduodenal artery (IPD). There is an aneurysm (arrow) on the posterior arcade artery. The celiac artery is occluded (shorter arrow). The posterior and anterior arcades are markedly dilated, and blood flows through these arteries to the gastroduodenal (GDA) and to the hepatic (HA) and splenic (SA) arteries.

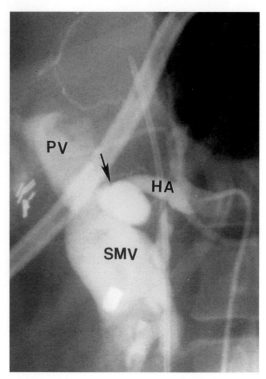

Figure 99.11 Arterioportal fistula that developed after a gunshot wound. Selective hepatic arteriogram (oblique view) demonstrates a large fistula (arrow) and aneurysm between the hepatic artery (HA) and portal vein (PV). SMV, superior mesenteric vein.

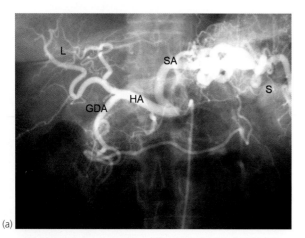

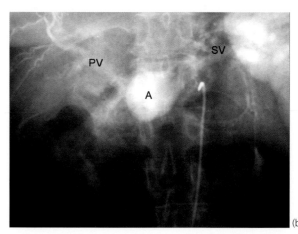

Figure 99.12 Portal venous aneurysm. **(a)** Celiac arteriogram shows tortuous splenic artery (SA), patent hepatic (HA) and gastroduodenal (GDA) artery. S, spleen, L, liver. **(b)** Venous phase of the celiac angiogram shows a portal vein aneurysm **(a)** arises from the junction of the splenic (SV) and portal (PV) veins. Venous aneurysms may occur in the splenic, superior mesenteric, and portal veins. Most portal vein aneurysms are found incidentally and cause no specific symptoms.

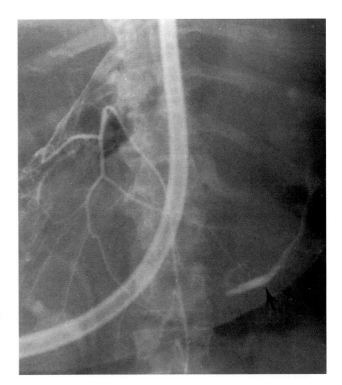

Figure 99.13 Arterial bleeding from peptic ulcer. The catheter has been selectively placed into the gastric artery. Angiogram shows extravasation of contrast medium in the body of the stomach near the greater curvature. The extravasated contrast medium gives the appearance of a vein ("pseudovein" sign) (arrow). The bleeding was successfully controlled by gelatin sponge (Gelfoam, Upjohn, Kalamazoo, MI) embolization.

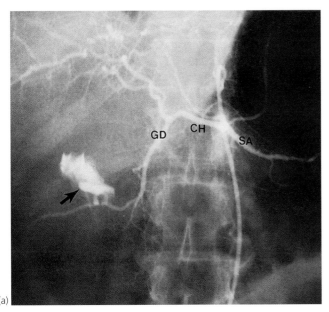

(a)

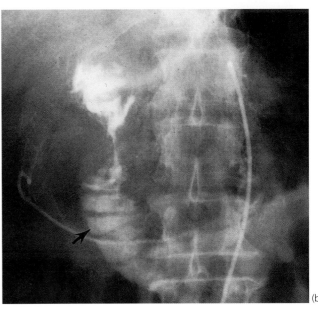

(b)

Figure 99.14 Massive arterial bleeding into the duodenum of a patient with peptic ulcer. **(a)** Celiac arteriogram (arterial phase) shows branches of the celiac artery with severe vasoconstriction caused by hypovolemic shock. Massive contrast extravasation is demonstrated in the duodenal bulb (arrow) from the proximal gastroepiploic artery. SA, splenic artery; CH, common hepatic artery; GD, gastroduodenal artery. **(b)** Venous phase of same angiogram shows extravasated contrast medium outlining the mucosal folds of the duodenum (arrow).

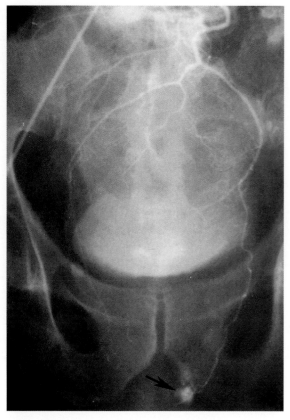

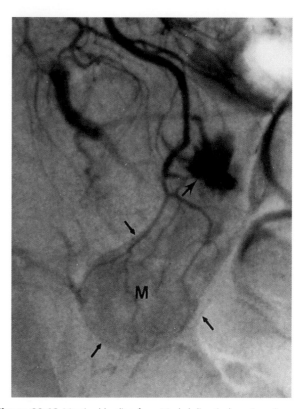

Figure 99.15 Rectal bleeding complicating rectal tube placement. Inferior mesenteric arteriogram shows active bleeding (arrow) into the distal rectum. Vasopressin infusion stopped the bleeding.

Figure 99.16 Massive bleeding from Meckel diverticulum. Superior mesenteric arteriogram of a 7-year-old girl with lower gastrointestinal bleeding shows Meckel diverticulum (M, small arrows) and extravasation of the contrast medium (large arrow) near its attachment to the ileum.

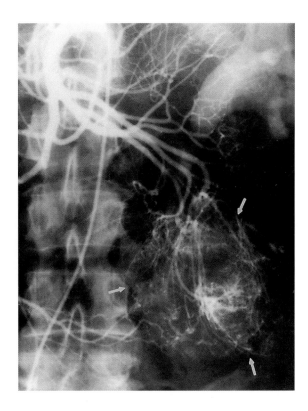

Figure 99.17 Intestinal leiomyosarcoma. Superior mesenteric arteriogram demonstrates a vascular tumor with dilated feeding arteries and tumor vessels (arrows). The inhomogeneous tumor blush and poor margin of the tumor suggest a malignant tumor.

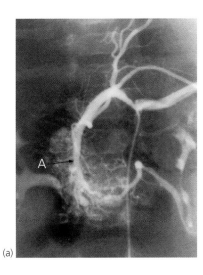

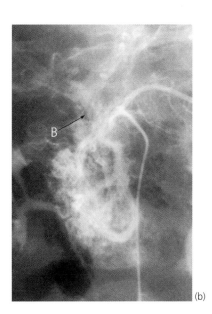

Figure 99.18 Pancreatic and duodenal arteriovenous malformations. **(a)** Arterial phase of a gastroduodenal angiogram of a 7-month-old boy with gastrointestinal hemorrhage demonstrates tortuous abnormal vascular channels in the duodenum and pancreas. The gastroduodenal artery (A) and its branches supply the malformations. **(b)** Parenchymal phase demonstrates mottled staining and early, dense venous opacification from the lesion. B, portal vein.

(a)

(b)

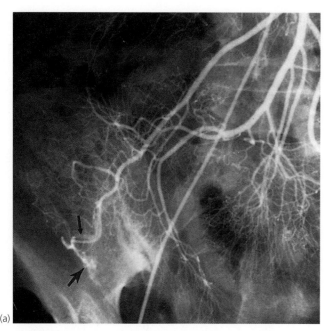

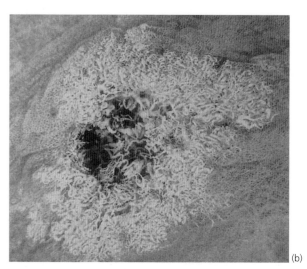

(a)

(b)

Figure 99.19 Vascular ectasia of the cecum. **(a)** Superior mesenteric arteriogram of a 70-year-old woman with recurrent lower gastrointestinal bleeding. Dilated cecal artery feeds a small mucosal vascular ectasia (large arrow). An early draining vein (small arrow) is beginning to fill. **(b)** The resected cecum has been injected with Microfil (Canton Bio-Medical Products, Inc., Boulder, CO) and has undergone the clearing process. Mucosal vascular ectasia is present.

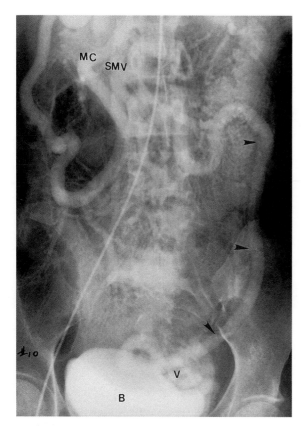

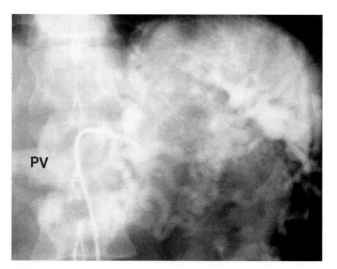

Figure 99.21 Isolated gastric varices of a patient with splenic vein occlusion associated with pancreatitis. Venous phase of splenic angiogram shows varices in the wall of the stomach and upper abdomen. Varices reconstitute the portal vein (PV). Splenectomy is curative for bleeding gastric varices. Partial splenic artery embolization is a safe, effective alternative to surgical treatment.

Figure 99.20 Varices in the wall of the urinary bladder of a patient with hematuria. Venous phase of superior mesenteric angiogram shows large varices (V) in the wall of the bladder (B) filled from the superior mesenteric vein (SMV) through the middle (MC) and left colic (arrowheads) veins.

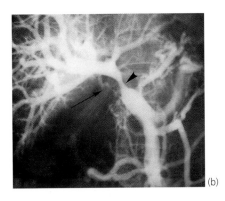

Figure 99.22 Invasion of common bile duct by gallbladder carcinoma. **(a)** Arterial phase of a hepatic angiogram demonstrates occlusion of the bile duct artery (arrow). **(b)** Portal venogram through the percutaneous transhepatic approach shows that vein of the bile duct (arrow) and portal vein (arrowhead) are encased, indicating unresectability of the tumor.

(a)

(b)

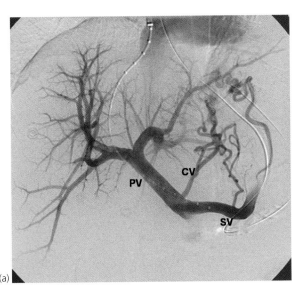

(a)

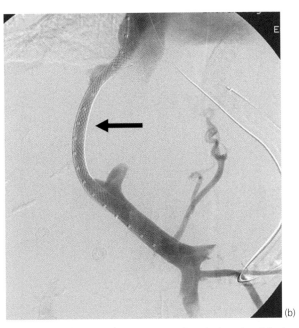

(b)

Figure 99.23 Transjugular portography in a patient with cirrhosis and portal hypertension. **(a)** Direct splenoportogram: the splenic and portal veins are patent, and portal blood flows toward the liver (hepatopetal). The coronary vein (CV) and gastric varices are filled. **(b)** After creation of a portosystemic shunt (TIPS), the TIPS stent (arrow) is patent, and blood flows through this TIPS stent and to the hepatic vein.

Figure 99.24 Ileal carcinoid tumor with mesenteric metastases. **(a)** Barium study of a 52-year-old woman with diarrhea and abdominal pain shows that loops of small bowel are retracted and their walls are thickened. **(b)** Superior mesenteric arteriogram shows that right colic and ileocolic arteries are encased and the mesenteric artery branches are retracted into a stellate pattern.

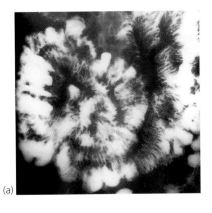

(a)

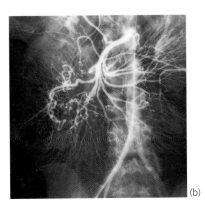

(b)

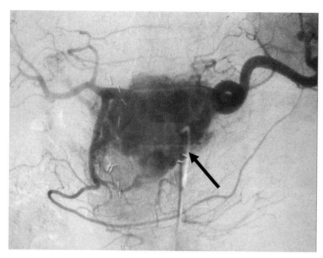

Figure 99.25 Pancreatic metastasis from renal cell carcinoma. Celiac angiogram shows a large hypervascular tumor (arrow) in the head and neck region of the pancreas.

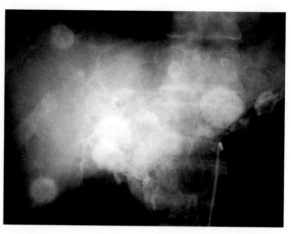

Figure 99.26 Liver metastases from renal cell carcinoma. Parenchymal phase of a hepatic angiogram shows multiple hypervascular metastases. Other vascular hepatic metastases are from pancreatic neuroendocrine tumors, carcinoid tumors, renal cell carcinoma, medullary thyroid carcinoma, and melanoma.

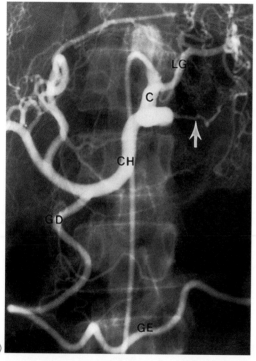

(a)

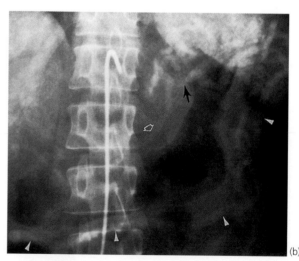

(b)

Figure 99.27 Splenic artery encasement and occlusion caused by pancreatic carcinoma. **(a)** Celiac angiogram (arterial phase) demonstrates encasement (arrow) and occlusion of the splenic artery. Collateral circulation toward the spleen is visible through the left gastric (LG) and right gastroepiploic (GE) arteries. C, celiac axis; CH, common hepatic artery; GD, gastroduodenal artery. **(b)** Venous phase of the same angiogram shows the splenic vein occluded (arrow) in the region of the body of the pancreas. Venous collateral vessels have developed through the gastroepiploic (arrowheads) and gastric (open arrow) veins.

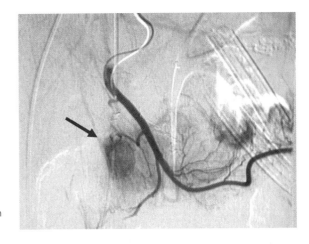

Figure 99.28 Insulinoma. Gastroduodenal arteriogram shows a vascular lesion in the head of the pancreas (arrow) representing an islet cell adenoma.

Figure 99.29 Glucagonoma. **(a)** Arterial phase of a celiac angiogram of a 64-year-old man with dermatitis, diabetes mellitus, and anemia. Hypervascular tumor (T) in the head of the pancreas is supplied by the pancreatic arcade arteries. A, common hepatic artery; B, gastroduodenal artery; C, posterior arcade artery; D, anterior arcade artery. **(b)** Parenchymal phase shows tumor has homogeneous dense contrast accumulation characteristic of an islet cell tumor.

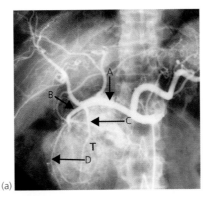

(a)

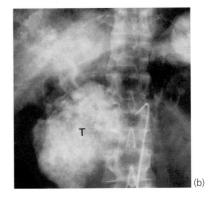

(b)

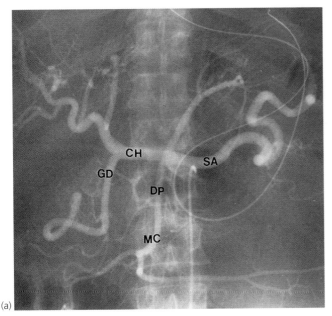

(a)

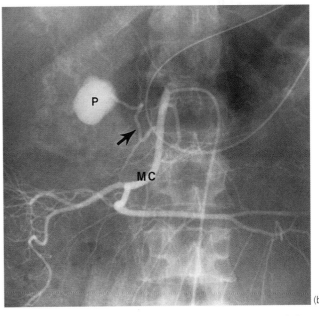

(b)

Figure 99.30 Bleeding into a pseudocyst. **(a)** Celiac angiogram (arterial phase) shows middle colic artery (MC) arising from the dorsal pancreatic (DP) artery that originates from the celiac axis. SA, splenic artery; CH, common hepatic artery; GD, gastroduodenal artery. **(b)** Selective injection into the dorsal pancreatic artery demonstrates a pseudoaneurysm (P) filled from a branch of the dorsal pancreatic artery (arrow).

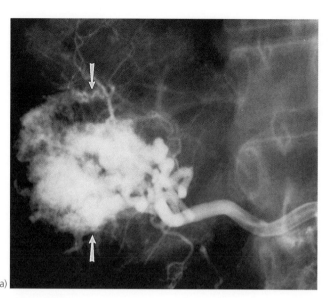
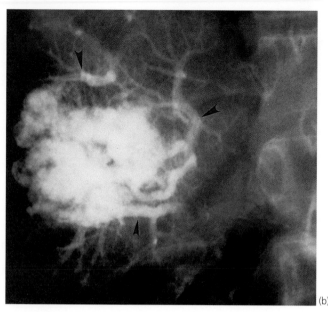

Figure 99.31 Cavernous hemangioma. **(a)** Hepatic angiogram (arterial phase) shows dilated hepatic artery and the vascular spaces of the hemangioma filled with contrast medium (arrows). **(b)** Vascular spaces have retained contrast medium through the venous phase, characteristic of hemangioma. Portal veins (arrowheads) are opacified, indicating arteriovenous shunting. Arteriovenous shunting is an unusual finding with hemangioma.

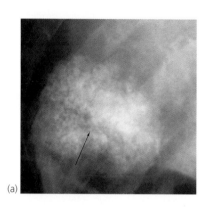
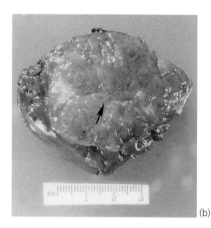

Figure 99.32 Focal nodular hyperplasia. **(a)** Parenchymal phase of a hepatic angiogram, magnification technique, of a 26-year-old woman demonstrates nodular accumulation of contrast medium with central scar formation (arrow) typical of focal nodular hyperplasia. **(b)** Section of the resected mass shows a nodular pattern, central scar (arrow), and radiating septa.

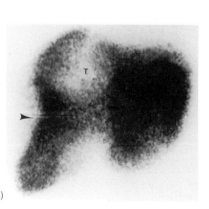
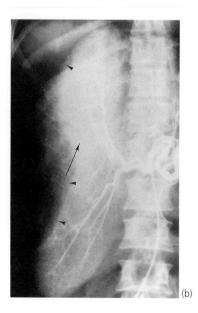

Figure 99.33 Ruptured hepatic adenoma with massive hemorrhage. **(a)** ^{99m}Tc sulfur colloid scan of a 30-year-old woman with a history of use of oral contraceptives demonstrates a photon-deficient area (T) and large subcapsular hematoma (arrowhead) in the right lobe of the liver. **(b)** Arterial phase of a hepatic angiogram demonstrates an avascular mass (arrow) associated with a large subcapsular hematoma (arrowheads). Liver is displaced from the lateral abdominal wall.

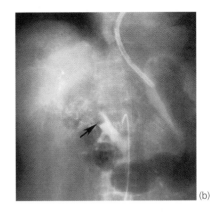

Figure 99.34 Invasion of the portal vein by hepatoma in a patient with esophageal variceal bleeding. **(a)** Arterial phase of a celiac angiogram shows linear abnormal vessels (arrow) running along the portal vein. **(b)** Venous phase of same angiogram demonstrates tumor thrombus (arrow) in the portal vein.

(a)

(b)

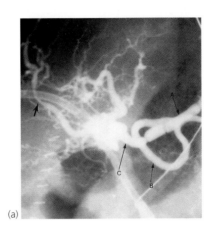
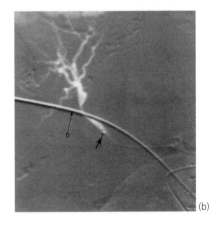

Figure 99.35 Superselective catheterization of a hepatic artery branch with a coaxial catheter system (Tracker-18, Boston Scientific Corporation, Natick, MA) in a patient with hemobilia subsequent to percutaneous biliary drainage. **(a)** Celiac arteriogram shows biliary catheter has injured a right hepatic arterial branch (arrow). **(b)** Digital subtraction arteriogram through a 3F catheter (arrow) in the bleeding artery demonstrates arterial injury. Hemobilia was controlled by means of embolization. A, celiac artery; B, splenic artery; C, hepatic artery; D, transhepatic biliary catheter.

(a)

(b)

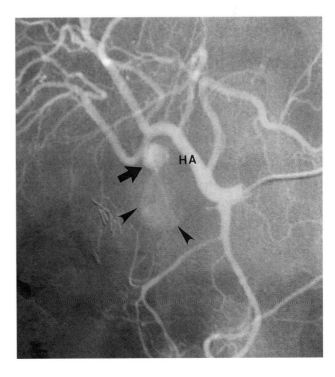

Figure 99.36 Massive bleeding complicating laparoscopic cholecystectomy. Hepatic angiogram (arterial phase) demonstrates bleeding (arrowheads) from pseudoaneurysm (arrow) of the right hepatic artery (HA).

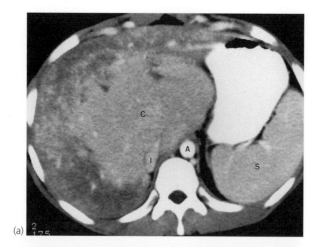

(a)

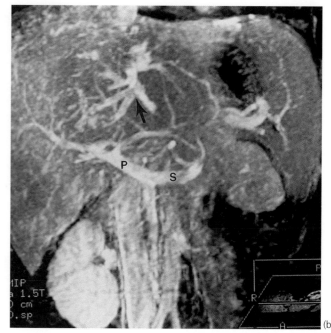

(b)

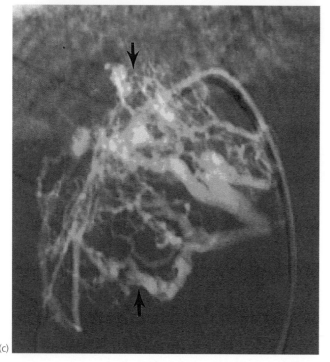

(c)

Figure 99.37 Budd–Chiari syndrome. **(a)** Computed tomographic scan of a 23-year-old woman with ascites and pulmonary embolism demonstrates an enlarged caudate lobe (C) and inhomogeneous perfusion in the periphery of the liver. A, aorta; I, inferior vena cava; S, spleen. **(b)** Three-dimensional contrast magnetic resonance angiogram demonstrates obliteration of the hepatic veins. The dilated accessory hepatic veins (arrow) drain from the caudate lobe into the inferior vena cava. The splenic (S) and portal (P) veins are patent. **(c)** Wedged hepatic venogram with injection of contrast medium through the occluded hepatic vein demonstrates typical spider web hepatic venous collateral vessels (arrows). The patient underwent orthotopic liver transplantation.

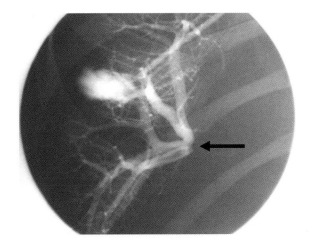

Figure 99.38 Portal vein occlusion. Wedged hepatic venogram with contrast medium shows occlusion of the portal vein (arrow) at the hilus.

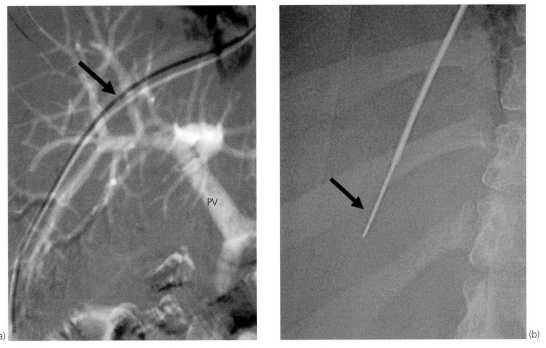

(a)

(b)

Figure 99.39 Transjugular liver biopsy. **(a)** CO_2 wedged hepatic venogram shows filling of the portal vein (PV). The right hepatic vein with the catheter in place (arrow) overlies the intrahepatic portal vein branches in the right hepatic lobe. **(b)** Digital image taken during liver biopsy shows a Quick-Core biopsy needle (arrow).

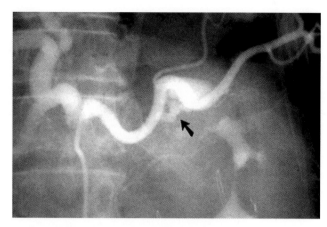

Figure 99.40 Splenic artery aneurysm bleeding into the pancreatic duct. Celiac angiogram shows an aneurysm in the mid part of the splenic artery from which contrast medium extravasates into the pancreatic duct (arrow).

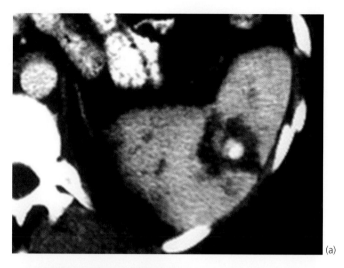

(a)

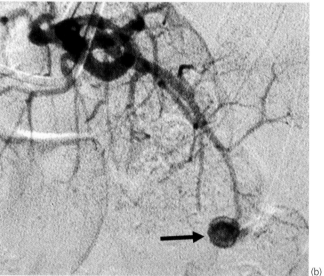

(b)

Figure 99.42 Traumatic splenic artery pseudoaneurysm. **(a)** CT taken after splenic injury shows a dense contrast collection within the spleen surrounded by a low density area. **(b)** Splenic arteriogram shows a discrete pseudoaneurysm in the lower pole of the spleen (arrow). The aneurysm was treated with transcatheter embolization.

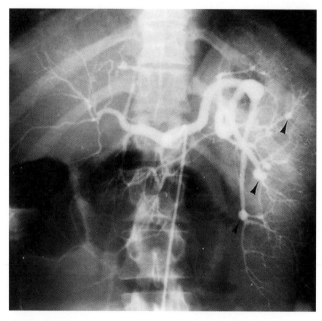

Figure 99.41 Splenic artery aneurysms associated with portal hypertension. Multiple aneurysms are present in the splenic artery branches (arrowheads). The spleen is enlarged because of portal hypertension.

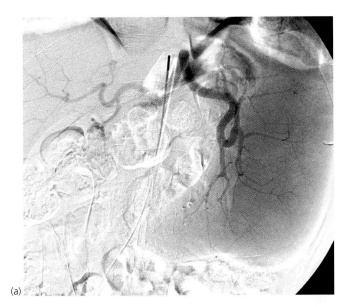

(a)

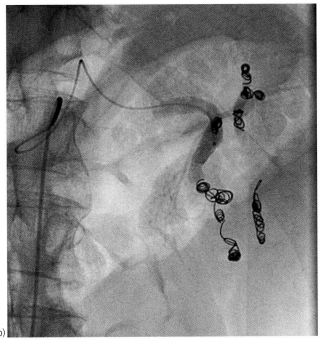

(b)

Figure 99.43 Splenic embolization prior to laparoscopic splenectomy in a 70-year-old man with chronic lymphocytic leukemia. **(a)** Splenic arteriogram shows massive splenomegaly. **(b)** After embolization of the segmental branches of the splenic artery and the distal main splenic artery with coils, an avascular segment is created in the splenic artery to facilitate laparoscopic splenectomy.

100

Interventional radiology

Kyung J. Cho

Interventional radiological techniques are used for the diagnosis and treatment of a variety of vascular and nonvascular disorders. They can be divided into vascular (infusion, occlusion, dilation) and nonvascular (biopsy, drainage, dilation, and ostomy formation) procedures. This chapter describes techniques and clinical applications of interventional radiology in the management of gastrointestinal disorders.

Vasopressin infusion

Intraarterial infusion of vasopressin is effective in controlling bleeding from hemorrhagic gastritis, Mallory–Weiss tears, and lower gastrointestinal bleeding (Figs 100.1 and 100.2). The method is less effective for bleeding caused by peptic ulcer disease. Once a bleeding site has been demonstrated, the catheter is placed in the bleeding artery. Vasopressin is infused into the left gastric artery for gastric bleeding, into the superior mesenteric artery for small bowel and right colonic bleeding, and into the inferior mesenteric artery for left colonic and rectosigmoidal bleeding. The vasopressin is mixed so that the perfusate has 0.2 pressor units per mL (100 units of vasopressin in 500 mL normal saline) or 0.4 pressor units per mL (100 units of vasopressin in 250 mL of normal saline). The infusion usually is started at the rate of 0.2 units/min. After 20 min the effectiveness of the infusion is assessed. If contrast medium still extravasates from the bleeding artery then the dosage should be increased to 0.4 units/min. The infusion should be continued for the next 12–24 h at the same rate. If the bleeding has stopped, the vasopressin dosage should be reduced to 0.1 units/min for additional 6–8 h. The most hazardous complication of vasopressin infusion is myocardial infarction. For patients with coronary artery disease, concomitant administration of nitroglycerin is required. The other potential risks include arrhythmia, bowel ischemia, and oliguria. The therapeutic role of this technique in the treatment of gastrointestinal (GI) bleeding has diminished as the more effective, relatively safe embolization method has become available.

Atlas of Gastroenterology, 4th edition. Edited by Tadataka Yamada, David H. Alpers, Anthony N. Kalloo, Neil Kaplowitz, Chung Owyang, and Don W. Powell. © 2009 Blackwell Publishing, ISBN: 978-1-4051-6909-7

Selective arterial embolization

Selective arterial embolization is effective treatment for patients with massive gastrointestinal hemorrhage and is the treatment of choice among patients with arterial bleeding if endoscopic treatment fails. The method is effective for both upper and lower gastrointestinal bleeding. It is essential to deliver the embolic agents as close to the bleeding site as possible to prevent embolization of normal tissue. The left gastric artery usually is embolized for gastric hemorrhage, the gastroduodenal artery for duodenal hemorrhage (Figs 100.3 and 100.4), mesenteric branches for small bowel (Fig. 100.5) or colonic bleeding (Fig. 100.6), and the inferior mesenteric artery for rectosigmoid bleeding. The embolic materials that have been used included Gelfoam, polyvinyl alcohol (PVA) particles, microcoil, and n-butyl cyanoacrylate.

The other uses of selective arterial embolization are control of hemobilia and obliteration of visceral artery aneurysms. Splenic artery embolization has been used as an alternative to splenectomy to treat patients with hypersplenism, splenic vein occlusion, and traumatic splenic bleeding. The risk of splenic artery embolization is formation of a splenic abscess. This complication can be avoided with occlusion of less than 80% of splenic arterial branches and use of antibiotic prophylaxis.

Variceal embolization

Percutaneous transhepatic variceal embolization is effective for bleeding from gastroesophageal varices or from varices at unusual sites. Rebleeding is common because of development of new collateral veins, which historically hampered enthusiasm for this technique. Variceal embolization is rarely used because of the availability of simpler (endoscopic) or more effective techniques, such as a transjugular intrahepatic portosystemic shunt (TIPS). Gastroesophageal varices can be embolized from the transhepatic, transjugular, or retrograde femoral vein approach (Fig. 100.7). Gelatin sponge (Gelfoam, Upjohn, Kalamazoo, MI) ethanol, and coils have been used as embolic agents. If communication between the gastroesophageal varices and the pulmonary vein is demonstrated, particulate embolic agents should not be used because of the risk of systemic arterial embolization.

Embolic therapy may be justified if bleeding persists despite endoscopic therapy and balloon tamponade, or if stabilization is required before a TIPS procedure, shunt operation, or liver transplantation.

Percutaneous translumenal angioplasty

Percutaneous translumenal angioplasty (PTA) is effective for treating patients with chronic mesenteric ischemia caused by atherosclerotic narrowing of the mesenteric vessels (Fig. 100.8). The use of PTA is justified in the treatment of patients at high surgical risk. It can be used to manage Budd–Chiari syndrome caused by occlusion or stenosis of the hepatic vein or hepatic segment of the inferior vena cava. Stents and PTA have been used in therapy for suprahepatic caval anastomotic stenosis complicating orthotopic liver transplantation (Fig. 100.9).

Insertion of TIPS is a widely accepted interventional radiological procedure for decompressing portal hypertension and for managing variceal bleeding. It has a lower mortality rate than emergency surgical shunting and is currently indicated for patients with variceal bleeding unresponsive to endoscopic therapy. The utility of TIPS as an effective bridge to treat patients with variceal bleeding while they await hepatic transplantation has been documented. It also is effective for managing intractable ascites in patients with cirrhosis and portal hypertension (Fig. 100.10). Shortening of the stent or biliary stent fistula may cause acute shunt thrombosis. Revision can be performed by means of balloon dilation, placement of metallic stents within the TIPS, or use of a mechanical thrombectomy device. The use of covered stents may be beneficial if a biliary-TIPS fistula is demonstrated. Unfortunately, development of neointimal hyperplasia leads to stenosis or occlusion of the TIPS among as many as 50% of patients within 1 year. Ultrasound surveillance is used to detect stenosis and correct the lesion to prevent occlusion. Balloon dilation or stent placement is effective management of stenosis of a TIPS (Fig. 100.11).

Percutaneous biliary drainage

Percutaneous transhepatic catheterization of the bile duct is an important interventional radiological procedure. The technique is used for biliary drainage, dilation of biliary strictures, stone extraction, and intraductal biliary biopsy. A right lateral approach is used for catheterization of the right hepatic duct (Fig. 100.12), and an anterior subxiphoid approach is used for the left hepatic duct (Fig. 100.13). To minimize risk for bleeding, a peripheral bile duct is punctured in patients who need a large catheter for drainage or stone extraction. Rarely peridochal varices associated with portal vein occlusion can compress the extrahepatic bile duct

and cause obstructive jaundice (Fig. 100.14). In patients with malignant obstruction of the extrahepatic duct, the obstruction can be effectively managed with placement of metallic stent so that the external drainage catheter can be removed (Fig. 100.15). Biliary fistulae can be caused by trauma, surgery, infection, tumors and liver transplantation. Biliary decompression by either transhepatic or endoscopic approach is required when the fistula is associated with common bile duct obstruction. Bile leak from a surgical biliary anastomosis or trauma is treated with percutaneous transhepatic biliary catheter (Fig. 100.16). The bronchobiliary fistula can be managed by embolization using the bronchial or transhepatic route (Fig. 100.17).

Percutaneous abscess drainage

Percutaneous techniques can be used to drain intraabdominal abscesses and fluid collections, including hepatic cysts, hydatid cysts, pyogenic abscess, and pancreatic pseudocysts. Successful drainage of an intraabdominal abscess (Fig. 100.18) requires accurate localization by means of computed tomography (CT) or ultrasound scanning. Follow-up sinograms document shrinkage of the abscess cavity and exclude an underlying fistula.

Percutaneous gastrostomy and gastrojejunostomy

Percutaneous gastrostomy is a safe and effective method for enteral feeding and decompression of intestinal obstruction. It is a simple technique used for nutritional support of patients unable to maintain oral intake because of neurological disorders or esophageal obstruction. Before puncture of the gastric lumen, a sufficient amount of air should be insufflated into the stomach to achieve gastric distention. This brings the anterior wall of the stomach to the abdominal wall and pushes the small bowel and colon away from the puncture site. Inserting suture anchors into the gastric lumen facilitates placement of a gastric tube (Fig. 100.19). The gastric tube is inserted between the two anchor sutures or adjacent to a single anchor, and the distal self-retaining loop is string-fixed to prevent dislodgment (Fig. 100.20). After the tube is drained for 24 h, feeding may be started. Among patients with gastroesophageal reflux or pyloric or duodenal obstruction, or gastric paresis, a gastrojejunostomy tube is placed with the tip beyond the ligament of Treitz. When percutaneous gastrostomy is not possible because of previous gastric operations, direct percutaneous jejunostomy can be performed for enteral feeding (Fig. 100.21). Percutaneous cecostomy is effective for colonic obstruction in the care of patients who are at poor surgical risk for surgical colostomy or resection of the underlying lesion.

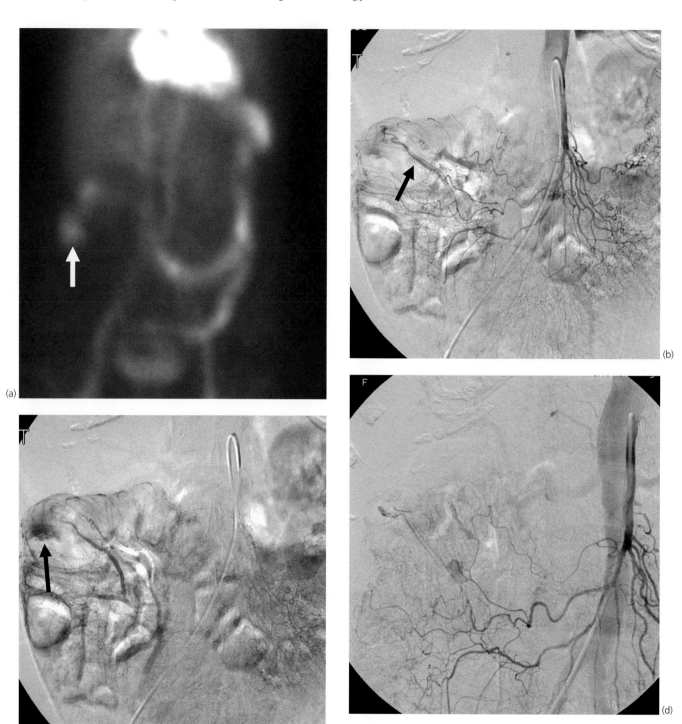

Figure 100.1 Vascular ectasia of the right colon. Superior mesenteric angiogram in a 73-year-old woman with recurrent lower GI hemorrhage. She was on Coumadin therapy following aortic valve replacement for aortic stenosis. **(a)** GI bleeding study with autologous red blood cell labeled with ^{99m}Tc pertechnetate. Radioactive tracer extravasates at the hepatic flexure of the right colon (arrow), which is transported to the transverse and descending colon. **(b)** Arterial phase of superior mesenteric angiogram. A vascular cluster is seen in the hepatic flexure of the colon. Early draining vein (arrow) is opacified. Contrast medium is beginning to extravasate. **(c)** Parenchymal phase. The dilated draining vein is densely opacified. The collection of extravasated contrast medium is clearly seen (arrow). **(d)** After intraarterial infusion of vasopressin the bleeding has stopped. The vascular ectasia is still seen but the draining vein is small owing to mesenteric vasoconstriction from the vasopressin infusion. One week later, right hemicolectomy was performed.

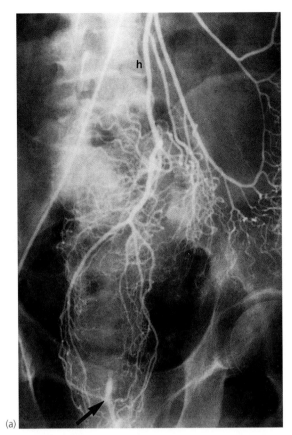

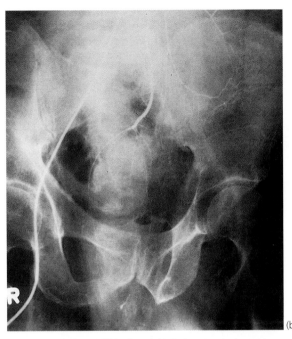

Figure 100.2 Vasopressin infusion into the inferior mesenteric artery in a patient with rectosigmoid bleeding. **(a)** Inferior mesenteric arteriogram shows extravasation (arrow) of contrast medium in the rectum. The bleeding artery is a branch of the superior hemorrhoidal artery (H). **(b)** Arteriogram 20 min after intraarterial infusion of vasopressin at 0.2 units/min. Most of the inferior mesenteric arterial branches reveal severe constriction. The bleeding has stopped.

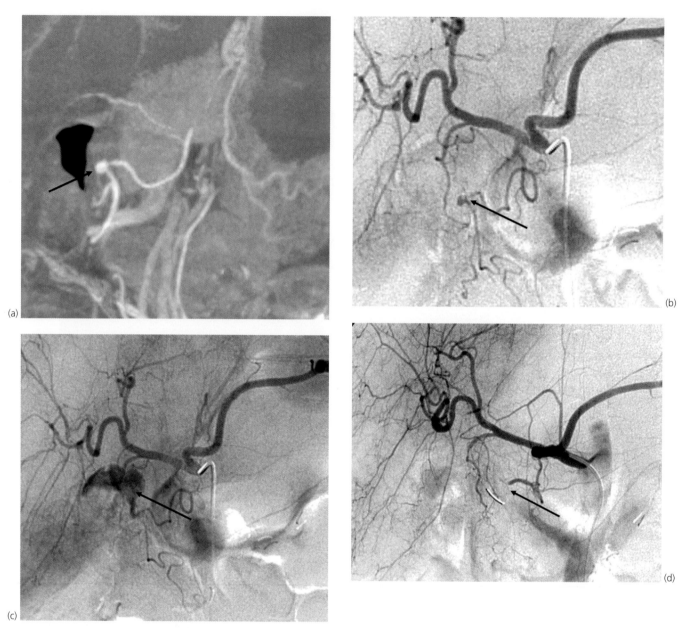

Figure 100.3 Bleeding from a duodenal ulcer. Celiac angiogram and CT arteriogram in a 52-year-old woman with massive upper GI hemorrhage. Her blood pressure was 60/40 mmHg and hemoglobin was 4.9 gm/dL when presented to the emergency room. She was resuscitated and transfused with 2 units of red blood cells. Endoscopy revealed a large duodenal bulb ulcer. **(a)** CT angiogram. A small aneurysm (arrow) is seen from the pancreatic arcade. **(b)** Celiac angiogram. The aneurysm arises from the anastomotic branch of the dorsal pancreatic artery that originates from the common hepatic artery. **(c)** Late phase of the celiac angiogram. Contrast medium (arrow) begins to extravasate from the aneurysm during the angiogram. **(d)** The bleeding artery was superselectively catheterized and embolized with microcoil (arrow). The bleeding has stopped.

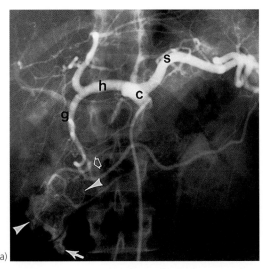

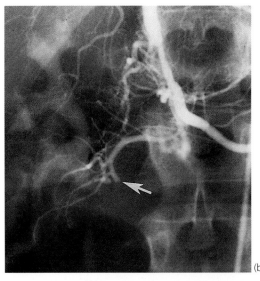

Figure 100.4 Control of bleeding from a duodenal leiomyoma with gelatin sponge (Gelfoam, Upjohn, Kalamazoo, MI) embolization in a 26-year-old woman. **(a)** Celiac arteriogram shows a vascular mass (arrowheads) in the second portion of the duodenum. The tumor receives its blood supply from the anterior superior pancreaticoduodenal branch (open arrow) of the gastroduodenal artery (g). Contrast extravasation from the tumor is indicated (arrow). The right hepatic artery arises from the superior mesenteric artery. c, celiac axis; s, splenic artery; h, hepatic artery. **(b)** Arteriogram after embolization with gelatin sponge pieces shows occlusion of the bleeding artery (arrow). The bleeding has stopped after embolization. One month later, the patient underwent surgical removal of a leiomyoma of the duodenum.

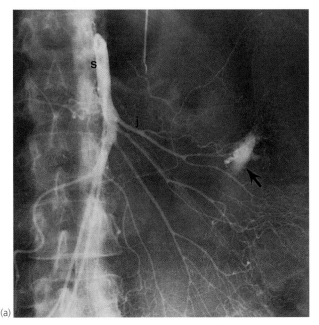

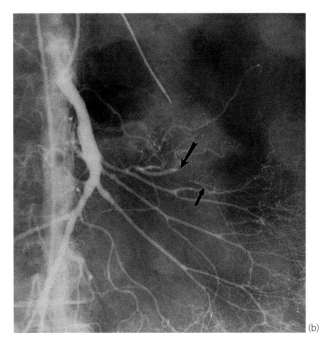

Figure 100.5 Jejunal bleeding controlled with Gelfoam (Upjohn, Kalamazoo, MI) embolization. **(a)** Superior mesenteric (s) arteriogram shows contrast extravasation (arrow) in the proximal jejunum. The bleeding artery is a proximal jejunal artery (j). **(b)** Arteriogram after embolization shows bleeding has stopped. Occlusion of the jejunal branches is indicated (arrows).

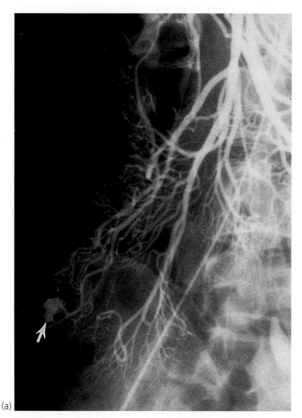

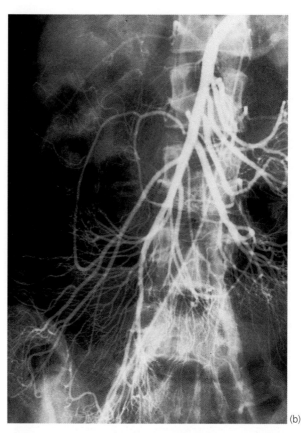

Figure 100.6 Embolic control of colonic bleeding in a 21-year-old woman with bright red blood per rectum. Flexible sigmoidoscopic examination showed blood in the colon. Technetium 99m–tagged red blood cell scan localized the bleeding to the right colon. After resuscitation, the patient underwent angiography and embolization. **(a)** Superior mesenteric arteriogram shows a collection of contrast medium (arrow) in the right colon. The bleeding artery was selectively catheterized with a 3F coaxial catheter system. Polyvinyl alcohol sponge particles (250–350 μm) were injected close to the bleeding site. **(b)** Arteriogram after embolization showed no contrast extravasation. The bleeding stopped. The patient underwent right hemicolectomy to prevent recurrent bleeding.

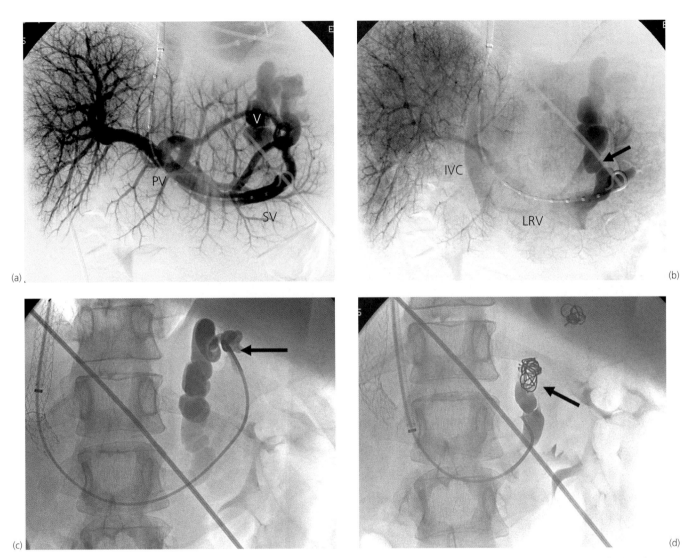

(a)

(b)

(c)

(d)

Figure 100.7 Embolization of gastric varices. TIPS placement and variceal embolization in a 58-year-old woman with alcoholic cirrhosis and portal hypertension, and recurrent variceal bleeding despite multiple banding procedures. **(a)** Transjugular splenoportogram. Large gastric varices (V) fill through the left gastric and short gastric veins from the splenic vein (SV). The portal vein (PV) is patent and its blood flow is hepatopetal. **(b)** Late phase of the splenic vein injection. The gastric varices drain through the left inferior phrenic (arrow) and left adrenal vein into the left renal vein (LRV) and inferior vena cava (IVC). **(c)** Occlusion of the short gastric vein. The short gastric vein (arrow) is catheterized through the TIPS stent and embolized with a large coil (Nester coil, Cook Inc.). **(d)** Occlusion of the inferior phrenic vein. The dilated inferior phrenic vein draining the gastric varices was embolized with a large Nester coil (arrow) close to the gastric varices.

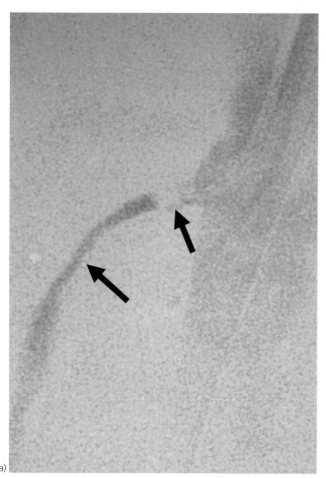

(a)

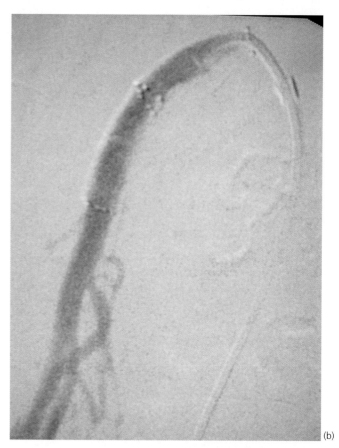

(b)

Figure 100.8 Superior mesenteric artery stenosis in a 69-year-old woman with abdominal angina. A CT scan demonstrated a heavily calcified aorta with high-grade stenosis of the celiac and superior mesenteric arteries. **(a)** Superior mesenteric arteriogram. The superior mesenteric artery stenosis was crossed using a 3F microcatheter to avoid dissection. Two stenoses (arrows) are present in the superior mesenteric artery. The lesions were predilated with a 4-mm angioplasty balloon to facilitate stent placement and 8-mm stents were deployed and dilated to 7-mm angioplasty balloon catheter. **(b)** After stent placement, her postprandial pain resolved.

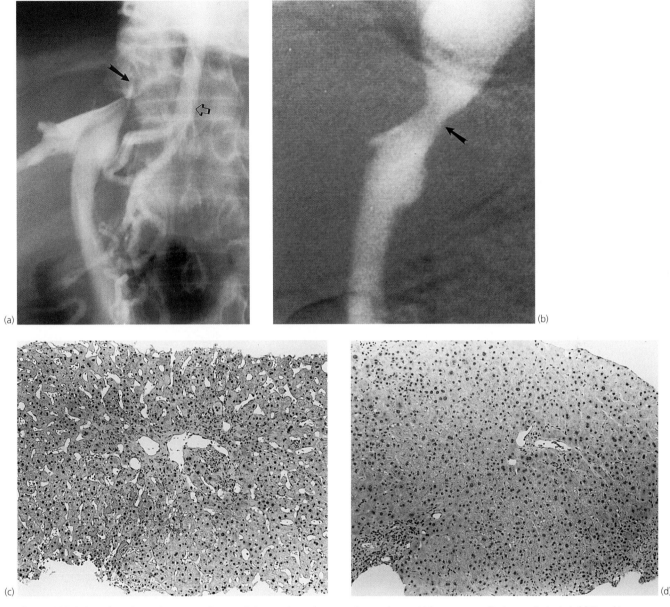

Figure 100.9 Suprahepatic caval anastomotic stenosis in a patient who, 6 months earlier, had undergone hepatic transplantation. **(a)** Inferior vena cavogram shows suprahepatic caval anastomosis (black arrow) is nearly occluded and collateral blood flows through the azygos vein (open arrow). **(b)** Digital subtraction venacavogram after angioplasty with 15-mm-diameter balloon catheter demonstrates substantial decrease in stenosis (arrow). The azygos venous collateral vessel disappeared and the abnormal cavoatrial pressure gradient was eliminated. **(c)** Liver biopsy specimen before angioplasty shows chronic congestive changes and profound sinusoidal dilation consistent with high-grade venous outflow obstruction (H & E stain; original magnification ×100). **(d)** Liver biopsy 2 months after angioplasty shows sinusoidal dilation has resolved (H & E stain; original magnification ×100).

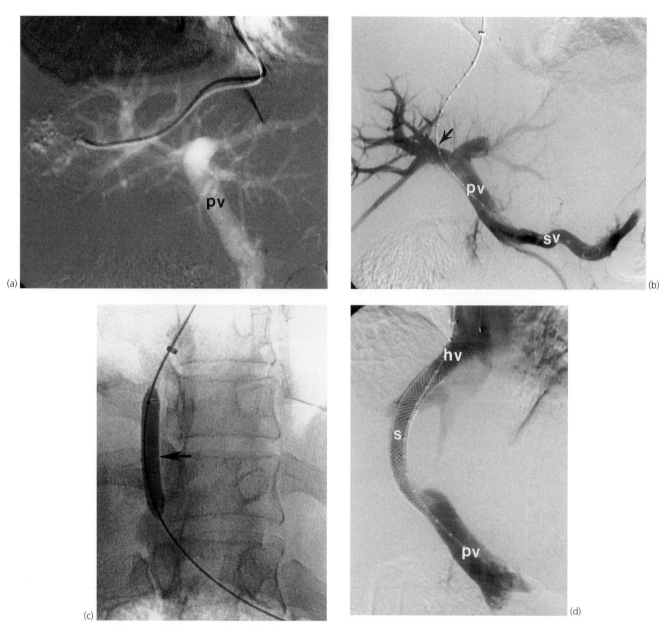

Figure 100.10 Transjugular intrahepatic portosystemic shunt (TIPS) placement in a patient with end-stage liver disease secondary to alcohol abuse, complicated by refractory ascites. **(a)** CO_2 wedge hepatic venogram from a right jugular approach shows patent portal vein (pv). **(b)** After successful puncture of the right main portal vein (arrow) using a Colapinto needle (Cook, Bloomington, Indiana), splenoportography was performed, which demonstrates patent splenic (sv) and portal vein (pv). The flow in the intrahepatic portal vein is hepatopetal. **(c)** The liver parenchymal tract is dilated with an angioplasty balloon (arrow). **(d)** After placement of a 10 mm-diameter Wallstent in the parenchymal tract, extending from the portal vein (pv) to the hepatic vein (hv), portogram demonstrates patent shunt (s) and reversal in the intrahepatic portal flow. Pressure gradient (portal pressure minus right atrial pressure) decreased from 20 mmHg (pre-TIPS) to 10 mmHg (post-TIPS). The patient's ascites has resolved but he developed mild encephalopathy.

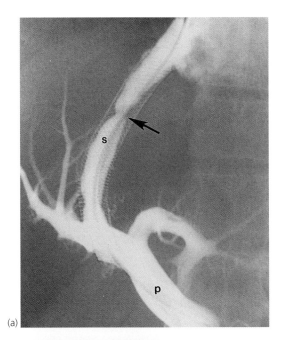

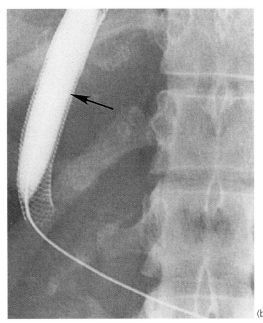

(a)

(b)

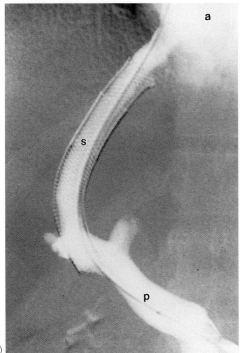

(c)

Figure 100.11 Stenosis of a transjugular intrahepatic portosystemic shunt (TIPS) in a 39-year-old woman who, 11 months earlier, had undergone a TIPS procedure for Budd–Chiari syndrome. Transjugular liver biopsy revealed chronic congestive changes and central hemorrhagic necrosis. **(a)** Transjugular catheterization of the shunt. The catheter has been passed through the shunt into the portal vein. Contrast medium fills the portal vein (p) and shunt (s). Moderate stenosis (arrow) is visible in the shunt consistent with neointimal hyperplasia. **(b)** The stenosis was dilated with a 10-mm-diameter balloon catheter (arrow) and stent placement. **(c)** Portal venogram after revision. The shunt (s) is widely patent. Portal blood (p) flows toward the shunt into the right atrium (a). The portosystemic gradient decreased from 15 to 6 mmHg. The patient's symptoms improved, and her liver function remained stable with patency of the shunt for 18 months.

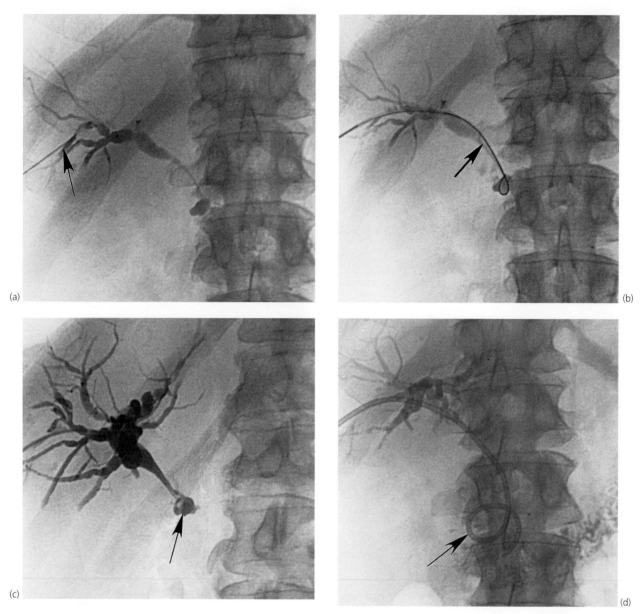

(a)

(b)

(c)

(d)

Figure 100.12 Percutaneous transhepatic biliary drainage in a patient with distal common bile duct obstruction caused by pancreatic cancer. **(a)** Peripheral bile duct branch is punctured with a 22-gauge needle (arrow). **(b)** The 0.018-inch diameter guidewire (arrow) is introduced through the needle. **(c)** After decompression of the bile duct with an introducer catheter, a 5F catheter was introduced into the bile duct. Contrast medium shows obstruction (arrow). **(d)** After the obstruction had been crossed, an 8.5F Cope loop catheter (arrow) (Cook Inc., Bloomington, IN) was introduced into the duodenum for external and internal drainage.

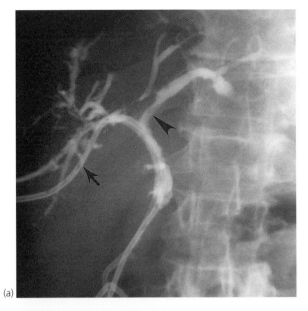

(a)

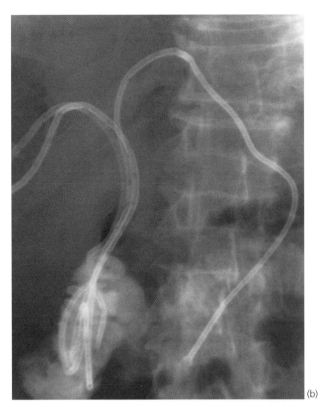

(b)

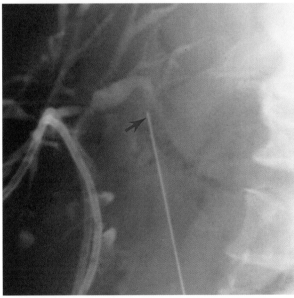

(c)

Figure 100.13 Percutaneous transhepatic drainage of left hepatic duct in a 53-year-old man who, 5 years earlier, had undergone orthotopic liver transplantation because of cryptogenic cirrhosis. The patient had recurrent cholangitis and multiple intrahepatic biliary strictures. **(a)** Two percutaneous transhepatic biliary catheters (arrow) have been placed for right hepatic biliary strictures. Moderate stricture is present in the left hepatic duct (arrowhead). **(c)** Opacification of the left hepatic duct with injection of contrast medium and air into the right biliary catheter in left anterior oblique view. A 22-gauge needle is placed into the left hepatic duct filled with air (arrow) under fluoroscopic guidance. **(b)** After a guidewire was advanced through the needle, the tract was dilated. An 8.5F Cope loop catheter was placed with its distal loop in the duodenum.

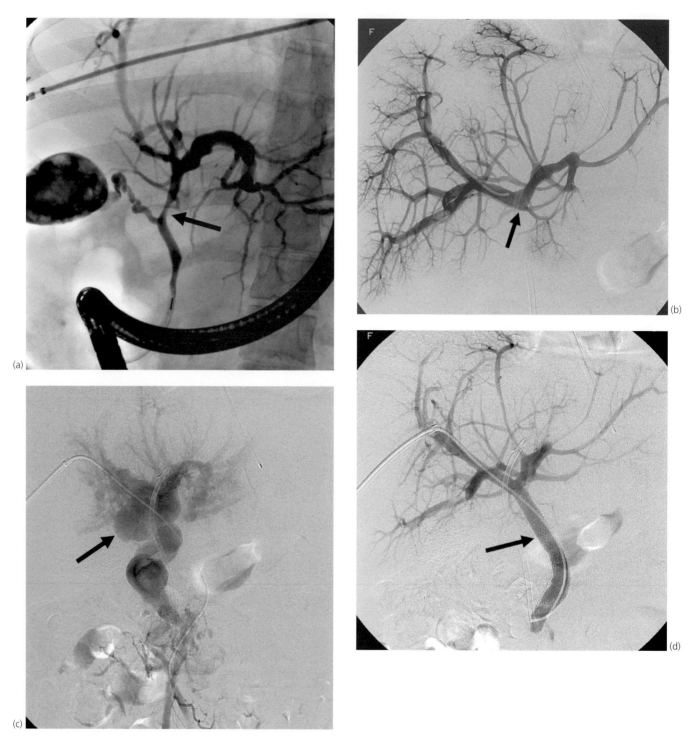

Figure 100.14 Extrahepatic biliary obstruction caused by choledochal varices. A 25-year-old man with Klippel–Trenaunay–Weber syndrome presents with jaundice (bilirubin 14.2 mg/dL). **(a)** Endoscopic retrograde cholangiopancreatography (ERCP) shows smooth compression of the bile duct (arrow). **(b)** Transhepatic portogram shows occlusion of the portal vein at the portal hepatis (arrow). **(c)** After crossing the occlusion, contrast-medium injection into the superior mesenteric vein shows markedly dilated collaterals (cavernomatous transformation) (arrow), which compress the bile duct. **(d)** After placement of a 12-mm diameter, self-expanding nitinol stent within the occluded portal vein, the portal vein is patent without filling collaterals. Three months later, his bilirubin was 1 mg/dL.

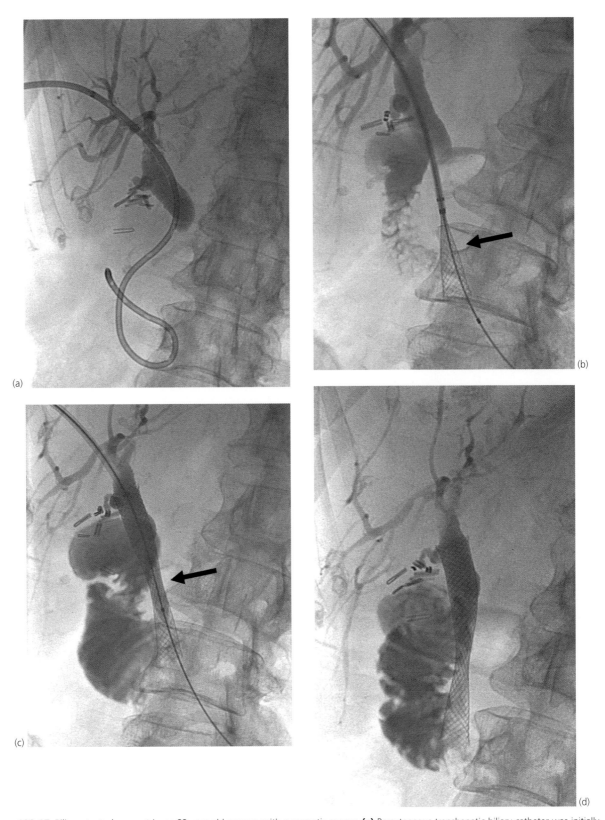

Figure 100.15 Biliary stent placement in an 82-year-old woman with pancreatic cancer. **(a)** Percutaneous transhepatic biliary catheter was initially placed to decompress biliary obstruction. **(b)** 10 mm diameter Wallstent is deployed from the duodenum (arrow). **(c)** After stent placement, the stent is dilated to 6 mm (arrow). **(d)** The external biliary catheter has been removed.

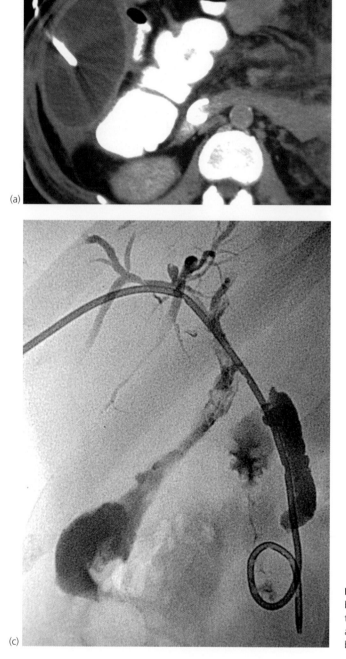

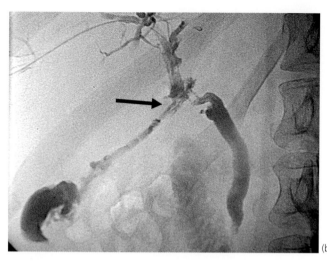

Figure 100.16 Bile leak in liver transplant. **(a)** CT scan shows subhepatic biloma, which has been drained percutaneously. **(b)** Percutaneous transhepatic cholangiogram. Bile leak is seen from the bile duct anastomosis (arrow). **(c)** Percutaneous transhepatic biliary drainage. An 8F biliary-drainage catheter is placed. One month later, no bile leak was seen.

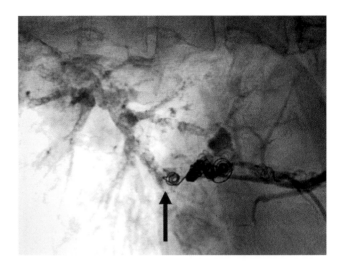

Figure 100.17 Bronchobiliary fistula. The fistula developed after a left hepatic lobectomy for bile duct carcinoma in a 44-year-old woman. The fistula was treated with transhepatic coil embolization.

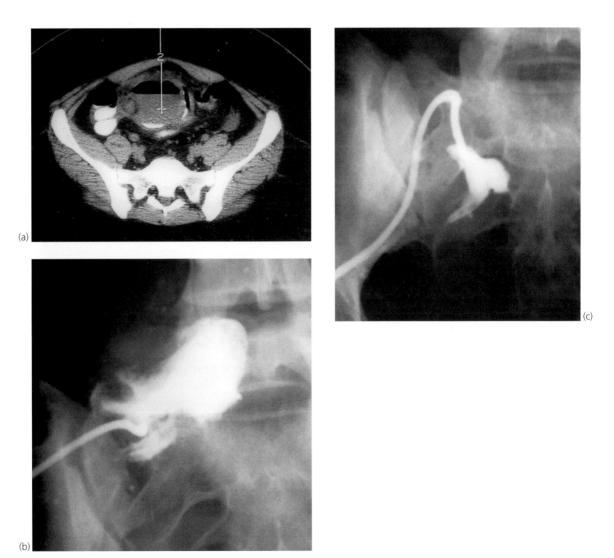

(a)

(b)

(c)

Figure 100.18 Successful percutaneous drainage of an intraabdominal abscess in a 24-year-old woman. With computed tomographic guidance **(a)**, a needle and then a catheter over a guidewire **(b)** were inserted into the fluid collection. **(c)** Follow-up contrast sinogram shows the cavity is smaller and there is no fistula. The abscess was successfully drained, and the catheter was removed after 10 days.

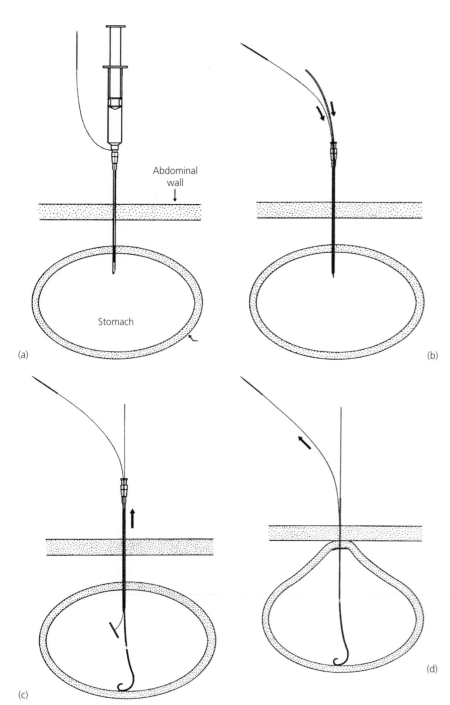

(a)

Abdominal
wall

Stomach

(b)

(c)

(d)

Figure 100.19 Suture anchor technique for percutaneous gastrostomy. **(a)** The stomach (arrow) is insufflated with air through a nasogastric tube. The introducer needle preloaded with the gastrointestinal suture anchor is thrust into the stomach under fluoroscopic guidance. **(b)** The guidewire is introduced through the needle, and the suture anchor is pushed into the gastric lumen. **(c)** The needle is removed while the wire is left in the stomach. **(d)** While the guidewire is in position, traction is applied to the suture to pull the anterior wall of the stomach against the abdominal wall. The guidewire is used to introduce a gastrostomy catheter. The suture may be left in place for 2 weeks, or it may be cut after placement of a gastrostomy tube.

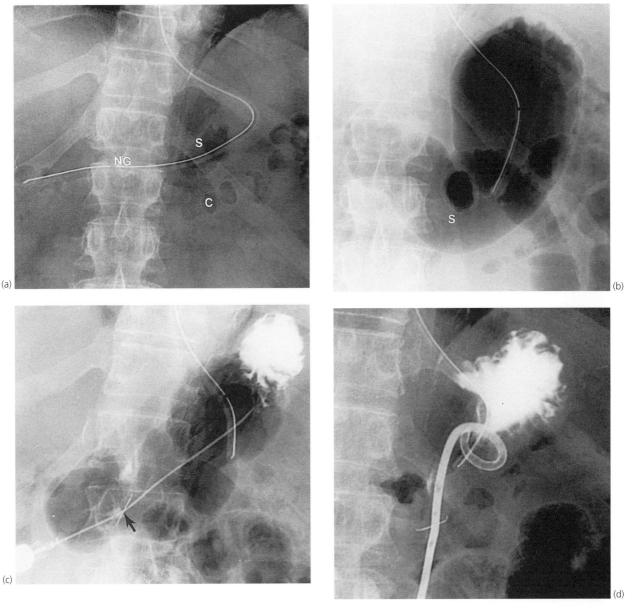

Figure 100.20 Percutaneous gastrostomy in a patient who is unable to swallow. **(a)** Plain abdominal radiograph shows nasogastric tube (NG) has been placed in the stomach. The stomach (S) is not distended, and the transverse colon (C) is near the stomach. **(b)** Air has been insufflated into the stomach (S) after intravenous administration of 1 mg of glucagon.

(c) After placement of a suture anchor (arrow) into the stomach, a 5F dilator was introduced into the stomach. Injection of contrast medium confirmed catheter position in the fundus of the stomach. **(d)** After dilation of the tract, a 12F Cope loop gastrostomy tube (Cook Inc., Bloomington, IN) was placed.

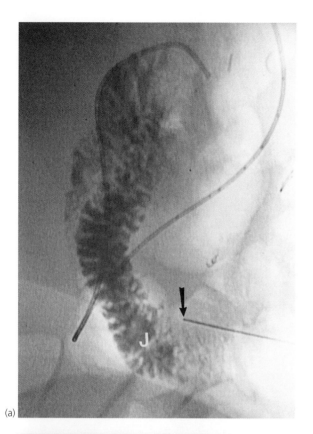

(a)

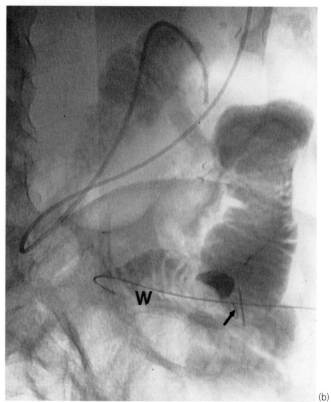

(b)

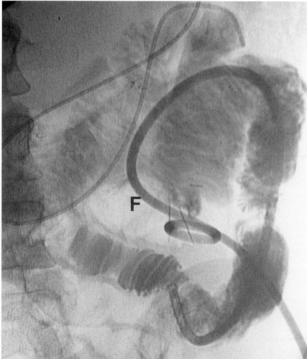

(c)

Figure 100.21 Percutaneous jejunostomy in a patient who is unable to swallow after esophagectomy and gastric pull-through for esophageal cancer. **(a)** After intravenous administration of 1 mg of glucagon, proximal jejunum (J) has been visualized with contrast medium. An 18-gauge needle (arrow) was then inserted into the jejunum under fluoroscopic guidance. **(b)** After placement of two suture anchors (arrow) to fix the wall of the jejunum to the abdominal wall, a wire (W) was introduced into the jejunum. **(c)** After dilation of the tract, a 12F loop jejunostomy tube (F) was placed.

C PATHOLOGY

101

Endoscopic mucosal biopsy: histopathological interpretation

Elizabeth Montgomery, Anthony N. Kalloo

The key principle of biopsy interpretation of the gastrointestinal tract is that it has a limited repertoire of responses to a host of injuries, and diagnosing the type of injury in any given biopsy often requires correlation with clinical details. When dealing with mucosal biopsies of the gastrointestinal (GI) tract, it should also be noted that they only display the mucosa (and possibly a small amount of submucosa), a feature that is obvious but sometimes forgotten by endoscopists and pathologists alike. Correlating endoscopic imaging with histopathological findings may be critical in establishing correct clinical diagnosis. This chapter matches pathology with endoscopy for many common and uncommon gastrointestinal conditions.

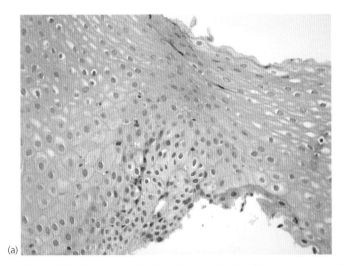

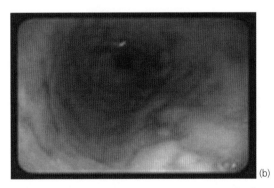

(a)

(b)

Figure 101.1 (a) Reflux esophagitis. **(b)** Reflux esophagitis with erosions. Savary–Miller Grade III (circumferential lesion, erosive or exudative) reflux-type esophagitis and multiple erosions in the lower third of the esophagus can be seen in this image.

Atlas of Gastroenterology, 4th edition. Edited by Tadataka Yamada, David H. Alpers, Anthony N. Kalloo, Neil Kaplowitz, Chung Owyang, and Don W. Powell. © 2009 Blackwell Publishing, ISBN: 978-1-4051-6909-7

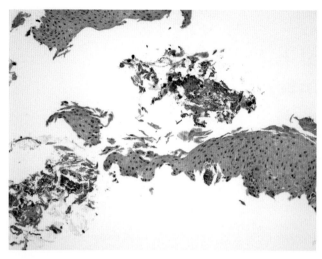

Figure 101.2 Iron pill esophagitis. The brown material in the image is iron pigment. The associated squamous epithelium shows reparative features.

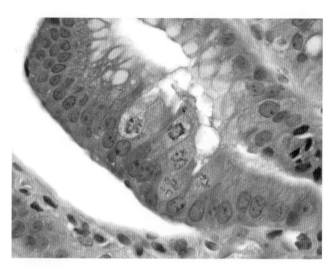

Figure 101.4 Taxol effect. This process involves metaplastic columnar mucosa in the esophagus. The ring mitoses are an indication of mitotic arrest.

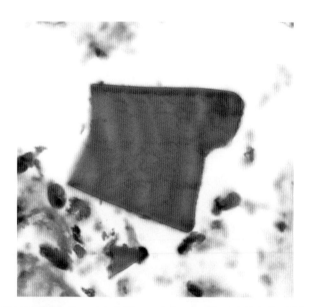

Figure 101.3 Kayexalate (sodium polystyrene sulfonate). Note the "fish scale"-like appearance of the crystalline material.

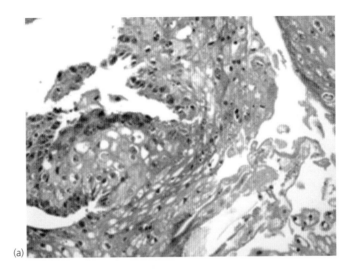

(a)

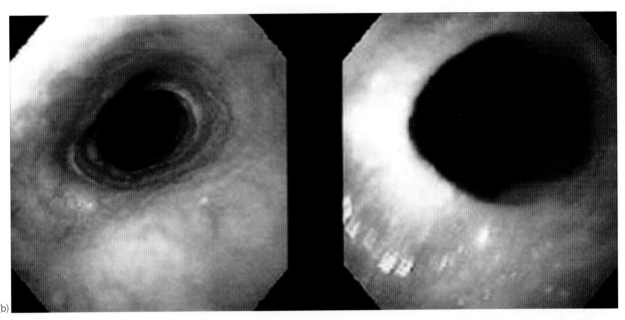

(b)

Figure 101.5 **(a)** Graft-versus-host disease (GVHD). There is extensive squamous epithelial apoptosis such that the nuclei resemble specks of dust. **(b)** GVHD of the esophagus with multiple fine mucosal webs present.

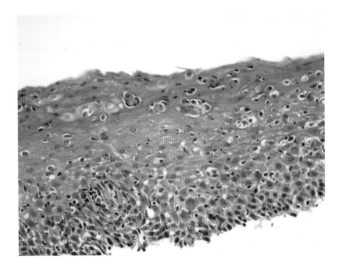

Figure 101.6 Lichen planus involving the esophagus. This field shows prominent intraepithelial lymphocytosis and necrotic squamous cells.

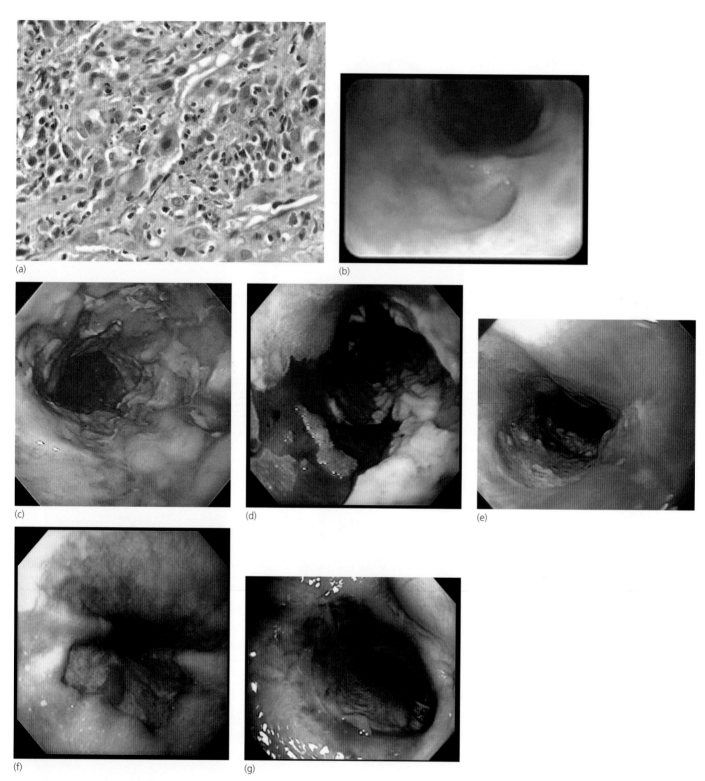

Figure 101.7 (a) Cytomegalovirus (CMV) esophagitis. An endothelial cell in the center of the field is affected. There is a large intranuclear inclusion. **(b)** Cytomegalovirus esophageal ulcer. Upper endoscopy in a patient with acquired immune deficiency syndrome (AIDS) and dysphagia revealed a distal esophageal ulceration. An immunohistochemical stain for CMV was positive. **(c)** Diffuse ulceration with a serpiginous appearance with overlying candidal debris. This patient with AIDS has CMV esophagitis and *Candida* coinfection. **(d)** Diffuse candidal plaque has been removed with the endoscope revealing a shallow serpiginous ulceration, which on biopsy confirmed CMV. **(e)** Large, deep ulceration in the proximal esophagus owing to CMV in a patient with AIDS. **(f)** Solitary, deep, well-circumscribed ulcer at the gastroesophageal junction caused by CMV. **(g)** Circumferential ulceration in the midesophagus as a result of CMV.

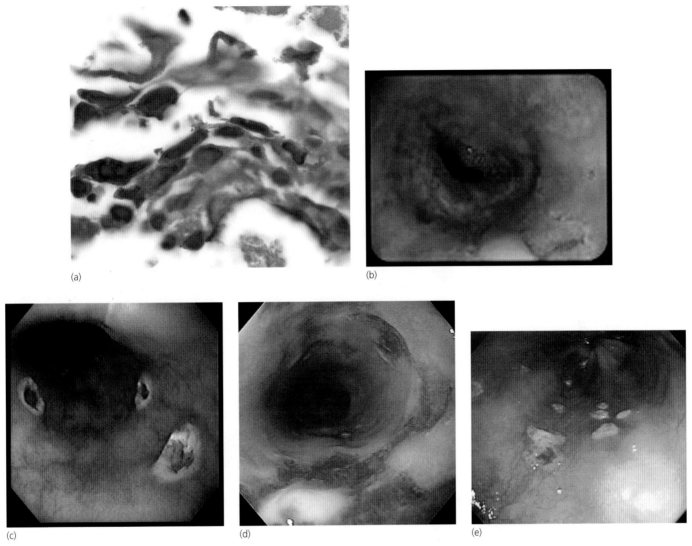

(a)

(b)

(c)

(d)

(e)

Figure 101.8 (a) Herpes simplex virus (HSV) esophagitis. The infected cells are multinucleated with "smudged" nuclei. **(b)** Herpetic esophageal ulcer. The earliest manifestation of herpes simplex esophagitis may be vesicular, though this is rarely seen. The herpetic lesions may coalesce. On endoscopy, a well-circumscribed, volcano-like appearance has been described. In this case, HSV-1 was cultured from esophageal biopsies. **(c)** Small volcano-like ulcers due to HSV. **(d)** Multiple well-circumscribed, shallow esophageal ulcers due to HSV esophagitis. **(e)** Small well-circumscribed areas of exudate resembling *Candida*. This is a classic appearance of mild HSV esophagitis. This patient had eutropenia.

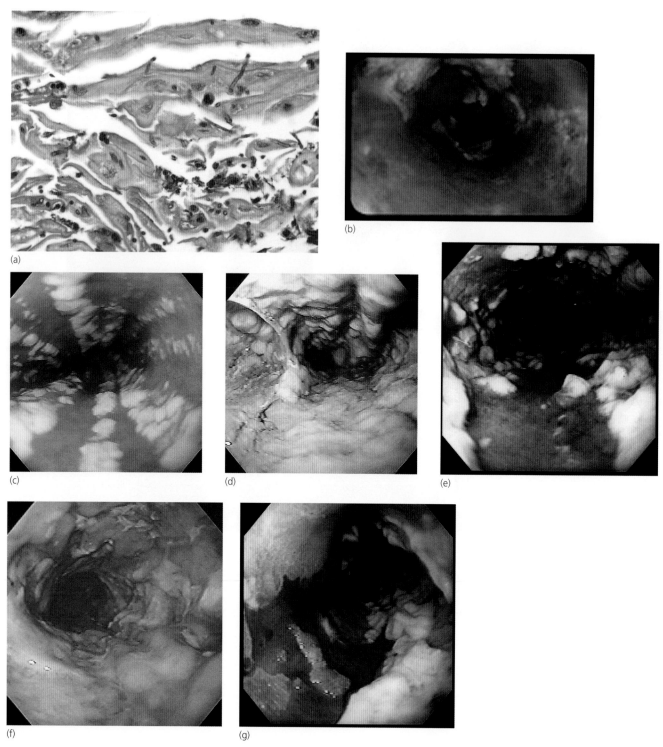

Figure 101.9 (a) *Candida* esophagitis. This periodic acid–Schiff (PAS) stain highlights pseudohyphal forms. **(b)** Candidal esophagitis. Inflammation with thick white adherent plaques in a patient with AIDS and candidal esophagitis. Fluconazole-sensitive *Candida albicans* was cultured from the esophageal brushing. **(c)** Multiple raised white plaques involving the esophagus with normal intervening mucosa. This would be classified as Grade II *Candida* esophagitis. **(d)** Exuberant yellow plaque material encroaching on the esophageal lumen typical for severe *Candida* esophagitis (Grade IV). **(e)** The plaque material has been removed with the endoscope revealing relatively normal underlying mucosa without ulceration. **(f)** Diffuse ulceration with a serpiginous appearance with overlying candidal debris. This AIDS patient has CMV esophagitis and *Candida* coinfection. **(g)** Diffuse candidal plaque has been removed with the endoscope revealing a shallow serpiginous ulceration, which on biopsy confirmed CMV.

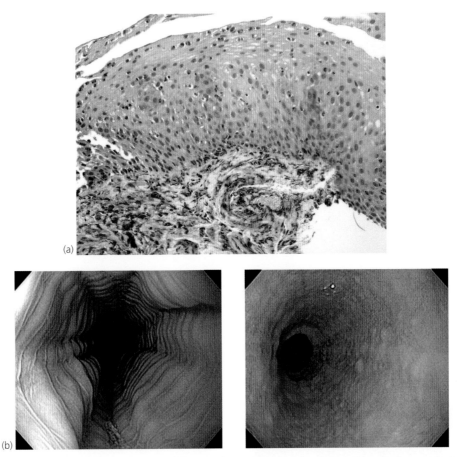

Figure 101.10 Eosinophilic esophagitis. **(a)** Numerous eosinophils, some degranulating, are seen in both the epithelium and the lamina propria. Far fewer eosinophils are seen in reflux esophagitis. Compare this image to Figure 101.1. **(b)** Feline esophagus demonstrating rippling or plications of the esophageal mucosa. This is a transient occurrence and disappears with continued observation, as shown in the right panel. Eosinophilic esophagitis can present with a similar appearance but the rings persist with air insufflation and are less tightly spaced apart (right panel).

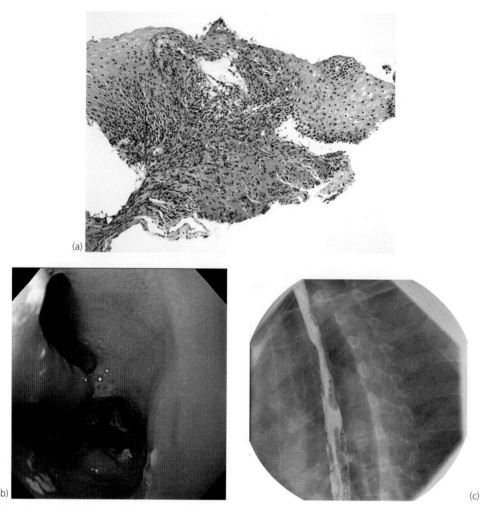

Figure 101.11 Crohn's disease. **(a)** Crohn's disease involving the esophagus. There is a prominent lymphoplasmacytic infiltrate. A granuloma is seen in the lower center portion of the field. **(b)** An endoscopic view of Crohn's disease of the esophagus with diffuse esophageal narrowing, a prominent sinus tract, and exudative plaques. **(c)** A barium swallow from the same patient shows esophageal narrowing, mucosal irregularity, ulceration, and nodularity, as well as sinus tracts parallel to the esophagus. (*Continued on next page.*)

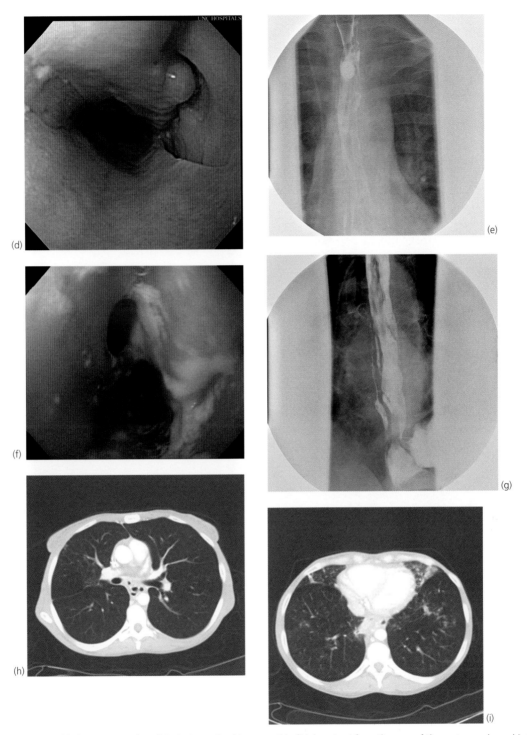

Figure 101.11 *Continued* **(d–i)** More examples of Crohn's esophagitis. Esophageal narrowing and deep sinus tracts again noted **(d)**, and on barium swallow, the barium tablet becomes lodged in the proximal esophagus **(e)**. Several fistulae with white exudate and possible *Candida* are seen opening from the esophagus **(f)**; barium swallow confirms a thin fistulous tract from the area of the gastroesophageal junction (GEJ) extending caudally to the right mainstem bronchus **(g)**. On CT scan, a thickened esophagus with multiple sinus tracts is readily apparent **(h)**, and just above the GEJ a fistulous tract is seen entering the lung **(i)**.

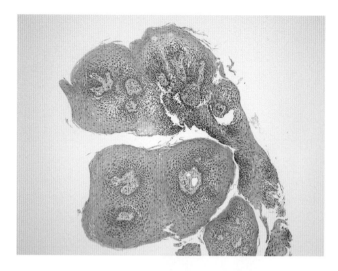

Figure 101.12 Squamous papilloma of the esophagus. Squamous mucosa coats fibrovascular cores.

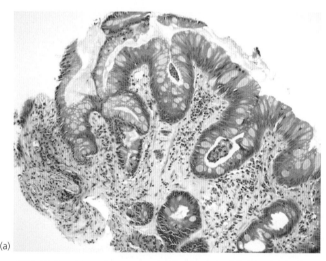

(a)

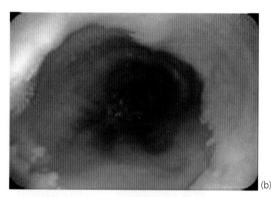

(b)

Figure 101.13 Barrett esophagus, negative for dysplasia. **(a)** Note the goblet cells. There is surface maturation of the metaplastic cells and abundant lamina propria. **(b)** This image demonstrates the characteristic salmon pink mucosa of Barrett esophagus extending proximally from the gastroesophageal junction. The normal esophageal squamous mucosa is pearly white and can be seen here in the proximal portion of the esophagus.

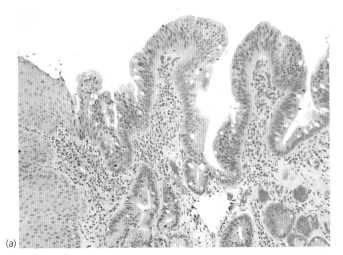

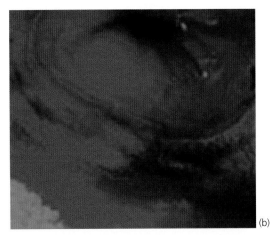

Figure 101.14 Low-grade dysplasia in Barrett esophagus. **(a)** The epithelial changes are seen both in deep glands and on the surface but the nuclei are aligned perpendicularly to the basement membrane (maintained nuclear polarity). **(b)** Chromoendoscopy. This involves staining the gastrointestinal mucosa for better endoscopic visualization, usually for the detection of malignant or premalignant lesions. In this image, Lugol solution has been used to stain the distal esophagus. Negative staining of nodular mucosa can be seen, and biopsy confirmed Barrett esophagus with mild dysplasia. Courtesy of Dr Moises Guelrud.

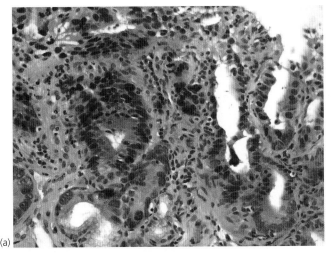

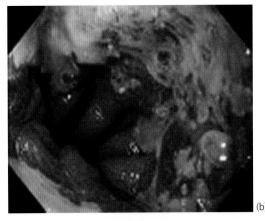

Figure 101.15 High-grade dysplasia and intramucosal carcinoma in Barrett esophagus. **(a)** Hyperchromatic nuclei have lost their polarity (relation to the basement membrane). **(b)** Narrow band imaging (NBI), Barrett esophagus with high-grade dysplasia. NBI is a high-resolution endoscopic technique that may enhance the visualization of the fine vasculature and mucosal morphology. In this patient with Barrett esophagus, high-grade dysplasia, and squamous overgrowth, NBI demonstrates dysmorphic glands and vasculature. Courtesy of Drs Herbert C. Wolfsen and Michael B. Wallace.

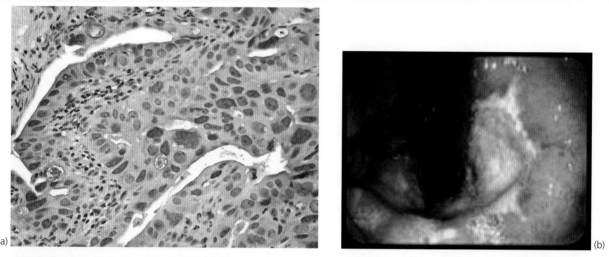

Figure 101.16 Esophageal adenocarcinoma. (a) In this field, the adenocarcinoma undermines adjoining squamous mucosa. (b) Endoscopic appearance of an ulcerated gastroesophageal junction mass, which revealed poorly differentiated esophageal adenocarcinoma on biopsy. In this image, the mass can be seen extending from the gastroesophageal junction in a retroflexed view.

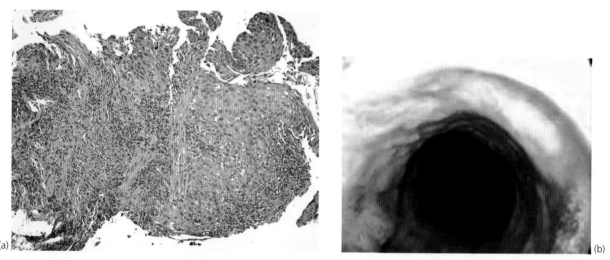

Figure 101.17 Esophageal squamous cell carcinoma. (a) There is a squamous pearl towards the right of the field. In this biopsy, the lesion has invaded the muscularis mucosae, seen as slender pink strips. (b) In the mid esophagus, an irregular nodular plaque was observed in a patient with a history of alcohol and tobacco use. Biopsies revealed moderately differentiated squamous cell cancer of the esophagus.

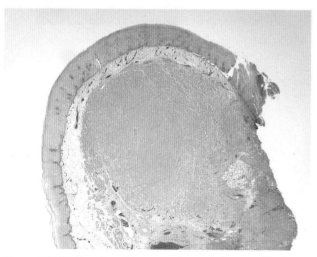

Figure 101.18 Granular cell tumor esophagus. At low magnification, a well-marginated nodule is seen in the lamina propria.

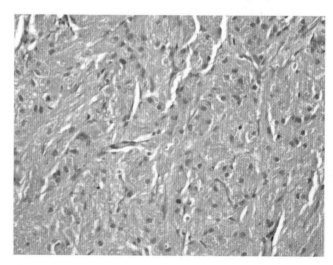

Figure 101.19 Granular cell tumor esophagus. Note the granular appearance of the eosinophilic proliferating cells.

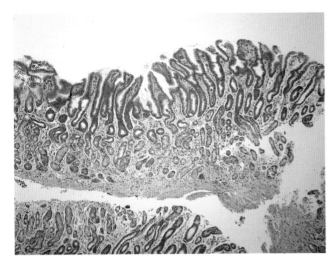

Figure 101.20 Chemical gastritis/reactive gastropathy. The antral mucosa has a villiform appearance and there is mucin loss in the epithelium. There is very little inflammation.

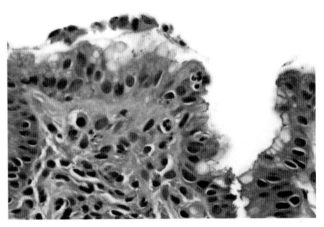

Figure 101.22 Active chronic *Helicobacter pylori* gastritis. At high magnification, neutrophils are seen in the epithelium. Organisms are easily identified on this hematoxylin and eosinstain but it is usually best to apply one of several other stains to detect them.

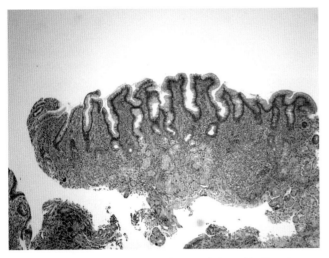

Figure 101.21 Active chronic *Helicobacter pylori* gastritis. Note the lymphoid follicles in this low-magnification field.

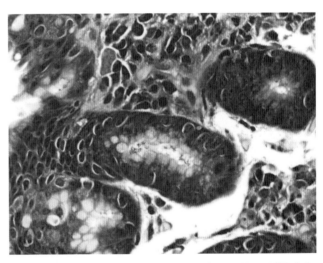

Figure 101.23 Active chronic *Helicobacter pylori* gastritis. A DiffQuik® stain highlights the organisms, seen as curved bacilli in the gland at the center of the field.

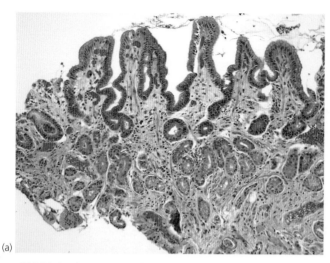

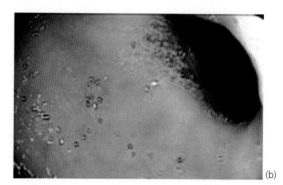

(a)

(b)

Figure 101.24 Autoimmune metaplastic atrophic gastritis. **(a)** The antrum from this patient shows chemical gastritis – there are few inflammatory cells. **(b)** This patient had diffuse atrophic gastritis. The image of the antrum reveals thin mucosa with visible submucosal vessels. Biopsy confirmed chronic antral gastritis with marked intestinal metaplasia consistent with atrophic gastritis.

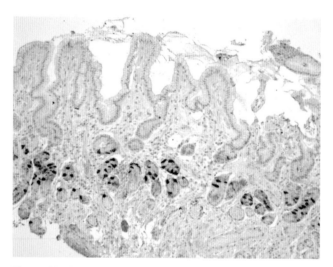

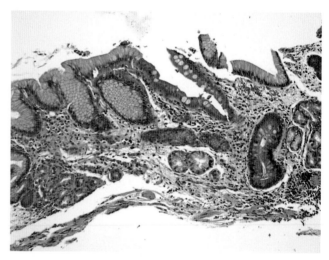

Figure 101.25 Autoimmune metaplastic atrophic gastritis. This is a gastrin stain from the field depicted in Figure 101.24. There are many gastrin-producing cells. The patient was probably hypergastrinemic.

Figure 101.26 Autoimmune metaplastic atrophic gastritis. This biopsy is from the gastric body but there are no acid-producing cells. There is intestinal metaplasia in the center portion of the field (goblet cells).

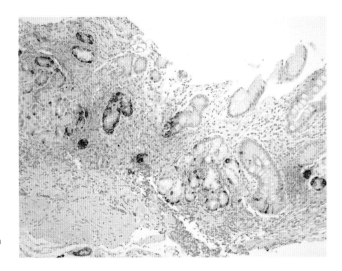

Figure 101.27 Autoimmune metaplastic atrophic gastritis. This chromogranin stain highlights endocrine cell hyperplasia in the area seen in Figure 101.26. Such proliferation can lead to Type 1 carcinoid tumors.

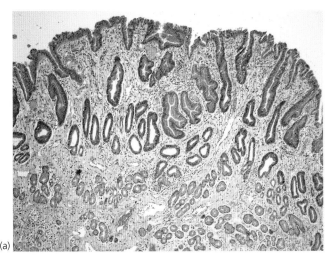

(a)

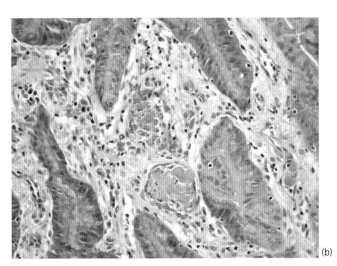

(b)

Figure 101.28 Gastric antral vascular ectasia (GAVE), "watermelon stomach". **(a)** Even at low magnification, many vascular thrombi are apparent. **(b)** High magnification of fibrin thrombi.

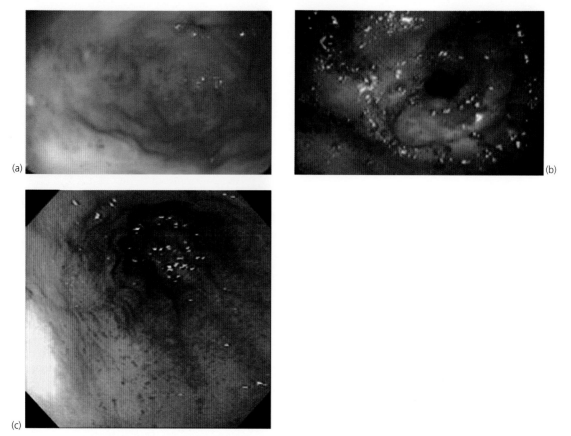

Figure 101.29 Gastric antral vascular ectasia (GAVE), "watermelon stomach". **(a)** GAVE presenting with typical erythematous lesions in the antrum of the stomach. These lesions may require repeated treatments with argon plasma coagulation or electrocautery to prevent recurrent GI bleeding. **(b)** Watermelon stomach. Another term for gastric antral vascular ectasia (GAVE), watermelon stomach refers to the watermelon-like appearance of the antrum in the presence of the striped lines of GAVE. In this patient, multiple bleeding angioectasias can be seen in the gastric antrum. These were treated with argon plasma coagulation with successful hemostasis. **(c)** Gastric antral vascular ectasia.

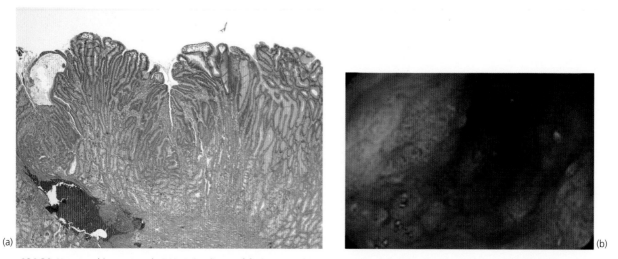

Figure 101.30 Hypertrophic gastropathy/Ménétrier disease. **(a)** There is striking hyperplasia of foveolar (mucin-producing cells). **(b)** Giant gastric folds/ Ménétrier disease. This patient with hypoalbuminemia presented with markedly enlarged gastric folds. Biopsies revealed edematous gastric mucosa with foveolar hyperplasia and no evidence of malignancy, confirming Ménétrier disease; however, years later he developed gastric leiomyosarcoma.

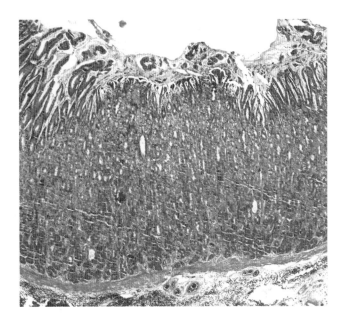

Figure 101.31 Gastric mucosa in Zollinger–Ellison syndrome. There is striking hyperplasia of parietal cells. Contrast this to Figure 101.30a.

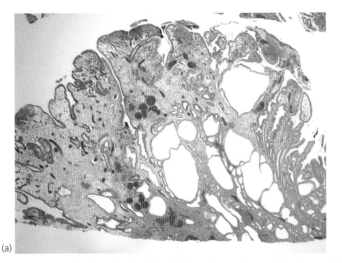

(a)

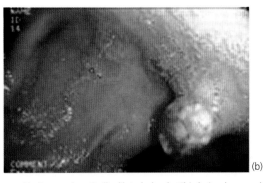

(b)

Figure 101.32 Gastric hyperplastic polyp. **(a)** There is prominence of mucin-producing epithelium and cystically dilated glands. This lesion has overlap with hypertrophic gastropathy and diagnosis of either condition requires correlation with the endoscopic appearance. **(b)** Gastric inflammatory polyp: hyperplastic polyp. An inflamed hyperplastic polyp is seen here in the antrum of the stomach. Hyperplastic polyps are the most common type of gastric polyp and, while they have a low malignant potential, should be removed at the time of endoscopy.

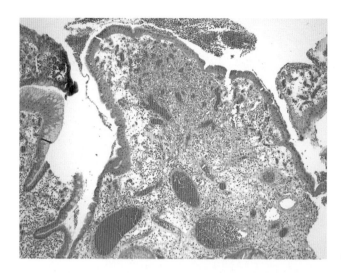

Figure 101.33 Gastric hyperplastic polyp: it is not uncommon for large hyperplastic polyps to display surface erosions or ulcers and reparative epithelial changes.

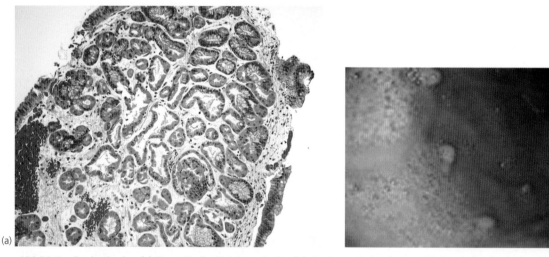

(a)

(b)

Figure 101.34 Fundic gland polyp. **(a)** The cystically dilated oxyntic (fundic) glands are the key feature. **(b)** Gastric fundic gland polyp: fundic gland polyps. These small sessile polyps that are distributed in the body and fundus in a patient with a history of proton pump inhibitor therapy are characteristic of fundic gland polyps.

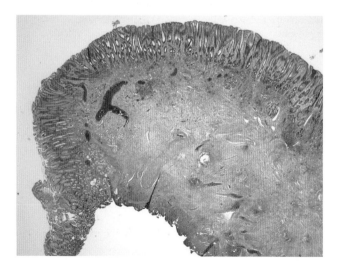

Figure 101.35 Inflammatory fibroid polyp. These tumors have their epicenters in the superficial submucosa.

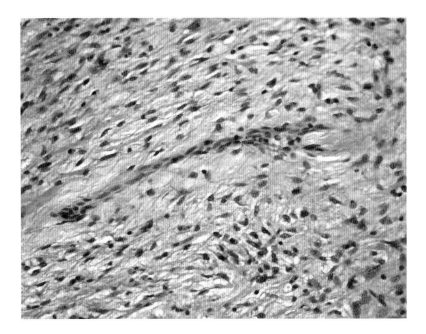

Figure 101.36 Inflammatory fibroid polyp. At higher magnification, there is a spindle cell lesion punctuated by many eosinophils.

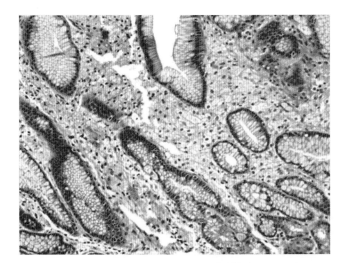

Figure 101.37 Gastric xanthoma. Numerous lipid-laden macrophages are seen in the lamina propria.

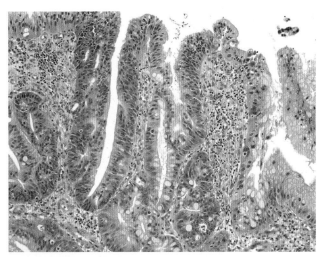

Figure 101.38 Gastric adenoma intestinal type. This example shows both intestinal metaplasia and high-grade dysplasia.

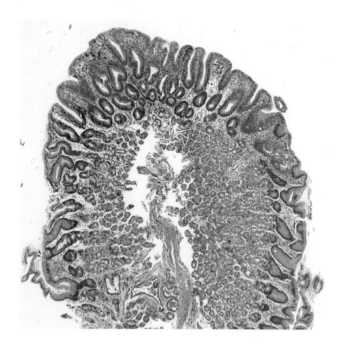

Figure 101.39 Gastric adenoma "gastric" type. Such a lesion, arising in normal background mucosa, is a "low-risk" lesion unlikely to be associated with either high-grade dysplasia or invasive carcinoma.

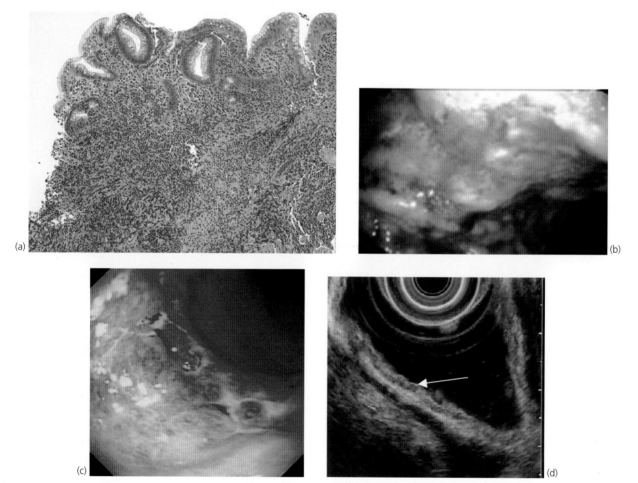

Figure 101.40 Mucosa-associated lymphoid tissue (MALT) lymphoma. **(a)** MALT lymphoma, also called extranodal marginal zone B-cell lymphoma. Note the "bottom-heavy" distribution of the lymphoid infiltrate. **(b)** Gastric MALT lymphoma. Friable ulcerated mucosa on the lesser curvature of the stomach. Biopsies revealed a dense lymphoid infiltrate with focal ulceration consistent with low-grade marginal zone MALT B-cell lymphoma. **(c)** MALT lymphoma: endoscopic appearance. **(d)** MALT lymphoma: thickened gastric mucosa without submucosa involvement (arrow) as shown by endoscopic ultrasonography (stage IE1).

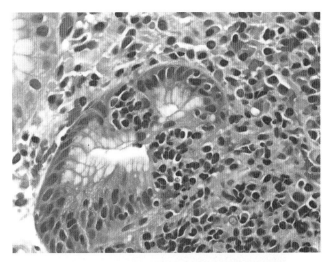

Figure 101.41 Mucosa-associated lymphoid tissue (MALT) lymphoma. This field shows a "lymphoepithelial lesion" in which lymphoid cells proliferate in the epithelium itself.

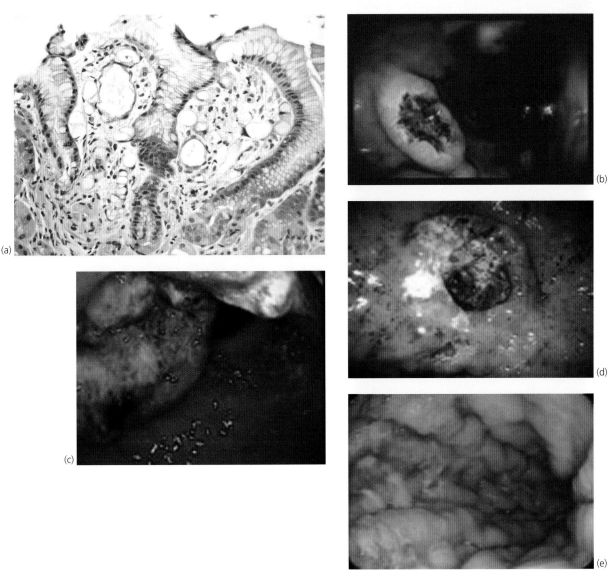

Figure 101.42 Gastric adenocarcinoma. **(a)** This subtle early lesion is seen only in the lamina propria of the stomach (intramucosal carcinoma). **(b)** Malignant gastric ulcer. This large cratered gastric ulcer had heaped margins and a chronic appearance. Biopsies from this ulcer revealed a signet ring cell adenocarcinoma with ulceration and candidal overgrowth. **(c)** Moderately differentiated invasive gastric adenocarcinoma. An ulcerated mass in the antrum of the stomach seen here in an 84-year-old woman from Korea with iron deficiency anemia. Stomach cancer is the most prevalent malignant neoplasm in Korea. **(d)** Advanced gastric carcinoma: irregular fungating ulcerated pyloric channel mass. The mass was an invasive, poorly differentiated adenocarcinoma on biopsy. **(e)** Linitis plastica. In this image, the rugal folds of the stomach are thickened diffusely. This patient was found to have poorly differentiated metastatic adenocarcinoma of the breast.

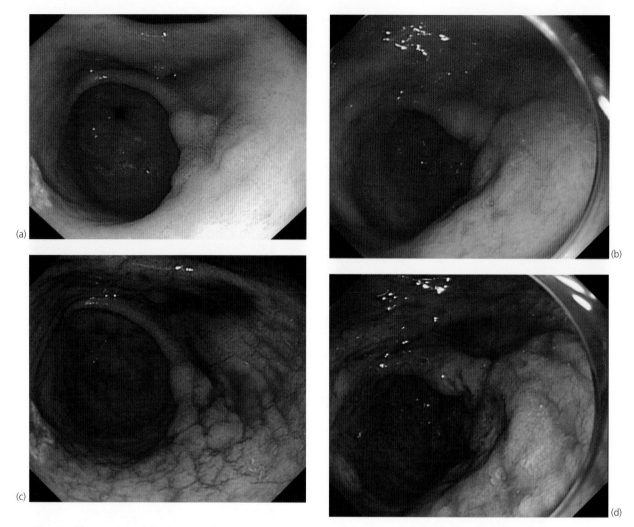

Figure 101.43 Chromoendoscopy for diagnosis of early gastric cancer. The use of indigocarmine can enhance the detection of early gastric cancer. **(a)** and **(b)**, Type I protruded gastric cancer; **(c)** and **(d)**, Type IIc depressed lesion.

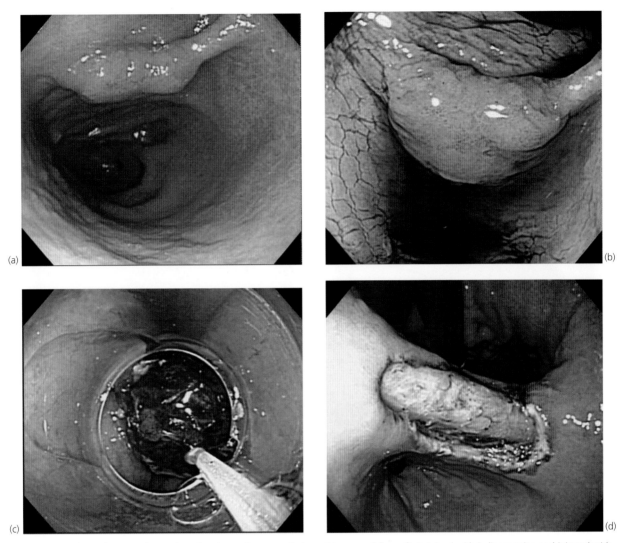

Figure 101.44 Endoscopic mucosal resection of early gastric cancer. Early gastric cancer **(a)** was first stained with indigocarmine and injected with normal saline to lift up the lesion **(b)**. The lesion was then sucked into the suction cap **(c)** and removed by an endoscopic mucosal resection snare **(d)**.

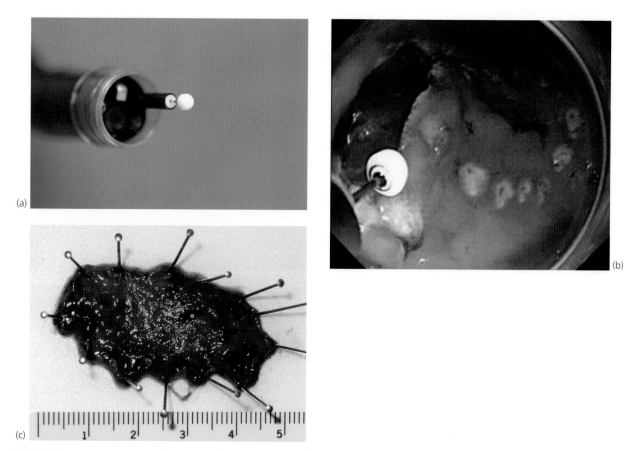

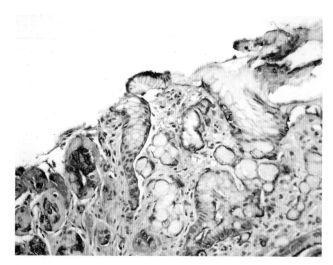

Figure 101.45 Endoscopic submucosal dissection of early gastric cancer. **(a)** The insulation-tipped needle knife consists of a conventional diathermic needle knife with a ceramic ball at the top to minimize the risk of perforation; **(b)** The knife can be used in submucosal dissection and complete en bloc resection of larger lesion; **(c)** One-piece removal of early gastric cancer.

Figure 101.46 Gastric adenocarcinoma. A keratin stain highlights the cancer cells from the field seen in Figure 101.42a.

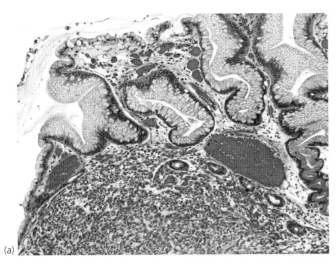

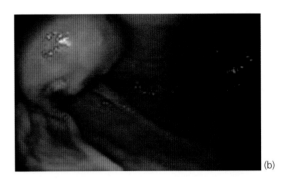

Figure 101.47 Gastrointestinal stromal tumor (GIST), spindle cell type. **(a)** This lesion displays mucosal invasion, a feature of malignant GIST. **(b)** Endoscopic appearance of a 3.4-cm GIST in the stomach. These submucosal tumors may have an overlying ulceration as seen here.

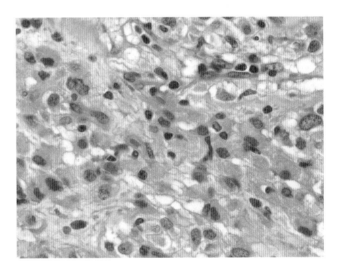

Figure 101.48 Gastrointestinal stromal tumor (GIST), epithelioid type. Note the eosinophilic appearance of the lesional cells. Such tumors were referred to as "leiomyoblastoma" in the past.

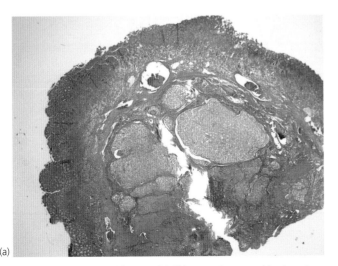

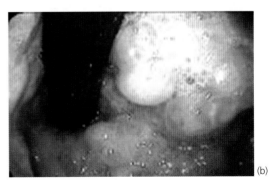

Figure 101.49 Gastric carcinoid tumor. **(a)** This tumor is centered in the submucosa. **(b)** A large fungating and submucosal noncircumferential mass was found in the cardia in this patient with multiple endocrine neoplasia type 1. Biopsies confirmed a low-grade carcinoid tumor.

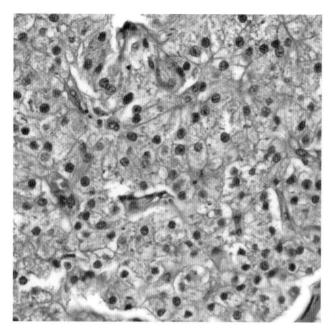

Figure 101.50 Gastric carcinoid tumor. Note the uniform nuclear features.

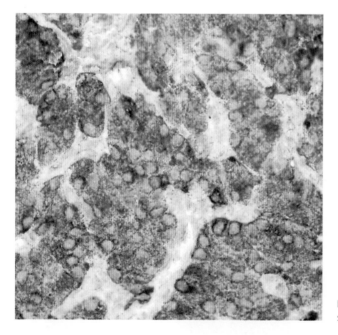

Figure 101.51 Gastric carcinoid tumor. The lesional cells are reactive with synaptophysin antibodies.

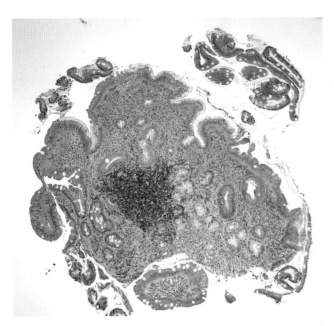

Figure 101.52 Chronic peptic duodenitis. At low magnification, normal duodenal mucosa is seen at the left (goblet cells are present) but the central portion shows gastric-type epithelium that is metaplastic.

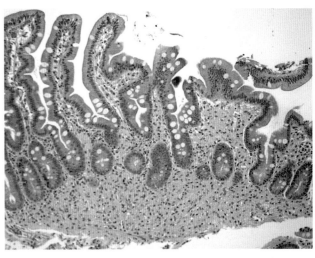

Figure 101.54 *Mycobacterium avium* intracellular duodenitis. The villi are expanded with macrophages.

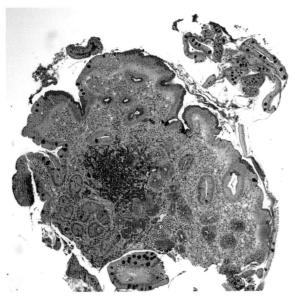

Figure 101.53 Chronic peptic duodenitis. A periodic acid Schiff stain with alcian blue shows the gastric metaplasia to advantage; it appears magenta.

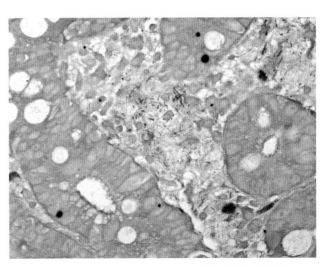

Figure 101.55 *Mycobacterium avium* intracellular duodenitis. This acid-fast stain highlights the organisms.

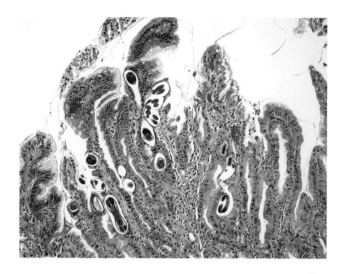

Figure 101.56 Strongyloidiasis. Multiple larval forms are seen in the small intestinal mucosa.

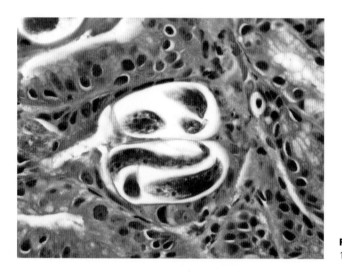

Figure 101.57 Strongyloidiasis. Higher magnification of image Figure 101.53.

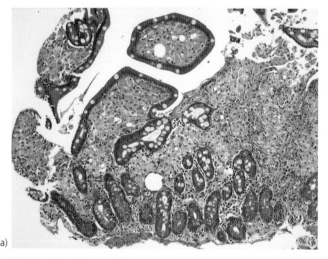

(a)

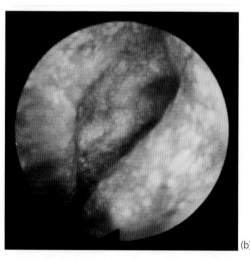

(b)

Figure 101.58 Whipple disease. **(a)** Like Figure 101.51, this image shows many foamy macrophages expanding the villi. In contrast, dilated lacteals are a feature of Whipple disease. **(b)** Characteristic duodenoscopic appearance of the duodenum of an untreated patient with Whipple disease. The folds are thickened and are covered with small yellowish-white plaques. This endoscopic appearance may be the first clue to the diagnosis.

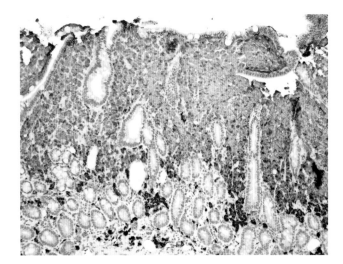

Figure 101.59 Whipple disease. This is an immunohistochemical preparation using an antibody directed against the organism.

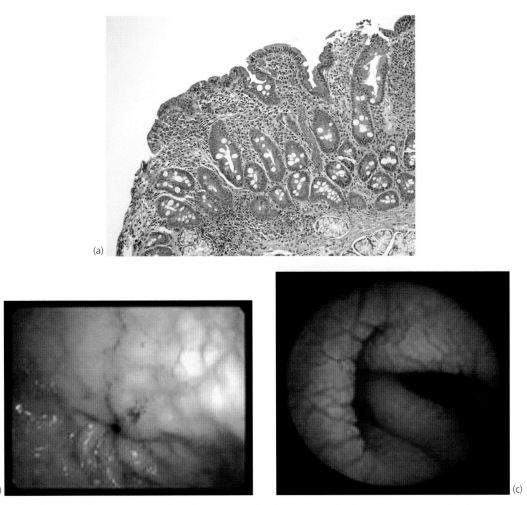

Figure 101.60 Celiac disease. **(a)** The villi in this duodenal biopsy are wholly attenuated. **(b)** Duodenal mucosa in the bulb with a scalloped mosaic appearance in a patient with celiac disease. This patient had a high titer of antiendomysial and tissue transglutaminase antibodies. Small bowel biopsies confirmed villous blunting, crypt hyperplasia, and markedly increased intraepithelial lymphocytes. **(c)** Capsule endoscopy in a patient with celiac disease reveals scalloping of the small intestinal mucosa. Courtesy of Dr Myles D. Keroack.

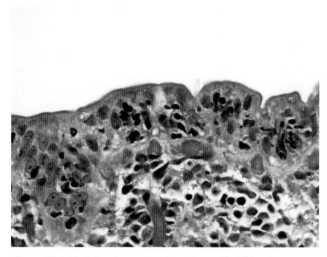

Figure 101.61 Celiac disease. Prominent intraepithelial lymphocytes are a key diagnostic feature.

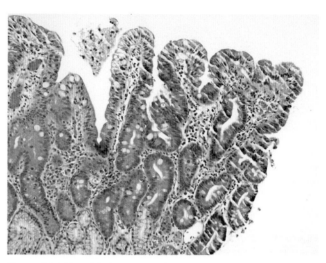

Figure 101.63 Colchicine toxicity. This patient's duodenal biopsy shows attenuated villi and an expanded proliferative compartment. Mitotic arrest is seen as ring mitoses.

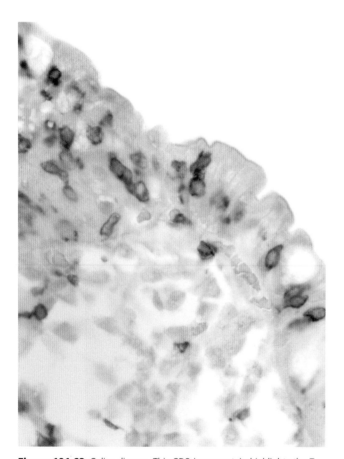

Figure 101.62 Celiac disease. This CD3 immunostain highlights the T cells in the epithelium.

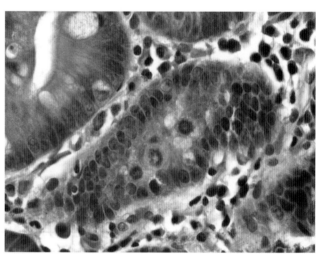

Figure 101.64 Colchicine toxicity. Higher magnification of arrested mitoses.

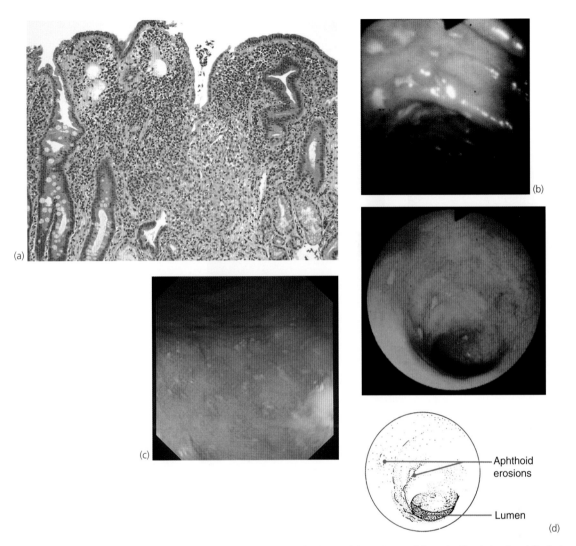

Figure 101.65 Crohn's disease. **(a)** Crohn's disease. A granuloma is seen in the center of the field. **(b)** Crohn's colitis with discrete small, round ulcers separated by normal mucosa. **(c)** Crohn's disease involving the transverse colon with multiple aphthous ulcers. A 26-year-old woman with Crohn's disease for 2 years has persistent symptoms despite prednisone 25 mg daily and sulfasalazine 3 g daily. Endoscopic image shows multiple aphthous ulcers; edematous and erythematous mucosa with a loss of normal vascular markings and mucous exudate. **(d)** Characteristic superficial aphthoid erosions in Crohn's disease have erythematous rings.

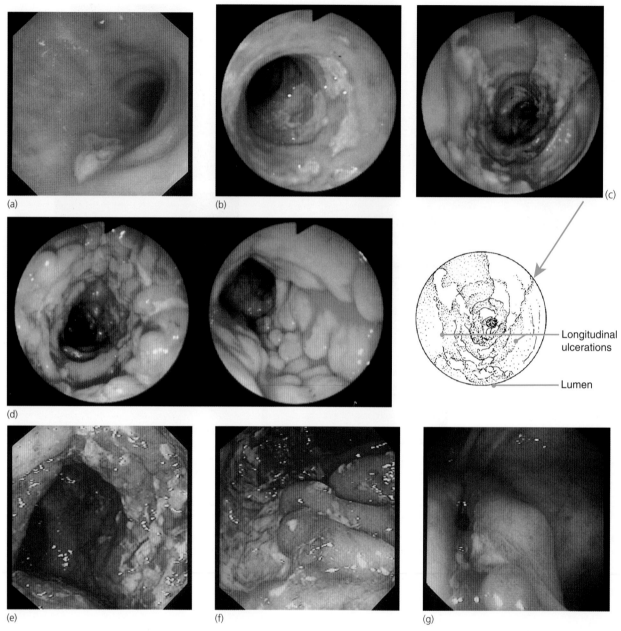

Figure 101.66 **(a)** Crohn's disease of the colon with focal ulcer. A 24-year-old man with Crohn's disease for 2 years currently has minimal symptoms while taking metronidazole 250 mg three times daily and mesalamine 2.4 g daily. There is a focal ulcer in the distal sigmoid colon, mild inflammatory changes of the surrounding mucosa, distortion of the vascular markings, mild granularity, and erythema. **(b)** Multiple large, deep, excavated ulcers in severe ulcerating Crohn's disease show distinct margins. This patient has concomitant sclerosing cholangitis. **(c)** Longitudinal alignment of ulceration causes a railroad-track appearance in Crohn's disease. **(d)** Active phase of Crohn's disease shows cobblestoning caused by interconnecting ulcerations (left). Area of cobblestoning after therapy (right). **(e)** Severely active Crohn's disease of the colon. A 22-year-old man with a 1-year history of Crohn's disease has severe diarrhea, a 19-pound weight loss, and continuing symptoms despite prednisone 60 mg daily. Colonoscopic image shows severe ulceration in the transverse colon with markedly edematous, granular, and friable mucosa. **(f)** Severely active Crohn's disease of the colon (same patient as in part [i]). Deep rake ulcer in middescending colon with surrounding mucosal edema, granularity, and friability. **(g)** Crohn's disease with ulceration at the ileocecal valve. A 26-year-old woman with a history of Crohn's disease for 4 years has involvement of the terminal ileum. The disease was previously controlled with mesalamine 4 g daily, with worsening cramping abdominal pain in recent weeks. Colonoscopy revealed ulceration at the ileocecal valve with stenosis of the valve, which could not be intubated with a colonoscope. The colon otherwise appeared normal.

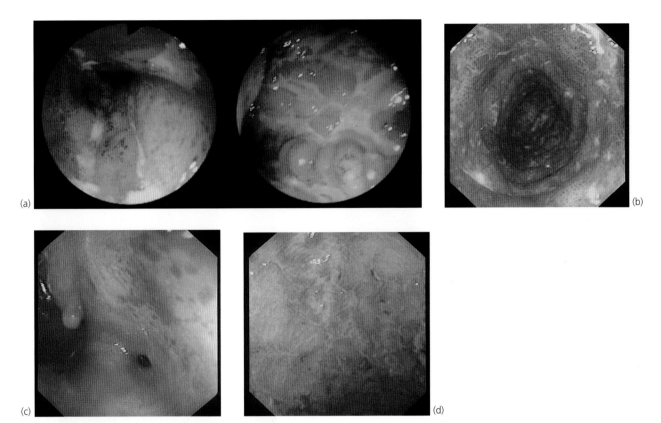

(a)

(b)

(c)

(d)

Figure 101.67 (a) Diffuse, concentric involvement of the distal terminal ileum in Crohn's disease presents itself as swelling, erythema, punctiform bleeding, and ulceration (left). Circumferential involvement of the distal terminal ileum with longitudinal ulcers and cobblestoning (right).
(b) Crohn's disease involving the neoterminal ileum with multiple superficial ulcers. A 29-year-old woman with a history of Crohn's disease for 6 years had undergone resection of the terminal ileum and cecum with ileal-ascending colonic anastomosis. Symptoms of recurrent Crohn's disease (cramping abdominal pain and malaise) developed 4 months after resection. Colonoscopic image with visualization of the neoterminal ileum shows multiple focal superficial ulcers with edema, erythema, and granularity of the intervening mucosa. **(c)** Crohn's disease – view of the rectum with rectovaginal fistula and prominent anal papilla. A 40-year-old woman has a 10-year history of Crohn's disease involving the colon. A symptomatic rectovaginal fistula developed with gas and stool passed per vagina. Retroflexed view of the rectum shows a central fistulous opening communicating with the vagina. The endoscope is in the left field of the photo, and a prominent anal papilla is present. The mucosa is granular, edematous, and friable. **(d)** Mildly active Crohn's disease of the sigmoid colon in a 51-year-old man with a 4-year history of Crohn's colitis, now controlled with azathioprine 175 mg daily and metronidazole 250 mg twice daily. The mucosa shows superficial scarring, loss of normal vascular markings, and slight mucous exudate.

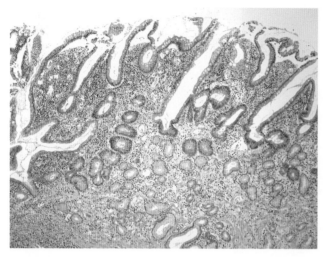

Figure 101.68 Crohn's disease. This ileal biopsy shows pyloric metaplasia – the metaplastic glands in the deep portion of the field lack goblet cells. (See also Fig. 101.67.)

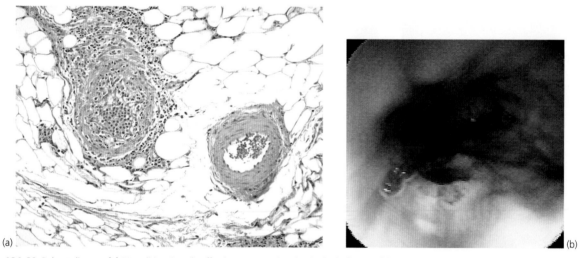

(a)

(b)

Figure 101.69 Behçet disease. **(a)** Vasculitis primarily affecting mesenteric veins is the hallmark. **(b)** An endoscopic view of esophageal ulceration in a patient with Behçet disease.

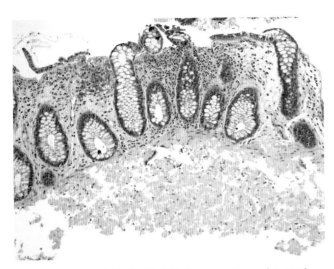

Figure 101.70 Amyloidosis. This field shows prominent submucosal deposits. This is from a colonic biopsy.

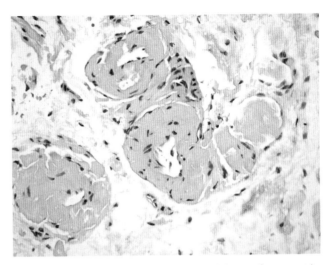

Figure 101.72 Amyloidosis. This vascular deposition was from a gastric biopsy.

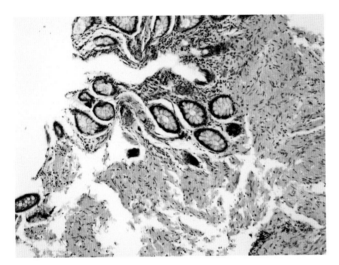

Figure 101.71 Amyloidosis. The Congo red preparation imparts an orange–brown color.

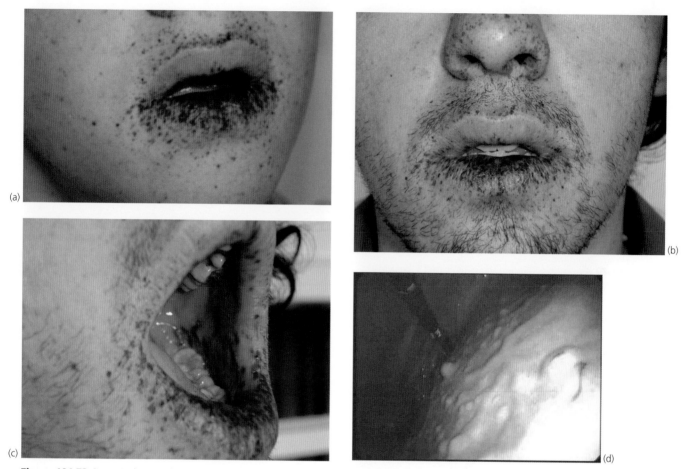

(a)

(b)

(c)

(d)

Figure 101.73 Peutz–Jeghers syndrome. **(a–c)** Perioral, lip, and buccal pigmentation. Courtesy of Dr Asadur J. Tchekmedyian. **(d)** Gastric Peutz–Jeghers polyps.

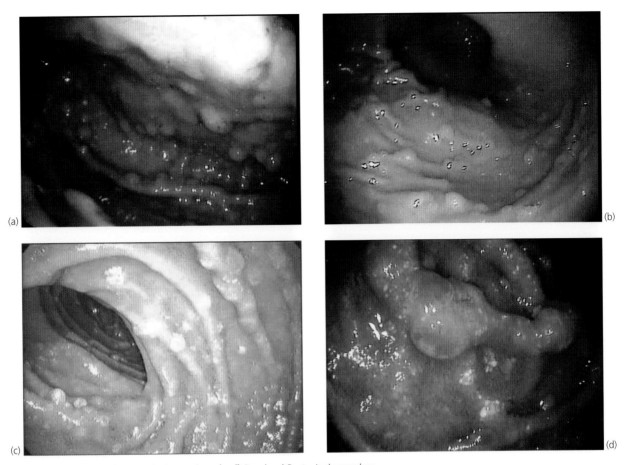

(a)

(b)

(c)

(d)

Figure 101.74 (a, b) Gastric Peutz–Jeghers polyps. **(c, d)** Duodenal Peutz–Jeghers polyps.

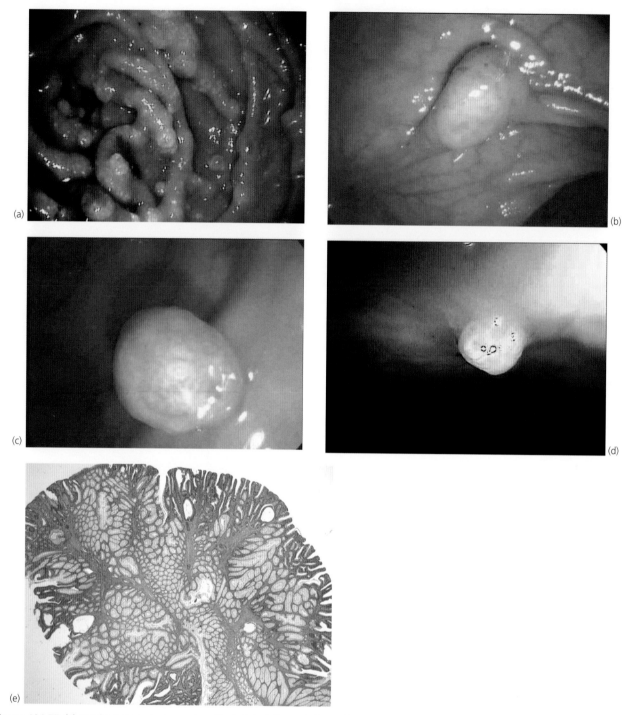

Figure 101.75 (a) Duodenal Peutz–Jeghers polyps. **(b–d)** Colonic Peutz–Jeghers polyps. **(e)** Peutz–Jeghers polyp. Note the striking muscular arborizing cores.

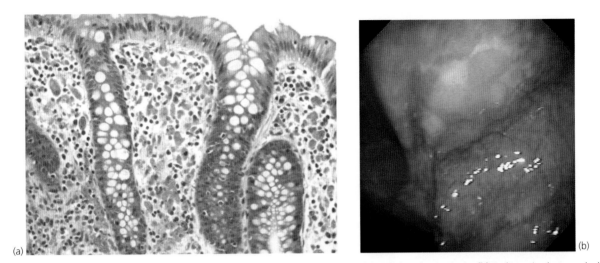

(a)

(b)

Figure 101.76 (a) Melanosis coli. The pigment in the lamina propria macrophages is lipofuscin rather than melanin. **(b)** Endoscopic photograph shows a 1-cm flat, multilobulated polyp adjacent to the cecal sling fold. The polyp is pale pink, whereas the surrounding mucosa is brown because of melanosis. Adenomas do not take up melanin and stand out in melanosis coli.

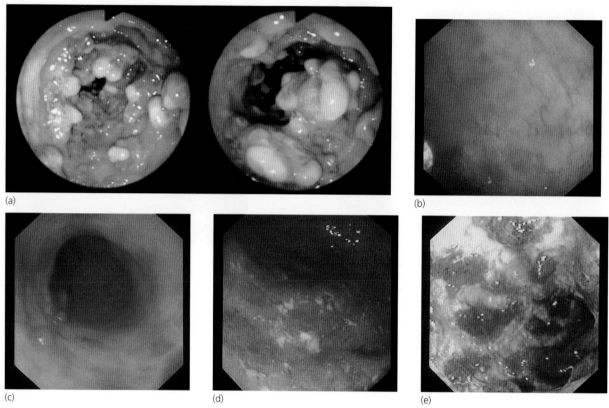

Figure 101.77 Ulcerative colitis. **(a)** Multiple pseudopolyps in ulcerative colitis. Their surface is smooth and glistening. Detailed view of exudate creating whitish caps. **(b)** Quiescent (inactive) ulcerative colitis in a 39-year-old woman with ulcerative pancolitis for 11 years, now asymptomatic. There is distortion of the vascular markings but no granularity, edema, friability, mucus exudate, or ulcerations. **(c)** Mildly active ulcerative colitis with pseudopolyps. Same patient as in part **(b)**, 1 year after the endoscopic examination in **(b)**, with a mild flare in symptoms. The disease now is responding to prednisone 20 mg daily and mesalamine 4 g daily. There are two small pseudopolyps; the mucosa is mildly granular and erythematous; and the vascular markings are distorted. **(d)** Moderately active ulcerative colitis in a 19-year-old woman with ulcerative pancolitis for 2 years. The patient has continuing symptoms despite oral mesalamine 4 g daily and prednisone 40 mg daily. Moderate granularity, edema, and mucus exudate is demonstrated. **(e)** Severely active ulcerative colitis in a 54-year-old woman with left-sided ulcerative colitis for 7 years. There is marked ulceration. At least half of the surface area depicted is denuded by ulcers, and there are intervening areas of edematous granular mucosa.

Figure 101.78 **(a)** Coarsely nodular deformity of mucosal contour in ulcerative colitis. Mucosa is intensely erythematous and friable. **(b)** Sharp transition from normal to inflamed bowel is discernible at the rectosigmoid junction. Erythema and superficial ulceration of diseased mucosa contrast to the normal vascular pattern. **(c)** Mildly active ulcerative colitis with multiple pseudopolyps. A 54-year-old woman (same patient as in Fig. 101.77d) about 1 year after a course of topical 5-ASA (mesalamine) and prednisone 60 mg daily tapered and discontinued 9 months previously. There is mild granularity and erythema; the vascular markings are distorted, and multiple small pseudopolyps are present. **(d)** Long-standing ulcerative colitis with scarring and pseudopolyps. A 25-year-old man had a 9-year history of ulcerative colitis. The patient is now asymptomatic with azathioprine 150 mg daily and mesalamine 2.4 g daily. There is scarring and loss of the normal vascular markings. Two small pseudopolyps are present. **(e)** Ulcerative colitis with bridging pseudopolyps. A 25-year-old man has had ulcerative colitis for 9 years (same patient as in part [d]) and the disease is asymptomatic with azathioprine 150 mg daily and mesalamine 2.4 g daily. Endoscopic picture shows bridging pseudopolyps in the transverse colon. **(f)** Sequential study of severe pancolitis. Massive ulceration of the colon was studied at intervals of 4–6 weeks after institution of medical therapy. A, view of the proximal sigmoid shows extensive ulceration before therapy. Some islands of remaining mucosa are visible; B, regression of inflammation and early reepithelialization; C, ulcers are regressing with pseudopolypoid elevation of nonulcerated mucosal islands; D, full reepithelialization and pseudopolypoid transformation characterize healing.

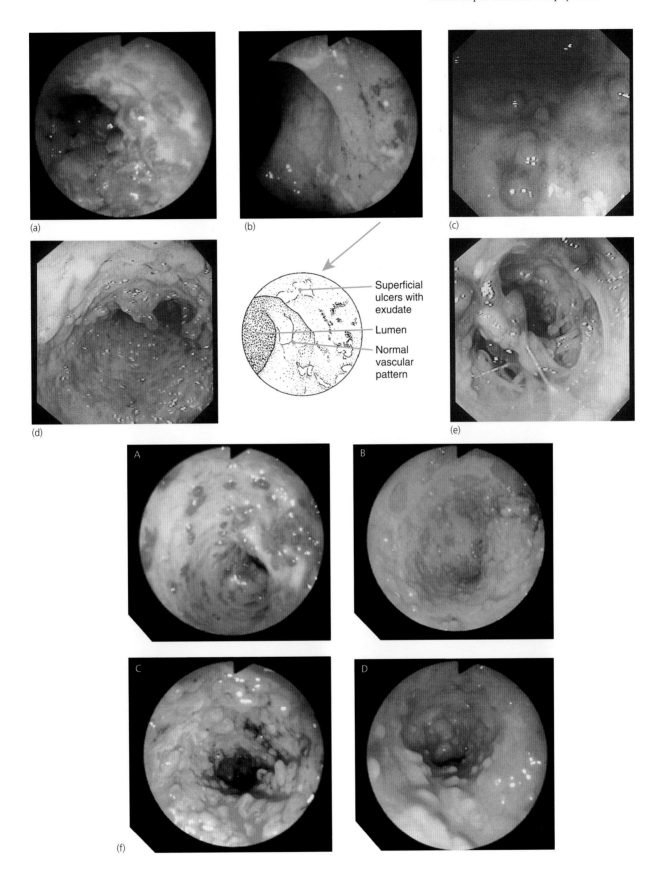

(a)

(b)

(c)

Superficial
ulcers with
exudate

Lumen

Normal
vascular
pattern

(d)

(e)

A

B

C

D

(f)

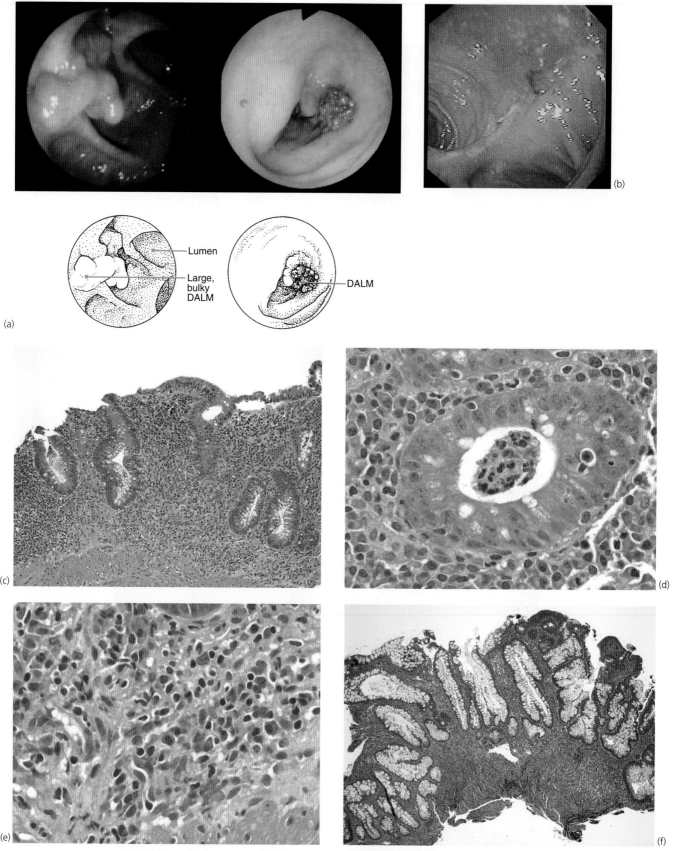

Figure 101.79 (a) Examples of dysplasia-associated lesions or masses in long-standing, inactive ulcerative colitis. **(b)** Mild to moderately active pouchitis. This 36-year-old woman has a history of ulcerative colitis for which she underwent colectomy with ileal J pouch-anal anastomosis 2 years previously. She had recurrent liquid stools and cramping discomfort relieved with bowel movements. Endoscopic image of the pouch, with views of the afferent limb of the neoterminal ileum in the left portion of the field and the blind end of the J pouch in the inferior aspect of the field, shows mucus exudate, superficial ulceration, and friability of the pouch mucosa but not of the mucosa in the neoterminal ileum. **(c–f)** Ulcerative colitis. In these fields, the crypts are distorted and do not reach the muscularis mucosae at the bottom of the fields.

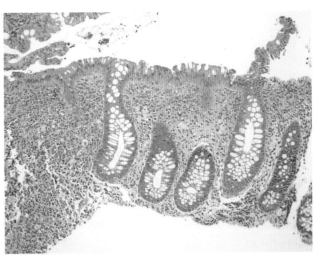

Figure 101.80 Schistosomiasis. Ova surrounded by eosinophils are seen in the submucosa.

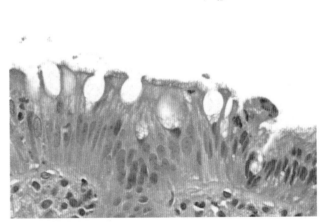

Figure 101.82 Spirochetosis. This biopsy was from an immunosuppressed person with diarrhea. The biopsy shows features of acute self-limiting colitis in that there is cryptitis without crypt distortion.

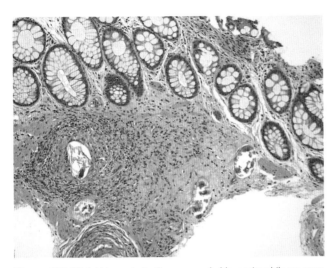

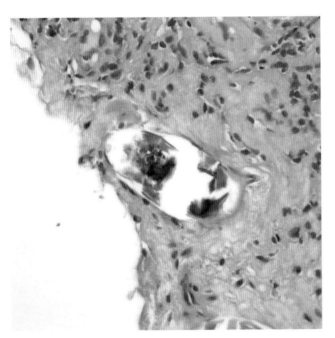

Figure 101.83 Spirochetosis. The hair-like structures emanating from the surface are the organisms.

Figure 101.81 Schistosomiasis. The lateral spine of this ovum is in keeping with schistosomiasis mansoni.

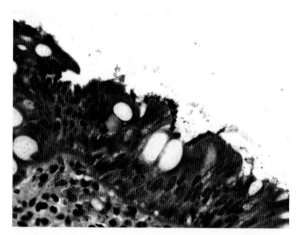

Figure 101.84 Spirochetosis. This Warthin-Starry silver stain highlights the organisms.

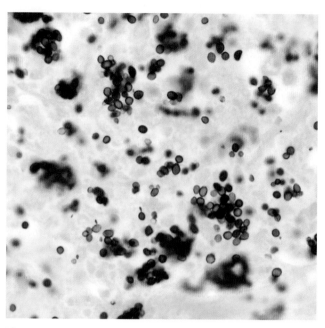

Figure 101.87 Histoplasmosis. A Gomori-methenamine silver stain from the image seen in Figure 101.80 shows budding yeast forms.

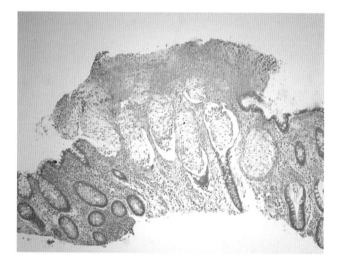

Figure 101.85 Pseudomembranous colitis. A pseudomembrane is seen at the center of the field.

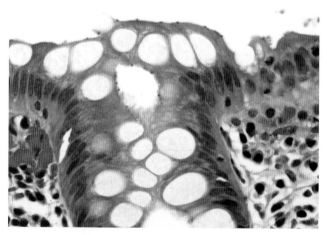

Figure 101.88 Cryptosporidiosis. Organisms appear as small beads at the epithelial surface.

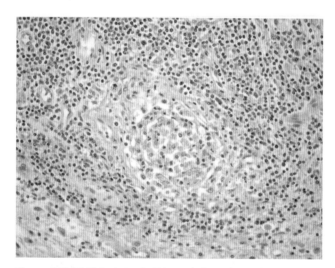

Figure 101.86 Histoplasmosis. This poorly-formed necrotizing granuloma was found in an immunosuppressed person and contained the organisms.

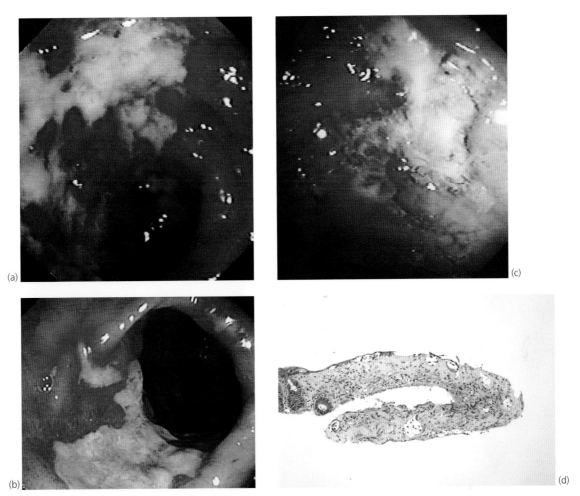

(a)

(c)

(b)

(d)

Figure 101.89 Ischemic colitis. **(a)** An 83-year-old female who presented with abdominal pain and bloody diarrhea. Colonoscopy revealed the presence of large ulcerations in the splenic flexure. Biopsies were compatible with the diagnosis of ischemic colitis. This region is commonly affected in colonic ischemia because of its relatively low perfusion (watershed area). Colonoscopy is the method of choice for the diagnosis of ischemic colitis, because it allows direct visualization of the mucosa and tissue sampling. **(b)** Large ulceration in the sigmoid region caused by ischemia. The sigmoid colon is another area that is particularly susceptible to ischemic lesions because of its relatively low perfusion.

Although this lesion can be reached by a sigmoidoscopy, complete colonoscopy should be performed in patients suspected of having ischemic colitis because 50% of the ischemic lesions are proximal to the sigmoid colon. **(c)** Endoscopic findings in a 62-year-old female with ischemic colitis associated with a low-flow state (sepsis). The mucosa of the affected segment appears edematous, hemorrhagic, friable, and ulcerated. **(d)** Ischemic colitis. This example is from an individual who was receiving Kayexalate® but the features are similar regardless of etiology. This biopsy shows atrophic microcrypts and lamina propria hyalinization.

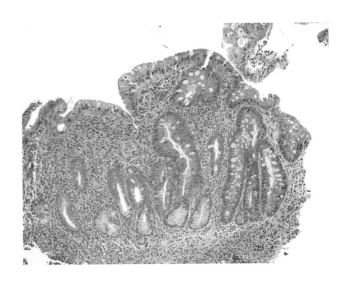

Figure 101.90 Common variable immunodeficiency. The features are similar to those of ulcerative colitis and it is easy for pathologists to make an incorrect diagnosis in such cases.

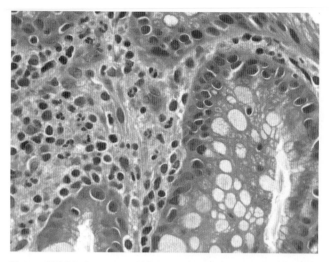

Figure 101.91 Common variable immunodeficiency. The key is the absence of plasma cells in the lamina propria; they would be a prominent constituent in the inflammatory backdrop of ulcerative colitis. The prominent lamina propria neutrophils in this biopsy are in keeping with an acute infection.

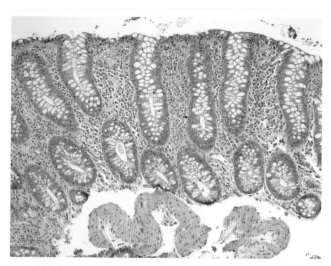

Figure 101.94 Lymphocytic colitis: note the intraepithelial lymphocytosis.

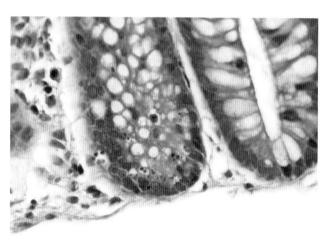

Figure 101.92 Graft-versus-host disease: note the crypt apoptosis. Crypt apoptosis may also result from phosphasoda bowel preparation so this method is not advised if assessing for graft-versus-host disease.

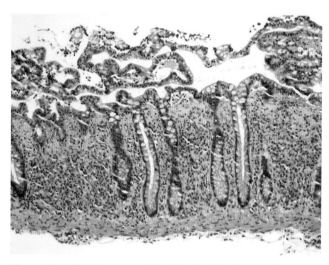

Figure 101.95 Collagenous colitis. Subepithelial collagen is the hallmark.

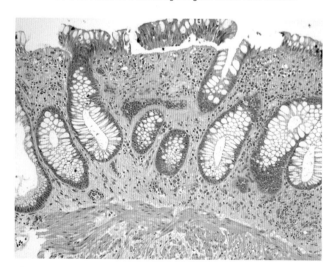

Figure 101.93 Radiation proctitis: note the prominent vessel parallel to the epithelial surface.

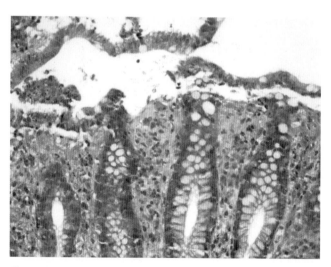

Figure 101.96 Collagenous colitis. This trichrome stain results in a blue color in the subepithelial collagen.

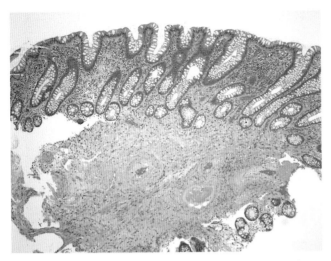

Figure 101.97 Elastosis. This process produced an "incidental" polyp.

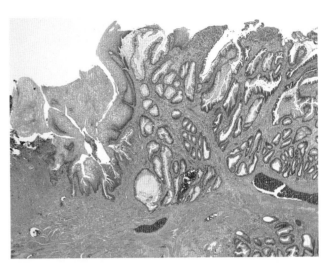

Figure 101.99 Inflammatory cloacogenic polyp. This prolapse lesion is found at the junction of anal squamous (left part of field) and rectal mucosa.

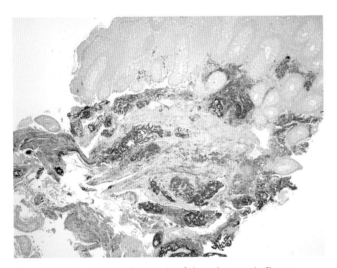

Figure 101.98 Elastosis. Elastic stain of the polyp seen in Figure 101.91.

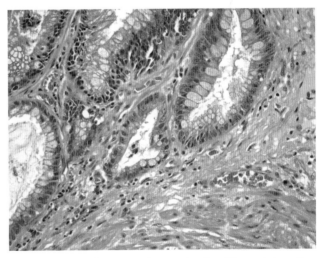

Figure 101.100 Inflammatory cloacogenic polyp. "Diamond-shaped" glands are a characteristic finding of colorectal prolapse lesions.

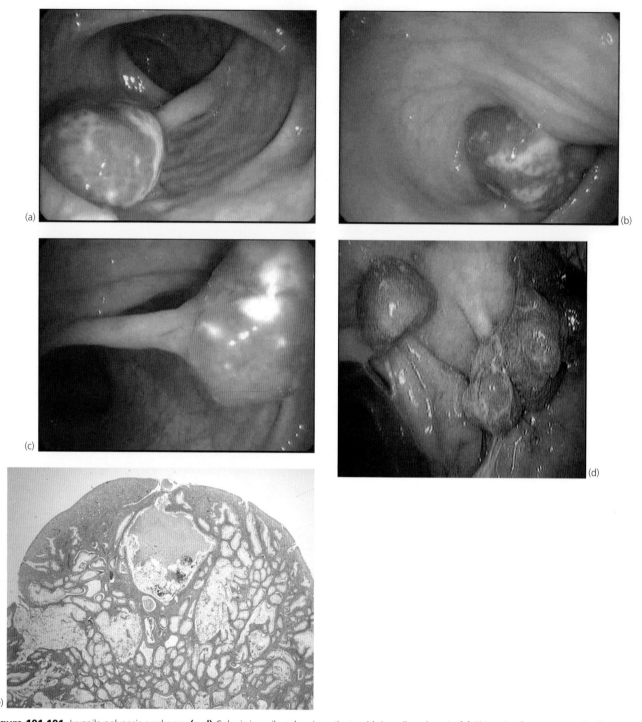

Figure 101.101 Juvenile polyposis syndrome. **(a–d)** Colonic juvenile polyps in patients with juvenile polyposis. **(e)** This polyp features cystically dilated glands, an expanded lamina propria and an eroded surface.

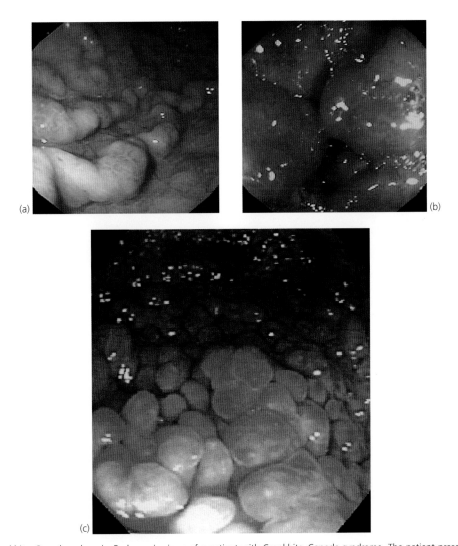

(a)

(b)

(c)

Figure 101.102 Cronkhite–Canada polyposis. Endoscopic views of a patient with Cronkhite–Canada syndrome. The patient presented with dysgeusia, alopecia, onychodystrophy, and diarrhea. **(a)** Stomach. **(b)** Colon: the largest polyp is a pedunculated adenomatous polyp; all other polyps shown exhibited histology typical of Cronkhite–Canada lesions. Courtesy of Dr Edward L. Krawitt. **(c)** Cronkhite–Canada polyposis. This endoscopic image is from the patient's cecum. He had polyps throughout his gastrointestinal tract, sparing only his esophagus.

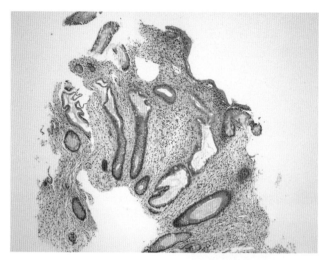

Figure 101.103 Cronkhite–Canada polyposis. This histological appearance of a colonic polyp is hardly specific – the polyp appears similar to a juvenile-type polyp. The distinction is made on clinicopathological grounds and by attention to the background flat mucosa, which is abnormal in Cronkhite–Canada polyposis but normal in juvenile polyposis.

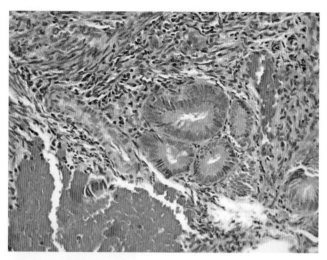

Figure 101.105 Colonic endometriosis. Higher magnification of the lesion seen in Figure 101.104.

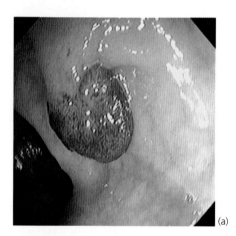

(a)

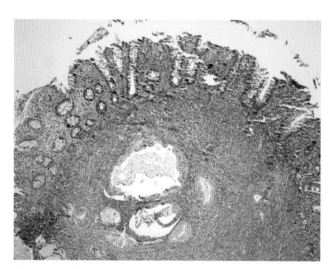

Figure 101.104 Colonic endometriosis. This is a diagnostic pitfall for endoscopists and pathologists alike. The key is for the pathologist to note the background stromal tissue accompanying the glands.

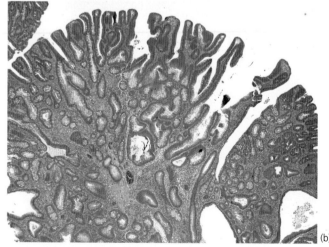

(b)

Figure 101.106 Tubular adenoma. **(a)** Colonoscopic photograph of an 8-mm tubular adenoma on a moderate sized stalk. **(b)** Histological appearance of a tubular adenoma. By definition, the epithelium is dysplastic (neoplastic) but not invasive carcinoma is evident.

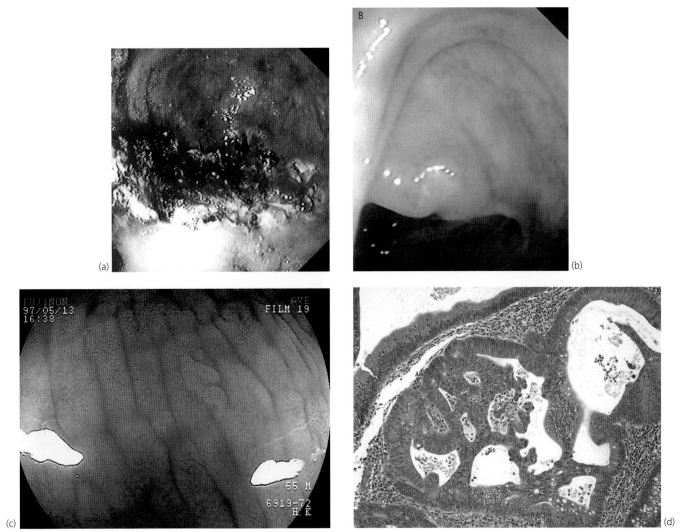

Figure 101.107 High-grade dysplasia in tubular adenoma.
(a) Colonoscopic photograph of a villous adenoma after polypectomy followed by destruction of residual adenoma at the margins by argon plasma coagulation. Close follow-up is required to check for recurrence because total destruction cannot be guaranteed. **(b)** Colonoscopic photograph of a flat adenoma with slight central depression on the edge of a fold in sigmoid colon. These are likely to show high-grade dysplasia. Flat adenomas are recognized more commonly in Japan, and a recent study has shown that they may be as common in Western countries such as the United Kingdom. Courtesy of Dr Michael Bourke. **(c)** Magnifying colonoscopic view of a cluster of aberrant crypts with histopathological features of dysplasia. These are the earliest stage of adenoma formation. *APC* or *Ras* mutations (or both) may already be established in these lesions. **(d)** High-grade dysplasia in a tubular adenoma. The gland in the center is complex with a cribriform architecture. However, the basement membrane around it is intact.

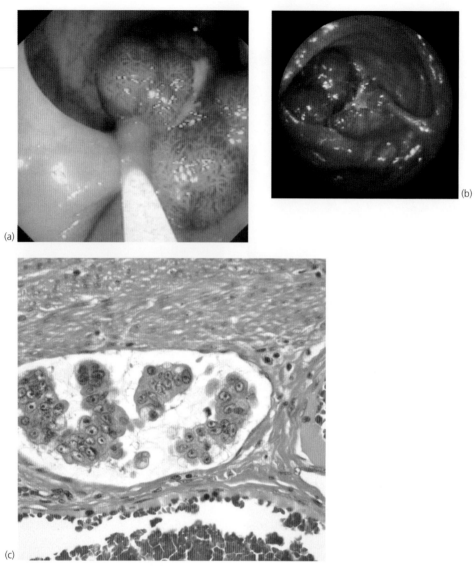

Figure 101.108 Carcinoma arising in adenoma. **(a)** Colonoscopic photograph of a large, multilobulated tubulovillous adenoma showing the diathermy loop secured to the stalk a good distance below the adenoma tissue. Histopathology confirmed total removal with a 4-mm margin. Such polyps have a chance of containing a focus of carcinoma and complete removal at the first attempt is desirable. Courtesy of Dr Michael Bourke. **(b)** Adenocarcinoma, sigmoid with synchronous (sentinel) adenoma. A cancer with an ulcerated mass appearance was found at the splenic flexure (in the distance at the 3 o'clock position). Just distal to this in the proximal descending colon, a pedunculated polyp is present as a sentinel neoplasm. The possibility that other adenomas or even cancers are present in this colon emphasizes the need to perform colonoscopy at the time of diagnosis to clear the colon of other lesions that could alter patient management. **(c)** Carcinoma arising in association with an adenoma; vascular space invasion. This is a feature that most authors believe should prompt resection following a diagnosis of "cancer in a polyp."

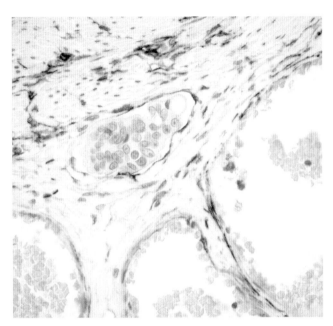

Figure 101.109 Carcinoma arising in association with an adenoma; vascular space invasion. This CD34 stain highlights endothelial cells lining the invaded vessel from the lesion seen in Figure 110.108.

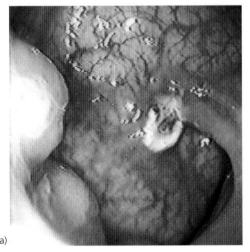

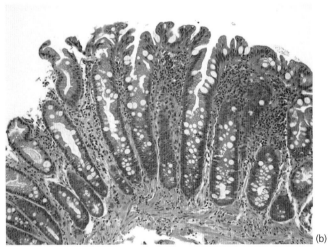

(a)

(b)

Figure 101.110 Hyperplastic polyp. **(a)** Colonoscopic photograph of hyperplastic polyps in the left colon of a patient with hyperplastic polyposis. These polyps are not distinguishable from adenomas without histological examination, preferably performed after polypectomy. **(b)** This serrated polyp shows cells with eosinophilic cytoplasm. Note that the bases of the glands are narrow.

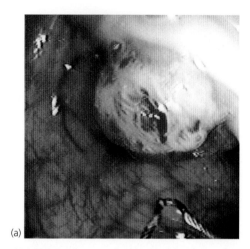

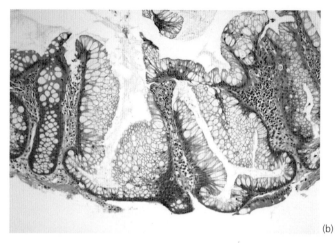

(a)

(b)

Figure 101.111 Sessile serrated adenoma. **(a)** Colonoscopic photograph of a large serrated adenoma about to be removed from a patient with hyperplastic polyposis. This lesion superficially resembles a hyperplastic polyp but differs **(b)** by having broad-based glands (compare to Figure 101.110). It lacks conventional dysplasia but is fully capable of progressing to invasive carcinoma.

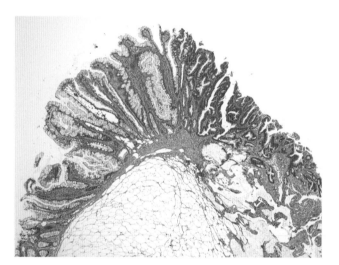

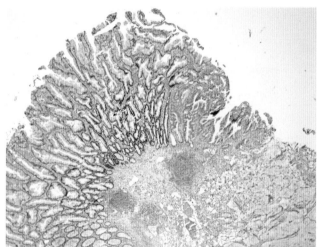

Figure 101.112 Sessile serrated adenoma with associated dysplasia and invasive carcinoma. The high-grade dysplasia and carcinoma component is at the right of the field.

Figure 101.113 Sessile serrated adenoma with associated dysplasia and invasive carcinoma. In this immunohistochemical preparation for the mismatch repair protein MLH1, there is (nuclear) loss in the high-grade dysplasia and carcinoma component.

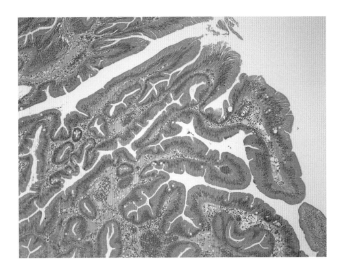

Figure 101.114 Traditional serrated adenoma. There is serrated architecture of the epithelial cells as well as traditional epithelial dysplasia like that of an ordinary adenoma.

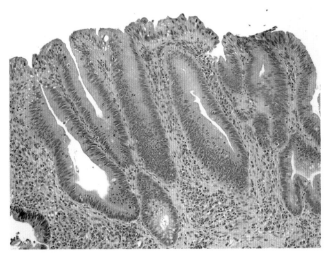

Figure 101.115 Dysplasia associated lesion or mass (DALM). This lesion has low-grade dysplasia and presented as an elevated visible lesion.

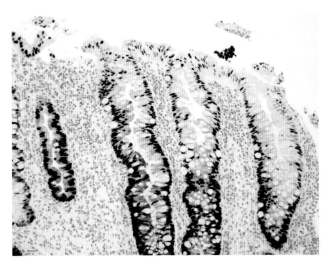

Figure 101.116 Dysplasia associated lesion or mass (DALM). A p52 stain can be useful in confirming an impression of DALM.

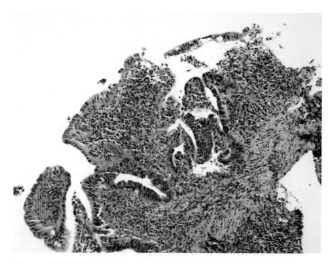

Figure 101.117 Dysplasia associated lesion or mass (DALM). This area shows high-grade dysplasia.

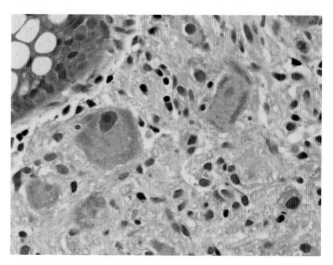

Figure 101.119 Ganglioneuroma. Aberrant ganglion cells and Schwann cells (bland spindled cells) proliferate in the colonic lamina propria. Most examples are isolated sporadic lesions.

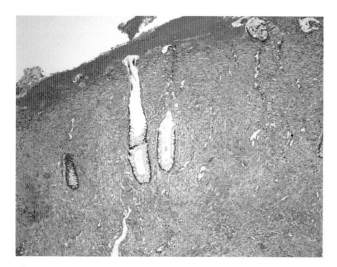

Figure 101.118 Benign fibroblastic polyp of the colon. The lamina propria is expanded by a benign spindle cell proliferation.

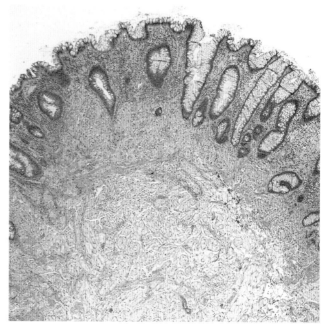

Figure 101.120 Benign epithelioid peripheral nerve sheath tumor. This lesion is centered around the lamina propria and superficial submucosa.

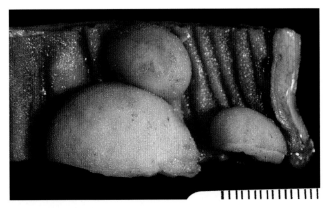

Figure 101.121 Colonic lipoma: surgical specimen.

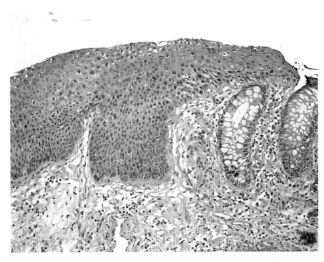

Figure 101.124 Anal intraepithelial neoplasia. This process often occurs at the anorectal transition.

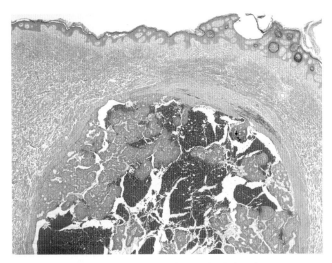

Figure 101.122 Hidradenoma papilliferum. This lesion shows differentiation along sweat gland lineage and is found in the perineum of females.

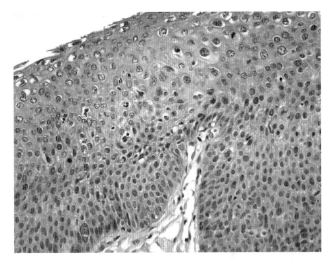

Figure 101.125 Anal intraepithelial neoplasia. The changes here are those of AIN 2 (moderate dysplasia) and would be subsumed under high-grade in situ lesions.

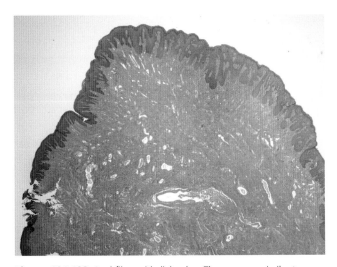

Figure 101.123 Anal fibroepithelial polyp. These appear similar to "skin tags" elsewhere.

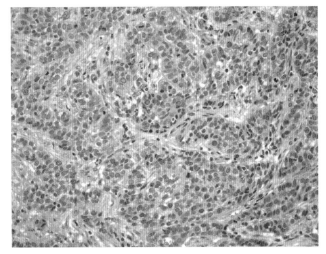

Figure 101.126 Anal squamous cell carcinoma. This example is basaloid (formerly "cloacogenic").

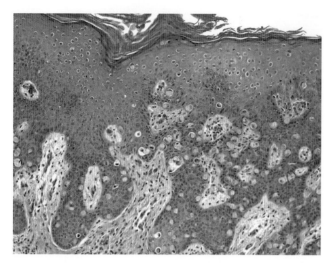

Figure 101.127 Anal Paget disease. Glandular cells proliferate in the squamous mucosa.

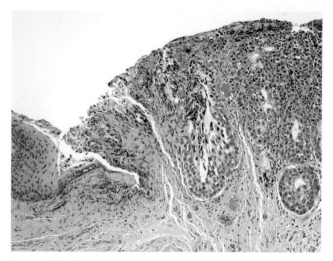

Figure 101.129 Anal melanoma: note the melanin pigment.

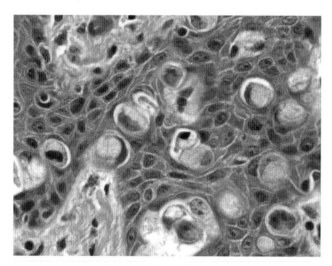

Figure 101.128 Anal Paget disease. At high magnification, intracellular mucin is apparent in these Paget cells.

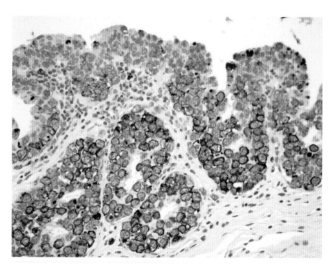

Figure 101.130 Anal melanoma. This immunohistochemical stain (HMB45) is for a relatively melanoma-specific antigen.

102

Evaluation of gastrointestinal motility: emerging technologies

John W. Wiley, Chung Owyang

Introduction

The objective of this chapter is to review selected emerging approaches for monitoring gastrointestinal motility and visceral sensation. We include assessment of visceral sensation because abnormalities in visceral sensory pathways are thought to be involved in a number of functional gastrointestinal motility disorders, such as the irritable bowel syndrome and nonulcer dyspepsia. Many of the emerging methods incorporate advances in volumetric measurements, endosonographic imaging technologies, and functional brain imaging to measure lumenal wall muscle structure and function and central nervous system (CNS) response to activation of sensory pathways innervating the viscera. The emerging methodologies to be discussed include:

- impedance planimetry (IP)
- intralumenal ultrasound applications to gastrointestinal motility
- motility measurements of the stomach: scintigraphic emptying, volumetric assessment [e.g., single photon emission computed tomography (SPECT), three-dimensional (3D) ultrasound, magnetic resonance (MR)] and combined emptying volume measurements
- motility measurements of the pelvic floor, especially with MR imaging (MRI); and assessment of visceral sensation using functional brain imaging techniques
- assessment of regional activation in the brain using positron emission tomography (PET) and functional magnetic resonance imaging (fMRI) in conjunction with visceral stimulation.

This chapter highlights examples of how these emerging technologies have been used in research studies involving human participants.

Atlas of Gastroenterology, 4th edition. Edited by Tadataka Yamada, David H. Alpers, Anthony N. Kalloo, Neil Kaplowitz, Chung Owyang, and Don W. Powell. © 2009 Blackwell Publishing, ISBN: 978-1-4051-6909-7

Impedance planimetry

Background

Recently, tools have been developed for studying both the active (phasic and tonic contractions) and passive function using impedance planimetry before and during administration of drugs that affect gastrointestinal (GI) motility. Measurements of interest include tension, stress and strain because these endpoints give information about the elastic properties of the gut wall and mechanoreceptors respond more directly to these parameters than to pressure and volume. Muscle function can be more accurately evaluated when force and tension are measured rather than the pressure generated by contractions. The most commonly employed bag distention technique is the barostat but techniques such as impedance planimetry and distention combined with imaging techniques give more detailed geometric information that more accurately represent the actual motility pattern. For example, rather than analyzing pressure–volume relationships based on the barostat, impedance planimetry generates data on the cross-sectional area (CSA) of the bag during distention. This method provides improved documentation of the dynamic changes in the alimentary lumen diameter during contraction and relaxation compared with volume measurements.

Applications of impedance planimetry to gastrointestinal motility

Data obtained using IP provide more detailed information than conventional manometry regarding the contractile patterns in the compartment of interest, particularly the elasticity of the gut wall. Changes in the elastic properties of the gut wall have been implicated in a variety of GI motility disorders. Some examples of how this technology has been employed to study disorders affecting GI motor function are provided below.

Systemic sclerosis (SS) is a connective tissue disease that affects the gastrointestinal (GI) tract. Previous studies have shown decreased and abnormal intestinal motility, dilation, and a stiffer wall. However, because of the limitations of conventional recording techniques, little is known about the underlying basis for altered muscle mechanics in this population. As discussed previously, impedance planimetry allows the study of several properties of muscle mechanics in vivo, including the wall–stretch ratio, tension, shortening velocity and muscle power, which can be calculated from pressure and cross-sectional area data. Patients with SS demonstrated increased wall stiffness and impaired muscle dynamics, including reduced power and decreased velocity of the duodenum, which correlated well with clinical symptoms (Fig. 102.1). The circumferential tension–stretch ratio diagrams showed a similar curve pattern for the controls and the patients with SS. Thus, the passive tension curves were exponential and the active tonic and phasic tension curves showed an ascending leg, a local maximum and the initial part of the descending leg in both the volunteers and patients. However, the tension–stretch ratio clearly decreased in the patients with SS compared with the volunteers. By comparing the tracings in the middle and the bottom curves, it appears that the duration of disease is important. The translation to the left on the stretch ratio axis indicates that the intestine becomes stiffer in the patients with SS and the low tension indicates that the muscle does not have the ability to contract with the same force as in the volunteers. Both in the patients and in the volunteers, the active tonic and phasic tension curves appear to peak at the same stretch ratio values. However, IP does not provide information regarding whether the impaired muscle function could result from reduced contractility of individual muscle cells, a reduced number of muscle cells or increased stiffness of the matrix surrounding the muscle. In addition, the reduced contractility may also be influenced by lumenal dilation, causing a shift of the tension–stretch curves.

The efficacy of potential therapeutic interventions has also been examined using IP. For example, theophylline has been proposed as a potentially effective treatment for noncardiac chest pain. The effects of intravenous theophylline or placebo were examined on esophageal sensorimotor function and chest pain, in patients with esophageal hypersensitivity, after intravenous theophylline or placebo. The CSA of the esophagus increased significantly after theophylline compared with the placebo. The tension–strain relationship shifted significantly to the right in the group of subjects who received i.v. theophylline but was unchanged in those who received placebo (Fig. 102.2). Based on these data, a second randomized 4-week cross-over study was performed. Oral theophylline and placebo were administered to patients with esophageal hypersensitivity. Frequency, intensity, and duration of chest pain episodes were evaluated. Theophylline relaxed the esophageal wall, decreased hypersensitivity, and decreased chest pain.

In another application, impedance planimetry was used to examine the sensory and biomechanical properties of the esophagus in patients with gastroesophageal reflux disease (GERD) before and after laparoscopic Nissen fundoplication compared with healthy controls. The pathophysiology of persistent GERD symptoms after antireflux surgery is unclear. At baseline, GERD patients had lower thresholds for first perception, discomfort, and pain compared with controls. The esophagus was more reactive and less distensible in patients compared with controls. In GERD patients, before Nissen fundoplication, the curve that expresses the relationship between tension and strain shifted significantly to the left compared with controls (Fig. 102.3). This suggested that the esophageal wall was less distensible, or stiffer, in GERD patients. After Nissen fundoplication, in patients with persistent symptoms, the curve shifted to the right and was similar to the curve for controls, suggesting that the distensibility of the esophageal wall had improved. Of interest, some patients demonstrated persistent symptoms after Nissen fundoplication. In this population the sensory thresholds were unchanged but esophageal wall reactivity decreased, and distensibility improved. The authors conclude that laparoscopic Nissen fundoplication improves esophageal biomechanical dysfunction but not the underlying hypersensitivity. These observations highlight the application of this technology to identify and differentiate between abnormalities in the biomechanical properties of gut wall and primary sensory mechanisms.

Summary

Current understanding of the "mechanical" physiology of the GI tract is based on measurement techniques such as manometry. The objective of techniques such as impedance planimetry is to better understand the muscle properties of the gut wall and how they relate to mechanisms involved in symptom generation. The advantage of the IP method is improved correlation of the measurements with lumenal wall elasticity based on assessment of changes in the balloon cross-sectional area compared with changes in the balloon volume. As an experimental tool for assessment of distention-induced responses, IP appears to be superior to other available distention techniques because the mechanoreceptors are most likely sensitive to mechanical parameters, such as force, tension, and strain, rather than to direct variation in pressure or volume. Direct comparisons with traditional barostat recording methods in specific patient populations in the absence and presence of interventions are required to establish the superiority of the impedance planimetric method in clinical research and before general acceptance of this approach as a diagnostic tool in the clinical setting. Similar to the barostat method this approach is relatively invasive requiring conscious sedation and intubation for positioning of the recording apparatus.

Application of endosonography to study anatomy and motor function in the gastrointestinal tract

Background

Endosonography has emerged as a useful tool for studying the visceral wall and adjacent structures in detail. This section focuses on the utility of endosonography to assess biomechanical and motor function of the gastrointestinal tract.

Echoendoscopes combine endoscopy with integrated ultrasound transducers. They may have radial or curvilinear array transducers using frequencies between 7.5 and 30 MHz. Typically, higher frequencies provide more anatomical detail but less penetration. Small transducers or miniprobes have been developed that have a diameter that allows the probe to be inserted through the biopsy channel of a conventional endoscope. The small diameter probes can be passed into stenotic areas or areas with smaller lumenal diameters, such as the biliary tree, not traversable with larger echoendoscopes. Ultrasound systems are available that combine linear compound scanning with mechanical sector scanning or M-mode. Doppler sonography can provide important information about vascular flow and separate vessels from other echo-poor structures.

Applications of endosonography in the clinical setting to study biomechanics and GI motility

Achalasia

Achalasia is a disorder in esophageal motility and is defined by its typical manometry pattern. The diagnosis can be supported by findings at barium radiography that may show delayed passage through the lower esophageal sphincter and dilation of the body of the esophagus. At manometry, achalasia is characterized primarily by aperistalsis of the esophageal body and incomplete relaxation of the lower esophageal sphincter. In autopsy studies of patients with achalasia, the thickness of the lower esophageal sphincter is increased. Using high frequency ultrasound probes, it has been shown that the thickening of muscularis propria mainly appear in the inner circular portion (Fig. 102.4). The available literature suggests that thickening of the circular layer of the muscularis propria at the gastric cardia may support the diagnosis of evolving achalasia. A study of the esophageal wall in patients with newly diagnosed achalasia was performed using a sector scanning echoendoscope with a 12 MHz transducer frequency. The endosonographic findings were correlated with manometric features and clinical symptoms and suggest that in these patients an increase in thickness of the muscularis propria occurs at the level of the lower esophageal sphincter and the proximal 5 cm of the sphincter. Miller et al. (Gastrointest Endosc 1995;42:545)

used a 20 MHz radial ultrasound transducer to examine the width of the total muscularis propria, and the circular and longitudinal smooth muscles at the lower esophageal sphincter in patients with achalasia, comparing them with 19 normal subjects. They found that the mean width of these muscles was increased in patients with achalasia. However, because of overlap in muscle width thicknesses between these groups it was noted that a thickened muscularis propria cannot be used to differentiate clinically between patients with achalasia and normal controls. Nevertheless, investigators observed that the mean diameter of both the longitudinal and the circular smooth muscle layers at the lower esophageal sphincter were wider in patients with achalasia than in normal subjects. Trowers et al. (Gastrointest Endosc 1992;38:244A) used a single crystal transendoscopic probe providing linear images and showed that patients with achalasia have a fourfold increase in the thickness of the muscularis propria compared with the control subjects.

Scleroderma

Patients suffering from systemic sclerosis frequently demonstrate clinical gastrointestinal manifestations, such as swallowing problems. Endosonography can be useful to define morphological as well as physiological abnormalities of the esophagus in patients with scleroderma of the esophagus. Lieu et al. (Radiology 1992;184:721) found that ultrasound images in patients with scleroderma correlated with established pathological descriptions, such as smooth muscle atrophy, variable fibrosis, and collagen deposition. Specifically, increased echogenicity and thinning of the muscularis propria, consistent with fibrosis and atrophy of the smooth muscle were observed. Miller et al. (Gastroenterology 1993;105:31) used a 20 MHz ultrasound transducer to evaluate patients with systemic sclerosis and healthy subjects. Postmortem autopsy studies were also performed to compare histopathological abnormalities with sonographic findings in the esophagus. Hyperechoic abnormalities were observed ultrasonographically in the muscularis propria in patients with scleroderma but not in normal controls. These findings corresponded to fibrosis noted in histological examinations. A positive correlation between esophageal hyperechoic and manometric abnormalities was also observed.

Nutcracker esophagus

Patients with nutcracker esophagus (NE) experience dysphagia or chest pain owing to strong peristaltic contractions. High-pressure amplitudes are found at manometry. Melzer et al. (Gastrointest Endosc 1997;46:223; 1995;42:366) used an echoendoscope to examine the thickness of the muscularis propria at the gastroesophageal junction and in the lower, middle, and upper esophagus in patients with NE. The muscularis propria was thickened in one-third of the patients. This thickening, however, did not correspond to the location and magnitude of the manometric abnormality and did not correlate with the clinical presentation. They also reported a patient with NE and esophageal pressures exceeding 800 mmHg in whom endoscopic ultrasonography demonstrated a markedly thickened esophageal muscularis propria. The hypertrophy of the muscularis propria extended from the gastroesophageal junction upwards to the midesophagus.

Gastroduodenal motility

Ultrasonography can provide both qualitative and quantitative information about motility, both in a fasting state and after meal ingestion. Gastric contractions and propagation of waves can be visualized and evaluated by ultrasound. Both frequency and amplitude can be monitored; the latter defined as the maximal reduction of antral area induced by a contraction, as a fraction of the relaxed area. High-resolution ultrasound using frequencies in the range of 7–15 MHz enables detailed studies of gastric wall-layer involvement during peristalsis (Fig. 102.5). Ultrasound is more sensitive than manometry in detecting antral contractions, particularly nonocclusive contractions.

Novel techniques and applications

Three-dimensional (3D) endoultrasonography (EUS) images are thought to be easier to understand and communicate than the mental reconstruction of two-dimensional (2D) images. Currently, 3D techniques are under development for most imaging modalities and 3D-EUS may be applied for improved recognition of the GI anatomy and pathological lesions. 3D-EUS images can be obtained using images acquired by echoendoscopes or miniprobes. Typically, a pullback device has been employed to obtain parallel 2D images that are reconstructed to a 3D image. Acquired ultrasound images can be stored and digitized using frame grabbing but direct digitizing of ultrasound raw data is increasingly being used in new scanners. Advanced software programs containing different rendering or other reconstruction algorithms are used for post processing and display of 3D ultrasound data, which can be studied using any plane slicing, segmentation, and volume calculation. The advanced programs enable the import of image data that are acquired both with mechanical devices and magnetic position sensors as well as with endosonographic acquisitions. Manual segmentation or semiautomatic rendering of structures in the 3D data set makes accurate volume estimation and reconstruction of organs or pathological tissue achievable. A representative display from a 3D ultrasound system is shown in Figure 102.6. Additional information regarding 3D ultrasound systems is available in the literature.

Strain rate imaging

Strain rate imaging (SRI) is a recently introduced technique to measure deformation of biological tissue. The technique is based on tissue velocity imaging, which is an ultrasound technique that provides quantitative information on velocities of deformation within a tissue. By color-coded tissue velocity imaging, velocity data from the whole field of view are available simultaneously. This allows extraction of other parameters through spatial and temporal processing of the velocity data. Strain and strain rate are examples of such parameters. The methods have primarily been used in echocardiography, but other uses have also been reported, including measurements of gastric motor function. For example, estimation of relative strain of the muscle layer of the gastric wall by Doppler ultrasonography is feasible (Fig. 102.7) and enables detailed mapping of local strain distribution. Even though the two layers cannot be separated visually in the 2D images, SRI is capable of distinguishing contractile activity of the longitudinal and circular muscle layers. It is anticipated that ongoing and future studies will determine whether SRI can be applied to evaluate the relation between symptoms and biomechanical factors in clinical disorders.

Assessment of gastric accommodation and volume

Recently, a novel method was reported that measures gastric "accommodation" as the percentage change in planar 2D gastric cross-sectional area, using a left anterior oblique planar projection, and the percentage change in total single photon emission computed tomography (SPECT) gastric voxel counts (by 3D imaging) compared with baseline fasting volume using NIH image software (http://rsb.info.nih.gov/ij/index.html). The procedure uses anterior and posterior images for estimation of gastric emptying, followed by SPECT imaging with a separate SPECT camera every 20 min. This approach is potentially significant because it allows simultaneous measurements of gastric emptying and volume, thereby, providing a means to noninvasively assess the pathophysiology of gastric motility disorders.

Other studies confirm the ability to measure the dynamics of gastric volume and emptying functions in health. One approach involves tomographic acquisition over 360° on a dual-head gamma camera SPECT (Fig. 102.8). Specialized software is used to acquire the required planar images from the tomographic data and integrate them into the gastric emptying study and to measure gastric accommodation (Fig. 102.9). The results suggest that the volume measured is not just the volume of the meal in the stomach.

Magnetic resonance imaging (MRI) of the stomach (Fig. 102.10) has the potential of being a safe, noninvasive test that measures emptying, volume change and wall motion as a surrogate of contractile activity without radiation exposure. It is noteworthy that MRI has the ability to separately assess the emptying of fat and water from the stomach. Additional validation is required for MRI of the stomach, e.g., comparison with barostat, including studies in disease and response to interventions, including but not limited to the effects of nutrients and response to prokinetic drugs. The ability to resolve wall movement and to apply acquisition and projection algorithms developed for dynamic imaging for other indications, such as MR angiography, and the absence of radiation exposure make MRI of gastric function a potentially attractive technology, as long as it is affordable. However, MR imaging of the small intestine is in the developmental stages. The resolution of abdominal organ imaging is enhanced with techniques such as respiratory gating and multiarray imaging using two surface MRI coils.

Motility measurements of the pelvic floor, pelvic organs, and anorectum

Pelvic floor MRI has the potential to characterize several components of continence and defecation simultaneously. Dynamic imaging (Fig. 102.11) and the use of magnets that allow for studies in the seated position provide detailed information about structure and integration with function that was not possible using a combination of techniques, such as barium defecography and endoanal ultrasound. For example, a recent report demonstrates the occurrence of different phenotypes of obstructed defecation, abnormal structure and function of the pelvic floor and anal sphincters in people with incontinence and physiological alterations associated with aging. Frokjaer et al. (Neurogastroenterol Motil 2007;19:253) used a flexible PVC catheter equipped with a bag for gut distention and a radiopaque ring allowing proper positioning of the probe to examine sigmoid colon biomechanics in conjunction with MRI (Fig. 102.12). The geometry of the distended sigmoid colon was complex and varied considerably between the subjects, as depicted in Figure 102.13. The circumferential radii of curvature increased, i.e., increase in diameter, during the sigmoid distention but showed a highly inhomogeneous spatial distribution that was observed in all subjects. Histograms illustrating the distribution (frequency diagram) of the circumferential wall stress and wall thickness throughout the sigmoid wall are shown in Figure 102.14. The histograms reveal "bell-shaped" distributions with an overall increase in wall stress and tendency of decrease in peak wall thickness during the distention. The sensation induced by distention before and after administration of the muscarinic receptor antagonist butylscopolamine is shown in Figure 102.15 as a function of bag volume, bag pressure and the average values of the 3D distribution of the circumferential strain, circumferential wall tension and stress. Administration of butylscopolamine did not affect the wall thickness, circumferential length and strain. Bag pressure and wall stress were reduced by smooth muscle relaxation. Therefore, sensory response decreased as a function of circumferential strain, i.e. right

shift of the stimulus–response curves in the presence of butylscopolamine. The nonhomogeneous and complex 3D sigmoid geometry suggest that this type of 3D modeling will likely be useful and provide reliable data for detailed studies of the biomechanical and mechanosensory properties. This technique may be useful in the clinical setting for understanding biomechanical properties and visceral perception in several hollow visceral organs.

The role of functional brain imaging in the assessment of visceral sensation in health and disease

We include a section on functional brain imaging because there is general acceptance that selective activation of brain regions occurs in response to regional distention of the gut in health and emerging data supporting differential activation of brain regions in patients with functional bowel disorders (FBDs), such as the irritable bowel syndrome (IBS) and nonulcer dyspepsia (NUD). For example, several reports suggest that the limbic and emotional motor system in the brain may be differentially activated on positron emission tomography (PET) or functional brain imaging (fMRI) in patients with functional gastrointestinal diseases. However, brain imaging in FBDs requires additional technical and methodological advances to clarify the reported differences in regional brain activation and their relationship to stress, pain and emotion. The regions of activation often involve neural circuitry of several interacting regions of the brain which is not addressed in some manuscripts. For example, regions in the cerebellum can be activated during rectal distention without any clear rationale regarding why this occurs. Other unresolved issues include the imaging differences between PET and fMRI and differences in brain regions activated in males and females in response to painful rectal distention. Methodological concerns include:
- the confounding effects of the distention itself vs anticipation of the distention on imaging
- the potentially significant central effects of placebo controls
- inclusion of clinically heterogeneous patients (e.g. diagnosis and severity of disease)
- existence of comorbidities such as fibromyalgia. For example, anterior cingulate cortex activation during somatic pain appears to reflect anticipation.

This was confirmed in patients with functional gastrointestinal disorders. However, it has also been reported that actual and anticipated esophageal pain elicits similar cortical responses.

The timing and intensity of brain activation may be different in health and disease. For example, cortical activity associated with perceived and unperceived esophageal acid exposure in patients with gastroesophageal reflux disease

(GERD) and healthy controls, respectively, involves multiple brain regions, but it occurs more rapidly and with greater intensity in patients with GERD than the activity in response to subliminal acid exposure in healthy controls. Another marker of hypersensitivity in IBS may be detected by an enhanced response to subliminal stimuli. A study in patients with IBS and age- and sex-matched healthy controls focused on fMRI activity using a computerized barostat-controlled rectal distention device that generated equal subliminal distention pressures (e.g. 10, 15 and 20 mmHg) in both controls and patients. In all three distention levels, the fMRI activity in IBS patients was significantly larger than in controls, supporting the existence of hypersensitivity in this patient group irrespective of stimulus-related cognitive processes (Fig. 102.16).

Summary

Further validation of the emerging technologies discussed in this chapter is required both for research purposes and

before their routine application in clinical practice. Validation should include critical appraisal of the:

• internal validity (accurately drawing conclusions about the source population based on information from the study population) and external validity (independent, blind comparison with a reference standard)

• technology's performance (in particular, reproducibility and coefficient of variation)

• technology's sensitivity (proportion of true positives of all positives) and specificity (proportion of true negatives of all negatives)

• likelihood ratios (that is the link between the pretest probability of the diagnosis of a disorder and the probability after the test)

• the responsiveness of the diagnostic test to change and the relationship between that change and a change in clinical outcome

• the cost-benefit of the technology, either as a diagnostic tool or therapeutic intervention, for acceptance in the clinical setting.

These are the standards to which diagnostic tests are held in other areas.

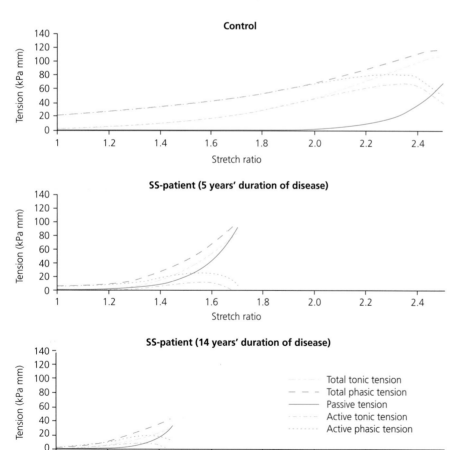

Figure 102.1 Representative length–tension curves including total phasic tension, total tonic tension, active phasic tension, active tonic tension, and passive tension obtained in a volunteer (top), a patient with duration of systemic sclerosis for 5 years (middle) and a patient with duration of systemic sclerosis for 14 years (bottom). The key identifying the meanings of the different lines in the third panel applies to all panels in this figure.

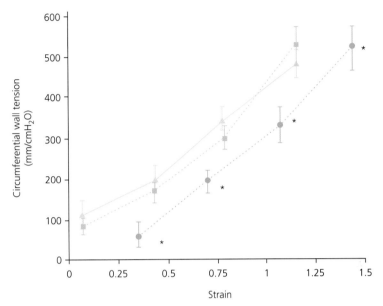

Figure 102.2 Effects of placebo and intravenous theophylline on circumferential wall tension–strain relationship. The curve in subjects that received theophylline (blue circle dotted line) is significantly shifted to the right when compared with placebo (blue squares dotted line). These data suggest that the esophageal wall relaxed and became more deformable or more compliant after theophylline infusion (mean ± SEM).

$*P < 0.05$ when compared to placebo

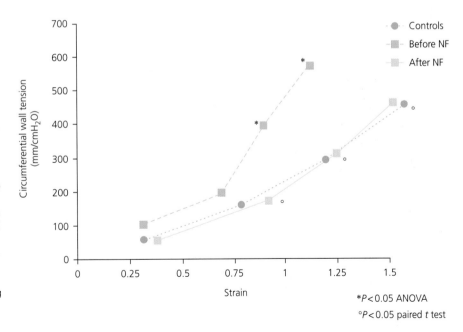

Figure 102.3 Relationship between circumferential wall tension and strain in response to graded balloon distention in controls and GERD patients before and after Nissen fundoplication (NF) (mean ± SEM). The curve in patients with GERD before surgery significantly shifted to the left compared with controls. This suggests that for the same level of tension (force), the degree of strain or the deformability of the esophageal wall was less in patients with GERD. However, after NF the curve shifted significantly to the right and was similar to that of the controls, suggesting that the deformability of the esophageal wall had improved after NF.

$*P < 0.05$ ANOVA
$°P < 0.05$ paired t test

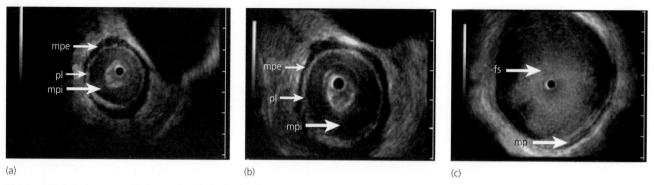

(a)   (b)   (c)

Figure 102.4 Endosonographic images **(a, b)** obtained with a 15 MHz miniprobe in a patient with achalasia showing the longitudinal, outer layer of the proper muscle (mpe) separated from a thickened circular, inner layer (mpi) by an echogenic layer corresponding to the localization of the plexus myentericus (pl). **(c)** This shows a dilated esophageal lumen with food content (fs). A normal aspect of the proper muscle is seen (mp).

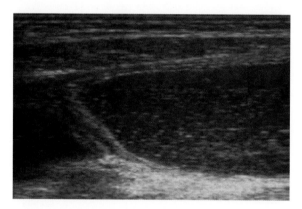

Figure 102.5 Ultrasonogram of the fluid-filled gastric antrum showing the different wall layers and a propagating contraction wave that occludes the lumen.

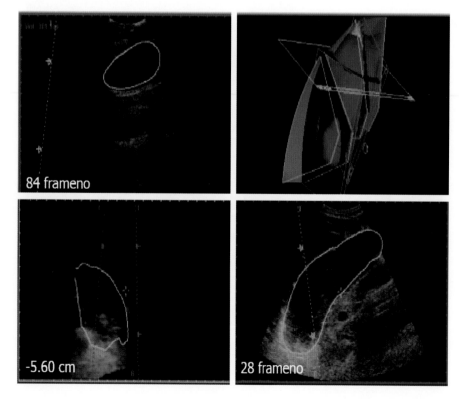

Figure 102.6 A 3D reconstruction of the total stomach volume (red) in the upper left panel. The acquisition is based on magnetic scanhead tracking. Three orthogonal orientation planes are shown in red, green, and blue. The upper left panel is a volume reconstruction window where manual outlining of the structures are made.

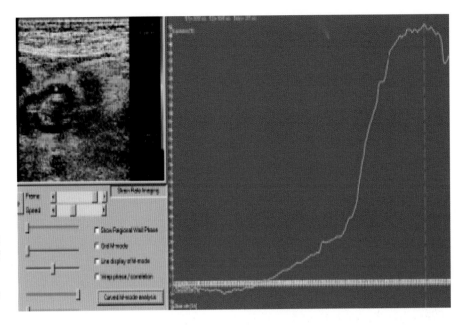

Figure 102.7 These graphics outline the relative radial strain of the circular muscle layer of the antral wall. The exact sampling point in the gastric wall is denoted with a red marker in the color Doppler ultrasonogram of the **left panel**. In the **right panel**, the positive strain curve with a maximum of 150% radial elongation of the muscle layer is demonstrated.

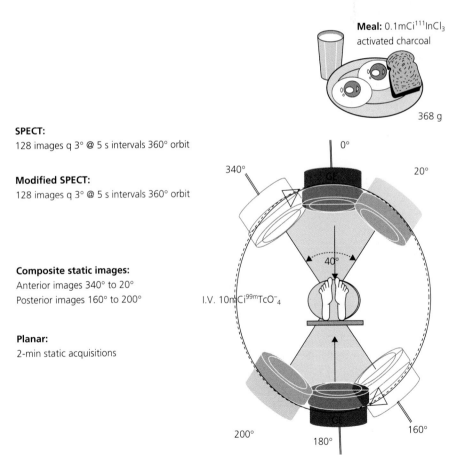

Meal: $0.1mCi^{111}InCl_3$ activated charcoal

368 g

SPECT:
128 images q 3° @ 5 s intervals 360° orbit

Modified SPECT:
128 images q 3° @ 5 s intervals 360° orbit

Composite static images:
Anterior images 340° to 20°
Posterior images 160° to 200°

Planar:
2-min static acquisitions

I.V. $10mCi^{99m}TcO_4^-$

0°
20°
340°
40°
160°
180°
200°

Figure 102.8 Method for combined measurements of gastric volume and emptying. SPECT, single photon emission computed tomography.

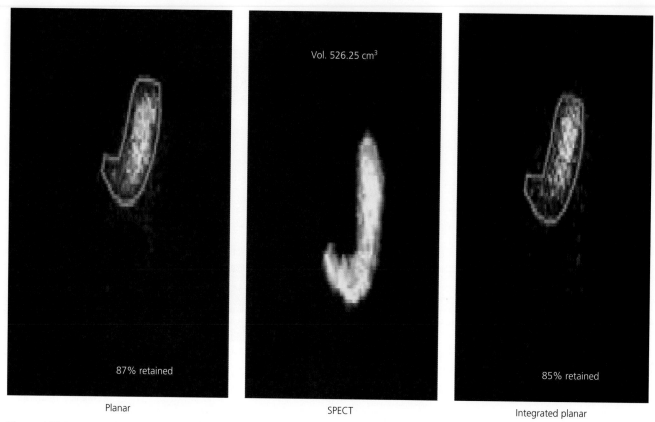

Figure 102.9 Images of the stomach by planar scans, single photon emission computed tomography (SPECT) and composite SPECT acquisition to construct anterior image using the method described by Burton et al. (Am J Physiol 2005;289:261). Note that the amount of food retained in the stomach is similar when calculated using the traditional two-dimensional or planar anterior and posterior gamma camera images. The central image demonstrates the stomach volume simultaneously estimated using SPECT.

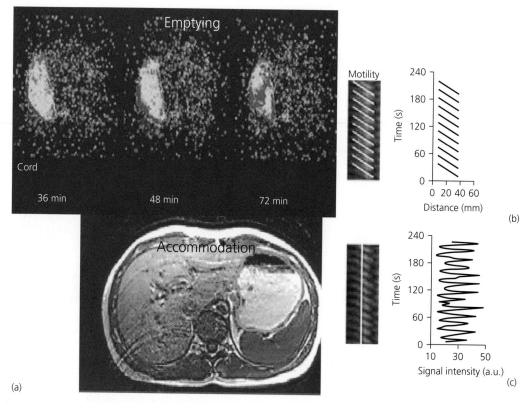

Figure 102.10 Magnetic resonance (MR) imaging provides the potential to estimate gastric emptying, accommodation, and wall motion in a noninvasive manner.

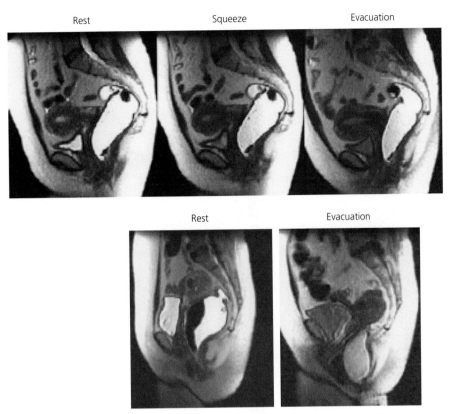

Rest   Squeeze   Evacuation

Rest   Evacuation

Figure 102.11 Defecation dynamics in patients with evacuation disorders owing to immobile perineum **(upper)** or descending perineum syndrome **(lower)** using magnetic resonance (MR) imaging.

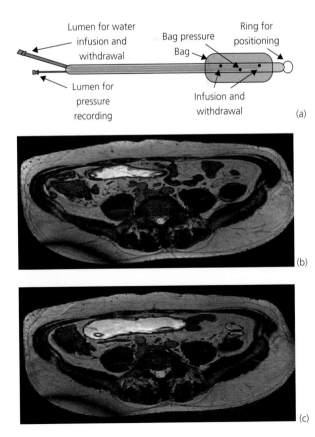

Lumen for water infusion and withdrawal

Bag pressure

Ring for positioning

Bag

Lumen for pressure recording

Infusion and withdrawal

(a)

(b)

(c)

Figure 102.12 The probe **(a)** allows bag distention and pressure measurements during magnetic resonance imaging (MRI). Transverse MRI shows the distended water-filled bag (high signal intensity) in the sigmoid colon at 100 mL **(b)** and 300 mL **(c)**.

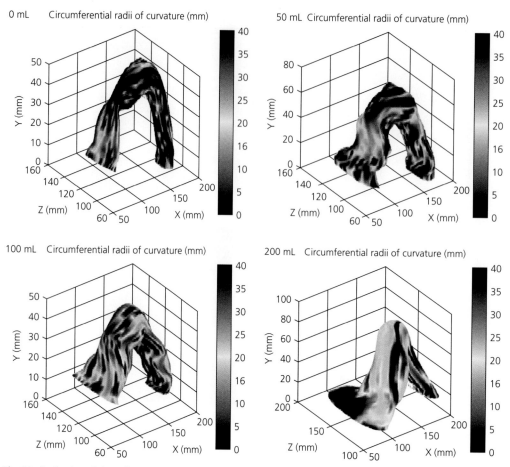

Figure 102.13 The 3D distribution of circumferential principal radii of curvatures in one volunteer before administration of butylscopolamine at infused volumes of 0, 50, 100 and 200 mL.

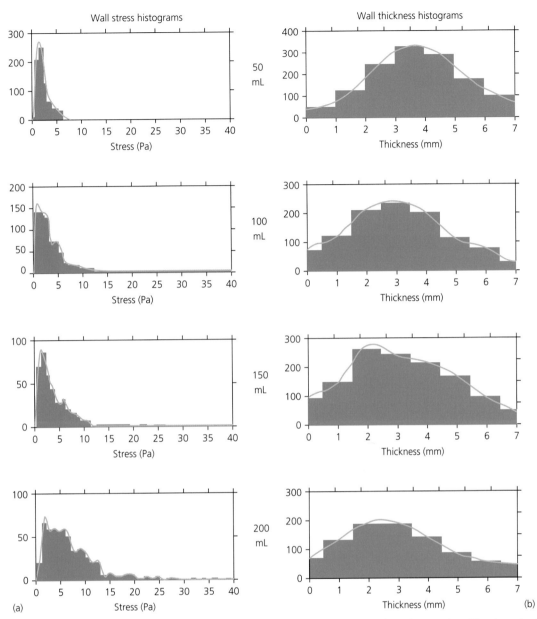

Figure 102.14 Histograms illustrating the distribution of the wall stress **(a)** and wall thickness **(b)** before administration of butylscopolamine throughout the 3D sigmoid surface in one subject are given. The y-axis indicates the number of surface squares. During distention, the distribution of stress clearly shifted to the right, while the distribution of wall thickness was not affected to the same degree. The same pattern was seen in all subjects.

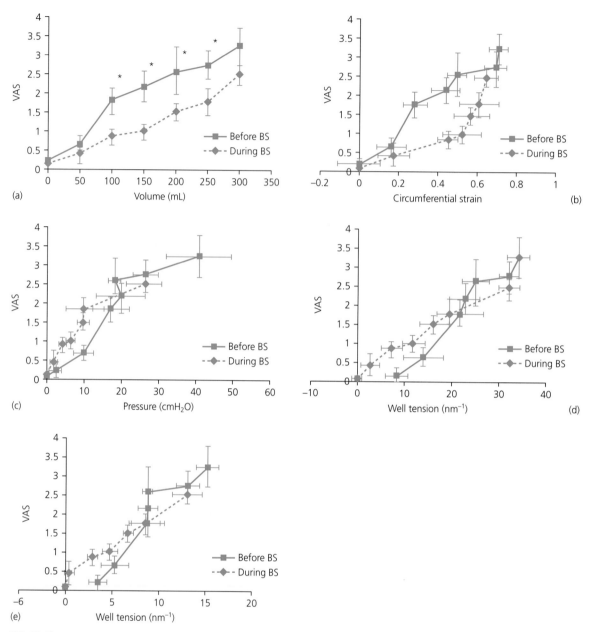

Figure 102.15 The sensory response rated on a visual analog scale (VAS) is illustrated as a function of infused bag volume **(a)**, average 3D circumferential strain **(b)**, bag pressure **(c)**, circumferential tension **(d)**, and stress **(e)** before and after administration of butylscopolamine. Asterisk (*) indicates significant difference for the volume data. BS, butylscopolamine. The error bars indicate standard error of the mean (SEM).

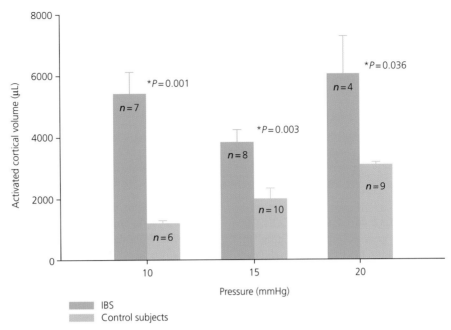

Figure 102.16 Total fMRI cortical activity volume response to three levels of subliminal rectal distention pressures in patients with IBS and controls. In all three subliminal distention pressures, the fMRI activity volumes in IBS patients were significantly larger than those of controls. Furthermore, fMRI cortical activity volumes showed a stimulus intensity-dependent relationship in controls ($P < 0.001$), but not in IBS patients for the three analyzed pressure levels.

Figure credits

Chapter 1
Figures 1.8, 1.9, 1.10, 1.11, 1.12 and 1.13 From Elta GH. Approach to the patient with gastrointestinal bleeding. In: Humes HD, DuPont HL, Gardner LP, et al. (eds). Kelley's Textbook of Internal Medicine, 4th edn. Philadelphia: Lippincott Williams & Wilkins, 1997.

Chapter 2
Figure 2.2 From Ali MA, Luxton W, Waller WH. Serum ferritin concentration and bone marrow iron stores: a prospective study. Can Med Assoc J 1978;118:945.
Figure 2.16 From Ahlquist DA, Wieand HS, Moertel CG, et al. Accuracy of fecal occult blood screening for colorectal neoplasia. A prospective study using Hemoccult and Hemo-Quant tests. JAMA 1993;269:1262.
Figures 2.17 and 2.21 From Stewart J, Ahlquist DA, McGill DB. Gastrointestinal blood loss and anaemia in runners. Ann Intern Med 1984;100:843.

Chapter 3
Figure 3.4 From Nussbaum MS. Diseases of the appendix. In: Bell RH Jr, Rikkers LE, Mulholland MW (eds). Digestive Tract Surgery: A Text and Atlas. Philadelphia: Lippincott-Raven, 1996.

Chapter 5
Figure 5.1 and 5.3 From Thillainayagam AV, Hunt JB, Farthing MJ. Enhancing clinical efficacy of oral therapy: is low osmolality the key? Gastroenterology 1998; 114:197.
Figure 5.2 From Kilgore PE, Holman RC, Clarke MJ, Glass RI. Trends of diarrheal disease-associated mortality in U.S. children,1968 through 1991. JAMA 1995;274:1143.
Figure 5.5 From Surawicz CM. Food poisoning: a practical approach to management. Gastrointest Dis Today 1997;6:12.
Figure 5.6 From Misiewicz JJ, Forbes A, Price A, et al. Atlas of clinical gastroenterology, 2nd edn. London: Wolfe, 1994.
Figures 5.7 and 5.8 From Dhouri MR, Huang G, Shiau YF. Sudden stain of fecal fat: new insight into an old test. Gastroenterology 1989;96:423.

Figure 5.9 From Hamilton J, Lunch MJ, Reilly BJ. Active celiac disease in children. Q J Med 38:142.
Figure 5.11 From Fine KD, Fordtran JS. The effect of diarrhea on fecal fat excretion. Gastroenterology 1989; 96:423.
Figure 5.12 From Jabbari M, Wild G, Goresky CA, et al. Scalloped valvulae conniventes: an endoscopic marker of celiac sprue. Gastroenterology 1988;95:1519.
Figure 5.13 From Myner TP, Moss AA. Radiologic evaluation of the malabsorption syndrome. Pract Gastroenterol 1980;4:25.
Figure 5.14 From Marsh MN (ed.). Coeliac Disease, Oxford: Blackwell Scientific, 1992.
Figure 5.15 From Bayless TM. Lactose deficiency and intolerance to milk. Viewpoints on Digestive Disease 1971;3:3.
Figure 5.16 From Silverstein FE, Tytgat GNJ. Gastrointestinal Endoscopy, 3rd edn. London: Mosby-Wolfe, 1997.
Figure 5.17 From Wrong O, Metcalfe-Gibson A, Morrison BIR, et al. In vivo dialysis of faeces as a method of stool analysis. Clin Sci 1965;28:357.
Figure 5.18 From Cutz E, Rhoads JM, Drumm B, et al. Microvillus inclusion disease: an inherited defect of brush-border assembly and differentiation. N Engl J Med 1989;320:646.
Figure 5.19 and 5.20 From Maton PN, O'Dorisio TM, Howe BA, et al. Effects of long-acting somatostatin analogue (SMS 201-955) in a patient with pancreatic cholera. N Engl J Med 312;18:1985.

Chapter 6
Figure 6.5 From Guerrant RL, Van Gilder T, Steiner T, et al. Practice guidelines for the management of infectious diarrhea. Clin Infect Dis 2001;32:331.
Figure 6.8 From Haque R, Huston CD, Hughes M, et al. Amebiasis. N Engl J Med 2003;348:1568.
Figure 6.9 From Warshauer DM, Napierkowski JJ, Sachar DS, et al. Image of the Month. Gastroenterology 2003; 125:8.
Figure 6.11 From Herwaldt BL. Cyclospora cayetanensis: a review, focusing on the outbreaks of cyclosporiasis in the 1990s. Clin Infect Dis 2000;31:1040.

Chapter 7

Figure 7.1 From Higgins PD, Johanson JF. Epidemiology of constipation in North America: a systematic review. Am J Gastroenterol 2004;99:4.

Figure 7.11 Rao SSC, Sadeghi P, Beaty J et al. Ambulatory 24-hour colonic manometry in slow-transit constipation. Am J Gastroenterol 2004;99:2405.

Chapter 8

Figures 8.2 and 8.3 Adapted from Lindsay KL, Hoofnagle JH. Serologic tests for viral hepatitis. In: Kaplowitz N (ed.). Liver and Biliary Disease, 2nd edn. Baltimore: Williams and Wilkins, 1996.

Chapter 11

Figure 11.7 From Rumack, BH. Acetaminophen hepatotoxicity: The first 35 years. Clinical Toxicology 2002;40:3.

Chapter 12

Figures 12.1 and 12.2 From Scott JD, Gretch DR. Molecular diagnostics of hepatitis C virus infection: a systematic review. JAMA 2007;297:724.

Figure 12.3 From Ferenci P, Fried MW, Shifman ML, et al. Predicting sustained virological responses in chronic hepatitis C patients treated with peginterferon alfa-2a (40KD)/ribavirin. J Hepatol 2005;43:425.

Figures 12.5 and 12.7 From Lok AS, McMahon BJ. Chronic hepatitis B. Hepatology 2007;45:507.

Figure 12.8 From Rapti I, Dimou E, Mitsoula P, et al. Adding-on versus switching-to adefovir therapy in lamivudine-resistant HBeAg-negative chronic hepatitis B. Hepatology 2007;45:307.

Chapter 15

Figure 15.3 From Kahrilas PJ, Lin S, Chen J, Logemann JA. Oropharyngeal accommodation to swallow volume. Gastroenterology 1996;111:297.

Figure 15.6 From Kahrilas PJ, Ergun GA. Evaluation of the patient with dysphagia. In: Bone R (ed.). Current Practice of Medicine, Philadelphia: Current Medicine, 1996.

Figure 15.12 From Hirano I, Tatum RP, Shi G, et al. Manometric heterogeneity in patients with idiopathic achalasia. Gastroenterology 2001;120:789.

Figure 15.14 From Kahrilas PJ, Dodds WJ, Hogan WJ. The effect of peristaltic dysfunction on esophageal volume clearance. Gastroenterology 1988;94:73.

Figure 15.20 From Stevoff C, Rao S, Parsons W, et al. Case report: endocsosonographic and histopathologic correlates in eosinophilic esophagitis. Gastrointest Endosc 2001;54:373.

Chapter 16

Figure 16.1 From Locke GR 3rd, Talley NJ, Fett SL, et al. Prevalence and clinical spectrum of GER: a population-based study in Olmsted County, Minnesota. Gastroenterology 1997;112:1448.

Figure 16.2 From Mittal RK, Balaban DH. The esophagogastric junction. N Engl J Med 1997;336:924.

Figure 16.2 From Helm JF, Dodds WJ, Pelc LR, et al. Effect of esophageal emptying and saliva on clearance of acid from the esophagus. N Engl J Med 1984;310:284.

Chapter 17

Figure 17.19 From DeSilva R, Stoopack P, Raufman JP. Esophageal fistulae associated with mycobacterial infection in patients at risk for AIDS. Radiology 1990;175:449.

Chapter 18

Figures 18.1, 18.2, 18.3, 18.7 and 18.15 From Eisenberg RL. Gastrointestinal Radiology: A Pattern Approach, 4th edn. Philadelphia: Lippincott Williams & Wilkins, 2003.

Figures 18.4 and 18.11 From Silverstein FE, Tytgat GNJ. Gastrointestinal Endoscopy, 3rd edn. London: Mosby-Wolfe, 1997.

Figures 18.5 and 18.10 Misiewicz JJ, Bartram CI, Cotton PB, et al. Atlas of Gastroenterology. London: Gower, 1988.

Figure 18.11 From Silverstein FE, Tygat GNJ. Gastrointestinal Endoscopy, 3rd edn. London: Mosby-Wolfe, 1997.

Chapter 19

Figure 19.12 Misiewicz JJ. Atlas of Gastroenterology, 2nd edn. London: Mosby-Year Book, 1994.

Figures 19.17, 19.20 and 19.21 From Eisenberg, RL. Gastrointestinal Radiology: A Pattern Approach, 4th edn. Philadelphia: Lippincott Williams & Wilkins, 2003.

Chapter 20

Figure 20.3 From Hollinshead WH, Rosse C. Textbook of Anatomy, 4th edn. Philadelphia: Lippincott Williams & Wilkins, 1985.

Figure 20.4 From Rosse C, Gaddum-Rosse P. Hollinshead's Textbook of Anatomy. Philadelphia: Lippincott-Raven, 1997.

Figure 20.5 From Gartner LP, Hiatt JL. Color Textbook of Histology. Philadelphia: WB Saunders, 1997.

Figure 20.7 From Ross MH, Romrell LJ, Kaye GI. Histology. Baltimore: Lippincott Williams & Wilkins, 1995.

Figure 20.8 From Digestive system. In: Sadler TW (ed.). Langman's Medical Embryology, 5th edn. Baltimore: Lippincott Williams & Wilkins, 1985.

Figure 20.10 From Eisenberg RL. Gastrointestinal Radiology: A Pattern Approach, 4th edn. Philadelphia: Lippincott Williams & Wilkins, 2002.

Chapter 21

Figure 21.2 From Guo JP, Maurer AH, Fisher RS, et al. Extending gastric emptying scintigraphy from 2 h to 4 h detects more patients with gastroparesis. Dig Dis Sci 2001;46:24.

Figure 21.3 From Gonlachanvit S, Maurer AH, Fisher RS, et al. Regional gastric emptying abnormalities in functional dyspepsia and gastroesophagal reflux disease. Neurogastroenterol Motil 2006;18:894.

Figure 21.4 From Knight LC, Parkman HP, Brown KL, et al. Delayed gastric emptying and decreased antral contractility in normal premenopausal woman compared to men. Am J Gastroenterol 1997;92:968.

Figure 21.5 From Simonian HP, Kantor S, Knight LC, et al. Simultaneous assessment of gastric accommodation and emptying: Studies with liquid and solid meals. J Nuclear Med 2004;45:1155.

Figures 21.7 and 21.8 From Parkman HP, Hasler WL, Barnett JL, et al. Electrogastrography: a document prepared by the gastric section of the American Motility Society Clinical GI Motility Testing Task Force. Neurogastroenterol Motil 2003;75:89.

Figure 21.9 From Simonian HP, Panganamamula K, Parkman HP, et al. Multichannel electrogastrography in normal subjects: A multicenter study. Dig Dis Sci 2004;49:594.

Chapter 25

Figures 25.3 and 25.5 From Debas HT, Orloff SL. Surgery for peptic ulcer disease and postgastrectomy syndromes. In Yamada T, Alpers DH, Owyang C, et al (eds). Textbook of Gastroenterology, 2nd edn. Philadelphia: JB Lippincott, 1995.

Chapter 27

Figure 27.1 Larsen WJ (ed.). Human Embryology, 2nd edn. New York: Churchill Livingstone 1997:241.

Figure 27.7 Langer JC. Gastroschisis and omphaocele. Semin Pediatr Surg 1996;5:124.

Chapter 28

Figure 28.1 From Grundy D, Camilleri M. Neurogastroenterology and motility: new millennium, new horizons. Neurogastroenterol Motil 2001;13:177.

Figure 28.2 From Mitros FA. Atlas of Gastrointestinal Pathology. London: Gower, 1988.

Figure 28.4 From Mueller LA, Camilleri M, Emslie-Smith AM. Mitochondrial neurogastointestinal encephalomyopathy: manometric and diagnostic features. Gastroenterology 1999;116:959.

Figures 28.6 and 28.7 From Bonsib SM, Fallon B, Mitros FA, et al. Urologic manifestations of patients with visceral myopathy. J Urol 1984;132:1112.

Figure 28.9 From Smith VV, Eng C, Milla PJ. Intestinal ganglioneuromatosis and multiple endocrine neoplasia type 2B: implications for treatment. Gut 1999; 45:143.

Figures 28.10 and 28.11 From Lee JC, Thuneberg L, Berezin I, et al. Generation of slow waves in membrane potential is an intrinsic property of interstitial cells of Cajal. Am J Physiol 1999;277:G409.

Figures 28.12 and 28.13 From He CL, Bugart L, Wang L, et al. Decreased interstitial cell of Cajal volume in patients with slow transit constipation. Gastroenterology 2000; 118:14.

Figure 28.14 From Ordog T, Takayama I, Cheung WK, et al. Remodeling of networks of interstitial cells of Cajal in a murine model of diabetic gastroparesis. Diabetes 2000; 49:1731.

Figure 28.15 From Mayer EA, Schuffler MD, Rotter JI, et al. Familial visceral neuropathy with autosomal dominant transmission. Gastroenterology 1986;91:1528.

Figure 28.17 From Camilleri M. Medical treatment of chronic intestinal pseudoobstruction. Pract Gastroenterol 1991;15:10.

Figure 28.19 From Choi MG, Camilleri M, O'Brien MD, et al. A study of motility and tone of the left colon in patients with diarrhea due to functional disorders and dysautonomia. Am J Gastroenterol 1997;92:297.

Chapter 29

Figure 29.9 Modified from Johnson S, Gerding D. Clostridium difficile-associated diarrhea. Clin Infect Dis 1998; 26:1027.

Chapter 30

Figure 30.6 From Fantry GT, James SP. Whipple's Disease. Dig Dis 1995;13:108.

Figures 30.11, 30.12, 30.13, 30.14 and 30.15 From Fenoglio-Preiser CM, Noffsinger AE, Stemmermann GN, et al. Nonneoplastic lesions of the small intestine. In: Gastrointestinal Pathology: An Atlas and Text, 2nd edn. Philadelphia: Lippincott-Raven, 1999.

Figure 30.16 From Shull HJ. Human histoplasmosis: a disease with protean manifestations, often with digestive system involvement. Gastroenterology 1953;25:389.

Figures 30.17 and 30.18 From Prescott RJ, Harris M, Banerjee SS. Fungal infections of the small and large intestine. J Clin Pathol 1992;45:806.

Chapter 36

Figures 36.1 and 36.2 From Kodner IJ, Fry RD, Fleschman JW, et al. Colon, rectum and anus. In: Schwartz SI (ed.). Principles of Surgery, 6th edn. New York: McGraw Hill, 1994.

Figures 36.5 and 36.6 Cohn SM, Birnbaum EH. Colon: anatomy and structural anomalies. In: Yamada T, Alpers DH, Owyang C, et al (eds). Textbook of Gastroenterology, 2nd edn. Philadelphia: JB Lippincott, 1995.

Chapter 37

Figures 37.1 and 37.6 From Stenson WF, MacDermott RP. Inflammatory bowel disease. In: Yamada T, Alpers DH, Owyang C, et al (eds). Textbook of Gastroenterology. Philadelphia: JB Lippincott, 1991.

Figures 37.4 and 37.10 From Mitros FA. Atlas of Gastrointestinal Pathology. London: Gower, 1988.

Figures 37.5, 37.40, 37.41, 37.45, 37.46, 37.50, 37.52, 37.53, 37.54 and 37.58 From Silverstein FE, Tytgat GNJ. Gastrointestinal Endoscopy, 3rd edn. London: Mosby-Wolfe, 1997.

Figure 37.16 From Misiewicz JJ, Forbes A, Price A, et al. Atlas of Clinical Gastroenterology, 2nd edn. London: Wolfe, 1994.

Figures 37.18, 37.22, 37.27 and 37.28 From Stenson WF, MacDermott RP. Inflammatory bowel disease. In: Yamada T, Alpers DH, Owyang C, et al (eds). Textbook of Gastroenterology. Philadelphia: JB Lippincott, 1991.

Chapter 38

Figures 38.1, 38.5, 38.6, 38.8, 38.9, 38.11 and 38.12 From Silverstein FE, Tytgat GNJ. Gastrointestinal Endoscopy, 3rd edn. London: Mosby-Wolfe, 1997.

Figures 38.2, 38.3, 38.4 and 38.7 From Blackstone MO. Postsurgical appearances and uncommon colonic conditions. In: Endoscopic Interpretation: Normal and Pathological Appearances of the Gastrointestinal Tract. New York: Raven Press, 1984.

Figure 38.10 From Eisenberg RL. Gastrointestinal Radiology: A Pattern Approach, 4th edn. Philadelphia: Lippincott Williams & Wilkins, 2003.

Figure 38.13 Misiewicz JJ, Bartram CI, Cotton PB, et al. Atlas of Clinical Gastroenterology. London: Gower, 1988.

Chapter 39

Figures 39.1 and 39.16 From Pemberton JH, Armstrong DN, Dietzen CD. Diverticulitis. In: Yamada T, Alpers DH, Owyang CO, et al (eds). Textbook of Gastroenterology, 2nd edn. Philadelphia: JB Lippincott, 1995.

Figure 39.2, 39.8, 39.10, 39.11, 39.12 and 39.17 From Young-Fadok TM, Pemberton JH. Colonic diverticular disease: epidemiology and pathophysiology. In: Rose BD (ed.). UpToDate in Medicine [CD-ROM]. Wellesley, MA, UpToDate, 1997.

Chapter 40

Figure 40.1 From Luk GD, Alousi MA, Jones LA Jr, et al. Colonic polyps: benign and premalignant neoplasms of the colon. In: Yamada T, Alpers DH, Owyang C, et al. (eds). Atlas of Gastroenterology. Philadelphia: JB Lippincott, 1992.

Chapter 41

Figures 41.4 and 41.5 From Gardener EJ, Burt RW, Freston JW. Gastrointestinal polyposis: syndromes and genetic mechanisms. West J Med 1980;132:488.

Figures 41.6 and 41.11 From Sogol PB, Sugawara M, Gorden HE, et al. Cowden's disease: familial goiter and skin haematomas. West J Med 1983;139:324.

Figure 41.7 From Traboulsi EI, Krush AJ, Gardner EJ, et al. Prevalence and importance of pigmented ocular fundus legions in Gardner's syndrome. N Engl J Med 1987; 316:661.

Figure 41.12 From Russell DM complete remission in Cronkhite-Canada syndrome, Bhathal PS, St John DJ. Gastroenterology 1983;85:180.

Figure 41.14 From Malhotra R. Cronkhite-Canada syndrome associated with colon carcinoma and adenomatous changes in C-C polyps. Am J Gastroenterol. 1988;83:722.

Chapter 42

Figure 42.1 From Miller AB. Trends in cancer mortality and epidemiology. Cancer 1983;51:2413.

Figure 42.2 Adapted from Greenwald P. Colon cancer overview. Cancer 1992;70:1206.

Figure 42.3 From Armstrong B, Doll R. Environmental factors and cancer incidences and mortality in different countries with special reference to dietary practices. Int J Cancer 1975;15:617.

Figure 42.4 From Boland CR, Sato J, Appelman HD, et al. Microallelotyping defines the sequence and tempo of allelic losses at tumour suppressor gene loci during colorectal cancer progression. Nat Med 1995;1:902.

Figure 42.6 From Winawer SJ, Fletcher RH, Miller L, et al. Colorectal cancer screening: clinical guidelines and rationale. Gastroenterology 1997;112:594.

Figure 42.8a From Fuchs C, Giovannucci EL, Colditz GA, et al. A prospective study of family history and the risk of colorectal cancer. N Engl J Med 1994;331:1669.

Figure 42.7b-d From Winawer SJ, Zauber AG, Gerdes H, et al. Risk of colorectal cancer in the families of patients with adenomatous polyps. N Engl J Med 1996;334:82.

Figure 42.8 From Boland CR. Malignant tumors of the colon. In: Yamada T, Alpers DA, Laine L, et al. (eds). Textbook of Gastroenterology, 3rd edn. Philadelphia: Lippincott Williams & Wilkins, 1999.

Figure 42.9 From Colon and rectum. In: Beahrs OH, Henson DE, Hutter RVP, et al. (eds). Manual for Staging of Cancer of the American Joint Committee on Cancer, 4th edn. Philadelphia: JB Lippincott, 1992.

Figure 42.10 From August DA, Ottow RT, Sugarbaker PH. Clinical perspectives on human colorectal cancer metastases. Cancer Metastasis Rev 1984;3:303.

Figure 42.17 From Lind DS, Souba WW. Neoplasms of the colon and rectum. In: Bell RH Jr, Rikkers LF, Mulholland MW (eds). Digestive Tract Surgery: A Text and Atlas. Philadelphia: Lippincott-Raven, 1996.

Figure 42.21 From Misiewicz JJ, Forbes A, Price A, et al. Atlas of Clinical Gastroenterology, 4th edn. London: Wolfe, 1994.

Figures 42.22, 42.23, 42.24, 42.25 and 42.26 Blackstone MO. Colonic malignancies. In: Endoscopic Interpretation: Normal and Pathologic Appearances of the Gastrointestinal Tract. New York: Raven Press, 1984.

Figures 42.27 and 42.28 From Corman ML, Veidenhelmer MC, Swinton NW. Diseases of the Anus, Rectum, and Colon. Part 1: Neoplasms. New York: Medcom, 1972.

Figures 42.30, 42.31 and 42.32 From Corman ML. Carcinoma of the colon. In: Colon and Rectal Surgery, 4th edn. Philadelphia: Lippincott-Raven, 1998.

Figure 42.33 From Milsom JW, Ludwig KA. Surgical management for rectal cancer. In: Wanebo HJ (ed.). Surgery for Gastrointestinal Cancer: A Multidisciplinary Approach. Philadelphia: Lippincott-Raven, 1997.

Chapter 43

Figure 43.1 From Bharucha AE. Fecal incontinence. Gastroenterology 2003;124:1672.

Figures 43.7, 43.8, 43.12 and 43.14 From Rios Magrina E. Color Atlas of Anorectal Diseases. Barcelona: Salvat Editores, 1980.

Figure 43.10 From Suppurative processes. In: Rios Margrina E. Atlas of Therapeutic Proctology. Philadelphia: WB Saunders, 1984.

Figure 43.16 From Bharucha AE, et al. Phenotypic variation in functional disorders of defecation. Gastroenterology 2005;128:1199.

Figure 43.17 From Wald A. Fecal incontinence in adults. N Engl J Med 2007;356:40.

Figures 43.18, 43.19, 43.20 43.21, 43.28 and 43.29 From Wald A and Schoendorf J. Rome III: The functional GI Disorders slide set. Courtesy of Dr Arnold Wald and Jerry Shoendorf, MAMS.

Figure 43.23 From Bharucha AE, Fletcher JG, Harper CM, et al. Relationship between symptoms and disordered continence mechanisms in women with idiopathic fecal incontinence. Gut 2005;54:546.

Figure 43.26 From Bharucha AE. Outcome measures for fecal incontinence: Anorectal structure and function. Gastroenterology 2004;126:S90.

Chapter 44

Figures 44.1, 44.3 and 44.4 From Misiewicz JJ, Forbes A, Price A, et al. Atlas of Clinical Gastroenterology, 4th edn. London: Wolfe, 1994.

Figures 44.5, 44.6, 44.7 and 44.8 From Skandalakis JE, Gray SW, Rowe JS. Anatomical Complications in General Surgery. New York: McGraw-Hill, 1983.

Figure 44.9 From Misiewicz JJ, Forbes A, Price A, et al. Atlas of Clinical Gastroenterology, 4th edn. London: Wolfe, 1994.

Figure 44.11 From Aram F. Hezel et al. Genetics and biology of pancreatic ductal adenocarcinoma. Genes Dev 2006;20:1218–249.

Chapter 45

Figures 45.5 and 45.6 From Misciewicz JJ, Forbes A, Price A, et al. Atlas of Clinical Gastroenterology, 4th edn. London: Wolfe, 1994.

Figure 45.8 From Banks PA, Burrell MI, Sweeting JG, et al. The American Gastroenterological Association Clinical Teaching Project, Unit 5, Pancreatitis. Bethesda, MD: American Gastroenterological Association, 1990.

Chapter 46

Figure 46.2 From Misiewicz JJ, Forbes A, Price A, et al. Atlas of Clinical Gastroenterology, 4th edn. London: Wolfe, 1994.

Figure 46.4 From Beger HG, Buchler M, Dischuneit H, et al. Chronic Pancreatitis. Heidelberg: Springer-Verlag, 1990.

Figure 46.5 Adapted from DiMagno EP, Go VL, Summerskill WH. Relations between pancreatic enzyme outputs and malabsorption in severe pancreatic insufficiency. N Engl J Med 1973;288:813.

Figures 46.7 and 46.24 From Banks PA, Burrell MI, Sweeting JG, et al. The American Gastroenterological Association Clinical Teaching Project, Unit 5, Pancreatitis.

Figure 46.8 From Eisenberg RL. Gastrointestinal Radiology: A Pattern Approach, 4th edn. Philadelphia: Lippincott Williams & Wilkins, 2003.

Figure 46.23 From Little AG, Moosa AR. Gastrointestinal hemorrhage from left-sided portal hypertension. An unappreciated complication of pancreatitis. Am J Surg 1981;141:153.

Figures 46.25 and 46.26 From Bengtsson M, Löftström JB. Nerve block in pancreatic pain. Acta Chir Scand 1990;156:285.

Figure 46.29 From Prinz R. Surgical drainage procedures. In: Howard JM, Idezuki Y, Ihse I, et al. Surgical Diseases of the Pancreas, 3rd edn. Baltimore: Williams and Wilkins 1998;30:130.

Chapter 49

Figure 49.1 Adapted from Serohijos AW, Hegedus T, Aleksandrov AA, et al. Phenylalanine-508 mediates a cytoplasmic-membrane domain contact in the CFTR 3D structure crucial to assembly and channel function. Proc Natl Acad Sci USA 2008;105:3256.

Figure 49.2a From Marino CR, Matovcik LM, Gorelick FS, et al. Localization of the cystic fibrosis transmembrane conductance regulator in pancreas. J Clin Invest 1991;88:712.

Figure 49.2b From Cohn JA, Strong TV, Picciotto MR, et al. Localization of the cystic fibrosis transmembrane conductance regulator in human bile duct epithelial cells. Gastroenterology 1993;105:1857.

Figure 49.3 Adapted from Marino CR, Matovcik LM, Gorelick FS, et al. Localization of the cystic fibrosis transmembrane conductance regulator in pancreas. J Clin Invest 1991;88:712.

Figure 49.10 Adapted from Whitcomb DC, Gorry MC, Preston RA, et al. Hereditary pancreatitis is caused by a mutation in the cationic trypsinogen gene. Nat Genet 1996;14:141.

Figure 49.12 Data from Howes N, Lerch MM, Greenhalf W, et al. Clinical and genetic characteristics of hereditary pancreatitis in Europe. Clin Gastroenterol Hepatol 2004;2: 252.

Chapter 50

Figures 50.1 and 50.6 From Pellegrini CA, Duh Q-Y. Gallbladder and biliary tree: anatomy and structural anomalies. In Yamada T, Alpers DH, Owyang C, et al (eds). Textbook of Gastroenterology, 2nd edn. Philadelphia: JB Lippincott, 1995.

Figures 50.4. 50.11 and 50.12 From Linder H. Embryology and anatomy of the billiary tree. In: Way LW, Pellegrini CA (eds). Surgery of the Gallbladder and Bile Ducts. Philadelphia: WB Saunders, 1987.

Figure 50.13 From Soper NJ. Cystic disease of the biliary tract. In: Bell RH, Rikkers LF, Mulholland MW (eds). Digestive Tract Surgery: A Text and Atlas. Philadelphia: Lippincott-Raven, 1996.

Chapter 52

Figure 52.2 From Angulo P, Pearce DH, Johnson CD, et al. Magnetic reesonance cholangiography in patients with biliary disease: its role in primary sclerosing cholangitis. J Hepatol 2000;33:520.

Figure 52.12 From Prytz H, Keiding S, Bjornsson E, et al. Dynamic FDG-PET is useful for detection of chlorangiocarcinoma in patients with PSC listed for liver transplantation. Hepatology 2006;44:1572.

Figure 52.13 From Moreno-Luna LE, Gores GJ. Advances in the diagnosis of cholangiocarcinoma in patients with primary sclerosing cholangitis. Liver Transpl 2006;17: 515.

Figure 52.15 From Tischendorf J, Krüger M, Trautwein C, et al. Cholangioscopic characterisation of dominant bile duct stenoses in patients with primary sclerosing cholangitis. Endoscopy 2006;38:665.

Chapter 53

Figure 53.4 From Dr. Morton I. Burrell, from the American Gastroenterological Association Clinical Teaching Project Unit 4, Hepatobiliary Disease and Jaundice, 1989.

Figure 53.5 From Hamlin JA. Anomalies of the biliary tract. In: Berk, JE (ed.). Bockus Gastroenterology. Philadelphia: WB Saunders, 1985.

Figure 53.6 From Dr Morton I. Burrell, American Gastroenterological Association Clinical Teaching Project Unit 4, Hepatobiliary Disease and Jaundice. Philadelphia: Lippincott Williams & Wilkins, 1989.

Figure 53.9 From Kaplowitz N (ed.). Liver and Biliary Diseases. Baltimore: Williams and Wilkins, 1992.

Chapter 55

Figures 55.4, 55.5 and 55.7 From Agur AMR, Lee MJ. Grant's Atlas of Anatomy, 10th edn. Philadelphia: Lippincott Williams & Wilkins, 1999.

Figure 55.6 From Moore KL, Dalley II AF. Clinically Oriented Anatomy, 4th edn. Philadelphia: Lippincott Williams & Wilkins, 1999.

Figures 55.8, 55.12 and 55.14 From Sherlock S, Dooley J. Diseases of the Liver and Biliary System, 11th edn. Oxford: Blackwell Science, 2002.

Figure 55.11 From Phillips MJ, Poucell S, Patterson J, et al. The Liver: An Atlas and Text of Ultrastructural Pathology. New York: Raven Press, 1987.

Chapter 57

Figure 57.7 Data from the World Health Organization and Centers for Disease Control and Prevention fact sheets, available at www.who.int and www.cdc.gov, respectively.

Chapter 61

Figure 61.15 Adapted from Heathcote J. AASLD practice guidelines: management of primary biliary cirrhosis. Hepatology 2000;31:1005.

Chapter 62

Figure 62.6 From Alexander J, Kowdley KV. Hereditary hemochromatosis: genetics, pathogenesis, and clinical management. Ann Hepatol 2005;4:240.

Chapter 65

Figure 65.22 Data from Volzke H, Robinson DM, Kleine V, et al. Hepatic steatosis is associated with an increased risk of carotid atherosclerosis. World J Gastroenterol 2005;11: 1848.

Figure 65.23 From Ramesh S, Sanyal AJ. Evaluation and management of non-alcoholic steatohepatitis. J Hepatol 2005;42:S2.

Figure 65.26 From Sanyal AJ, Mofrad PS, Contos MJ, et al. A pilot study of vitamin E versus vitamin E and pioglitazone for the treatment of nonalcoholic steatohepatitis. Clin Gastroenterol Hepatol 2004;2:1107.

Chapter 66

Figure 66.1 From Weissenborn K, Rückert N, Hecker H, Manns MP. The number connection tests A and B: interindividual variability and use for the assessment of early hepatic encephalopathy. J Hepatol 1998;28:646.

Figure 66.2 From Amodio P, Gatta A. Neurophysiological investigation of hepatic encephalopathy. Metab Brain Dis 2005;20:369.

Figure 66.3a Adapted from Norenberg MD. The role of astrocytes in hepatic encephalopathy. Neurochem Pathol 1987;6:13.

Figure 66.3b From Swain MS, Blei AT, Butterworth RF, Kraig RP. Intracellular pH rises and astrocytes swell after portacaval anastomosis in rats. Am J Physiol 1991;261: R1491.

Figure 66.4 Adapted from Pomier-Layrargues G, Spahr L, Butterworth RF. Increased manganese concentrations in pallidum of cirrhotic patients. Lancet 1995;345:735.

Figure 66.5 From Lockwood AH, Yap EWH, Wong W. Cerebral ammonia metabolism in patients with severe liver disease and minimal hepatic encephalopathy. J Cereb Blood Flow Metab 1991;11:337.

Figure 66.10 From Abrams GA, Nanda NC, Dubovsky EV, et al. Use of macroaggregated albumin lung perfusion scan to diagnose hepatopulmonary syndrome: A new approach. Gastroenterology 1998;114:305.

Figure 66.11 From Passarella M, Fallon MB, Kawut SM. Portopulmonary hypertension. Clin Liver Dis 2006;10:653.

Chapter 67

Figures 67.1, 67.2, 67.3 and 67.6 From 2006 Annual report of the US Organ Procurement and Transplantation Network and Scientific Registry of Transplant Recipients: Transplant Data 1996–2005. Health Resources and Services Administration, Healthcare Systems Bureau, Division of Transplantation, Rockville, MD.

Chapter 69

Figure 69.4 From Reynolds TB. Liver abscess. In: Kaplowitz N (ed.). Liver and Biliary Diseases, 2nd edn. Baltimore: Williams and Wilkins, 1996.

Chapter 73

Figure 73.6b From Knechtges P, Buchanan GN, Willatt J, et al. Fistula-in-ano: The role of imaging in diagnosis and presurgical planning. Semin Colon Rectal Surg 2007;18: 111.

Chapter 74

Figures 74.15 and 74.16 From Ros PR, Olmsted WW, Moser RP Jr, et al. Mesentric and omental cysts: histologic classification with imaging correlation. Radiology 1987; 164:327.

Chapter 75

Figure 75.4 From Smith PD, Saini SS, Raffield M, et al. Cytomegalovirus induction of tumor necrosis factor-alpha by human monocytes and mucosal macrophages. J Clin Invest 1992;90:1642.

Chapter 76

Figures 76.3, 76.5 and 76.6 From Mitros FA. Atlas of Gastrointestinal Pathology. London: Gower, 1988.

Chapter 77

Figure 77.2 From Sepulveda B, Manzo N. Clinical manifestations and diagnosis of amebiasis. In: Martinez-Palomo A (ed). Amebiasis. Amsterdam: Elsevier, 1986.

Figure 77.5 From Healy GR, Garcia LS. Intestinal and urogenital protozoa. In: Murray PR (ed.). Manual of Clinical Microbiology. Washington, DC: ASM Press, 1995.

Figure 77.6 From Case records of the Massachusetts General Hospital. Weekly clinicopathological exercises. Case 8-1997. A 65-year-old man with recurrent abdominal pain for five years. N Engl J Med 1997;336:786.

Figure 77.9 From Healy GR, Garcia LS. Intestinal and urogenital protozoa. In: Murray PR (ed.). Manual of Clinical Microbiology. Washington, DC: ASM Press, 1995.

Figure 77.10 From Farar WE, Wood MJ, Innes JA, et al. Infectious Diseases: Text and Color Atlas. St Louis: Mosby-Year Book, 1992.

Figure 77.11 From Guerrant RL, Petri WA, Wanke CS. Parasitic causes of diarrhea. In: Lebenthal E, Duffey M (eds). Paraphysiology of Secretory Diarrhea. Boston: Raven Press, 1990.

Figure 77.12 From Soave R, Weikel CS. *Cryptosporidium* and other protozoa including *Isospora, Sarcocystis, Balantidum coli,* and *Blastocystis.* In: Mandell GL, Douglas RG Jr, Bennett JE (eds). Principles and Practice of Infectious Diseases, 3rd edn. New York: Churchill Livingstone, 1990.

Chapter 78

Figure 78.9 From Smith JW, Thompson JH Jr, et al. Intestinal helminths. In: Atlas of Diagnostic Medical Parasitology Series. Chicago: American Society of Clinical Pathologists, 1984.

Figure 78.6 From Gryseels B, Polman K, Clerinx J, et al. Human schistosomiasis. Lancet 2006;368:1106.

Figure 78.10a From Smith JW, Ash LR, Thompson JH Jr, et al. Intestinal helminths. In: Atlas of diagnostic medical parasitology series. Chicago: American Society of Clinical Pathologists, 1984.

Figure 78.12 From WHO Informal Working Group on Echinococcosis. International classification of ultrasound images in cystic echinococcosis for application in clinical and field epidemiological settings. Acta Trop 2003;85: 253.

Chapter 80

Figures 80.5, 80.6, 80.21, 80.25, 80.27, 80.28, 80.35, 80.53, 80.55 and 80.56 From Sherertz EF, Jorizzo JL. Skin lesions associated with gastrointestinal diseases. In: Yamada T, Alpers DH, Owyang C, et al(eds). Textbook of Gastroenterology. Philadelphia: JB Lippincott, 1991.

Chapter 81

Figures 81.4 and 81.5 From Bresalier RS. Neoplasia of the colon and rectum. In: Feldman M (ed.). Gastroenterology and Hepatology: the Comprehensive Visual Reference. Philadelphia: Current Medicine, 1997.

Figures 81.7, 81.8, 81.11, 81.12, 81.13 and 81.14 From Allison MC. Diagnostic Picture Tests in Gastroenterology. London: Mosby-Wolfe, 1991.

Figure 81.9 From Habif TP. Superficial fungal infections. In: Baxter S (ed.). Clinical Dermatology: A Color Guide to Diagnosis and Therapy, 3rd edn. St. Louis: Mosby, 1996.

Figures 81.10, 81.15, 81.16, 81.17 and 81.18 From Briggaman R. Clinical Nutrition Slideset. American Gastroenterological Association, Bethesda, MD: 2000.

Chapter 82

Figure 82.1 From Eidus LB, Rasuli P, Manion D, et al. Caliberpersistant artery of the stomach (Dieulafoy's vascular malformation). Gastroenterology 1990;99:1507.

Figure 82.2 From Scheider DM, Barthel JS, King PD, et al. Dieulafoy-like lesion of the distal esophagus. Am J Gastroenterol 1994;89:2080.

Figure 82.5 From Boley SJ, Sammartano R, Adams A, et al. On the nature and etiology of vascular ectasias of the colon: degenerative lesions of aging. Gastroenterology 1977;72:650.

Figure 82.6 From Foutch PG. Angiodysplasia of the gastrointestinal tract. Am J Gastroenterol 1993;88:807.

Figures 82.8 and 82.9 From Cappell MS. Spatial clustering of simultaneous nonhereditary gastrointestinal angiodysplasia: small but significant correlation between nonhereditary colonic and upper gastrointestinal angiodysplasia. Dig Dis Sci 1992;37:1072.

Figure 82.10 From Boley SJ, Sprayregen S, Sammartano RJ, et al. The paraphysiologic basis for the angiographic signs of vascular ectasias of the colon. Radiology 1977;125:615.

Figure 82.11b From Savides TJ, Jensen DM. Therapeutic endoscopy for nonvariceal gastrointestinal bleeding. Gastroenterol Clin North Am 2000;29:465.

Figure 82.13 From Haitjema T, Westermann CJ, Overtoom TT, et al. Hereditary haemorrhagic telangiectasia (Osler–Weber–Rendu disease): new insights into pathogenesis, complications, and treatment. Arch Intern Med 1996;156:174.

Figure 82.16 From Watson M, Hally RJ, McCue PA, et al. Gastric antral vascular ecstasia (watermelon stomach) in patients with sytemic sclerosis. Arthritis Rheum 1996;39:341.

Figure 82.19 From Cappell MS, Price GB. Characterization of the syndrome of small and large intestinal variceal bleeding. Dis Dig Sci 1987;32:422.

Figure 82.21 From Sandhu KS, Cohen H, Radin R, et al. Blue rubber bleb nevus syndrome presenting with recurrences. Dig Dis Sci 1987;32:214.

Figure 82.22 From Weinstein EC, Moertel CG, Waugh JM. Intussuscepting hemangionomas of the gastro-intestinal tract: report of a case and review of the literature. Ann Surg 1963;157:265.

Figure 82.24 From Bak YT, Oh CH, Kim JH, et al. Blue rubber bleb nevus syndrome: endoscopical removal of the gastrointestinal hemangiomas. Gastrointest Endosc 1997;45:90.

Figure 82.25a From Stratte EG, Tope WD, Johnson CL, et al. Multimodal management of diffuse neonatal hemangiomatosis. J Am Acad Derm 1996;34:337.

Figure 82.25b From McCauley RG, Leonidas JC, Bartoshesky LE. Blue rubber bleb nevus syndrome. Radiology 1979;133:375.

Figure 82.26 From Brandt LJ. Gastrointestinal Disorders of the Elderly. New York: Raven Press, 1984:5.

Chapter 83

Figure 83.1 From Schlossberg L, Zuidema GD. The Johns Hopkins Atlas of Human Functional Anatomy, 3rd edn. Baltimore: The Johns Hopkins University Press, 1986.

Figures 83.5a, 83.5b, and 83.6 From Bastidas JA, Reilly PM, Bulkley GB. Mesenteric vascular insufficiency. In: Yamada T, Alpers DH, Owyang C, et al (eds). Textbook of Gastroenterology. Philadelphia: JB Lippincott, 1995.

Chapter 93

Figures 93.1 and 93.3 From Levine MS. Plain radiograph diagnosis of the acute abdomen. Emerg Med Clin North Am 1985;3:541.

Figures 93.4 and 93.7 From Rubesin SE, Glick SN. The tailored double-contrast pharyngogram. CRC Crit Rev Diagn Imaging 1988;28:133.

Figure 93.9 From Levine MS, Rubesin SE, Herlinger H, et al. Double contrast upper gastrointestinal examination: technique and interpretation. Radiology 1988;168:593.

Figure 93.11 From Levine MS, Creteur V, Kressel HY, et al. Benign gastric ulcers: diagnosis and follow-up with double contrast radiography. Radiology 1987;164:9.

Chapter 99

Figure 99.18 From Chuang VP, Pulmano CM, Walter JF, et al. Angiography of pacreatic arteriovenous malformation. AJR Am J Roentgenol 1977;129:1015.

Figures 99.24, 99.32 and 99.33 From Inflammatory Disease. In: Reuter SR, Redman HC, Cho KJ. Gastrointestinal Angiography, 3rd edn. Philadelphia: WB Saunders, 1986.

Figure 99.29 From Cho, KJ, Wilcox CW, Reuter SR. Glucagon-producing islet cell tumor of the pancreas. AJR Am J Roentgenol 1977;129:159.

Index

Note: page numbers in *italics* refer to figures, those in **bold** refer to tables